Rotator Cuff Disorders

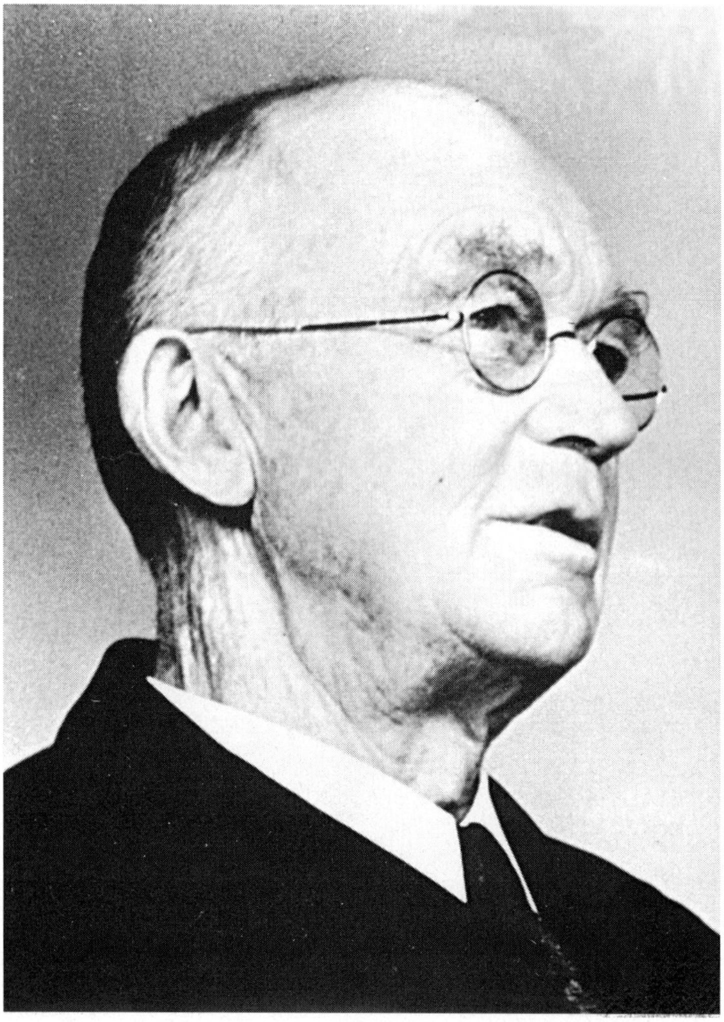

Earnest Amory Codman, circa 1934, at the Massachusetts General Hospital. (Courtesy of Carter R. Rowe.)

Rotator Cuff Disorders

Wayne Z. Burkhead, Jr., M.D.
Clinical Associate Professor
University of Texas Southwestern Medical School
Attending Physician
W.B. Carrell Memorial Clinic
Dallas, Texas

SANS TACHE
Williams & Wilkins
A WAVERLY COMPANY
BALTIMORE • PHILADELPHIA • LONDON • PARIS • BANGKOK
BUENOS AIRES • HONG KONG • MUNICH • SYDNEY • TOKYO • WROCLAW
1996

Editor: Darlene B. Cooke
Managing Editor: Fran Klass
Production Coordinator: Marette D. Magargle
Book Project Editor: Susan Sfarra
Typesetter: University Graphics, Inc.
Printer: Maple Press
Binder: Maple Press

ISBN 0-683-01215-0

9 780683 012156 90000

351 West Camden Street
Baltimore, Maryland 21201-2436 USA

Rose Tree Corporate Center
1400 North Providence Road
Building II, Suite 5025
Media, Pennsylvania 19063-2043 USA

Accurate indications, adverse reactions, and dosage schedules for drugs are provided in this book, but it is possible that they may change. The reader is urged to review the package information data of the manufacturers of the medications mentioned.

Printed in the United States of America

Library of Congress Cataloging-in-Publication Data

Rotator cuff disorders / edited by Wayne Z. Burkhead, Jr.—1st ed.
p. cm.
Includes index.
ISBN 0-683-01215-0
1. Shoulder joint—Rotator cuff—Diseases. 2. Shoulder joint—Rotator cuff—Wounds and injuries. 3. Shoulder joint—Rotator cuff—Surgery. I. Burkhead, Wayne Z.
[DNLM: 1. Rotator Cuff—injuries. 2. Rotator Cuff—physiopathology. 3. Rotator Cuff—pathology. WE 810 R842 1996]
RD557.5.R67 1996
617.5′72—dc20
DNLM/DLC
for Library of Congress 95-14112
CIP

The Publishers have made every effort to trace the copyright holders for borrowed material. If they have inadvertently overlooked any, they will be pleased to make the necessary arrangements at the first opportunity

96 97 98 99
1 2 3 4 5 6 7 8 9 10

Reprints of chapters may be purchased from Williams & Wilkins in quantities of 100 or more. Call Isabella Wise in the Special Sales Department, (800) 358-3583.

DEDICATION

To all of my teachers: my father, who taught me love of science; my mother, who taught me love of art; Harold Jeskey, who taught me love of "cultural material;" Vert Mooney, who taught me love of orthopaedics; Charlie Rockwood, who taught me love of the shoulder; Ray Lawson and Dickie Jones, who taught me love of self; and my wife and children, who taught me love is more important than anything else.

Foreword

Dr. Burkhead has done a superb job in bringing to us "Everything you ever wanted to know about the rotator cuff"—and then some! He has collaborated with a very distinguished group of nationally and internationally known physicians and shoulder surgeons and has written nine of the chapters himself. As we sometimes swallow a bitter pill with ice cream, he has skillfully blended the important basic science issues into multiple chapters that are quite palatable. The chapters, beginning with the history of the rotator cuff, flow smoothly through anatomy, imaging, types of lesions, conservative treatment, types of surgical repairs and reconstructions, and what you do when you run into a massive defect that is difficult to repair or reconstruct.

Now that I have given you the general glowing comments about this fine text, let me tell you something about the editor-in-chief, Buzz Burkhead. Following his residency in the Department of Orthopaedics at the University of Texas Health Science Center in Dallas in 1983, we were delighted to have Buzz as our Shoulder Fellow in the Department of Orthopaedics in San Antonio. During his stay with us, he became a friend of all of the staff, residents, and hospital personnel. He has a winning, pleasing, and happy personality and is always quick with his smile. He is a popular educator and has served as the guest of many national, local, state, and international orthopaedic and shoulder societies. This includes visiting professorships to Brazil, Germany, Japan, France, and England. Buzz is a superb teacher that stimulates his audience through wit, humor, and helpful information.

He has a successful shoulder practice in Dallas, Texas and we share consultations on the management of difficult problems. In addition to his busy practice, Buzz plays guitar in a Dallas group of musicians called "Doctor – Doctor." His group has cut records for "Bone Tone" record company, and I have a copy of his hit record entitled "Baby Ain't Got No Tan Lines." I admire the enthusiasm of Dr. Burkhead and consider him a close friend. He has a lovely family, a beautiful wife and three children. I consider Dr. Burkhead as one of the bright stars of American orthopaedics and especially a star in the care of shoulder problems.

Charles A. Rockwood, Jr., M.D.
Professor and Chairman Emeritus
Department of Orthopaedics
University of Texas Health Science Center
San Antonio, Texas

Preface

"No one is obliged to read a preface, but in it the author should introduce himself to the reader and give him a glimpse of his own personality, amusement, and intellectual processes."

Codman, 1934

Since Codman was so right about the shoulder so long ago, I can only assume that he is right about the preface of a book, in that the editor or author should introduce himself to his readers and give them, as Codman described, a glimpse of himself. Most would say that I have an unusual personality. Entertaining others has always been important to me, whether it involves playing an original humorous song on my guitar or creating a funny slide or video presentation at an otherwise austere meeting. As for intellectual processes, I am sure there are many who would say that I have little or no capacity in that regard. Fortunately, over the years I have come in contact with many who possess a tremendous degree of intellect and who share my interest in the shoulder. Many of these contributors are entertaining in their own right. These contributors will entertain and educate you with their wonderful work.

Although the importance of shoulder pain can be overshadowed in the grand scheme of things by the problems that face medicine, society, and our interface today, these same problems faced the surgeons in the past. Codman's 1904 description of rotator cuff tears occurred next to an article on transmission of the plague. K.G. Smith's article on rotator cuff tears found at autopsy occurred next to an article critical of midwifery, and many of Codman's patients saw chiropractors prior to seeing him. Harrison McLaughlin's report in 1943 came at the height of World War II.

While the practitioners of other specialties and subspecialities, especially those that deal with the quantity of life such as cardiology, oncology, thoracic, and general surgery, might discount the importance of shoulder pain, the number of patients who experience and suffer through misdiagnosis and mistreatment of common shoulder conditions do not. The quality of life provided by a good night's sleep is never discounted by a patient who has had a torn rotator cuff left untreated for several years. This disturbance in the quality of a patient's life can lead to depression and in some extreme examples, leads patients to consider terminating their lives. If a single patient sleeps better and is able to enjoy their life more fully because of this book, I will feel all the hard work by the contributors and myself will be justified.

Life-threatening epidemics, controversies in the division of labor within medicine, and wars of much greater proportion than exist today did not stop our forebearers from trying to understand this complex joint, nor should they stop us now or in the future.

Dallas, Texas

Wayne Z. Burkhead, Jr.

Acknowledgment

A special thanks to Karen Lozano, who typed this manuscript, my shoulder fellows, James Shankwiler, Jeff Cantrell, Mike Ciepiela, and John Itamura, all of my employees who bore the brunt of my mood swings related to this project, and the contributors and their families. I would also like to thank Williams and Wilkins, especially Darlene Cooke and Fran Klass. They believed in this project when others did not.

Contributors

Evan J. Bachner, MD
Orthopaedic Surgeon
West Valley Orthopaedics and Sports Medicine
West Hills, California
Former Fellow in Sports Medicine and Arthroscopic Surgery
Southern California Orthopaedic Institute
West Hills, California

Carl Basamania, MD
Chief Orthopaedic Surgery Service
Womack Army Medical Center
Fort Bragg, North Carolina
Clinical Assistant Professor
Department of Orthopaedic Surgery
Duke University
Durham, North Carolina

Stephen S. Burkhart, MD
Clinical Associate Professor
Department of Orthopaedic Surgery
University of Texas Health Science Center at San Antonio
San Antonio, Texas

Wayne Z. Burkhead, Jr., MD
Clinical Associate Professor
University of Texas Southwestern Medical School
Attending Physician
W.B. Carrell Memorial Clinic
Dallas, Texas

Jeffrey S. Cantrell, MD
Orthopaedic Associates
Lewisville, Texas

Michael D. Ciepiela, MD
Teaching Faculty Orthopaedic Residency
Georgia Baptist Medical Center
Atlanta, Georgia

John M. Clark, MD, PhD
Associate Professor
Department of Orthopaedics
University of Washington
Seattle, Washington

Timothy P. Codd, MD
Attending Staff Physician
Department of Orthopaedics
Children's Hospital and Center for Reconstructive Surgery
Bennett Institute for Sports Medicine
Baltimore, Maryland

Edward V. Craig, MD
Attending Surgeon
Hospital for Special Surgery
Professor of Clinical Surgery (Orthopaedics)
Cornell University Medical Center
New York, New York

Sanjay S. Desai, MD
Assistant Clinical Professor of Orthopaedic Surgery
Medical College of Virginia
Richmond, Virginia
West End Orthopaedic Clinic
Richmond, Virginia

Marybeth Ezaki, MD
Department of Orthopaedics
University of Texas Health Science Center at Dallas
Dallas, Texas

Evan L. Flatow, MD
Herbert Irving Associate Professor of Orthopaedic Surgery
Associate Chief, The Shoulder Service
New York, New York

Richard J. Friedman, MD, FRCS(C)
Professor of Orthopaedic Surgery
Medical University of South Carolina
Charleston, South Carolina

Hiroaki Fukuda, MD
Professor and Chairman
Department of Orthopaedic Surgery
Tokai University School of Medicine
Bohseidai, Isehara, Japan

J. Mark Fulmer, MD
Diagnostic Radiology
Baylor University Medical Center
Dallas, Texas

Dominique F. Gazielly, MD
Staff Orthopaedic Surgeon
Active Member of European Society for
Surgery of the Shoulder and Elbow
Corresponding Member of American Shoulder and Elbow Surgeons
Saint Etienne, France

Thomas P. Goss, MD
Professor of Orthopaedic Surgery
Department of Orthopaedic Surgery
University of Massachusetts Medical Center
Worchester, Massachusetts

Guerdon Greenway, MD
Attending Physician, Department of Radiology
Baylor University Medical Center
Dallas, Texas
Associate Clinical Professor, Department of Radiology
University of California
San Diego School of Medicine
San Diego, California
Clinical Associate Professor, Department of Orthopaedic Surgery
University of Texas Southwestern Medical Center at Dallas
Dallas, Texas

Peter Habermeyer, MD
Assistant Professor of The University in Munich
Director of the Sportklinik Stuttgart
Member of the International Board of Shoulder Surgery
Stuttgart, Germany

Kazutoshi Hamada, MD
Assistant Professor
Department of Orthopaedic Surgery
Tokai University, School of Medicine
Boseidai, Iseharashi, Kanagawa, JAPAN

Phillip E. Hansen, MD
Attending Orthopoedic Surgeon,
Section of Shoulder and Elbow Surgery
Baylor University Medical Center
Clinical Assistant Professor
University of Texas Southwestern Medical School at Dallas and Parkland Medical Hospital
Attending Surgeon, Humana Hospital–Medical City Dallas
Dallas, Texas

Douglas T. Harryman II, MD
Associate Professor of Orthopaedic Surgery
Director, Shoulder and Elbow Service
University of Washington
Seattle, Washington

John M. Itamura, MD
Assistant Professor of Orthopaedic Surgery
University of Southern California
Los Angeles, California

Frank W. Jobe, MD
Associate, Kerlan–Jobe Orthopaedic Clinic
Clinical Professor, Department of Orthopaedics
USC School of Medicine
Los Angeles, California
Orthopaedic Consultant To
Los Angeles Dodgers, PGA Tour, and Senior PGA Tour

Sumner E. Karas, MD
Clinical Instructor
Boston University
Boston, Massachusetts

Paulo Kechele, MD
Orthopaedic Surgeon
Chairman Upper Extremity Surgery
Hospital Regional Sao Jose
Florianopolis, Brazil

Robert P. Knetsche, MD
Department of Surgery
Dwight D. Eisenhower Army Medical Center
Fort Gordon, Georgia

Ronald S. Kvitne, MD
Associate, Kerlan–Jobe Orthopaedic Clinic
Inglewood, California
Assistant Clinical Professor, Department of Orthopaedics
University of Southern California
Los Angeles, California

Motohiko Mikasa, MD
Director, Department of Orthopaedic Surgery
Tokyo Metropolitan Ohkubo Hospital
Tokyo, Japan

David S. Morrison, MD
Director of Shoulder and Elbow Surgery
Southern California Center for Sports Medicine
Long Beach, California

Katsuya Nobuhara, MD
Director, Nobuhara Hospital and Institute of Biomechanics
President, Asian Shoulder Association
Hyogo, Japan

Jiro Ozaki, MD
Director and Chairman, Department of Orthopaedic Surgery
Nara Prefectural Hospital
Assistant Professor, Department of Orthopaedic Surgery
Nara Medical University
Nara, Japan

Pekka Paavolainen, MD, PhD
Associate Professor, Head of Surgery
The Jorvi Hospital
Espoo, Finland

Charles A. Rockwood, Jr., MD
Professor, Chairman Emeritus
Department of Orthopaedics
University of Texas Health Science Center
San Antonio, Texas

Patrick A. Ruwe, MD
Assistant Professor
Department of Orthopaedics and Rehabilitation
Section of Sports Medicine
Yale University School of Medicine
Co-Director, Yale Shoulder Center
New Haven, Connecticut

K. Sarkar, MD*
Professor of Pathology
Ontario, Canada

Dana G. Seltzer, MD
Chief, Sports Medicine and Shoulder Surgery
Maricopa Medical Center
Phoenix, Arizona
Assistant Professor of Orthopaedic Surgery
Mayo Graduate School of Medicine
Rochester, Minnesota
Assistant Professor of Orthopaedic Surgery
University of Arizona School of Medicine
Tucson, Arizona

James A. Shankwiler, MD
Pasadena, California

James F. Silliman, MD
Clinical Assistant Professor
University of Texas Southwestern Medical Center
Dallas, Texas

Stephen J. Snyder, MD
Orthopaedic Surgeon Specializing in Arthroscopy and Reconstructive Surgery of the Shoulder
Van Nuys, California

*Deceased

William F. Tucker, Jr., MD
Dallas, Texas

Hans K. Uhtoff, MD
Professor of Surgery (Orthopaedics)
Ottawa General Hospital
Department of Orthopaedics
Ottawa, Ontario, Canada

Gilles Walch, MD
Lyon, France

Michael Watson, MD, MA, MRCP, FRCS
Consultant Orthopaedic Surgeon
Guy's Hospital
Shoulder and Elbow Surgeon
London, England

Gerald R. Williams, Jr., MD
Assistant Professor of Orthopaedic Surgery
Director, Shoulder Study Group
Department of Orthopaedic Surgery
Hospital of the University of Pennsylvania
Philadelphia, Pennsylvania

Kaoru Yamanaka, MD
Department of Orthopaedic Surgery
Shizuoka Red Cross Hospital
Shizuoka, Shizuoka Pref., Japan

Contents

Section 1

History of Cuff Repair

Chapter 1

The Rotator Cuff: A Historical Review of Our Understanding

Wayne Z. Burkhead, Jr. and Peter Habermeyer

For their work continueth and their work continueth. Broad and deep continueth. Greater than their knowing.

Rudyard Kipling

History seems to justify the importance placed on the rotator cuff by surgeons around the world today, as the earliest descriptions of rotator cuff injury are found in the oldest of medical writings, *Edwin Smith's Surgical Papyrus* (Fig. 1–1).[1] Fortunately, in this day and age, most injuries to the soft tissues around the shoulder are less severe, and the results of treatment more rewarding.

The ancient Asian contribution to anatomy is detailed in a wonderful chapter on gross anatomy of the shoulder by Christopher Jobe.[2] The bony anatomy of the shoulder was understood by Sustruta and Atroya in the sixth century B.C., 150 years before Hippocrates.[3,4]

The relationship of the tendons around the shoulder, their displacement, and possible role in instability of the shoulder were discussed by Hippocrates in the third century B.C.[5,6] He discussed the fact that patients can be attacked with inflammation of surrounding tendons, stressed the importance of gentle early motion, and noted a variability in rate and success of healing.[7]

SECOND CENTURY A.D. TO 1400

Galen, sometimes referred to as the father of both clinical anatomy and sports medicine, wrote "that the best physician is also a philosopher." [2,8] His discourse represents the earliest effort at detailed functional shoulder anatomy and the shoulder's important linked relationship to the elbow and wrist. Because of the prevailing Roman laws, Galen's dissections were limited to animals. Therefore, he perpetrated the erroneous notion that the acromion was a separate bone.

The christianization of the Roman Empire intensified the already existing laws against human dissection, and it was not until the thirteenth century that necropsy was allowed,[2] permitting Ruggerio of Palermo to observe capsular rupture in acute dislocations.[9]

THE RENAISSANCE

Leonardo da Vinci brought to the world his concept that every phenomenon perceived became an object of knowledge.[10]

Saper Vedere, "knowing how to see," became the great theme of his blend of science and art. The notebook of da Vinci reveal drawings of several shoulders from several different directions. In some specimens the acromion is fused and in some it is unfused (Fig. 1–2). Rather than speculate (an activity that he scorned) on the normality of this variation, da Vinci merely drew what he saw. Rather than assume, da Vinci was able to record irrefutable facts gained from experience, facts that we today take for granted (i.e., the acromion can exist in a fused and unfused state).

The teaching of anatomy was codified by Pope Clement in 1537.[2] At the age of 28 the physician, anatomist, and entrepreneur Andreas Vesalius of Brussels changed the course of anatomy as a scientific discipline with the publication of his epochal work, *De Humanis Corporis Fabrica Libri Septem.*[11] The muscles of the rotator cuff and the biceps, as well as their origins and insertions, are well presented in this work (Fig. 1–3). With Vesalius there was

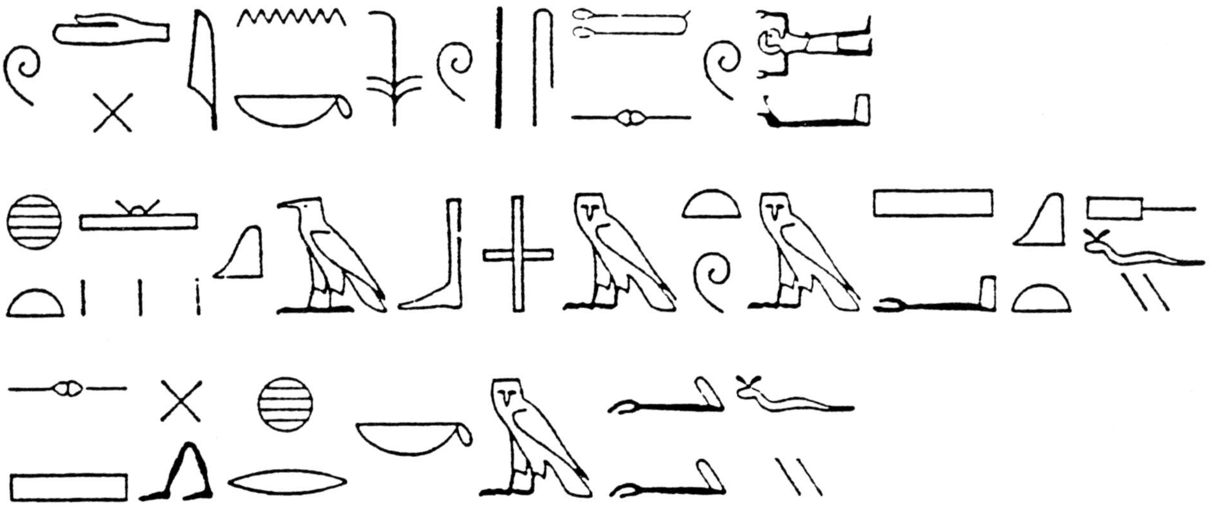

Fig. 1–1. **An open fracture of the proximal humerus. The result, death, is depicted in the top right corner. One wonders if the snake indicated that an attorney was involved. (From Smith E. *Edwin Smith's Surgical Papyrus.* Chicago, IL: University of Chicago Press; 1930.)**

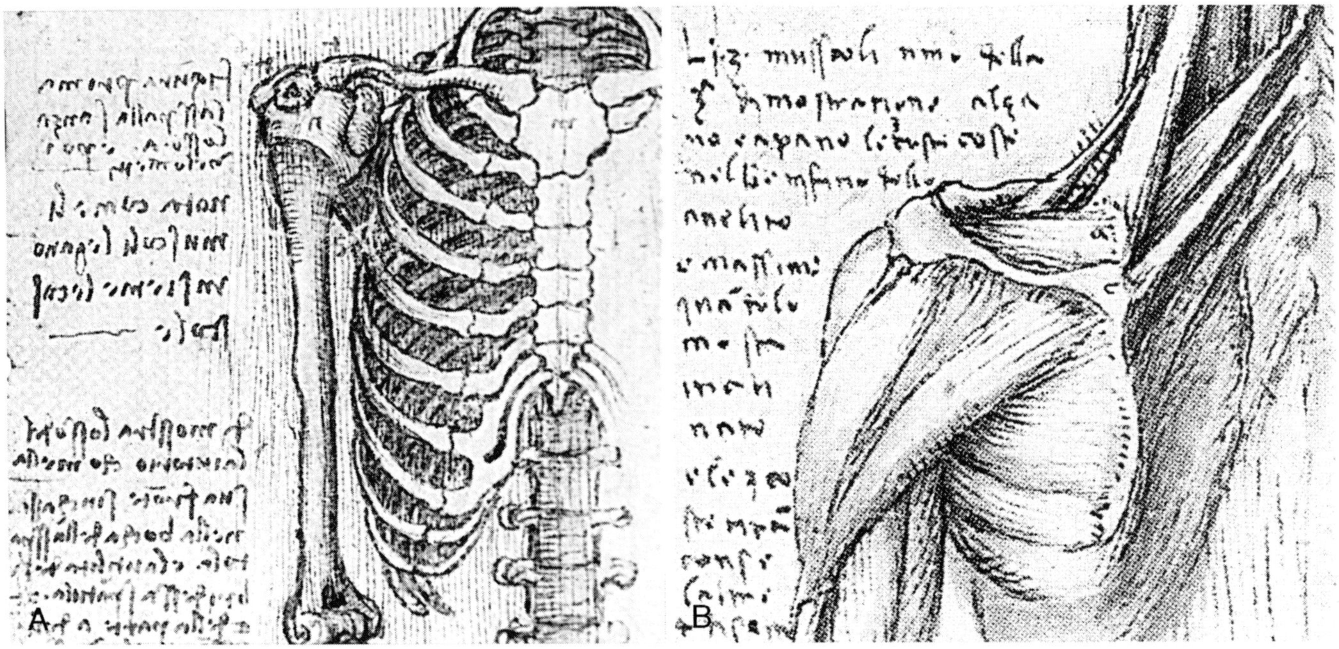

Fig. 1–2. ***A,* An illustration from Leonardo's notebook. The acromion is unfused in this specimen and labeled A. (From da Vinci L. *The Anatomy of Man. Drawings From the Collection of Her Majesty, Queen Elizabeth II.* Boston: Little, Brown & Co; 1992). *B,* An illustration from Leonardo's notebook. In this specimen the acromion is fused to the scapula. (From Clark Kenneth. *Leonardo da Vinci.* New York: Penguin; 1988.)**

a return to the organized teaching of medicine, especially anatomy.

SEVENTEENTH TO NINETEENTH CENTURY

Perhaps because the strong cowl of the deltoid prevented inspection, or because the bodies were obtained illegally from grave-snatching, the necropsy and drawings were hurriedly done; and the biceps received much more attention in the early literature than did the tendons that we now refer to as the rotator cuff.[12–17] In fact, the bicep was surgically repaired by Morton 25 years prior to the first rotator cuff repair.[17] Moseley discovered that in 1788, in a book entitled *A Description of all the Bursae Mucosa of the Human Body;* Monro illustrated a rent in the supraspinatus (Fig. 1–4).[18,19]

On Saturday, May 24 1834, in the *London Medical Gazette,* the first detailed series of rotator cuff ruptures was published in the form of a letter to the editor.[20] John

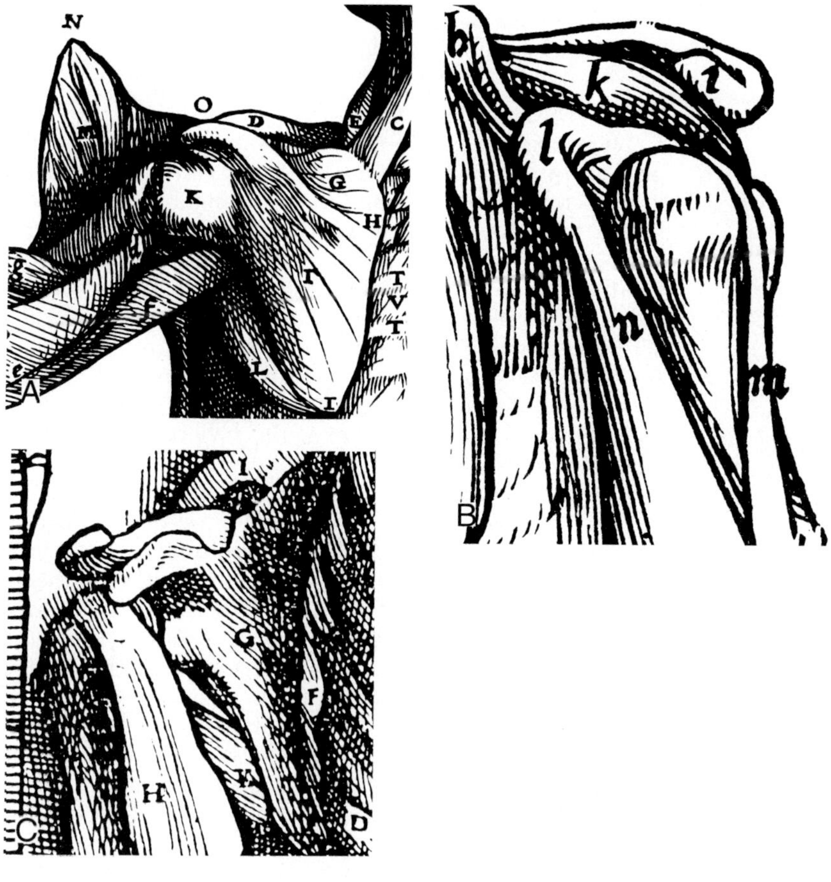

Fig. 1–3. *A,* While the infraspinatus and teres minor are shown as one muscle they blend into a common tendon (K) with the supraspinatus. (From Saunders JB de CM, O'Malley CD. *The Illustrations From the Works of Andreas Vesalius of Brussels.* Cleveland: The World Publishing Co; 1950.) *B,* The sixth plate of muscles. The supraspinatus (k) is showing coursing beneath the acromion (i). (From Saunders JB de CM, O'Malley CD. *The Illustrations From the Works of Andreas Vesalius of Brussels.* Cleveland: The World Publishing Co; 1950.) *C,* The sixth plate of muscles. The subscapularis (H) removed from the scapula (G). (From Saunders JB de CM, O'Malley CD. *The Illustrations From the Works of Andreas Vesalius of Brussels.* Cleveland: The World Publishing Co; 1950.)

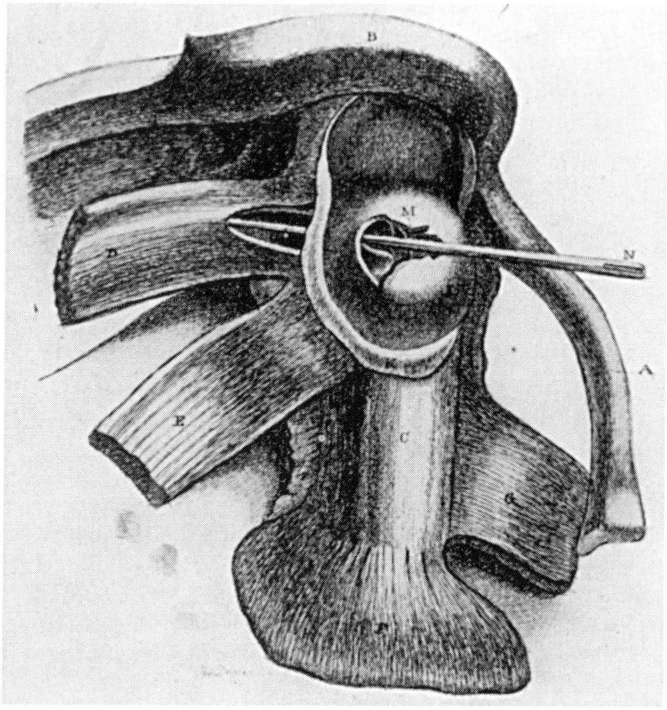

Fig. 1–4. The first illustration of a rotator cuff tear, 1788. From a posterior angle with the humerus in flexion, Monro draws a probe (N) going through a tear in the supraspinatus and infraspinatus. (From Moseley HF. Ruptures of the rotator cuff. *Br J Surg.* 1951;38:340–369.)

Gregory Smith, writing from the *Hunterian Theatre of Anatomy*, had discovered seven cases of tears in the rotator cuff in specimens obtained by grave robbing. In this report Smith described many of the variations recognized today, ranging from the small tear involving the subscapularis (resulting from dislocation of the shoulder) to the massive degenerative tear with an associated biceps dislocation.

Ashurst,[21] writing in 1869 in the *Science and Art of Surgery*, described tears of the rotator cuff associated with dislocations. However, with the exception of the discussions by Smith and Adams on what is now referred to as rotator cuff tear arthropathy, a full 70 years passed before anything of significance was written about tears of the rotator cuff.[22–24] Even then the significance of Smith's contribution went unrecognized until 1935, when his work was rediscovered by Haldeman and Soto-Hall.[25] Codman, who was introduced to Smith's work by Soto-Hall wrote in 1937, "My eyes have now been opened by a paper, written over 100 years ago, which seems to me so good that I have requested the Editor of this Journal to reprint it in full."[26] Smith, long dead, couldn't have rolled over in his grave too much, for he had missed Monro's illustration from a generation earlier than his own. Thus is the history of science and medicine; until the zeitgeist is correct, discoveries and their discoverers will, like Sustruta and the concept of the one bone scapula, be buried together.

The following is a reproduction of the first of seven cases reported by Smith in 1834.

> Case I. In the body of a man brought to the dissecting-room, under the old system of violation of the grave, in the month of February 1832, the following pathological condition of the left shoulder-joint was observed:
>
> On making transverse section in the centre of the deltoid muscle, for the purpose of reflecting it, the bursa situated beneath was observed to be much larger than usual, very much thickened, and communicating with the general cavity of the shoulder-joint by a large irregular opening. On further examination, it was noticed that the tendinous insertion of the subscapularis muscle had been entirely torn away from the lesser tubercle; the supra spinatus, infra spinatus, and the teres minor muscles, had likewise been completely detached from the greater tubercle. The tendon of the long head of the biceps had been torn away from the upper part of the glenoid cavity, and entirely withdrawn from the joint.

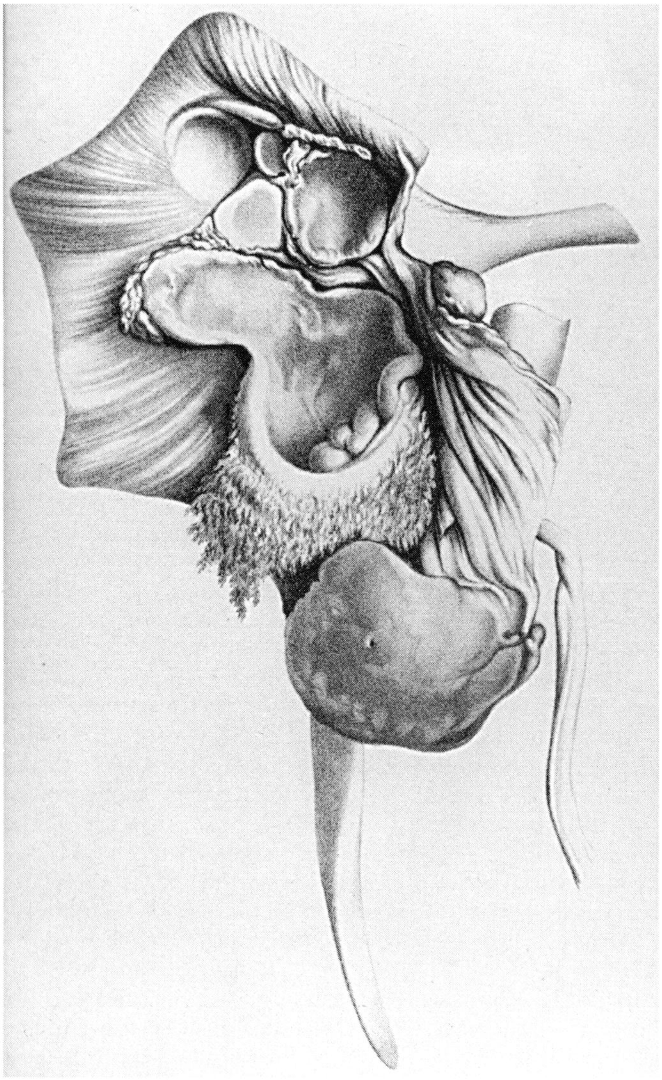

Fig. 1–5. Chronic rheumatic arthritis of the shoulder is illustrated by Robert W. Smith. Note polished acromial surface from articulating with the head devoid of rotator cuff. Erosion into the coracoid, AC joint, and the proliferative bursa is well demonstrated. (From Smith RW. Observations upon chronic rheumatic arthritis of the shoulder. II. *Dublin Quarterly J Med Sci.* 1853;XV:343–358.)

The debate over whether the findings of superior migration of the humeral head with a destructive arthritis is directly related to trauma and mechanical factors rather than a resultant rheumatic condition is not a new one. Long before the *Milwaukee Shoulder,* Robert W. Smith, writing in the *Dublin Quarterly Journal of Medical Science* in 1853, felt that John Smith had gratuitously described his cases as related to trauma when in actuality they were the "well known results of chronic rheumatic arthritis upon the structures of the shoulder joint."[23] John Smith describes in detail the pathoanatomy of an elderly woman's shoulder who had suffered from shoulder pain for years and who had no history of trauma. "Upon removing the deltoid muscle, the naked head of the humerus, elevated to the acromion process, came into view the centre of its summit was devoid of cartilage over a space as large as a shilling, and covered with ivory-like deposit . . . The remainder of the socket presented the appearance of ivory, which manifestly must have been established before the head of the bone had perforated the capsule" (Fig. 1–5). Adams, in a wonderful atlas of arthritis of all the joints, demonstrates superior subluxation and acetabularization of the acromion, meso, and basi os acromiale, as well as biceps rupture and dislocation (Fig. 1–6).

Subsequent to the reports by Smith and Adams, a number of European surgeons reported autopsy studies documenting avulsion of the rotator cuff with impingement.[27–31] In 1861 Flower concluded that "ruptures of the tendons inserting on the greater tuberosity are rather common."[32]

Von Pitha[33] described the function of the rotators as a "tendinous glenoid cavity," noting that "the supraspinatus, infraspinatus, and teres minor muscles limit the excursions of the humeral head to the boundaries of the small, shallow glenoid."

Konig stated that shoulder dislocations were caused "mainly by extensive lacerations of tendons and tendon insertions"[34] while Kornlein, in his 1882 textbook, *Lehre von den Luzationen,* was among the first to note the importance of a functionally and anatomically correct reconstruction of the injured structures.[31] In 1882 Cramer,[35] following a proposal by Huter,[36] resected the humeral head in a dislocated shoulder. He suggested that the surgical repair of tendon ruptures in this context.

In 1866 Bardenheuer noted a supraspinatus tendon rupture while performing anatomic studies and stated that avulsed rotators could and should be reattached with sutures.[37] Finney, a colleague of Halstead in Boston,[38] reported in 1894 on "a very interesting shoulder injury that is not described in the textbooks" and whose pathology could not be adequately explained. This injury involved "one of the most common shoulder injuries seen in daily practice." Finney proceeded to describe the classic clinical symptoms in his patients, which today would be interpreted as a rotator cuff tear.

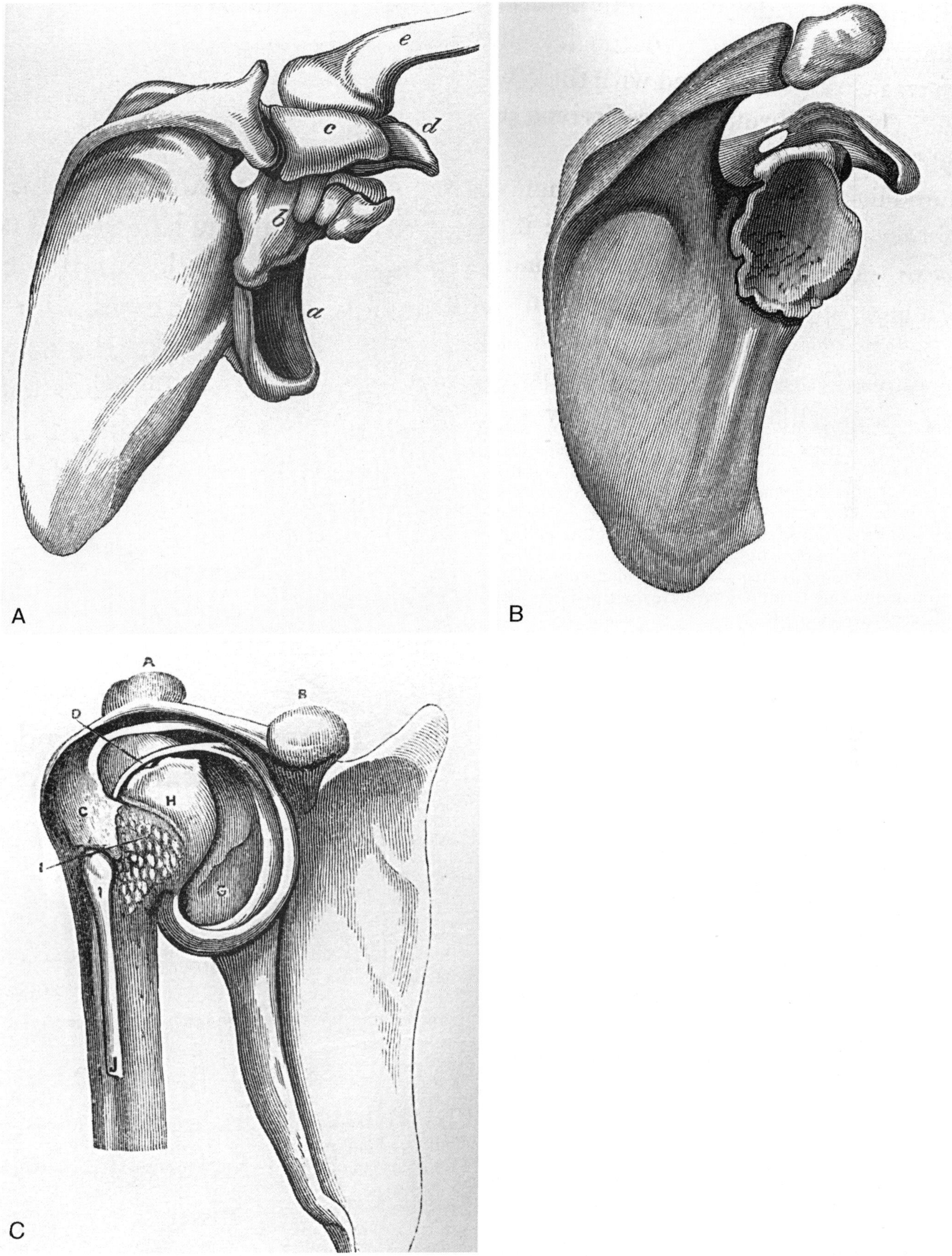

Fig. 1–6. *A,* Meso and *B,* basi acromial unfused os acromiale are demonstrated in this specimen of a right scapula along with medial dislocation of the biceps, *C.* (From Adams R. *A Treatise of Rheumatic Gout, or Chronic Rheumatoid Arthritis of all the Joints.* 2nd ed. London: John Churchill & Sons. Edinburgh: Maclachlan & Stewart; 1873:1–568.)

1900 TO 1940

Carter Rowe's Codman lecture given in Toronto, Canada during the Second International Symposium on Surgery of the Shoulder, describes Codman as a man of intellect, courage, conviction, controversy, and irrepressible honesty, in fact, at times, too much honesty for his own good. "Codman, who stood 6 feet 2 inches, a true Bostonian, carved from stubborn New England granite, was born on the 30th of December, 1869 and died on the 23rd of November, 1940. He graduated from Harvard College and entered Harvard Medical School in 1891 at the age of 22."[39]

Codman dated his interest in the subacromial bursa to his third year of medical school when he was allowed to travel to Vienna.[40] There, the subdeltoid bursa was unveiled in a text by Albert.[41] His first report mentioning the subject was in April of 1904. Codman's maverick antiestablishment personality resulted in his temporary "separation" from the Massachusetts General Hospital and led to the founding of his own hospital. Codman's influence on the development of surgery ranks with those of Pean, Halstead, and Cushing, and Codman goes beyond their technical contributions by introducing the end result idea or the notion, now taken for granted, that hospitals and the doctors that work in them should follow their patients long term to determine the true benefit of their medical treatment.

In 1904, describing the shoulder, Codman stated that, "No surgeon can practice long without seeing certain puzzling cases of lesions in this region that defy his diagnosis and treatment." He further remarked that "such lesions, when we know more about them, will be separated into more distinct anatomical entities." Codman eschewed the use of such terms as periarthritis, which he described as a "surgical wastebasket in which we throw our diagnostic failures."[42]

In 1906 Codman described the anatomy of the subdeltoid bursa and its clinical importance.[43] He discussed the treatment of partial tears of the supraspinatus by manipulation and abduction bracing (Fig. 1–7) in 1908.[44] His admonition that unless the brace was comfortable it was useless should be remembered today.

Goldthwait offered a mechanical/attritional theory to explain shoulder pain and bursitis. He pointed out the importance of the length and slope of both the acromion and the coracoid as possible etiologies for painful shoulders.[45] The biomechanics of the rotator cuff tendons and their contribution to subacromial bursitis was discussed by Stevens in 1909.[46]

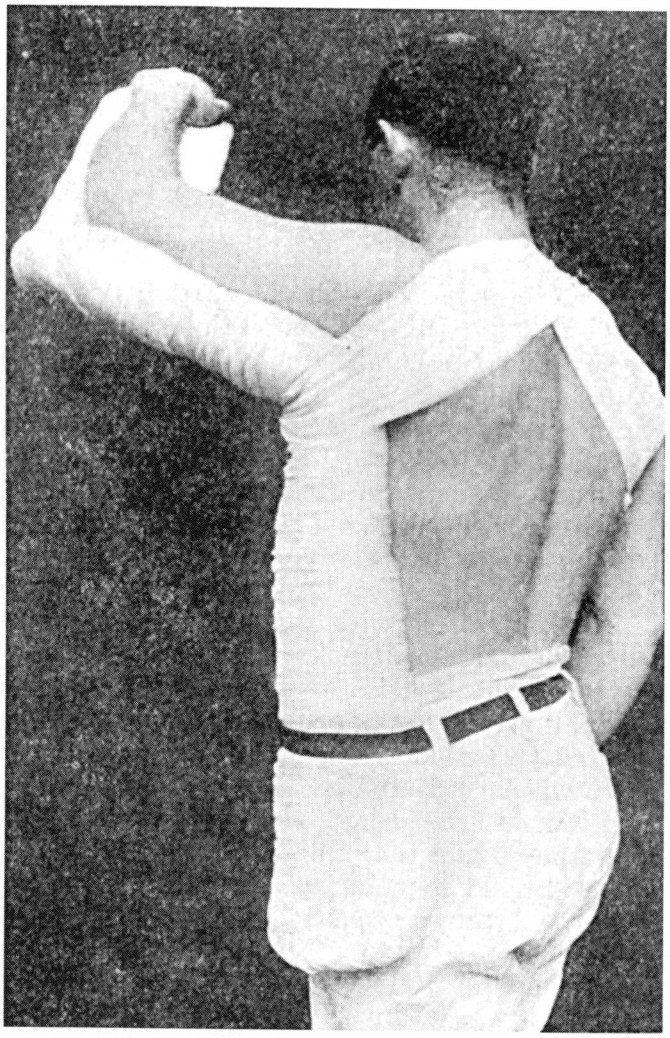

Fig. 1–7. Codman wrote, "when properly adjusted it is perfectly comfortable. Unless it is comfortable it is useless." Fortunately, belts were fashionable at the time. (From Codman EA. Bursitis subacromialis or periarthritis of the shoulder joint (subdeltoid bursitis). *Bost Med J.* 1908; 159:533–537, 576–578, 615–616, 677–680, 723–726.)

THE FIRST REPAIRS

According to Perthes, the first repair of the rotator cuff appears to have been performed in 1889 by Muller.[47] Muller reports repairing both the supraspinatus and infraspinatus with cat gut sutures in the context of instability repair.[48] Perthes himself would later reattach avulsed muscles in three patients, using U-pins rather than sutures, and he was the first investigator to describe partial ruptures (Fig. 1–8).[47]

Codman's first repair is described in detail in 1911:[49] "By holding the bursa wide open, pulling down on the arm and raising the elbow from the table, the retracted end of the supraspinatus could be seen. This was caught with a tenaculum and pulled down enough to suture with four heavy silk threads to the remaining portion still attached to the tuberosity. This could not be done exactly, but was done merely enough so that it seemed possible for repair to take place along the silk sutures. A little gap was also left on each side, which was not covered with tendon substances. It was in a sense a 'suture-á-distance'." The young surgeon facing his first large rotator cuff tear should take heart that even Codman could not get his first supraspinatus tear totally repaired. The patient's excellent result as well as the result of his second

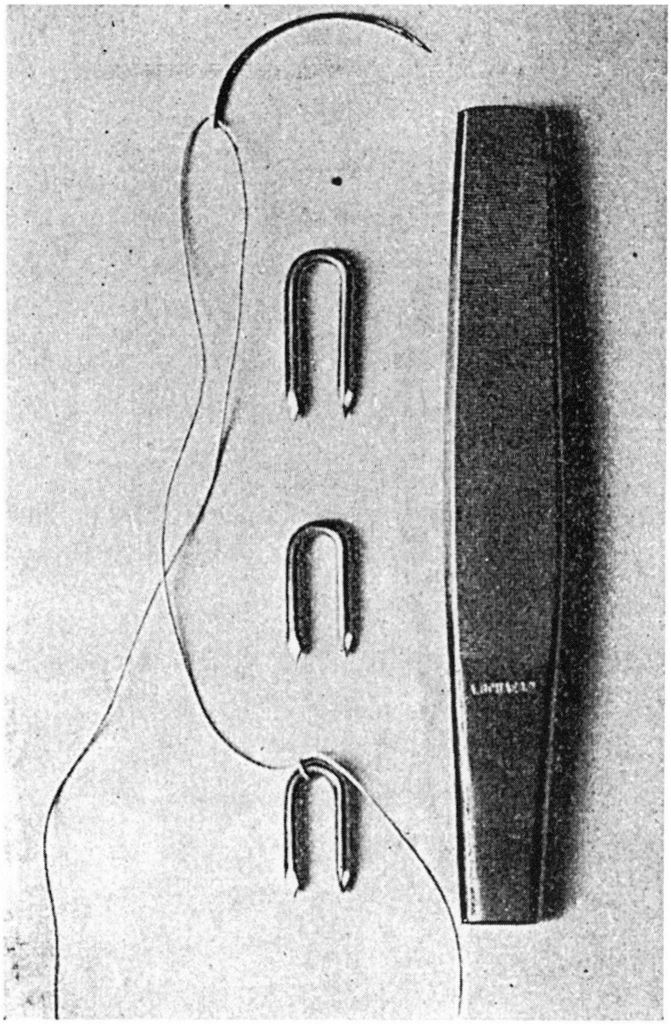

Fig. 1–8. Perthes' staple and suture anchor. (From Bergmann EV, ed. *Deutsche Zeitschift fur Chirurgie.* Leipzig: Verlag Von F.C.W. Vogel; 1906:103.

repair done almost 2 years later (he didn't get this one closed either) when compared with the poor result in a patient with an unrepaired tendon, encouraged him to recommend aggressive diagnosis and surgical treatment of these lesions for the duration of his career.

Baer and Painter described the symptoms of rotator cuff tears as a feature of subdeltoid bursitis.[50,51] Baer observed functional recovery in cases treated by excision of the bursa and suture repair.[50] Dawburn described a clinical sign for bursitis.[52]

Bergemann[53] and Stieda[54] were the first German writers to describe calcific densities on radiographs of the shoulder joint in 1908, 1 year after Painter[51] of the U.S. had described similar densities. Codman believed that the calcified deposits found in the tendons signified deficient tendon healing caused by an insufficient blood supply.[44] In 1912 Wrede, who like Stieda was a pupil of Lexer, definitively localized the calcified masses to the supraspinatus tendon.[55] Prompted by this finding, in 1915 Moschcowitz performed a histologic study of the calcium deposits occurring in bursitis.[56] He found that the deposits formed in necrotic tissue.

The traumatic entrapment of the supraspinatus and subacromial bursa between the acromion and humerus during abduction was recognized as a cause of bursitis by Brickman[57] and Buchholz.[58] They found that the most common intraoperative findings were tendon rupture and bleeding into the tendon substance.

In 1922 Buchholz, a student of Codman, published the first report in Germany describing avulsion of the supraspinatus tendon as a severe, separate pathologic entity.[59] There was a general consensus on the traumatic etiology of tendon lesions prior to 1923, but in that year Meyer noted that partial or complete tendon rupture can result from friction against the bone.[60] In 1924 Meyer published his theory on the degenerative nature of rotator cuff tears,[61] describing attritional wear of the supraspinatus tendon caused by entrapment between the humeral head and acromion.

Burman introduced diagnostic arthroscopy of the shoulder in 1931 based on studies in Dresden and New York and even noted the feasibility of arthroscopic surgery once suitable instruments could be developed.[62] Interestingly, the German surgeon Bircher had already performed successful arthroscopic examinations of the knee joint in 1922 using a laparoscope,[63] but cadaveric studies led him to conclude that the shoulder joint was inaccessible to this procedure.

Payr[64] and Dollinger[65] assumed that supraspinatus lesions were the cause of shoulder pain in bursitis and periarthritis. Payr recommended surgery, while Dollinger recommended massage as the only therapy.

Keyes' studies of supraspinatus tendon ruptures in cadaveric specimens confirmed the results of Codman, Wilson, and other investigators.[66] Keyes found that these ruptures were frequent and tended to attract older individuals. He concluded that age was the main predisposing factor for the occurrence of the defects.

In 1993 Ohnsorge investigated the importance of the external rotators for elevation of the arm.[67] In the same year Oberholzer used pneumoarthrography to investigate recurrent shoulder dislocations.[68,69]

While not considered epochal at the time of it's publication in 1934, Codman's text *The Shoulder* synthesizes his best work garnered over a 30-year span. The depth of his understanding is well illustrated. This includes his knowledge of anatomy, including obscure bursa that might mimic cuff disease (Fig. 1–9). He pointed out the importance of examining the shoulder from all sides.

In *The Shoulder*, Codman demonstrates his awareness that tears may develop as a result of degeneration, attritional wear, or trauma (Fig. 1–10). He also describes in detail, with the technology of the time, the transition zone from tendon to bone, the critical zone of hypovascularity, and the spectrum of tears from articular side tears or "rim rents" (Fig. 1–11) to massive avulsions or "insubstance tears" (Fig. 1–12), including tears of the rotator interval. Although articular side tears and rotator interval lesions are popular topics of discussion today, one has to merely reread Codman to become a believer

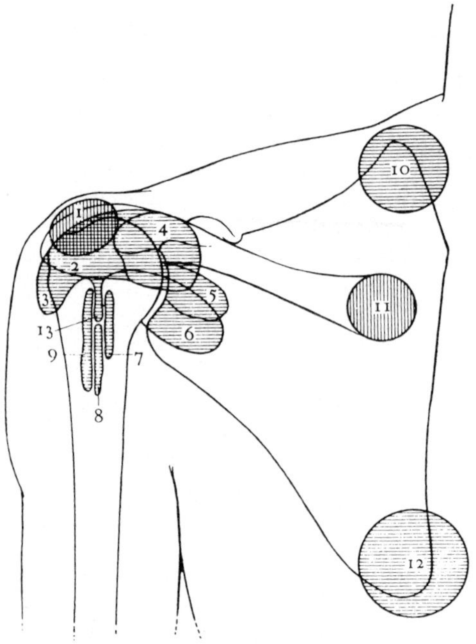

Fig. 1–9. Bursa of the shoulder girdle. (From Codman EA. *The Shoulder, Rupture of the Supraspinatus Tendon and Other Lesions in or About the Subacromial Bursa.* Malabar, FL: RE Krieger; 1984.)

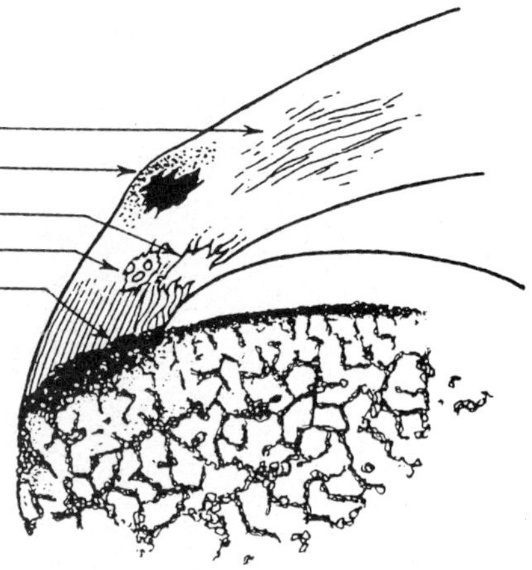

Fig. 1–10. Degenerative changes. (From Codman EA. *The Shoulder, Rupture of the Supraspinatus Tendon and Other Lesions in or About the Subacromial Bursa.* Malabar, FL: RE Krieger; 1984.)

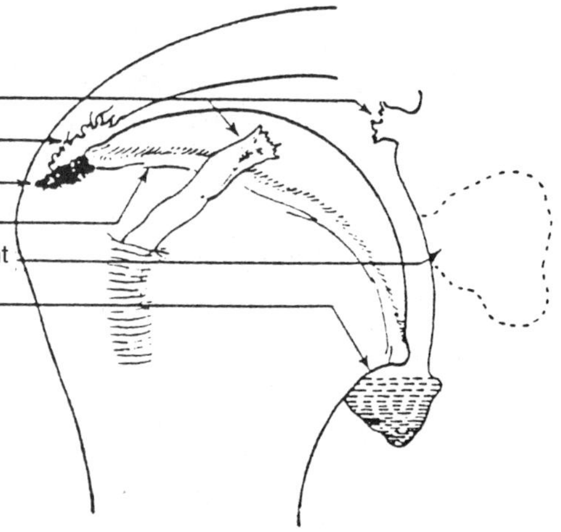

Fig. 1–11. The articular side rim rent. (From Codman EA. *The Shoulder, Rupture of the Supraspinatus Tendon and Other Lesions in or About the Subacromial Bursa.* Malabar, FL: RE Krieger; 1984.)

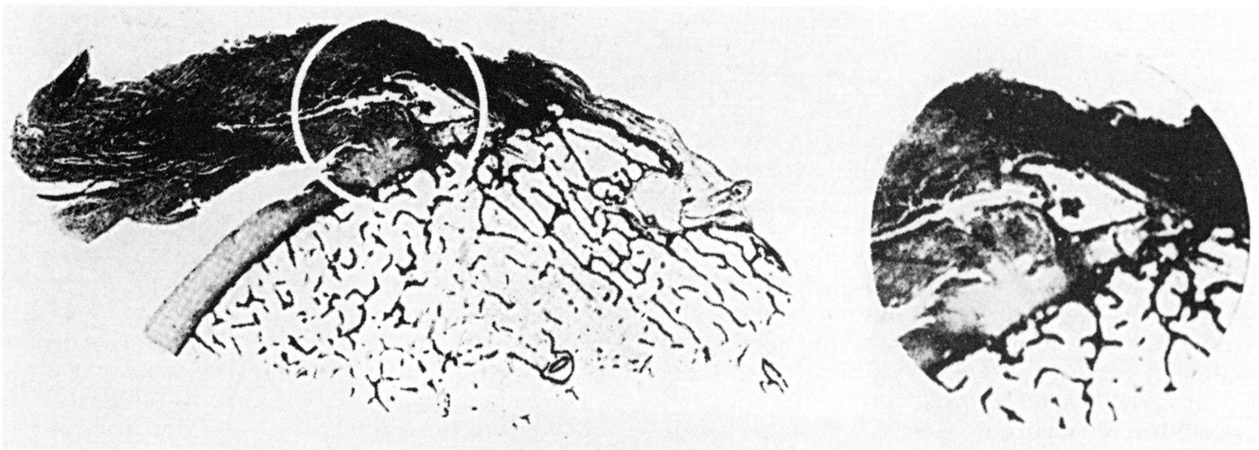

Fig. 1–12. In substance tearing of the rotator cuff. (From Codman EA. *The Shoulder, Rupture of the Supraspinatus Tendon and Other Lesions in or About the Subacromial Bursa.* Malabar, FL: RE Krieger; 1984.)

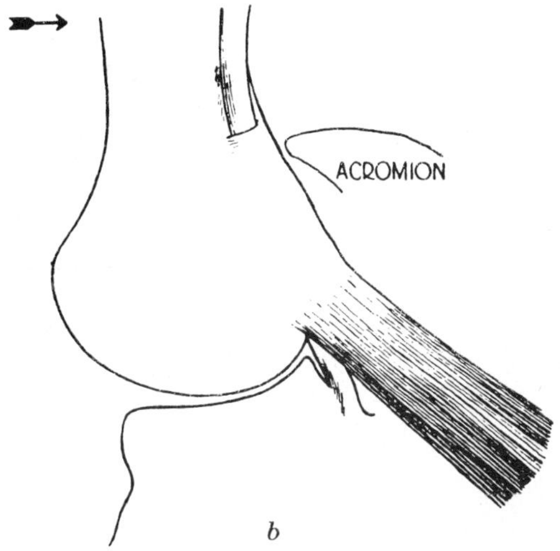

Fig. 1–13. **Posterior superior impingement of the glenoid against the tuberosity and cuff insertion. Note the proximity of the biceps to the acromion in this position. (From Codman EA. *The Shoulder, Rupture of the Supraspinatus Tendon and Other Lesions in or About the Subacromial Bursa.* Malabar, FL: RE Krieger; 1984.)**

in the concept that nothing is truly new or unrecognized. This includes the ''newer'' concepts of posterior-superior or internal impingement of the greater tuberosity against the glenoid in (Fig. 1–13) creating articular side tears.

In regards to surgical treatment, Codman realized early that proper positioning of the shoulder improved exposure of the rotator cuff where he had found the calcium deposits. He realized that the Saber incision, initially described by Gill[70] for glenohumeral fusion (Fig. 1–14), while providing excellent exposure, carried with it the morbidity of nonunion of the transacromial approach. He realized that the surgery could be done through a smaller deltoid splitting incision and arm rotation would deliver the pathoanatomy into the wound (Fig. 1–15). Codman offered several suggestions on how the tendon could be repaired (Fig. 1–16). Perhaps the most important illustration to reproduce Figure 1–17 shows the interlocking of articulations from the shoulder girdle to the fingers. The analogy of trying to back up as a series of trailers, the last one containing boards, would have been lost on Galen, who commented on these articulations 1700 years before. However, the philosophical aspects of this, i.e. that the most important ''articulation'' of all is with the brain, would surely have placed Codman among those that Galen said were best (i.e., the physician who is also a philosopher).

Codman's lectures, 11 articles, and his book, ''The Shoulder,'' stimulated many other researchers in the 1930s.[26,40,42–44,49,71–76] Wilson in his 1931 article described Codman's contributions as splendid and felt surgeons owed all that was known at that time about the subacromial bursa and supraspinatus tendon to him.[77] Codman was grateful, but frustrated; when he wrote, ''A dog may bark up a tree for a long time before anyone comes to see what is up in the branches. For 20 years I bayed out not continuously about the importance of rupture of the supraspinatus and I owe a debt to Dr. Philip Wilson, the

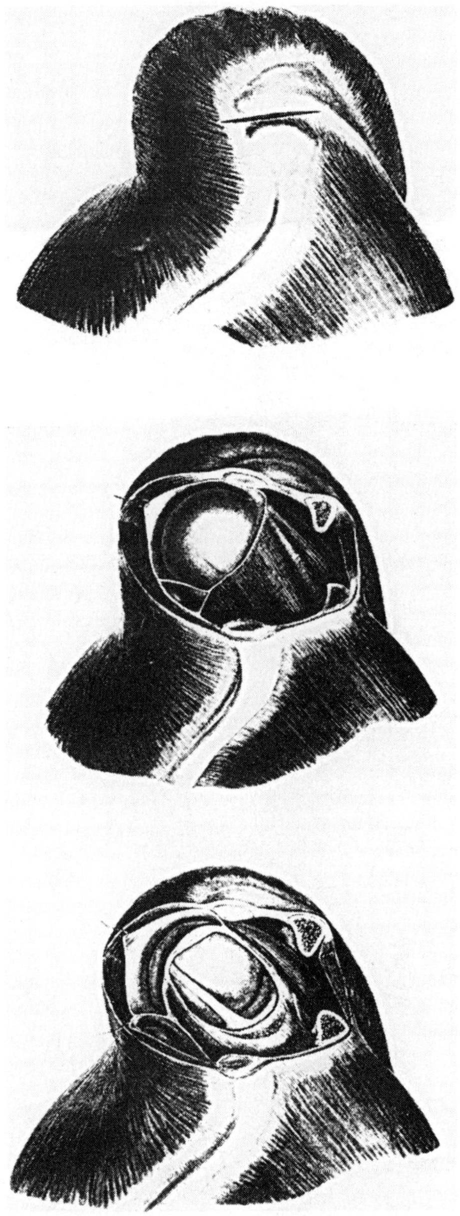

Fig. 1–14. **The Saber incision. (From Codman EA. *The Shoulder, Rupture of the Supraspinatus Tendon and Other Lesions in or About the Subacromial Bursa.* Malabar, FL: Robert E. Krieger Publishing Co; 1984.)**

first prominent surgeon to take time enough to study the evidence that there was something at which to bay.''[40]

In 1932 Fowler was apparently the first to repair what he felt was an acute tear.[78] Moseley, writing from Montreal on rupture of the supraspinatus in 1939, was inspired by a visit to Codman in Boston.[79] His work confirmed that partial and complete ruptures of the supraspinatus account for the majority of cases involving a painful shoulder following injury. He pointed out the value of early motion over the internally rotated posture provided by a sling, pleaded for practitioners to make an accurate diagnosis, and realized that the prognosis was determined by the interval between the accident and the initiation of ''intelligent treatment.''

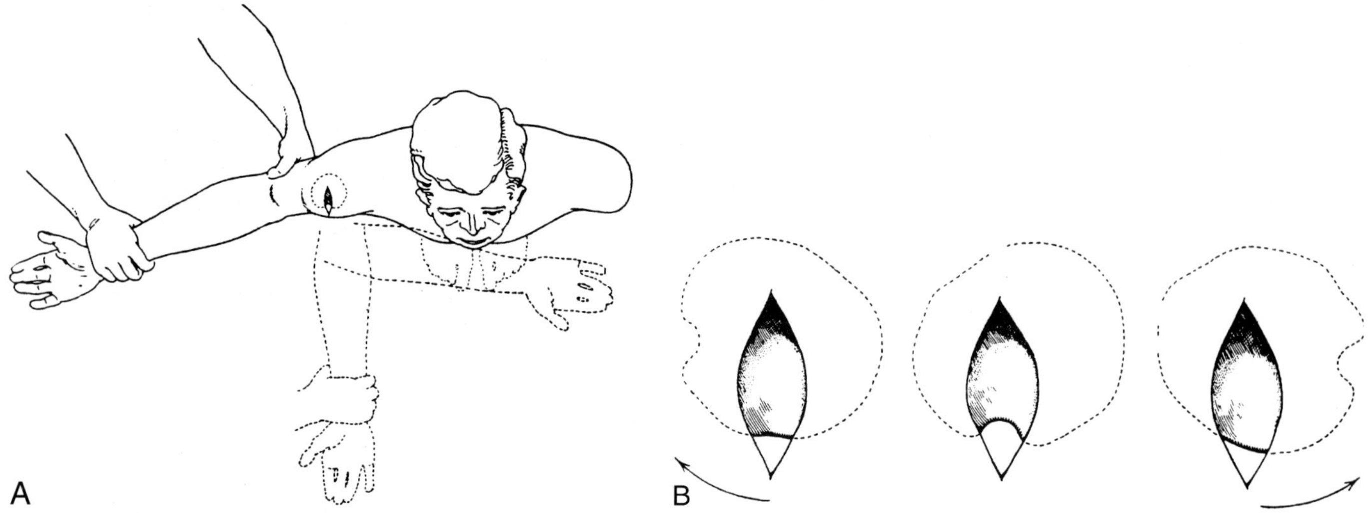

Fig. 1–15. *A,B,* The pathology can be rotated into the wound. (From Codman EA. *The Shoulder, Rupture of the Supraspinatus Tendon and Other Lesions In or About the Subacromial Bursa.* Malabar, FL: RE Krieger; 1984.)

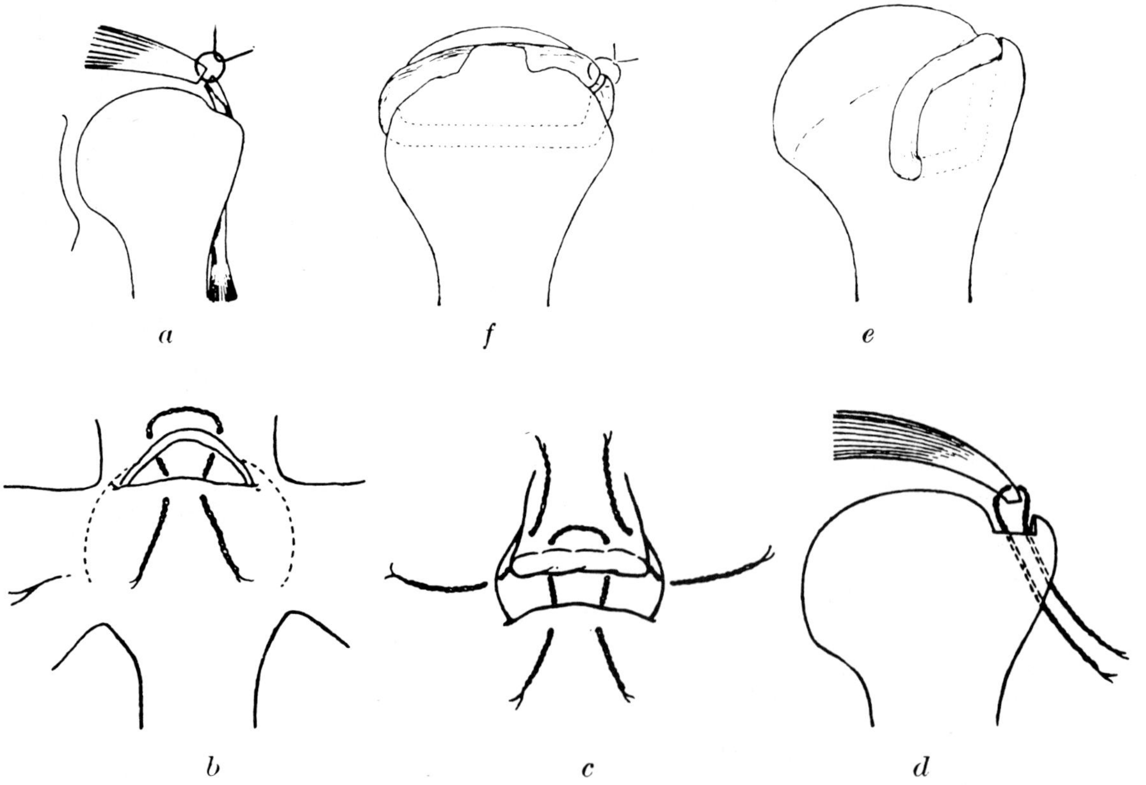

Fig. 1–16. Methods of tendon repair. (From Codman EA. *The Shoulder, Rupture of the Supraspinatus Tendon and Other Lesions in or About the Subacromial Bursa.* Malabar, FL: RE Krieger; 1984.)

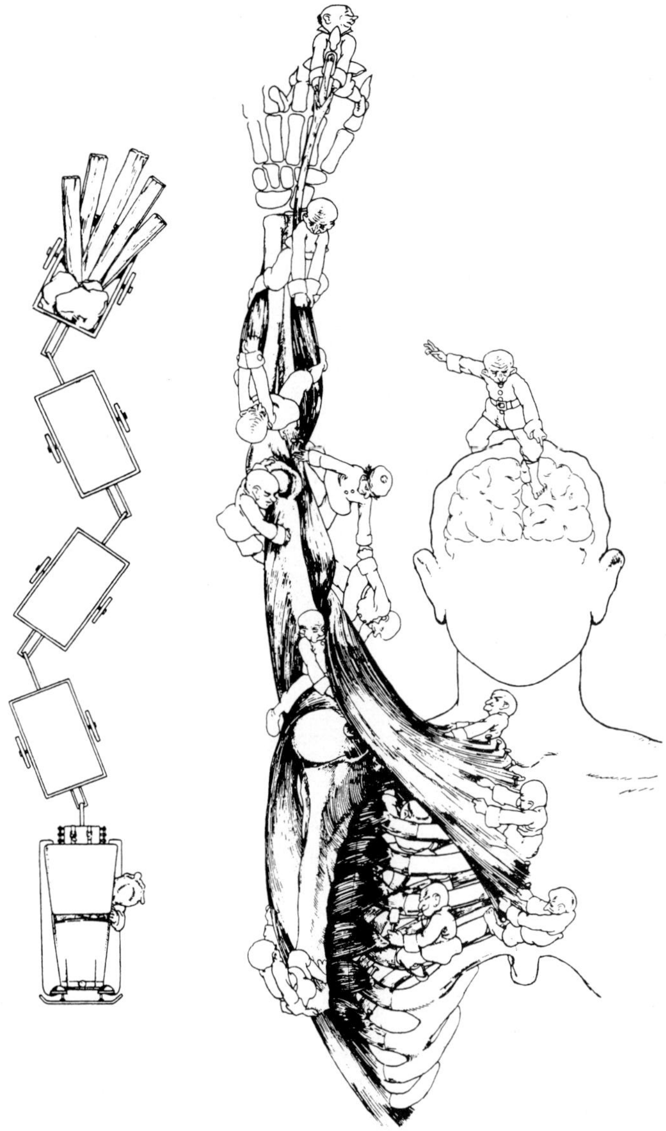

Fig. 1–17. Codman's chain of command for the delicate balance of articulation. (From Codman EA. *The Shoulder, Rupture of the Spraspinatus Tendon and Other Lesions in or About the Subacromial Bursa.* Malabar, FL: RE Krieger; 1984.)

However, not everyone agreed with Codman. Haldeman and Soto-Hall,[20] writing in the *Journal of the American Medical Association* in 1935, felt that Codman confused certain anatomic changes in the shoulder (that were a result of senile wear) with purely traumatic conditions and, contrary to Wilson, who diagnosed ruptures of the supraspinatus in 10 patients in an 18-month period after reading Codman's book, they still were under the impression that supraspinatus tendon tears were infrequent. However, even these doubters recognized the advantages of Codman's saber incision and repair of the rotator cuff into a bony trough. They described fixing or repairing the acromial process back in place with a beef bone peg.

In his thesis on humeroscapular periarthritis in 1936, Schaer recognized supraspinatus tendon defects as one of the accompanying features of this disorder and claimed that a completely healthy tendon cannot rupture.[80] The same recommendation was offered by Davis and Sullivan, who believed that the tendon was predisposed to rupture by age and exertion.[81] Ferguson considered the differential diagnosis of bursitis and tendon ruptures to be unimportant, because the treatment for both conditions was practically the same.[82]

Also in 1937, Sandstrom[83] reported on calcium deposits in the tendons secondary to circulatory impairment and necrosis, and Ferguson[82] made an early reference to the "wringer effect" of the humeral head on the supraspinatus tendon. Ellis also noted that the supraspinatus can easily become entrapped between the humerus and acromion.[84]

CADAVERIC STUDIES

By 1931 Codman and Akerson had evaluated 100 shoulders.[74] They discussed 4 hypotheses to explain the observed incidence of 39% full-thickness tears: (1) trauma; (2) result of weakness from old calcific deposits; (3) the result of constitutional necrosis, i.e. aging and degeneration analogous to degenerative arthritis in weightbearing joints; and (4) attritional wear, the theory popularized by Meyer.[79,85–89] Codman stated that of all the theories, attritional wear against the acromion was the least likely. In 1933 Lawrence Keyes confirmed the work of Codman and Akerson on the prevalence of supraspinatus tears, and their relative increase with the age of the specimen.[90] This same type of study has been repeated numerous times over the years by many investigators such as Horowitz,[91] Skinner,[92] Grant and Smith,[93] Wilson,[94,95] Cotton and Rideout,[96] Yamanaka,[97] DePalma,[98] Fukuda et al.,[99] Uhthoff,[100] and Neer.[101] The ranges of incidence of full-thickness tears in these series varies from 5 to 26.5%, with incidence and bilaterality increasing with age. Partial-thickness tears exceed full-thickness tears. The debate over the etiology primarily centering on hypotheses 1, 3, and 4, described by Codman, continues to this day.

ACUTE ROTATOR CUFF REPAIRS

Fowler[75] and Ferguson[102] reported early repair with encouraging results. Mayer reported a further four cases with early operation. In three, silk sutures and a deltoid-splitting incision that was too long resulted in poor function secondary to axillary nerve injury. In a fourth patient the deltoid was detached and the deltopectoral interval used. In this case he used fascia with gallie needles to repair the cuff (Fig. 1–18) and obtained an excellent result.[103] These investigators reiterated what Codman had speculated for over 30 years and that was the belief that early treatment would give better results.

In 1938 the first case of rotator cuff debridement was performed by Outland and Shepherd[104] when, in a series of 12 cases they reported 1 case in which a tear with wide retraction made suturing impossible. Remnants of the

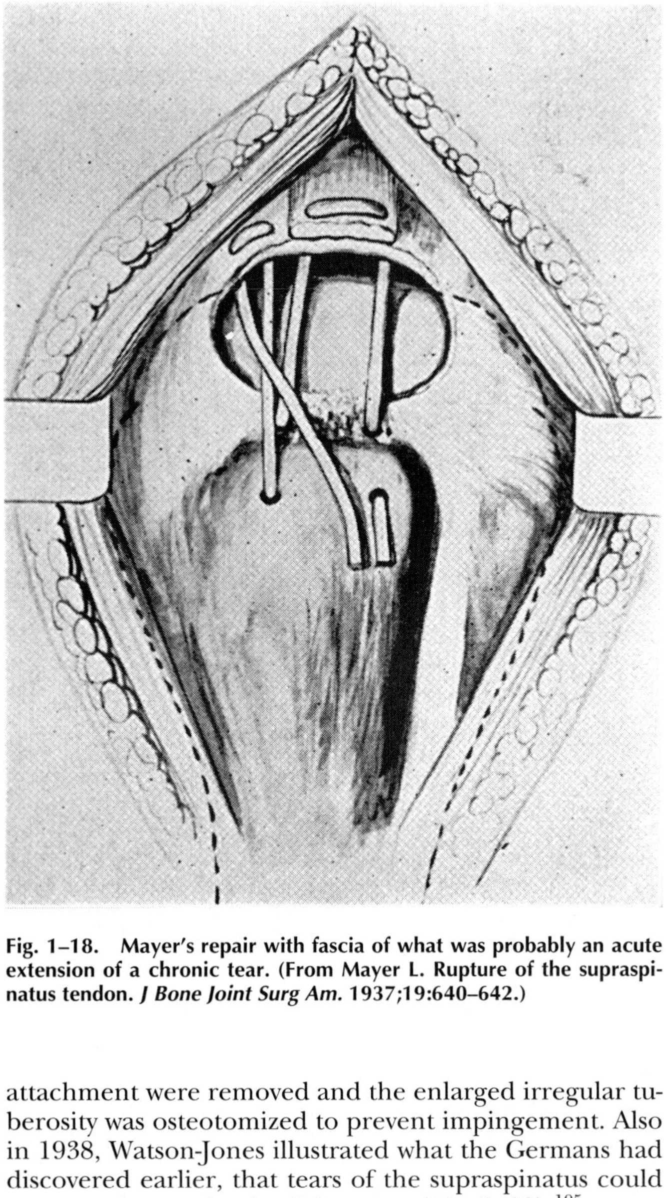

Fig. 1–18. Mayer's repair with fascia of what was probably an acute extension of a chronic tear. (From Mayer L. Rupture of the supraspinatus tendon. *J Bone Joint Surg Am.* 1937;19:640–642.)

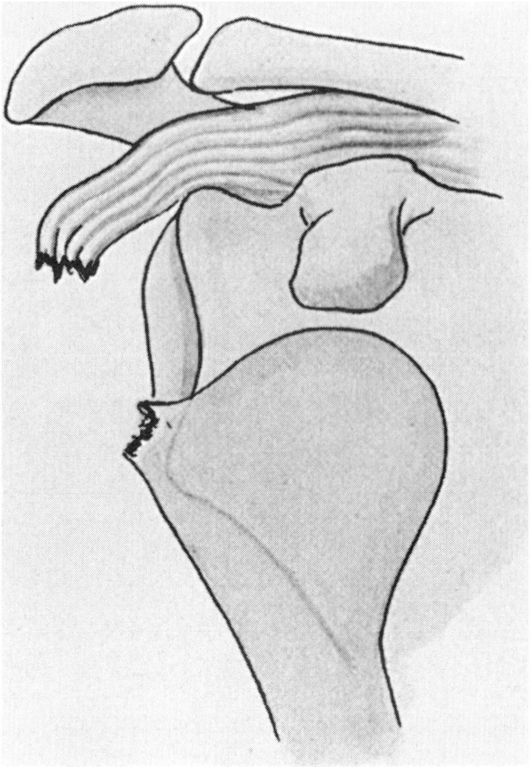

Fig. 1–19. Supraspinatus tearing as a result of anterior inferior glenohumeral dislocation. (From Watson-Jones R. Injuries in the region of the shoulder joint, (II) Bone and joint injuries. *Brit Med J.* 1938;2:80–83.)

attachment were removed and the enlarged irregular tuberosity was osteotomized to prevent impingement. Also in 1938, Watson-Jones illustrated what the Germans had discovered earlier, that tears of the supraspinatus could occur as the result of a dislocation (Fig. 1–19).[105]

It is in David Bosworth's article from 1940 that the first use of the term rotator cuff is found.[106] Prior to this time, the individual tendons were mentioned or were referred to in a group as the short rotators. In his follow-up review, Bosworth described just about every lesion and a complete classification was offered.[107,108]

RADIOLOGY OF THE ROTATOR CUFF

Plain film radiology was used to demonstrate the calcifications seen by Painter in 1907.[51] Air arthrography was first carried out by Oberholtzer in 1933.[109] Radiographic contrast was used by Lindblom and Palmer.[110] A more detailed study of the evaluation of radiographic techniques is beyond the scope of this chapter.

In 1937 Frank Liberson[111] reported on 25 cases of os acromiale, following a study of routine roentgenographic examinations of 1,800 shoulder girdles (Fig. 1–20). His stimulus for this work was a workmen's compensation case in which it was alleged that an os acromiale was a fracture. In reviewing the literature, he found that Kohler[112] made reference to the radiographic appearance of the os acromiale in 1928.

1941 TO 1972

The relationship of rotator cuff disease in the throwing athlete and a description of coracoid impingement was discussed by Bennett in two reports in 1941.[113,114] With World War II, the necessity and use of the fracture service became apparent. Under the leadership of Darrach, the now famous fracture service at the Columbia Presbyterian Hospital was formed. According to Neer, Darrach (whose anatomical retractors we use today to mobilize the rotator cuff) hired Harrison McLaughlin as his assistant in 1934. Both Darrach and McLaughlin were interested in Codman's book published that same year.

Harrison McLaughlin, writing in 1944, gave Codman credit for repeatedly pointing out the importance of the subacromial structures and stimulating vis a vis his teachings, the study of these cases at the fracture service of Presbyterian Hospital in New York.[115] Initially labelling sore shoulders by the then fashionable term bursitis, he would later state that "bursitis was no more a diagnosis than headache or jaundice and that when present usually constituted a second condition, having no connection with the primary lesion other than proximity." McLaughlin was critical of the deltoid-splitting approach, which resulted in his opinion, in inadequate exposure, poor cosmesis, and frequent axillary nerve injury. He described a new incision beginning just lateral to the acromioclavicular (AC) joint (Fig. 1–21). He recommended deltoid splitting be near the anterior border from proximal to distal. For complete exposure of the joint region, an acromial osteotomy was performed.

McLaughlin, like Brown,[116] used local anesthetic as a guide to treatment.[117,118] McLaughlin's experience was extensive at the time, having treated over 3,000 painful

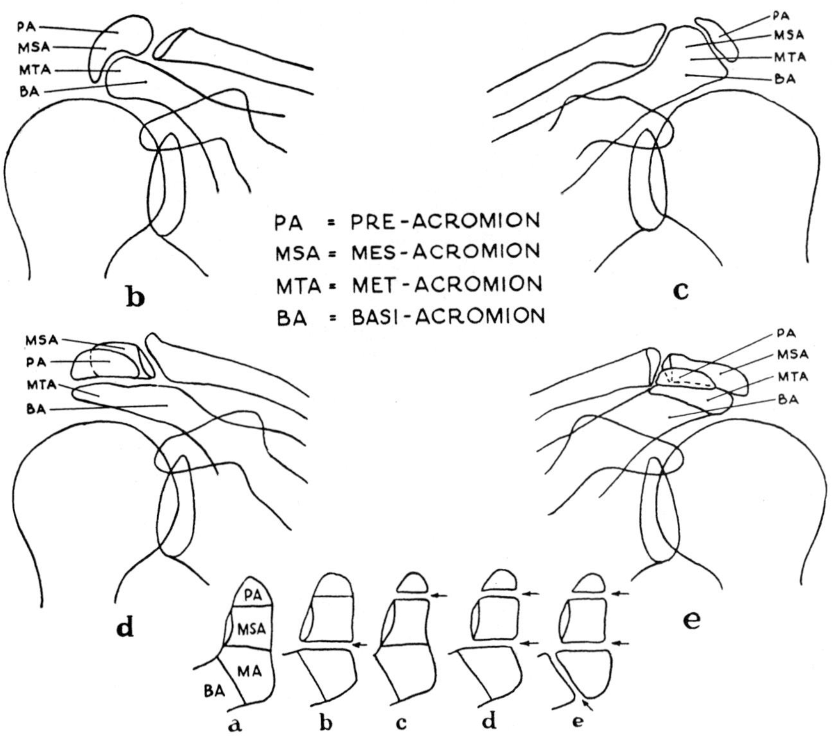

Fig. 1–20. Description of the different types of un4fused acromion as found by Liberson. (From Liberson F. Os acromiale—A contested anomaly. *J Bone Joint Surg.* 1937;19: 683–689.)

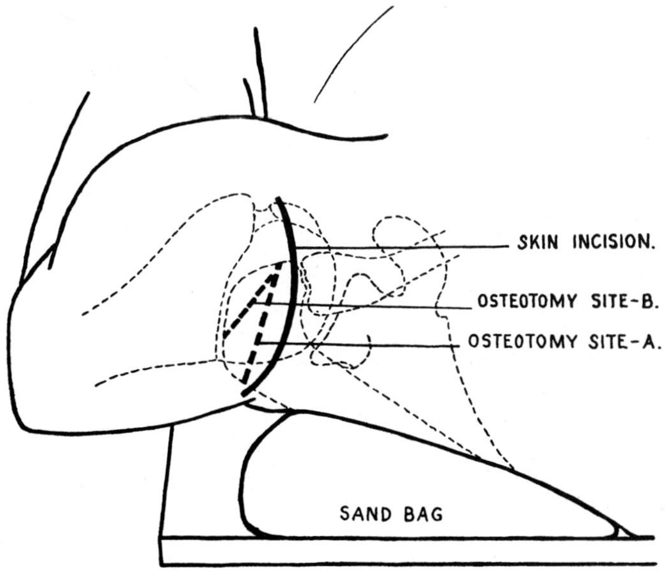

Fig. 1–21. McLaughlin's exposure for rotator cuff tears. Two different osteotomies were proposed based on the exposure requirements. (From McLaughlin HL. Lesions of the musculotendinous cuff of the shoulder. The exposure and treatment of tears with retraction. *J Bone Joint Surg.* 26:31–51.)

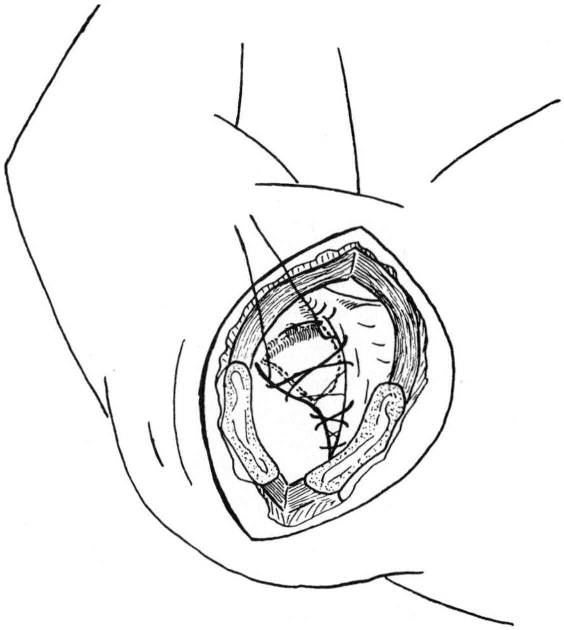

Fig. 1–22. The classic shoe lace stitch of McLaughlin. (From McLaughlin HL. Lesions of the musculotendinous cuff of the shoulder. The exposure and treatment of tears with retraction. *J Bone Joint Surg.* 1944; 26:31–51.)

shoulders with 275 operations being performed over a 10-year period. He reminded his readers that: "No two lesions are ever alike and no two lesions ever call for identical operative technique."[119]

The general conception of the tear with retraction as a pure transverse tear was challenged by McLaughlin. He noted that such ruptures seldom occurred except in tendinous cuffs that had been subjected to sufficient attritional wear to make them weak. He likened the cuff to a sheet of cellophane, which as long as it remained intact had great tensile strength, but once a tear occurred, the tear would propagate and progressively tear more and more. He also recognized that concomitant to the transverse tear, a longitudinal tear occurred, commencing usually at one end of the original transverse rupture.

Because of the difficulty of obtaining end-to-end repair in chronic cases, he developed what he called the shoelace repair (Fig. 1–22), in which the shoe-lace type of continuous suture begins medially, pulling the two edges together. Eventually, only a small V-shaped opening of the humeral head would remain. He recommended repairing the tendons at the point at where they came to lie without tension, with the arm at the side, into a V-shaped trough (Fig. 1–23).

A "simplified" operation was offered by Laurence Jones in 1944.[120] He was the first to recommend infraspinatus and subscapularis transposition for massive tears and used infraspinatus advancement for supraspinatus tears with retraction as opposed to McLaughlin's shoelace repair (Fig. 1–24).

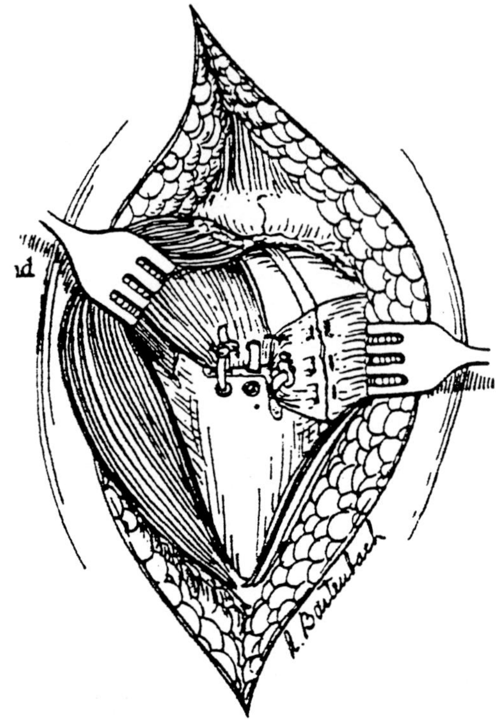

Fig. 1–24. *A,B,* Subacromial and infraspinatus transposition as described by Jones for massive rotator cuff tear. (From Jones L. Complete rupture of the supraspinatus tendon. A simplified operative repair. *Arch Surg.* 1944;49:390–398.)

In 1963 in a follow-up article for *Surgical Clinics of North America,* McLaughlin stated his requisites for successful repair. These included snug apposition of healthy tissues, a tension-free repair with the arm at the side, restoration of continuity, a smooth surface repair, a water tight repair, removal of an abnormal biceps tendon, release of the coracoacromial ligament, and operation only by necessity.[121] The striking difference between his 1963 article and the one written in 1943 is his enthusiasm for the operation had waned somewhat. He stated that there were "cogent" contraindications to early operation and recommended that the concept of "operation by necessity" be used, i.e. the operation was not indicated by the diagnosis as much as it was by continuing pain and disability. Although he formerly favored early operation, experience demonstrated that the results of early and late repair were essentially the same. This correlates with Rowe's later statement that "the more experienced the surgeon, the more conservative he will be with this entity."[122]

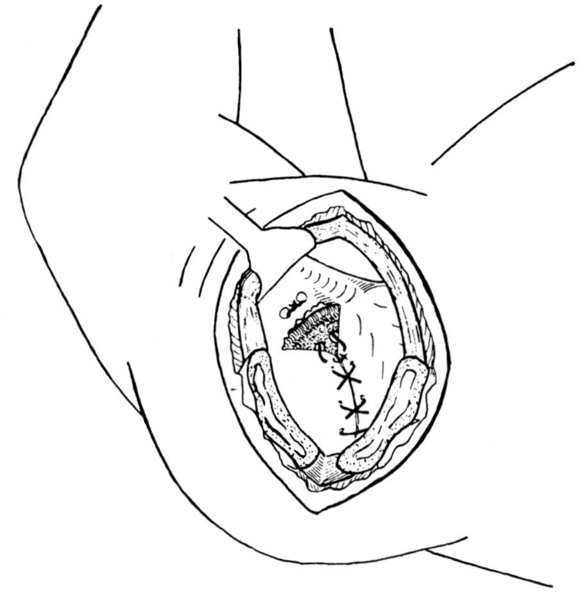

Fig. 1–23. With McLaughlin's technique, the rotator cuff is advanced as far as possible and then sutured into the humeral head at whatever point it reaches without tension. (From McLaughlin HL. Lesions of the musculotendinous cuff of the shoulder. The exposure and treatment of tears with retraction. *J Bone Joint Surg.* 1944;26:31–51.)

In the late 1940s Julius Neviaser, who coined the term adhesive capsulitis, wrote about the treatment of this entity.[123] Later he would offer unique techniques for repair of the rotator cuff.[124] Not only did he leave a legacy of literature, but also a legacy of life through his three sons, who all contributed to our understanding of the shoulder literature. His work is discussed in detail in Chapter 17.

EVOLUTION OF THE ACROMIOPLASTY

The evolution of the acromioplasty is depicted in Figure 1–25. Codman's saber incision involved an osteotomy

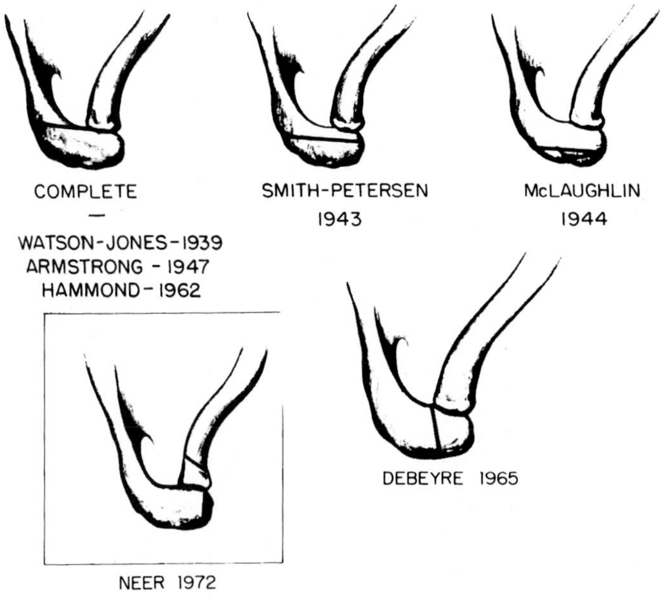

Fig. 1–25. The evolution of acromioplasty. Reproduced with deletion of Stamms glenoplasty. (From Neer CS II. *Shoulder Reconstruction.* Philadelphia: WB Saunders; 1990.)

at the base of the acromion; however, there is no record that he ever removed the fragment. He did, however, later in his career, favor a less extensive deltoid splitting approach.[76] Armstrong[125] credits Watson-Jones with describing excision of the acromion in the treatment of supraspinatus tendon lesions at a meeting of the British Orthopaedic Association in Oswestry in 1939.[126] However, Smith Petersen reports the first operation of acromioplasty was performed by him in 1935 for an exostosis.[127] He subsequently performed the operation on 11 patients with rheumatoid arthritis. In 1943, Watson-Jones described his first acromionectomy done for heterotopic ossification and calcification.[128] Armstrong reported on 95 patients after acromionectomy, with satisfactory results occurring in 84.2%. He noted that patients who had complete acromionectomies fared better than those who had the AC joint left in place. He should know; in 1944 Watson-Jones had excised Armstrong's own acromion.[126]

Moseley offered a slightly more oblique osteotomy, which was less aggressive than the Saber approach. Moseley noted that more rapid recovery occurred when the acromion was not sectioned and only the distal clavicle removed. As late as 1962, acromionectomy was alive and well in the "City of Healing,"[129] and it wasn't until Neer's classic article in 1972 that focused the attention to the anterior aspect of the acromion that an alternative form of surgical approach that could improve the exposure, treat a component of the underlying pathology, and cause less harm to the deltoid was available.[130]

In France, Debeyre, disappointed with the results he obtained with McLaughlin's technique; but convinced of the need to repair the cuff, developed the idea of muscle advancement in 1961.[131]

1972 TO PRESENT

Charles S. Neer

Neer's initial interest in the shoulder began as a resident under Darrach on the fracture service at Columbia, when he first witnessed the poor outcome from treatment of displaced proximal humeral fracture-dislocations by head excision and hypothesized that a metallic humeral head replacement could be created to improve the results. Darrach encouraged this endeavor and, after returning from World War II, Neer designed a prosthesis and published his initial findings in 1953.[132] McLaughlin and Neer were colleagues and friends who spoke frequently at meetings together (Fig. 1–26). Neer concentrated at that time primarily on arthroplasty and fractures, while McLaughlin's interest was in rotator cuff tears, glenohumeral dislocations, and trauma in general.

Neer's first article on rotator cuff tears appeared in 1972. From 1975 until 1990, his ideas evolved with regard to the etiology, pathoanatomy, surgical treatment, and rehabilitation of rotator cuff tears. Twenty-five years of careful observation in the operating room, anatomy lab, and clinic and over 20 publications on cuff disease alone, coupled with numerous presentations culminated in the publication of his book *Shoulder Reconstruction* in 1990.

In addition to introducing the anterior acromioplasty,[130] Neer coined the term "rotator cuff tear arthropathy,"[133] pointed out the relationship between impingement and biceps tendon ruptures,[134] decried radical acromionectomy,[135] and developed treatment options for the unfused acromial epiphysis.[136] Neer classified impingement lesions, defined the supraspinatus outlet, and recommended earlier passive motion as an important part of rehabilitation.[137,138] The long term results of cuff repair, as well as rerepair of rotator cuff tears, were reported in the late 1980s, along with the useful technique of coracohumeral ligament incision.[137,140–143] Neer's system to repair outlet impingement is discussed in detail in Chapter 10.

Patients and physicians around the world owe a tremendous debt to Neer, the son of a general surgeon from Vinita, Oklahoma. Although retired from practice, his system of evaluating and treating outlet impingement continues to allow countless patients and, therefore, their physicians to sleep well at night.

The remainder of this book is devoted to advances in diagnostic and therapeutic techniques over the last 30 years. Neer's techniques and reliance on the impingement/attritional theory have been challenged in recent years by other investigators, some of whom have contributed to this book. The historical significance of their work will not be judged solely by peer reviewed journals, but by the physicians who adopt their philosophy and the patients on whom their hypotheses and procedures are tested.

Many of the contributors to shoulder surgery over the years trace the development of their interest to a book they read sometime in their career. I can only hope that someday a reader of this book will be stimulated to con-

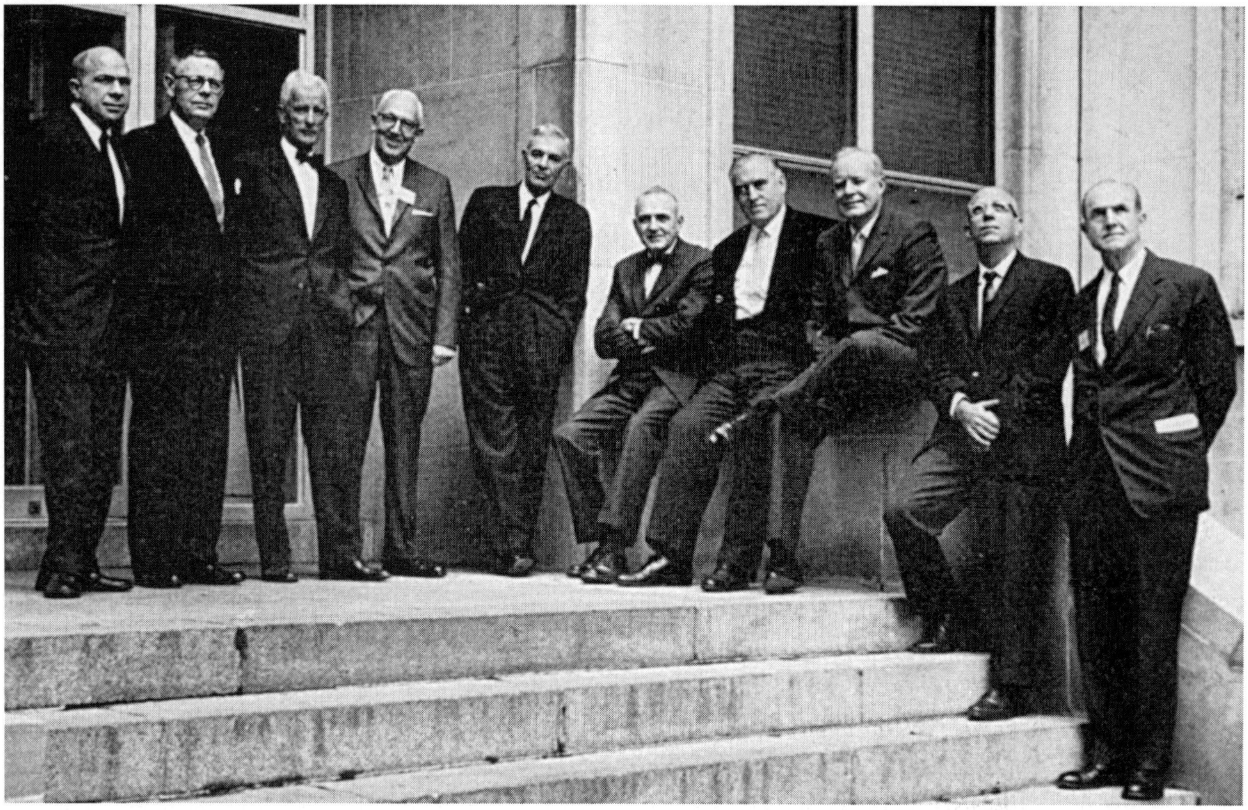

Fig. 1–26. The faculty of the first course dedicated to the shoulder in North America (Montreal) Left to right: Charles S. Neer II, MD; Thomas B. Quigley, MD; Professor R. Merle d'Aubigne; Julius S. Neviaser, MD; Harrison L. McLaughlin, MD; Alexander P. Aitken, MD; H. Fred Moseley, DM; James E. Bateman, MD; Anthony F. DePalma, MD; and Carter R. Rowe, MD. (From Forward. *Surg Clin N Am.* 1962; 43:1463–1780.)

tribute further to our understanding and treatment of rotator cuff disease, which is, like history itself, a continuum with an unintelligible beginning and an imperceivable end.

REFERENCES

1. Smith E. *Edwin Smith's Surgical Papyrus.* Chicago: University of Chicago Press; 1930.
2. Jobe CM. Gross anatomy of the shoulder. In: Rockwood CA, Matsen FA, eds. *The Shoulder.* Philadelphia: WB Saunders; 1990:34–89.
3. Hoernle AFR. *Studies in the Medicine of Ancient India. Part I. Osteology of the Bones of the Human Body.* Oxford, England: Clarendon Press; 1907.
4. Persaud TVN. *Early History of the Human Anatomy. From Antiquity to the Beginning of the Modern Era.* Springfield, IL: Charles C. Thomas; 1984.
5. Adams FL. *The Genuine Works of Hippocrates.* New York: William Wood & Co; 1886; Vol. 1 & 2.
6. Rang M. Reductions. In: *Anthology of Orthopedics.* Edinburgh: Churchill Livingstone; 1966:225–226.
7. Hippocrates. Hippocratic writings translated by Francis Adam. In: Adler MJ, ed. *The Great Books.* Chicago: Encyclopedia Britannica; 1972:197.
8. Galen. On the works of natural faculties. In: Adler MJ, ed. *The Great Books.* Chicago: Encyclopedia Britannica; 1992:343–449.
9. Reeves B. Experiments on the tensile strength of the anterior capsular structures of the shoulder region. *J Bone Joint Surg Br.* 1928; 50:858.
10. da Vinci L. *The Anatomy of Man.* Drawings from the collection of Her Majesty, Queen Elizabeth II. Houston, Texas: Museum of Fine Arts and Bulfinch Press, 1992.
11. Saunders JB de CM, O'Malley CD. *The Illustrations From the Works of Andreas Vesalius of Brussels.* Cleveland: The World Publishing Company; 1950.
12. Cowper W. *Myotomia Reformata.* London: 1694:75.
13. Bromfield W. *Chirgical Observations and Cases.* London:1773:76.
14. Monteggia GB. *Instituzioni Chirurgiche.* Milan: G. Truffi, T.V, 1830, p. 179; also Part II, p. 334, 1803.
15. Pouteau C. *Melanges de Chirurgie.* Lyons: G. Regnault; 1760:433.
16. Soden J. Two cases of dislocation of the tendon of the long head of the biceps. *Med Chir Tr.* 1841;14:2.
17. Morton. Rupture of long tendon of the biceps muscle due to muscular effort—suture, and successful result—antiseptic appliances. *Philadelphia Medical Times.* 1886;17:120–121.
18. Monro A. *A Description of All the Bursae Mucosae of the Human Body.* Edinburgh: Elliott Kay; 1788.
19. Moseley HF. Ruptures of the rotator cuff. *Br J Surg.* 1951; 38:340–369.
20. Smith JG. Pathological appearances of seven cases of injury to the shoulder-joint; with remarks. Letter to the Editor. *London Med Gazette.* (Being a Weekly Journal of Med and Collateral Sciences) pp. 0–5; Saturday, May 24, 1834.
21. Ashurst J. *Science and Art of Surgery.* Erickson E, Ashurst J Jr, eds. A.M.D.D. Philadelphia: Henry C. Lee; 1869:302.
22. Adams R. *A Treatise of Rheumatic Gout or Chronic Rheumatoid Arthritis of All the Joints.* 2nd ed. London: John Churchill & Sons. Edinburgh: Maclachlan & Stewart; 1873:1–568.
23. Smith RW. Observations upon chronic rheumatic arthritis of the shoulder. I. *Dublin Quarterly J Med Sci.* 1853;15:1–16.

24. Smith RW. Observations upon chronic rheumatic arthritis of the shoulder. II. *Dublin Quarterly J Med Sci.* 1853;15:343–358.
25. Haldeman KO, Soto-Hall R. Injuries to muscles and tendons. *J Am Med Assoc.* 1935;104:2319–2324.
26. Codman EA. Rupture of the supraspinatus- 1834–1934. *J Bone Joint Surg Am.* 1937;19:643–652.
27. Malgaigne JF (1840) zit. In: Jossel G. Uber die recidive der humerusluxationen. *Dtsch Z Chir.* 1880;13:167–184.
28. Jossel G. Anatomische Beitrage zur Kenntnis der humerusluxationen mit fractur der tuberkel. *Dtsch Z Chir.* 1871;4:124–129.
29. Jossel G. Uber die recidive der humerusluxationen. *Dtsch Z Chir.* 1880;13:167–184.
30. Jossel G. Lenrbuch der topographisch-chirurgischen. *Anatomie.* 1884;1:17–22.
31. Kronlein RU. *Die Lehr von Den Luxationen.* Stuttgart: Verlag F. Enke; 1882.
32. Flower WH. On pathological changes produced in the shoulder joint. *Trans Path Sac London.* 1861:12:179–200.
33. Von Pitha. Lehrbuch der chirurgie. zit. In: Jossel G, ed. *Lehrbuch der Topographisch-Chirurgischen.* Anatomie 1884: 1:17–22.
34. Konig. Lehrbuch. 2.Aufl. II. S. 601 zit in: Cramer F: Resection des oberarmkopfos wegen habitueller luxation. *Berl klin Wschr.* 1882; 19:21–25.
35. Cramer F. Resection des oberamkopfes wegen habitueller luxation. *Berl klin Wschr.* 1882;19:21–25.
36. Hueter (1870), zit in: Cramer F: Resection des oberamkopfes wegen habitueller luxation. *Berl klin Wschr.* 1882;19:21–25.
37. Bardenheuer B. Die verletzungen der oberen extremitaten. *Reihe Deutsche Chirurgie.* 63, 1886.
38. Finney. Injury to the shoulder. *Johns Hopkins Hosp Bull.* 1891;5:83.
39. Rowe CR. Codman—His influence on the development of surgery of the shoulder. In: Bateman JE, Welsh RP, eds. *Surgery of the Shoulder.* Philadelphia: BC Decker; 1984:1–6.
40. Codman EA. *The Shoulder, Rupture of the Supraspinatus Tendon and Supraspinatus Tendon and Other Lesions in or About the Subacromial Bursa.* Malabar, FL: Robert E Krieger Co; 1984.
41. Albert E. Diagnostik der chirugischer krankheiten. Weiss, 1893.
42. Codman EA. Some points on the diagnosis and treatment of certain neglected minor surgical lesions. *Bost Med Surg J.* 1904; 150:371–374.
43. Codman EA. On stiff and painful shoulders. The anatomy of the subdeltoid or subacromial bursa and its clinical importance. Subdeltoid bursitis. *Bost Med Surg J.* 1906;154:613–616.
44. Codman EA. Bursitis subacromialis or periarthritis of the shoulder joint (subdeltoid bursitis). *Bost Med Surg J.* 1908;159:533–537, 576–578, 615–616, 677–680, 723–727.
45. Goldthwait JE. An anatomic and mechanical study of the shoulder-joint, explaining many of the cases of painful shoulder, many of the recurrent dislocations, and many of the cases of brachial neuralgias or neuritis. *Am J Ortho Surg.* 1909;6:579–606.
46. Stevens HH. The action of the short rotators on normal abduction of the arm, with a consideration of their action on some cases of subacromial bursitis and allred conditions. *Am J Med Science.* 138:870, 1909.
47. Perthes G. Uber operationen bei habitueller schulterluxation. *Deutsch Z Chir.* 1906;85:199–227.
48. Muller W. Uber habituelle schulterluxationen. XXVII. *Chirurg (Berlin).* 1898.
49. Codman EA. Complete rupture of the supraspinatus tendon. Operative treatment with report of two successful cases. *Bost Med Surg J.* 1911;164:708–710.
50. Baer WS. Operative treatment of subdeltoid bursitis. *Johns Hopkins Hosp Bull.* 1907;18:2–4.
51. Painter CF. Subdeltoid bursitis. *Bost Med J.* 1907;156:345–349.
52. Dawburn RHM. Subdeltoid bursitis—A pathognomonic sign for its recognition. *Bost Med Surg J.* 1906;154:691.
53. Bergemann A, Stieda A. Uber die mit kalkelnlagerungen einhorgehende entzundung der schulterschleimbeutel. *MMW* 1908; 52:99–2702.
54. Stieda A. Zur pathologie der schultergelenkschleimbeutel. *Arch klin Chir.* 1908;85:910–919.
55. Wrede L. Ueber kalkablagerungen in der umgebung des schultergelenkes und ihre bezlehung zur periarthritis scapulohumeralas. *Arch klin Chir.* 1912;79:259–272.
56. Moschcowitz. Histopathology of calcification of the spinatus tendons as associated with subacromial bursitis. *Am J Med Sci.* 1915; 150:115–126.
57. Brickner WM. Pain in the arm: Subdeltoid (subacromial) bursitis. *JAMA.* 1917;69:1237–1243.
58. Buchholz H. Therapeutic exercise and massage. Philadelphia: Lea & Febiger; 1917:231.
59. Buchholz H. Der abrib der supraspinatussehne. *Arch klin Chir.* 1922;1:255–264.
60. Meyer AW. Evidence of attrition in the human body. *Anat Rec.* 1923;25:142.
61. Meyer AW. Further evidence of attrition in the human body. *Am J Anat.* 1924;34:241–267.
62. Burman MS. Arthroscopy or the direct visualization of joints. *J Bone Joint Surg Am.* 1931;13:669–695.
63. Bircher E. Beltrag zur pathologie (arthritis deformans) und diagnose der meniscus-verletzungen (arthroendoskopie). *Beltrag klin Chir.* 1922;127:239–250.
64. Payr E. Gelenk "Sperren" und "Ankylasen;" uber die schultersteifen verschiedener ursache und die sogenannte "Periarthritis humeroscapularis." *Zbl Chir.* 1931:58:2993.
65. Dollinger J. Die anatomische lokalisation des irrtumlich bursitis chronica subacromialis Duplay usw, genannten schulterschmerzes und seine behandlung. *Zbl Chir.* 1932;10:579–583.
66. Keyes EL. Observations on rupture of the supraspinatus tendon. *Ann Surg.* 1933;97:849–856.
67. Ohnsorge K: Die bedeutung der oberamauswartsroller fur die hebung des armes in der frontalebene. *Dtsch Z Chir.* 1933;58:382–389.
68. Oberholzer J. Die arthro-pneumoradiographie bei habitueller schulterluxation. *Roentgenpraxis.* 1933;5:589–590.
69. Bircher E. Beitrag zur pathologie (arthritis deformans) und diagnose der meniscus-verietzungen (arthroendoskopic). *Boitr klin Chil.* 1922;127:239–250.
70. Gilli AB. A new operation for arthrodesis of the shoulder. *J Bone Joint Surg.* 1931;13:287–295.
71. Codman EA. On stiff and painful shoulders, as explained by subacromial bursitis and partial rupture of the tendon of the supraspinatus. *Bost Med Surg J.* 1912;165:115–120.
72. Codman EA. The pathology and treatment of lesions in and about the shoulder joint. *Industrial Doctor.* 1926;4:121–131.
73. Codman EA. Obscure lesions of the shoulder. Rupture of the tendon of the supraspinatus. *Bost Med Surg J.* 1927;196:381–387.
74. Codman EA, Akerson TB. The pathology associated with rupture of the supraspinatus tendon. *Ann Surg.* 1931;93:348–359.
75. Codman EA. Rupture of the supraspinatus tendon. *Surg Gynecol Obstet.* 1931;52:579–586.
76. Codman EA. Rupture of the supraspinatus. *Am J Surg.* 1938; 42:603–606.
77. Wilson PD. Complete rupture of the supraspinatus tendon. *J Am Med Assoc.* 1931;96:433–438.
78. Fowler EB. Rupture of the spinati tendons and capsule, repaired by a new operation. *Ill Med J.* 1932;61:332–334.
79. Moseley HF. Rupture of supraspinatus tendon. *Can Med Assoc J.* 1939;41:280–282 .
80. Schaer H. Die periarthritis humeroscapularis. *Ergebn Chir Orthop.* 1936;29:221–309.
81. Davis T, Sullivan E. Rupture of the supraspinatus tendon. *Ann Surg.* 1937;106:1059–1069.
82. Ferguson LK. Painful shoulder arising from lesions at the subacromial bursa and supraspinatus tendon. *Ann Surg.* 1937;105:243–256.
83. Sandstrom C, Wahlgren F. Beitrag zur kenntnls der "peritendinitis calcarea" (sogen. "bursitis calculosa") speziell vorn pathologisch-histologischen Gasichtspunkt. *Acta Radiol (Stockh).* 1937; 18:263–296.
84. Ellis VH. Lesions of the supraspinatus. *Proc Roy Soc Med.* 1938; 31:451–453.
85. Meyer AW: Unrecognized occupational destruction of the tendon of the long head of the biceps brachii. *Arch Surg.* 1921; 2:130–144.
86. Meyer AW. Further observations upon use destruction in joints. *J Bone Joint Surg.* 1922;4:491–511.
87. Meyer AW. Spontaneous dislocation of the tendon of the long

head of the biceps brachii. Report of four cases. *Arch Surg.* 1926; 13:109–119.
88. Meyer AW. Spontaneous dislocation and destruction of the tendon of the long head of the biceps brachii. Fifty-nine incidences. *Arch Surg.* 1928;17:493–506.
89. Meyer AW. The minute anatomy of attrition lesions. *J Bone Joint Surg.* 1931;13:341.
90. Keyes EL. Observations on rupture of supraspinatus tendon. Based upon a study of 73 cadavers. *Ann Surg.* 1933;97:849–856.
91. Horowitz MT. Lesions of the supraspinatus tendon and associated structures. Investigation of comparable lesions in the hip joint. *Arch Surg.* 1939;38:990–1003.
92. Skinner HA. Anatomical consideration relative to ruptures of the supraspinatus tendon. *J Bone Joint Surg Am.* 1937; 19:137–151.
93. Grant JCB, Smith CG. Age incidence of rupture of the supraspinatus tendon (abstract). *Anat Rec.* 1948;100:666.
94. Wilson CL. Lesions of the supraspinatus tendon: Degeneration, rupture, and calcification. *Arch Surg.* 1943;46:307–325.
95. Wilson CL, Duff GL. Pathologic study of degeneration and rupture of the supraspinatus tendon. *Arch Surg.* 1943; 47: 121–135.
96. Cotton RE, Rideout DF. Tears of the humeral rotator cuff. A radiological and pathological necropsy survey. *J Bone Joint Surg Br.* 1964;46:314–328.
97. Yamanaka K, Fukuda H, Hamada K, Mikasa M. Incomplete thickness tears of the rotator cuff. *Orthop Traumatol Surg (Tokyo).* 1983; 26:713.
98. DePalma AF. *Surgery of the Shoulder.* 2nd ed. Philadelphia: JB Lippincott; 1973.
99. Fukuda H. Rotator cuff tears. *Geka Chiryo. (Osaka)* 1980;43:28.
100. Uhthoff HK, Loehr J, Sarkar K. *The pathogenesis of rotator cuff tears.* In: Proceedings of the Third International Conference on Surgery of the Shoulder. Fukuoka, Japan, October 27, 1986.
101. Neer CS II, Poppen NC. Supraspinatus outlet. *J Bone Joint Surg Am.* 1987;11:234.
102. Ferguson LK. Suture of ruptured supraspinatus tendon four days after surgery. *J Surg.* 1935;29:384–386.
103. Mayer L. Rupture of the supraspinatus tendon. *J Bone Joint Surg Am.* 1937;19:640–642, 1937.
104. Outland TA, Shepherd WF. Tears of the supraspinatus tendon. Resume of twelve operated cases. *Ann Surg.* 1938;107:116–121.
105. Watson-Jones R. Injuries in the region of the shoulder joint, (II) Bone and joint injuries. *Brit Med J.* 1938;2:80–83.
106. Bosworth DM. An analysis of consecutive cases of incapacitating shoulder lesions radically explored and repaired. *J Bone Joint Surg Am.* 1940;22:369–392.
107. Bosworth DM. The supraspinatus syndrome. Symptomatology, pathology, and repair. *JAMA.* 1941;117:422–428.
108. Bosworth DM. Muscular and tendinous defects of the shoulder and their repair. In: *American Academy of Orthopaedic Surgeons: Lectures on Reconstruction Surgery of the Extremities.* Ann Arbor, Michigan: JW Edwards;1944:380–390.
109. Oberholtzer J. Die arthropneumoradiographe bei habitueller schulterluxatio. *Roentgenpraxis.* 1933;5:589–590.
110. Lindblom K, Palmer I. Ruptures of the tendon aponeurosis of the shoulder joint—the so-called supraspinatus ruptures. *Acta Chir Scand.* 1939;82:133–142.
111. Liberson F. Os acromiale—A contested anomaly. *J Bone Joint Surg Am.* 1937;19:683–689.
112. Kohler A. *Roentgenology: The borderland of the normal and early pathological in the skiagram.* 6th ed., New York: William Wood & Co; 1937.
113. Bennett GE. Shoulder and elbow lesions of professional baseball pitchers. *J Am Med Assoc.* 1941;117:510–514.
114. Bennett GE. Shoulder and elbow lesions distinctive of baseball players. *Ann Surg.* 1947;1:107–110.
115. McLaughlin HL. Lesions of the musculotendinous cuff of the shoulder. The exposure and treatment of tears with retraction. *J Bone Joint Surg Am.* 1944;26:31–51.
116. Brown JT. Early assessment of supraspinatus tears. Procaine infiltration as a guide to treatment. *J Bone Joint Surg Br.* 1949;31:423–425.
117. McLaughlin HL. Common shoulder injuries. Diagnosis and treatment. *Am J Surg.* 1947;74:282–295.
118. McLaughlin HL, Asherman EG. Lesions of the musculotendinous cuff of the shoulder IV: Some observations based upon the results of surgical repair. *J Bone Joint Surg Am.* 1951; 33:76–86.
119. McLaughlin HL. Rupture of the rotator cuff. *J Bone Joint Surg Am.* 1962;44:979–983.
120. Jones L. Complete rupture of the supraspinatus tendon. A simplified operative repair. *Arch Surg.* 1944;49:390–398.
121. McLaughlin HL. Repair of major cuff ruptures. *Surg Clin North Am.* 1963;43:1535–1540.
122. Rowe CR. Ruptures of the rotator cuff. Selection of cases for surgical treatment. *Surg Clin North Am.* 1976;43:176.
123. Neviaser JS. Adhesive capsulitis of the shoulder. A study of the pathological findings in periarthritis of the shoulder. *J Bone Joint Surg.* 1945;27:211–222.
124. Neviaser JS. Arthrography of the shoulder joint. Study of the findings in adhesive capsulitis of the shoulder. *J Bone Joint Surg Am.* 1962;44:1321–1330.
125. Armstrong JR. Excision of the acromion in treatment of the supraspinatus syndrome: Report of ninety-five excisions. *J Bone Joint Surg Br.* 1949;31:436–442.
126. Watson-Jones R. *Excision of acromion for supraspinatus tendinitis.* Demonstration of cases at meeting of British Orthopaedic Association, Oswestry, 1939.
127. Smith-Petersen MX, Aufranc OE, Larson CB. Useful surgical procedures for rheumatoid arthritis involving joints of the upper extremity. *Arch Surg.* 1943;46:764–770.
128. Watson-Jones R. *Fractures and Joint Injuries.* 2nd ed. Baltimore: Williams & Wilkins; 1960.
129. Hammond G. Complete acromionectomy in the treatment of chronic tendinitis of the shoulder. *J Bone Joint Surg Am.* 1962; 44:494–503.
130. Neer CS II. Anterior acromioplasty for the chronic impingement syndrome in the shoulder. *J Bone Joint Surg Am.* 1972; 54:41–50.
131. Debeyre J, Patte D. Une technique de reparation de la coiffe musculo-tendineuse de l'epaule. Voie d'aboul trans-acromiale et desinsertion du corps charnu du punscle dus epineux. *Presse Medicale.* 1959;69:2019.
132. Neer CS II, Brown TH Jr, McLaughlin HL. Fracture of the neck of the humerus with dislocation of the head fragment. *Am J Surg.* 1953;85:252.
133. Neer CS, Cruess RL, Sledge CB, Wilde AH. Total glenohumeral replacement. A preliminary report. *Orthop Trans.* 1977; 2:244–245.
134. Neer CS, Bigliani LU, Hawkins RJ. Rupture of the long head of the biceps related to subacromial impingement. *Orthop Trans.* 1977;1:111.
135. Neer CS, Marberry TA. On the disadvantages of radical acromionectomy. *J Bone Joint Surg Am.* 1981;63:416–419.
136. Norris TR, Fisher J, Bigliani LU, Neer CS II. The unfused acromial epiphysis and its relationship to impingement syndrome. *Orthop Trans.* 1983;7:505.
137. Neer CS II, Poppen NK. Supraspinatus outlet. *Orthop Trans.* 1987; 11:234.
138. Neer CS II, McCann PD, MacFarlane EA, Padilla N. Earlier passive motion following shoulder arthroplasty and rotator cuff repair. A prospective study. *Orthop Trans.* 1987;11:231.
139. Neer CS II, Flatow EL, Lech O. Long term results of anterior acromioplasty and repair of cuff tears. *Orthop Trans.* 1988;12:735.
140. Neer CS II, Satterlee CC. Re-operation for failed cuff repairs. *Orthop Trans.* 1988.
141. Neer CS II, Satterlee CC, Dalsey RM, Flatow EL. On the value of coracohumeral ligament release. *Orthop Trans.* 1989;13:235.
142. Neer CS II, Satterlee CC, Dalsey RM, Flatow EL. On the value of coracohumeral ligament release. In: Post M, Morrey B, Hawkins RJ, eds. *Surgery of the Shoulder.* St. Louis: Mosby-Year Book; 1990:44–46.
143. Neer CS II, Satterlee CC, Dalsey RM, Flatow EL. The anatomy and potential effects of contracture of the coracohumeral ligament. *Clin Orthop.* 1992;286:13–16.

Section 2

Basic Science and the Rotator Cuff

Chapter 2

Anatomy of the Rotator Cuff

Douglas T. Harryman II and John M. Clark, Jr.

Anatomy is the gateway to medicine. It is the queen of the basic sciences and is the sine qua non for entry into the field of medicine.
Crocco, 1977

The rotator cuff is a composite of tendons from the four scapulohumeral rotator muscles conjoined with the glenohumeral joint capsule and its ligaments. Among its functions, this structure contributes to glenohumeral joint stability and humeral head positional control. As orthopaedic surgeons, we must diagnose and treat pathological conditions affecting our patient's shoulders. Understanding each anatomic component as it relates to and functions in the rotator cuff complex benefits our surgical skills as well as our patients' outcomes.

During our lifetime, the rotator cuff endures wedged between the proverbial rocklike humeral head and the unforgiving hard place of the coracoacromial arch. Although these rigid anatomic confines appear to present an austere environment in which to perform, this architecture also serves to protect these vital tissues. Together, the coracoid process, the coracoacromial ligament, the AC joint, the acromion, and the scapular spine form a congruent contact roof that shields the musculotendinous junctions and the contiguous tendinous connections to the tuberosities. Although we assume most readers know a great deal about the surgical anatomy of the rotator cuff, for the purpose of this chapter, we will review the gross anatomy and delve into the detailed complex interrelationships among the musculotendinous and capsular structures, in order to better understand their functional association.

THE GROSS MACROSTRUCTURE OF THE ROTATOR CUFF

Four muscle tendon units originating from the blade of the scapula reach out to hold the humeral head in its proper relationship to the scapula. Unlike other articulations with a rigid articular enclosure or true connecting ligaments, the glenohumeral joint is almost totally dependent on the dynamic strength of the musculotendinous units and the static capsular containment to stabilize the joint. The interlocking fibers of the rotator cuff complex are strong, capable of resisting forceful torsional rotatory motions and eccentric shear loads that attempt to displace the humeral head from its shallow glenoid fossa.

Approximately three-fourths of the glenohumeral articular perimeter is surrounded by the combined attachment of the tendinous rotator cuff and the adjoining articular capsule (Fig. 2–1). The remaining one fourth is enclosed solely by the articular capsule and its thickened ligamentous modulations. The synergistic action of the four rotator cuff muscles reflexively adjust length and tension in application of torsional and compressive forces for stable humeral head motion. The strong and disciplined grasp of these four tendons reach out from their muscular origin on the scapula like the trained fingers of a baseball pitcher (Fig. 2–2). The use of the extremity for the graceful execution of a pitch or a powerlifter's press depends on the coordinated exertion of the cuff muscles. The cuff tendons are linked intimately with the articular capsule. Together these structures influence key functions of motion and stability, such as restraining humeral head translation, limiting glenohumeral rotation, and providing control of scapulohumeral position.[1]

We will now pursue a detailed inspection of the gross anatomy and function of the four musculotendinous rotator cuff components before delving into histological microstructure.

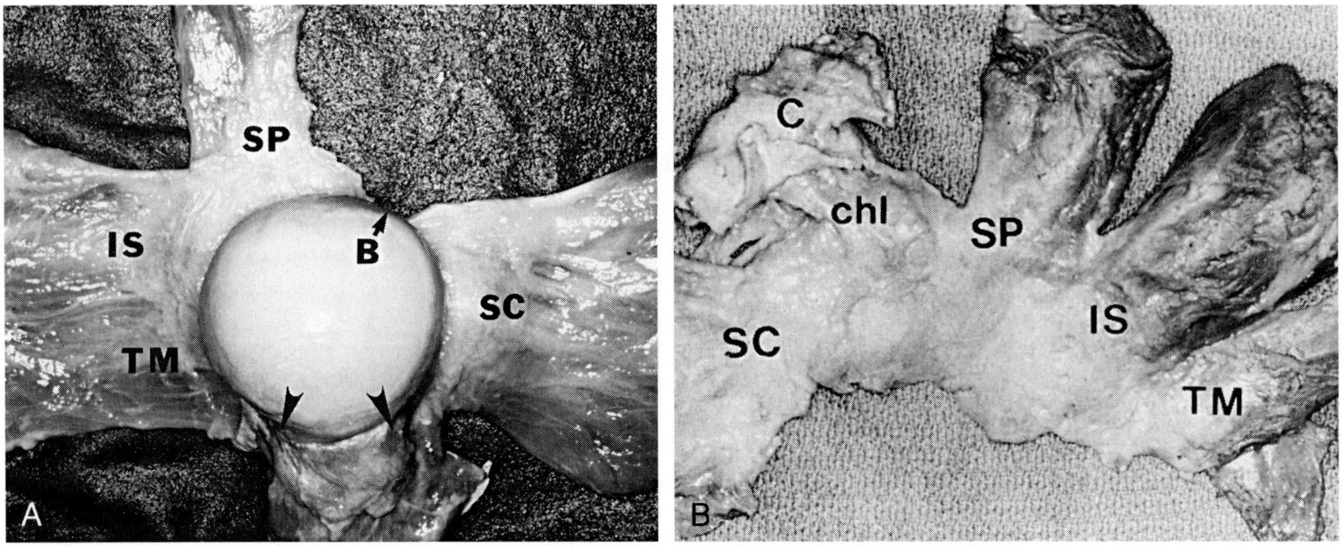

Fig. 2–1. ***A,*** **Anatomic view of the humeral head displaying the four rotator cuff tendons, (SP = supraspinatus, SC = subscapularis, IS = infraspinatus, and TM = teres minor), which surround the perimeter of the anatomic neck adjacent to the articular surface. The rotator cuff tendons enclose approximately 75% of the humeral head articular surface; notable exceptions are where the biceps (B) tendon exits and the capsule attaches adjacent to the humeral shaft (between arrowheads).** ***B,*** **The complete myotendinous cuff and capsule complex form a continuous sheet of tissue which is shown after it has been incised in the axillary pouch and peeled from the humeral head and scapula. The structures shown are the subscapularis (SC), the osteotomized coracoid process (C) with the attached rotator interval capsule (RIC), the supraspinatus (SP), the infraspinatus (IS), and the teres minor (TM). Also note the fleshy insertion of the teres minor and the subscapularis that have been detached from the humeral shaft. (From Clark JM, Harryman DT II. Tendons, ligaments, and capsule of the rotator cuff.** ***J Bone Joint Surg Am.*** **1992;74:713–725.)**

Anatomic Form and Function of the Musculotendinous Units

THE SUBSCAPULARIS

The subscapularis muscle is the largest and most powerful rotator of the four cuff muscles. Its broad, triangular, multipennate origin, arising from the subscapularis fossa, occupies greater than 90% of the anterior scapular surface. As the muscle funnels laterally toward the humerus, it covers the entire anterior scapular neck inferior to the coracoid base (Fig. 2–3). Only about 15 mm of the terminal subscapularis is compact tendon, but distinct tendinous bands are apparent in each pennate unit as they taper toward the scapular neck.[2] The tendinous insertion into the lesser tuberosity is supplemented inferiorly by muscular insertions along the surgical neck of the humerus.

The rounded superior border of the subscapularis glides immediately beneath the coracoid process as the proximal humerus is rotated. The coracoid splits the continuity of the rotator cuff anterosuperiorly to form an important capsular interval between the borders of the subscapularis and the supraspinatus muscles (Fig. 2–4). Although it is often unrecognized, the subscapularis and supraspinatus tendons actually interconnect across shared fibers of the rotator interval capsule and join terminally via indirect tendinous insertions that continue laterally into the periosteum.[2,3] The subscapularis extends lateral to the lesser tuberosity to form a sheath around the long head of the biceps tendon, which also links it secondarily to the tendons attached to the greater tuberosity (Fig. 2–5).

The subscapularis receives its innervation from the upper and lower subscapular nerves, which branch off the posterior cord of the brachial plexus. The majority of the muscle is innervated by the upper subscapular nerve.[4] A rich vascular network literally surrounds and permeates the subscapularis with a plethora of collateral circulation from the subscapular, circumflex scapular, suprascapular, and dorsal scapular vessels.

Functionally, the subscapularis is best known as a powerful internal rotator of the humerus. It's force vector has been recognized as a humeral head depressor, but more accurately, its function is clearly a compressive joint stabilizer.[5,6] It also serves actively to reposition the humeral head and guide motion during sporting activities that demand strength and rapid motion combinations.[7] Investigators have also documented its passive role as a stabilizer to anterior and posterior translation when wrapped around the humeral head under tension.[8]

THE SUPRASPINATUS

The fusiform supraspinatus muscle originates superiorly on the scapula from the fossa for which it is named. Laterally, the muscle fibers and tendinous junction glide through an elliptical osseous boundary, the supraspinatus outlet (Fig. 2–6). The confines of this outlet include the acromial roof and AC joint superiorly, the coracoid base anteriorly, the spine of the scapula posteriorly, and the superior glenoid and humeral head inferiorly. Throughout life, the supraspinatus tendon glides

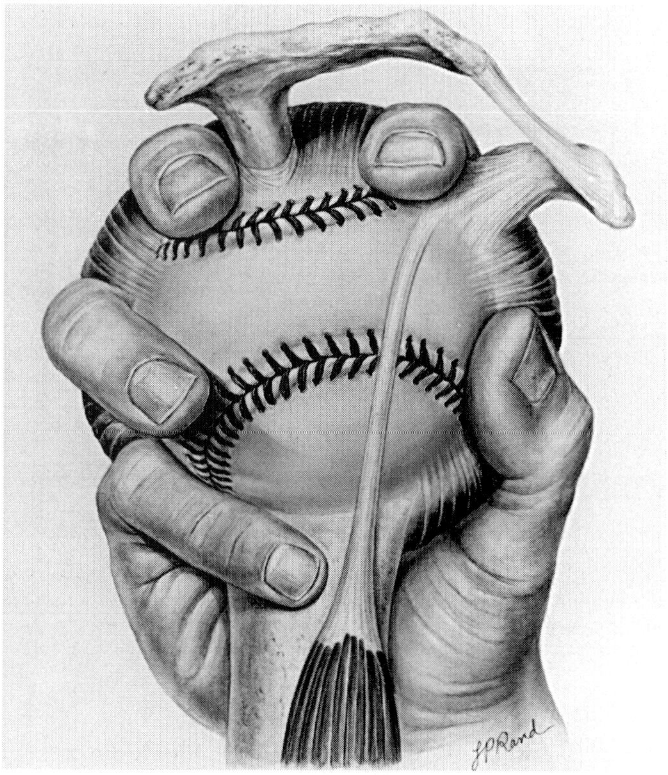

Fig. 2–2. Each of the four muscles about the rotator cuff reach out from the scapula like well-coordinated fingers of a baseball pitcher to control positional orientation of the humeral head and that of the upper extremity. Synergistic concentric or eccentric contraction of the four musculotendinous units will not only maintain balanced stability of the humeral head on the glenoid but also govern the position of the extremity and guide motion for use of the hand.

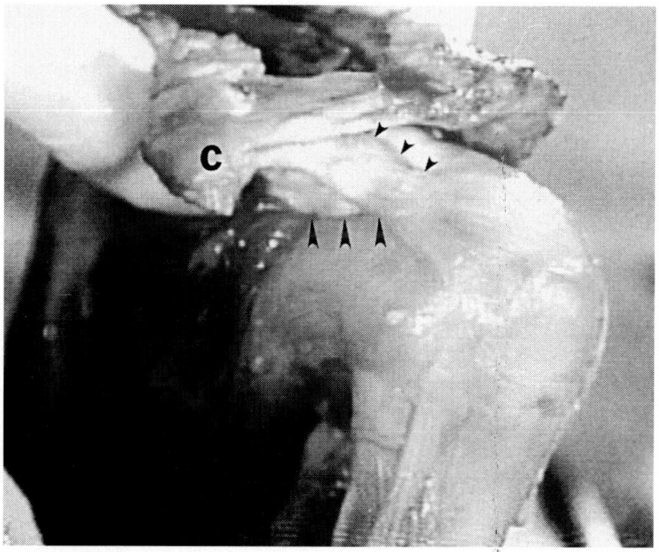

Fig. 2–4. The coracoid process of the scapula naturally divides the bulk of the rotator cuff, creating an important interval between the superior border of the subscapularis (large arrowheads) and the anterior border of the supraspinatus (small arrowheads) tendons. Ligamentous thickenings of the articular capsule, which fill the rotator interval, have specialized functions. Superficially, the coracohumeral ligament originates along the base of the coracoid, has two main folds that insert into the greater and lesser tuberosities, and suspends the cuff with fibers along the tendinous borders.

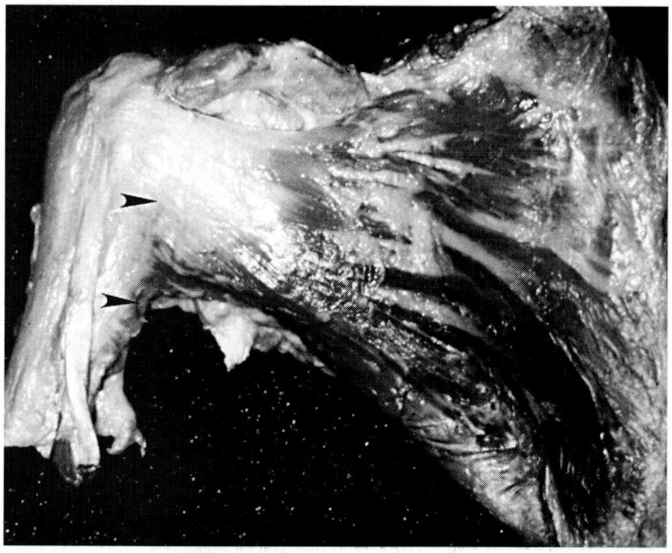

Fig. 2–3. The subscapularis, the largest of the scapulohumeral muscles, becomes tendinous at the level of the glenoid rim, where it can actively serve as a powerful anterior buttress to the glenohumeral joint. Note how the lower fleshy half (between arrowheads) combines obliquely with the direct transverse fibers of the tendon and contributes to a large inferior muscular insertion on the humeral shaft below the lesser tuberosity. The coracoid and acromion have been osteotomized to enhance visualization.

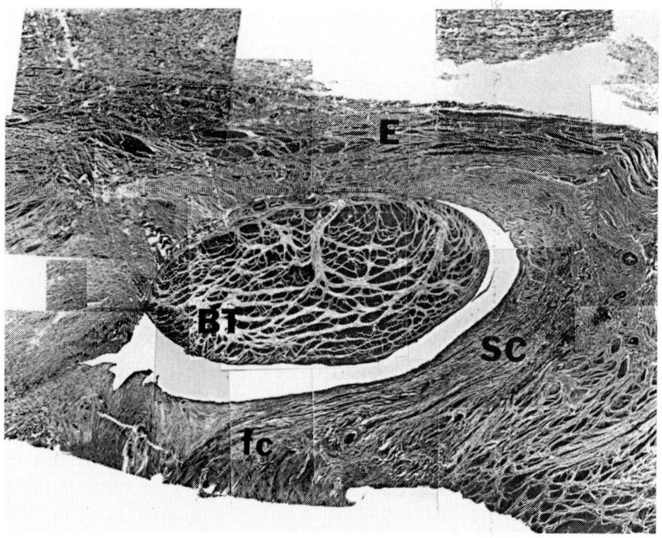

Fig. 2–5. This is a composite vertical section dissected away from the bone and cut through the biceps tendon (BT) adjacent to the opening of the bicipital groove showing fibers of the supraspinatus, subscapularis, and intertubercular ligament (Masson trichrome, ×38). The fibers crossing horizontally over the tendon are an extension (E) of the supraspinatus tendon. The floor of the bicipital sheath is composed primarily of fibers from the subscapularis (SC) which attaches to fibrocartilage (FC) at the bone level. (Courtesy of Clark JM, Harryman DT II. Tendons, ligaments, and capsule of the rotator cuff. *J Bone Joint Surg Am.* 1992; 74:713–725.)

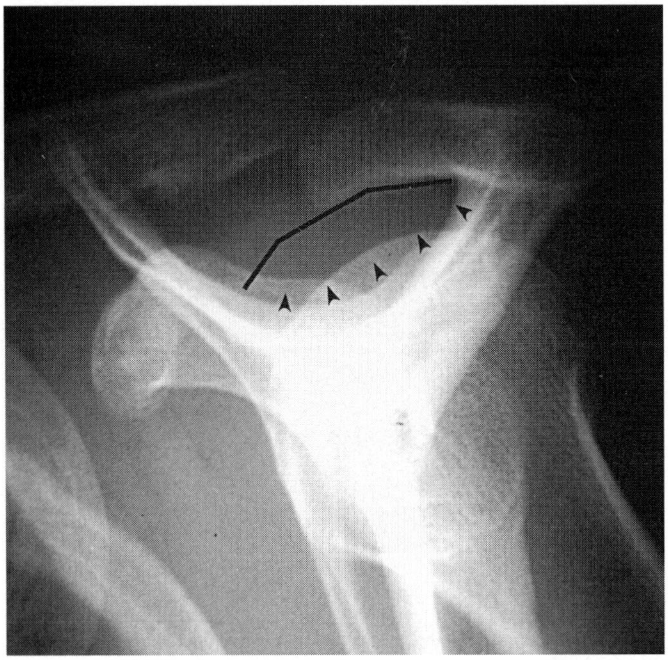

Fig. 2–6. Radiographic view looking directly through the supraspinatus outlet. The extra-articular, (coracoacromial ligament surface—heavy outline) and the intra-articular (glenohumeral surface—arrowheads) borders of the outlet are described in the text. The rotator cuff holds the humeral head securely within the glenoid by compressing it into the concave fossa. If the humeral head subluxates superiorly, as a result of rotator cuff weakness or a tendon tear, then the remaining tendons are compressed and abraded against the arch.

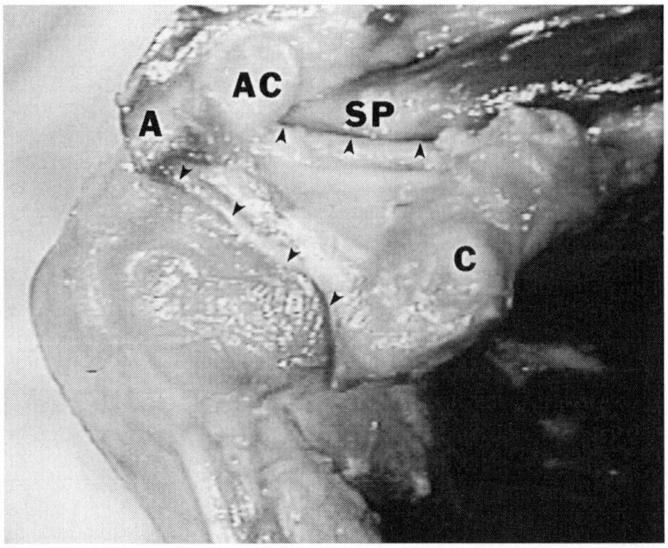

Fig. 2–7. The tendinous portion of the supraspinatus and the musculotendinous junction (1.5 to 2.0 cm) must glide without restriction under the acromion (A), the acromioclavicular joint (AC), and the coracoacromial ligament (anterior/posterior borders—arrowheads).

through this outlet for all planes of humeral elevation (Fig. 2–7).

Although the bulk of the supraspinatus tendon fibers appear oriented directly into the superior facet of the greater tuberosity, there are indirect linkages with neighboring structures. Notably, the anterior tendon border blends with the rotator interval capsule, and the posterior border becomes indistinguishable with the infraspinatus tendon near its insertion. As we age, the deep surface of the supraspinatus insertion into the tuberosity may retract without evidence of fiber disruption from the articular surface.[9] When this occurs, a periarticular sulcus along the anatomic neck of the humerus may develop (Fig. 2–8). For some shoulders, this periarticular gap may help accommodate coaptation of the glenoid articular rim at extremes of joint motion thereby avoiding contact against the deep surface of the rotator cuff.[10,11]

The nutrition and innervation of the supraspinatus muscle is derived from the suprascapular artery and nerve. Not all of the tendon, however, is supplied by the suprascapular artery; later in this chapter we will discuss an anatomic vascular "watershed" portion of the supraspinatus adjacent to the insertion of the tendon.[12–14]

At least three functions of the supraspinatus have been documented. These include its contributions to active scapulohumeral elevation,[15,16] derotation when the arm is elevated and rotated on the humeral axis,[17] and compressive stabilization of the humeral head.[18] Contraction of the supraspinatus muscle produces tension in the superior capsulo-cuff tendon complex, which serves not only to compress the humeral head into the concavity of the glenoid but also, as forces are applied tangential to the glenoid, the supraspinatus resists superior and inferior head translation.[6,19]

THE INFRASPINATUS

The bipennate infraspinatus muscle is the second largest rotator cuff muscle. It originates from the posterior scapular surface of the shallow infraspinatus fossa inferior to the scapular spine. The midportion of the infraspinatus muscle is divided by a longitudinal tendinous raphe that when sectioned axially divides the muscle into a superior and inferior half. Clinicians have found that this raphe can be used for surgical access to the posterior midaxial glenohumeral joint without compromise to its innervation (Fig. 2–9).[20] The tendon of the infraspinatus muscle joins the posterior border of the supraspinatus tendon lateral to the scapular spine approximately 1.5 cm from its insertion into the greater tuberosity. The fibers of the inferior border of the infraspinatus tendon blend with that of the teres minor in a similar way to their interdigitation with the supraspinatus tendon. The terminal branch of the suprascapular nerve arborizes soon after it passes through the spinoglenoid notch and enters the deep surface of the infraspinatus muscle belly. The vascular supply to the infraspinatus is shared by the suprascapular and circumflex scapular arteries.

The infraspinatus muscle is the most powerful scapulohumeral external rotator. It also serves to restrain the humeral head actively in the "cocked-arm" position reducing the load on the anterior capsular ligaments.[7] The tendon of the infraspinatus muscle functions actively as a barrier to humeral head translation.[21] when the arm is elevated in the anterior plane or When adducted across

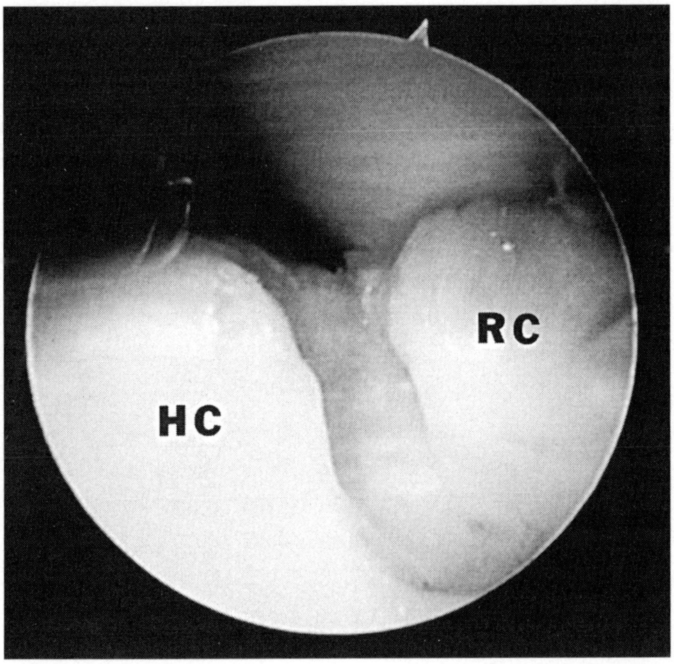

Fig. 2–8. Arthroscopic view of the rotator cuff deep surface and its periarticular attachment to the anatomic neck of the humeral head. Notice the bony rim between the smooth humeral articular cartilage (HC) and the smooth undersurface of the rotator cuff insertion (RC). The presence of this rim may result from attrition of the articular capsule.

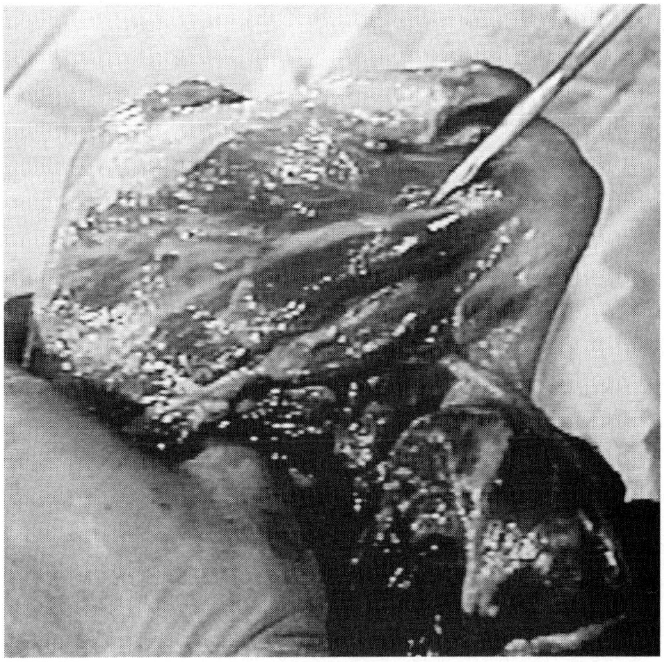

Fig. 2–9. The fat streak on the posterior surface of the infraspinatus tendon (indicated at the tip of the scissors) can be confused with the internervous plane between the infraspinatus and teres minor muscle. However, if the surgeon were to approach the joint posteriorly by incising along this raphe, splitting the muscle into a superior and inferior half actually provides good access to the posterior midaxial glenohumeral joint without denervation.

the body, it assists the posterior and superior capsule to provide posterior glenohumeral stability in accordance with the capsular constraint mechanism.[22]

THE TERES MINOR

The fusiform teres minor, the smallest of the rotator cuff muscles, originates along the inferolateral border of the posterior scapula adjacent to the margin of the infraspinatus fossa (Fig. 2–10). It inserts on the most inferior facet of the greater tuberosity after it has been joined by the posterior capsule. Like the subscapularis insertion, the tendinous insertion of the teres minor is short and is supplemented by muscular fibers that attach directly to the posterior surgical neck and extend inferiorly for a length of up to 2 cm below the tuberosity.

As the axillary nerve exits the quadrangular space, it gives off a short branch which divides to innervate the teres minor. The posterior branches of the circumflex scapular and branches of the suprascapular arteries supply vascularity to the teres minor muscle.

Although its size is diminutive when compared with the infraspinatus muscle, the teres minor is positioned favorably to generate a considerable external rotatory force of up to 40% of the total effort.[23] Its orientation couples with the lower fibers of the subscapularis to harness the humeral head and resist the upward pull of the deltoid by exerting a medial force with an inferior directed component. Coupling with the other cuff muscles, the teres minor compresses the humeral head into the glenoid concavity to stabilize the joint.[6,18,23]

THE MUSCULOTENDINOUS ROTATOR CUFF

When relaxed, the four muscular units of the rotator cuff are loosely applied to the superficial surface of the articular capsule medial to the capsulotendinous junction. With active rotation in the midrange of motion; the cuff muscles glide freely, accommodating capsular retraction, and folding into the recesses adjacent to the musculotendinous junction, glenoid rim, and scapular neck. In positions of capsular laxity, we can be certain that the capsule derives support from the cuff muscles. This way only a residual, finite joint volume of 1 to 2 cm^3 is maintained in the glenohumeral joint, and compliant capsular areas such as the subcoracoid recess present only a potential space.

The orientation of the rotator cuff tendon fibers must bend to accommodate extreme scapulo-humeral positions, such as maximal adduction and overhead elevation. Fibers of the supraspinatus adjacent to its insertion must flex adequately to tolerate an angular deviation in fiber direction in order to accommodate the total arc of internal and external rotation, as well as a range of planes of elevation anterior and posterior to the body for elevation arcs of greater than 180° around the torso (Fig. 2–11).[24] Given this degree of tendon excursion over millions of cycles, we can predict the area at which structural failure would be most likely to occur. Fortunately, the capsular ligaments reinforce the tendinous insertions, es-

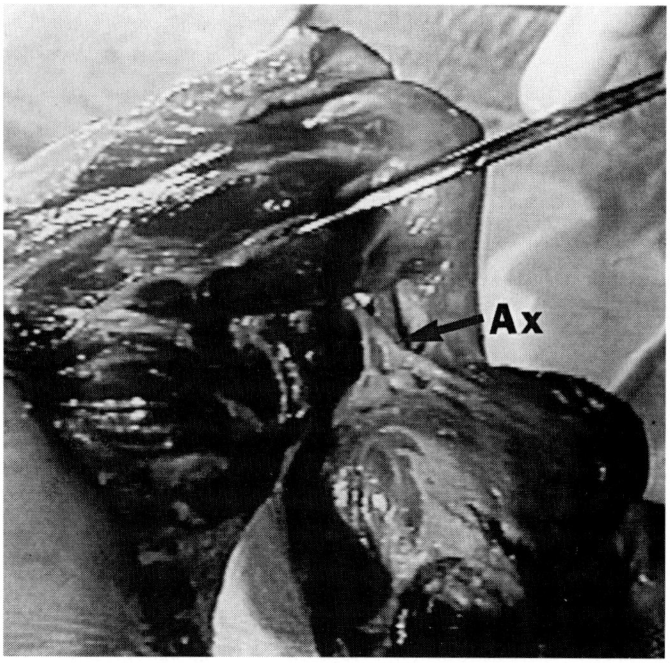

Fig. 2–10. The teres minor is the muscle seen just below the internervous plane (indicated by the scissors). At its inferior border, the axillary nerve exits the quadrangular space and is seen branching to the teres minor and the deltoid (reflected inferiorly).

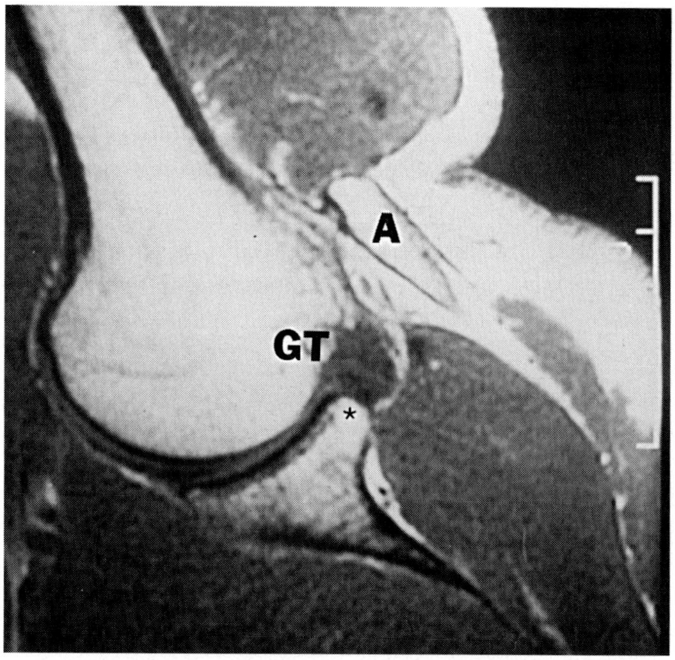

Fig. 2–11. The glenohumeral joint is positioned in maximum elevation for this coronal plane MRI section, which shows the supraspinatus tendon of the rotator cuff retracted on itself as the greater tuberosity (GT) passes under the acromion (A) and comes into close approximation with the postero-superior glenoid rim (*). The tendon fiber orientation at the insertion has angulated greater than 90° from the anatomic alignment when the arm is positioned at the side.

pecially the supraspinatus, to redistribute the tensile and compressive forces and diminish excessive stress.[2,25]

If the surgeon divides the cuff 1 cm medial to the greater tuberosity, it becomes obvious how difficult it is to differentiate grossly between the cuff tendons and the applied capsule. In this region, the tendinous fibers of the supraspinatus, infraspinatus, and the teres minor fuse with the articular capsule into a thick collagenous rind of compact cuff tissue. Blunt capsular dissection is not possible closer than approximately 1.5 cm to the insertion of the tendon into the greater tuberosity. When looking at this area of the rotator cuff arthroscopically, we recognize that the articular side of the rotator cuff appears bandlike, resembling an arch over the humeral head in the region where the capsulotendinous junction is devoid of synovial tissue (Fig. 2–12). On the superficial side of the same portion of the rotator cuff, the subacromial bursae can be separated only by sharp dissection. The bursal lining on this surface is normally only one to two cell layers thick. However, in the presence of a stenotic supraspinatus outlet, the bursal layer may become abraded, inflamed, and thickened.

Now, let us go back and take a closer look at the articular surface of the rotator cuff in the area where the synovium is absent. The surgeon recognizes the presence of thick transverse capsular fibers that span from the anterior border of the supraspinatus tendon to the posterior border of the infraspinatus fibers. Recently, this crescent-shaped arch has been the subject of intense scrutiny and will become our concern at a later time.

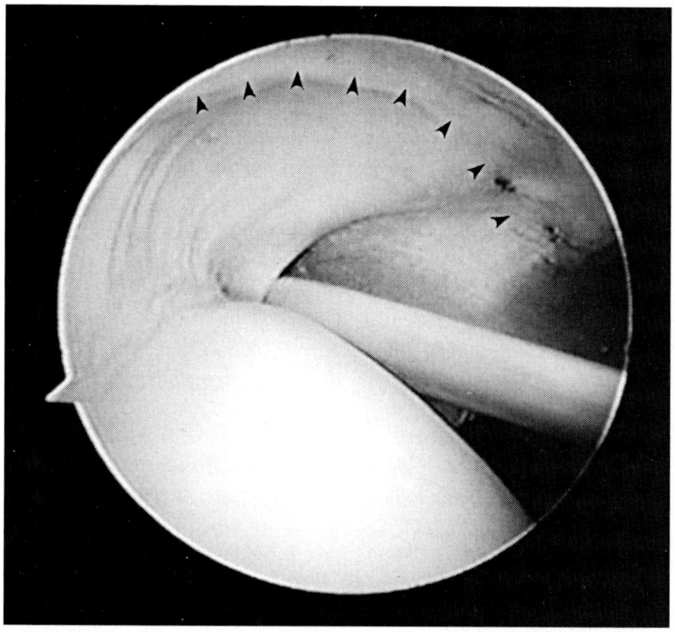

Fig. 2–12. Arthroscopic view of the undersurface of the superior capsule, which is applied to the deep surface of the rotator cuff. The arthroscopist can see that the synovium ends approximately 2 cm away from the insertion into the greater tuberosity. The superior arch of the capsule-cuff complex is consistently devoid of synovial tissue on its deep surface.

MICROSTRUCTURE OF THE ROTATOR CUFF

Layers of the Rotator Cuff

Clark dissected 32 intact cadaveric shoulders to evaluate the histological structure of the rotator cuff.[2] From these sections, we were able to determine the distinct fiber bundle orientation and visualize the discrete blood supply to the layers of the rotator cuff. The total thickness of the rotator cuff sections averaged between 9 and 12 mm. The sections made in the region of the supraspinatus and infraspinatus tendons were clearly delineated into five layers comprising the cuff-capsule complex. Below, we present a detailed description of the five rotator cuff layers that were identified (Fig. 2–13).

LAYER 1

After resection of the superficial subacromial bursae, we find the thinnest layer of the rotator cuff, which is typically less than 1 mm. This superficial collagenous layer is oriented obliquely with respect to the axis of the tendon. These fibers are contiguous with the superficial layers of the coracohumeral ligament and extend laterally into the periosteum, adjacent to the tuberosities and the bicipital groove. These fibers contribute to the indirect fiber insertions of the rotator cuff. Often, large arterioles are present in this layer.

LAYER 2

The thickness of the second layer ranges between 3 to 5 mm. The collagenous tendon fibers are grouped into large, densely organized parallel bundles. Each collagen bundle is 1 to 2 mm in cross-section and represents the direct insertion of the musculotendinous unit into the tuberosities. As expected, this layer is absent in the rotator interval and is less prominent in the interval between the supraspinatus and the infraspinatus tendons. Arterioles from the first layer enter between the fascicles to supply interstitial tendon nutrition.

LAYER 3

The third layer of the rotator cuff has smaller fascicles and less uniform density of collagen bundles. Here the tendon fibers within and among each musculotendinous unit interdigitate as their fibers splay. Vessels in this layer are small. The larger arterioles that have passed through the second layer now course between the second and third layers.

LAYER 4

The fourth layer is thin, approximately 1 mm, and is composed of predominately loose connective tissue interspersed by a few thick collagenous bands that are located on the extra-articular surface of the capsule. These ligamentous bands appear to represent ligamentous extensions from the rotator interval capsule with which they merge. This layer is a transitional zone between the articular capsule and the deep surface of the rotator cuff tendons. In this layer only capillaries that penetrate the articular capsule are found.

The first and fourth layers are similar in that they are thin extensions of the rotator interval capsule and appear to enclose the thicker tendinous fascicles of the second and third layers.

LAYER 5

The articular capsule (1.5 to 2 mm thick) is a continuous sheet of interwoven collagen fibrils. This layer becomes part of the rotator cuff complex when united with the rotator tendons and inserts as Sharpey fibers into the bone. This is the portion of the articular capsule that is not covered by synovium and appears to have an anterior to posterior fiber orientation that we have termed the transverse capsulo-tendinous ligament.

The Subscapularis Tendon

Histological sections in the region of the subscapularis tendon display a different layering pattern. The more superficial collagen bundles are tightly packed and well organized. The direct tendinous bundles reveal less distinct layering and are stacked into bundles of four to six collagen fibrils parallel to each other. As described by Benjamin et al., we also found that the terminal fibers angulate and splay to distribute their insertion over a broad surface area of fibrocartilage at the tendon insertion into the lesser tuberosity.[25] The articular capsule remains the deepest layer, with the anterior glenohumeral ligaments interspersed between the deepest tendon layer of the subscapularis and the thinnest lamination of the joint capsule.[26]

COMMENT

Although most anatomy texts[27,28] indicate separate insertional facets for each rotator cuff tendon, only the direct tendon fibers from each muscle tendon unit appear to attach at the facetal bony protuberances. A significant portion of each muscle tendon unit has fibers that intermingle confluently in the deeper layers of the cuff. Also, the lateral 1.5 cm of these tendon fibers blend inseparably with the articular capsule and its thickened ligamentous modulations. The tensile strength and resilience of every part of the rotator cuff depends on the organization and density of the collagenous layers and the supportive junction with cuff tendon layers and the capsule above and below. For this reason, certain portions of the cuff may be easier to disrupt traumatically. For example, a high stress area at the junction of the rotator interval and the supraspinatus tendon, immediately adjacent to the bicipital groove, may represent a weaker region of the cuff complex than the junction between the supraspinatus and infraspinatus tendons, which not only join to reinforce each other but are bound together securely by the transverse capsulo-tendinous ligament.[2]

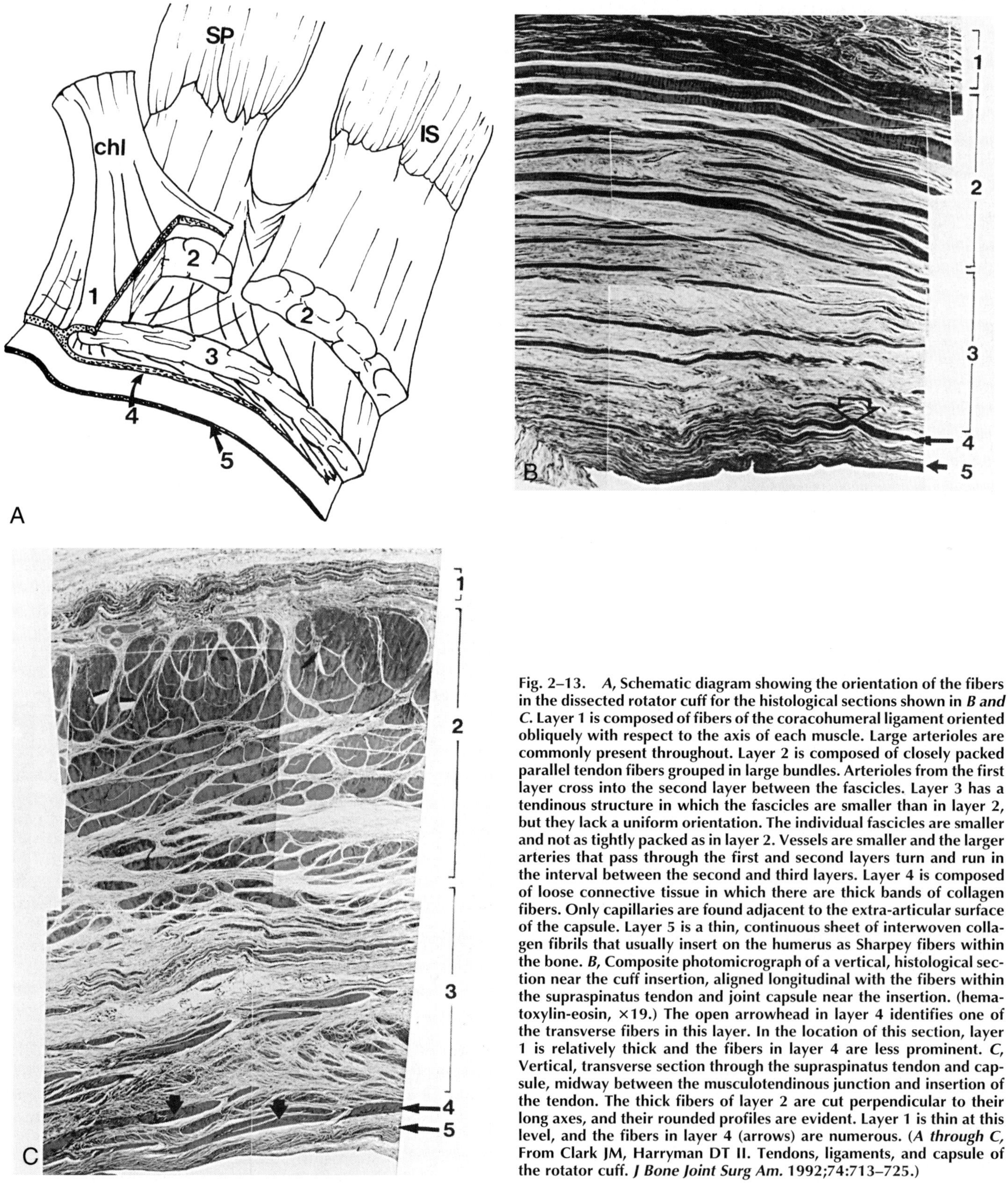

Fig. 2–13. *A,* Schematic diagram showing the orientation of the fibers in the dissected rotator cuff for the histological sections shown in *B and C.* Layer 1 is composed of fibers of the coracohumeral ligament oriented obliquely with respect to the axis of each muscle. Large arterioles are commonly present throughout. Layer 2 is composed of closely packed parallel tendon fibers grouped in large bundles. Arterioles from the first layer cross into the second layer between the fascicles. Layer 3 has a tendinous structure in which the fascicles are smaller than in layer 2, but they lack a uniform orientation. The individual fascicles are smaller and not as tightly packed as in layer 2. Vessels are smaller and the larger arteries that pass through the first and second layers turn and run in the interval between the second and third layers. Layer 4 is composed of loose connective tissue in which there are thick bands of collagen fibers. Only capillaries are found adjacent to the extra-articular surface of the capsule. Layer 5 is a thin, continuous sheet of interwoven collagen fibrils that usually insert on the humerus as Sharpey fibers within the bone. *B,* Composite photomicrograph of a vertical, histological section near the cuff insertion, aligned longitudinal with the fibers within the supraspinatus tendon and joint capsule near the insertion. (hematoxylin-eosin, ×19.) The open arrowhead in layer 4 identifies one of the transverse fibers in this layer. In the location of this section, layer 1 is relatively thick and the fibers in layer 4 are less prominent. *C,* Vertical, transverse section through the supraspinatus tendon and capsule, midway between the musculotendinous junction and insertion of the tendon. The thick fibers of layer 2 are cut perpendicular to their long axes, and their rounded profiles are evident. Layer 1 is thin at this level, and the fibers in layer 4 (arrows) are numerous. (*A through C,* From Clark JM, Harryman DT II. Tendons, ligaments, and capsule of the rotator cuff. *J Bone Joint Surg Am.* 1992;74:713–725.)

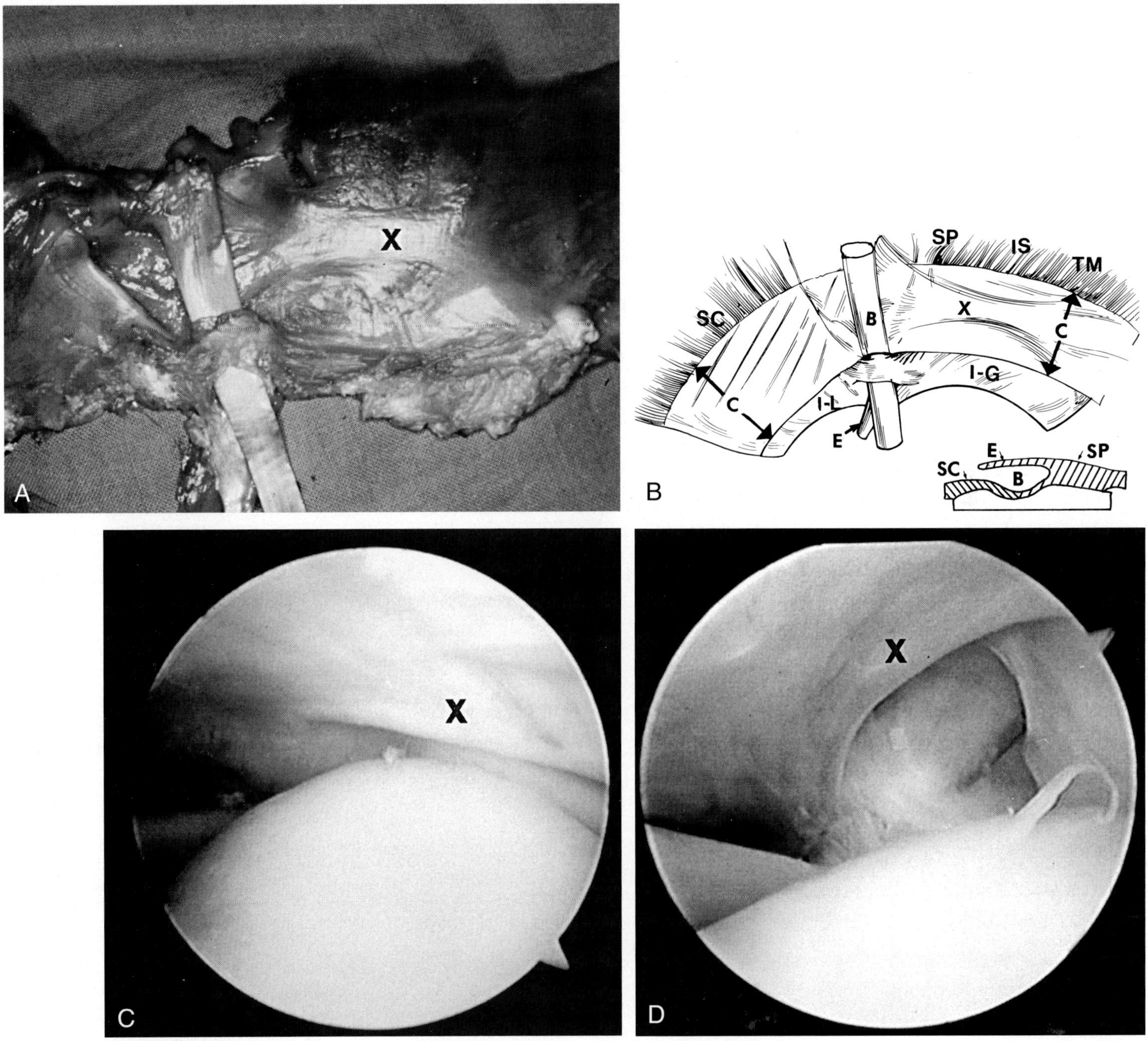

Fig. 2–14. *A,* Photograph of the deep (articular) aspect of the cuff-capsule complex after it was dissected off the humerus and the scapula. In this specimen, the cuff muscles have been divided near their musculotendinous junctions. A band of fibers (X) extends transversely from the rotator interval capsule in continuity with the coracohumeral ligament into the plane between the capsule and tendon fibers. This ligament courses posteriorly, where it ends or blends with the capsule approximately at the superior edge of the teres minor. *B,* Drawing of the deep surface of the rotator cuff-capsule complex after it has been detached from the humerus, as shown in *A.* The diagram in the inset is a cross section of the bicipital groove and related structures. Note the relationships of the capsule (C), subscapularis (SC), supraspinatus (SP), infraspinatus (IS), and teres minor (TM) tendons, as well as the confluence of the supraspinatus and subscapularis tendons proximal to their insertions on the lesser (I-L) and greater (I-G) tuberosities. In the inset, the complex sheath surrounding the biceps tendon (B) is shown diagrammatically in cross section. The deep portion of this sheath is formed by the subscapularis tendon, and a slip (E) from the supraspinatus tendon forms a roof over the biceps tendon. Also shown is the transverse capsulo-tendinous ligament (X) seen in *A,C, and D. C,* Arthroscopic in vivo view of the intact transverse capsulo-tendinous ligament (X) on the deep surface of the normal rotator cuff complex. *D,* Arthroscopic view of an intact transverse capsulo-tendinous ligament (X) on the deep surface of a recurrent rotator cuff tear. Note that the ligament has retracted medially from the normal humeral insertion forming a gap between the capsule-cuff tissue and the greater tuberosity. The anterior to posterior fiber orientation extending from the rotator interval capsule can be seen clearly. (*A and B,* From Clark JM, Harryman DT II. Tendons, ligaments, and capsule of the rotator cuff. *J Bone Joint Surg Am.* 1992;74:713–725.)

THE RELATIONSHIP OF CAPSULAR LIGAMENTS TO THE ROTATOR CUFF

The composition of the glenohumeral joint capsule is similar to other joints in that it is primarily composed of type I collagen (typical of bone, tendon, skin, and other connective tissues), with intermixed portions of type III (also found in muscular and elastic tissues) and type V (associated with smooth muscle, fibroblasts and chondrocytes).[29] Kaltsas has also reported[29] that the capsule becomes thin and perforated near the insertion of the rotator cuff and loses up to 25% of its tensile strength and resiliency to stretch with age. Therefore, collagenous degeneration of the capsule may help explain degenerative tears within the supraspinatus tendon associated with aging.

Clark, Sidles, and Matsen reported on the capsule as it relates to its attachment on the deep surface of the rotator cuff tendons near their humeral insertions.[26] In contrast to other reports, the capsule could always be identified as a separate continuous layer connecting the glenoid to the anatomic neck of the humerus. Although sharp dissection was required, a consistent plane could be developed even in the thick or thin capsular regions. The capsule was 1 to 2 mm thick on the deep surface of the rotator cuff where it was most firmly attached. The capsule was thinnest, less than 1 mm, where it had no attachment to the tendons. Adjacent to the rotator cuff, the thick capsule could be separated into two layers which were divided by the collagenous orientation. The first layer, 0.3 to 0.5 mm thick, forms a continuous lining that faces the joint surface. The second layer, on the tendinous side, corresponds to the regions of ligamentous hypertrophy. The transverse capsular fiber layer extends posteriorly from the lesser tuberosity, perpendicular to the direct fiber orientation of the rotator cuff tendons, and parallel to the superior anatomic neck of the humeral head. This band was identified in all specimens (Fig. 2–14).

Burkhart hypothesized that the fiber arrangement, which is perpendicular to the direct tendon fibers, binds the rotator cuff together to function as a loaded cable that resists humeral head displacement even in the presence of a rotator cuff tear.[30] Normally, the transverse capsulo-tendinous ligament may act as a sling or tension cable to partly unload the rotator cuff tendons and protect them from stresses, which attempt to tear the fibers apart.

The coracohumeral ligament is the only capsular ligament visible from outside the rotator cuff. This thin expansive ligament originates along the base of the coracoid. It can be thought of as a roof to the capsular interval between the rotator cuff tendons.[31] As the coracohumeral ligament courses laterally toward the tuberosities, some of its fibers splay and blend into the borders of the subscapularis and supraspinatus tendons. These fibers extend into the first and fourth layers of the rotator cuff.[2] We hypothesize that these extensions of the coracohumeral ligament help to protect and reinforce the cuff tendons again by distributing tensile forces. The direct, thicker portions of the coracohumeral ligament insert into the greater and lesser tuberosities adjacent to the intertubercular ligament (Fig. 2–15). The anatomy of the rotator interval is best visualized arthroscopically. The superior glenohumeral ligament, the most consistent of the anterior capsular ligaments, reinforces the floor of the rotator interval. This ligament originates just anterior to the biceps tendon in continuity with the superior labrum, capsule, and periosteum of the superior glenoid (Fig. 2–16). The ligament courses obliquely across the rotator interval capsule to insert on the humerus at the humeral fovea capitus, just superior to the lesser tuberosity. The rotator interval and its two ligaments, the coracohumeral and the superior glenohumeral, perform critical functions in glenohumeral stability and motion. Without these interval capsular ligaments, the humeral head would exhibit deficient restraint to posterior and inferior translation and humeral rotation would not be statically restrained at the limit of external rotation, forward elevation, extension, and adduction.[31,32]

Nearly a century ago, Poirier and Charpy stated that the musculotendinous cuff, which covers and reinforces the anterior, superior, and posterior aspects of the glenohumeral joint, acts as "true active ligaments."[33] Because the rotator cuff is joined inseparably with specific portions of the joint capsule, tension in the ligaments is shared within the musculotendinous insertion. Most notable is the subscapularis anteriorly, for positions of external rotation and coronal plane elevation, and the infraspinatus and teres minor posteriorly, for positions of

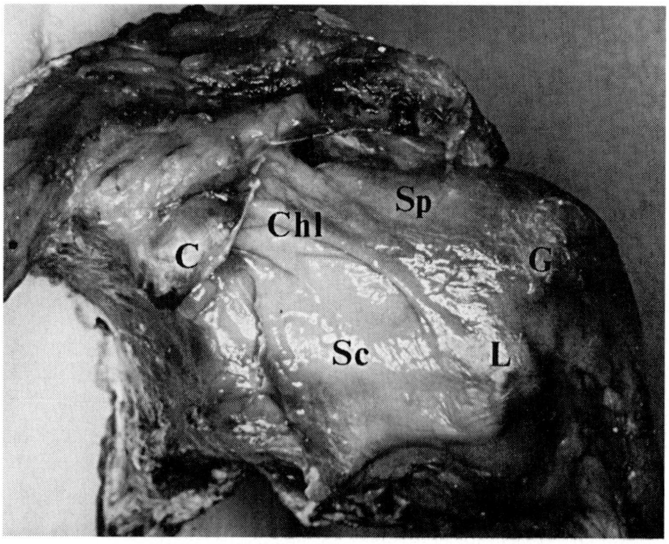

Fig. 2–15. The coracohumeral ligament (Chl) is an extension of the articular capsule which spans the interval between the anterior border of the supraspinatus (Sp) and the superior border of the subscapularis (Sc) tendon. The ligament originates along the base of the coracoid (C) and inserts primarily into the greater (G) and lesser (L) tuberosities. It is thin and contiguous with layers 1 and 4 of the rotator cuff. When shoulders become stiff and contracted or loose and unstable, this ligament may play a significant role in pathologic shoulder motion and/or stability. (From Harryman DT II, Sidles JA, Harris SL, Matsen FA III. The role of the rotator interval capsule in passive motion and stability of the shoulder. *J Bone Joint Surg Am.* 1992;74: 53–66.)

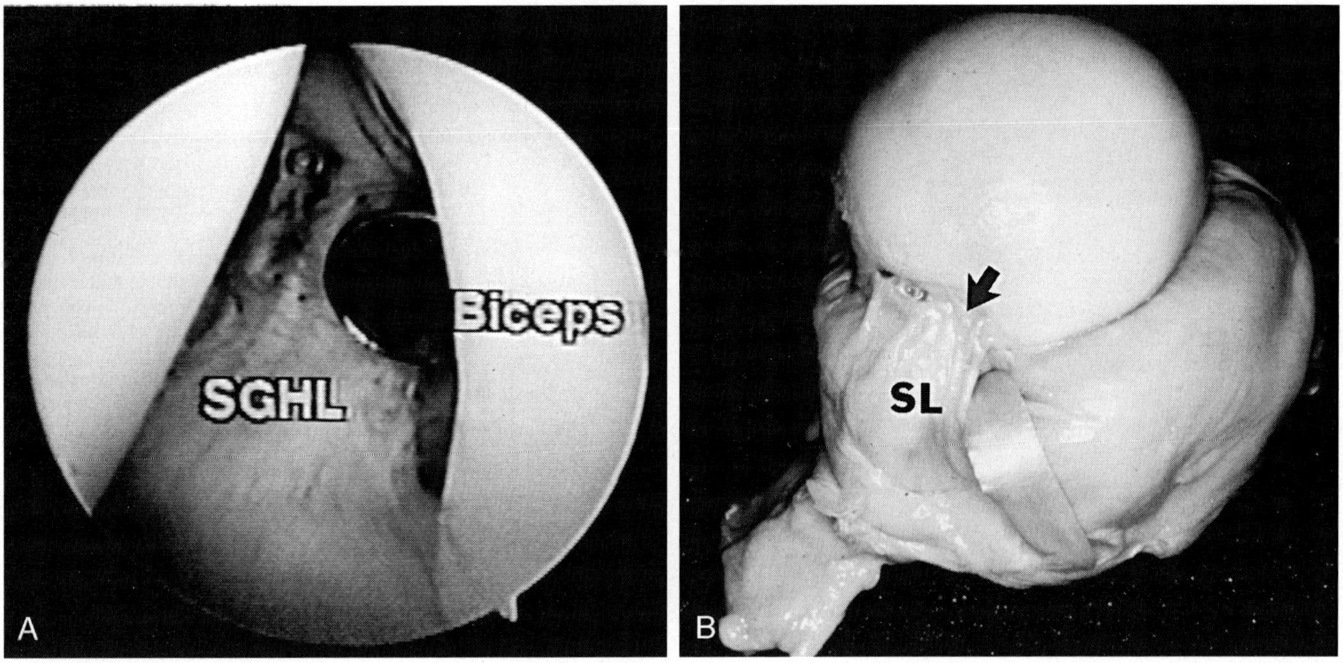

Fig. 2–16. *A,* Arthroscopic in vivo view of the superior glenohumeral ligament (SGHL), originating immediately anterior to the biceps tendon in continuity with the antero-superior labrum. *B,* The superior glenohumeral ligament crosses the rotator interval capsule on deep surface to insert at the humeral fovea capitus (arrow), which is adjacent to the superior margin of the lesser tuberosity and the medial border of the biceps tendon. This ligament plays a critical role in superior-inferior and posterior stability of the glenohumeral joint.

sagittal plane elevation and internal rotation. Tears of the humeral musculotendinous insertion would, therefore, contribute to instability in these positions.

VASCULAR SUPPLY TO THE ROTATOR CUFF

In elderly shoulders with intact rotator cuffs, such as those used for our anatomic dissections, degeneration was absent histologically, especially in the middle layers in which a natural paucity of vascularity is found. Therefore, we assume that perfusion to the middle layers of the rotator cuff is generally adequate to maintain tendon nutrition well beyond the sixth or seventh decade of life.

Overall, three sets of vessels supply the rotator cuff tendons, the capsule, and their bony insertions. These vessels include the osseous, muscular, and tendinous vessels. Gerber has shown that the osseous network is derived primarily from the anterolateral branch of the anterior humeral circumflex, which is also named the arcuate vessel.[34] This vessel ascends along the lateral border of the bicipital groove. Moseley and Goldie delineated the main blood supply to the rotator cuff tendons.[35] They found that the supraspinatus tendon and its insertion were dependent primarily on the anterior humeral circumflex, the suprascapular and the subscapular arteries. Gerber also studied the vascularization of the rotator cuff. He found that all of the supraspinatus tendon was supplied by the suprascapular artery, except for the insertion that received its blood supply from the posterior humeral circumflex (Fig. 2–17).[34] This region of the cuff has intrigued many investigators since it corresponds to a constant area that appears to have a vascularity radically different from the other tendons of the rotator cuff.[12,13] This "critical zone" corresponds to the anastomoses between the osseous and tendinous vessels (derived from the suprascapular and subscapular arteries). Although this tendinous region actually has a rich capillary network,[14] investigators found that when the tendon was subjected to normal bending, tensile and compressive forces within the tendon compromised its blood flow.[13] Likewise, attenuation of rotator cuff tendon fibers may apply excessive load to adjacent fibers that can impede the flow through the vascular network and compromise the nutritional supply.[36]

THE TENDINOUS INSERTION

The insertion of tendons and ligaments into bone is quite unique. The insertion is well adapted to dissipate force over an increasing gradient of stiffness from the transition of tendon to bone.[3] In the rotator cuff, this phenomenon is illustrated across four histological zones. The four zones include (1) the tendon, (2) uncalcified fibrocartilage, (3) calcified fibrocartilage, and (4) bone (Fig. 2–18). The intervening zones of fibrocartilage, between tendon and bone, serve to absorb impact loading and to protect the insertion against excessive shear, compression, and tension for positions of acute repetitive

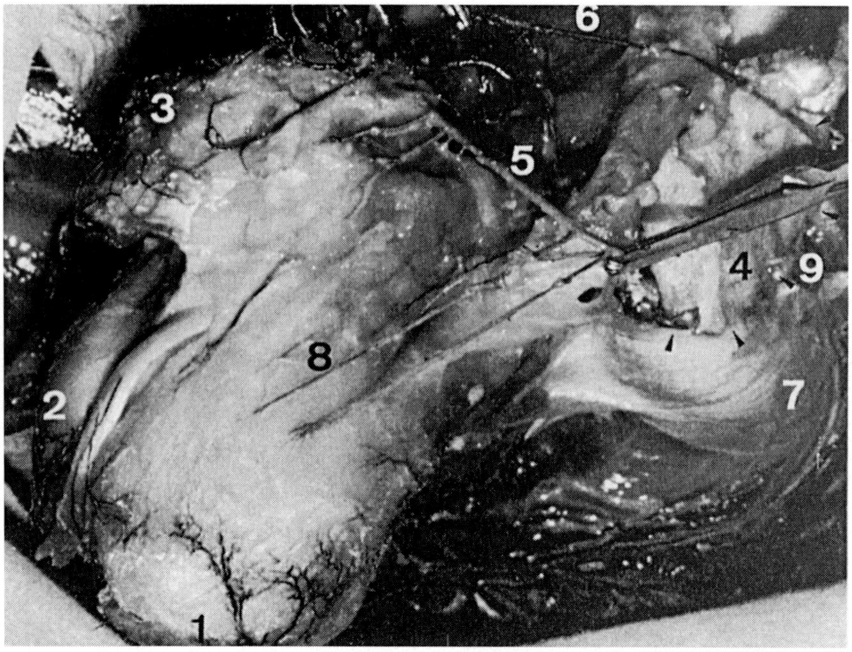

Fig. 2–17. The supraspinatus muscle and tendon are exclusively vascularized by the suprascapular artery, with the exception of the most lateral aspect (greater tuberosity), which is supplied by a few branches of the anterolateral branch of the anterior curcumflex artery and by branches of the posterior circumflex artery. The watershed between the territories of the anterior circumflex and posterior circumflex arteries is the middle of the greater tuberosity; 1 = greater tuberosity and 2 = lesser tuberosity (between the tuberosities lies the tendon of the long head of the biceps, with its vessels from the arteria profunda brachii); 3 = coracoid process; 4 = undersurface of the acromion; 5 = branch of the suprascapular artery anastomosing at (9) the inferior border of the acromion with (6) the acromial branch of the thoracoacromial artery; 7 = deltoid muscle; and 8 = branches of the suprascapular artery for the supply of the supraspinatus tendon. (From Gerber C, Schneeberger AG, Vinh T-S. The arterial vascularization of the humeral head. *J Bone Joint Surg Am.* 1990; 72:1486–1494.)

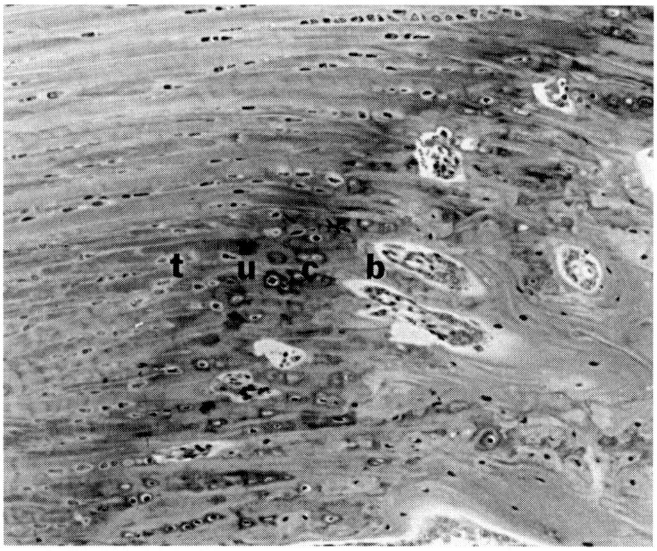

Fig. 2–18. Photomicrograph of the supraspinatus tendon insertion into the greater tuberosity. The tendon insertion is highly specialized to dissipate stress at the tendon-bone interface. The insertion is divided into four zones each having greater stiffness in the following order: (1) tendon (t); (2) uncalcified fibrocartilage (u); (3) calcified fibrocartilage (c); and (4) bone (b). This arrangement protects the cuff insertion from tearing, thereby increasing the durability of the tendon to bone junction.

bending. The terminal fibers of the rotator cuff tendon are seen to criss-cross on transverse section; this design not only helps bind the longitudinal fibers together but shares loads to protect the direct fiber insertion.[25] As mentioned previously, the nutrition to the cells within the tendon insertion are supplied by the osseous network on the one side and the tendinous network on the other.

SUMMARY

Understanding the anatomical arrangement of the rotator cuff provides the treating physician with information that helps explain delamination within the layers of the rotator cuff, which is often seen arthroscopically or at an open repair. Structural failure within any portion of the rotator cuff tendon complex or the capsular contribution causes additional stress on neighboring fibers. During surgery, restoration of the normal rotator cuff architecture will help insure longevity of the repair. Hopefully, this review of the anatomic structure prepares the reader for an investigation of pathologic conditions and provides insight into the natural history of rotator cuff failure. Although we may be unable to identify the initial event leading to degeneration of the rotator cuff, we know that compromise of capsule or cuff tendon integrity will lead to pathological alteration of the normal nutrition and affect the shared functions of stability and strength in critical positions.

REFERENCES

1. Matsen FA III, Thomas SC, Rockwood CA. Glenohumeral Instability. In: Rockwood CA Jr, Matsen FA III, eds. *The Shoulder.* Philadelphia: WB Saunders; 1990;1:547–551.
2. Clark JM, Harryman DT II. Tendons, ligaments, and capsule of the rotator cuff. *J Bone Joint Surg Am.* 1992;74:713–725.
3. Woo S, Maynard J, Butler D, et al. Ligament, tendon, and joint capsule insertions to bone. In: Woo SL-Y, Buckwalter JA, eds. *Injury and Repair of the Musculoskeletal Soft Tissues.* Savannah: American Academy of Orthopaedic Surgeons; 1987:133–166.
4. Jobe CM. Gross anatomy of the shoulder. In: Rockwood CA Jr, Matsen FA III, eds. *The Shoulder.* Philadelphia: WB Saunders; 1990; 1:50–62.

5. Perry J. Biomechanics of the shoulder. In: Rowe CR, ed. *The Shoulder.* New York: Churchill Livingstone; 1988:12–15.
6. Vanderhooft JE, Lippitt SB, Harris SL, Sidles JA, Harryman DT II, Matsen FA III. Glenohumeral stability from concavity-compression: A quantitative analysis. *Orthop Trans* 1992; 16:774.
7. Gowan ID, Jobe FW, Tibone JE, Perry J. A comparative electromyographic analysis of the shoulder during pitching. Professional versus amateur pitchers. *Am J Sports Med.* 1987;15:586–590.
8. Ovesen JO, Nielsen S. Stability of the shoulder joint. Cadaver study of stabilizing structures. *Acta Orthop Scand.* 1985;56:149–151.
9. DePalma AF, Callery G, Bennett GA. Shoulder joint: Variational anatomy and degenerative lesions of the shoulder joint. *AAOS Instructional Course Lectures.* 1949;6:255–281.
10. Walch G, Boileau P, Noel E, Donell ST. Impingement of the deep surface of the supraspinatus tendon on the posterosuperior glenoid rim: An arthroscopic study. *J Shoulder Elbow Surg.* 1992; 1:238–245.
11. Jobe CM, Walch G, Sidles JA. Evidence for a superior glenoid impingement upon the rotator cuff. *Orthop Trans.* 1992;16:763.
12. Rothman RH, Parke WW. The vascular anatomy of the rotator cuff. *Clin Orthop.* 1965;41:176–186.
13. Rathbun JB, Macnab I. The microvascular pattern of the rotator cuff. *J Bone Joint Surg Br.* 1970;52:540–553.
14. Swiontkowski MF, Iannotti JP, Boulas HJ, Esterhai JL. Intraoperative assessment of rotator cuff vascularity using laser doppler flowmetry. In: Hawkins RJ, Morrey BF, Post M, eds. *Surgery of the Shoulder.* St. Louis: Mosby-Year Book; 1990:208–212.
15. Colachis Jr SC, Strohm BR. Effects of suprascapular and axillary nerve block on muscle forces in the upper extremity. *Arch Phys Med Rehabil.* 1971;52:22.
16. Howell SM, Imobersteg AM, Segar DH, Marone PJ. Clarification of the role of the supraspinatus muscle in shoulder function. *J Bone Joint Surg Am.* 1986;68:398–404.
17. Dempster WT. Mechanisms of shoulder movement.*Arch Phys Med Rehab.* 1965;46A:49.
18. Sarrafian SK. Gross anatomy and kinesiology. In: Post M, ed. *The Shoulder: Surgical and Nonsurgical Management.* 2nd ed. Philadelphia: Lea & Febiger; 1988:51.
19. Basmajian JV, Bazant FJ. Factors preventing downward dislocation of the adducted shoulder joint. *J Bone Joint Surg Am.* 1959;41:1182–1186.
20. Bowen MK, Warren RF, O'Brien SJ, Altchek DW. Posterior subluxation of the glenohumeral joint treated by posterior stabilization.*Orthop Trans.* 1991;15:3:764.
21. Morrey BF, An KN. Biomechanics of the shoulder. Rockwood CA Jr, Matsen FA III, eds. *The Shoulder.* Philadelphia: WB Saunders; 1990;1:228–229.
22. Harryman DT II, Sidles JA, Clark JM, Gibb TD, Matsen FA III. Translation of the humeral head on the glenoid with passive glenohumeral motion. *J Bone Joint Surg Am.* 1990;72:1288–1298.
23. Colachis Jr SC, Strohm BR, Brecher VL. Effects of axillary nerve block on muscle force in the upper extremity. *Arch Phys Med Rehabil.* 1969;50:645–647.
24. Pearl ML, Harris SL, Lippitt SB, Sidles JA, Harryman DT II, Matsen FA III. A system for describing positions of the humerus relative to the thorax and its use in the presentation of several functionally important arm positions. *J Shoulder Elbow Surg.* 1992;1:2:113–118.
25. Benjamin M, Evans EJ, Copp L. The histology of tendon attachments to bone in man. *J Anat.* 1986;149:89–100.
26. Clark J, Sidles JA, Matsen FA III. The relationship of the glenohumeral joint capsule to the rotator cuff. *Clin Orthop.* 1990;254:29–34.
27. Grant JCB. *An Atlas of Anatomy.* Baltimore: Williams & Wilkins; 1972; 6:26.
28. Gray H. *Anatomy of the Human Body.* Goss CM, ed. 29th ed. Philadelphia: Lea & Febiger; 1973:455–458.
29. Kaltsas DS. Comparative study of the properties of the shoulder joint capsule with those of other joint capsules. *Clin Orthop.* 1983; 173:20–26.
30. Burkhart SS. Fluoroscopic comparison of kinematic patterns in massive rotator cuff tears. *Clin Orthop.* 1992; 4:144–152.
31. Harryman DT II, Sidles JA, Harris SL, Matsen FA III. The role of the rotator interval capsule in passive motion and stability of the shoulder. *J Bone Joint Surg Am.* 1992;74:53–66.
32. Warner JJP, Deng X-H, Warren RF, Torzilli P. Static capsuloligamentous restraints to superior-inferior translation of the glenohumeral joint. *Am J Sports Med.* 1992;20:675–685.
33. Poirier P, Charpy A. *Traite' d' Anatomie Humaine.* Vol 1. Paris: Masson; 1899:6.
34. Gerber C, Schneeberger AG, Vinh T-S. The arterial vascularization of the humeral head. *J Bone Joint Surg Am.* 1990;72:1486–1494.
35. Moseley HF, Goldie I. The arterial pattern of the rotator cuff of the shoulder. *J Bone Joint Surg Br.* 1963;45:780–789.
36. Matsen FA III, Arntz CT. Rotator cuff tendon failure. In: Rockwood CA Jr, Matsen FA III, eds. *The Shoulder.* Philadelphia: WB Saunders; 1990:647–649.

Chapter 3

Pathophysiology of Rotator Cuff Degeneration, Calcification, and Repair

K. Sarkar and Hans K. Uhthoff

Even such is time, that takes in trust our youth, our joys, our all we have and pays but with age and dust.

Raleigh

Degeneration of rotator cuff tendons is defined as structural alterations in the tendon proper and/or in the zone of attachment. Although degeneration is inevitable in every individual surviving to or beyond the fifth decade, these degenerative changes do not necessarily cause functional impairment. In many individuals, however, the degeneration may lead to painful shoulder syndromes including various degrees of tendon tears.

SOFT TISSUES AROUND THE GLENOHUMERAL JOINT

The glenohumeral joint, formed between a shallow glenoid cavity of the scapula and the head of the humerus, is constructed in such a way as to allow a maximum range of motion at the expense of stability. Many of the degenerative changes that are seen in the soft tissues of the shoulder, including the rotator cuff tendons, may be attributed to the vulnerability inherent in the anatomy of this joint and its surrounding structures. We begin with a brief review of the soft tissues that are associated with the glenohumeral joint.

The Glenoid Labrum

The edge of the glenoid cavity is rimmed by the glenoid labrum. It consists mostly of dense fibrous tissue but becomes fibrocartilaginous near the articular cartilage.[1] Rare elastin fibers are present in the adult labrum. The labrum is vascularized, especially at its peripheral attachment to the capsule. The vascularity tends to decrease with increasing age.[2] Trauma, frequently caused by athletic activities, can inflict labral damage, even avulsion, inducing degenerative changes that may set the stage for partial tears and attenuation of the cuff.

The Capsule

Because the capsule is intimately related to the tendon of the long head of the biceps and the tendons forming the rotator cuff (Fig. 3–1), there must be a significant interplay between the cuff tendons and the capsule biomechanically. It is generally acknowledged that the capsule has wide anatomical variations. The use of arthroscopic visualization of the capsule and its ligamentous thickenings has elucidated the anatomic variability and also added to the knowledge of its function.

The capsule is lax, being much larger than the entire surface area of the humeral head. It extends from the labrum, even from the anterior aspect of the neck of the scapula,[3] to the anatomical neck and proximal shaft of the humerus. It is reinforced above and in front by ligamentous thickenings known as the superior, middle and inferior glenohumeral ligaments, and the coracohumeral ligament. All of these capsular structures are believed to be involved with the stabilization of the glenohumeral joint.

The integrity of the capsule is affected by aging, which seems to decrease the tensile strength of the capsule.[4] The capsule has also been largely implicated in the

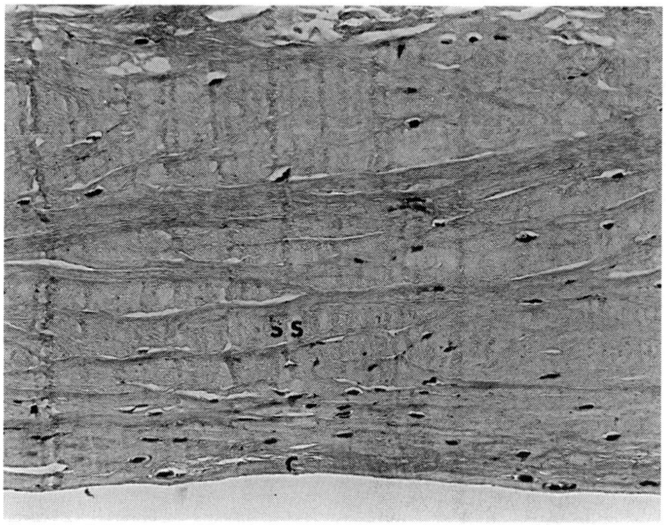

Fig. 3–1. Capsule (C) covering the inferior aspect of the supraspinatus tendon (SS) is not demarcated from the tendon (azan, ×66).

pathogenesis of frozen shoulder. Although the name "adhesive capsulitis" has been suggested as a more specific alternative to frozen shoulder,[5] the presence of adhesions as such has not been found with certainty.[6] Ozaki et al.[7] found histologic changes (including fibrosis, hyalinization, and fibrinoid degeneration) causing contracture of the coracohumeral ligament and the rotator cuff interval, which produced the characteristic decrease in external rotation seen in frozen shoulder. They also observed an absence of the synovial lining and fibrosis of the subsynovial tissue.[7] We feel, however, that these features suggest permanent tissue damage and, therefore, do not explain how in many cases a "frozen" shoulder spontaneously "thaws" with the return of normal function. We do recognize that the capsule with its ligaments is primarily involved, but to us, the term "retractile capsulitis" appears more suitable than "adhesive capsulitis."[8]

The Subacromial Bursa

The subacromial bursa overlies the rotator cuff tendons and is continuous with the subdeltoid bursa. The bursa is bounded superiorly by the coracoacromial arch and deltoid muscle. Like any other bursa of the body, its cavity is lined by one or more layers of synovial cells. The wall of the bursa may vary in thickness and is composed of fibrofatty tissue with numerous blood vessels. The wall seems to blend with the peritenon of the supraspinatus tendon with no line of cleavage between them (Fig. 3–2). Complete tears of the rotator cuff connect the subacromial bursa with the glenohumeral joint, producing changes that are often called bursitis. The bursa, however, does not show the usual features of inflammation. A primary bursitis without an underlying cuff tendinopathy is, in our opinion, a rarity.

The Rotator Cuff Tendons

The tendons of the subscapularis, supraspinatus, infraspinatus, and teres minor muscles conjoin to form the rotator cuff, which overlies the humeral head. Extensions of the subscapularis and supraspinatus tendons surround the biceps tendon like a sheath at the proximal end of the bicipital groove.[9] The capsule is intimately attached to the cuff tendons at the lateral aspects but is clearly separated from the tendons more medially. At the lateral aspect, a distinction between the capsule and the tendons cannot be made, even histologically.

The cuff tendons, like many other tendons of the body, include a tendon proper and a zone of attachment or area of insertion into bone. The tendon proper consists of bundles of collagen type I fibers, but the endotenon surrounding the bundles is mainly composed of collagen type III. No collagen type II fibers are present in a normal tendon proper. In the zone of attachment, on the other hand, the fibrocartilage is primarily composed of collagen type II fibers, with the presence of collagen types I and II being less conspicuous. This area is divided into four parts: (1) a nonmineralized fibrocartilage adjoining the tendon proper, (2) the blue line, (3) the zone of mineralized fibrocartilage, and (4) the bone (Fig. 3–3). The mineralized fibrocartilage has a varying thickness, and the border separating the mineralized fibrocartilage from the bone is irregularly undulated. Pathologic changes inevitably develop with aging in the zone of attachment of cuff tendons, and it seems likely that the changes could give rise to symptoms of enthesopathy.

The Coracoacromial Ligament

The coracoacromial ligament spans the interval between the acromion and the coracoid process. The three structures together form the coracoacromial arch. Dur-

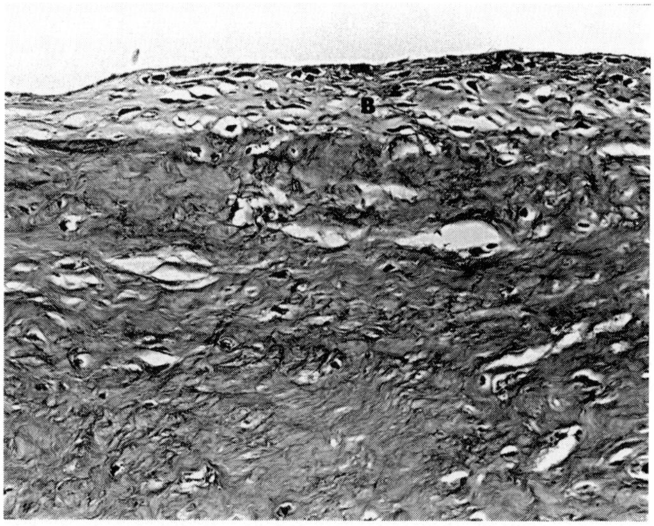

Fig. 3–2. The wall of the subacromial bursa (B) overlies the tendon and appears in continuity with the epitenon (azan, ×66).

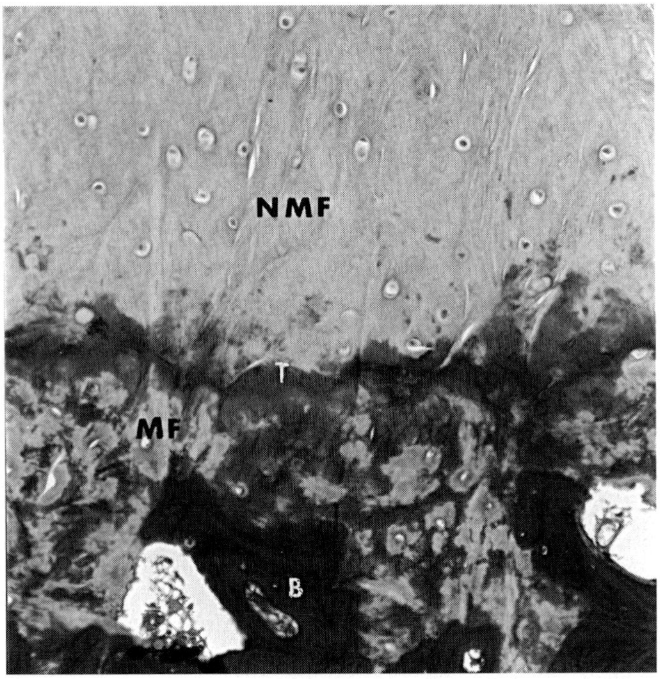

Fig. 3–3. The zone of attachment of the supraspinatus tendon showing four parts: nonmineralized fibrocartilage (NMF), the tidemark (T), mineralized fibrocartilage (MF), and bone (B) (azan, ×33).

ing movements of the shoulder, the humeral head, with the overlying cuff and the bursa, must glide under this rigid, unyielding arch. The insertion of the ligament into the coracoid process is somewhat broad. At the acromion, the more superficial part of the ligament inserts into the anteromedial aspect, whereas the deeper part inserts into the undersurface of the acromion (Fig. 3–4). Spur formation of the acromion occurs at the anteromedial corner through a process of endochondral ossification.[10] In cases of long-standing, large rotator cuff tears or those of cuff arthropathy, the undersurface of the acromion becomes devoid of any ligamentous structures.

PATHOPHYSIOLOGY OF DEGENERATIVE CHANGES

Some systemic diseases, such as diabetes mellitus and rheumatoid arthritis, and occupations that require heavy manual work have been reported to cause degenerative changes in rotator cuff tendons. The present discussion will be limited to local causes producing cuff tendon degeneration. The local causes involving the supraspinatus tendon (the involvement of which occurs more often than any other cuff tendon) may be intrinsic, arising within the substance of the tendon, or extrinsic, when abnormalities in structures outside the tendon induce degenerative changes because of their proximity to the tendon. As examples of intrinsic causes, we will discuss the concept of the "critical zone," tendon vascularity, wear-and-tear effect, and aging; and, as an example of extrinsic cause, we will discuss the process of impingement. However, it is understood that extrinsic and intrinsic causes may coexist. Tears of the supraspinatus tendon may be accompanied by lesions of the coracohumeral ligament, the superior glenohumeral ligament, and the superior portion of the subscapularis tendon, structures which belong to the rotator interval.[10a]

The factors mentioned above induce degeneration of cuff tendons mostly in middle-aged and elderly individuals. In young persons it appears that athletic activities involving overuse of above-the-shoulder movement have emerged as a significant cause of degenerative rotator cuff tendinopathy.

The Concept of the Critical Zone and Tendon Vascularity

Codman[11] noted that in the supraspinatus tendon both complete tears and calcifying tendinitis, the two major symptom-producing lesions of cuff tendons, tend to occur in one particular area. Codman called it "the critical portion." It is a "half inch proximal to the palisades," that is, the row of cells in the fibrocartilage that constitutes the zone of insertion. With respect to any structural peculiarity of this area, Codman felt that "even under the microscope one cannot distinguish, in this part of tendon, between joint membrane, capsule, tendon substance, and bursal floor because they are welded into one single structure."[11] The vulnerability of the "critical portion" for developing lesions is generally recognized, and many investigators since Codman have spent considerable effort in elucidating the anatomical peculiarity of this area.

The delineation of vascular arrangement in the "critical portion" has been the principal target of investigation. Using both microangiography and histology, Moseley and Goldie[12] found that the tendon was generously

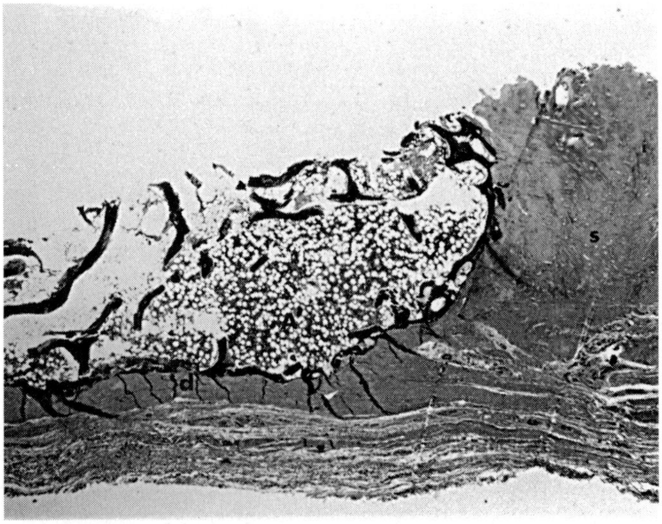

Fig. 3–4. Insertion of the coracoacromial ligament into the acromion (A). One part (s) inserts into the antero-medial edge while the other (d) attaches to the undersurface where it serves as a cushion (azan, ×5).

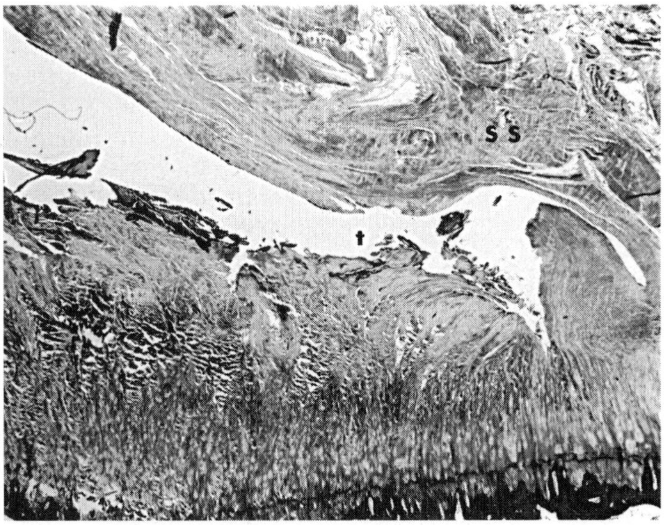

Fig. 3–5. Incomplete tear (t) at the articular aspect of the supraspinatus tendon (SS) insertion (goldner, ×15).

supplied by a network of vessels originating at both the muscular and the osseous ends of the tendon. Vessels from these two sources anastomosed in an area corresponding to Codman's "critical portion." The investigators called it the "critical zone," a term which has been popular since then. This area, however, was found to be no less vascularized than any other part of the tendon.[12] Rothman and Parke,[13] on the other hand, showed in their microangiographic studies that the critical zone was markedly "undervascularized." According to these investigators, a poor blood supply was of prime importance for the development of lesions in the critical zone. Rathbun and Macnab[14] were enthusiastic proponents of the idea that hypoxia in the critical zone was the principal factor responsible for the occurrence of lesions. The hypoxia, however, was not caused by the anatomic distribution of the vessels, but was dependent upon the position of the arm. They demonstrated in cadavers that when micropaque was injected into the shoulder vessels with the arm in the position of adduction, the critical zone as well as the area of tendon insertion did not fill. In the contralateral shoulder, the vessels filled completely throughout the tendon when the arm was placed in a position of abduction. The investigators therefore concluded that the zone of avascularity was a wringing-out effect, resulting from pressure exerted by the head of the humerus on the supraspinatus tendon. According to Macnab,[15] repeated bouts of hypoxia lead to degenerative changes in the critical zone that are characterized by separation and fragmentation of collagenous fascicles and loss of tenocytes, with the possible consequence of developing tears or calcification.

There is no doubt that the neighborhood of the junctional area between the tendon proper and the bony attachment zone is the critical site in which complete tears generally occur, usually involving the zone of attachment as well. We believe, however, that the pattern of vascular distribution is crucial only at the articular aspect near the insertion where there is a lack of perfusable vascular channels. That is, vascular compromise does not extend throughout the whole area of the critical zone. Our microangiographic studies consistently showed an area of underfilling near the insertion at the articular side.[16]

Histologically, there are no areas in the supraspinatus tendon devoid of vascular channels except the fibrocartilage in the zone of attachment. We have observed that there are more vessels at the bursal side than at the articular side. It appears that the tendon is most likely to tear at its articular aspect near the zone of attachment where vascularity is deficient. This area suffers from impaired perfusion regardless of the position of the arm. Moreover, the joint side layer of the supraspinatus tendon is weaker in tension than the bursal side layer.[16a] Incomplete tears are commonest in this area (Fig. 3–5), and it is conceivable that many of the tears that become complete might begin in this area as partial tears. A widening of the sulcus (i.e., the interval between the articular cartilage of the humeral head and the insertion of the supraspinatus tendon) is often seen in older subjects and is possibly the consequence of an incomplete tear, the distal stump of which had undergone resorption (Fig. 3–6).

Wear-and-Tear Effect and Aging

Meyer[17] introduced the concept of wear-and-tear effects on the soft tissues of the shoulder. He believed that even the ordinary use of the shoulder "hour to hour, day to day, month to month, year to year and decade to decade" would induce degenerative changes, and "it is the repetition and not the range of motion that counts." Meyer's concept is easy to appreciate because the shoulder is the most used joint of the body. In Meyer's descrip-

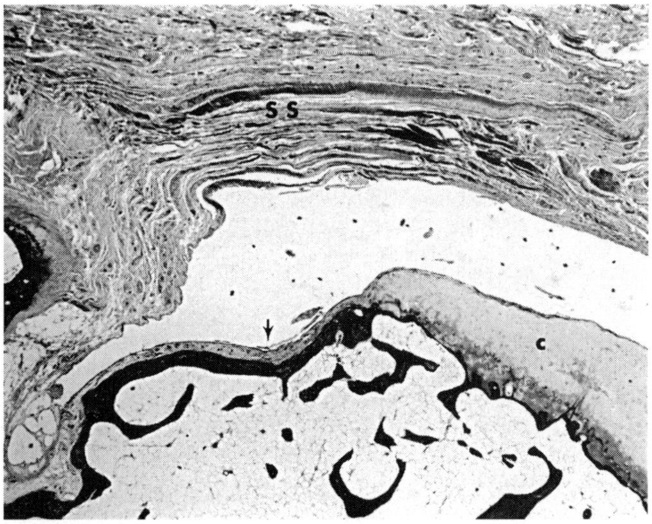

Fig. 3–6. Widened sulcus. The supraspinatus tendon (SS) does not insert close to the articular cartilage (c) and the bone at this interval is covered with a thin layer of granulation tissue (arrow). The tendon shows signs of fibrillation (goldner, ×5).

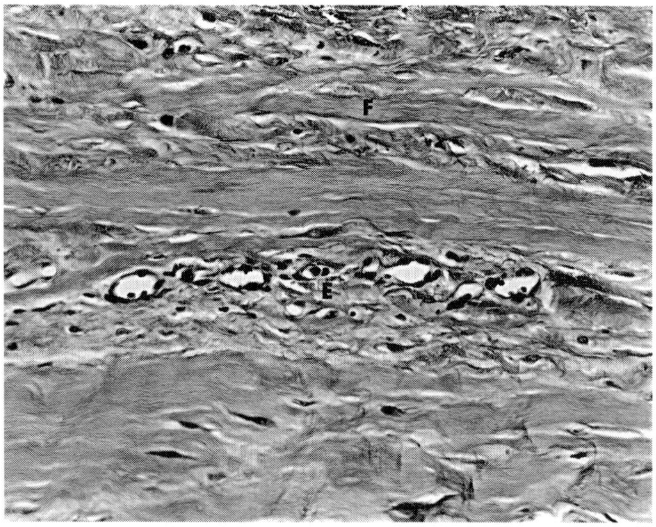

Fig. 3–7. The supraspinatus tendon of an elderly male shows widening of the endotenon (E) space and thinning of fascicle (F) (azan, ×66).

tion, the changes in the soft tissues begin in a milder way and progress to become destructive lesions. The capsule becomes thin and then perforates; the subacromial bursa loses the smooth lining and becomes roughened and frayed, and the tendons show separation and thinning of fascicles with destruction of a part or whole of the width.[17]

Many of the changes that Meyer described have been attributed to aging in later studies. Aging of the cuff tendons happens independently of chronological old age, and histologically identifiable degenerative changes seem to appear as early as the third decade.[18,19] In general, the distal part of the tendon, including the zone of attachment, appears to get more involved than the proximal part.[19] Wilson and Duff[20] found that the earliest features of tendon aging was altered staining of fiber bundles followed by fibrillation. The number of blood vessels appear to increase with age. The fibrocartilage in the attachment zone is broadened and fibrillated with splitting of the tidemark.[20–22] There are ''flamelike offshoots'' into the fibrocartilage.[19] Brewer,[23] examining autopsy specimens from 20-, 50-, and 70-year-old subjects, showed that the cuff tendons gradually lost the integrity in the arrangement of fibers and staining properties with aging. Concurrently, there was loss of cellularity and deformity of the articular surface. In an immunohistochemical study of the zone of an attachment of cuff tendons in postmortem cases ranging in age from 52 to 90 years, we could show that in the presence of the degenerative lesions staining with collagen type III was more prominent than in the absence of such lesions. This could explain the impairment of mechanical properties of the tendon of its zone of attachment.[23a]

It is not uncommon to find various degrees of cuff tear in random samplings of elderly human cadavers. Yamanaka and Fukuda[24] studied the aging changes in the supraspinatus tendon of human cadavers ranging in age from the first to the ninth decade, with 89% of the cases being over 50 years of age. The investigators found an incidence of 7.9% complete tears and 14.5% incomplete tears in individuals older than 40 years of age, all involving the critical zone.

If complete or incomplete tears are not included in the survey of aging changes, the histologic findings in the supraspinatus tendon from cadavers of elderly humans who had no known history of shoulder ailments appear to consist of (1) thinning and fibrillation of fascicles in the tendon proper, resulting in broadening of the endotenon spaces (Fig. 3–7); (2) irregular thickening of the blue line, with calcific deposits straying into the nonmineralized fibrocartilage and distorting its architecture (Fig. 3–8); (3) microtears involving the fibrocartilage; and (4) disruption of the blue line by fibrovascular tissue.

The area of insertion and the critical zone are most conspicuously affected by aging. Further from these areas the fascicular thinning and fibrillation in the tendon proper are extremely variable. It is surprising that despite all the changes that occur in the distal part of the tendon, the possibility of enthesopathy relating to the glenohumeral joint is not commonly entertained by clinicians in the differential diagnosis of painful shoulder syndromes of elderly individuals. With improvement of noninvasive imaging procedures, enthesopathy of cuff tendons may yet emerge as a diagnosis worth considering. Finally, it must be emphasized that although some of the changes in cuff tendons can be attributed to aging, it is difficult and unreliable to estimate the patient's age by histologic examination of the tendon.[25]

The Process of Impingement

The smooth gliding of the supraspinatus tendon in the subacromial space may be impeded by the process of impingement. The process may originate either in the tendon itself or in the coracoacromial arch. We have classified the sources of problems in the shoulder as intrinsic if they originate in the tendon or extrinsic if they are

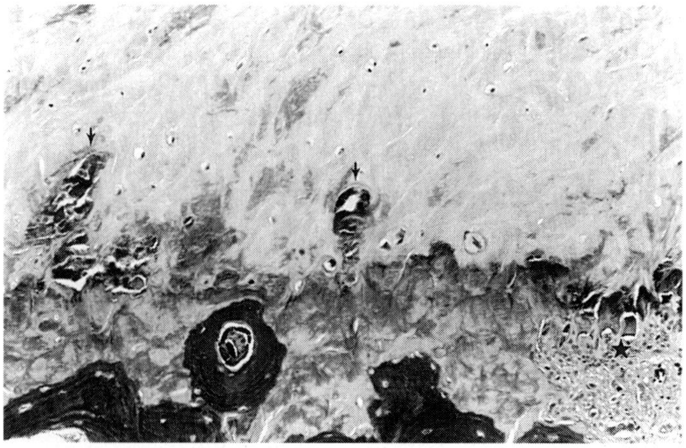

Fig. 3–8. The tidemark (T) in the attachment zone of the supraspinatus tendon from an elderly man shows irregular thickening, disruption by fibrovascular tissue (asterisk), and calcific excrescences (arrows) (goldner, ×33).

caused by anatomic variations or pathologic changes in the components of the coracoacromial arch.[26] The impingement syndrome has become relevant to rotator cuff tears since Neer[27] contended that "95% of tears of the rotator cuff are initiated by impingement wear rather than circulatory impairment or trauma." Neer[27] has proposed an elaborate hypothesis on the impingement syndrome describing how degenerative changes in the tendon and the subacromial bursa lead to tear in three sequential stages. These stages merit description because they are widely followed in the formulation of treatment for the impingement syndrome.

According to Neer, the Stage I is primarily seen in individuals less than 25 years of age and is characterized by edema, hemorrhage, and inflammation that swell the bursa and make it less compliant. The changes are not detectable by radiography and are reversible if activities that are usually athletic in nature are suspended until symptoms improve. Patients between 25 and 40 years of age demonstrate Stage II lesions, consisting of fibrosis and thickening of the bursa and scarring and disassociation of fibers in the supraspinatus and biceps tendons. At this stage the disorder has reached a chronic state, is no longer reversible, and has become progressive. Radiographs still fail to show any abnormality. Patients in Stage III are over 40 years of age and have a long history of symptoms. Bony and tendinous lesions are identifiable by radiologic and arthroscopic examinations. There are bony alterations of the anterior acromion and greater tuberosity and a partial or complete rupture of the tendon initially evident on the bursal aspect of the tendon.[27] An anterior acromioplasty is necessary to decompress the rotator cuff to relieve the impingement.

One can appreciate the clinical aspect of Neer's staging of the impingement syndrome in the throwing arm of a young athlete, but in the vast majority of nonathletic patients, neither the pathogenesis nor the structural changes are readily explained by Neer's hypothesis. According to Neer, abnormalities in the shape and slope of the acromion, along with the coracoacromial ligament, constitute the principal causative factor for the impingement syndrome. However, we believe that in the majority of cases, because of the presence of an intrinsic lesion, the tendon is expanded and the symptoms of impingement appear because it occurs within the unyielding subacromial space.

In support of Neer's contention about the importance of the slope of the acromion, Bigliani et al.[28] found that a hooked (type III) acromion was associated with as many as 70% of the cases with tears secondary to the impingement syndrome. However, the number of patients with the impingement syndrome with a type III acromion but no tear has not been documented. It should also be noted that the difference in the degrees of slope between type III and type II acromion (0.7 vs 22.7) was small, and the latter was involved with a minority of cases with tears. Furthermore, acromial spurs, another assumed factor for the impingement syndrome, might be a consequence rather than a primary cause of impingement.[10,29]

Other extrinsic causes have been implicated as causative factors for the impingement syndrome. Watson[30] considered thickening or stiffening of the coracoacromial ligament. However, morphological studies of the ligament mainly show fatty changes or microtears without any evidence of excessive collagen production that would increase the caliber or rigidity of the ligament.[31] Osteophytes of the AC joint can conceivably result in impingement,[30] but the arm has to sustain a position of extreme internal rotation or one of maximal abduction with internal rotation for impingement of the tendon to occur. Anatomical abnormalities of the coracoid process have been reported to cause impingement,[32,33] but the conditions are rare. We feel that these extrinsic causes of impingement are insignificant for the pathogenesis of degenerative tendinopathy.

We believe, then, that tendinopathies resulting from intrinsic causes are primarily responsible for impingement, and that any suggestion that chronic impingement syndrome without an underlying tendinopathy would eventually lead to tear is misleading. The first two stages proposed by Neer[27] are clearly open to question because the structural changes of these stages have never been substantiated by soft-tissue imaging or histopathological studies. We have failed to find extensive fibrosis that is supposed to occur in the subacromial bursa in chronic impingement syndrome.[34] No morphological studies of the supraspinatus tendon have been possible, because the tendon is not biopsied during surgery for chronic impingement syndrome.

Not infrequently, the term impingement is used inappropriately and indiscriminately. There should be an awareness of this problem among the surgeons to avoid unnecessary or even harmful surgical interventions.

Sports and Cuff Tendinopathy

Forceful swinging of the arm above the level of the shoulder in sporting activities, such as throwing a baseball or serving in tennis, creates abnormally high demands on the soft tissues of the glenohumeral joint. The overuse of the shoulder during these activities produces injuries to the glenoidal labrum, to the capsule, and to the rotator cuff tendons.[35,36] In an athlete with a subluxing shoulder, impingement occurs secondarily to instability.[36] Shoulder instability as such may accelerate the progression of structural changes. Fraying is frequently mentioned among the changes that might also include features that are similar to the degenerative changes seen in nonathletic, elderly adults. Young athletes, however, form a unique population, and we feel that, along with the study of biomechanics, special efforts should be made to characterize the pathological changes so that strain-induced damage could be distinguished from degeneration induced by the factors that we have discussed previously.

Calcification

Abnormal deposition of calcium in soft tissues that are injured or dead is not an uncommon pathologic finding and is known as dystrophic calcification.[37] It is limited to

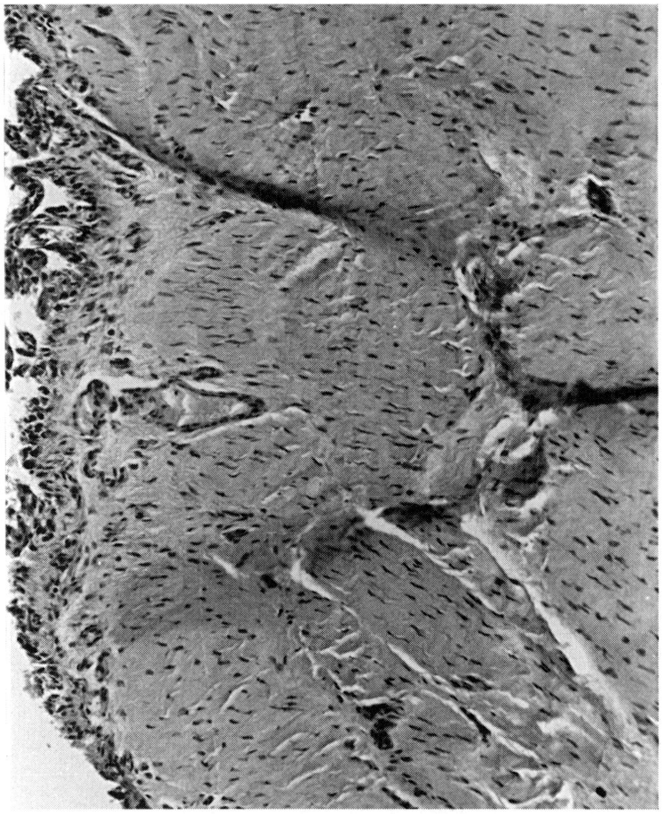

Fig. 3–9. Marked cellular proliferation at the margin of a torn tendon represents a repair cap (hematoxylin-eosin, ×33).

the severely damaged or necrotic tissue without spreading to surrounding viable structures and is not dependent on elevated serum calcium. Long-standing cases of rotator cuff tear may develop radiologically visible calcifications that appear as stippled opacities overlying the greater tuberosity, corresponding to the site of cuff tendon insertion. Sometimes calcification is detected only microscopically in tendinous tissues removed during surgical repair or at autopsy. The presence of calcification generally denotes a poor prognosis in rotator cuff injuries.[38]

Calcification in degenerative rotator cuff tears should be carefully distinguished from calcifying tendinitis, a nondegenerative disorder of uncertain etiology in which calcium tends to disappear spontaneously with time and the tendon undergoes natural healing. In contrast, dystrophic calcification does not resorb but tends to progress with time.

REPAIR

Considering how pervasive the degenerative changes in cuff tendons are, it is pertinent to ask (a) how much of the degeneration in cuff tendons is reversible, (b) do cuff tendons have the potential to repair, and (c) are the soft tissue structures in contiguity to the tendon of any assistance when repair of the tendon is needed?

Historically, tendon repair has been studied extensively in the tendons of the palm and digits but seldom in rotator cuff tendons. The principal issues to determine are the source(s) of cells that would produce collagen to reconstitute the tendon and the supply of nutrition during the period of repair.

In the course of studies on the implication of adhesion formation in flexor tendon injuries, it was argued that tendon healing occurs essentially with the help from an extrinsic source, the tendon sheath.[39] The sheath was believed to provide both vascular and cellular components for healing as granulation tissue derived from the sheath migrated into the wound gap. Although fibrovascular proliferation in the endotenon was seen at a later stage, the predominant mechanism of repair was believed to be mediated by the sheath.[39]

In recent times, a considerable number of publications have demonstrated the intrinsic capability of tendons to heal themselves.[40] By using in vitro methods in which human flexor tendons were cleanly isolated, it was shown that the cut ends were covered by migrating elongated fibroblasts that proliferated in the epitenon or the endotenon. Some of these cells phagocytosed collagen debris. Ultrastructural examinations of the fibroblasts showed extensive rough endoplasmic reticulum and secretory vesicles participating in protein synthesis.[41,42]

In a morphological study of human surgical biopsies comparing the repair process of calcifying tendinitis with that of rotator cuff tear, we have shown that repair in calcifying tendinitis, following spontaneous removal of calcium, demonstrates an outstanding example of intrinsic healing.[43] In rotator cuff tears, on the other hand, fibrovascular proliferation comprising granulation tissue is more conspicuous in the bursa, which is extrinsic to the tendon, than within the substance of the tendon.[44] The expanded bursal wall encroaches upon the area of rupture and the torn edge of the tendon very often shows

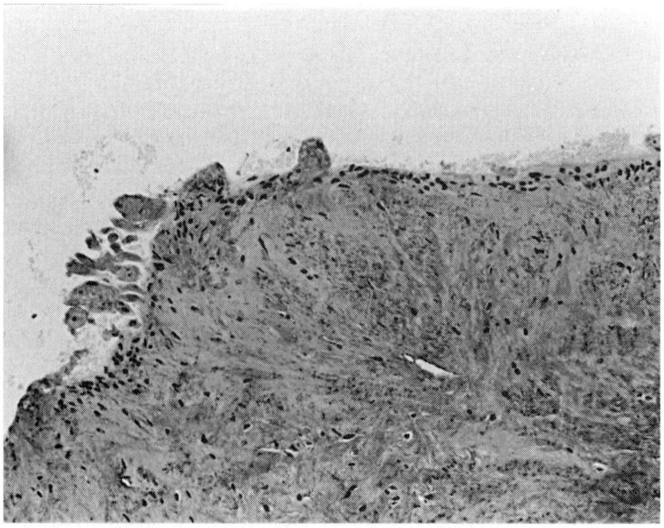

Fig. 3–10. Immunohistochemical labeling of collagen type III appearing as dark gray streaks in a ruptured supraspinatus tendon. The cellular proliferation at the margin of the tear represents a repair cap (×33).

accumulation of cells that represents a repair cap (Fig. 3–9). Thus, repair reaction characterized by granulation tissue and cellular cap was constantly found in the area of the tear regardless of the age of the patient and the duration of preoperative conservative treatment.[44] It is interesting to note that when Swiontowski and his co-workers[45] used intraoperative laser Doppler flowmetry to assess cuff vascularity in patients with cuff tears, they found that all 3 patients with partial tears and 6 out of 8 patients with complete tears had a hyperemic response.

Further evidence of repair activity is the presence of a considerable amount of collagen type III in the healing tendon.[46] A normal tendon is primarily composed of collagen type I. A small amount of collagen type III is preferentially located in the endotenon.[47] In cuff tears, however, an abundant amount of collagen type III is found in perivascular areas of the bursal wall as well as in the tendon where it is no longer limited to endotenon spaces (Fig. 3–10). It is also seen in the fronds of the tendon tissue in the vicinity of the torn edge, even in the absence of vessels in the neighborhood.[46] It is well known that the collagen type III increases significantly during the healing of a wound and that it is the principal collagen component of granulation tissue. It is replaced by the collagen type I as the scar matures.[48,49] It is intriguing to note that morphological evidence of the early stage of repair can persist in torn cuff tendons and the adjacent bursal wall for as long as several years.

CONCLUDING REMARKS

Degenerative changes are inevitable and inexorably progressive in rotator cuff tendons. However, assuming that all cuff tendinopathies, no matter how severe, are caused by underlying degenerative changes is a mistake. Degenerative tendinopathies, such as tears, deteriorate with age, whereas calcifying tendinitis, a self-healing condition, usually has an excellent prognosis. Therefore, it should not be classified along with the degenerative tendinopathies, nor should all calcification be grouped with dystrophic calcification, which worsens the prognosis of cuff tears. Some degenerative cuff tendinopathies are related to impingement, a diagnosis that tends to be overused. Misdiagnosis of this syndrome subjects patients to unnecessary operative intervention, such as anterior acromioplasty, which may prove to be ineffective.

Although the intrinsic ability of a tendon to repair has been convincingly demonstrated by a large number of laboratory studies, its practical use has been ignored by surgeons repairing rotator cuff tears. Moreover, an injury to the cuff tendon elicits intensive reparative response in the subacromial bursa that, in all likelihood, might contribute to the repair of the tendon. Neither the tendon nor the bursa remains inert when a repair of the cuff tendon is needed. Therefore, any intervention to restore continuity in a torn tendon should include a plan for how to integrate the participation of the innate repair capability of the tendon and of the bursa into surgical measures.

We hope that by developing further means to improve our clinical diagnosis and an understanding of pathophysiologic changes we will increase the efficiency of the management of degenerative tendinopathies.

ACKNOWLEDGEMENT

Work in the authors' laboratory has been supported by the Medical Research Council of Canada. We thank J. Wiley, MD for his helpful advice.

REFERENCES

1. Cooper DE, Arnoczky SP, O'Brien SJ, Warren RF, DiCarlo E, Allen AA. Anatomy, histology, and vascularity of the glenoidal labrum. An anatomical study. *J Bone Joint Surg Am.* 1992;74:46–52.
2. Prodromos CC, Ferry JA, Schiller AL, Zarins B. Histological studies of the glenoid labrum from fetal life to old age. *J Bone Joint Surg Am.* 1990;72:1344–1348.
3. Uhthoff HK, Piscopo M. Anterior capsular redundancy of the shoulder: Congenital or traumatic? An embryologic study. *J Bone Joint Surg Br.* 1985;67:363–365.
4. Reeves B. Experiments on tensile strength of the anterior capsular structures of the shoulder in man. *J Bone Joint Surg Br.* 1968;50:858–865.
5. Neviaser JS. Adhesive capsulitis of the shoulder. *J Bone Joint Surg.* 1945;27:211–222.
6. Baslund B, Thomson BS, Jenson EM. Frozen shoulder: Current concepts. *Scand J Rheumatol.* 1990;19:321–325.
7. Ozaki J, Nakagawa Y, Sakurai G, Tamai S. Recalcitrant chronic adhesive capsulitis of the shoulder. *J Bone Joint Surg Am.* 1989; 71:1511–1515.
8. Uhthoff HK, Sarkar K. Periarticular soft tissue conditions causing pain in the shoulder. *Curr Opin Rheumatol.* 1992;4:241–246.
9. Clark JM, Harryman DT II. Tendons, ligaments, and capsule of the rotator cuff. Gross and microscopic anatomy. *J Bone Joint Surg Am.* 1992;74:713–725.
10. Ogata S, Uhthoff HK. Acromial enthesopathy and rotator cuff tear: A radiologic and histologic postmortem investigation of the coracoacromial arch. *Clin Orthop.* 1990;254:39–48.
10a. Walch G, Nove-Josserand L, Levigne C, Renaud E. Tears of the supraspinatus tendon associated with "hidden" lesions of the rotator interval. *J Shoulder Elbow Surg.* 1994;3:347–352.
11. Codman EA. *The Shoulder.* Boston: Thomas Todd; 1934:98.
12. Moseley HF, Goldie I. The arterial pattern of the rotator cuff of the shoulder. *J Bone Joint Surg Br.* 1963;45:780–789.
13. Rothman RH, Parke WW. The vascular anatomy of the rotator cuff. *Clin Orthop.* 1965;41:176–186.
14. Rathbun JB, Macnab I. The microvascular pattern of the rotator cuff. *J Bone Joint Surg Br.* 1970;52:540–553.
15. Macnab I. Rotator cuff tendinitis. *Ann R Coll Surg Engl.* 1973; 53:271–287.
16. Uhthoff HK, Lohr J, Hammond I, Sarkar K. Atiologie und Pathogenese von Rupturen der Rotatormanschette. In: Helbig B, Blauth W, eds. *Schulterschmerzen und Rupturen der Rotatormanschette.* Berlin: Springer-Verlag; 1986:3–9.
16a. Nakajima T, Rokuuma N, Hamada K, Tomatsu T, Fukuda H. Histologic and biomechanical characteristics of the supraspinatus tendon: Reference to rotator cuff tearing. *J Shoulder Elbow Surg.* 1994; 3:79–87.
17. Meyer AW. Chronic functional lesions of the shoulder. *Arch Surg.* 1937;35:646–674.
18. DePalma AF. *Surgery of the Shoulder.* Philadelphia: JB Lippincott; 1950.
19. Olssen O. Degenerative changes of the shoulder joint and their connection with shoulder pain. A morphological and clinical investigation with special attention to the cuff and biceps tendon. *Acta Chir Scand Suppl.* 1953;181:1–130.

20. Wilson CL, Duff GL. Pathologic study of degeneration and rupture of the supraspinatus tendon. *Arch Surg.* 43;47:1–135.
21. Schaer H. Die Periarthritis humeroscapularis. *Ergebn Chir Orthop.* 1936;29:211–309.
22. Glatthaar E. Zur Pathologie der Periarthritis humeroscapularis. *Dtsch Z Chir.* 1938;251:414–434.
23. Brewer BJ. Aging of the rotator cuff. *Am J Sports Med.* 1979;7: 102–110.
23a. Kumagai J, Sarkar K, Uhthoff HK. The collagen types in the attachment zone of rotator cuff tendons in the elderly: An immunohistochemical study. *J Rheumatol.* 1994;21:2096–2100.
24. Yamanaka K, Fukuda H. Aging process of the supraspinatus tendon with reference to rotator cuff tears. In: Watson MS, ed. *Surgical Disorders of the Shoulder.* New York: Churchill Livingstone; 1991:247–258.
25. Uhthoff HK, Sarkar K. Pathology of rotator cuff tendons. In: Watson MS, ed. *Surgical Disorders of the Shoulder.* New York: Churchill Livingstone; 1991:259–270.
26. Uhthoff HK, Sarkar K. Classification and definition of tendinopathies. *Clin Sports Med.* 1991;10:707–720.
27. Neer CS. Impingement lesions. *Clin Orthop.* 1983;173:70–77.
28. Bigliani LU, Ticker JB, Flatow EL, Soslowsky LJ, Mow VC. The relationship of acromial architecture to rotator cuff disease. *Clin Sports Med.* 1991;10:823–838.
29. Matsen FA III, Arntz CT. Rotator cuff tendon failure. In: Rockwood CA Jr, Matsen FA III, eds. *The Shoulder.* Philadelphia: WB Saunders; 1990;2:647–677.
30. Watson M. The impingement syndrome in sportsmen. In: Bateman JE, Welsh RP, eds. *Surgery of the Shoulder.* Philadelphia: BC Decker; 1984:140–142.
31. Sarkar K, Taine W, Uhthoff HK. The ultrastructure of the coracoacromial ligament in patients with chronic impingement syndrome. *Clin Orthop.* 1990;254:49–54.
32. Gerber C, Terrier F, Ganz R. The role of the coracoid process in the chronic impingement syndrome. *J Bone Joint Surg Br.* 1985; 67:703–708.
33. Dines DM, Warren RF, Inglis AE, et al. The coracoid impingement syndrome. *J Bone Joint Surg Br.* 1990;72:314–316.
34. Uhthoff HK, Sarkar K, Hammond DI. The subacromial bursa: A clinicopathological study. In: Bateman JE, Welsh RP, eds. *Surgery of the Shoulder.* Philadelphia: BC Decker; 1984:121–125.
35. Abrams JS. Special shoulder problems in the throwing athlete: Pathology, diagnosis, and nonoperative management. *Clin Sports Med.* 1991;10:839–861.
36. Jobe FW, Tibone JE, Jobe CM, Kvitne RS. The shoulder in sports. In: Rockwood CA Jr, Matsen FA III, eds. *The Shoulder.* Philadelphia: WB Saunders; 1990:961–990.
37. Earnshaw P, Desjardins D, Sarkar K, Uhthoff HK. Rotator cuff tears: The role of surgery. *Can J Surg.* 1982;25:60–63.
38. Scarpelli DG, lannaccone PM. Cell injury and errors of metabolism. In: Kissane JM, ed. *Anderson's Pathology.* Vol 1, St. Louis: CV Mosby; 1990:36.
39. Peacock EE Jr. *Wound Repair.* Philadelphia: WB Saunders; 1984:271.
40. Manske PR. Flexor tendon healing. *J Hand Surg.* 1988;13: 237–245.
41. Mass DP, Tuel RJ. Human flexor tendon participation in the in vitro repair process. *J Hand Surg.* 1989;14:64–72.
42. Mass DP, Tuel RJ. Participation of human superficialis flexor tendon segments in repair in vitro. *J Orthop Res.* 1990;8:21–34.
43. Uhthoff HK, Sarkar K, Lohr J. Repair in rotator cuff tendons. In: Post M, Morrey BF, Hawkins RJ, eds. *Surgery of the Shoulder.* St. Louis: Mosby-Year Book; 1990:6–9.
44. Uhthoff HK, Sarkar K. Surgical repair of rotator cuff ruptures. The importance of the subacromial bursa. *J Bone Joint Surg. Br.* 1991; 73:399–401.
45. Swiontkowski MF, Iannotti JP, Boulas HJ, Esterhai JL. Rotator cuff repairs: Healing and function. Intraoperative assessment of rotator cuff vascularity using laser Doppler flowmetry In: Post M, Morrey BF, Hawkins RJ, eds. *Surgery of the Shoulder.* St. Louis: Mosby-Year Book; 1990:208–212.
46. Kumagai J, Uhthoff HK, Sarkar K, Murnaghan JP. Collagen type III in rotator cuff tears: An immunohistochemical study. *J Shoulder Elbow Surg.* 1992;1:187–192.
47. Duance VC, Restall DJ, Beard H, Bourne FJ, Bailey AJ. The location of three collagen types in skeletal muscle. *FEBS Lett.* 1977;79:248–252.
48. Clore JN, Cohen IK, Diegelmann RF. Quantitation of collagen types I and III during wound healing in rat skin. *Proc Soc Exp Biol Med.* 1979;161:337–340.
49. McPherson JM, Piez KA. Collagen in dermal wound repair. In: Clark RAF, Henson PM, eds. *The Molecular and Cellular Biology of Wound Repair.* New York: Plenum; 471–496.

Chapter 4

Biomechanics of the Rotator Cuff

Richard J. Friedman and Robert P. Knetsche

A man ought to read just as inclination leads him; for what he reads as a task will do him little good.

James Boswell, Life of Johnson

The glenohumeral joint has the greatest range of motion of any joint in the body. This degree of freedom is caused by the minimal containment provided by the bony anatomy and the multiple supporting joints and musculotendinous rotator cuff, which act in concert with the glenohumeral joint articulation. There is a delicate balance between this excessive range of motion and the resulting decreased ability to restrict undesirable and, therefore, potentially damaging movements.

The prime stabilizing elements during motion of the glenohumeral joint are the muscles of the rotator cuff. Their biomechanical properties and actions are important knowledge in performing any type of shoulder repair, because the final success or failure of many shoulder procedures rests on the ability of the surgeon to restore or repair the biomechanical properties of the rotator cuff muscles. This chapter on rotator cuff biomechanics will examine the stabilizing factors of the glenohumeral joint, forces and motion across the shoulder joint, and finally pathologic biomechanics caused by rotator cuff injury.

The shoulder joint is the developmental equivalent of the hip joint in the upper extremity. The hip joint is a true ball and socket design, with a great deal of bony stability between two conforming surfaces and little stability contributed by the surrounding soft tissues. As a result, motion is limited in this joint. The glenohumeral joint, on the other hand, has little inherent bony stability.[1] A soft-tissue socket provides the necessary stability to the joint, thus allowing for a wide range of motion. This soft-tissue socket includes (1) the capsular-ligamentous complex, consisting of the superior, middle, and inferior portions and the coracohumeral ligament, all of which are static stabilizers,[2] and (2) the rotator cuff and the surrounding shoulder muscles, which are dynamic stabilizers.[3]

There are five main elements necessary for stability of the glenohumeral joint: (1) adequate size of the glenoid fossa. Saha found that if the longitudinal diameter of the glenoid fossa was less than 75% and the transverse diameter less than 57% that of the humeral head, the joint was more likely to be unstable; [1] (2) posterior tilt to the glenoid fossa. Found in only 27% of normal shoulders, anteriorly tilted or severely anteverted glenoid fossae occur in approximately 80% of shoulders with anterior instability;[4,5] (3) humeral head retroversion is the third element of stability for the shoulder joint; (4) an intact capsule and glenoid labrum are also necessary, with younger persons more likely to have a glenoid labrum injury and older persons more likely to have a stretched capsule injury; and (5) proper function of the rotator cuff muscles in order to control the anteroposterior and superior-inferior translation of the humeral head during movement.[4–6]

STATIC STABILITY OF THE GLENOHUMERAL JOINT

Bony Articulations of the Glenohumeral Joint

The glenohumeral joint is a synovial articulation between the humeral head and the glenoid fossa of the scapula, consisting of a nearly hemispherical convex humeral articular surface and a relatively flat glenoid articulation surrounded by a soft-tissue socket. As a minimally constrained ball-and-socket joint, it allows much greater freedom of motion than does a more rigid ball-and-socket joint, such as the hip; but in the minimally constrained joint there is much less inherent stability.

The articular surface of the glenoid cavity subtends an arc of enclosure of 76° in the coronal plane, and a some-

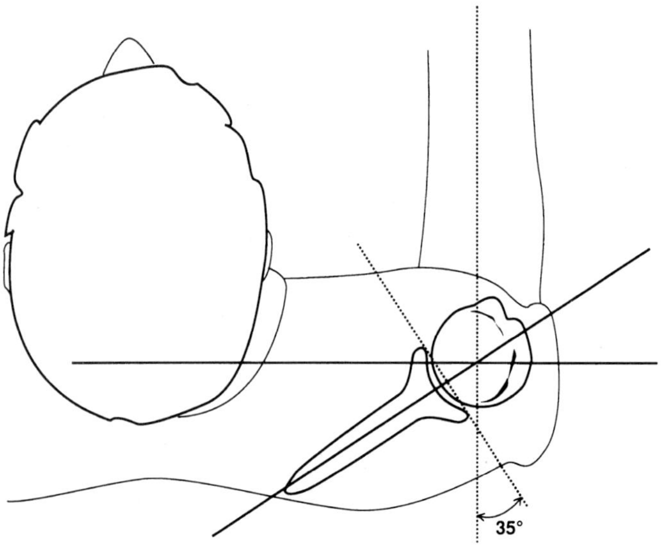

Fig. 4–1. Transverse view of the right shoulder from above, demonstrating the relationship of the humeral head and glenoid to the body. With the shoulder in neutral rotation, the humeral head is retroverted 35°, while the face of the glenoid cavity lies off the coronal plane of the body a similar amount, such that the two articular surfaces line up.

what lesser arc (62°) in the transverse plane.[7] This means that the glenoid cavity is flatter in the transverse plane and, therefore, has a larger radius of curvature compared to the coronal plane. With the arm at the side, the scapula angles downward approximately 5°. However, the relationship of the articular surface to the body of the scapula is highly variable and difficult to define precisely. Other investigators have found that the glenoid faces 3° to 5° superiorly.[8] In the transverse plane, the glenoid fossa in normal individuals lies in a slightly anteverted position (2°), relative to the long axis of the scapula in normal individuals, while other investigators have reported a slightly retroverted position.[9]

The articular surface of the humeral head, defined by the anatomic neck, encloses an arc of 155° and is oriented upwards 47°.[7] The axis of the humeral shaft lies 2.5° off the vertical in a resting position. The relationship between the two articular surfaces allows for 79° of glenohumeral elevation in the scapular plane, and combined with 41° of scapulothoracic motion, the arm can elevate 120° before the greater tuberosity impinges on the acromion. At this point, the humerus externally rotates to expose more of the humeral articular surface to the glenoid fossa for further elevation to 180° to occur.

The diameter of the humeral head ranges from 37 mm to 55 mm, with a mean of 48 mm.[10] The mean humeral head-shaft angle is 141°, and the head itself is retroverted about 32° with respect to the axis of flexion at the elbow.[5] The articular surface of the humerus constitutes approximately one-third the surface of a sphere, with retroversion of approximately 30° relative to the condylar axis of the distal humerus.[11–13]

The scapula, and therefore the plane of the glenoid articular surface, lies on the posterior chest wall, inclined approximately 30° to 40° anterior to the coronal plane of the body when viewed in the transverse plane, and is rotated 3° superiorly (Fig. 4–1).[14,15] The plane of the glenoid articular surface lies slightly anteverted to the longitudinal axis of the scapula in normal individuals.[16] The humeral head, and its articular surface, is retroverted a corresponding amount, so that the articular surfaces of the glenoid and humeral head line up.[1]

The glenoid fossa is pear shaped, measuring on average 41 mm in height and 25 mm in width. The height of the glenoid fossa is therefore about 75% and its width approximately 60% of the articulating surface of the humeral head.[1] Therefore, in any given anatomical position, the contact area between the two articulating surfaces is small, and the glenoid fossa only covers 25 to 30% of the humeral head.[10,11,13] Consequently, the articular surfaces provide little inherent bony stability to the joint.[17]

The perimeter of the glenoid fossa is lined by the fibrocartilaginous reflections of the joint capsule, the glenoid labrum, the glenohumeral ligaments, and the tendon of the long head of the biceps. The glenoid labrum serves to deepen the shallow glenoid fossa, which helps to minimize movement of the humeral head on the glenoid surface and therefore decrease susceptibility to instability and rotator cuff damage.[5]

The conformity between the humeral head and glenoid cavity in the transverse plane has only recently been examined; [1,4,10,17,18] three possible situations can exist. In type A, the radius of curvature of the humeral head is less than that of the corresponding glenoid, such that the glenoid is flatter and the humeral head rounder. Type B has equal radii of curvature between the two surfaces, and they conform exactly to each other. In type C, the radius of curvature of the humeral head is greater than the glenoid; therefore, it appears flatter compared to a more rounded glenoid (Fig. 4–2).

Type B would theoretically have 100% contact between the two surfaces, with the joint forces evenly distributed. Type C would have the humeral head contacting and loading the glenoid peripherally on its rim, without any central contact. Type A would allow the humeral head to contact the middle portion of the glenoid, with the forces concentrated over a smaller area. Anteroposterior translation could also occur with this configuration. This dimensional relationship can be quantified as the glenohumeral or conformity index, defined as the radius of

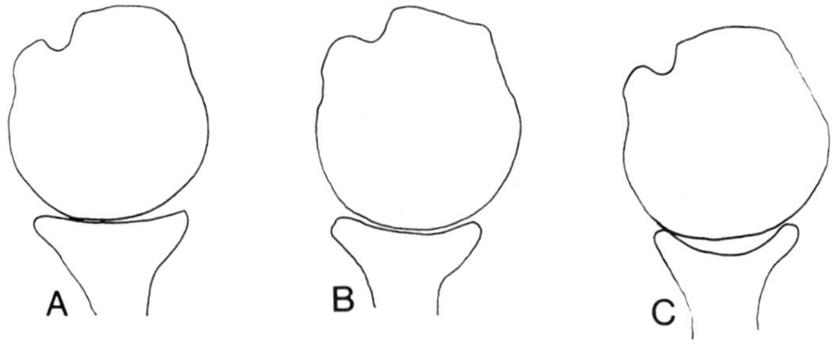

Fig. 4–2. Three types of glenohumeral configurations: *A*, shallow, narrower glenoid with respect to the humeral head; *B*, glenoid and humeral head of equal size and conformity; and *C*, deeper glenoid with decreased conformity.

the humeral head/the radius of the glenoid for both the anteroposterior and lateral planes. These ratios have been reported as 0.75 in the coronal plane (as viewed on an anteroposterior radiograph) and 0.6 in the sagittal plane (as viewed on the axillary radiograph) by Saha,[1] and 0.86 and 0.58, respectively, by Maki.[18]

A more recent study using a highly accurate, reproducible computer analysis technique defined these values as 0.67 (coronal plane) and 0.39 (sagittal plane).[10] Only 9% had radii that matched (type B). The vast majority had a more curved humeral head and flatter glenoid (type A), with less conformity in the sagittal versus the coronal plane. A constraint index, defined as the arc of enclosure/360, had a value of 0.18 in the coronal plane and 0.10 in the sagital plane, meaning that there was more curve to the glenoid in the coronal vs. sagittal plane. These anatomic features help to keep the humeral head from translating in a superior-inferior direction, but allow translation in an anteroposterior direction.

The relationship between the contact area and the radius of curvature has recently been examined.[19] Ninety-three percent of the shoulders studied were type A, where the rounder humeral head articulated with a flatter glenoid surface and resulted in a mean contact area of 30%. It is over this area that the forces across the glenohumeral joint are transmitted. The contact area was found to decrease in certain positions, such as abduction and external rotation, resulting in a greater force per unit area across the joint. These anatomic features may contribute to wear patterns, impingement, and subsequent rotator cuff tears. In order for any rotator cuff repair to be successful, these anatomic features should be restored as much as possible, so that the soft tissues and surrounding musculotendinous cuff are properly balanced and the normal kinematics of the glenohumeral joint are restored.

Soft-Tissue Structures of the Glenohumeral Joint

Unlike other ball and socket joints that rely on inherent bony stability, the glenohumeral joint relies primarily on the surrounding soft-tissue structures for stability, because of the smaller percentage of bone to bone articulation. The glenohumeral joint capsule is a thin, redundant structure composed of types I, III, and V collagen that is important for stability of the glenohumeral joint. The capsular-ligamentous complex is composed of the joint capsule plus the superior, middle, and inferior glenohumeral ligaments with the coracohumeral ligament (Fig. 4–3).

The coracohumeral ligament originates from the anterolateral base of the coracoid process and extends as two bands over the top of the shoulder to blend with the capsule and attach to the greater and lesser tuberosities.[20] This ligament is a fairly consistent finding, and has been shown to become taut during external rotation and resist inferior subluxation of the humeral head.[21]

The superior glenohumeral ligament is a constant structure arising from the tubercle of the glenoid anterior to the origin of the long head of the biceps tendon and running inferior and lateral to insert on the head of the humerus near the proximal tip of the lesser tuberosity. Its function is to provide passive resistance to infe-

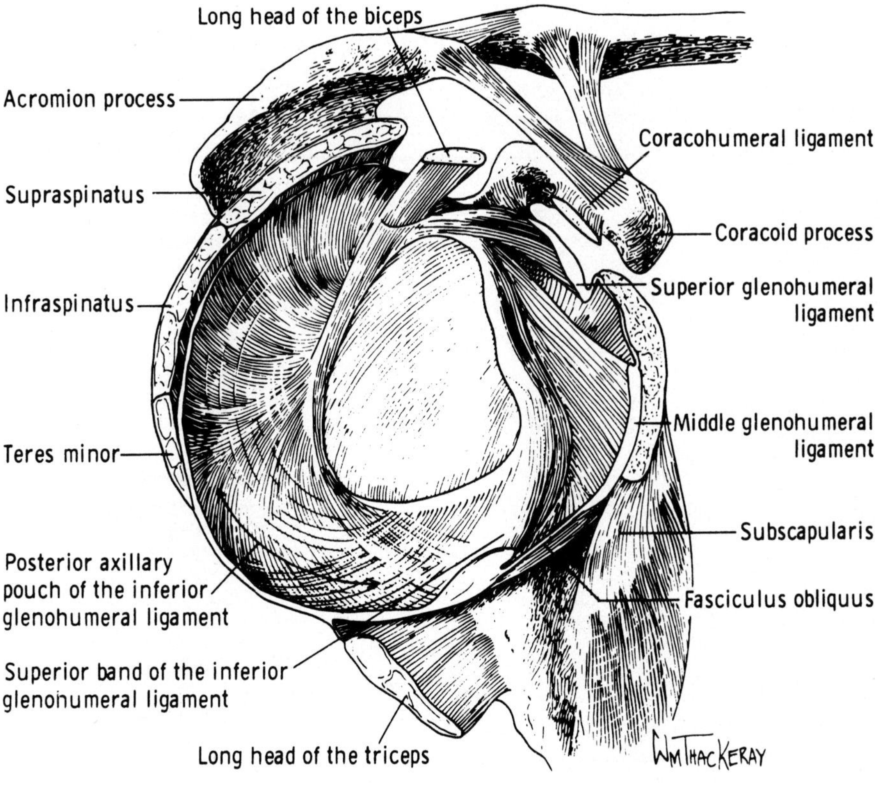

Fig. 4–3. Anatomic configuration of the soft-tissue structures about the glenohumeral joint. (From Turkel SJ, Panio MW, Marshal JL, Girgis FG. Stablilizing mechanisms preventing anterior dislocation of the glenohumeral joint. *J Bone Joint Surg Am.* 1981;63:1209.)

rior subluxation of the humerus, and an intact superior glenohumeral ligament prevents posterior and inferior translation of the humeral head even in the absence of the inferior ligament and capsule.[22]

The middle glenohumeral ligament originates from the supraglenoid tubercle at the superior aspect of the glenoid and from the anterior aspect of the labrum, and extends laterally and inferiorly to blend with the subscapularis tendon approximately two centimeters medial to its insertion on the lesser tuberosity. It is a relatively large structure measuring 2 cm in length and 4 mm in thickness and acts as a major restraining factor in anterior humeral displacement, becoming taut when the shoulder is abducted and externally rotated.[23] Although this is not the sole structure that resists anterior translation with abduction and external rotation, it is a major contributor to anterior stability of the glenohumeral joint.[24]

The inferior glenohumeral ligament is considered to be the most important component of the capsular-ligamentous complex for preventing anterior and inferior subluxation of the humerus, as well as acting as a restraining factor in elevation of the arm. The inferior glenohumeral ligament originates from almost the entire anterior glenoid labrum and courses laterally and inferiorly to insert on the inferior margin of the humeral articular surface and then down and around the anatomical neck of the humerus. Glenoid labrum tears are often associated with recurrent anterior dislocations, because the inferior glenohumeral ligament is disrupted at its origin.

Thus, the major static stabilizer of the glenohumeral joint is the capsular-ligamentous complex. A proposed mechanism of load sharing, describing how the capsule functions in a coordinated manner to resist joint translation, was first described in 1965.[25] Load sharing occurs primarily by resisting displacement because of the tautness of the capsular-ligamentous complex, particularly the superior and inferior ligaments. Secondarily, this tautness imparts increased joint contact pressure opposite to the direction of the displacement, thus further mechanically enhancing stability.

As stated, studies of the capsular-ligamentous complex show the inferior glenohumeral ligament to be the major static stabilizer of the shoulder joint.[6,23] However, the capsule itself is often thin and redundant, which may represent a congenital variation in normal individuals or may be secondary to an underlying disease process, such as inflammatory arthritis.[26] The static elements contributing to the stability of a total shoulder arthroplasty are, therefore, minimal.[24] On the other hand, if the disease process results in scarring and contracture of the capsule, this may well interfere postoperatively following a rotator cuff repair.

Atmospheric Pressure and Stability

Another factor influencing glenohumeral stability is the intra-articular atmospheric pressure. Recently, investigators have noted an intra-articular pressure of −82 cm H_2O in loaded arms, with the shoulder tending to subluxate inferiorly as much as 2 cm after capsular puncture and demonstrating marked alteration in joint constraint during passive motion.[27] These studies confirm earlier work done by Kumar and then by Harryman et al. on the subject of atmospheric pressure's contribution to glenohumeral joint stability.[28,29]

DYNAMIC STABILITY OF THE GLENOHUMERAL JOINT

In the face of dynamic movement, the glenohumeral bony articulation and the capsular-ligamentous complex play minor supporting roles in stabilization. The primary dynamic stabilizing factor is the musculotendinous cuff about the glenohumeral complex. These muscles of the shoulder can be grouped into three anatomical categories: scapulohumeral, axioscapular, and axiohumeral. The latter two groups include the trapezius, rhomboids, serratus anterior, and levator scapulae (axioscapular) and the latissimus dorsi and pectoralis major muscles (axiohumeral). These muscle groups are important because of their contributions toward motion and the forces generated about the glenohumeral joint.

The scapulohumeral muscle group, consisting of the supraspinatus, infraspinatus, teres minor, subscapularis, and deltoid muscles, play the most significant role in dynamic stabilization of the glenohumeral joint. During motion of the shoulder joint, of the 26 separate muscles controlling movements of the shoulder girdle, only the four rotator cuff muscles plus the three heads of the deltoid play any significant role in overall dynamic gleno-

Table 4–1. Motion at the Glenohumeral Joint

Movement	*Muscles*
Flexion	Pectoralis major, clavicular part Deltoid, clavicular part Biceps, short head Coracobrachialis
Extension	Deltoid, posterior part Latissimus dorsi Teres major
Abduction	Deltoid, acromial part Supraspinatus
Adduction	Pectoralis major, sternal part Latissimus dorsi Teres major
External rotation	Infraspinatus Teres minor Deltoid, posterior part
Internal rotation	Subscapularis Pectoralis major Latissimus dorsi Deltoid, clavicular part Teres major
Stabilization	Subscapularis Supraspinatus Infraspinatus Teres minor Triceps, long head Biceps, long head

humeral stability (Table 4–1).[30] Electromyography (EMG) studies have shown that the supraspinatus functions both as a humeral head compressor and arm abductor.[31,32] The subscapularis and infraspinatus, in addition to being internal and external rotators, respectively, both act as compressors of the humeral head when abduction, or elevation, is initiated. The deltoid muscle appears to function strictly as an abductor, or elevator, of the upper extremity. In general, the stability and mobility of the shoulder is maintained by a well-functioning scapulohumeral musculature. The necessity of a properly functioning rotator cuff to the clinical success of both operative and conservative treatment of shoulder pathology has been recognized since the early development of shoulder surgery.[11]

The rotator cuff muscles act as stabilizers through four different mechanisms: (1) passive muscle tension from the bulk effect of the muscles, (2) contraction causing compression of the articular surfaces, (3) joint motion that causes secondary tightening of the ligamentous restraints, and (4) the barrier effect of the contracted muscle.[33]

1. Passive muscle tension: the passive role played by muscle bulk in joint stability is demonstrated by the increased passive arc of motion when the muscle is removed. It has been demonstrated that up to 10 mm of additional superior and inferior translation may occur with the removal or release of the rotator cuff muscles. There is also greater inferior translation caused by the effect of gravity when muscles are resected or removed in cadaver preparations.[6,28,34,35]
2. Compression of the articular surface: various studies have demonstrated that stimulation of the rotator cuff muscles causes a centering of the humeral head without balanced muscle activity. This is thought to be caused by the secondary obligatory tightening of the ligaments supporting the glenohumeral joint, causing increased contact area and pressure along the entirety of the capsular-ligamentous complex and thereby centering the humeral head in the glenoid fossa.[33]
3. Dynamic elements causing secondary tightening of static constraints: the supraspinatus muscle has the action of simultaneously elevating and externally rotating the arm. This external rotation tightens the inferior glenohumeral ligament and limits elevation. The rotator cuff musculature has thus rotated the shoulder into a more stable configuration by tightening the ligaments in the direction opposite the rotation.[25]
4. Barrier effect: the rotator cuff muscles serve as dynamic and well-balanced stabilizers of the humeral head, while also controlling fine rotational motion of the glenohumeral joint. Stabilizing the humeral head reduces the sheer strain on the joint by maintaining close proximity between the humeral head and the glenoid fossa during arm movement.

The supraspinatus muscle is active in all patterns of arm elevation, primarily functioning to initiate arm abduction to approximately 30° of elevation by compressing the humeral head against the glenoid fossa. The short lever arm and small size of the supraspinatus limit the torque it can generate and prevent any further elevation of the arm beyond 30° without assistance from the deltoid muscle.

The infraspinatus muscle is the second most active muscle of the rotator cuff and is stimulated to act during arm elevation with some degree of elbow flexion. It contributes to glenohumeral joint stability, but its prime function is external rotation of the humeral head on the glenoid fossa, while providing a counterforce to prevent excessive external rotation and hyperextension from posterior deltoid action.

The subscapularis muscle is an internal rotator of the humerus, acting in concert with the pectoralis major, teres major, and latissimus dorsi. Its activity in providing internal rotation serves to decelerate external rotation by the deltoid, thereby contributing to overall stability by providing anterior restraint.

The teres minor serves as an external rotator of the humeral head on the glenoid, acting in concert with the infraspinatus. Oppositional inferior stability is provided by opposing the superior forces of the middle deltoid.[36]

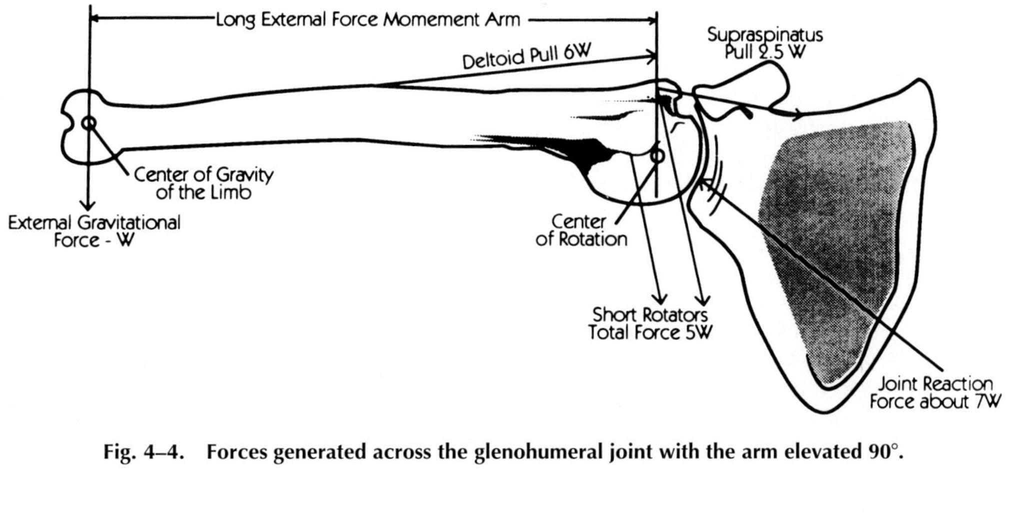

Fig. 4–4. Forces generated across the glenohumeral joint with the arm elevated 90°.

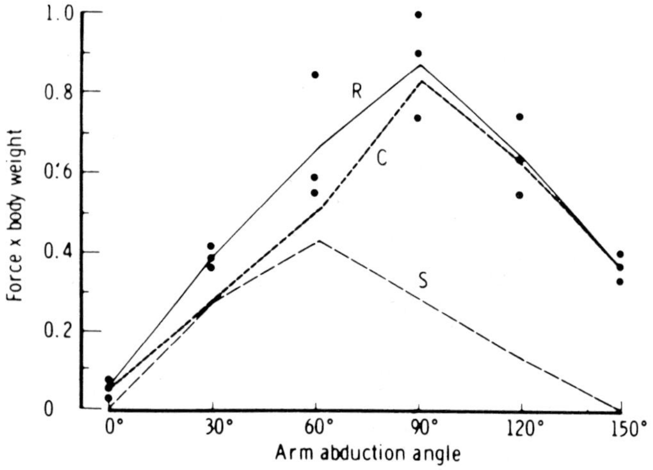

Fig. 4–5. The resultant force (R) of the glenohumeral joint is a combination of the compressive component (C) perpendicular to the face of the glenoid and the shear force (S) up the face of the glenoid. (From Poppen N, Walker P. Forces at the glenohumeral joint in abduction. *Clin Orthop.* 1978;135:165–170.)

The rotator cuff muscles, which are responsible for kinematic stability through four different mechanisms (both direct and indirect) serve to limit translation of the humerus on the glenoid by causing increased compressive forces between the articular surfaces and thereby enhancing the stability of the glenohumeral joint.

FORCES AT THE GLENOHUMERAL JOINT

The forces across the glenohumeral joint are complex, varying not only with the load applied, but also with the position of the arm.[7,37,38] While the glenohumeral joint is often referred to as non-weight-bearing, this does not mean that significant forces are not transmitted across the joint.

With simple arm elevation to 90°, a force of one times body weight is generated. Lifting an object weighing only 5 kg held in the laterally extended hand generates a force of approximately 2.5 times body weight across the joint, similar to loads that act across the hip joint.[37] However, this load is transmitted across a significantly smaller articular surface area in the shoulder as compared to the hip, meaning that the magnitude of mechanical stresses the glenohumeral joint is subjected to is substantial.

The forces to consider around the glenohumeral joint include the weight of the extremity and any external forces, the abducting muscles (deltoid and supraspinatus), the muscles pulling in a downward direction (subscapularis, infraspinatus, teres minor), and the resultant vector of the compression and shear forces of the humeral head on the glenoid.[39] Studies have shown that the deltoid muscle itself can generate a maximum force of 6 times limb weight, the supraspinatus 2.5 times limb weight, the rotators 5 times limb weight, and a joint reaction force of 7 times limb weight (Fig. 4–4).[38,40]

When abduction of the arm is initiated, compressive forces are generated by the rotator cuff muscles to hold the humeral head against the glenoid fossa and counter the shear forces up the face of the glenoid being created by the abducting muscle forces. This allows the extremity to abduct efficiently and prevents the humeral head from simply sliding up the face of the glenoid. The combination of compressive forces and shear forces gives the resultant force. Up to 60°, the compression and shear forces are roughly equal. After this, the shear force decreases as abduction increases. The compressive force continues to increase to a maximum at 90° of abduction and then it decreases as abduction continues to increase (Fig. 4–5).[41] The resultant force also peaks at 90° of abduction, and then it decreases at the same rate it increased as abduction increases. For example, considering the weight of the arm as the only load, the resultant force is 0.4 times body weight at both 30° and 150° of abduction and 0.8 times body weight at 60° and 120° of abduction. At 90° abduction, the joint force is approximately one times body weight.

In addition to the magnitude, the direction of the resultant force vector is also important. For the humeral head to remain in the glenoid cavity with abduction, the resultant force vector must lie within the angle, or arc of safety of the glenoid (Fig. 4–6).[41] During abduction of the arm in the scapular plane with neutral rotation, the initial force is directed downward and contained within the inferior border of the glenoid. As the arm abducts to

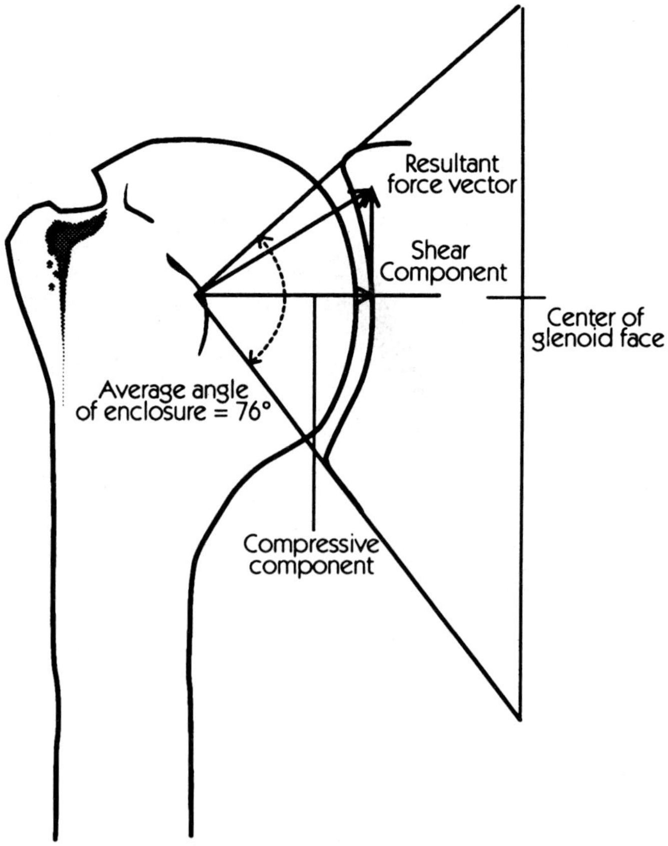

Fig. 4–6. The compressive and shear forces comprise the resultant force vector, which must fall within the glenoid angle of enclosure for elevation to occur.

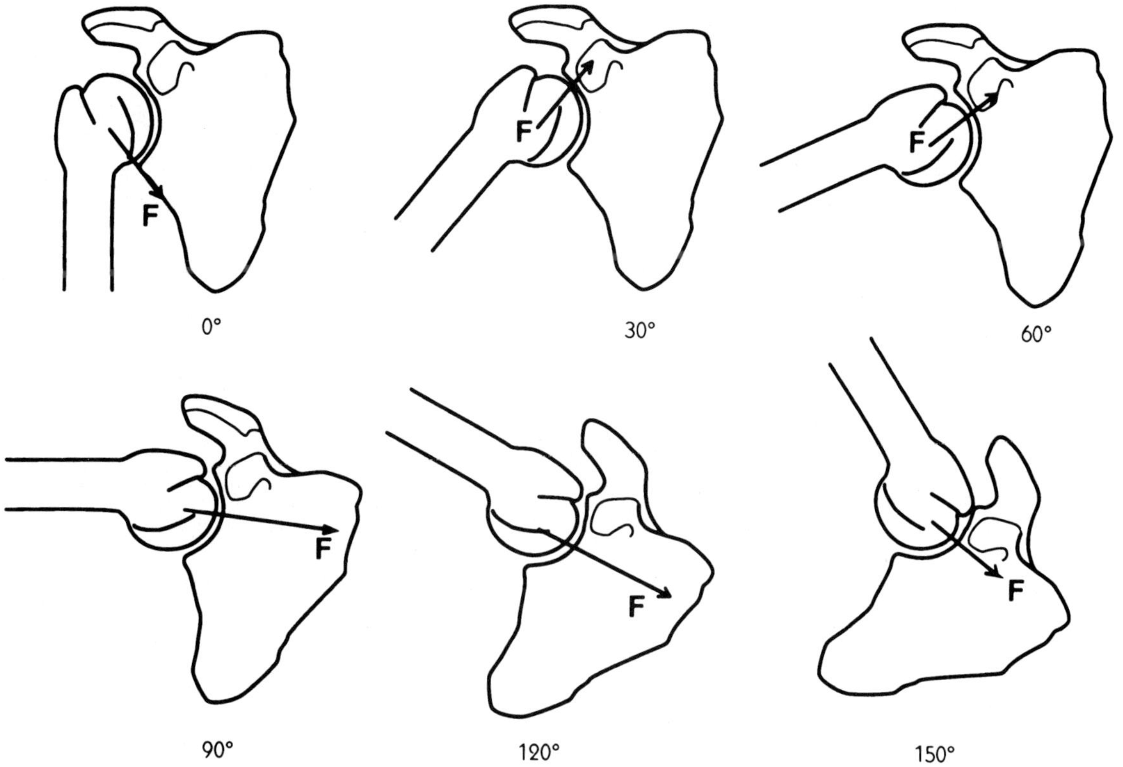

Fig. 4–7. **The resultant force vectors change with relation to their direction in the glenoid cavity as the arm is abducted. Stability increases with abduction.**

30° and 60°, the force moves to the superior edge of the glenoid, consistent with the high shear forces generated, and then moves back towards the center of the glenoid as abduction continues to increase (Fig. 4–7).[42]

Similar calculations with the arm in internal and external rotation show that muscle efficiency and stability are superior in external rotation compared to internal rotation.[41] Forces in external rotation are similar to those in neutral rotation, but the resultant force vector is directed more centrally into the glenoid cavity, because of the deltoid muscle increasing its contribution to compressive forces and decreasing the shear component.

The force vector for internal rotation is larger than in neutral or external rotation and directed more superiorly, because of an increased shear force. The resultant joint forces in internal rotation are twice that in external rotation at 90° of abduction. This is easily demonstrated by an individual abducting both arms to 90°, with one in maximum internal rotation and the other in maximum external rotation. The arm in internal rotation will fatigue and become painful much more quickly than the arm in external rotation.

In neutral rotation with abduction to 60°, the resultant force vector of the humeral head is contained just within the arc of enclosure of the glenoid. The loss of a functioning rotator cuff mechanism, particularly the supraspinatus, causes a decrease in the compressive forces and an increase in the shear forces, shifting the resultant force vector superiorly out of the arc of enclosure of the glenoid. The resulting instability is seen clinically with superior subluxation of the humeral head on the glenoid.

The significant forces across the glenohumeral joint mentioned above are also transferred to the prosthetic interface in a total shoulder arthroplasty. While the humeral component has a large surface area and a canal-filling stem over which the forces can be distributed, the fixation of the glenoid component is much more tenuous. Forces greater than one times body weight are transmitted across a small surface area, such that the load per unit area is high, possibly surpassing that of the fixation and leading to failure.

SHOULDER KINEMATICS

Planes of Reference for Shoulder Motion

Elevation of the arm, one of the most important functions of the shoulder joint, results from a combination of glenohumeral and scapulothoracic motion. This has been studied extensively in normal individuals, initially examining the question referable to the coronal plane but more recently referencing the scapular plane.[11,38,42–44] Many investigators have stressed the importance of using the scapular rather than the coronal plane, because the true plane of the glenohumeral joint is 30 to 40° an-

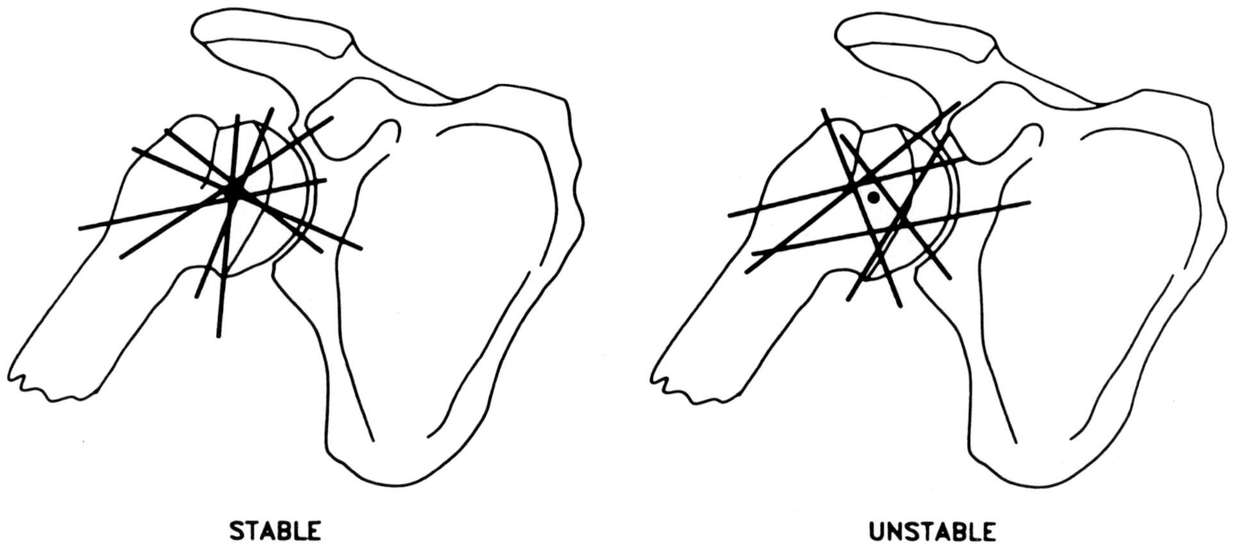

Fig. 4–8. The point of intersection of the screw axis of the glenohumeral joint provides an anatomically stable pivot point for joint motion. Rotator cuff tears cause translation that serves to disrupt the screw axis, leading to wide dispersion of the pivot centers, which in turn creates inefficient and unstable biomechanics of the glenohumeral joint.

terior to the coronal plane.[14,15] The plane of scapular abduction in which maximum glenohumeral elevation occurs has recently been defined as 23° anterior to the plane of the scapula.[45] However, neither reference system is ideal, because scapular rotation is not taken into account.[46]

Glenohumeral Motion

The instant centers of rotation of the glenohumeral joint have been shown to lie close to each other and to the center of the humeral head itself in normal subjects.[7,46] In contrast, patients with rotator cuff pathology demonstrated instant centers that deviated considerably from the center of the humeral head.

A correlation exists between the instant centers of rotation and excursion (or translation) of the humeral head in a superior-inferior direction. A small amount of superior translation averaging 3 mm has been found to occur during the first 30° of elevation.[47] Thereafter, approximately 1 mm of further excursion in an upwards or downwards direction occurs between positions measured. In patients with rotator cuff tears, significantly more excursion occurs, which tends to disperse the points of intersection of the screw axis of the humerus. This dispersion displaces the pivotal point of the three-dimensional center of rotation for the shoulder musculature and results in an unstable biomechanical situation at the glenohumeral joint (Fig. 4–8).

The above discussion deals with motion in the coronal plane. Differences exist when studying motion of the glenohumeral joint in the lateral or transverse plane. With less conformity in the transverse compared to the coronal plane, a variety of motions (translation, rotation, and rolling) are possible.[5] Translation is defined as motion of a moving segment against the surface of a fixed segment. The contact point of the moving segment does not change, while its mating surface has a constantly changing contact point. Rotation is the exact opposite of translation; the moving segment rotates and the contact point on the fixed surface does not change. Rolling motion is motion between fixed and moving segments in which the contact points on each surface are constantly changing. The arc length of the moving surface matches the path on the fixed surface so that the two surfaces have point to point contact without slippage. Thus, the relative motion of rolling is a combination of translation and rotation (Fig. 4–9).[33]

Surface motion of the normal glenohumeral joint is primarily rotation in the transverse plane, with very little translation occurring. A study of 20 normal individuals demonstrated that the humeral head remained centered in the glenoid cavity throughout the range of horizontal flexion, except in a position of maximum extension and external rotation, when 4 mm of posterior translation occurred.[48] In patients with anterior instability, translation of the humeral head on the glenoid occurred, indicating a significant disruption of the structures responsible for anterior stability.

Recent studies have suggested that anteroposterior translation can occur in normal, asymptomatic shoulders.[29,49] While the amount of translation varied between individuals, all exhibited some degree of glenohumeral translation in the anteroposterior direction during clinical testing for instability. The translation was also found to be reproducible in each subject. None of the normal subjects studied had any symptoms consistent with shoulder instability.

As discussed, cadaveric studies examining the glenohumeral joint have shown that the glenoid and humeral head do not have equal radii of curvature, but in the majority of cases, the radius of curvature of the normal glenoid is larger than that of the corresponding humeral

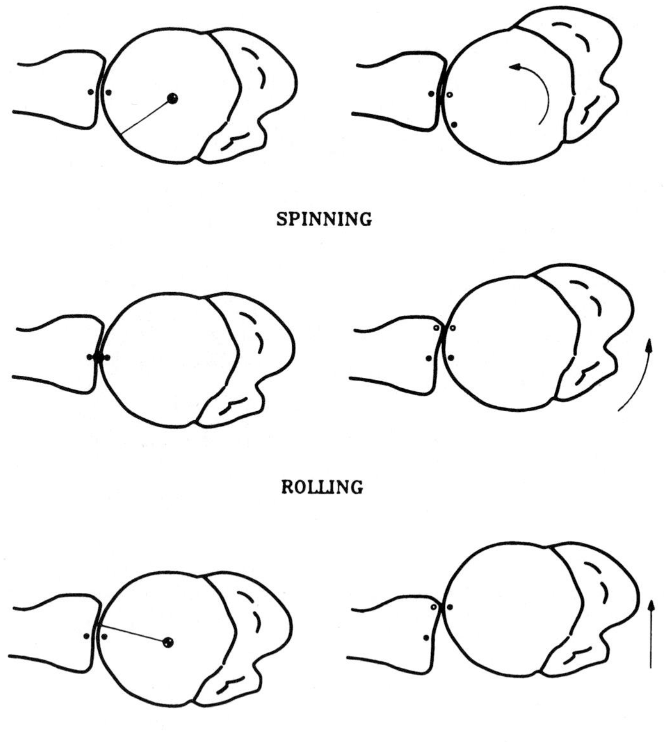

Fig. 4–9. Three types of motion, rotation, translation, and rolling occur at the glenohumeral joint.

head.[10] With the glenoid flatter and the humeral head more rounded, there is little inherent bony stability, and this anatomic relationship allows translation in the anteroposterior direction to occur.

Scapulothoracic Motion

Early studies defined the relative contributions of glenohumeral and scapulothoracic motion to shoulder abduction in the coronal plane as being a 2:1 ratio throughout.[11,38] In other words, for every 2° of glenohumeral motion, there is 1° of scapulothoracic motion contributing to shoulder abduction. In abducting the arm to 120°, 80° would come from the glenohumeral joint and 40° from the scapulothoracic joint. Following external rotation of the humeral head to clear the greater tuberosity from the undersurface of the acromion and expose more articular surface to the glenoid, abduction proceeds to 180°, resulting from 120° of glenohumeral motion and 60° of scapulothoracic motion.[7,42]

More recent studies of abduction in the scapular plane have confirmed this ratio throughout the full range of motion, but it appears to vary during the first 25 to 30° of abduction. [43,44,47] These and other studies have been summarized in Figure 4–10. Greater motion occurs at the glenohumeral joint during the first 30° of elevation. An equal contribution of glenohumeral and scapulothoracic motion occurs in the last 60° of elevation, but the overall ratio remains approximately 2:1 throughout the entire arc of elevation.

Abduction

The full range of humeral abduction is 180°, and the prime movers are the supraspinatus and deltoid muscles. Both are active throughout abduction, as demonstrated by EMG studies, reaching maximal activity between 90 and 180°. The trapezius and serratus anterior muscles are synergistic in scapular rotation, providing full mechanical advantage to the deltoid and supraspinatus. A suprascapular nerve block, thereby eliminating the active contribution of the supraspinatus and infraspinatus muscles, causes a reduction in the force of elevation in the scapular plane by 35% at 0° elevation and 60% at 60°. Above 60° the loss of force was less significant, resulting in only a 30% reduction at 150°. An axillary nerve block, eliminating the active contribution of the deltoid muscle, reduced the force of elevation by 35% at 0° elevation and by 60 to 80% at 150°.[50,51]

Nerve stimulation studies have demonstrated that stimulation of the axillary nerve (deltoid, teres minor) resulted in only 40° of abduction.[29] Suprascapular nerve stimulation (supraspinatus, infraspinatus) resulted in abduction to 90° and external rotation to 45°. Patients with isolated paralysis of the supraspinatus and infraspinatus muscles could achieve no more than 45° of active abduction, thus demonstrating the importance of these muscles for shoulder abduction.[31]

The subscapularis, infraspinatus, and teres minor muscles are known collectively as the short rotators and play an essential biomechanical role in humeral abduction. During abduction, the directional force of the short rotators is directed downward and inward, serving to depress the humeral head into the glenoid fossa and thereby opposing the upward and outwardly directed force of the deltoid and supraspinatus from superiorly subluxing the humeral head against the acromion process.[3] The horizontal force of the deltoid acts below the center of rotation of the humeral head and is opposite to the direction of the short rotators that act at the center of rotation. This action of the short rotators provides a fixed fulcrum and allows elevation of the humerus to occur through the resultant force couple. The deltoid acting alone elicits only an upward subluxation of the humeral head because the fulcrum is lost (Fig. 4–11). If the short rotators act alone, they depress the humeral head and may cause inferior subluxation of the humeral head. Studies using EMG confirm continuous activity during abduction by the short rotators.

Adduction and Extension

The main muscles involved in these movements are the latissimus dorsi, teres major, lower portion of the pectoralis major, posterior deltoid, and the long head of the triceps, with the latissimus and pectoralis major acting as the prime movers. The posterior deltoid is also active, partly to resist the internal rotation that the main adductors would produce if unresisted. The teres major acts only if there is a resistance to movement. The rotator cuff

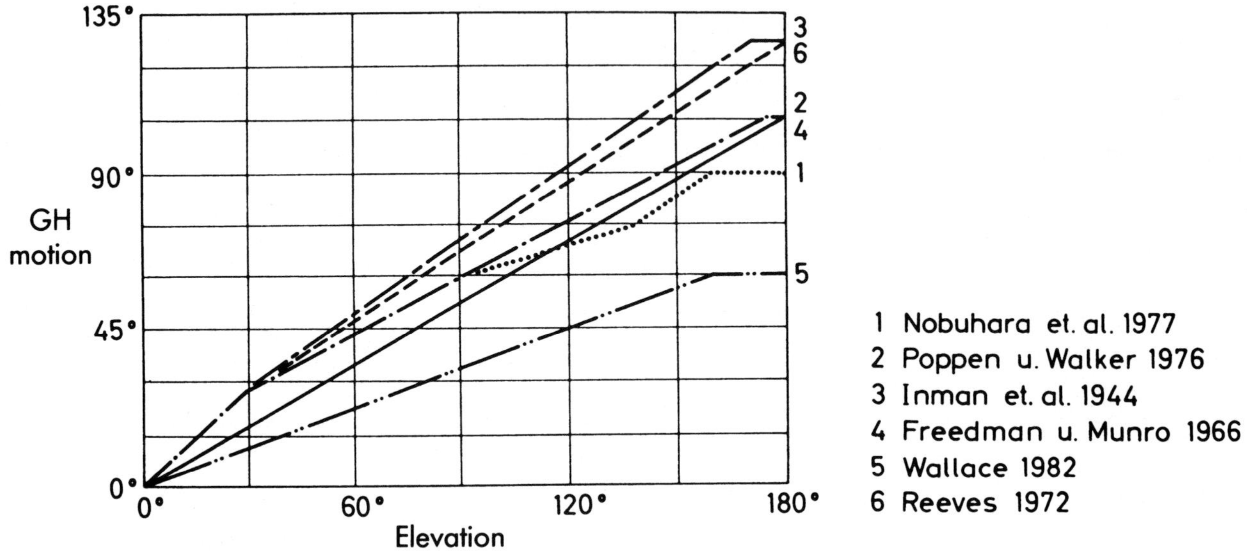

Fig. 4–10. Various studies showing the relationship of glenohumeral to scapulothoracic motion with increasing elevation of the arm. In general, the ratio of glenohumeral to scapulothoracic motion is 2:1 in the normal shoulder. (From Bergmann G. Biomechanics and pathomechanics of the shoulder joint with reference to prosthetic joint replacement. In: Kobel R, Helbi B, Blanth W, eds. Shoulder Replacement. Berlin: Springer-Verlag; 1987:33.)

plays little part in these movements as demonstrated by EMG analysis.[8,17]

Flexion

Flexion of the arm is accomplished primarily through the actions of the anterior head of the deltoid and the clavicular portion of the pectoralis major, which operate throughout the full range of motion. The coracobrachialis and biceps brachii act mainly through the first 90° of flexion, but their actions decline or cease altogether in flexion beyond 90°. The terminal range of shoulder flexion is the same as that for shoulder abduction, in that it depends on upward rotation of the scapula and external rotation at the glenohumeral joint.[8,17,52] As in abduction, the short rotators depress the humerus, which along with the upward force of action of the deltoid creates a force couple that elevates the humerus. The infraspinatus and teres minor also provide the necessary external rotation for complete elevation of the arm.

Internal Rotation

Internal rotation is accomplished with the subscapularis, teres major latissimus dorsi, pectoralis major, and anterior deltoid. The subscapularis acts as a pure internal rotator, and with the hip and trunk flexed to a right angle and the arm relaxed and hanging, the subscapularis can internally rotate with little or no assistance from the other four muscles. The pectoralis major combines internal rotation with adduction of the shoulder so that its action carries the arm in front of the body. The anterior deltoid flexes the shoulder as it internally rotates, while the latissimus dorsi and teres major muscles combine internal rotation with adduction and extension. A useful way to test subscapularis function is the lift off test, in which the patient has the shoulder internally rotated and the elbow flexed so that the back of the hand rests on the lower lumbar region. The patient then actively lifts the hand away from the lower back. The starting position for this action has the shoulder at approximately 100° of internal rotation, in which the only internal rotator is the subscapularis. If the subscapular nerve is electrically stimulated, the arm will internally rotate 25° and flex 20° from the action of the subscapularis acting alone.[31]

External Rotation

The muscles responsible for active external rotation are mainly the infraspinatus and teres minor, with the infraspinatus being active throughout the entire 70° of

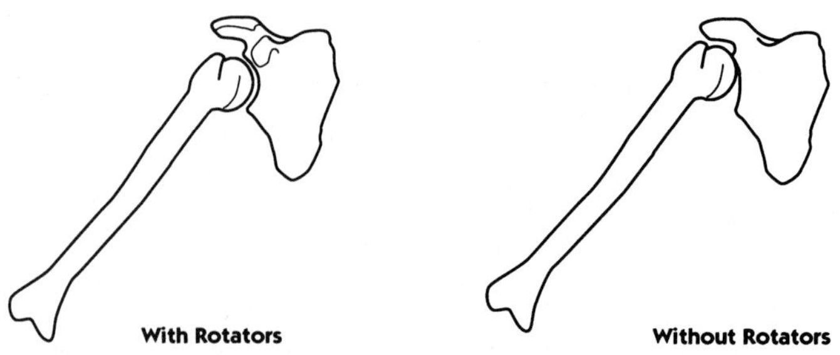

Fig. 4–11. With the rotator cuff intact, the resultant force vector lies within the arc of enclosure and the humeral head remains centered as the arm is elevated (left). When a large rotator cuff tear is present, the resultant vector lies outside the glenoid articular surface, causing the humeral head to sublux superiorly when the deltoid muscle initiates elevation (right).

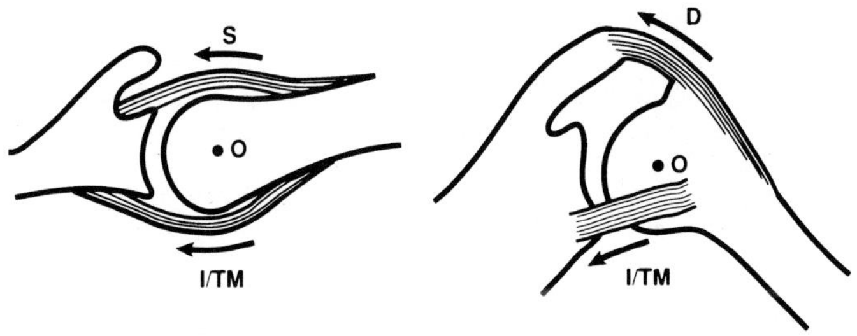

Fig. 4–12. The schema of intact force couples in the transverse and coronal planes: O—screw axis, S—subscapularis, D—deltoid, I—infraspinatus, and TM—teres minor.

Table 4–2. Kinematic Patterns and Location of Rotator Cuff Tears

Kinematic Pattern	*Tear Location*
Stable fulcrum kinematics	Supraspinatus and part of infraspinatus
Unstable fulcrum kinematics posterior cuff tear pattern	Supraspinatus and all of posterior cuff (infraspinatus and teres minor)
Captured fulcrum kinematics	Supraspinatus and all of posterior cuff and at least 50% subscapularis tear
Unstable fulcrum kinematics subscapularis tear pattern	Supraspinatus and complete subscapularis tear

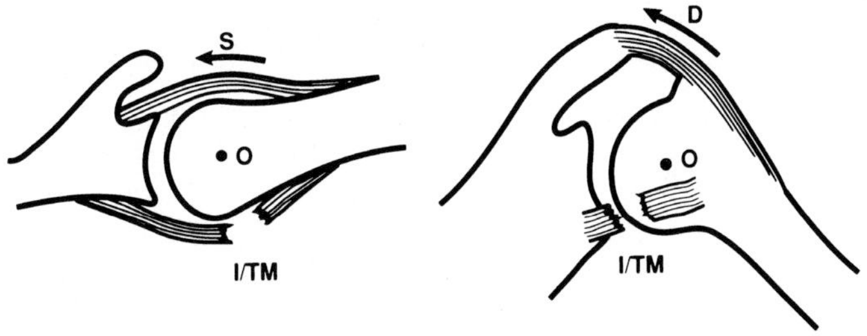

Fig. 4–13. Uncoupling of the force couples in both the coronal and transverse planes via posterior rotator cuff tears resulting in disruption of the glenohumeral fulcrum.

motion and the teres minor assuming an active role after 30° of external rotation. The deltoid also externally rotates, primarily at initiation until 30° external rotation. Scapular stabilizers during external rotation include the supraspinatus, upper trapezius, serratus anterior, biceps, and the deltoid after 30° of external rotation. Electrical stimulation of the suprascapular nerve alone causes external rotation of 45° from infraspinatus action and 90° abduction from supraspinatus action.[8,31,33]

Rotator Cuff Mechanics During Throwing

The rotator cuff plays a crucial role in the actions of throwing a ball, because a wide range of dynamic stabilization is necessary to prevent subluxation of the humeral head secondary to the increased stresses put on the glenohumeral joint complex. The rotator cuff muscles must act in synchrony to provide a tense forceful unit ready for accelerated release, respond to decelerate the limb, reduce residual force, and thereby avoid injury. Overhead throwing is divided into five phases: (1) the windup or preparatory phase, which ends when the ball leaves the gloved or non-throwing hand; (2) early cocking with shoulder abduction and external rotation, ending with contact of the forward foot on the ground; (3) late cocking phase that continues until maximum external rotation of the shoulder is achieved; (4) the acceleration phase that starts with internal rotation of the humerus and ends with ball release; and (5) the follow-through phase that starts with ball release and ends with the cessation of motion.

During throwing the deltoid is responsible for arm elevation with active forward flexion and abduction of the humerus. The supraspinatus also plays a role in humeral abduction, with its EMG action at peak activity in the late cocking phase in which the arm is already abducted and most vulnerable to subluxation. The supraspinatus also serves to draw the humeral head closer to the glenoid, increasing joint stability. The infraspinatus and teres minor muscles are responsible for external rotation and stability of the shoulder by depressing the head of the humerus toward the glenoid fossa. The activity patterns for both muscles are similar, with peak activity occurring during late cocking and follow-through, though both lag behind the supraspinatus in timing. The subscapularis has its peak activity in late cocking when it contracts eccentrically to protect the anterior joint, which at this point is under extreme tension. It then functions as an internal rotator to help carry the arm across the chest during acceleration and follow-through.[53]

PATHOMECHANICS OF THE ROTATOR CUFF

Tears of the rotator cuff muscles typically produce abnormal and unstable mechanical action at the glenohumeral joint, because of the disruption of the force couples either in the coronal plane, transverse plane, or both (Figs. 4–12 and 4–13). Burkhart has identified four separate patterns of abnormal rotator cuff kinematics based on the location of the tears that provide a useful classification for the pathomechanics of rotator cuff injury (Table 4–2).[54]

SUMMARY

To perform a successful rotator cuff repair, it is essential to understand the normal anatomy and biomechanics of the shoulder joint. Despite the clinical successes to date, improvements in the current state of the art are still needed and will result from increasing our understanding of the complex biomechanics of the rotator cuff muscles about the glenohumeral joint.

REFERENCES

1. Saha A. Dynamic stability of the glenohumeral joint. *Acta Orthop Scand.* 1971;42:491–505.
2. Black J, Dumbleton J. *Clinical Biomechanics.* 2nd ed. New York: Churchill Livingstone; 1988.
3. Lucas D. Biomechanics of the shoulder joint. *Arch Surg.* 1973; 107:425–432.
4. Saha A. Mechanics of elevation of glenohumeral joint. *Acta Orthop Scand.* 1973;44:668–678.
5. Zuckerman J, Matsen F. Biomechanics of the shoulder. In: Goldberg V, Nordin M, eds. *Biomechanics.* Philadelphia: Lea & Febiger; 1990:225–247.
6. Ovesen J, Nielsen S. Anterior and posterior shoulder instability. *Acta Orthop Scand.* 1986;57:324.
7. Walker P. *Human Joints and Their Artificial Replacements.* Springfield, IL: Charles C. Thomas; 1977.
8. Basmajian J, Bazan F. Factors Preventing Downward Dislocation of the Adducted Shoulder. *J Bone Joint Surg Am.* 1959;41:1182.
9. Friedman R, LaBerge M, Dooley R, O'Hara A. Finite element modeling of the glenoid component: Effect of design parameters on stress distribution. *J Shoulder Elbow Surg.* 1992; 1:261–270.
10. McPherson E, Friedman R, Dooley R. Anatomic basis of total shoulder design. *J Shoulder Elbow Surg.* 1993;2:S28.
11. Codman E. *The Shoulder.* Boston, Thomas Todd; 1934.
12. Dempster W. Mechanisms of shoulder movement. *Arch Phys Med Rehab.* 1970;51:711.
13. Steindler A. *Kinesiology of the Human Body Under Normal and Pathological Conditions.* ed, Springfield, IL: Charles C. Thomas; 1955.
14. Saha A. Mechanism of shoulder movements and a plea for the recognition of "zero position of the glenohumeral joint. *Indian J Surg.* 1950;12:153–165.
15. Johnston T. The movements of the shoulder joint. A plea for the use of the 'plane of the scapula' as the plane of reference for movements occurring at the humero-scapular joint. *Br J Surg.* 1937; 25:252–260.
16. Friedman R, Hawthorne K, Genez B. Evaluation of glenoid bone loss with computerized tomography. *J Bone Joint Surg Am.* 1992; 74:1032–1037.
17. Sarrafian S. Gross and functional anatomy of the shoulder. *Clin Orthop.* 1983;173:11–19.
18. Maki S, Gruen T. Anthropometric study of the glenohumeral joint. *Trans Orthop Res Soc.* 1976;1:173.
19. Friedman R, An Y, Chokeski R, Kessler L. Anatomic and biomechanical study of glenohumeral contact. *J Shoulder Elbow Surg.* 1994; 3:535.
20. Kapandji I. *The Physiology of Joints.* ed. Baltimore: Williams & Wilkins; 1970.
21. Neer C, Satterlee C, Dalsey R, Flatow E. The anatomy and potential effects of contracture of the coracohumeral ligament. *Clin Orthop.* 1992;280:182–185.
22. Schwartz E, Warren R, O'Brien S, Fronek J. Posterior shoulder instability. *Orthop Clin North Am.* 1987;18:409.
23. Turkel S, Panio M, Marshall J, Girgis F. Stabilizing mechanisms preventing anterior dislocation of the glenohumeral joint. *J Bone Joint Surg Am* 1981;63:1208–1217.
24. An K, Morrey B. Biomechanics of the shoulder. In: Morrey B, eds. *Joint Replacement Arthroplasty.* New York: Churchill Livingstone; 1990:397–405.
25. Dempster W. Mechanisms of shoulder movement. *Arch Phys Med Rehabil.* 1965;46:49.
26. Uhthoff H, Piscopo M. Anterior capsular redundancy of the shoulder: Congential or traumatic? *J Bone Joint Surg Br.* 1985; 67:363–366.
27. Browne A, Hoffmeyer P, An K, Morrey B. The influence of atmospheric pressure on shoulder stability. *Orthop Trans* 1990; 14:759.
28. Kumar V, Balusubramaniam P. The role of atmospheric pressure in stabilizing the shoulder: An experimental study. *J Bone Joint Surg.* 1985;67:719.
29. Harryman D, Sidles J, Clark J, McQuade K, Gibb T, Matsen F. Translation of the humeral head on the glenoid with passive glenohumeral motion. *J Bone Joint Surg Am.* 1990;72:1334–1343.
30. Spiegelmann J, Woo S-Y. A rigid-body method for finding centers of rotation and angular displacements of planar joint motion. *J Biomech.* 1987;20:715.
31. Celli L, Balli A, de Luise G, Rovesta C. Some new aspects of the functional anatomy of the shoulder. *Ital J Orthop Traumatol.* 1985; 11:83–91.
32. Ito N. Electromyographic study of shoulder joint. *J Jap Orthop Assoc* 1980;54:53–64.
33. An K, Morrey B. Biomechanics of the shoulder. In: Rockwood CA, Matsen FA, eds. *The Shoulder.* Philadelphia: WB Saunders; 1990: 208–247.
34. Howell S, Galinat B. The containment mechanism: The primary stabilizer of the glenohumeral joint. *Orthop Trans* 1987; 11:458.
35. Ohwovoriole E, Mekow C. A technique for studying the kinematics of human joints. Part II: The humeroscapular joint. *Orthopaedics.* 1987; 10:457.
36. Merrill K, Knetsche R, Friedman RJ. Sports medicine. In: Skinner HB, ed. *Current Diagnosis and Treatment in Orthopaedics.* East Norwalk, CT: Appleton-Lange; 1994:116–164.
37. Bergmann G. Biomechanics and pathomechanics of the shoulder joint with reference to prosthetic joint replacement. In: Kobel R, Helbig B, Blauth W, eds. *Shoulder Replacement.* Berlin: Springer-Verlag; 1987:33–43.
38. Inman V, Saunders M, Abbot L. Observations on the function of the shoulder joint. *J Bone Joint Surg Am.* 1944; 26:1–40.
39. Buechel F, Pappas M, DePalma A. "Floating socket" total shoulder replacement: Anatomical, biomechanical, and surgical rationale. *J Biomed Mater Res.* 1977;12:89–114.
40. de Luca C, Forrest W. Force analysis of individual muscles acting simultaneously on the shoulder joint during isometric abduction. *J Biomech.* 1973;6:385–393.
41. Poppen N, Walker P. Forces at the glenohumeral joint in abduction. *Clin Orthop.* 1978;135:165–170.
42. Walker P, Poppen N. Biomechanics of the shoulder joint during abduction in the plane of the scapula. *Bull Hosp Joint Dis.* 1977; 38:107–111.
43. Doody S, Freedman L, Waterland J. Shoulder movements during abduction in the scapular plane. *Arch Phys Med Rehabil.* 1970; 51:595–604.
44. Freedman L, Munro R. Abduction of the arm in the scapular plane: Scapular and glenohumeral movements. *J Bone Joint Surg Am.* 1966; 48:1503–1510.
45. Browne A, Hoffmeyer P, Tanaka S, An K, Morrey B. Glenohumeral elevation studied in three dimensions. *J Bone Joint Surg Br.* 1990; 72:843–845.
46. Laumann U. Kinesiology of the shoulder joint. In: Kobel R, Helbig B, Blauth W, eds. *Shoulder Replacement.* Berlin: Springer-Verlag; 1987:23–31.
47. Poppen N, Walker P. Normal and abnormal motion of the shoulder. *J Bone Joint Surg Am.* 1976;58:195–201.
48. Howell S, Galinat B, Renzi A, Marone P. Normal and abnormal mechanics of the glenohumeral joint in the horizontal plane. *J Bone Joint Surg Am* 1988;70:227–232.
49. Sidles J, Harryman D, Harris S, Matsen F. In vivo quantification of glenohumeral stability. *Trans Orthop Res Soc.* 1991;16:646.
50. Colachis S, Strohm B. Effects of suprascapular and axillary nerve blocks on muscle force in the upper extremity. *Arch Phys Med Rehabil.* 1971;52:22–29.
51. Colachis S, Strohm B, Brechner V. Effects of axillary nerve blocks on muscle force in the upper extremity. *Arch Phys Med Rehabil.* 1969; 50:647–654.
52. Lehmkul L, Smith L. *Clinical Kinesiology.* Philadelphia: FA Davis; 1983:219–258.
53. Glousman R. Instability versus impingement in the throwing athlete. *Orthop Clin North Am.* 1993;24:89–93.
54. Burkhart S. Arthroscopic debridement and decompression for selected rotator cuff tears. *Orthop Clin North Am.* 1993; 24:111–123.

Section 3

Evaluation and Classification of Cuff Lesions

Chapter 5

Evaluation of Painful Shoulders: Entities That May Be Confused With Rotator Cuff Disease

James A. Shankwiler and Wayne Z. Burkhead, Jr.

There are more things in heaven and earth than are dreamt of in your philosophy my dear Horatio.

Shakespeare, Julius Caesar

Man who jump to conclusions usually land at bottom of cliff.

Charlie Chan

What makes accurate diagnosis of shoulder pain difficult? Several factors are involved: (1) the shoulder serves as a crossroads of the body. It is traversed by muscle, bone, tendon, nerve, and vessels, all of which may be potential sources of both local and referred pain; (2) it is a watershed area of multiple nerves, the roots of some contributing to visceral innervation; (3) it is often difficult to discern the exact etiology of shoulder pain in which any one or a combination of conditions may interrelate to cause disability; (4) the circular nature of the glenohumeral joint allows pathology on one side of the shoulder to manifest itself prominently as pain on the opposite side; (5) secondary effects of primary conditions can cause greater symptomatology and may represent the patient's chief complaint (i.e., tendinitis features are more prominent than the subtle instability that may have caused it or conversely instability symptoms are noticed more than cuff weakness); and (6) many painful conditions around the shoulder tend to evolve over time. What may look like an easy to treat tendinitis may progress to an adhesive capsulitis. Patients with adhesive capsulitis may recover only to remain symptomatic from a partial-thickness cuff tear. Finally, the diagnostic process, when done methodically, takes time. Repeated visits, interpretation, and correlation of diagnostic tests with symptoms and response to selective injection are the rule rather than the exception. However, the more time you spend with the patient in the office, the less likely it is you will spend time with them in court.

An increase in our medical knowledge in general has furthered our appreciation of the complexity in evaluating patients with shoulder pain and our ability with appropriate diagnostic testing to make accurate diagnoses. Care must be taken in the initial evaluation of these patients to discern other possible etiologies in regard to their symptomatology, because many conditions may present in a similar fashion to impingement and rotator cuff tendinopathy. The fact that many chronic degenerative rotator cuff tears are asymptomatic makes it even more important to diagnose other conditions that can result in more serious disability or death.

We are taught early in our careers to interpret a chest radiograph by focusing not on the lung but on the soft tissues and bones, so as not to miss a subtle lesion. The patient with a painful shoulder in my opinion should be approached the same way (i.e., with the shoulder as the last point of focus). This approach can avoid the assumption that a subacromial click is the source of pain in a patient with lung cancer, which is a conclusion that, if jumped to, will wind you up, not at the bottom of a cliff, but in front of a jury of your peers.

On the other hand, acute full-thickness rotator cuff tears continue to be overlooked. Because this book is devoted to rotator cuff tears, Codman's clinical description

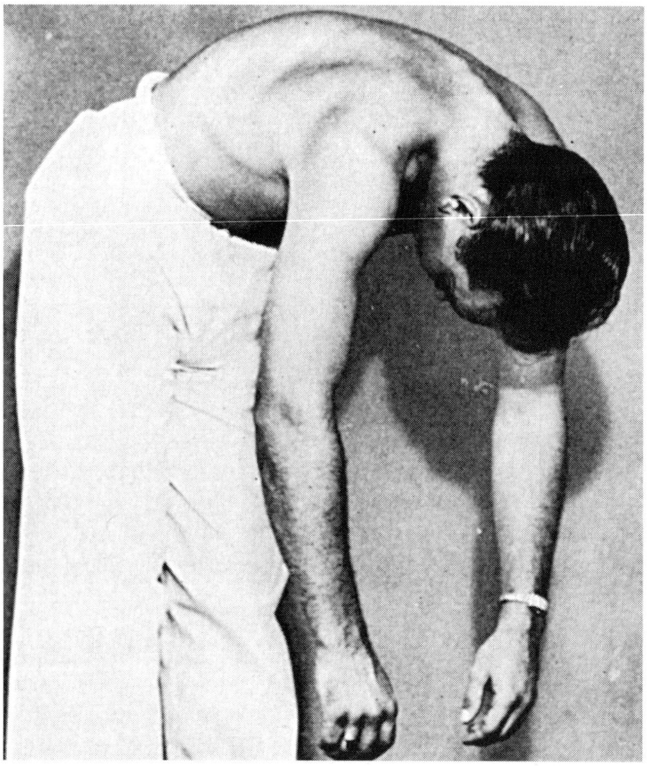

Fig. 5–1. Examination of the patient with an acute rotator cuff tear may be facilitated by examining them in the stooping position, as described by Codman. Moseley would refer to this as "the relaxed muscle position." (From Moseley HF. Examination of the shoulder. In: Moseley HF, ed. *Shoulder Lesions.* 3rd ed. Edinburgh: Churchill Livingstone; 1972:22–30.)

of the 18 conditions, symptoms, and signs seen with complete rupture of the supraspinatus tendon bear repeating. The occupation of the patient is usually a type of job that involves manual labor. He observed that rotator cuff injuries were rare under age 25, increase after age 30, and dramatically rise with complete tears after age 40. He felt a history of a previously painless and useful arm was unreliable because of a patient "working through" the pain and forgetting the causative event or concealing the injury. An adequate injury or event significant enough to cause the tear is important. He noted that patients complained of a sharp pain at the time of the tear, elicited voluntarily or involuntarily. Codman noted patients complained of increased pain at night, and there was an interim period between injury and the development of severe pain. He felt the patient's inability to raise the arm was constant but unreliable, as other causes of shoulder pain have the same effect. Also the patient may be able to elevate the arm with compensatory mechanisms. He noted a negative radiograph to be a constant finding. He observed no lack of restriction of motion (i.e., frozen shoulder) in patients with a supraspinatus tear. He stated the *sine qua non* for a supraspinatus tear to be faulty scapulohumeral rhythm with the patient exhibiting scapular compensation for glenohumeral motion. He defined the eminence as a more than normally palpable greater tuberosity with variable tenderness. He also noted palpable tenderness at the insertion sites of other cuff tendons, if they too were torn. A jog occurs because of faulty scapulohumeral rhythm noticeable to the patient and often to the examiner. The patient winced during the jog, although they may not wince with chronic tears. He observed a "velvety, gristally" soft crepitance with motion. He noted that palpation of the greater tuberosity caused pain that would disappear as it passed under the acromion (Dawbarn's sign). Codman stated the tendon stump could be palpated on the tuberosity with motion as a "palisade-hummock," as it moves under the examiner's finger. For the patient with too much spasm, the arm can be evaluated in the stooping position (Fig. 5–1), or alternatively with downward traction on the head of the humerus during abduction (Fig. 5–2).

In addition to the above 18 signs and symptoms, Codman also observed a relative hypertrophy of the deltoid, primarily caused by atrophy of the spinati. He described an auxiliary sign as fluid would flow through the tear into the subacromial space with arm elevation. A difference in shoulder contour can be noted by the observer while standing behind the patient. He termed this the "fluid sign."

Although Codman felt that there was no sharp anatomic distinction between complete and incomplete rupture, he felt the diagnosis of a complete rupture was important, as it would not heal "in the natural manner," as would incomplete rupture. Unfortunately, most patients who present to the doctor's office do not present in the acute or subacute phase following rotator cuff injury and as Neer has pointed out, many rotator cuff tears

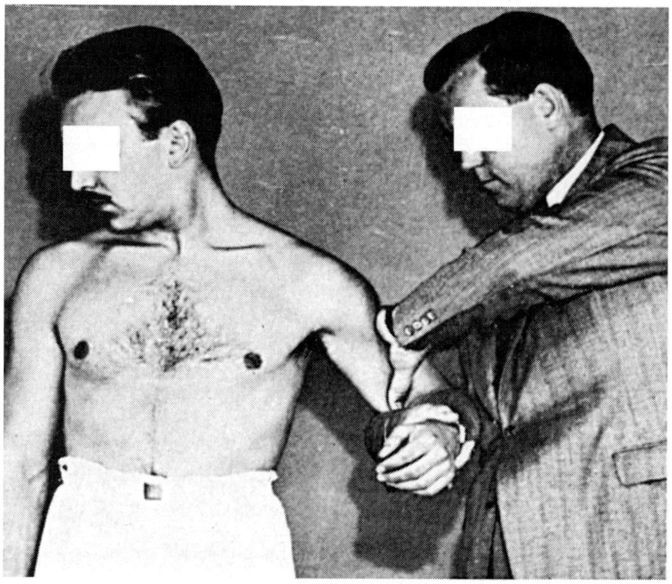

Fig. 5–2. The depression of the head test. When evaluating the patient with an acutely painful shoulder, downward pressure applied to the humeral head relieves the pain by moving the injured area from impingement on the coracoacromial arch. (From Moseley HF. Examination of the shoulder. In: Moseley HF, ed. *Shoulder Lesions.* 3rd ed. Edinburgh: Churchill Livingstone; 1972:22–30.)

occur in the absence of trauma. Therefore, it is important to develop a system for evaluating the painful shoulder in your own practice. The following is one we have found helpful.

CLASSIFICATION

Shoulder pain can generally be attributable to intrinsic (local) or extrinsic (remote) factors; extrinsic factors being those that occur outside the shoulder girdle with secondary pain being referred to the region and intrinsic factors being of primary origin within the shoulder girdle itself. Occasionally, often in the chronic pain patient, both intrinsic and extrinsic conditions interact to magnify the production of shoulder pain and morbidity. A prime example of this is the patient with cervical disc disease, C5–6 weakness, a degenerative tear in the rotator cuff, intrinsic impingement tendinitis, and acromioclavicular arthritis. On the other end of the spectrum, a patient with an unrepaired distal rotator cuff tear and altered scapulohumeral mechanics may develop neck pain, fibromyalgia, and fibrositis type symptoms because of the excess stress placed on the scapular support musculature from the intrinsic shoulder problem. A third category, systemic, can effect both intrinsic and extrinsic shoulder pain (i.e., the patient with rheumatoid arthritis and a painful glenohumeral joint has a systemic intrinsic lesion, while the patient with polymyalgia rheumatica has a systemic extrinsic etiology for their shoulder pain). Intrinsic shoulder pain and its relationship to rotator cuff disease is discussed thoroughly in Chapters 8–17 in Section IV of this book, in which not only the clinical diagnosis but the treatment of these entities are presented.

For the purposes of this discussion, the remainder of this chapter will center on extrinsic lesions, including the ultimate extrinsic lesion, malingering, and a method for evaluating shoulder pain. However, the evaluation of shoulder pain is no different than evaluation techniques that were drilled into our heads as junior medical students on the Internal Medicine Service. One should elicit the chief complaint, the history of the present illness, the past medical history, the social history, the family history, perform a thorough physical examination, create a list of diagnostic entities for a differential diagnosis, and create a plan for working through that differential diagnosis to come up with the patient's correct diagnosis.

FIRST IMPRESSION

A certain gestalt can be gleaned shortly after entering the examination room. Is the first thing the patient hands you a letter from a referring doctor or a disability insurance form? Does the spouse, if present, seem supportive and genuinely concerned (enabling) or counterproductive (disabling)? Does the patient eagerly shake your hand despite discomfort, hoping you will be the one to help, or does the patient draw the wounded wing beneath his/her shirt or gown? Is there a discrepancy between arm movement as the patient relates his/her history and your focused examination? Does the patient look you in the eye when telling his/her story?

PAST MEDICAL HISTORY

How did it start? Was the onset sudden and memorable and related to a particular activity or did it begin insidiously? Does the patient remember what he/she was doing or where he/she was the first time discomfort was experienced? Was there a temporal relationship to any viral illnesses, new medications, or injections given to the patient at the time of the onset of their shoulder pain? **What is the quality of the pain?** Is it diffuse, dull, and aching in nature, as one would expect with tendinitis, or is it sharp lancinating pain? Burning pain often indicates a neurogenic source typical of cervical radiculopathy or the pain caused by sudden motion in a patient with adhesive capsulitis. **Is it constant or intermittent?** Do specific motions, activities, or phases of activities produce the pain? If so, which ones? Intermittent shoulder pain radiating down the arm that occurs during walking and diminishes with rest over several minutes is more likely cardiac than cuff in origin. Patients who have pain in their parascapular region after eating fatty foods are seldom relieved of that discomfort with an arthroscopic acromioplasty.

The first clue that one is dealing with a symptom magnifier or malingerer may well be in the description of their pain. Hyperbole is the rule with inferences to penetrating wounds by ancient weapons and ripping or tearing by wild animals, which were often followed by the application of ground glass, salt, cayenne pepper, or all three. "Just take the arm off" may be their proposed solution.

Where do you feel the bulk of your pain? Pain locale is an important point in the differential. Pain in the trapezius and rhomboid area (Fig. 5–3), is seen commonly with cervical disc disease, fibrositis, fibromyalgia, and referred pain of neurogenic or visceral origin, while pain at the deltoid insertion is more common with intrinsic shoulder problems (Fig. 5–4). Levine's sign of the shoulder is atypical of rotator cuff pathology. Pain at the superior aspect of the shoulder emanates not only from intrinsic lesions of the AC joint, but also ulnar nerve neuritis. Posterior joint line pain may represent capsular tightness or osteoarthritis, but can also be seen in neurogenic pain, especially pain just below the posterolateral corner of the acromion.

Where does the pain go? Although radiating pain from the neck to the shoulder is most commonly associated with extrinsic neurogenic compressive lesions or degenerative changes of the cervical spine, one must keep in mind that referred pain can travel from distal to proximal. Moseley found that injecting the supraspinatus tendon with a small volume of saline caused pain localized to the deltoid insertion. Larger volumes increased the intensity of the pain and caused pain radiating to the neck and down to the thumb and index.[1] Finally, it has

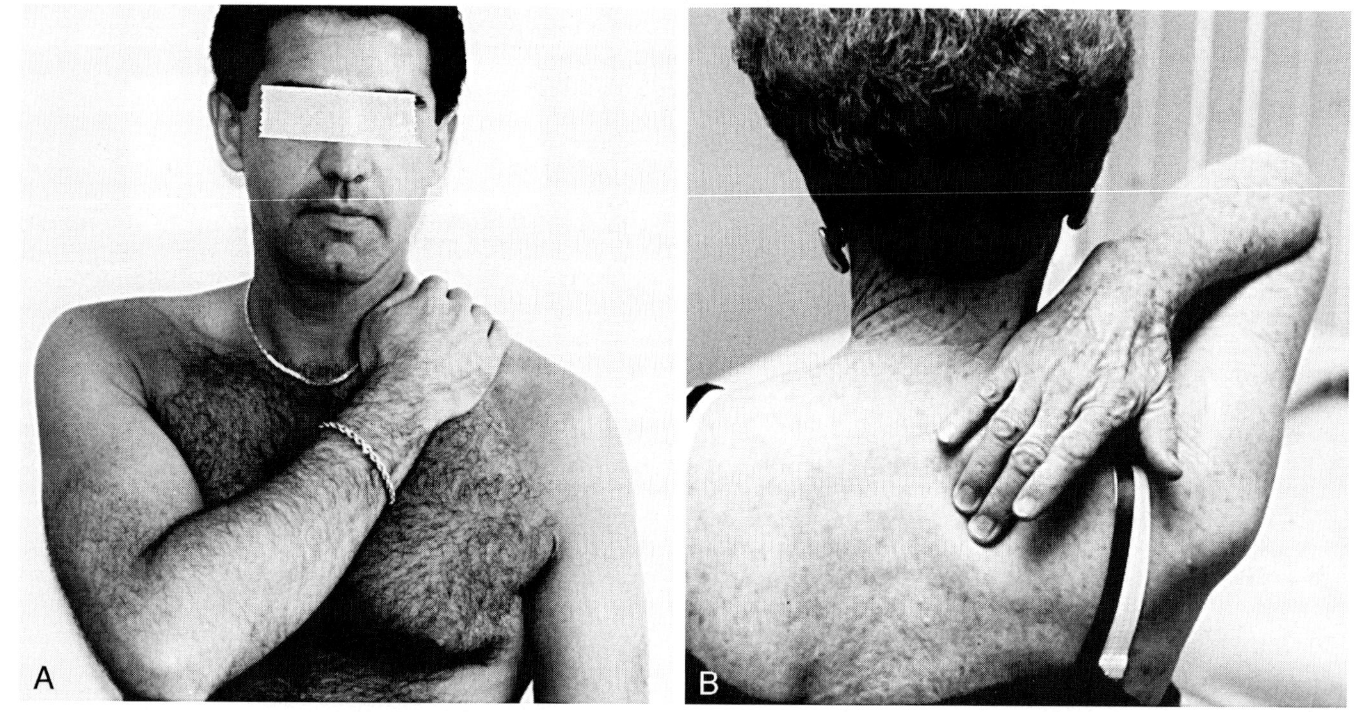

Fig. 5–3. *A,* Pain in the trapezius is typical of cervical radicular pain, fibromyalgia, fibrositis, and referred pain of visceral origin (rarely AC joint pain). *B,* As with trapezius pain, pain along the parascapular border in the region of the rhomboids is generally indicative of referred pain from the cervical spine, fibrositis, fibromyalgia, and scapulothoracic disorders. Intrinsic shoulder conditions, such as adhesive capsulitis or rotator cuff tearing, can cause increased stress on the scapular musculature and give pain in this region also.

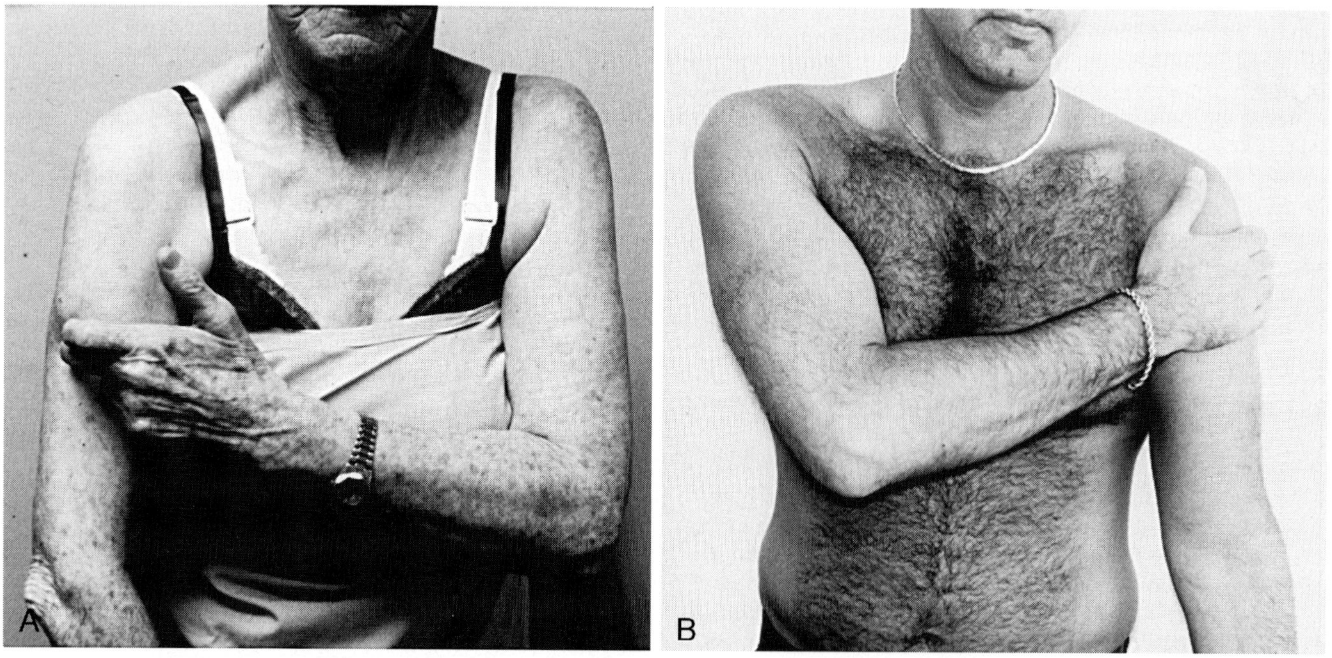

Fig. 5–4. *A,* Pain at the deltoid insertion. Commonly seen in patients with adhesive capsulitis and referred pain of intrinsic shoulder origin. *B,* Levine's sign of the shoulder (primarily pathognomonic sign) for rotator cuff pathology when the patient is asked where his/her pain is.

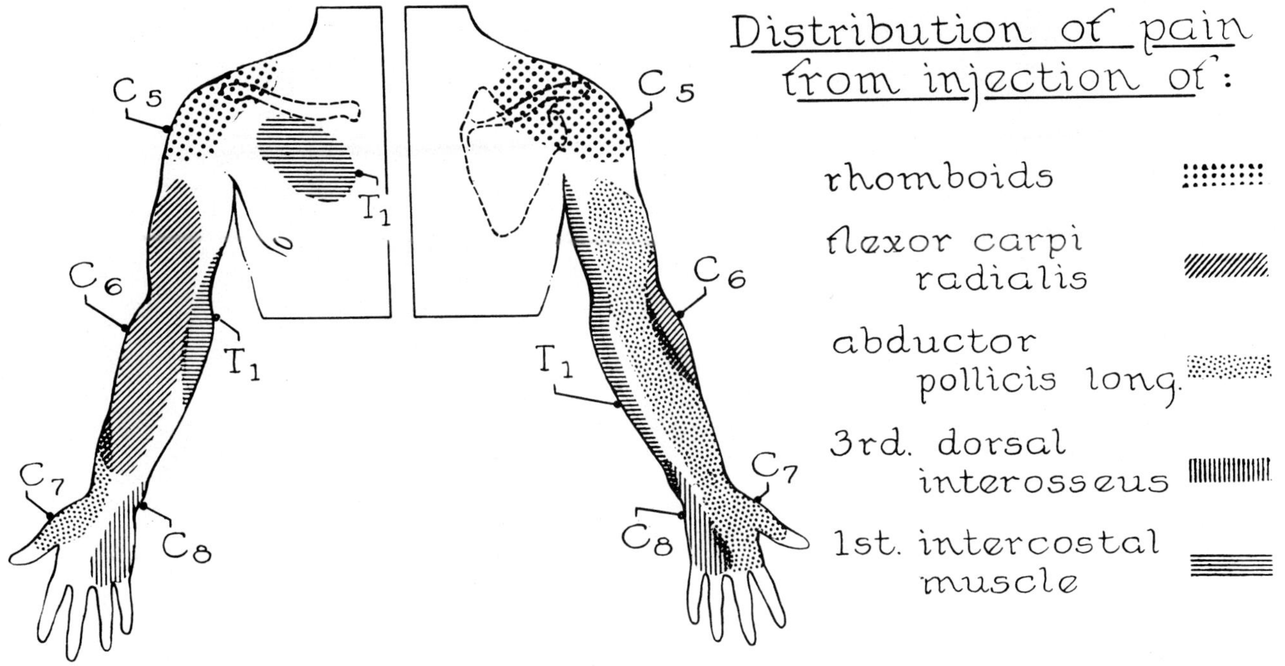

Fig. 5–5. Deep segmental pain indicating distal to proximal referred pain patterns from hypertonic saline injections. (From Moseley HF. Examination of the shoulder. In: Moseley HF, ed. *Shoulder Lesions.* 3rd ed. Edinburgh: Churchill Livingstone;1972:22–30.)

been our experience that the AC joint, because of its triple innervation and perhaps because of its proximity to the trapezius, seems to cause referred neck pain (as well as occasional pectoral and axillary pain) much more commonly than do lesions of the cuff per se. Lesser recognized causes of neurogenic compressive shoulder pain include the common peripheral nerve entrapment syndromes such as carpal tunnel, ulnar nerve neuritis, or radial nerve entrapment, as well as the less common but more proximate entities of suprascapular nerve entrapment, thoracic outlet, and the ultimate rarity, quadrilateral space syndrome. Kellgren and Lewis have mapped pain emanating from the muscles supplied by the brachial plexus[2] using local injections of hypertonic saline to map deep pain segments of the upper limb with surprising accuracy (Fig. 5–5).

Specific provocative questions should include the following: **What makes the pain worse and what makes it better? What is the effect of arm position and motion?** Patients who have no pain with shoulder motion whatsoever seldom have an intrinsic lesion in the shoulder. Abducting the shoulder occasionally helps the patient with cervical nerve root irritation but exacerbates thoracic outlet and intrinsic shoulder pain.

What is the effect of neck position and motion? The patient should be asked specifically about the effect of Valsalva maneuvers, coughing, and sneezing. Neck rotation and lateral bending towards the painful shoulder should increase the pain in cervical disc disease and radiculopathy, while rotating towards the opposite side exacerbates the pain from brachial plexus irritation. Neurogenic compressive-type pain unaffected by cervical rotation should make one suspicious of peripheral nerve involvement and/or visceral (phrenic nerve mediated) pain.

Is the pain significant to disturb ones' sleep? Although night pain is typical of rotator cuff tears, with the exception of cervical disc disease, most disorders that cause shoulder pain seem to be worse at night.

What medications have been tried by the patient to control the pain? It is always amazing to us when patients who have shoulder pain wait weeks to be seen without ever having tried treating themselves with over-the-counter analgesia or anti-inflammatory medication. On the other hand, some patients have pain that even oral narcotic agents do not seem to control. Pain at that end of the spectrum should raise the possibilities of calcific tendinitis, neurogenic compressive pain, or systemic intrinsic problems such as metastases. A visual analog rating scale of 1 to 10 is helpful in determining the degree of pain on presentation and whether or not an increase or decrease in that pain is occurring with treatment and/or time.

Review of Systems

General systemic symptoms such as weight loss, fever, chills, or change in appetite, as well as a thorough review of systems, are mandatory in the patient with hard to explain shoulder pain. The presence or absence of paresthesia, weakness, or discoordination are important. A generalized slowing of mentation and gait may be the earliest manifestation of Parkinsonism. The past medical

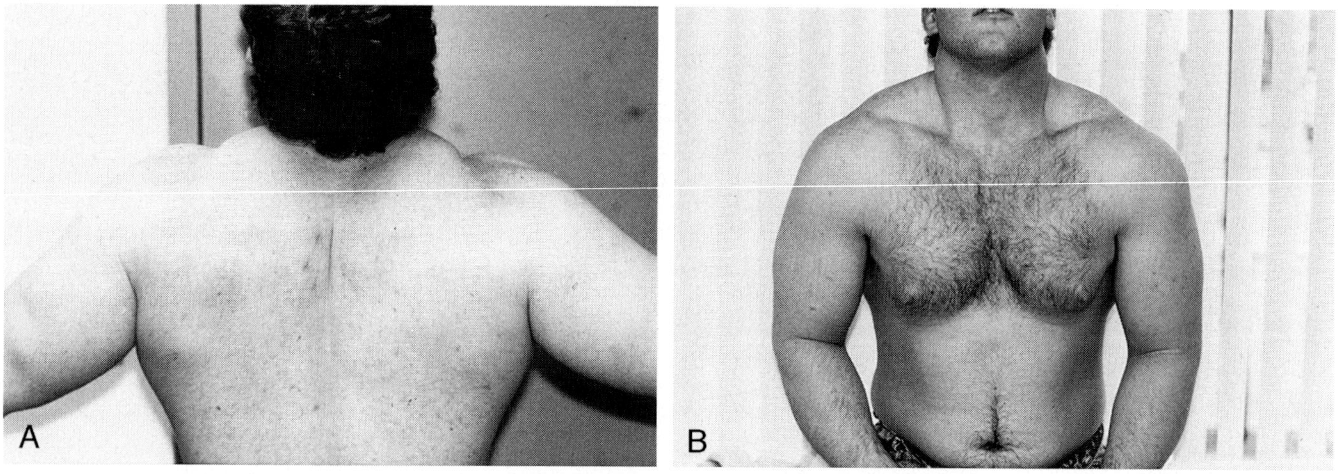

Fig. 5–6. *A and B,* **Format for evaluation of the male patient. Note diagnosis was combined AC joint osteolysis and thoracic outlet syndrome from muscular hypertrophy, both secondary to weightlifting.**

history is important for previous history of carcinoma, cardiac disease, endocrine, gastrointestinal, or rheumatologic history.

Social History—Family History

Social history is important. Occupation or leisure activities that can contribute to shoulder pain range from repetitive use at the computer terminal with thoracic outlet and fibrositis to occupational exposure to carcinogens. Stress is an important factor, not only in the production of certain syndromes, but also in their maintenance. A family history of carcinoma, heart disease, or abdominal disorders might lead one to a more exacting diagnosis.

Finally, after all these questions, prior to the physical, ask perhaps the most important question of all. **Where does the patient think the pain is coming from?**

PHYSICAL EXAMINATION

A good general physical exam should be recommended to every patient with unexplained shoulder pain if the following shoulder/neck exam fails to provide a diagnosis.

Inspection

Physical examination should be done from the front and the back from both sides with the shoulders exposed (Fig. 5–6). Female patients' modesty can be protected and their shoulders evaluated using commercially available velcro fastening halter tops (Fig. 5–7). Many patients we see tell us, "You're the first doctors that really looked at my shoulder." Examination techniques as illustrated in Figure 5–8 are the reason why. A general impression should be obtained including the patient's facies (affect), posture, muscular development, and nutritional status. One should inspect for atrophy, skin lesions, striae, scars, deformity, hypertrophy, muscle rupture, and swelling. Range of motion of the cervical spine and shoulder should be accurately recorded along with any tendency towards joint laxity.

Range of Motion

Range of motion of the shoulder should be done actively and passively (the American Shoulder and Elbow Surgeons' standard) and elevation, external rotation, and internal rotation to the spinous process should be measured. During passive elevation, the malingerer will often forcefully contract their triceps and latissimus dorsi to prevent elevation. Rather than free motion up to a solid end point, as seen in frozen shoulder, the malingerer will exhibit progressively increased resistance applied to your hand.

Palpation

Bony prominences, joint lines, the location, course, excursion of tendons, and areas of crepitance should be palpated. Palpate lastly the patient's tender areas that they have pointed out, so as not to miss other areas of tenderness. The supraclavicular fossa, axillary, and anterior and posterior cervical chains of lymph nodes should be evaluated. For the symptom magnifier palpate areas that should not be tender: midclavicle, midaspect spine of scapula, and midacromion.

Neurologic Examination

Deep tendon reflexes, in both the upper and lower extremities, should be performed. Remember that in cer-

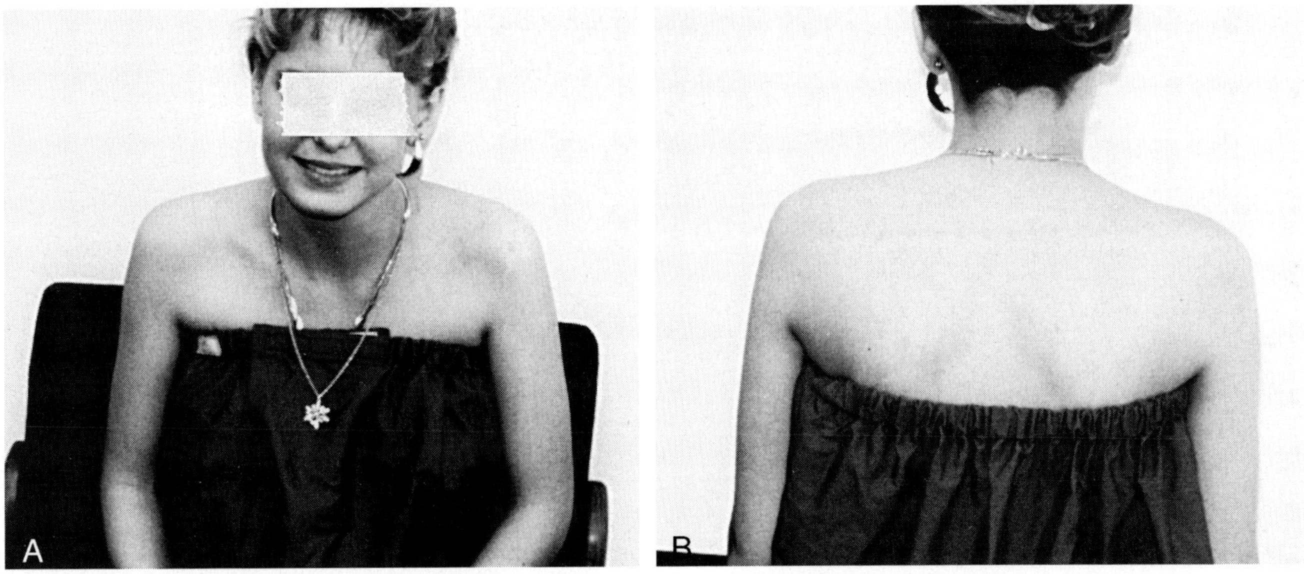

Fig. 5–7. *A,* Commercially available velcro fastening halter top allows the female patient to protect her modesty while both shoulders can be examined. Note: Despite the different body habitus from the patient in Figure 5–6, this patient had thoracic outlet syndrome as well, primarily on a postural basis. *B,* The hair must be placed up so that the neck can be visualized as well.

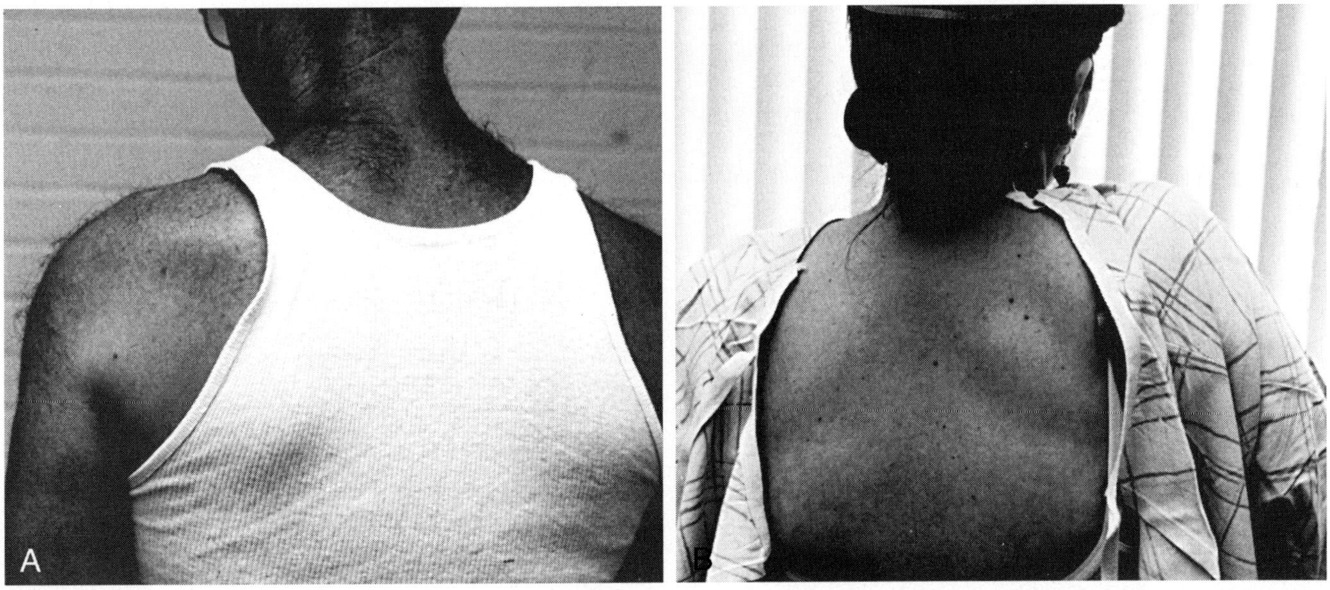

Fig. 5–8. *A,* How not to evaluate patients in your office. While the patient's supraspinatus and infraspinatus atrophy are observed in this patient, what is not clear is that the neck, trapezius, and rhomboids are atrophic in this patient with viral brachial neuritis. *B,* How not to evaluate patients with shoulder pain. With a gown on like this, one cannot determine whether the scapular hiking seen in this patient's right shoulder is related to pain and splinting or altered scapulothoracic mechanics on initiation of abduction.

vical myelopathy, upper extremity reflexes may be normal or hyporeactive, whereas lower extremity reflexes are spastic and associated pathologic reflexes often present.

Careful motor and sensory examination to determine the dermatomal level should be performed (Fig. 5–9). Motor testing offers you another opportunity to determine malingering. If one is testing abduction strength, palpate the deltoid at the same time. During a valid attempt at abduction against resistance, the deltoid should palpably contract in the absence of an axillary nerve lesion. Provocative tests for peripheral nerve entrapment such as the elbow compression test, Phalen's test, and third finger extension test should be done.

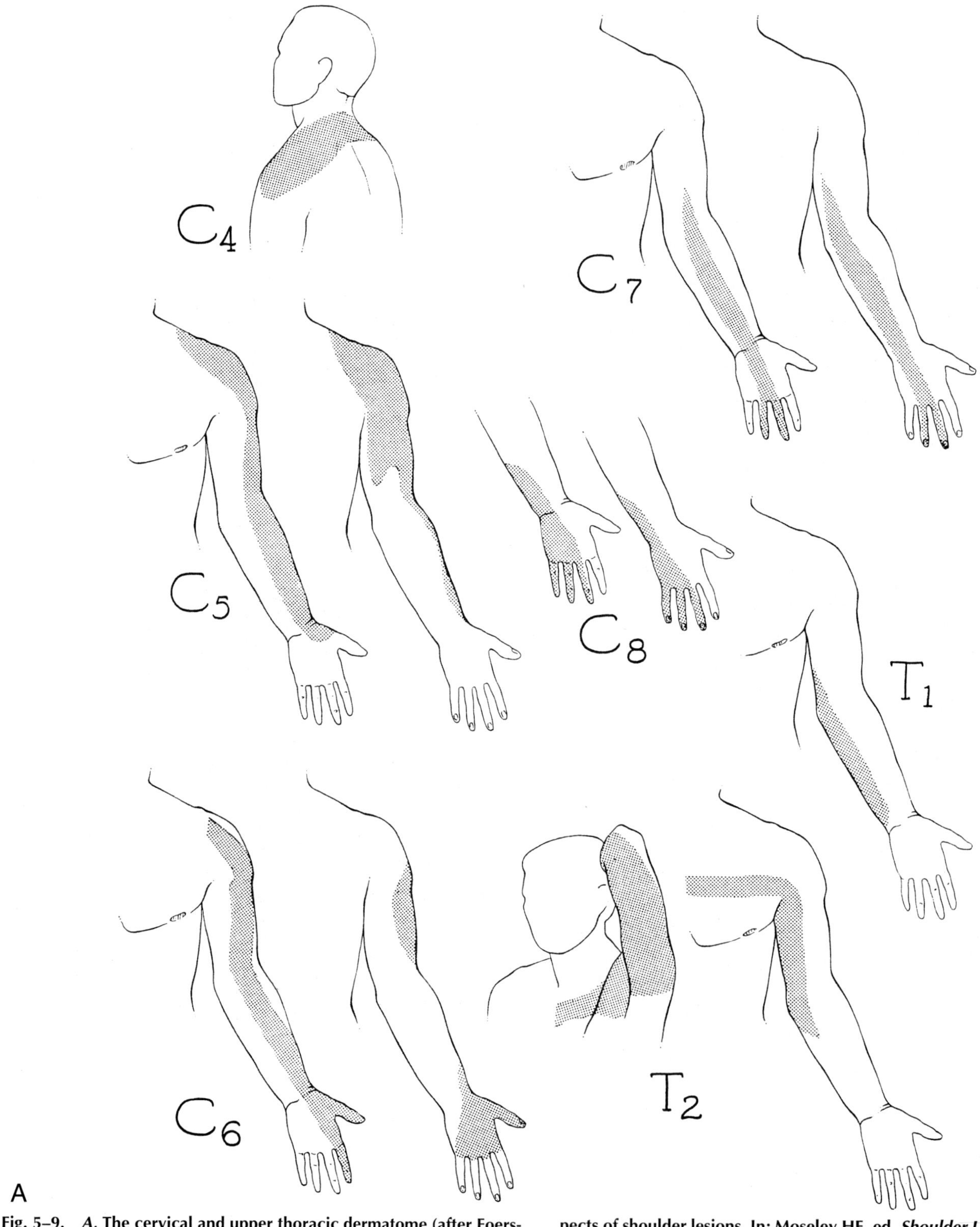

Fig. 5–9. *A,* The cervical and upper thoracic dermatome (after Foerster, 1933 and Brock, 1938). (From McNaughton FL. Neurological aspects of shoulder lesions. In: Moseley HF, ed. *Shoulder Lesions.* 3rd ed. Edinburgh: Churchill Livingstone; 1972:22–30.)

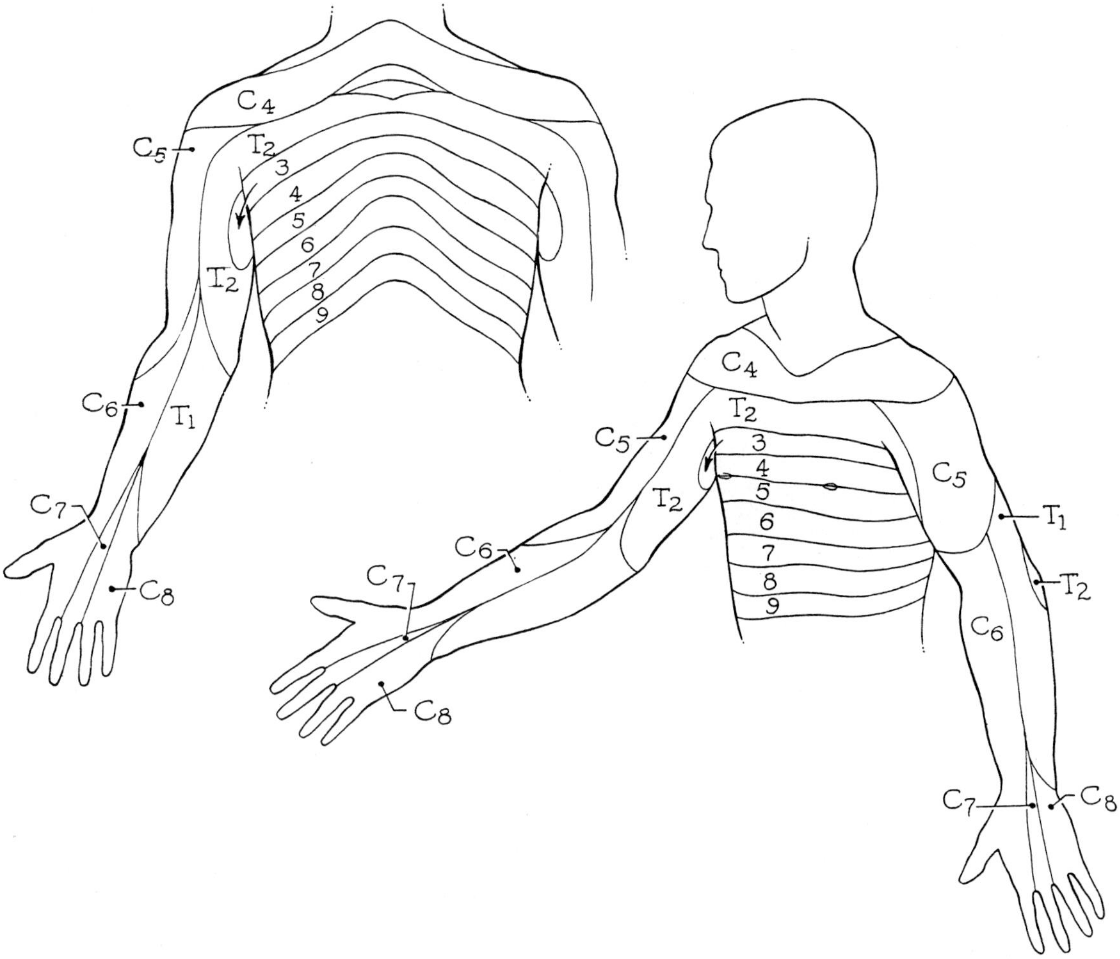

B

Fig. 5–9. ***Continued. B,*** **The composite dermatome map of Foerster for the trunk and upper limbs. (From McNaughton FL: Neurological aspects of shoulder lesions. In: Moseley HF, ed.** ***Examination of the Shoulder.*** **In: Moseley HF, ed.** ***Shoulder Lesions.*** **3rd ed. Edinburgh: Churchill Livingstone;1972:22–30.)**

Vascular Exam

Thoracic outlet maneuvers, Wright, Adson, and Roos' overhead exercise tests should be performed (Figs. 5–10 through 5–12).

Provocative maneuvers for various intrinsic shoulder lesions can be found in Chapters 8 through 11.

Last Impression

The last impression you make on a patient with shoulder pain should be the importance of following through with the treatment or diagnostic regimen you have recommended and the importance of repeat follow-up if symptoms change. Your last impression of the patient should be garnered as the patient gets dressed. You are likely dealing with a malingerer if at the termination of the interview and examination, the patient who grimaced, groaned, and said "you're killing me, doc" while you tried to passively elevate their arm, appears incredibly gracile when putting on a sleeve while they think you are preoccupied with paperwork.

With this method a differential diagnosis can be made and appropriate diagnostic testing ordered. For a detailed description of plain film radiology and advanced imaging techniques for the rotator cuff, see Chapter 6.

Injections

Selective injections are an incredibly important part of our evaluation. Selective injections serve three purposes: (1) as confirmatory evidence that the abnormality seen on clinical examination and diagnostic testing are indeed the primary pain generators; (2) some idea as to the patient's overall pain threshold and response to pain can be obtained by the injection process itself; and (3) this injection gives the patient with intrinsic shoulder pain an idea of what they will feel like at the end of successful conservative or operative care. Following diagnostic tests, selective diagnostic lidocaine (Xylocaine) or bupivacaine hydrochloride (Marcaine) blocks can be performed in the AC joint, subacromial bursa, glenohumeral joint, or bicipital groove to rule out a component of intrinsic shoulder pathology and diagnostic blocks of the median,

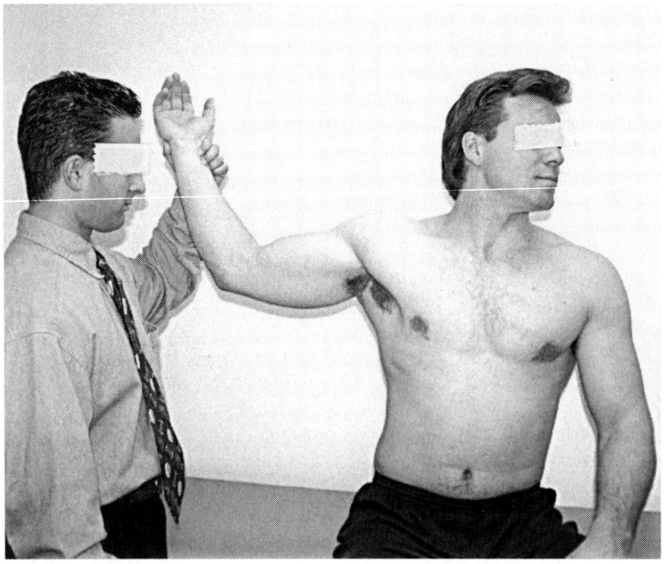

Fig. 5–10. Wright's hyperabduction maneuver. The patient's arm is placed in abduction-external rotation and he is asked to look away from the side of the lesion. Diminishment of pulse, combined with reproduction of the patient's symptoms, is considered a positive test for thoracic outlet. It should be noted that 20% of individuals have a positive Wright's maneuver without symptoms of thoracic outlet.

ulnar, posterior interosseous, or suprascapular nerve to determine what component of pain is emanating from peripheral nerve entrapment. The subscapular bursa and cervical facets help elucidate the source of parascapular and neck discomfort. Trigger points can be injected to determine the extent to which they contribute to the constellation of the patient's pain.

EXTRINSIC CONDITIONS

Cervical Origin

Cervical pathology may commonly present with associated shoulder discomfort. The area of referred pain will often assume a dermatomal pattern consistent with the involved nerve roots. Therefore, evaluation of pain patterns is important in discerning the type and location of associated cervical pathology. Pain over the trapezius and lateral shoulder and brachium is often caused by discogenic radicular pain originating in the C5-C6 region. Cervical radicular pain often may also radiate over the occiput and posterior midline of the neck and upper thoracic spine. Inspection will occasionally reveal dysymmetry by craning of the head and neck and/or hiking of the shoulder on the affected side. Cervical range of motion may be limited, especially with extension and lateral rotation toward the affected side. Spurling's test can be performed to evaluate for underlying discogenic or radicular pain by rotating and deviating the patient's head toward the affected side with gentle axial compression applied by the examiner (Fig. 5–13), with exacerbation or recreation of the patient's pain complaints being considered a positive test result. Occasionally, cervical traction applied gently by the examiner may be noted to improve the patient's pain, because this may decrease pressure on the involved nerve roots (Fig. 5–14). Muscular atrophy and weakness are also important to note on the initial inspection of patients with shoulder pain. Inspection and strength testing may reveal atrophy of the spinati and deltoid with weakness on resisted shoulder abduction and/or external rotation testing with C5-C6 lesions that may mimic tears of the rotator cuff; however, a decreased biceps reflex will usually be present.

Thoracic outlet syndrome is a condition in which compression occurs to the nerves and vessels to the arm as they pass through the interval created by the anterior and middle scalene muscles and the first rib. The presence of cervical ribs and/or hypertrophy of the scalene muscles has been related to its onset.[3–5] In addition, scapular ptosis and poor posture have also been noted to be associated with its occurrence. Occasionally, clavicular fractures may narrow the interval between the clavicle and the first rib, causing significant compression of the nerves and vessels in the region.[6] Patients often give a history of vague shoulder pain that may appear consistent with rotator cuff pathology. The pain is typically seen in the anterior aspect of the shoulder, especially in the region of the coracoid and/or supra and infraclavicular fossae. Paresthesias are usually experienced in the ulnar two digits, because these are innervated by the lower trunk of the plexus that is more commonly involved. Provocative maneuvers such as Wright's and Adson's tests have been discussed. Roos' overhead grip test can be performed to evaluate for this condition. Positive tests will confirm the diagnosis by recreating the patient's symptomatology with associated diminution of peripheral pulses caused by vascular compression. The patient with

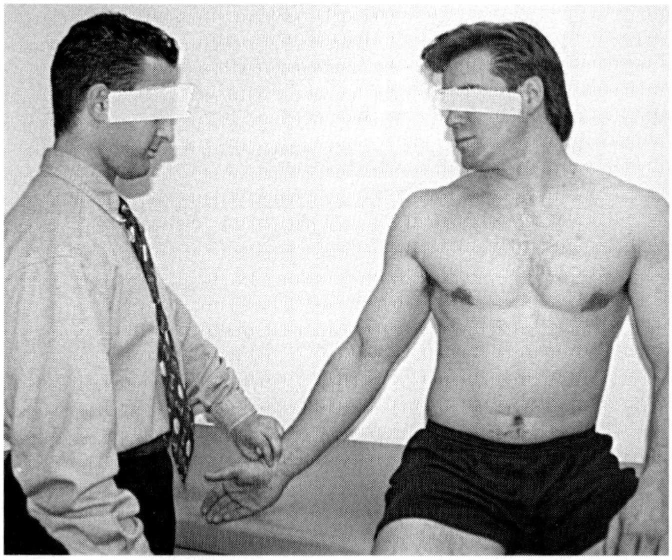

Fig. 5–11. Adson's maneuver for scalenus medius syndrome. The patient is asked to look towards the involved shoulder and upward. Again, as in Wright's maneuver, a positive test is present if the maneuver reproduces the patient's symptoms consistently.

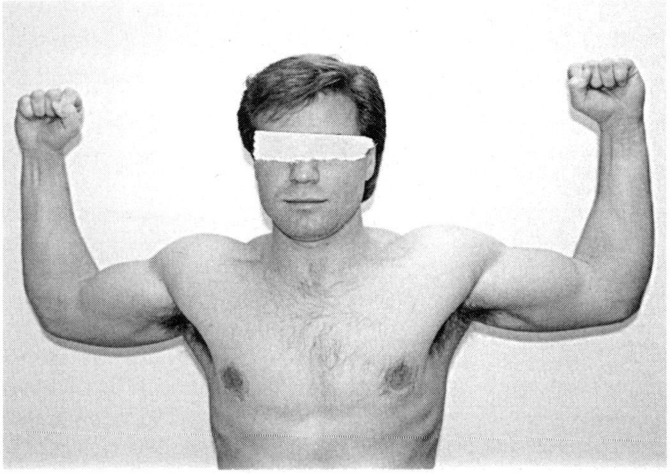

Fig. 5–12. With both arms held overhead, the patient is asked to rapidly flex and extend the fingers. Aching fatigue in the forearm and hand with reproduction of pain in the shoulder within 20 to 30 seconds is the rule in patients with thoracic outlet syndrome and constitutes a positive test.

true vascular compromise will have symptoms begin within seconds of starting Roos' overhead grip test. Acute traction injuries to the arm may also injure the brachial plexus with subsequent pain, paresthesias, and weakness.[7–9] Often a history of lifting or catching a heavy object will be related by the patient, with an onset of burning dysesthesias into the arm and hand. Pain patterns and symptoms are extremely similar to those seen with thoracic outlet syndrome. Tenderness may often be elicited on palpation in the supra and infraclavicular fossae, with occasional recurrence of paresthesias. Often Wright's and/or Adson's maneuvers may exacerbate the patient's discomfort without any change in peripheral pulses being noted by the examiner. The apprehension maneuver may also cause significant discomfort in this patient group, leading the examiner to consider a diagnosis of subtle instability. However, the relocation maneuver, as described by Jobe, will not alleviate the patient's discomfort as it does in the presence of instability.

In addition to the above mentioned pathology, idiopathic brachial plexus neuropathy may also occur.[10,11] This is more commonly seen in males than females and in individuals in their second and third decades of life. The onset of this has been associated with a recent history of immunizations and/or viral illnesses. Associated pain complaints may often be severe with atrophy and/or weakness that often involves the shoulder. Atrophy of the shoulder musculature may lead to scapular dysrhythmia with secondary mechanical impingement occurring (Fig. 5–15). Treatment is supportive and often takes as much as 2 or 3 years for resolution of symptomatology to occur.

In addition to brachial plexus pathology, injury to the peripheral innervation of the shoulder musculature may also lead to pain and disability that is similar in presentation to rotator cuff tendinopathy. Injury to the suprascapular nerve that innervates both the supraspinatus and infraspinatus muscles may cause weakness and shoulder pain, as in tearing of the rotator cuff. The suprascapular nerve arises from the upper trunk of the brachial plexus and passes through the suprascapular notch separated from its accompanying artery by the transverse scapular ligament, which in turn may cause compression of the nerve. Scapular fractures and congenital narrowing of the scapular notch may also lead to entrapment neuropathy of the suprascapular nerve.[12] In addition, ganglions have also been reported to occur in the spinoglenoid notch with subsequent compression of the nerve and isolated infraspinatus weakness.[13] Patients with this condition typically present with pain complaints centered over the trapezius and posterior aspect of the shoulder overlying the scapula. Significant atrophy of the spinati with weakness in abduction and external rotation of the arm may be noted on examination. In these cases, EMG results will usually show latency from stimulus to response in the supraspinatus consistent with compression neuropathy of the suprascapular nerve. Occasionally surgical decompression of the nerve by release of the overlying transverse scapular ligament is necessary for treatment.[14,15]

Injury to the axillary nerve may also mimic rotator cuff pathology. The axillary nerve derives from the posterior cord of the brachial plexus and lies adjacent to the subscapularis muscle under which it passes posteriorly to exit the quadrangular space, with motor distribution being given to both the teres minor and deltoid muscles with sensation to the lateral aspect of the deltoid. The nerve is at risk for injury with shoulder dislocations, fractures of the proximal humerus, and iatrogenic injuries from surgical procedures as well.[16,17] Typically, injury secondary to fractures and dislocations causes a transient neuropraxia that often resolves completely over time. Most investigators recommend surgical exploration of the axillary nerve if no return has occurred by 3 to 4 months. It is important to remember in the context of anterior

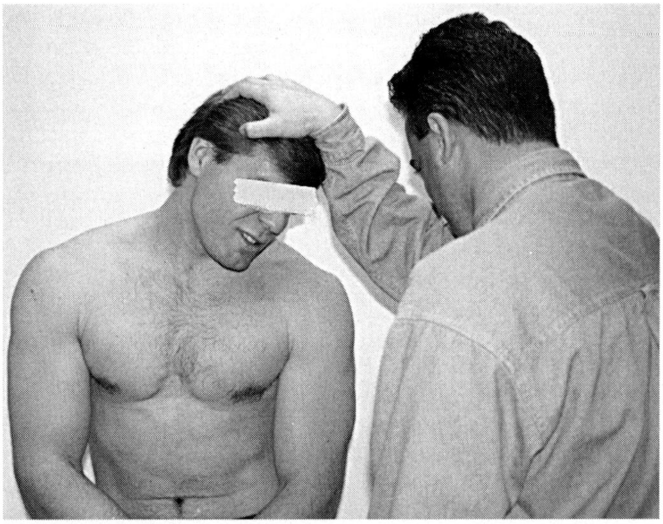

Fig. 5–13. Spurling's test. The patient's neck is compressed towards the side of the complaints. Reproduction of radicular symptoms is a positive test.

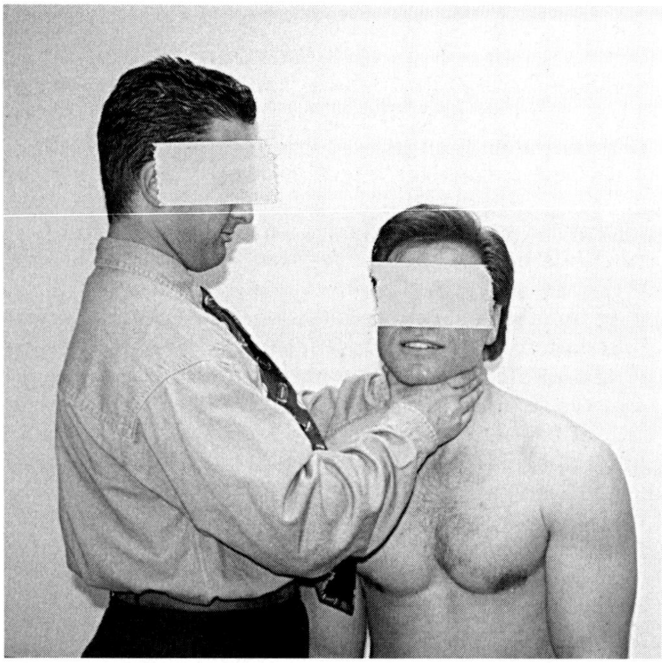

Fig. 5–14. Office traction test. Often pain from cervical disc disease will be improved by application of gentle cervical traction in the office.

dislocation in patients over 40 years old that rotator cuff tears are more common than axillary nerve injury.[18]

A quadrilateral space syndrome has also been described that may lead to compression and injury to the axillary nerve.[19,20] In this rare condition, the nerve is compressed by fibrous bands in the quadrilateral space. This typically occurs when the arm is held in abduction and external rotation with subsequent tightening of the fibrous bands across the nerve. Neurologic and EMG tests are usually within normal limits and are not helpful. Diagnosis in this case is made by performance of an arteriogram of the subclavian artery to visualize the posterior humeral circumflex artery as it passes through the quadrangular space. The arteriogram will often reveal compression of the artery as it traverses the quadrangular space when the arm is in the abducted and externally rotated position. However, vascular radiologists note this not uncommonly on asymptomatic individuals.[21] Surgical intervention with decompression of the region by exploration and release of fibrous bands and/or the tendon of the teres minor is indicated in indolent cases.[21,22]

Injuries to the spinal accessory nerve may also cause weakness and discomfort in the shoulder consistent with impingement; pathology usually can occur from an acute traction injury to the neck and/or arm or direct blow or pressure in the base of the neck, with injury to the nerve with subsequent denervation of the trapezius. Surgical procedures, such as lymph node biopsy in the neck, also place the nerve at risk for iatrogenic injury.[22] Associated pain that radiates from the neck into the trapezius and shoulder with weakness in abduction occurs as a result of these injuries.

Subsequent progressive atrophy of the trapezius is seen with dysymmetry and ptosis of the involved shoulder. This may lead to narrowing of the supraspinatus outlet with possible secondary impingement. EMG examination is usually diagnostic in these cases. If no evidence of return is noted at 6 months, surgical treatment can consist of exploration of the nerve with possible tendon transfer as in the Eden-Lange procedure for irreparable conditions.[23] Paralysis of the serratus anterior muscle may also lead to scapular dysrhythmia and pain reminiscent of rotator cuff pathology.[22] The serratus anterior is innervated by the long thoracic nerve which derives from the fifth, sixth, and seventh cervical roots. Injury to the nerve causes subsequent winging of the scapula with discomfort on active forward flexion of the shoulder. In persistently painful lesions without evidence of recovery, surgical treatment with scapulothoracic fusion or stabilization by tendon transfer using either the pectoralis minor or major have all been described.[24,25]

Finally, peripheral compression neuropathies in the arm may also give referred pain to the shoulder. Both carpal tunnel and cubital tunnel syndromes may present with pain similar to that of impingement. Associated numbness and paresthesias in the appropriate dermatomal distribution will often direct the examiner toward the appropriate diagnosis. Often an associated sensation of clumsiness with the hand will be voiced by the patient

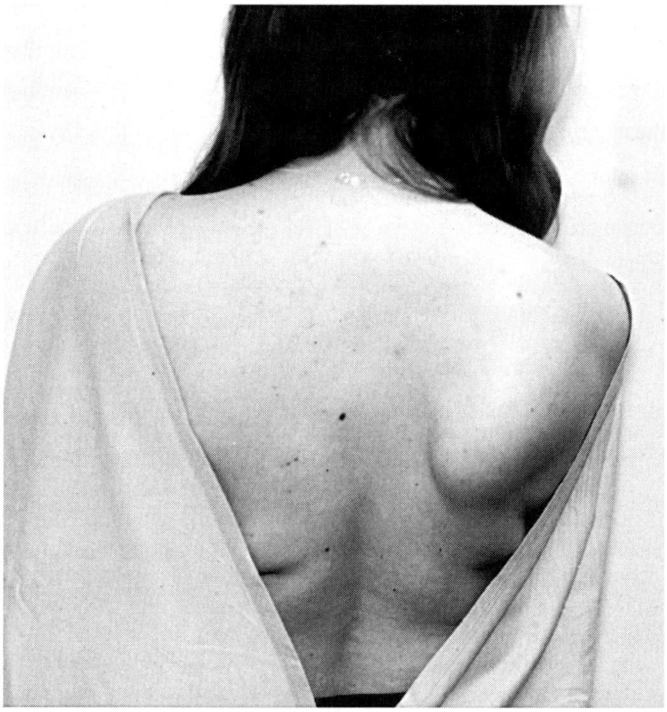

Fig. 5–15. Scapular winging with secondary nonoutlet impingement. Brachial plexus traction injury resulted in this lesion. Note that the gown has slipped off her ptotic shoulder. Had this not occurred, this type of inappropriate exam-wear might have precluded the diagnosis. Her hair, which should have been tied up, hides the scar from an unsuccessful cervical disc surgery done for brachial plexus traction injury.

with a frequency of dropping objects. Tinel's sign may be present over the region of the cubital and/or carpal tunnels with recreation of the patient's paresthesias in the ulnar and median nerve distributions respectively. Provocative maneuvers such as prolonged elbow flexion, Phalen's, and reverse Phalen's tests can be performed to elucidate the presence of these conditions. Decreased two-point discrimination and intrinsic atrophy are usually late findings with regard to peripheral compression neuropathies.[26] Diminished vibratory sense is felt to be a subtle finding present early on in the course of these syndromes and is an easily reproducible test with the use of a tuning fork.[26,27] EMG and nerve conduction velocity examination may show evidence of slowed conduction and latency at the appropriate anatomic levels to help in diagnosis. However, EMG testing may often be nonspecific in relation to these conditions. The diagnosis is often made on the preponderance of clinical evidence in this regard, with the exclusion of other possible etiologies.

In addition to neurologic disease, neoplasms may also primarily involve the shoulder or subsequently metastasize to the region. An associated history of carcinoma, especially with tumors that have a predilection for metastasis to bone (thyroid, renal, lung, prostate, and breast), should make the examiner highly suspect. Care must therefore be taken to obtain a full past medical history. Pain complaints are often present at rest, with exacerbation at night. Atypical pain patterns without relief by selective injection with local anesthetic to the region should alert the examiner to other possible underlying pathology. Plain radiographs often demonstrate evidence of bony changes and should be carefully examined for subtle lytic and/or destructive changes. Bone scanning, CT, and MRI studies can be obtained as indicated for further evaluation of the lesion. Typically, if indicated, biopsy should be deferred to the treating oncologic surgeon. The admonition that dogs can have ticks and fleas at the same time is illustrated by a patient with a positive arthrogram as well as metastatic disease in the scapula.

Rheumatologic conditions may also involve the shoulder and have symptomatology that mimics primary rotator cuff disease. Polymyalgia rheumatica (PMR) is a rheumatologic condition that may involve the shoulder and may present in a fashion similar to rotator cuff tearing. Typically, patients with PMR are men in the fifth or sixth decade of life. Patients complain of pain and stiffness in the shoulder and/or pelvic girdles of insidious onset. Associated fever, weight loss, anorexia, and malaise may be present. Symmetric shoulder synovitis is common. Sternoclavicular and acromioclavicular pain may occur in as many as 15% of patients. Physical examination may reveal atrophy with diffuse tenderness to palpation over the muscle mass. Generalized, rather than isolated, muscle weakness is the usual feature of PMR and can be used as a delineating factor from primary rotator cuff disease. Temporal arteritis commonly occurs in association with PMR and may exist in those patients with complaints of headaches in association with shoulder pain. Radiographic evaluation often is unremarkable. Laboratory findings will show an elevated sedimentation rate, normochromic-normocytic anemia, and, occasionally, an elevated alkaline phosphatase.[28]

Fibromyalgia is another rheumatologic entity that has gained significant recognition in recent years as a cause of myofascial pain. Patients with fibromyalgia may present with complaints of vague shoulder pain reminiscent of a primary shoulder etiology. However, multiple diffuse trigger points are noted on examination that usually assume a typical pattern overlying the shoulders, back, and pelvic girdle. Pain may be worse at night with a history of sleep disturbance. Fibromyalgia may occur secondary to an acute traumatic event or be of idiopathic onset. Patients will often improve with gentle antidepressant medication and sedatives to aid in normalization of their sleep patterns coupled with a gentle aerobic exercise program.[29–31]

Systemic pathology may also be an extrinsic cause of shoulder pain that may present in a similar fashion to that of rotator cuff pathology. Care must be taken with the initial history not to ignore other systemic complaints in favor of focusing solely on the shoulder when more grave pathology may be present elsewhere. Some conditions that may have referred visceral pain to the shoulder that may mimic rotator cuff pathology are cholecystitis, coronary artery disease, and apical pulmonary disease. Suspicion of the presence of these conditions often leads to their discovery rather than their misdiagnosis.

CONCLUSION

The shoulder can be affected by both intrinsic and extrinsic conditions that may mimic rotator cuff pathology on initial presentation. Care must be taken in obtaining a medical history and with evaluation of the patient who presents with a complaint of shoulder pain similar to impingement and rotator cuff tendinopathy, because many more serious and/or unrelated conditions may be easily overlooked.

REFERENCES

1. Moseley HF. Ruptures of the rotator cuff. *Br J Surg.* 1951;38:340–369.
2. Lewis T. *Pain.* New York: McMillan; 1942.
3. Roos DB. Congenital anomalies associated with thoracic outlet syndrome. Anatomy, symptoms, diagnosis, and treatment. *Am J Surg.* 132:771–778, 1976.
4. Leffert RD. Thoracic outlet syndrome. In: Gelberman RH, ed. *Operative Nerve Repair and Reconstruction.* New York: JB Lippincott; 1991:1177–1195.
5. Urschel HC, Paulson DL, MacNamara JJ. Thoracic outlet syndrome. *Ann Thorac Surg.* 1968;6:1.
6. Jupiter J, Leffert RD. Non-union of the clavicle: Associated complications and surgical management. *J Bone Joint Surg Am.* 1987;69:753–760.
7. Leffert RD, Seddon HJ. Infraclavicular brachial plexus injuries. *J. Bone Joint Surg Br.* 1965;47:9.

8. Leffert RD. Thoracic outlet and the shoulder. In: Jobe F, ed. *Clinics in Sports Medicine. Symposium on Injuries to the Shoulder in the Athlete.* Philadelphia: WB Saunders; 1983.
9. Urschel HC, Rossuk M. Management of thoracic outlet syndrome. *N Eng J Med.* 1972;286:1140.
10. Spinner M. Correspondence club newsletter. 1977:32
11. Parsonage MJ, Turner JWA. Neurologic amyotrophy. The shoulder girdle syndrome. *Lancet.* 1948;1:973–978.
12. Solheim LF, Roaas A. Compression of the suprascapular nerve after fracture of the scapular notch. *Acta Orthop Scand.* 1978;49:338.
13. Ogino T, Minami A, Kato H, et al. Entrapment neuropathy of the suprascapular nerve by a ganglion: A report of three cases. *J Bone Joint Surg Am.* 1991;73:141–147.
14. Post M, Mayer J. Suprascapular nerve entrapment: Diagnosis and treatment. *Clin Orthop.* 1987;223:126.
15. Rengachary SS, Burr D, et al. Suprascapular entrapment neuropathy: Diagnosis and treatment. Parts I, II, and III. *Neurosurg.* 1979; 5:447–451.
16. Burkhead WZ, Scheinberg RR, Box G. Surgical anatomy of the axillary nerve. *J Shoulder Elbow Surg.* 1992;1:31–36.
17. Cooper DE, O'Brien SJ, Warren RF. Supporting layers of the glenohumeral joint. *Clin Orthop.* 1993;289:144–155.
18. Neviaser RJ, Neviaser TJ, Neviaser JS. Anterior dislocation of the shoulder and rotator cuff rupture. *Clin Orthop.* 1993;291:103–106.
19. Cahill BR, Palmer RE. Quadrilateral space syndrome. *J Hand Surg.* 1983;8:65–69.
20. Jobe FW, Tibone JE, et al. The shoulder in sports. In: Rockwood CA, Matsen FA, eds. *The Shoulder.*. Philadelphia: WB Saunders; 1990:961–990.
21. Greenway G. Personal communication, 1992.
22. Narakas AO. Compression and traction neuropathies about the shoulder and arm. In: Gelberman RH, ed. *Operative Nerve Repair and Reconstruction.* New York: JB Lippincott Co; 1991:1147–1175.
23. Bigliani L, Perez-Sanz JR, Wolfe IN. Treatment of trapezius paralysis. *J Bone Joint Surg Am.* 1985;67:871–877.
24. Chavez JP. Pectoralis minor transplanted for paralysis of the serratus anterior. *J Bone Joint Surg Br.* 1951;33:2128.
25. Marmor L, Bechtal CO. Paralysis of the serratus anterior due to electric shock relieved by transplantation of the pectoralis major muscle. A case report. *J Bone Joint Surg Am.* 1983;45:156–160.
26. Szabo RM. Carpal tunnel syndrome—general. In: Gelberman RH, ed. *Operative Nerve Repair and Reconstruction.* New York: JB Lippincott Co;1991:869–888.
27. Slater RR, Bynum DK. Diagnosis and treatment of carpal tunnel syndrome. *Orthop Rev.* 1993;22:1095–1105.
28. Curran JF, Ellman MH, Brown NL. Rheumatologic aspects of painful conditions affecting the shoulder. *Clin. Orthop.* 1983;173:27–37.
29. Goldenberg DL. Fibromyalgia syndrome: An emerging but controversial condition. *J Am Med Assoc.* 1987;257:2782–2787.
30. Fan TP, Blanton ME. Clinical features and diagnosis of fibromyalgia. *J Musculo Med.* 1992;24–42.
31. Nies KM. Treatment of the fibromyalgia syndrome. *J Musculo Med.* 1992;20–26.

Chapter 6

Imaging of the Rotator Cuff

Guerdon Greenway and J. Mark Fulmer

The past two decades have witnessed rapid growth in the clinical understanding of lesions of the rotator cuff and in the concepts underlying the pathophysiology of rotator cuff disease. Paralleling this expansion of clinical knowledge, the radiographic evaluation of rotator cuff pathology has advanced, as well, largely as the result of the introduction of new technology. Currently, physicians treating patients with lesions of the rotator cuff may complement their clinical evaluation with multiple radiographic modalities, including plain films, arthrography, ultrasonography, scintigraphy, computed tomography (CT), computed arthrotomography, and, most recently, magnetic resonance imaging (MRI). Although most of these examinations are not routinely indicated, often, one or more of these imaging modalities may provide significant information in the clinical evaluation of suspected lesions of the rotator cuff.

PLAIN FILM RADIOGRAPHY

Technique

The radiographic evaluation of the shoulder should begin with a plain film examination. Indeed, most physicians interested in the diagnosis and treatment of shoulder pain incorporate plain radiographs into their initial evaluation. The traditional plain film examination usually includes two frontal views of the shoulder, with the humerus in internal and external rotation.[1] The anteroposterior (AP) view of the shoulder, however, is not a true AP view of the scapula, and the glenohumeral joint is viewed obliquely. A true AP radiograph of the scapula is obtained with the patient in the 40° posterior oblique position.[2,3] This view provides the optimal projection for evaluation of the glenohumeral joint, as the articulation is projected tangentially and the osseus glenoid is printed. In order to view the glenoid at right angles to the frontal view, either an axillary view or a lateral scapular view should be obtained. The axillary view is obtained with the arm abducted and with the humerus in external rotation. The cassette is placed adjacent to the superior aspect of the shoulder, and the radiographic beam is directed through the glenohumeral joint angled 15 to 30° toward the midline in the coronal plane (Fig. 6–1).[4,5] In addition to visualizing the glenoid and assessing glenohumeral relationships, the axillary view displays the lateral extent of the coracoid process and provides the best evaluation of an os acromiale. It is also the most appropriate projection to assess an anterior acromial protuberance, as described by Gartsman.[6] The lateral scapular view is obtained with the patient in a 60° anterior oblique position.[7–9] This view may be obtained with the patient upright or recumbent. In this projection, the scapula appears as a "Y," with the body of the scapula forming the vertical limb and the acromion and coracoid processes each forming an upper limb. The glenoid fossa is visualized as a circular density at the junction of these three limbs. Normally, the humeral head is directly superimposed over this junction. In addition to defining glenohumeral relationships, the lateral scapular view provides excellent assessment of the anterior acromion and the AC joint.

In the classical shoulder impingement syndrome, pain is elicited by comparison of the supraspinatus tendon and the subacromial bursa, between the greater tuberosity of the humerus and one or more components

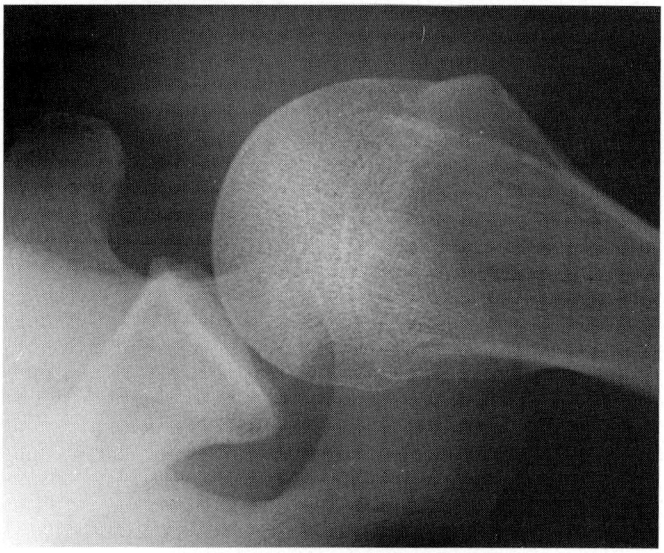

Fig. 6–1. Normal axillary view.

of the coracoacromial arch superiorally. This long, bony-ligamentous arch consists of the AC joint, the anterior third of the acromion, the coracoacromial ligament, and the anterior portion of the coracoid process.[10–12] Congenital variations or acquired abnormalities of this arch may narrow the supraspinatus outlet and, thus, predispose the development of the impingement syndrome. Consequently, additional radiographic views have been developed to evaluate the coracoacromial arch.

Subacromial spurs arise in the insertion of the coracoacromial ligament.[13–15] These spurs are best evaluated with the subacromial or "caudal tilt" view, an AP radiograph of the shoulder centered over the acromion with the beam angled 30° in the caudal direction (Fig. 6–2).[11,14,16–20] In this view, the radiographic beam passes parallel to the inferior surface of the acromion, permitting inferiorly projecting spurs to be more easily visualized (Fig. 6–3).

The anterior portion of the acromion is also well demonstrated on the supraspinatus outlet view, a modified lateral scapular or scapular "Y" view (Fig. 6–4). This view is obtained with the patient placed in the 60° anterior oblique position, which places the blade of the scapula perpendicular to the film. The radiographic beam is centered at the AC joint and is angled 10° caudally.[6,11,18,20–22] When properly positioned and exposed, this view clearly demonstrates the anterior projection of the acromion. The combination of the subacromial (caudal tilt) view with the supraspinatus outlet view provides near orthogonal projections of the anterior one-third of the acromion. A modification of the axillary view, described by Andrews et al., has also been used to provide a sagittal view of the anterior acromion.[23]

There is substantial variation in the configuration of the acromion. Morrison and Bigliani have defined three types of acromia based on the slope of the undersurface of the acromion (Figs. 6–5 and 6–6).[24,25,63] Type I has a flat undersurface; Type II has a concave, curved undersurface; Type III has an anteroinferior hook at the anterior edge of the undersurface. Type III acromia were found in 40% of the general population but were evident in 70 to 80% of patients with rotator cuff tears.[24,25] This

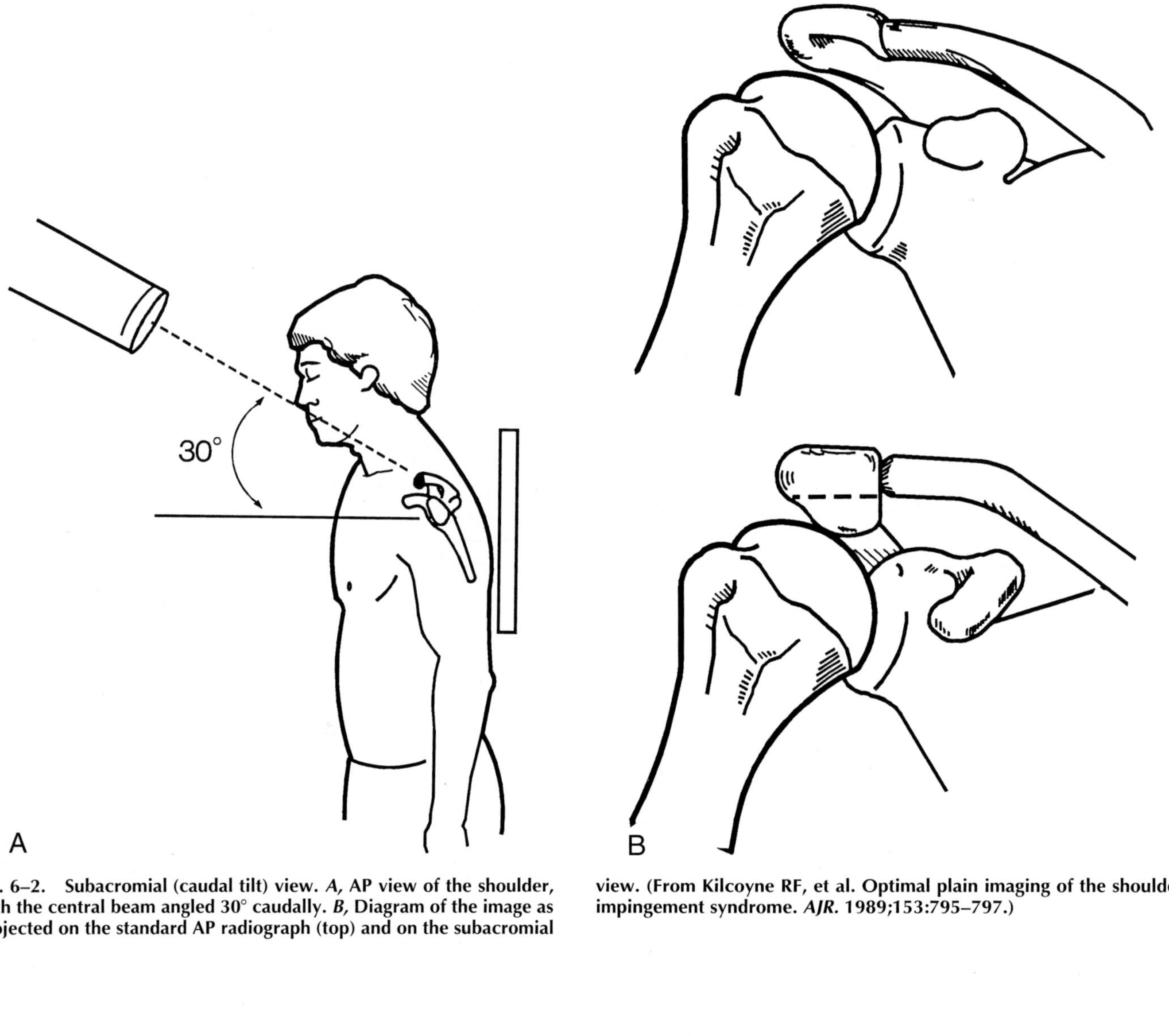

Fig. 6–2. Subacromial (caudal tilt) view. *A,* AP view of the shoulder, with the central beam angled 30° caudally. *B,* Diagram of the image as projected on the standard AP radiograph (top) and on the subacromial view. (From Kilcoyne RF, et al. Optimal plain imaging of the shoulder impingement syndrome. *AJR.* 1989;153:795–797.)

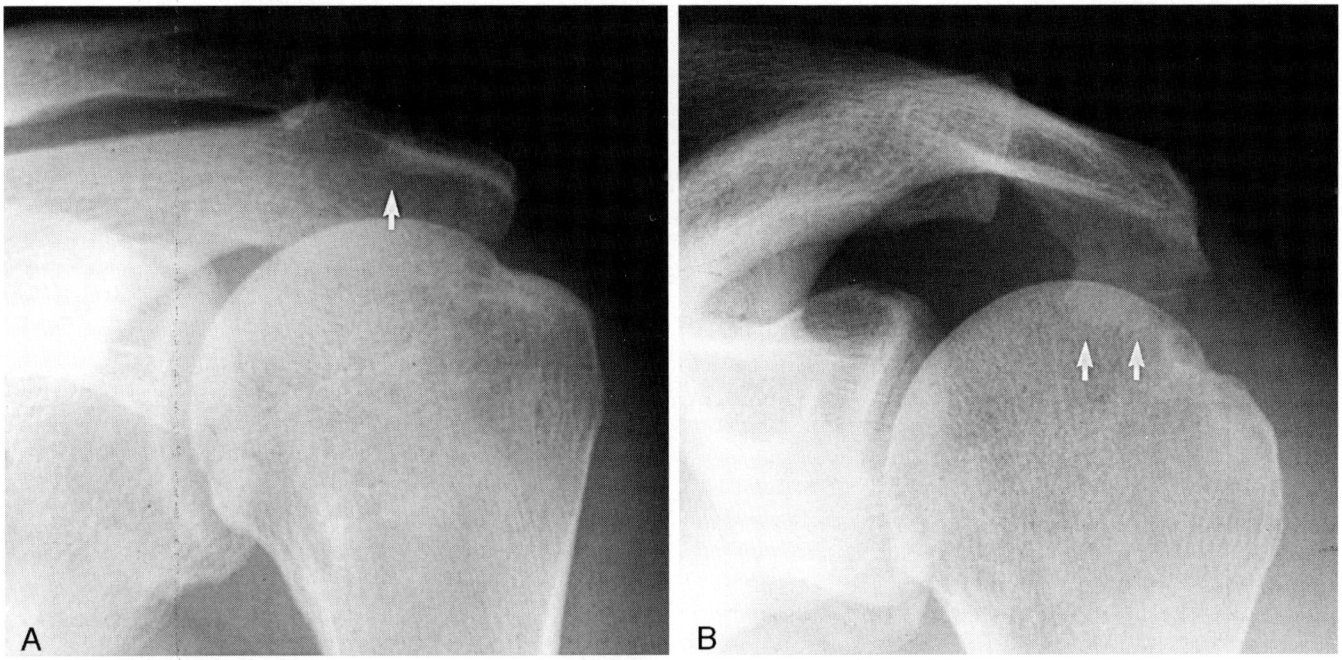

Fig. 6–3. Radiographic evaluation of subacromial spurs. *A,* Conventional AP radiograph of the shoulder. The anterior subacromial spur is superimposed over the acromion itself and is difficult to visualize (arrow). *B,* Subacromial view on the same patient, demonstrating a large acromial spur (arrows).

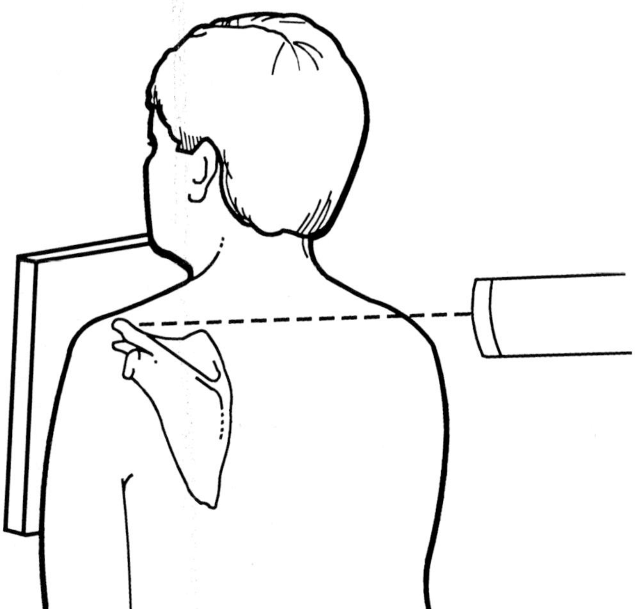

Fig. 6–4. The supraspinatus outlet view. This represents a modified lateral scapular view, with 10° of caudal angulation of the central beam, profiling the supraspinatus outlet. (From Kilcoyne RF, et al. Optimal plain film imaging of the shoulder impingement syndrome. *AJR.* 1989; 153:795–797.)

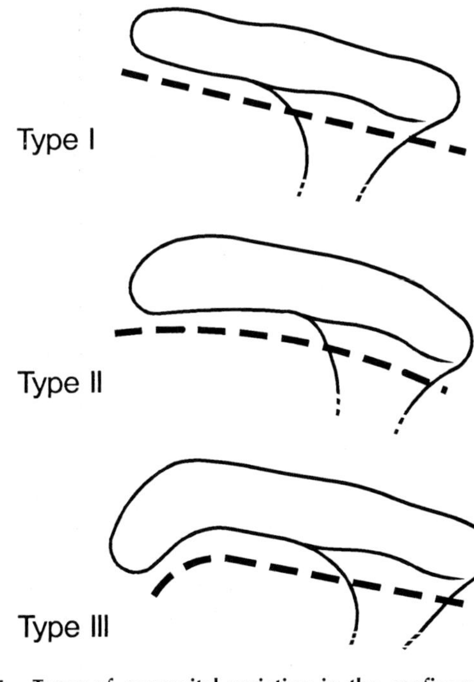

Fig. 6–5. Types of congenital variation in the configuration of the acromion. Type III results in narrowing of the supraspinatus outlet.

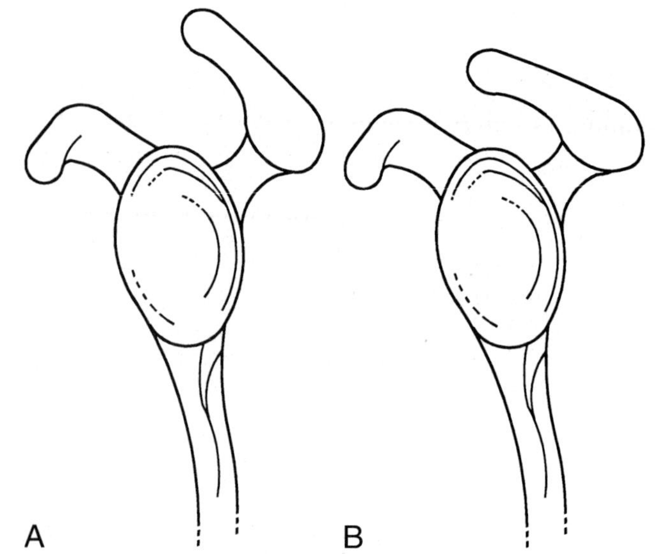

Fig. 6–6. *A,* **Congenital variations in the slope of the acromion. Note that a more horizontal orientation of the acromion results in narrowing of the supraspinatus outlet** ***(B).***

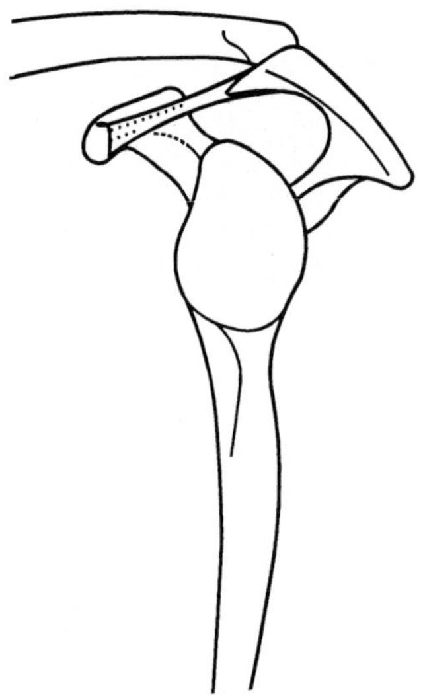

Fig. 6–7. Subacromial spur. This represents ossification in the acromial insertion of the coracoacromial ligament.

acromial morphology is best assessed on the supraspinatus outlet view. MRI has also been used to evaluate acromial shape.[26] Edelson and Taitz evaluated scapular specimens using lateral scapular radiographs and assessed degenerative changes in the anterior third of the acromion.[27] They noted that the more horizontal the acromion, the greater the incidence of degeneration. No acromion with a slope of 41° had degenerative changes (Figs. 6–7 and 6–8). However, 75% of acromia with slope angles of 35° or less manifested degenerative changes. The length of the acromion and the height of the coracoacromial arch also correlated with the incidence of degenerative change.

Osteoarthritis of the AC joint may result in osteophytes, which extend inferiorly and impinge on the rotator cuff.[10,11,28,29,63] As such, their preoperative identification is significant. Although the AC joint is usually adequately evaluated on routine AP radiographs of the shoulder, specific views of the joint may be indicated in special circumstances. These consist of an AP view centered at the joint, with 15° of cephalic angulation of the central ray, as well as a lateral view.[30,31] The lateral view is obtained with the patient in the posteroanterior projection and turned in a 35° antero-oblique position. The central ray is directed at the coracoid process, with 15° of caudal angulation.

Biceps tenosynovitis and rupture are related to subacromial impingement.[10,12,63] The long head of the biceps tendon is particularly vulnerable in the presence of a shallow intertubercular sulcus.[14,32] Plain film evaluation of the biceps groove is accomplished with the tangential view of the intertubercular sulcus.[32,33] With the patient supine and with the arm in external rotation, the cassette is placed perpendicular to the superior aspect of the shoulder. The central beam is directed parallel to the coronal axis of the humerus and angled 15° medially.

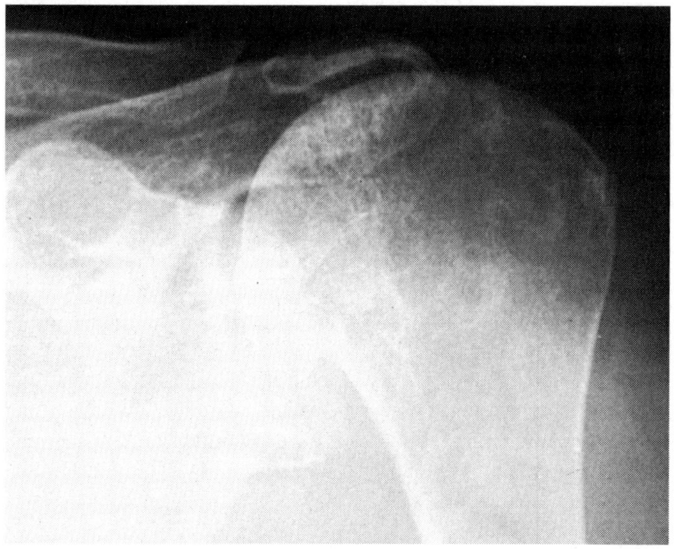

Fig. 6–8. Changes in the glenohumeral joint secondary to a chronic complete rotator cuff tear. Note the cyst formation around the greater tuberosity, the prominent narrowing of the acromiohumeral distance, and the concave erosion of the undersurface of the acromion.

Recommended Views

Physicians evaluating patients with impingement syndrome have multiple radiographic options. The recommended orthopaedic shoulder series is as follows:[22]

1. Posterior oblique AP projection, with external rotation of the humerus.

2. Standard AP projection of the shoulder, with the humerus in internal rotation.
3. Supraspinatus outlet view.
4. Axillary view.
5. Subacromial or caudal tilt view.

Findings

In the early stages of the impingement syndrome, plain radiographs of the shoulder are often normal.[34] Indeed, some patients with rotator cuff tears, especially those with tears of a single tendon, often demonstrate no radiographic abnormality.[35] As the impingement process progresses, however, the rotator cuff tears become more extensive, and radiographic changes become increasingly evident.[35]

Subacromial spurs represent one of the most common radiographic abnormalities noted in patients with rotator cuff lesions. In patients with the impingement syndrome, these spurs were identified radiographically in 68% of patients and operatively in 81% of patients.[35,36] In a series of 100 patients, subacromial spurs were identified on AP radiographs made with the standing patient rotated until the scapula was parallel to the film and using 22 to 25° of caudal beam angulation (modified subacromial view). The study demonstrated a direct correlation between the incidence of rotator cuff tears and the size of the subacromial spur.[19]

Subacromial spurs represent ossification in the acromial insertion of the coracoacromial ligament.[12–14,27,63] These spurs are thought to result from the transmission of tensile forces through the ligament, secondary to repetitive impingement of the greater tuberosity of the humerus on the ligament.[12,14,27] Indeed, Cone et al. believe that the presence of a subacromial spur is presumptive evidence of shoulder impingement.[14] The absence of spurs at the coracoid insertion of the coracoacromial ligament is caused by the triangular shape of the ligament, which has a wide base attached to the coracoid. Tensile forces are thus distributed over a broad area, and osteophyte formation does not occur.[27]

Degenerative change of the greater tuberosity, including osseous proliferation, sclerosis, and cortical cystic change, is common.[14,34,35,38–40] Hardy et al. noted these findings in 66% of patients with impingement syndrome, and Norwood et al. identified an even higher incidence of these changes in patients with rotator cuff tears.[34,35]

Narrowing of the acromial-humeral interval is frequently noted in patients with impingement syndrome.[11,34,35,40] This is the result of both attritional changes within the substance of the cuff and loss of the depressor function of the rotator cuff. The acromiohumeral interval is defined as the shortest distance between the superior aspect of the humeral head and the inferior cortical surface of the acromion and normally measures 6 to 14 mm on an AP supine film.[41–44] Acromiohumeral measurements of less than 7 mm are associated with an increased incidence of rotator cuff tear.[35,40] A reduction of the acromiohumeral distance to less than 6 mm is generally agreed to be indicative of a rotator cuff pathology.[44] When measuring the acromiohumeral distance, the rotation of the humerus must be taken into consideration, as external rotation of the humeral head normally results in a decrease in the acromiohumeral interval.[37]

Bloom has advocated the use of the active abduction view in the evaluation of rotator cuff tears.[45] A standing AP radiograph of the shoulder is obtained as the patient actively abducts the shoulder to 90° from the horizontal or, if this is not possible, to the maximum extent. Reduction of the acromiohumeral distance to 2 mm or less occurred only in those patients with complete rotator cuff tears.

As the rotator cuff atrophies, superior migration of the humeral head occurs. Ultimately, pressure by the unopposed humeral head causes pressure atrophy and concavity of the undersurface of the acromion.[35,38,40] This finding is strongly indicative of an associated rotator cuff tear.[35]

Osteoarthritis of the AC joint, often associated with inferiorly oriented osteophytes, is a frequent finding in patients with both the impingement syndrome and with rotator cuff tears.[28,34,35]

A distinctive form of shoulder arthropathy, associated with massive, longstanding rotator cuff tears, has been described by Neer and termed "cuff tear arthropathy."[46] This condition has also been reported in the medical literature as Milwaukee shoulder,[47] apatite-associated destructive arthritis,[48] and idiopathic destructive arthritis of the shoulder.[49] The patients are classically elderly females with joint instability, massive rotator cuff tears, large, blood-stained joint effusions containing basic calcium phosphate crystals, decreased mobility, and marked osseous resorption.[49] The radiologic findings include prominent, smooth pressure-type erosions of the humeral head and neck, greater tuberosity, glenoid, and anterior acromion and AC joint. Osteophyte formation is unusual, although subchondral sclerosis is frequently present. Subluxation of the humeral head superiorly or superomedially is a prominent finding (Fig. 6–9).[46,49] Periarticular calcification is occasionally present. The radiographic differential diagnosis includes rheumatoid arthritis, neuroarthropathy, and pyrophosphate arthropathy. Interestingly, some of these patients exhibit destructive arthritis in other articulations, indicating that the shoulder may not be a unique location for this process.[50,51]

An os acromiale represents a failure of fusion of one or more of the three ossification centers of the acromial epiphysis: the meta-acromion (proximal center), the mesoacromion, and the preacromion (distal center) (Fig. 6–10). The most common site of nonunion is between the mesoacromion and the meta-acromion.[52] This ossification variant, bilateral in over 65% of individuals, is best demonstrated on the axillary view. Instability resulting from the fibrous union may contribute to the impingement syndrome.[52,53] However, the incidence of unfused acromial epiphysis is no greater in patients with

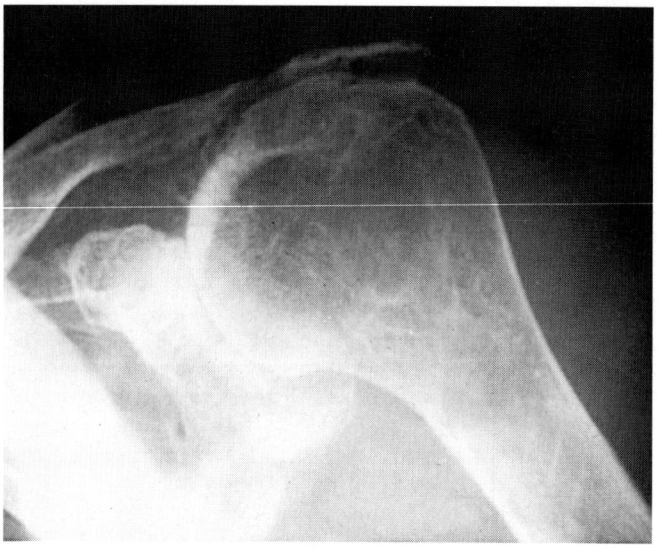

Fig. 6–9. Cuff-tear arthropathy. *A,* AP radiograph of the shoulder demonstrating changes of a chronic rotator cuff tear.

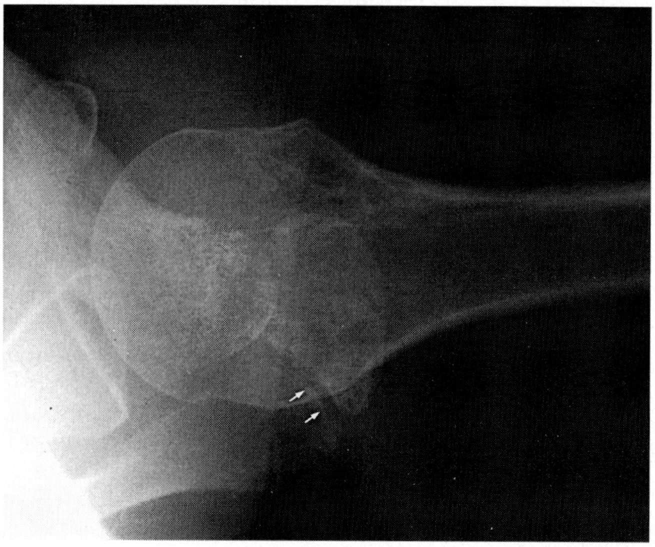

Fig. 6–10. Os acromiale. Axillary view demonstrating a large os acromiale (arrows).

tears of the rotator cuff,[10] and the anomaly is often asymptomatic.[54]

Calcium hydroxyapatite crystal deposition disease or calcific tendinitis is discussed thoroughly in Chapter 16.

Osseous Scintigraphy

Osseous scintigraphy is used primarily as a screening examination and has high sensitivity but relatively low specificity. Bone scanning is almost exclusively performed using Technetium-99m-labeled phosphate esters, either polyphosphates or diphosphonates. These radiotracers localize preferentially in bone through the phenomenon of chemisorption, during which the tracer is adsorbed on the hydration shell of hydroxyapatite.[64] Two processes facilitate the increased uptake of these imaging tracers:

1. Increased blood flow
2. Increased bone turnover

Areas of high osteoblastic activity and newly deposited bone mineral contain smaller crystals with greater surface area, which results in increased adsorption of the radiotracer.[64] Thus, osseous lesions, characterized by either hyperemia or mineralization of osteoid, demonstrate increased scintigraphic uptake.

In evaluating patients with suspected lesions of the rotator cuff, scintigraphy often directs clinical attention to specific or unsuspected skeletal lesions. Osteoarthritis of the glenohumeral or AC joints may be identified and unsuspected neoplastic lesions of the shoulder girdle detected. Scintigraphy also provides confirmation of the clinical diagnosis of adhesive capsulitis, revealing diffuse scintigraphic uptake without focal abnormality.

SONOGRAPHY

Sonographic evaluation of the rotator cuff became a clinically viable tool in the mid-1980s.[65,66] More recently, newer modalities have risen to prominence. However, the widespread availability and comparatively low cost of sonograms make this tool a powerful part of the imaging armamentarium.

Technique

As with all sonographic imaging, shoulder sonography necessitates that the appropriate equipment be used and that meticulous scanning technique be employed. These must be combined with a thorough knowledge of the sonographic appearance of the normal and abnormal rotator cuff.

High-frequency linear array transducers provide the near-field resolution required in rotator cuff sonography. Most investigators advocate 5-MHz, 7.5-MHz, or 10-MHz transducers, sometimes referred to as "small parts" transducers.[67,68] Real-time gray-scale imaging is used, with static or video images used for documentation.

A complete sonographic examination includes both shoulders. The examiner can evaluate the anterior and posterior musculotendinous junctions, the biceps tendon structures, and tendon motion during abduction, internal rotation, and external rotation (Fig. 6–11). A bedside study can be performed.

The biceps tendon groove of the humerus is the landmark for evaluation of anterior shoulder structures. Scanning in the transverse plane, the examiner identifies the biceps tendon as an echogenic structure within the humeral groove (Fig. 6–12). This tendon is traced superiorly to identify the rotator cuff (Fig. 6–13).

An oblique sagittal orientation of the transducer allows

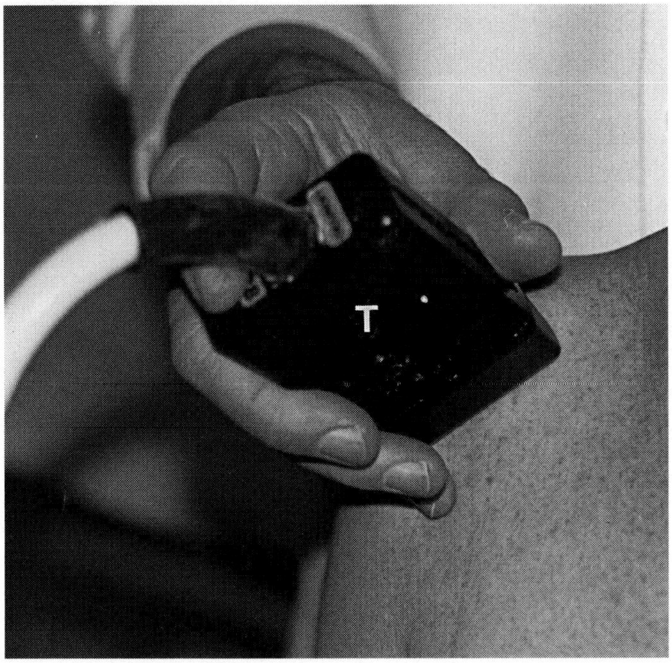

Fig. 6–11. Patient positioning for a sonographic examination. The patient is seated, facing away from the examiner. The sonogram transducer (T) is positioned to allow evaluation of the rotator cuff. The examination begins with the patient's arm in neutral position.

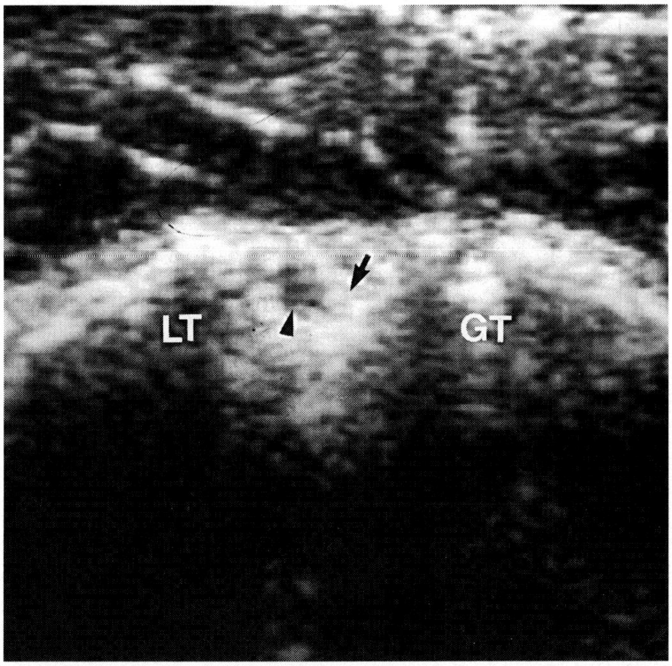

Fig. 6–12. Normal sonography appearance of biceps tendon. The biceps tendon groove of the humerus is defined by the brightly reflecting greater tuberosity (GT) and lesser tuberosity (LT) of the humerus. The normal biceps tendon (arrow) is an echogenic structure within the groove. There is normally a small amount of fluid (arrowhead) around the tendon.

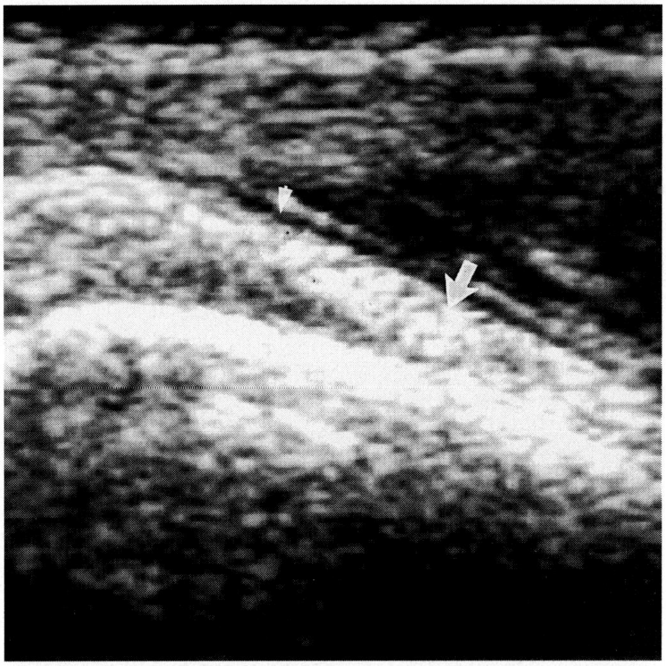

Fig. 6–13. Longitudinal evaluation of the biceps tendon. The biceps tendon (arrow) is identified in its long axis. A small amount of fluid is seen superiorly (arrowhead).

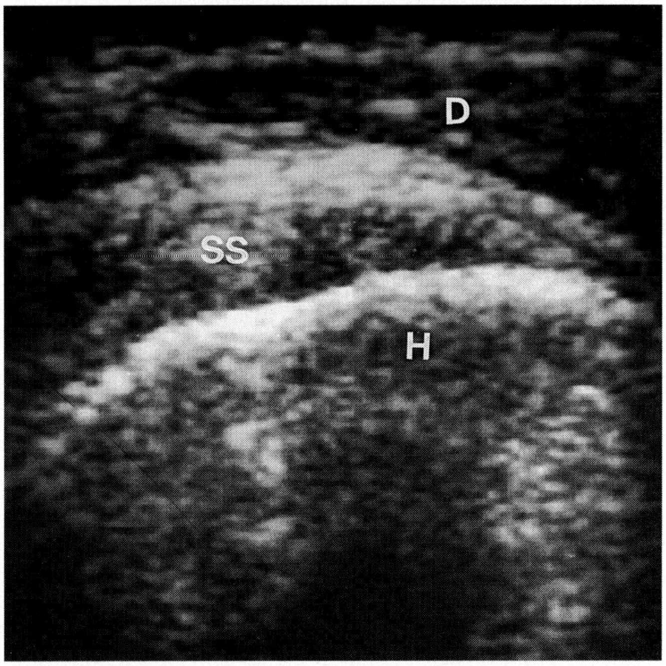

Fig. 6–14. Evaluation of the long axis of the supraspinatus muscle. The distal supraspinatus muscle (SS) is beak-shaped and homogeneous in echo texture. The deltoid (D) is shown more superficially, and the brightly reflecting humerus is visualized (H).

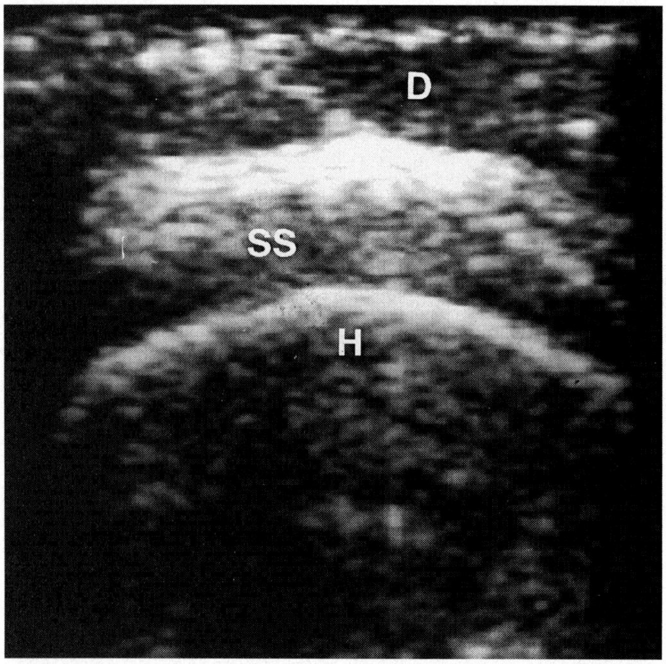

Fig. 6–15. Transverse evaluation of the distal supraspinatus muscle. The supraspinatus muscle (SS) is homogeneous in echo texture and crescent-shaped in the transverse orientation. The humeral head (H) and deltoid muscle (D) are also seen.

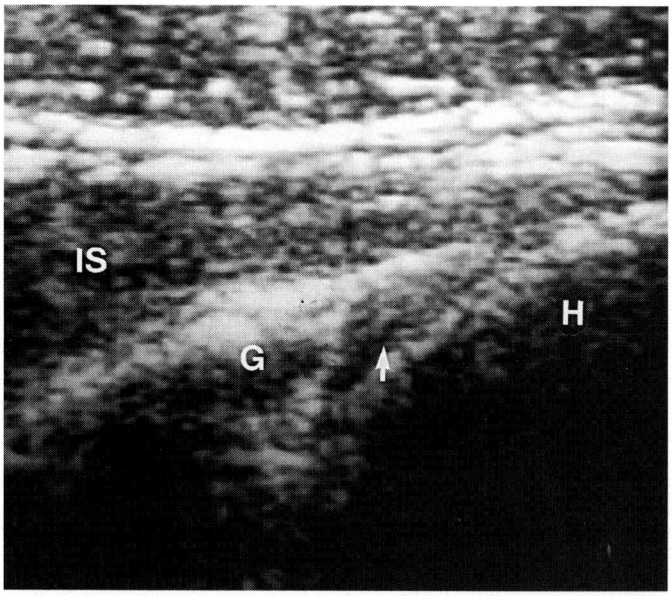

Fig. 6–16. Posterior structures of the shoulder. The osseous glenoid (G) and glenoid cartilage (arrow) can be identified posteriorly. The infraspinatus muscle (IS) and trapezius muscle are shown. The posterior humeral head (H) is also identified.

identification of the distal supraspinatus muscle, the supraspinatus tendon, and the greater tuberosity of the humerus (Fig. 6–14). Transverse scanning of the supraspinatus muscle and tendon is achieved by orienting the transducer 90° (Fig. 6–15).

The anterior portion of the examination also includes assessment of the subacromial and subdeltoid bursae. These structures are visualized in a para-sagittal orientation, slightly lateral to the distal supraspinatus muscle.[69] These potential spaces are normally not discernible as separate structures. However, fluid accumulation can be indirect evidence of rotator cuff disease.

In the posterior aspect of the shoulder, the posterior cartilaginous glenoid is seen as an echogenic triangle adjacent to the posterior aspect of the humeral head. The infraspinatus muscle is usually visible and is identified as an hypoechoic structure with a rhomboid shape (Fig. 6–16).

Assessment of tendon dynamics is performed by aligning the transducer along the long axis of the biceps tendon. The patient is then asked to flex the elbow against resistance supplied by the examiner. A similar maneuver is performed by aligning the transducer along the supraspinatus musculotendinous junction and by allowing the patient to abduct the humerus against resistance. In each case, attention is directed to the ease of tendon motion and the homogeneity of tendon texture. These maneuvers may display previously undetected inhomogeneities, particularly when compared to the asymptomatic shoulder.

Pathology

Abnormalities of the rotator cuff may demonstrate a variety of appearances on the sonographic examination.[70–72] Absence of the supraspinatus muscle and tendon is the most definitive finding of a rotator cuff tear. This is usually seen in elderly patients (older than 60 years of age) with a chronic tear in which the deltoid muscle is visible along with the greater tuberosity of the humerus but no supraspinatus structures can be identified. This is evidence of complete rotator cuff disruption, with retraction of the supraspinatus muscle beneath the clavicle.

Partial tears of the rotator cuff demonstrate more subtle sonographic abnormalities. The hallmark of a partial tear is the finding of fluid within the distal supraspinatus muscle or tendon. This manifests as a focus of echo loss, usually seen centrally in the distal muscle bundle at the musculotendinous junction. A focal gap may also be noted along the superior or inferior surface of the distal supraspinatus tendon. Partial rotator cuff tears have also been described as focal areas of increased echogenicity within the supraspinatus muscle.

The diagnosis of rotator cuff tendinitis has received less attention in the sonography literature, but both thinning and thickening of the supraspinatus tendon have been reported as evidence of tendon abnormality.

Irregularity in the contour of the muscle is a manifestation of impingement, and echogenic shadowing foci are seen in calcific tendinitis. Although less commonly demonstrated, similar areas of irregularity or alterations in echo texture can be found in the other muscles of the rotator cuff. Figure 6–17 demonstrates the spectrum of

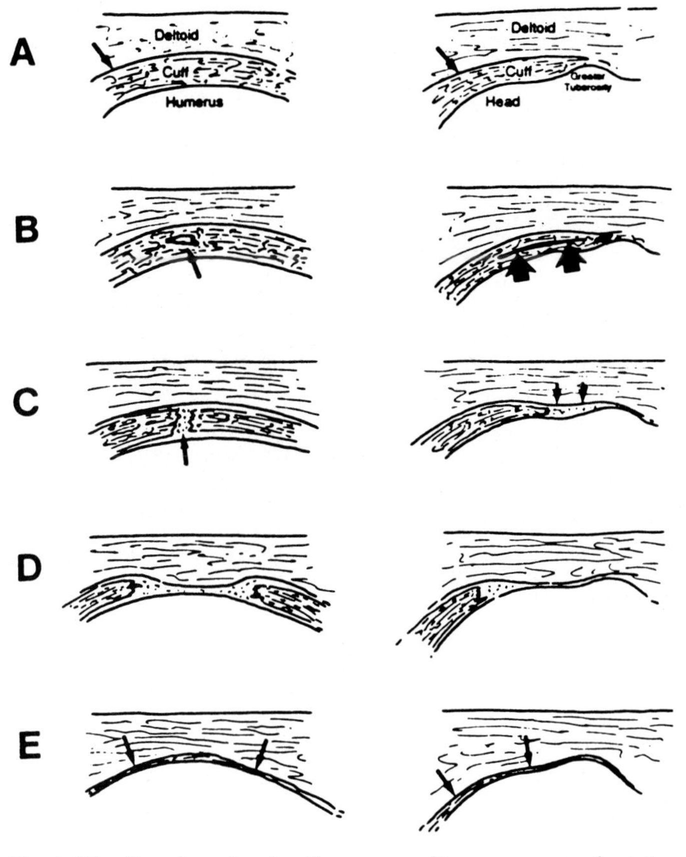

Fig. 6–17. Drawings showing the sonographic appearance of rotator cuff integrity in axial (left) and sagittal (right) planes. *A,* Normal rotator cuff with preserved anterior echogenic arc (arrow) of subdeltoid fascia and peritendinous fat. *B,* Partial-thickness tear appearing as intratendinous hypoechoic (thin arrow) or dominant echogenic (thick arrows) focus. *C,* Small full-thickness tear appearing as hypoechoic area of cuff discontinuity (long arrow) and loss of anterior arc and cuff substance at junction of cuff with greater tuberosity (short arrows). *D,* Large full-thickness tear. *E,* Massive tear. The rotator cuff is not visualized, and the subdeltoid fascia (arrow) "approximates" the humeral head.

sonographic abnormalities that may be demonstrated at the time of rotator cuff sonography.

Indirect evidence of rotator cuff disruption is seen as fluid accumulation in the subacromial and subdeltoid bursae. Dynamic maneuvers are particularly important, and any alteration in the shape and degree of distention during humeral rotation and abduction must be noted.

In the setting of shoulder trauma, sonography may allow demonstration of tendon avulsion, biceps tendon dislocation, and hemarthrosis. Similarly, evaluation of the postoperative shoulder may demonstrate recurrent disruption or focal hematoma.[73,74]

Pitfalls

There are innumerable pitfalls in the sonographic evaluation of the rotator cuff.[75–77] The normal biceps tendon is hyperechoic when compared to the supraspinatus muscle and tendon. Care must be taken not to mistake the crossing biceps tendon for focal increased echogenicity in the supraspinatus muscle (Fig. 6–18). Also, there is a normal focus of decreased echogenicity immediately posterior to the biceps tendon representing a small volume of fluid that normally surrounds the tendon. It can easily be mistaken for focal muscle disruption. Posterior thinning of the supraspinatus muscle is a normal finding and should not be ascribed to impingement. Glenohumeral instability has been shown to result in artifactual thickening of the supraspinatus muscle, because of subluxation of the humerus inferiorly. In many cases, comparison of the asymptomatic shoulder will prevent misinterpretation of normal structures or demonstrate symmetric variability in the echogenicity of the supraspinatus structures. Sonography may be impossible because of overlying bone, if the patient's acromion is large or there is clavicular deformity.

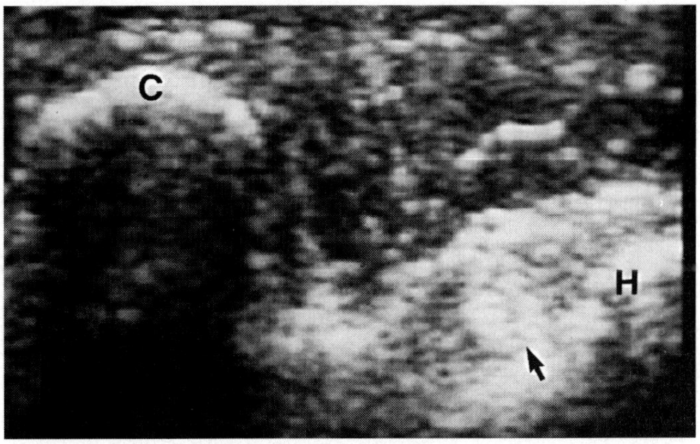

Fig. 6–18. Intra-articular biceps tendon. The crossing biceps tendon (arrow) demonstrates an hyperechoic focus in the more proximal supraspinatus muscle. This should not be ascribed to focal abnormality of the supraspinatus muscle. The coracoid process (C) and humeral head (H) demonstrate intense reflections.

SUMMARY

In the hands of experienced sonographers, shoulder sonography has been successful in evaluating rotator cuff pathology. The sensitivity for diagnosing cuff tears compares well with arthrography, approaching 95% in some series.[78,79] If no supraspinatus muscle or tendon is identified, the positive predictive value of complete tear is 100%. The major drawback of rotator cuff sonography is the expertise required to perform the study, particularly when more subtle abnormalities are sought. The range of reported sensitivities extends as low as 37% when comparing sonography to other modalities.[80,81] This has resulted in wide variation in the exuberance with which shoulder sonography has been embraced. In subspecialty practices with high volume shoulder referrals, one can expect a high accuracy rate in sonographic diagnoses. For the practice with only occasional opportunity to perform shoulder sonography, more uncertainty can be anticipated. The learning curve for rotator cuff sonography requires frequent and complete correlation of imaging and operative findings. Sonography of the shoulder will therefore find its greatest use in tertiary or quaternary musculoskeletal practices with a large case load of rotator cuff disease.

Arthrography and Bursography

Arthrography, with either the single or double-contrast technique, has been used in the evaluation of rotator cuff lesions for over 50 years. To perform the study, a 22- or 25-gauge needle is directed, under fluoroscopic control, into the glenohumeral joint from an anterior approach. The joint is then distended with radiographic contrast alone or with both radiographic contrast and air. Collections of contrast within the undersurface of the supraspinatus tendon indicate a partial tear of that structure, while communication with the subacromial-subdeltoid bursae confirms the presence of a full-thickness rotator cuff tear.

Recently, double-contrast arthrography has largely supplanted the single-contrast method in the evaluation of most lesions of the rotator cuff.[82–84] Advantages of the double-contrast method include evaluation of the width of the tear in the supraspinatus tendon, assessment of the quality of the remaining tendon, and visualization of the intra-articular portion of the long head of the biceps tendon (Fig. 6–19).[82–83] Most studies using carefully performed double-contrast arthrography demonstrate good accuracy, sensitivity, and specificity of the examination in the evaluation of rotator cuff tears.[22] Mink et al. demonstrated 100% sensitivity and 96% specificity in the diagnosis of complete rotator cuff tears using this technique.[22,83] However, partial tears of the bursal side of the supraspinatus tendon are not evaluated by glenohumeral arthrography.

Subacromial bursography is infrequently performed, although some investigators have advocated this technique for the evaluation of patients with the impingement syndrome and partial rotator cuff tears.[14,85,88,89] With this technique, a 22- or 25- gauge needle is directed immediately beneath the anterior acromion, using either an anterior or lateral approach, 6 to 10 mL of contrast are then injected. Fluoroscopic views of the bursa are then obtained, with the humerus in abduction and external rotation. The examination is completed with overhead films[14,88] (Fig. 6–20). The radiographic contrast can be diluted with local anesthetic to evaluate pain ablation.

Findings

The diagnosis of a complete rotator cuff tear is confirmed at arthrography by demonstrating opacification of the subacromial bursa. Frequently, the subdeltoid bursa and, occasionally, the subcoracoid bursa are also opacified, as the subacromial bursa usually communicates with the subdeltoid bursa in 80% of individuals and with the subcoracoid bursa in 10% of individuals.[85] Additionally, the anatomic deficit in the supraspinatus tendon is usually evident, as the insertion of this tendon is profiled using the upright double-contrast technique. Although isolated tears of the infraspinatus and

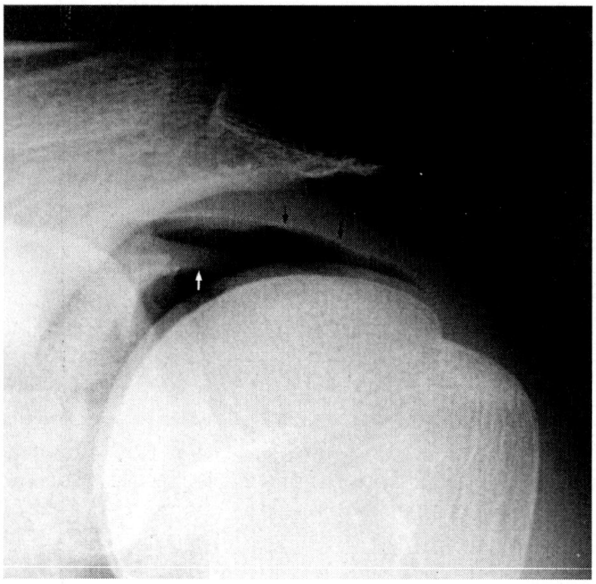

Fig. 6–19. Normal double-contrast arthrogram of the glenohumeral joint. Note the smooth undersurface of the supraspinatus tendon (black arrows), as well as the intra-articular portion of the long head of the biceps tendon (white arrow).

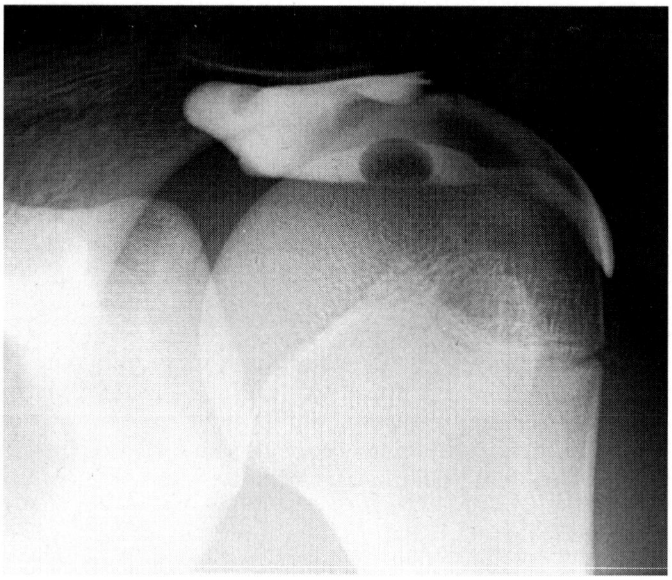

Fig. 6–20. Normal subacromial bursogram.

subscapularis tendons result in opacification of the subacromial bursa, establishing the diagnosis of a rotator cuff tear, their specific localization cannot be ascertained unless the study is followed by a CT examination. The gross width of the supraspinatus tear is generally well demonstrated using double-contrast arthrography, and, usually, the quality of the remaining tendon and the degree of retraction can be assessed. (Figs. 6–21 through 6–23). Degeneration of the rotator cuff tendon results in irregularity of the surface of the tendon and dissection of air and contrast into the substance of the fragments.[82]

Double-contrast arthrography of the glenohumeral joint following repair of a rotator cuff tear often reveals communication with the subacromial bursa.[84] Although this indicates a persistent defect in the rotator cuff tear, many of these patients are free of pain, with a full range of motion.[84] Arthrographic evidence of a rotator cuff tear in the postoperative patient must then be interpreted in the appropriate clinical context.

Partial tears of the supraspinatus tendon are demonstrated as focal, intraendogenous collections of contrast, without opacification of the subacromial bursa (Figs. 6–24 and 6–25).

Lesions of the intra-articular portion of the long head of the biceps tendon can also be demonstrated. Complete rupture of this tendon, medial dislocation, and attritional changes are often evident arthrographically (Fig. 6–26).[82,83]

Adhesive capsulitis is best demonstrated using single-contrast arthrography. With this technique, pain is elicited following the injection of less than 10 mL of radiographic contrast, and a decreased capacity of the joint capsule is evident (Fig. 6–27).[82] Double-contrast arthrography in these cases usually results in dissection of air

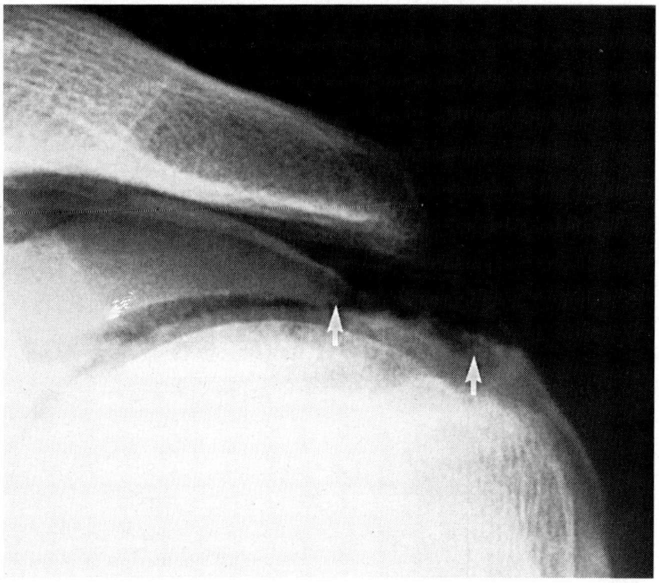

Fig. 6–22. Rotator cuff tear, supraspinatus tendon. There is a focal, 1-cm defect in the insertion of the supraspinatus tendon (arrows). Mild retraction of the supraspinatus muscle is apparent.

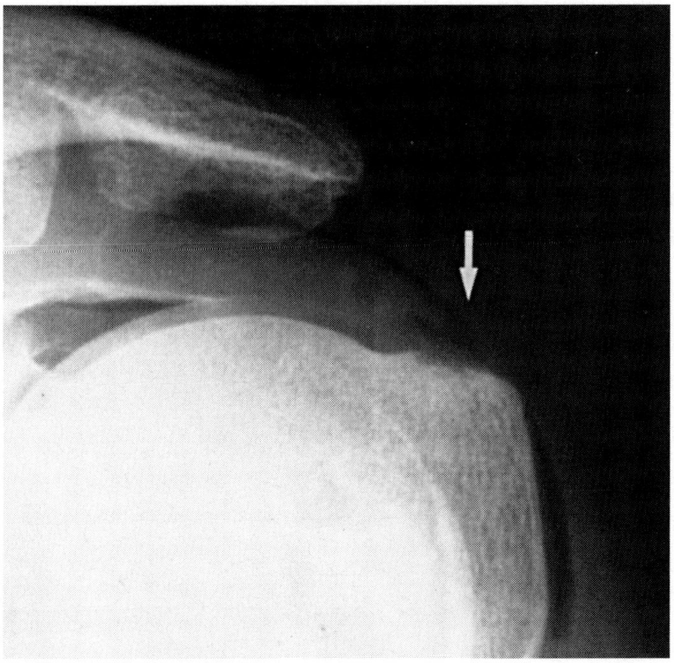

Fig. 6–21. Rotator cuff tear, supraspinatus tendon insertion. Double-contrast arthrography reveals a focal disruption of the insertion of the supraspinatus tendon (arrow). There is no arthrographic evidence of tendon degeneration, and no retraction of the supraspinatus tendon is present.

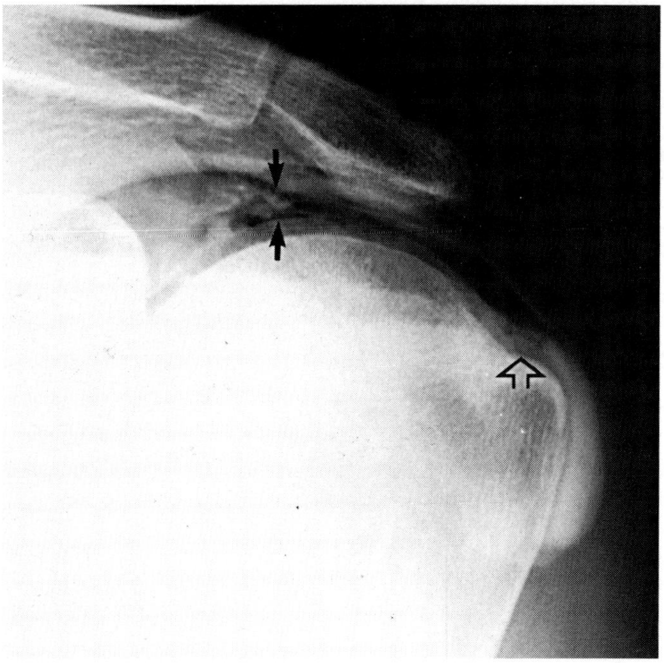

Fig. 6–23. Chronic rotator cuff tear, with prominent retraction of the supraspinatus tendon and degeneration of the tendon fragments. Note the air and contrast within the proximal portion of the supraspinatus tendon (arrowheads). (Open arrow denotes tendon insertion.)

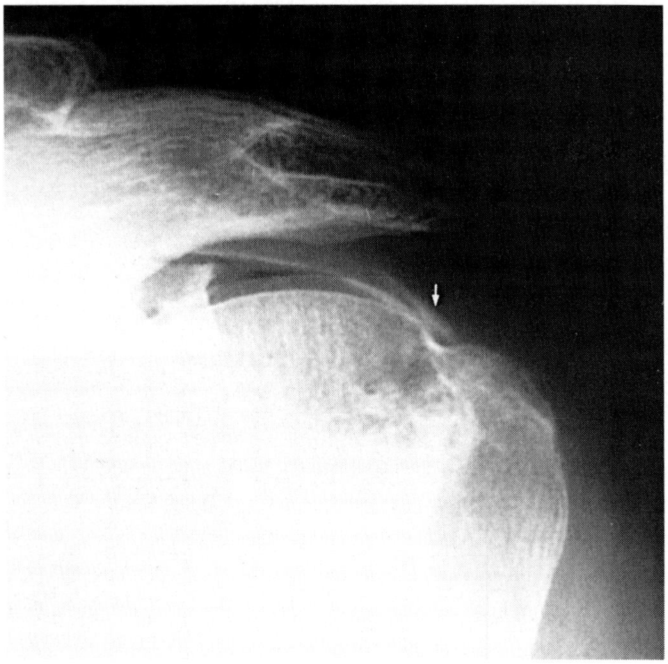

Fig. 6–24. Partial tear, supraspinatus tendon. Double-contrast arthrography demonstrates a focal collection of radiographic contrast within the insertion of the supraspinatus tendon (arrow). The contrast remains localized to the tendon, and there is no opacification of the subacromial bursa.

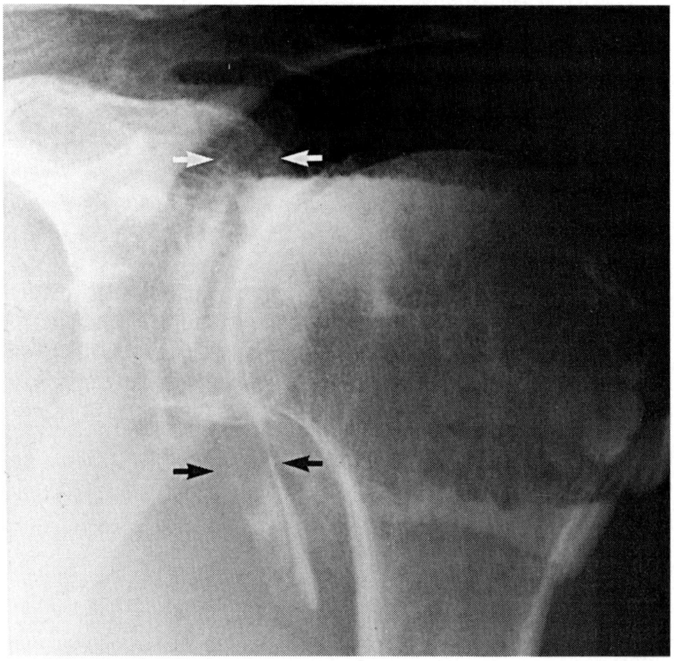

Fig. 6–26. Massive rotator cuff tear and medial dislocation of the long head of the biceps tendon (arrowheads), demonstrated on double-contrast arthrography.

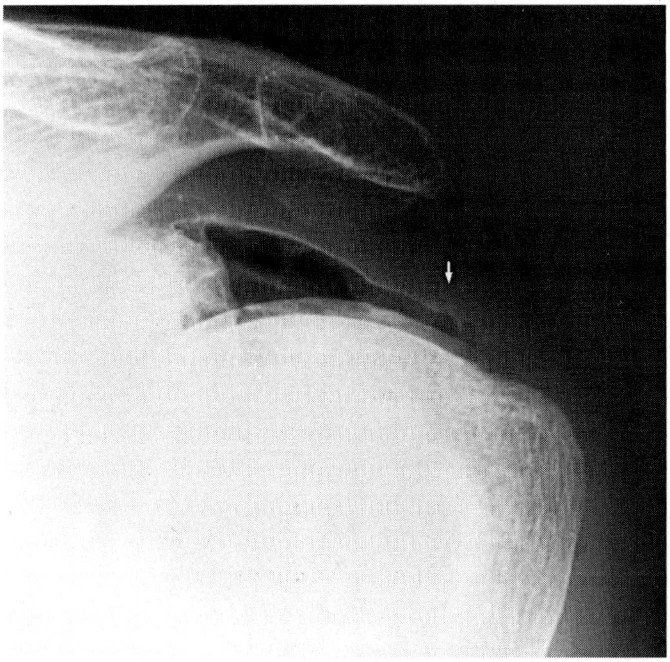

Fig. 6–25. Partial tear, supraspinatus tendon. A more subtle tear in the undersurface of the insertion of the supraspinatus tendon is evident (arrow).

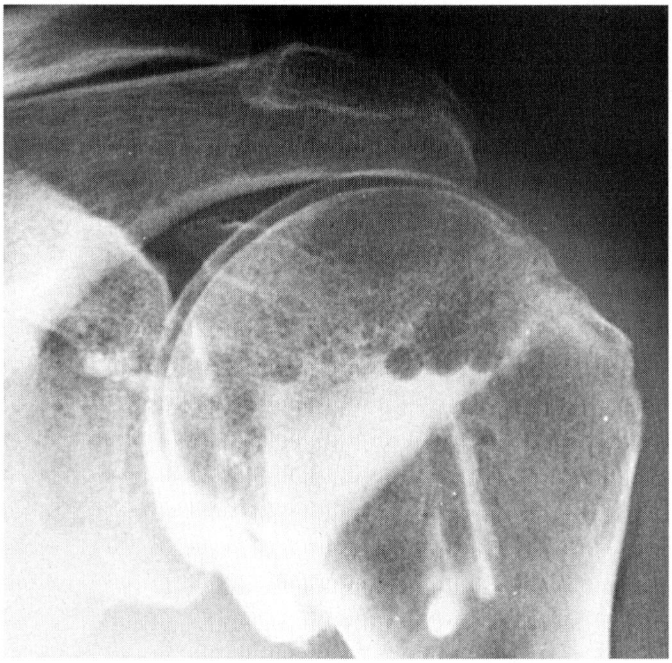

Fig. 6–27. Adhesive capsulitis. Note the markedly reduced volume of the glenohumeral joint, with obliteration of the axillary recess and contrast passing down the sheath of the long head of the biceps tendon.

from the subscapularis bursa and biceps tendon sheath, resulting in decompression of the capsule. The addition of local anesthetic and cortisone to the radiographic contrast may permit increased mobilization of the joint in subsequent physical therapy.

Nobuhara et al. have reported a series of patients with lesions of the rotator interval.[86] Arthrography in these patients is normal. However, when the arm is actively elevated in external rotation, contrast can be identified bulging into the rotator interval.[86]

The subcoracoid bursa lies anterior to the subscapularis tendon and may be inadvertently opacified during double-contrast arthrography. The unwary arthrographer may misinterpret this finding as evidence of filling of the subacromial bursa, thus indicating the presence of a rotator cuff tear (Fig. 6–28).[87] The absence of contrast outlining the articular surface of the glenohumeral joint, however, indicates that the injection is extra-articular.

Subacromial bursography has been primarily used in the evaluation of the impingement syndrome.[14,88,90,91] Signs of impingement include compression of the subacromial bursa by the greater tuberosity of the humerus with the arm in abduction, with associated distention of the subdeltoid bursa. However, Uthoff et al. noted that subacromial bursography may not be reliable when the coracoacromial ligament is the source of impingement.[91] Other signs of impingement at bursography include a diminished volume and synovial proliferation of the bursa.[88]

Subacromial bursography has also identified partial tears of the bursal aspect of the supraspinatus tendon.[89] Complete tears of the rotator cuff are evident when the glenohumeral joint is opacified on a subacromial bursal injection.

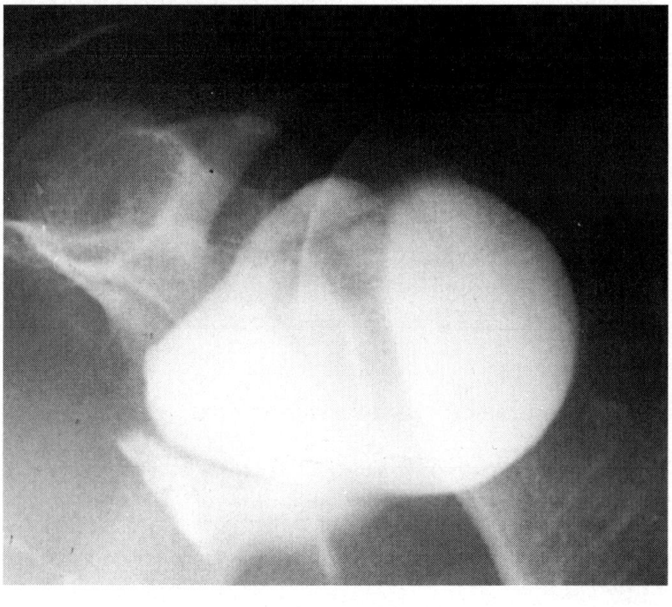

Fig. 6–28. Injection of the subcoracoid bursa. Note the lack of radiographic contrast outlining the articular surface of the humeral head.

COMPUTED TOMOGRAPHY AND COMPUTED ARTHROTOMOGRAPHY

Impingement of the tendinous cuff beneath the coracoacromial arch classically involves the anterior acromion, coracoacromial ligament, and, occasionally, the undersurface of the AC joint.[10,28,29] However, on rare occasions the subcoracoid bursa may be compressed between the coracoid process and the lesser tuberosity of the humerus.[92,95] Clinically, these patients have anterior shoulder pain exacerbated by forward flexion and medial rotation of the humerus. Conditions that narrow the coracohumeral distance predispose to this form of impingement and include prominence of the coracoid process, fractures of the coracoid process or lesser tuberosity, calcification within the subscapularis tendon, abnormal glenoid orientation secondary to a glenoid osteotomy, and operative changes of the coracoid process.[93,95] CT has been used in the evaluation of the coracoid impingement syndrome. The coracohumeral distance is minimized when the patient is positioned with the arm in forward flexion and internal rotation in the CT scanner.[93] Dines et al. studied normal patients with CT.[95] They determined a "coracoid index" by constructing a line tangent to the osseous glenoid and measuring the lateral extent of the coracoid process beyond this line. As determined by this method, the average coracoid index measured 8.2 mm (range −2.5 to +25 mm).[95]

In addition to primary impingement, caused by mechanical and anatomic factors resulting in outlet stenosis, impingement syndromes may also be caused by gleno-

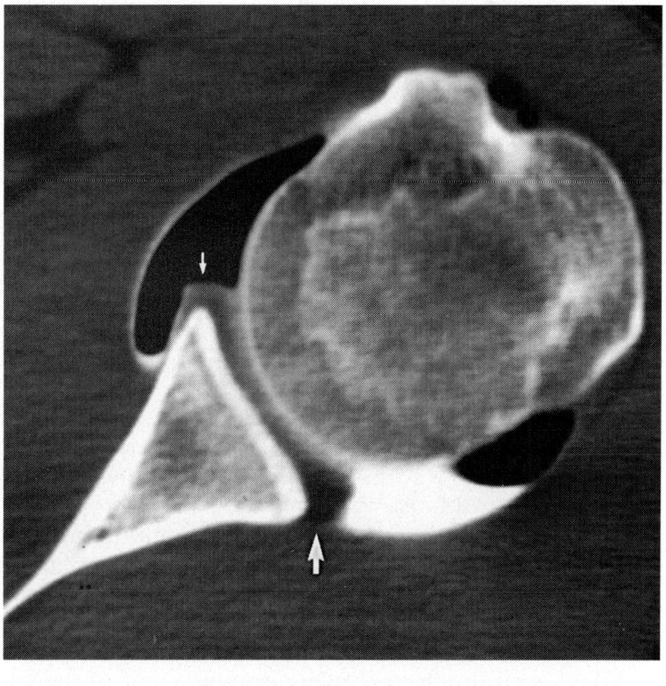

Fig. 6–29. Normal computed arthrotomography of the glenohumeral joint. Note the excellent depiction of the anterior (small arrow) and posterior (large arrow) cartilaginous glenoid labra, as well as the anterior and posterior capsule.

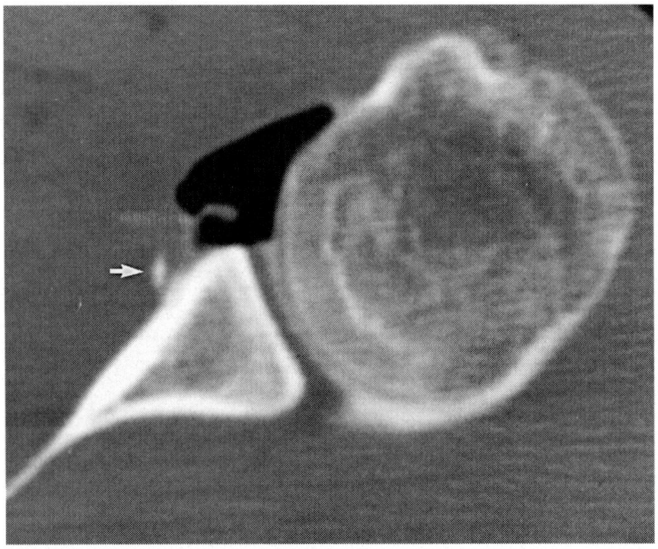

Fig. 6–30. Anterior glenohumeral instability. The anterior cartilaginous glenoid labrum has been avulsed, and the periosteum has been stripped from the anterior osseous glenoid (arrowhead).

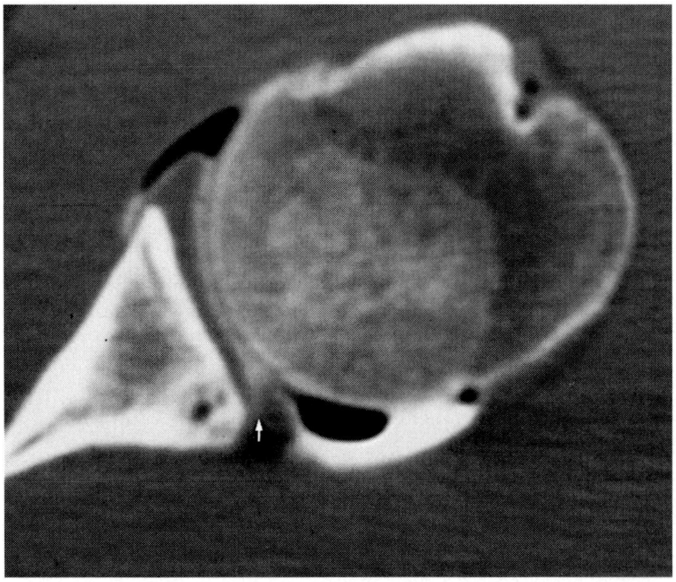

Fig. 6–32. Tear, posterior cartilaginous glenoid labrum. A focal collection of radiographic contrast is present within a tear of the posterior cartilaginous labrum (arrow). Note the subchondral cyst formation in the subjacent posterior osseous glenoid.

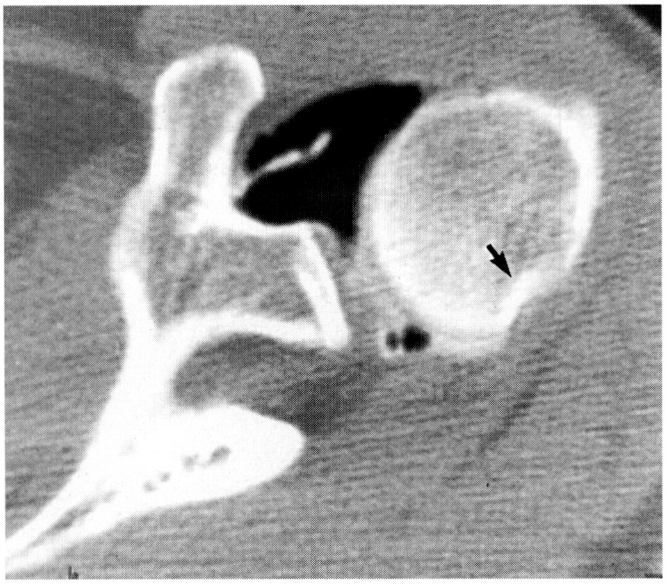

Fig. 6–31. Hill-Sachs lesion. Computed arthrotomography demonstrates the impaction fracture in the posterior lateral aspect of the articular portion of the humeral head (arrowhead).

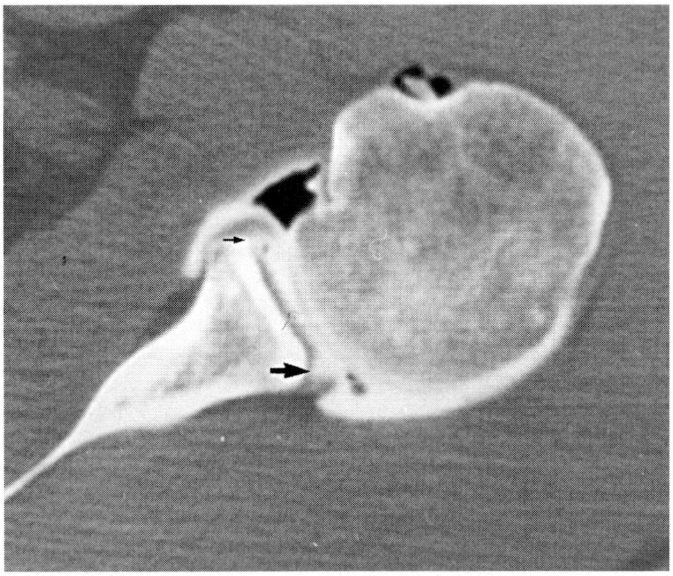

Fig. 6–33. Multidirectional instability. Note the focal tears of both the anterior (small arrow) and posterior (large arrow) cartilaginous glenoid labra.

humeral joint instability. This form of secondary impingement is more common in younger patients, especially throwing athletes.[12,96,97] In these patients, repetitive stress results in microtrauma to the glenohumeral ligaments, eventually resulting in attenuation of these structures. An anterior or multidirectional instability pattern results, placing increased stress on the rotator cuff. Fatigue of the rotator cuff permits the humeral head to translate, resulting in secondary impingement of the supraspinatus tendon beneath the coracoacromial arch.[97] Treatment of the impingement syndrome in these patients is directed at the underlying glenohumeral instability.

Computed arthrotomography is an excellent method of evaluating glenohumeral instability.[98,99] The anterior and posterior cartilaginous glenoid labrae are well demonstrated, as are the underlying osseous glenoid and the humeral head (Fig. 6–29). The capsule and its scapular insertion are also displayed well. Tears of the cartilaginous labrae, fractures of the osseous glenoid, and impaction fractures of the humeral head (Hill-Sachs lesion) are elegantly demonstrated with this technique (Figs. 6–30 through 6–33). Wilson et al. evaluated glenoid labral tears with computed arthrotomography and demonstrated a sensitivity of 100% and a specificity of 97% in the detection of these lesions with this technique.[99] Stripping of the scapular insertion of the capsule, intra-articular bodies, and fractures of the osseous glenoid labrae are also demonstrated well (Figs. 6–34 and 6–35).[22]

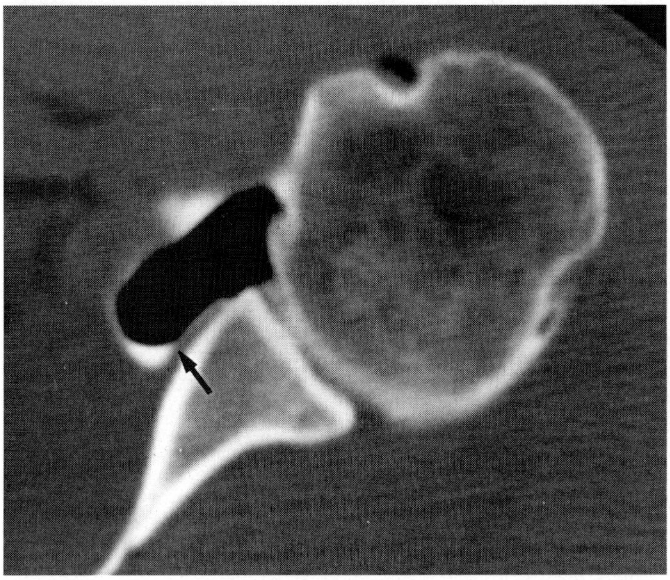

Fig. 6–34. Anterior glenohumeral instability. The scapular insertion of the anterior capsule has been stripped (arrow), and the anterior cartilaginous glenoid labrum has been avulsed.

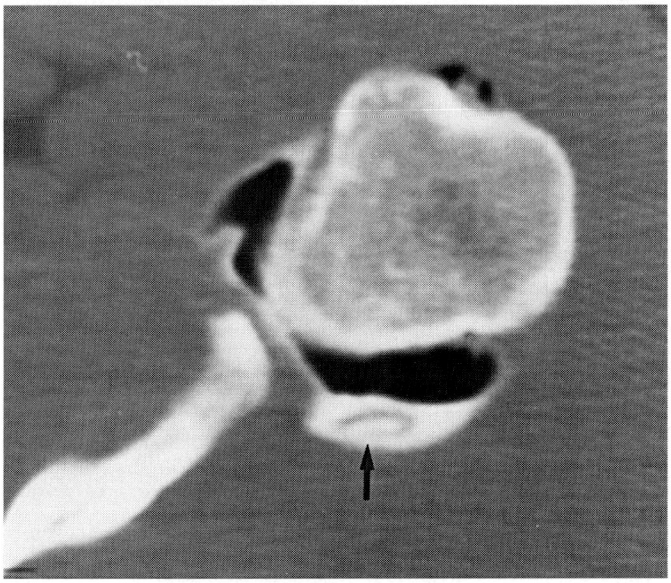

Fig. 6–35. Intra-articular body. Computed arthrotomography demonstrating an intra-articular body, with central calcification lying within the posterior aspect of the axillary recess (arrow).

Computed arthrotomography also displays less common rotator cuff lesions, including tears of the subscapularis tendon and dislocation of the intra-articular portion of the long head of the biceps tendon[22,39,100] (Figs. 6–36 through 6–38). Computed arthrotomography of the shoulder, using direct sagittal and coronal views, has been described and may permit more thorough evaluation of the supraspinatus tendon.[101,102] These techniques, however, require complicated and often uncomfortable positioning of the patient, as well as specifically constructed supports. The multiplanar reconstruction ability of the newly introduced spiral CT scanning technique may provide a quick and comfortable alternative to these techniques.

MAGNETIC RESONANCE IMAGING

MRI of the rotator cuff was initially heralded as the definitive modality in shoulder imaging. With its ability to image in multiple planes, lack of ionizing radiation, and exquisite soft-tissue delineation, MRI was embraced with great enthusiasm.[103–106] Many of the promises have been kept. As experience with MRI has grown, however, many diagnostic pitfalls have become evident. The early champions of this noninvasive tool have recognized that MRI must be used judiciously, and that it does not offer all the answers in every case of rotator cuff disease. Yet, when applied appropriately and interpreted carefully, shoulder MRI is unequaled in the wealth of information it provides.

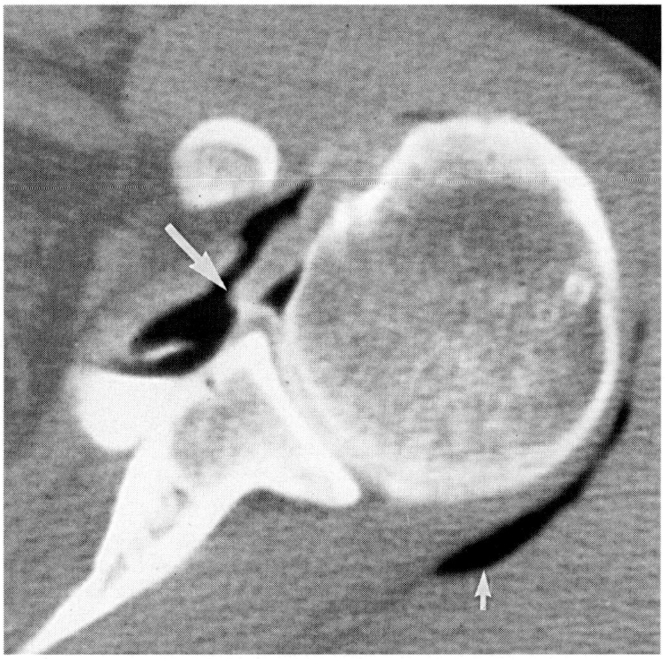

Fig. 6–36. Tear of the subscapularis tendon. Note the discontinuity of the subscapularis tendon (large arrow). Air is present within the subdeltoid bursa (small arrow), indicating a complete rotator cuff tear.

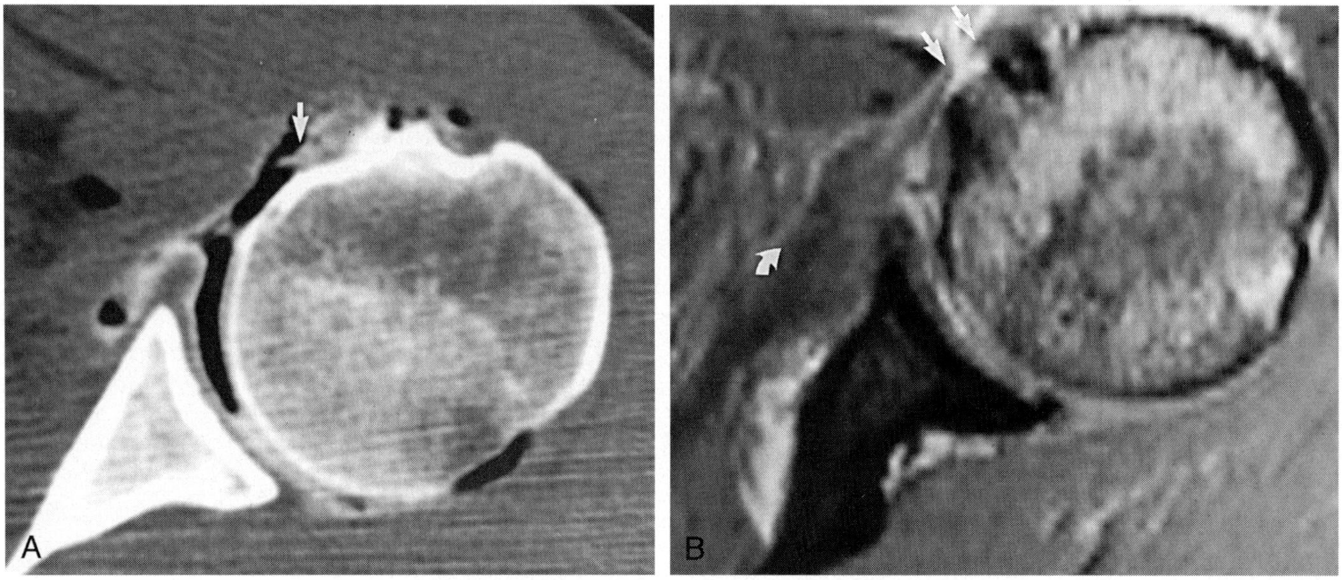

Fig. 6–37. Tear of the subscapularis tendon. *A,* Computed arthrotomography demonstrates disruption of the subscapularis tendon, with air and radiographic contrast evident at its insertion (arrowhead). *B,* Gradient echo magnetic resonance imaging in the same patient, demonstrating the defect in the tendon (arrowheads) and retraction of the subscapularis muscle (curved arrow).

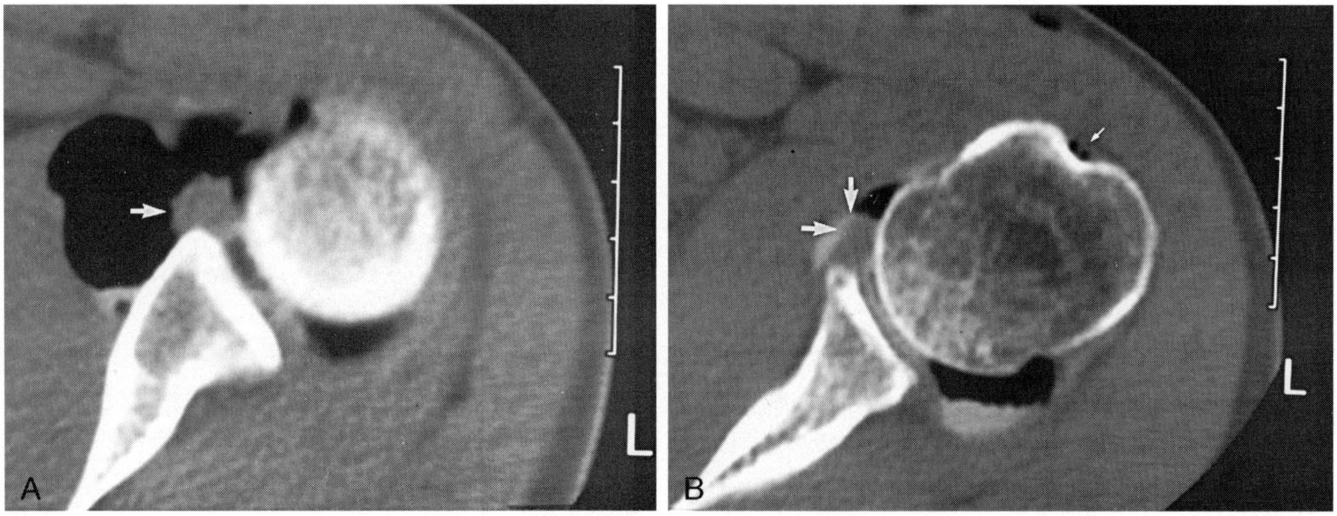

Fig. 6–38. Dislocation of the long head of the biceps tendon. *A,* Computed arthrotomography at the level of the superior aspect of the humeral head demonstrates the biceps tendon lying immediately adjacent to the anterior aspect of the glenohumeral joint (arrowhead). *B,* At the level of the mid glenoid, the tendon again is evident immediately adjacent to the anterior cartilaginous glenoid labrum (large arrows). Note the absence of the tendon in the intertubercular groove (small arrow).

Technique

MRI is a pictorial representation of the way a tissue responds in a strong external magnetic field. That magnetic field is perturbed in a controlled manner by the application of radio-frequency energy. The tissues under investigation absorb energy from the radio-frequency pulses. Those tissues then return to their ground state by two fundamental mechanisms, T1 relaxation and T2 relaxation. The rate of relaxation determines the relative brightness, or signal intensity, on the MRI images. When MRI is performed, the operator must determine which relaxation parameter to accentuate. Consequently, the images produced may be T1 weighted (T1WI) or T2 weighted (T2WI), depending on the scan technique. Images may also be produced by balancing the T1 and T2 information. These are referred to as proton-density weighted images, because the signal intensities reflect the relative number of mobile hydrogen protons in the tissue. In general, the T1WI provides exquisite anatomic detail, while the T2WI provides high contrast between normal and abnormal tissues. As fluid or edema accumulate in the tissues, the signal intensity increases on the T2WI images. The complex topic of clinical MRI physics is discussed more fully in other literature.[107–109]

A basic strength of MRI is the ability to image in multiple planes. This is particularly important in shoulder imaging, because MRI can provide direct visualization of the rotator cuff in spite of the obliquity of the tissues. Consequently, most imaging protocols include a series of images in an oblique coronal plane aligned along the long axis of the supraspinatus muscle (Fig. 6–39). Axial images are performed to evaluate the glenoid and capsular structures. A series of images is usually performed in an oblique sagittal plane as well. This allows direct visualization of the long axis of the acromion (Fig. 6–40). The oblique coronal plane is usually a T2WI sequence, with the axial and oblique sagittal images performed with T1 weighting. In some protocols, a series is acquired with three-dimensional technique to allow postacquisition manipulation of the data into various obliquities. Gradient echo techniques have also been employed in shoulder imaging, predominately in an attempt to shorten the exam time. Even with these gradient echo techniques, tissue contrast is based on differences of T1 and T2 relaxation.

Table 6–1 outlines the imaging parameters for a typical MRI evaluation of the shoulder. The values for repetition time (TR) and echo time (TE) are selected by the operator to produce images with the desired contrast char-

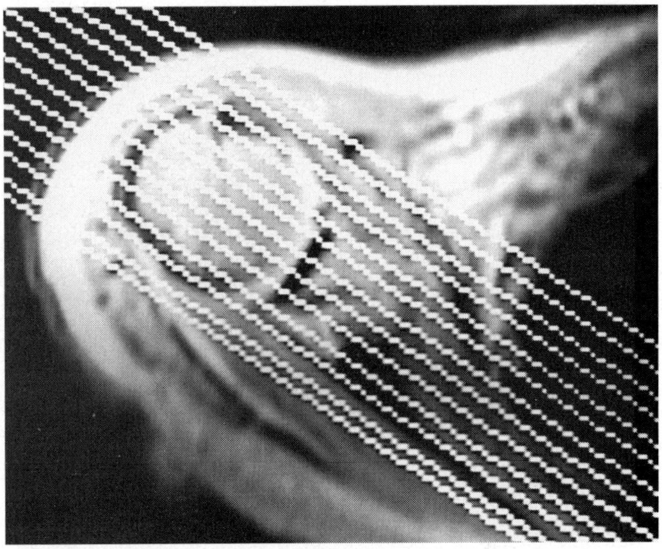

Fig. 6–39. **Oblique coronal orientation. An axial scout view of the shoulder is used to prescribe the oblique coronal sequence of images. The obliquity should match the orientation of the supraspinatus muscle.**

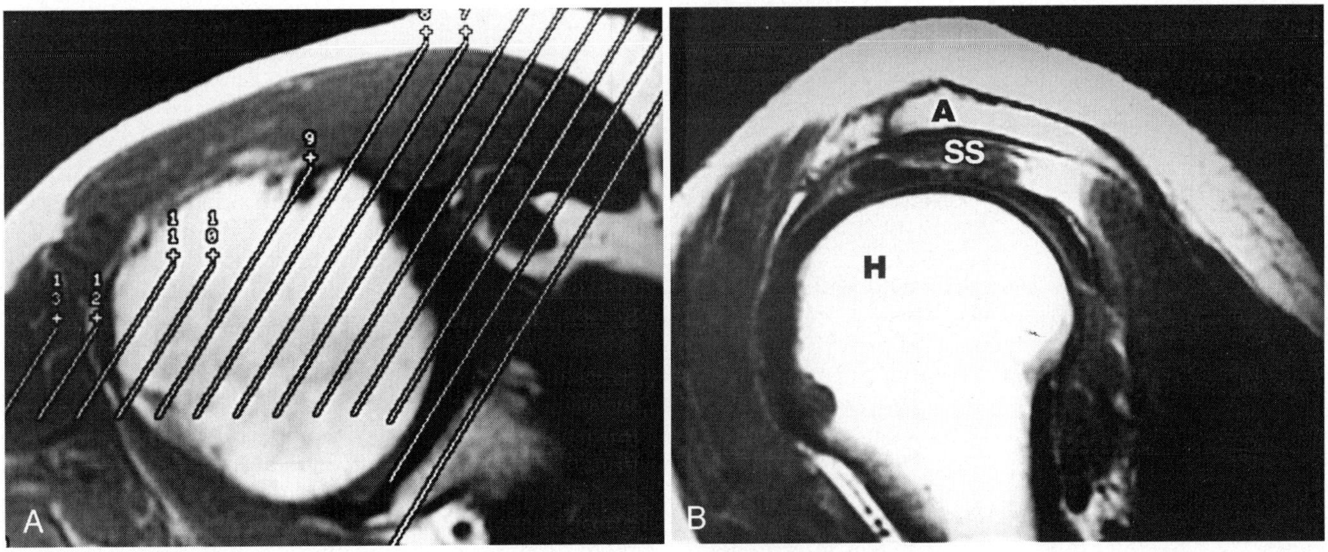

Fig. 6–40. ***A,*** **Oblique sagittal orientation. The oblique sagittal images are aligned perpendicular to the long axis of the supraspinatus muscle. This displays the long axis of the acromion.** ***B,*** **Oblique sagittal T1WI of the shoulder. The sagittal sequence of images allows direct visualization of the acromion (A) and its relationship to the distal supraspinatus muscle (SS) and humeral head (H).**

Table 6–1. MRI Shoulder Protocol*

Series	*Imaging Plane*	*Slice Thickness(mm)*	*TR(msec)*	*TE(msec)*
T1WI	Axial	4–5	300–450	15–30
T2WI	Oblique coronal	5	2000	30/80
T1WI	Oblique sagital	5	300–450	15–30

*This is a typical protocol utilizing spin-echo technique. See references for description of three-dimensional and gradient echo techniques.

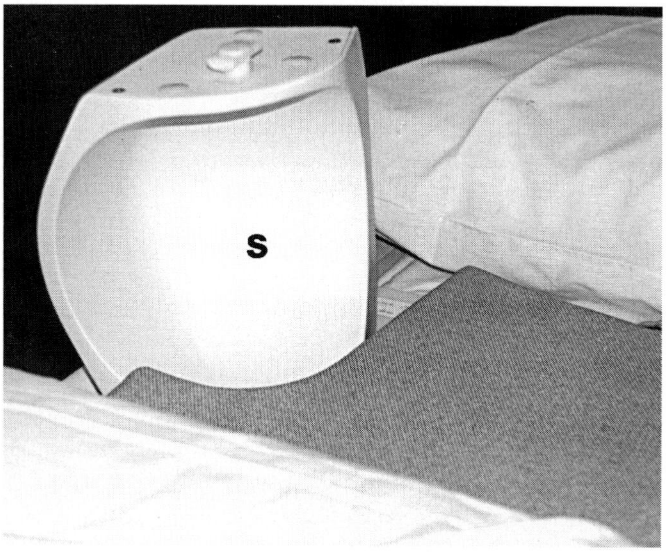

Fig. 6–41. Dedicated shoulder surface coil. A surface coil (S) is designed to be placed in close proximity to the area of interest. This improves the amount of signal received from the tissues. Most shoulder examinations are performed with the arm in a neutral position.

Table 6–2. MRI Signal Contrast Relationships*

Tissue	*T1WI*	*N(H)*	*T2WI*
Fat	High	Moderate	Moderate
Skeletal muscle	Moderate	Low	Very low
Tendons	Low	Low	Very low
Fluid	Very low	Moderate	High
Cortical bone	Very low	Very low	Very low

*These are relative signal intensities of the tissues in the shoulder.

acteristics. All sequences are performed with a surface coil on the shoulder (Fig. 6–41). This coil receives the signal from the underlying tissues and provides the high signal-to-noise ratio required in rotator cuff studies.

Normal Anatomy

The normal rotator cuff is demonstrated well on MRI images.[110,111] Skeletal muscle demonstrates intermediate signal intensity on the T1WI and decreasing signal on T2WI. Tendons are very low signal on both T1WI and T2WI sequences. Fat, whether in the marrow cavity of the humerus or subcutaneous tissues, is high signal on T1WI images and falls to intermediate signal on the T2WI sequences. Fluid is very dark on the T1 sequences and very bright on the T2WI scans. Because it contains few mobile protons, the osseous cortex returns almost no signal on any sequence. The cartilaginous glenoid and capsular ligaments are also of low signal intensity on both T1WI and T2WI sequences. These signal relationships are summarized in Table 6–2.

The multiple oblique planes in the typical protocol provide excellent delineation of anatomic relationships in and around the rotator cuff. The supraspinatus muscle is visualized along its long axis on the oblique coronal images (Fig. 6–42). This structure should taper smoothly as it traverses the humeral head to insert on the greater tuberosity. Axial images are best for evaluation of the humeral head and the shape and size of the cartilaginous glenoid. The anatomic relationships depicted in the axial plane are analogous to the axial depiction on CT. The normal cartilage of the glenoid fossa is seen as a triangular structure closely apposed to the humeral head and osseous glenoid (Fig. 6–43). On the MRI images, there may normally be a thin line of intermediate signal between the glenoid cartilage and osseous cortex. Axial images also demonstrate the infraspinatus and subscapularis muscles. The oblique sagittal plane demonstrates the shape of the acromion and the acromiohumeral distance. As has been previously discussed, the acromial shape is usually described as one of three types, based on the configuration of its undersurface. The type I acromion shows a flat surface. A type II shape is less common and shows a smoothly curved configuration. The type III acromion demonstrates caudal angulation of its anterior tip. These latter two shapes may narrow the supraspinatus inlet and thereby predispose to rotator cuff impingement. The marrow of the scapula and humerus is seen on all sequences and should be of homogeneous texture.

Rotator Cuff Disease

The MRI diagnosis of a complete rotator cuff tear is based on the demonstration of fluid signal within the tendons of the distal rotator cuff muscles. There is interruption of the normal tendon by a gap of high signal intensity, which is best seen on the T2WI (Fig. 6–44). Additional findings include retraction of the supraspinatus muscle beneath the clavicle (Fig. 6–45) and fluid within the subacromial or subdeltoid bursae. In massive tears or longstanding disruption, it may be impossible to identify the distal supraspinatus tendon (Fig. 6–46). Although many cases of complete rotator cuff tear will not show evidence of muscle retraction, high signal intensity in the distal supraspinatus tendon on the T2WI and fluid within the subacromial bursa are the hallmarks of complete disruption of the rotator cuff.[112–114]

The feature most characteristic of a partial rotator cuff tear is the presence of vertically oriented fluid within one

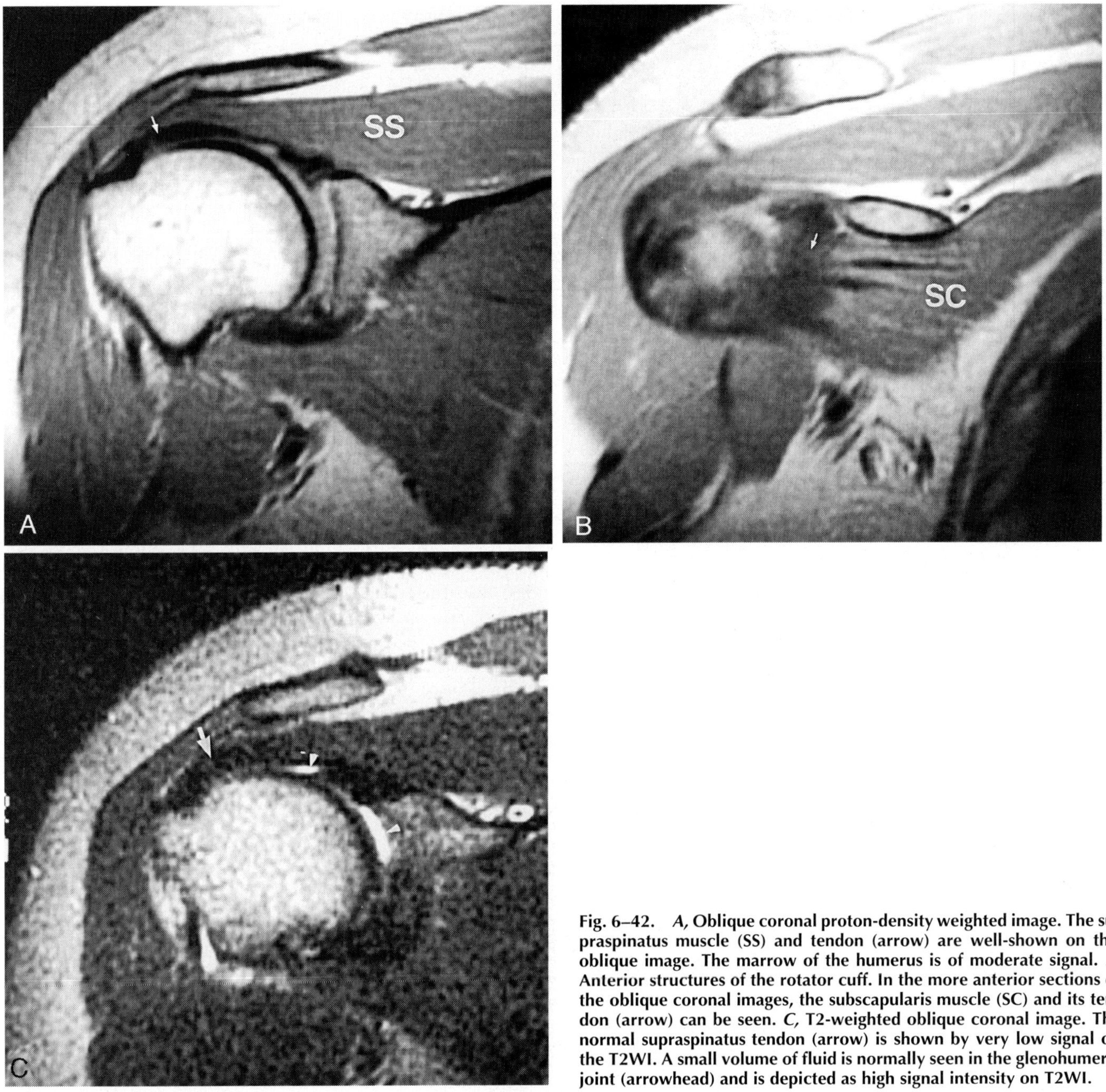

Fig. 6–42. ***A,*** **Oblique coronal proton-density weighted image. The supraspinatus muscle (SS) and tendon (arrow) are well-shown on this oblique image. The marrow of the humerus is of moderate signal.** ***B,*** **Anterior structures of the rotator cuff. In the more anterior sections of the oblique coronal images, the subscapularis muscle (SC) and its tendon (arrow) can be seen.** ***C,*** **T2-weighted oblique coronal image. The normal supraspinatus tendon (arrow) is shown by very low signal on the T2WI. A small volume of fluid is normally seen in the glenohumeral joint (arrowhead) and is depicted as high signal intensity on T2WI.**

surface of the distal supraspinatus tendon (Fig. 6–47). This may be seen either inferiorly or superiorly but does not extend from the glenohumeral joint to the subacromial space.[115] Therefore, partial tears of the rotator cuff do not demonstrate fluid in the subacromial or subdeltoid bursae.

Rotator cuff tendinitis has also been described as demonstrating increased signal in the supraspinatus tendon, predominately on the T1 weighted and proton-density weighted sequences. This is associated with loss of anatomic definition in the musculotendinous junction (Fig. 6–48). The distorted tendon shows only moderate or decreased signal on the T2WI images, in distinction to the high signal usually reported in true tears of the tendon.[116,117]

Controversy has arisen regarding the ability of MRI to distinguish partial rotator cuff tears from the degeneration associated with chronic impingement. In cadaveric studies, tendinous degeneration identified on histologic examination has been shown to demonstrate increased signal on proton-density weighted images.[118,119] Similar findings have been reported in partial tears of the distal

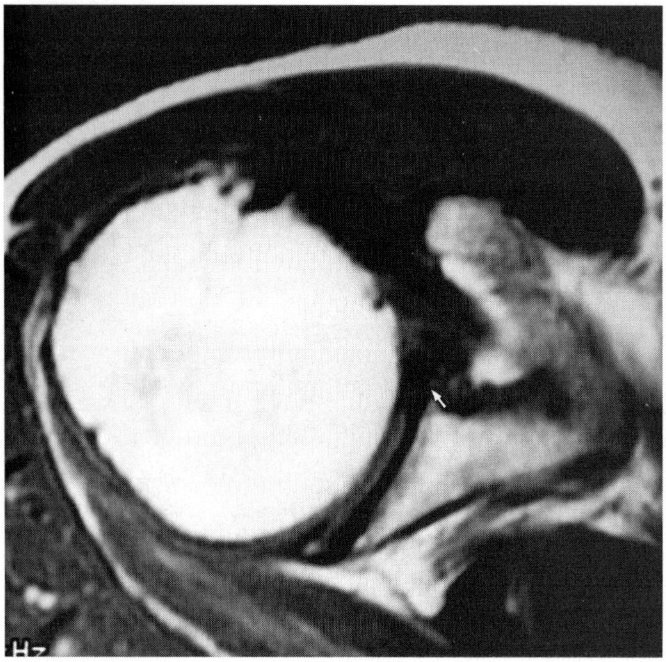

Fig. 6–43. Axial T-weighted image. The cartilage of the glenoid (arrow) is demonstrated as a low signal intensity triangular structure closely apposed to the humeral head.

supraspinatus tendon. The distinguishing feature of a partial rotator cuff tear is the demonstration of intratendinous fluid, seen as focal increased signal on the T2WI. The changes of tendinitis tend to be a loss of anatomic sharpness without a definable intratendinous cleft or gap.

Rotator cuff impingement is demonstrated as deformity along the superior surface of the supraspinatus muscle or narrowing of the acromiohumeral distance (Fig. 6–49). The superior deformity may be caused by alterations at the AC joint, such as a subacromial spur or AC joint hypertrophy. When the altered shape of the distal supraspinatus muscle is associated with ill-defined increased signal on the T2WI (Fig. 6–50), this is evidence of acute inflammation or severe degeneration and supports the diagnosis of symptomatic rotator cuff impingement.[120–122]

Although the muscles and tendons of the rotator cuff are the primary focus of most MRI studies of the shoulder, surrounding structures may be abnormal and mimic the clinical findings of rotator cuff impingement or tear. Dislocation of the long biceps tendon (Fig. 6–51)[123,124] and abnormalities of the cartilaginous glenoid are well shown. These abnormalities include the changes of multidirectional instability, as well as more recent reports of superior labral tears (SLAP lesions).[125–128] There has also been recent interest in the MRI diagnosis of tears in the rotator cuff interval (the ligamentous region between the supraspinatus and subscapularis tendons).[139]

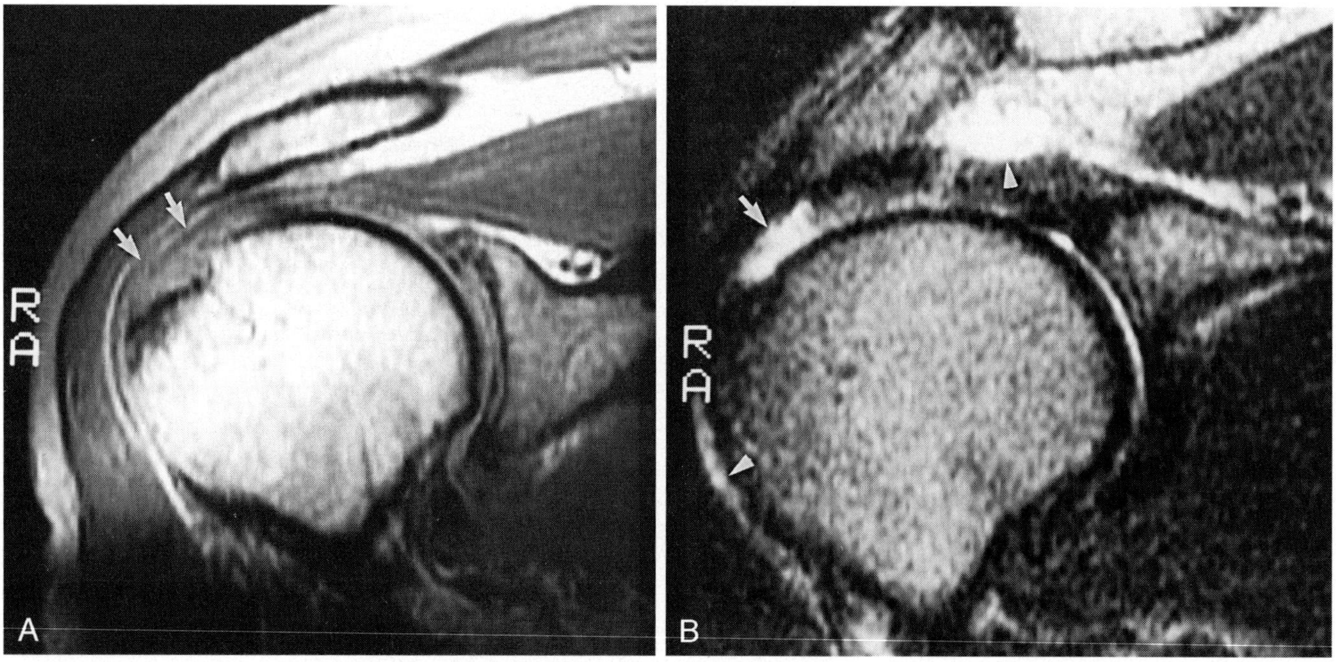

Fig. 6–44. Rotator cuff tear. *A*, Proton-density weighted oblique coronal image demonstrates loss of anatomic definition in the distal supraspinatus tendon (arrows), with abnormal increased signal. *B*, T2-weighted oblique coronal image. On the T2WI, a high signal intensity gap can be seen in the distal supraspinatus tendon (arrow). Fluid is noted in the subdeltoid bursa (arrowhead). These are the classic MRI findings of complete rotator cuff tear.

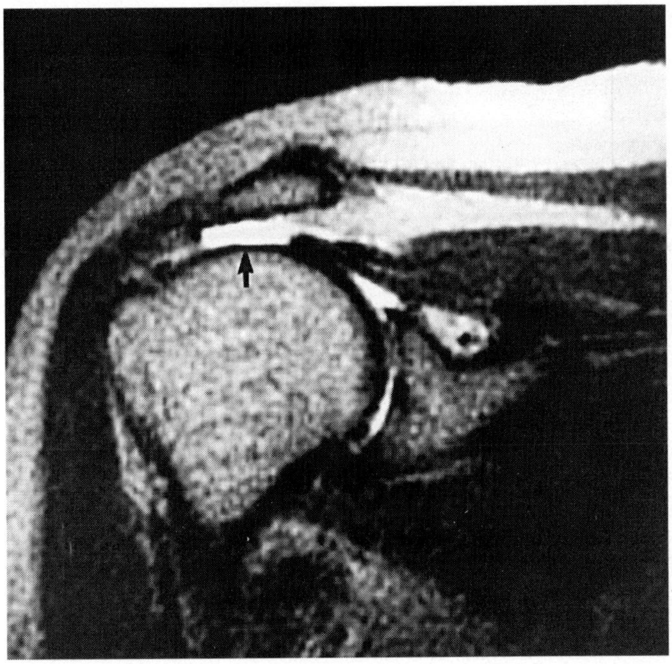

Fig. 6–45. Complete rotator cuff tear. The T2WI demonstrates high signal intensity gap (arrow) in the distal supraspinatus tendon. The tendon is retracted.

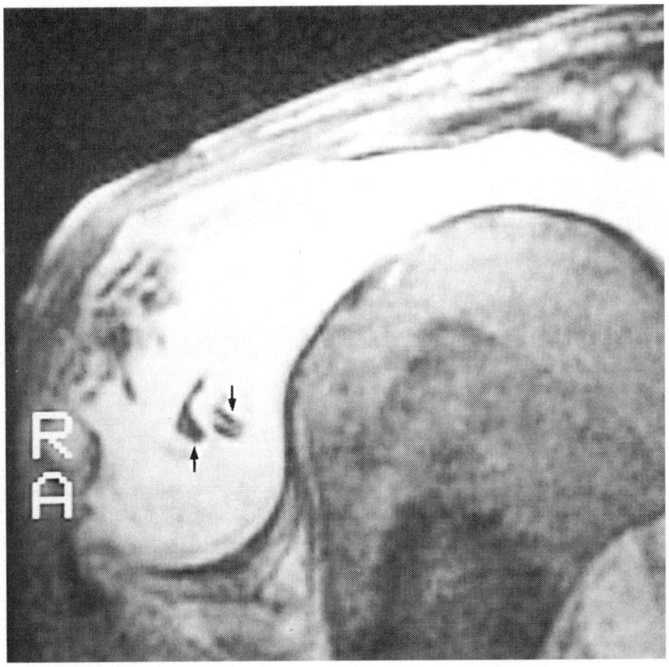

Fig. 6–46. Massive rotator cuff disruption. This T2-weighted oblique coronal image demonstrates complete loss of supraspinatus structures. There is a large joint effusion, with hemorrhagic debris (arrows).

Pitfalls

MRI is exquisitely motion sensitive. Therefore, patient cooperation is essential for the performance of a diagnostic study. A complete evaluation requires the patient to lie still for 30 to 45 minutes, a difficult task for some. Claustrophobia may also pose difficulty for some patients. The bore of the clinical imager is a close space, and sedation may be required for patient tolerance. Patients with a cardiac pacemaker or with intracerebral vascular clips cannot be scanned. Similarly, any patient who has metallic foreign bodies in the orbits must not be subjected to the strong magnetic flux of the MR imager.

As experience with shoulder MRI has grown, so has the number of reported imaging pitfalls.[129,130] Studies in asymptomatic volunteers demonstrated increased signal in the distal supraspinatus tendon on T1WI and proton-density weighted images.[131] This may result from including a small amount of normal fat in the imaging volume. The supraspinatus tendon can demonstrate artifactually increased signal because of its oblique course through the magnetic field lines in the imager. The resultant spurious increase in signal is seen only on the heavily T1WI and is referred to as "magic-angle" artifact.[132] This can be overcome by changing the direction of the tendon relative to the main magnetic field. If the shoulder is imaged in internal rotation, the overlapping tendons may cause increased signal on the T1WI and proton-density weighted series. Whatever the cause, it has become clear that the normal shoulder demonstrates variable signal in the distal supraspinatus tendon on the T1WI. Care must

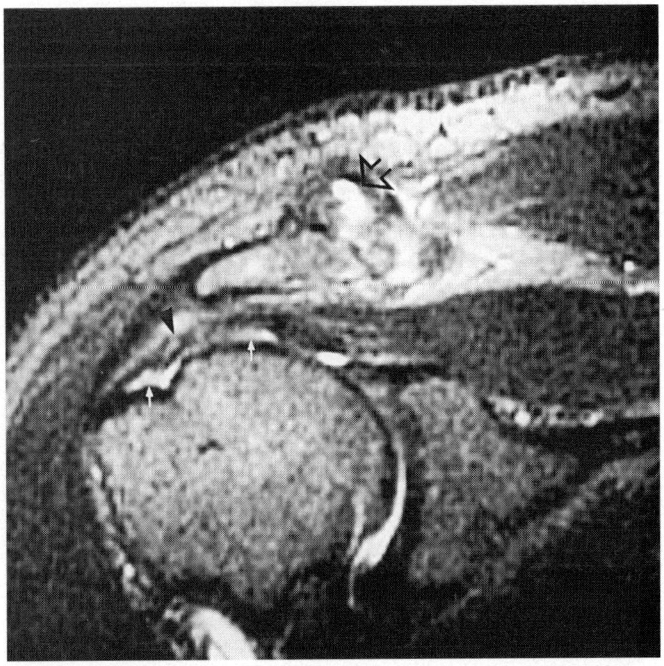

Fig. 6–47. Partial rotator cuff tear. Oblique coronal T2WI demonstrates fluid signal along the undersurface of the distal supraspinatus tendon (arrows). The distal tendon is distorted (arrowhead) but not completely disrupted. No subacromial or subdeltoid fluid is seen. There is fluid in the AC joint (open arrow).

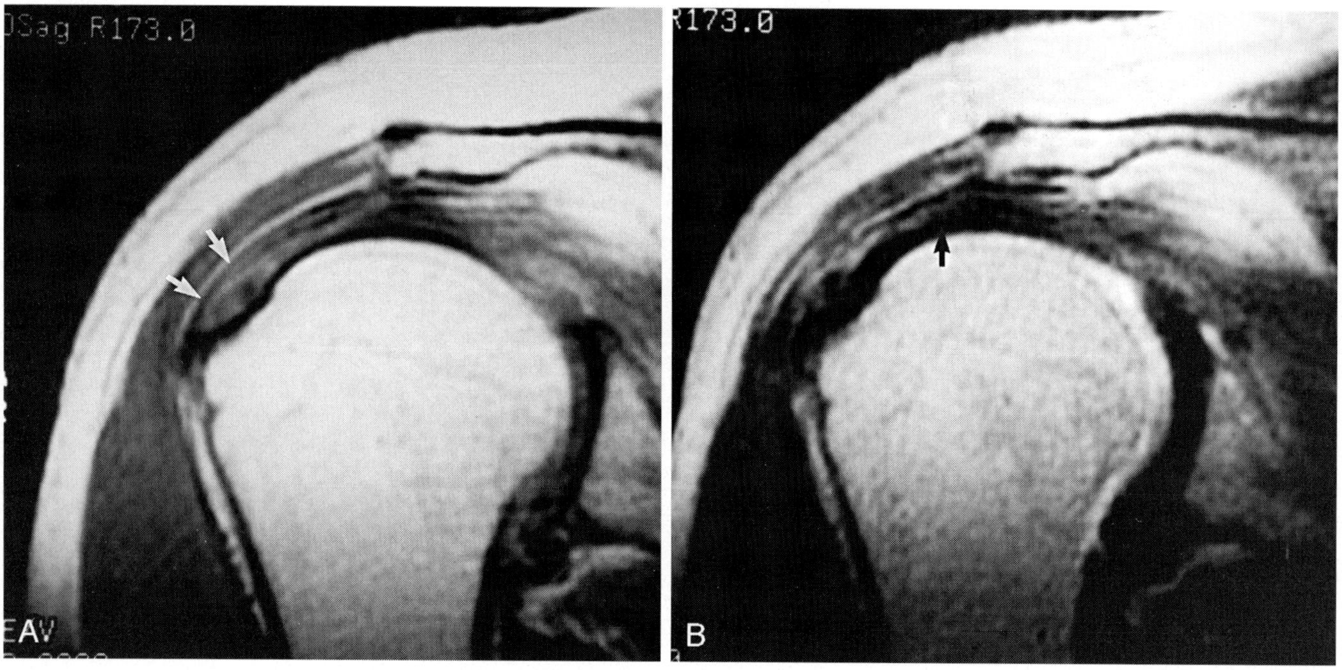

Fig. 6–48. **Supraspinatus tendinitis.** ***A,*** **This N(H)-weighted image demonstrates increased signal in the distal supraspinatus tendon (arrow), with loss of anatomic definition.** ***B,*** **On the T2WI, the distal supraspinatus tendon demonstrates moderate signal (arrow).**

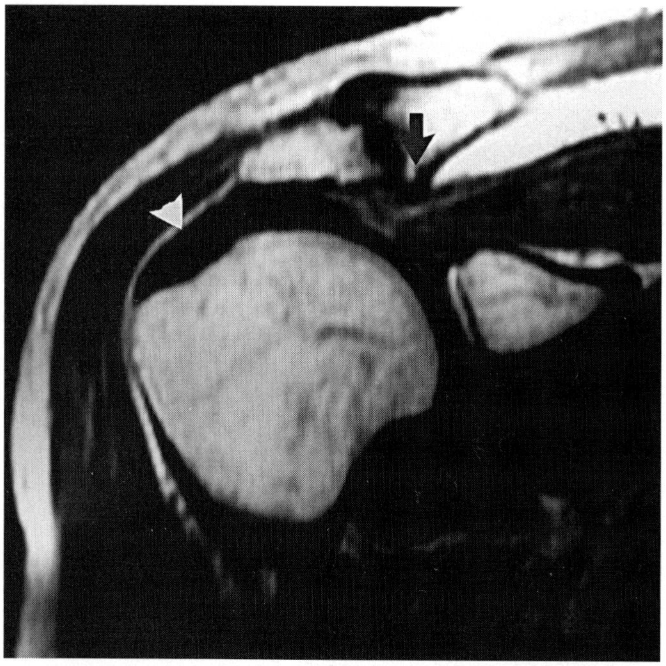

Fig. 6–49. **Rotator cuff impingement. A distal clavicular spur (arrow) deforms the supraspinatus muscle. The supraspinatus tendon (arrowhead) maintains its normal low signal intensity on this T2WI.**

be taken not to base the MRI diagnosis of rotator cuff tendinitis solely on the presence of increased signal in the supraspinatus tendon on the T1 or proton-density weighted images.

The magnetic field will be distorted by metal contained within the imaging volume. The metal may not be detectable with plain radiographs, but will result in areas of signal void on the images. The signal void is accentuated on the more T2WI scans and will obscure the surrounding anatomy. Such metallic artifact is frequently seen in postoperative patients.[133,134]

Calcifications are difficult to detect because of extremely low signal on all MR imaging sequences. This limits the usefulness of MRI as the single imaging modality in the detection of calcific tendinitis (Fig. 6–52). Similarly, in the patient with shoulder trauma, detection of small osseous fragments can be impossible. Radiographic or CT correlation is essential in those cases in which periarticular or intra-articular calcification is suspected.

MAGNETIC RESONANCE ARTHROGRAPHY

Contrast material for MRI was approved for clinical use in 1989. The agents are gadolinium-based chelates, initially introduced as intravenous agents for use in cerebral imaging. Contrast quickly became widely used in musculoskeletal, spine, and body applications as well, all with intravenous administration.

Recent reports have emphasized the clinical use of gadolinium contrast injected into the glenohumeral joint to create MRI arthrograms.[135,136] The joint is usually injected under fluoroscopic guidance, with a small amount of iodinated contrast used to confirm needle placement. The shoulder joint is distended with installation of 12 to 20 mL of dilute contrast. The patient is then imaged in the typical fashion with a standard MR imaging protocol. The gadolinium produces high signal intensity on the

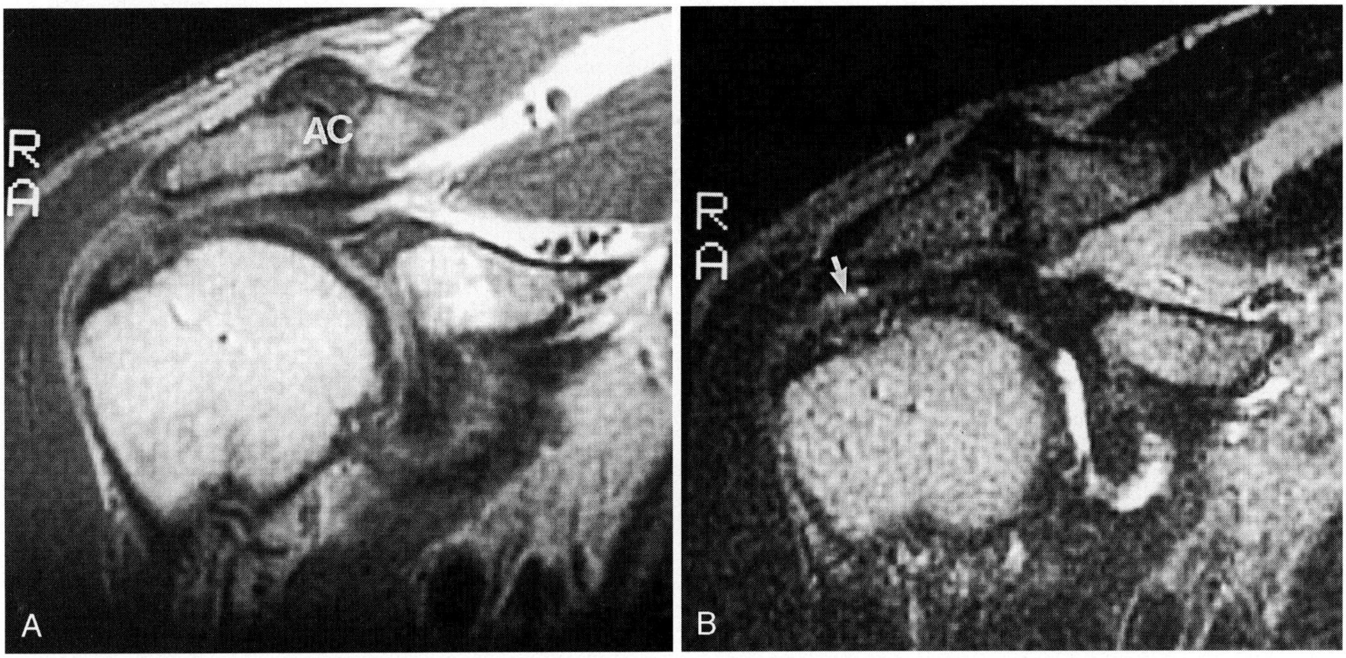

Fig. 6–50. *A,* Rotator cuff impingement, with inflammation. The supraspinatus muscle is deformed by the AC joint (AC). The joint is enlarged, due to osteoarthritis. *B,* Rotator cuff inflammation is seen as increased signal (arrow) in the distal supraspinatus tendon.

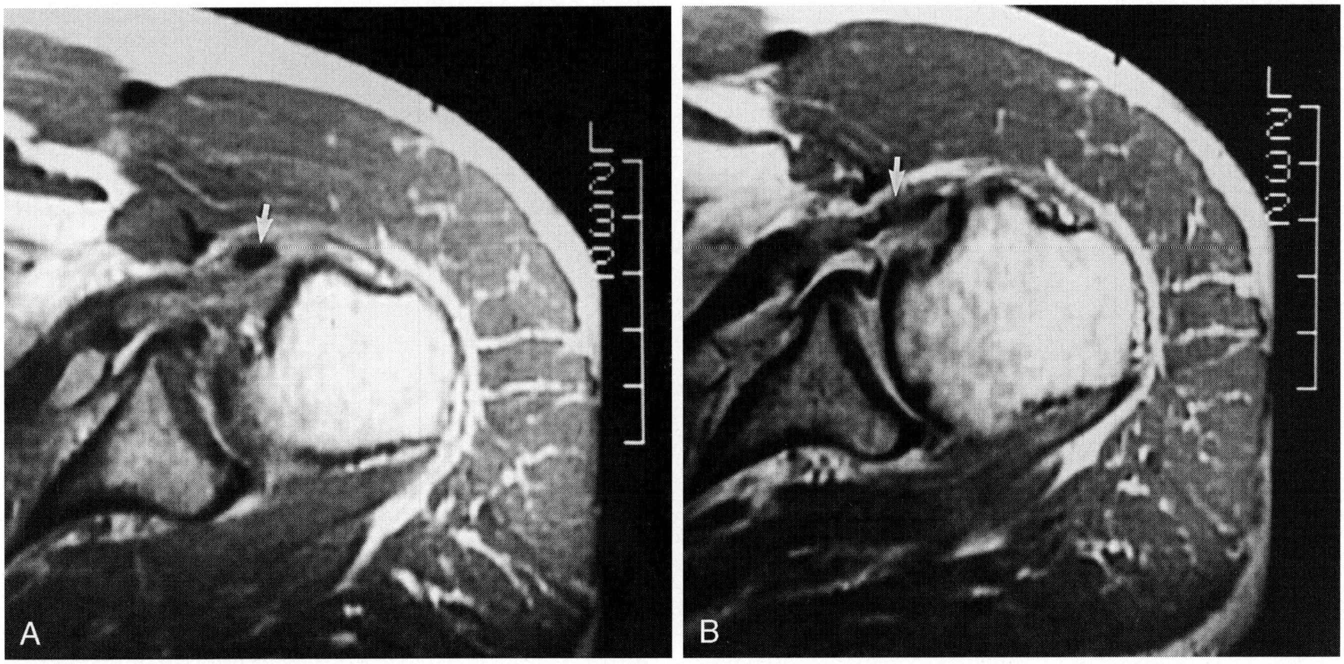

Fig. 6–51. Biceps tendon dislocation. *A,* The long biceps tendon (arrow) is dislocated medially. This may manifest clinically as pain on external humeral rotation. *B,* There is associated deformity of the subscapularis tendon (arrow).

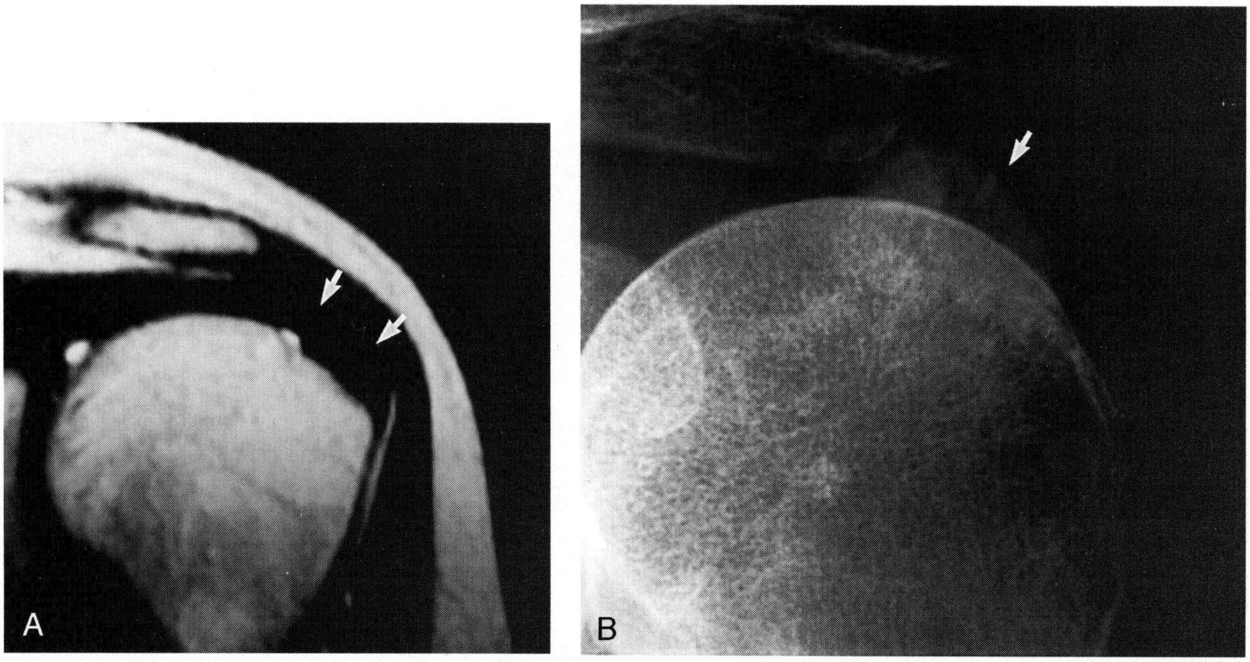

Fig. 6–52. Calcific tendinitis. ***A,*** **The distal supraspinatus tendon (ST) demonstrates enlargement and distortion of shape but no abnormal increased signal (arrows).** ***B,*** **The radiograph clearly demonstrates a large calcification in the location of the distal supraspinatus tendon (arrow).**

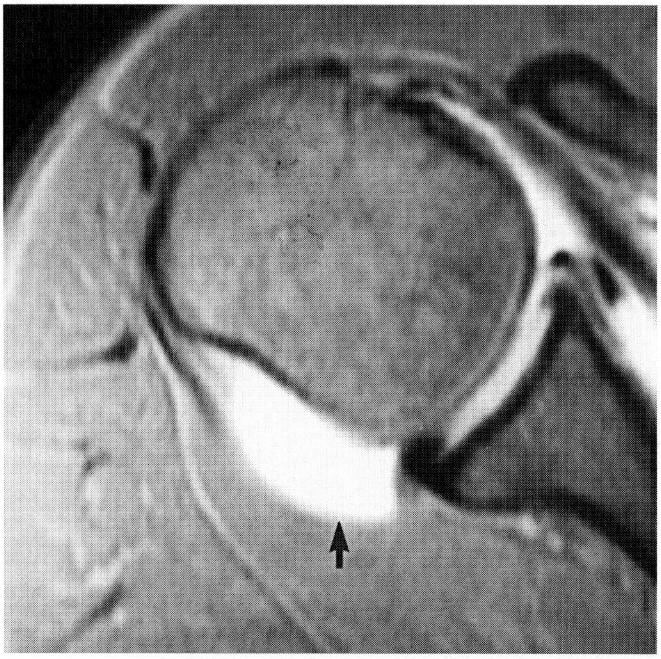

Fig. 6–53. MRI arthrogram. Dilute Gadolinium contrast material has been injected into the shoulder joint. This results in high signal intensity on the T1WI (arrow). This T1WI was also modified by reducing the signal from fat, a technique referred to as "fat pre-saturation."

T1WI, while the dilutant increases the signal on T2WI (Fig. 6–53). Thus, this technique allows joint distension with positive contrast, resulting in increased sensitivity for capsular and glenoid abnormalities. Leakage of contrast through the supraspinatus tendon is evidence of rotator cuff tear, as with the traditional arthrogram. Magnetic resonance arthrography is a significant advance in the MRI shoulder protocol.

The main disadvantage of intra-articular injection of gadolinium contrast is that it requires a needle puncture. The MRI is then no longer a noninvasive exam. Preliminary work done in knee imaging suggests that gadolinium injected intravenously accumulates in joint fluid.[137] This has led some to advocate the intravenous injection of contrast followed by joint exercise to achieve the arthrogram effect without direct contrast injection.[138] This technique is promising, but is presently undocumented in routine shoulder imaging.

SUMMARY

The diagnosis of lesions of the rotator cuff is generally established on the basis of a careful clinical history and examination. However, in those instances when the diagnosis remains uncertain, multiple imaging modalities are available, permitting more precise characterization of the underlying lesion.

Stiles et al. provide a comprehensive overview of the role of imaging techniques in shoulder disorders.[22]

For the diagnosis of rotator cuff tears, conventional arthrography is accurate and inexpensive. Ultrasound is noninvasive and inexpensive, but it is difficult to learn to perform accurately. MRI offers multiplanar depiction of the anatomy and superb soft-tissue contrast, but it is rather expensive. Furthermore, the interpretation of tendinous signal characteristics is in the evolutionary stage, resulting in diagnostic errors. As the era of cost contain-

Table 6–3. Shoulder Imaging Fees

Imaging Study	*Professional Fees (dollars)*	*Technical Fees (dollars)*	*Total Charge (dollars)*
Radiography, complete series	29.00	78.00	107.00
Shoulder arthrography	121.00	172.00	293.00
Shoulder arthrography with CT	165.00	480.00	635.00
Shoulder MR imaging	250.00	988.00	1,238.00
Shoulder US	74.00	109.00	183.00

Note: These fees represent an average of the fees from two different hospitals in the same metropolitan area. The fees from the two hospitals varied by as much as 78%. (From Stiles RG, Otte MT. Imaging of the shoulder. *Radiology*. 1993; 188:603–613.)

ment approaches, standard arthrography and ultrasound would seem to become increasingly attractive options. (Table 6–3). However, ultimately the appropriate examination should be the one that is most likely to answer the specific clinical question.

REFERENCES

1. Ballinger PW. *Merrill's Atlas of Radiographic Positions and Radiologic Procedures*. 7th ed. St. Louis: Mosby; 1991;1:116–117.
2. Slivka J, Resnick D. An improved radiographic view of the glenohumeral joint. *J Can Assoc Radiol.* 1979;30:83–85.
3. Ballinger PW. *Merrill's Atlas of Radiographic Positions and Radiologic Procedures*. 7th ed. St. Louis: Mosby; 1991;1:132–133.
4. DeSmet AA. Axillary projection in radiography of the nontraumatized shoulder. *AJR.* 1980;134:511–514.
5. Ballinger PW. *Merrill's Atlas of Radiographic Positions and Radiologic Procedures*. 7th ed. St. Louis: Mosby; 1991;1:120–121.
6. Gartsman GM. Arthroscopic acromioplasty for lesions of the rotator cuff. *J Bone Joint Surg Am.* 1990;72:169–180.
7. Rubin SA, Gray RL, Green WR. The scapular "Y": A diagnostic aid to shoulder trauma. *Radiology*. 1974;110:725–726.
8. DeSmet AA. Anterior oblique projection in radiography of the traumatized shoulder. *AJR.* 1980;134:515–518.
9. Ballinger PW. *Merrill's Atlas of Radiographic Positions and Radiologic Procedures*. 7th ed. St. Louis: Mosby; 1991;1:128–129.
10. Neer CS II. Impingement lesions. *Clin Orthop.* 1983;173:70–77.
11. Gold RH, Seeger LL, Yao L. Imaging shoulder impingement. *Skeletal Radiol.* 1993;22:555–561.
12. Burns WC II, Whipple TL. Anatomic relationships in the shoulder impingement syndrome. *Clin Orthop.* 1993;4:96–102.
13. Berens DL, Lockie LM. Ossification of the coraco-acromial ligament. *Radiology*. 1960;74:802–805.
14. Cone RO II, Resnick D, Danzig L. Shoulder impingement syndrome: Radiographic evaluation. *Radiology*. 1984;150:29–33.
15. Ogata S, Uhthoff HK. Acromial enthesopathy and rotator cuff tear. *Clin Orthop.* 1990;254:39–48.
16. Kitchel SH, Butters KA, Rockwood CA. The shoulder impingement syndrome. *Orthop Trans.* 1984;8:510.
17. Butters KP, Rockwood CA Jr. Office evaluation and management of the shoulder impingement syndrome. *Orthop Clin.* 1988; 19:755–765.
18. Kilcoyne RF, Reddy PK, Lyons F, Rockwood CA Jr. Optimal plain film imaging of the shoulder impingement syndrome. *AJR.* 1989; 153:795–797.
19. Jim YF, Chang CY, Wu JJ, Chang T. Shoulder impingement syndrome: Impingement view and arthrography study based on 100 cases. *Skeletal Radiol.* 1992;21:449–451.
20. Rockwood CA Jr, Lyons FR. Shoulder impingement syndrome: Diagnosis, radiographic evaluation, and treatment with a modified Neer acromioplasty. *J Bone Joint Surg Am.* 1993;75:409–423.
21. Neer CS II, Poppen NK. Supraspinatus outlet. *Orthop Trans.* 1987; 11:234.
22. Stiles RG, Otte MT. Imaging of the shoulder. *Radiology*. 1993; 188:603–613.
23. Andrews JR, Byrd JWT, Kupferman SP, Angelo RL. The profile view of the acromion. *Clin Orthop.* 1991;3:142–146.
24. Bigliani LU, Morrison DS, April EW. The morphology of the acromion and its relationship to rotator cuff tears. *Orthop Trans.* 1986; 10:2.
25. Morrison DS, Bigliani LU. The clinical significance of variations in acromial morphology. *Orthop Trans.* 1987;11:234.
26. Epstein RE, Schweitzer ME, Frieman BG, Fenlin JM, Mitchell DG. Hooked acromion: Prevalence on MR images of painful shoulders. *Radiology*. 1993;187:479–481.
27. Edelson JG, Taitz C. Anatomy of the coraco-acromial arch. *J Bone Joint Surg Br.* 1992;74:589–594.
28. Kessel L, Watson M. The painful arc syndrome: Clinical classification as a guide to management. *J Bone Joint Surg Br.* 1977;59:166–172.
29. Peterson CJ, Gentz CF. The significance of distally pointing acromioclavicular osteophytes in ruptures of the supraspinatus tendon. In: Bateman JE, Welsh RP, eds. *Surgery of the Shoulder.* Philadelphia: BC Decker; 1984:129–133.
30. Alexander OM. Radiography of the acromioclavicular articulation. *Med Radiography Photography.* 1954;30:34–39.
31. Ballinger PW. *Merrill's Atlas of Radiographic Positions and Radiologic Procedures.* 7th ed. St. Louis: Mosby; 1991;1: 140–141.
32. Cone RO, Danzig L, Resnick D, Goldman AB. The bicipital groove: Radiologic, anatomic and pathologic study. *AJR.* 1983;141:781–788.
33. Ballinger PW. *Merrill's Atlas of Radiographic Positions and Radiologic Procedures.* 7th ed. St. Louis: Mosby; 1991;1:130–131.
34. Hardy DC, Vogler JB II, White RH. The shoulder impingement syndrome: Prevalence of radiographic findings and correlation with response to therapy. *AJR.* 1986;147:557–561.
35. Norwood LA, Barrack R, Jacobson KE. Clinical presentation of complete tears of the rotator cuff. *J Bone Joint Surg Am.* 1989; 71:499–505.
36. Bjorkenheim J, Paavolainen P, Ahovuo J, Slatis P. Subacromial impingement decompressed with anterior acromioplasty. *Clin Orthop.* 1990;252:150–162.
37. Kotzen LM. Roentgen diagnosis of rotator cuff tear. *AJR.* 1971; 112:507–511.
38. Neer CS II. Anterior acromioplasty for the chronic impingement syndrome in the shoulder. *J Bone Joint Surg Am.* 1972;59: 41–50.
39. Bernageau J. Roentgenographic assessment of the rotator cuff. *Clin Orthop.* 1990;254:87–91.
40. Ellman H, Hanker G, Bayer M. Repair of the rotator cuff. *J Bone Joint Surg Am.* 1986;68:1136–1144.
41. Golding FC. The shoulder–The forgotten joint. *Brit J Radiol.* 1962; 35:149–158.
42. Cotton RE, Rideout DF. Tears of the humeral rotator cuff. *J Bone Joint Surg Br.* 1964;46:314–328.
43. Weiner DS, Macnab I. Superior migration of the humeral head. *J Bone Joint Surg Br.* 1970;52:524–527.
44. Petersson CJ, Redlund-Johnell I. The subacromial space in normal shoulder radiographs. *Acta Orthop Scand.* 1984; 55:57–58.
45. Bloom RA. The active abduction view: A new maneuvre in the diagnosis of rotator cuff tears. *Skeletal Radiol.* 1991; 20:255–258.
46. Neer CS II, Craig EV, Fukuda H. Cuff-tear arthropathy. *J Bone Joint Surg Am.* 1983;65:1232–1244.
47. McCarty DJ, Halverson PB, Carrera GF, Brewer BJ, Kozin F. "Milwaukee Shoulder"–Association of microspheroids containing hydroxyapatite crystals, active collagenase and neutral protenase with rotator cuff defects. 1. Clinical Aspects. *Arthritis Rheum.* 1981; 24:464–473.
48. Dieppe PA, Doherty M, Macfarlane DG, et al. Apatite associated destructive arthritis. *Brit J Rheumatol.* 1984; 23:84–91.
49. Campion GV, McCrae F, Alwan W, Watt I, Bradfield J, Dieppe PA. Idiopathic destructive arthritis of the shoulder. *Semin Arthritis Rheum.* 1988;17:232–245.
50. Halverson PB, McCarty DJ, Cheung HS, Ryan LM. Milwaukee

shoulder syndrome: Eleven additional cases with involvement of the knee in seven (basic calcium phosphate crystal deposition disease). *Semin Arthritis Rheum.* 1984;14:36–34.
51. Bock GW, Garcia A, Weisman MH, et al. Rapidly destructive hip disease: Clinical and imaging abnormalities. *Radiology.* 1993; 186:461–466.
52. Mudge MK, Wood VE, Frykman GK. Rotator cuff tears associated with os acromiale. *J Bone Joint Surg Am.* 1984; 66:427–429.
53. Norris TR, Fischer J, Bigliani LU, Neer CS II. The unfused acromial epiphysis and its relationship to impingement syndrome. *Orthop Trans.* 1983;7:505–506.
54. Burkhart SS. Os acromiale in a professional tennis player. *Am J Sports Med.* 1992;20:483–484.
55. Hayes CW, Conway WF. Calcium hydroxyapatite deposition disease. *Radiographics.* 1990;10:1031–1048.
56. Pedersen HE, Key JA. Pathology of calcareous tendinitis and subdeltoid bursitis. *Arch Surg.* 1951;62:50–63.
57. Uhthoff HK, Sarkar K, Maynard JA. Calcifying tendinitis: A new concept of its pathogenesis. *Clin Orthop.* 1976;118:164–168.
58. Moseley HF. *Shoulder Lesions.* 3rd ed. Baltimore: Williams & Wilkins; 1969:99–118.
59. Vigario GD, Keats TE. Localization of calcium deposits in the shoulder. *AJR.* 1970;108:806–811.
60. Goldman AB. Calcific tendinitis of the long head of the biceps brachii distal to the glenohumeral joint: Plain film radiographic findings. *AJR.* 1989;153:1011–1016.
61. Jim YF, Hsu HC, Chang CY, Wu JJ, Chang T. Coexistence of calcific tendinitis and rotator cuff tear: An arthrographic study. *Skeletal Radiol.* 1993;22:183–185.
62. Penny JN, Welsh RP: Shoulder impingement syndromes in athletes and their surgical management. *Am J Sports Med.* 1981;9:11–15.
63. Neer CS II. *Shoulder Reconstruction.* Philadelphia: WB Saunders; 1990:46–48.
64. Holder LE. Clinical radionuclide bone imaging. *Radiology.* 1990; 176:607–614.
65. Mack LA, Matsen III FA, Kilcoyne RF, et al. Ultrasound evaluation of the rotator cuff. *Radiology.* 1985;157:205–209.
66. Middleton WD, Edelstein G, Reinus WR, et al. Ultrasonography of the rotator cuff: Technique and normal anatomy. *J Ultrasound Med.* 1984;3:539–544.
67. Vick CW, Bell SA. Rotator cuff tears: Diagnosis with sonography. *AJR.* 1990;154:121–123.
68. Middleton WD, Reinus WR, Totty WG, et al. Ultrasonographic evaluation of the rotator cuff and biceps tendon. *J Bone Joint Surg Am.* 1986;68:440–450.
69. Holsbeeck MV, Strouse PJ. Sonography of the shoulder: Evaluation of the subacromial-subdeltoid bursa. *AJR.* 1993;160:561–564.
70. Middleton WD, Edelstein G, Reinus WR. Sonographic detection of rotator cuff tears. *AJR.* 1985;144:349–353.
71. Wiener SN, Seitz WH Jr. Sonography of the shoulder in patients with tears of the rotator cuff: Accuracy and value for selecting surgical options. *AJR.* 1993;160:103–107.
72. Mack LA, Rogers JV, Winter TC, et al. Ultrasound of the rotator cuff. In: Seeler LL, ed. *Diagnostic Imaging of the Shoulder.* Baltimore: Williams & Wilkins; 1992:96–118.
73. Mack LA, Nyberg DA, Matsen III FR, et al. Sonography of the postoperative shoulder. *AJR.* 1988;1089–1093.
74. Crass JR, Carig EV, Feinberg SB. Sonography of the postoperative rotator cuff. *AJR.* 1986;146:561–564.
75. Middleton WD, Reinus WR, Melson GL, et al. Pitfalls of rotator cuff sonography. *AJR.* 1986;146:555–560.
76. Middleton WD. Sonographic detection and quantification of rotator cuff tears. *AJR.* 1993;160:109–110.
77. Brandt TD, Cardone BW, Grant TH, et al. Rotator cuff sonography: A reassessment. *Radiology.* 1989;173:323–327.
78. Drakeford MK, Quinn MJ, Simpson SL, et al. A comparative study of ultrasonography and arthrography in evaluation of the rotator cuff. *Clin Orthop.* 1990;253:118–122.
79. Olive Jr RJ, Marsh HO. Ultrasonography of rotator cuff tears. *Clin Orthop.* 1992;2:110–113.
80. Miller CL, Karasick D, Kurtz AB, et al. Limited sensitivity of ultrasound for the detection of rotator cuff tears. *Skeletal Radiol.* 1989; 18:179–183.
81. Misamore GW, Woodward C. Evaluation of degenerative lesions of the rotator cuff. *J Bone Joint Surg Am.* 1991;73:704–706.
82. Goldman AB, Ghelman B. The double contrast shoulder arthrogram. *Radiology.* 1978;127:655–663.
83. Mink JH, Harris E, Rappaport M. Rotator cuff tears: Evaluation using double-contrast shoulder arthrography. *Radiology.* 1985; 157:621–623.
84. Calvert PT, Packer NP, Stoker DJ, Bayley JIL, Kessel L. Arthrography of the shoulder after operative repair of the torn rotator cuff. *J Bone Joint Surg Br.* 1986;68:147–150.
85. Mikasa M. Subacromial bursography. *J Jap Orthop Assoc.* 1979; 53:225–231.
86. Nobuhara K, Ikeda H. Rotator interval lesion. *Clin Orthop.* 1987; 223:44–50.
87. DeSmet AA. Arthrographic demonstration of the subcoracoid bursa. *Skeletal Radiol.* 1982;7:275–276.
88. Strizak AM, Danzig L, Jackson DW, Greenway G, Resnick D, Staple D. Subacromial bursography. *J Bone Joint Surg Am.* 1982; 64:196–201.
89. Fukuda H, Mikasa M, Yamanaka K. Incomplete thickness rotator cuff tears diagnosed by subacromial bursography. *Clin Orthop.* 1987;223:51–58.
90. Lie S, Mast WA. Subacromial bursography. *Radiology.* 1982; 144:626–630.
91. Uhthoff HK, Hammond DI, Sarkar K, Hooper GJ, Papoff WJ. The role of the coracoacromial ligament in the impingement syndrome. *Int Orthop.* 1988;12:97–104.
92. Goldthwait JE. An anatomic and mechanical study of the shoulder-joint, explaining many of the cases of painful shoulder, many of the recurrent dislocations and many of the cases of brachial neuralgias or neuritis. *Am J Orthop Surg.* 1909;6:579–606.
93. Gerber C, Terrier F, Ganz R. The role of the coracoid process in the chronic impingement syndrome. *J Bone Joint Surg Br.* 1985; 67:703–708.
94. Patte D. The subcoracoid impingement. *Clin Orthop.* 1990; 254: 55–59.
95. Dines DM, Warren RF, Inglis AE, Pavlov H. The coracoid impingement syndrome. *J Bone Joint Surg Br.* 1990;72:314–316.
96. Neviaser RJ, Neviaser TJ. Observations on impingement. *Clin Orthop.* 1990;254:60–63.
97. Fu FH, Harner CD, Klein AH. Shoulder impingement syndrome. *Clin Orthop.* 1991;9:162–173.
98. Rafii M, Minkoff J, Bonamo J, et al. Computed tomography (CT) arthrography of shoulder instability in athletes. *Am J Sports Med.* 1988;16;352–361.
99. Wilson AJ, Totty WG, Murphy WA, Hardy DC. Shoulder joint: Arthrographic CT and long term follow-up, with surgical correlation. *Radiology.* 1989;173:329–333.
100. Gerber C, Krushell RJ. Isolated rupture of the tendon of the subscapularis muscle. *J Bone Joint Surg Br.* 1991;736:389–394.
101. Beltran J, Gray LA, Bools JC, Zuelzer W, Weis LD, Unverferth LJ. Rotator cuff lesions of the shoulder: Evaluation by direct sagittal CT arthrography. *Radiology.* 1986;160:161–165.
102. Blum A, Boyer B, Regent D, Simon JM, Claudon M, Mole E. Direct coronal view of the shoulder with arthrographic CT. *Radiology.* 1993;188:677–681.
103. Huber DJ, Sauter R, Mueller E, et al. MR imaging of the normal shoulder. *Radiology.* 1986;158:405–408.
104. Kieft GJ, Bloem JL, Obermann WR, et al. Normal shoulder: MR imaging. *Radiology.* 1986;159:741–745.
105. Middleton WD, Kneeland JB, Carrera GF, et al. High resolution MR imaging of the normal rotator cuff. *AJR.* 1987;148: 559–564.
106. Iannotti JP, Zlatkin MB, Esterhai JL, et al. Magnetic resonance imaging of the shoulder. *J Bone Joint Surg Am.* 1991; 73:17–29.
107. Bushong SC: *Magnetic Resonance Imaging: Physical and Biological Principles.* St. Louis: Mosby; 1988.
108. Sprawls Jr P. *Physical Principles of Medical Imaging.* Rockville, MD: Aspen Systems; 1987.
109. *Christensen's Physics of Diagnostic Radiology.* Avery TS III, Dowdey JE, Marry RC Jr, eds. 4th ed. Philadelphia: Lea & Febiger; 1990.
110. Seeger LL. Magnetic resonance imaging of the shoulder. *Clin Orthop.* 1989;4:48–59.
111. Petersilge CA, Witte DH, Sewell BO, et al. Normal regional anatomy of the shoulder. *MRI Clin North America.* 1993; 1:1–18.

112. Burk DL Jr, Karaskck D, Kurtz AB, et al. Rotator cuff tears: Prospective comparison of MR imaging with arthrography, sonography, and surgery. *AJR.* 1989:153:87–92.
113. Evancho AM, Stiles RG, Fajman WA. MR imaging diagnosis of rotator cuff tears. *AJR.* 1988;151:751–754.
114. Farley TE, Neumann CH, Steinbach LS. Full thickness tears of the rotator cuff of the shoulder: Diagnosis with MR imaging. *AJR.* 1992;158:347–351.
115. Kneeland JB, Middleton WD, Carrera GF, et al. MR imaging of the shoulder: Diagnosis of rotator cuff tears. *AJR.* 1987;149: 333–337.
116. Recht MP, Resnick D. Magnetic resonance imaging studies of the shoulder. *J Bone Joint Surg Am.* 1993;75:1244–1253.
117. Stoller DW, Fritz RC. Magnetic resonance imaging of impingement and rotator cuff tears. *MRI Clin North Am.* 1993;1:47–63.
118. Seeger LL, Ruszkowski JT, Bassett LW. MR imaging of the normal shoulder: Anatomic correlation. *AJR.* 1987;148:83–91.
119. Kjellin I, Ho CP, Cervilla V, et al. Alterations in the supraspinatus tendon at MR imaging: Correlation with histopathologic findings in cadavers. *Radiology.* 1991; 181:837–841.
120. Kieft GJ, Bloem JL, Rozing PM, et al. Rotator cuff impingement syndrome: MR imaging. *Radiology.* 1988;166:211–214.
121. Seeger LL, Gold RH, Bassett LW, et al. Shoulder impingement syndrome: MR findings in 53 shoulders. *AJR.* 1088;150:343–347.
122. Crues JV III, Fareed DO. Magnetic resonance imaging of shoulder impingement. *Top Magn Reson Imaging.* 1991;3:39–49.
123. Chan TW, Dalinka MK, Kneeland JB, et al. Biceps tendon dislocation: Evaluation with MR imaging. *Radiology.* 1991; 179:649–652.
124. Cervills V, Schweitzer ME, Ho CP, et al. Medial dislocation of the biceps brachii tendon: Appearance at MR imaging. *Radiology.* 1991;180:523–526.
125. Kieft GJ, Sartoris DJ, Bloem JL, et al. Magnetic resonance imaging of glenohumeral joint diseases. *Skeletal Radiol.* 1987; 16:285–290.
126. Rafii M, Firooznja H, Golimbu C, et al. Magnetic resonance imaging of glenohumeral instability. *MRI Clin North Am.* 1993; 1:87–104.
127. Cartland JP, Crues JV III, Stauffer A, et al. MR imaging in the evaluation of SLAP injuries of the shoulder: Findings in 10 patients. *AJR.* 1992;159:787–792.
128. Hodler J, Kursunoglu-Brahne S, Flannigan B, et al. Injuries of the superior portion of the glenoid labrum involving the insertion of the biceps tendon: MR findings in nine cases. *AJR.* 1992;159:565–568.
129. Liou JTS, Wilson AJ, Totty WG. The normal shoulder: Common variations that simulate pathologic conditions at MR imaging. *Radiology.* 1993;186:435–441.
130. Kaplan PA, Bryans KG, Davick JP, et al. MR imaging of the normal shoulder: Variants and pitfalls. *Radiology.* 1992; 184:519–524.
131. Newmann CH, Holt RG, Steinbach LS, et al. MR imaging of the shoulder: Appearance of the supraspinatus tendon in asymptomatic volunteers. *AJR.* 1992;158:1281–1287.
132. Erickson SJ, Cox IH, Hyde JS, et al. Effect of tendon orientation on MR imaging signal intensity: A manifestation of the "Magic Angle" phenomenon. *Radiology.* 1991;181:389–392.
133. Owen RS, Iannotti JP, Kneeland JB, et al. Shoulder after surgery: MR imaging with surgical validation. *Radiology.* 1993;186:443–447.
134. Haygood TM, Oxner KG, Kneeland JB, et al. Magnetic resonance imaging of the postoperative shoulder. *MRI Clin North Am.* 1993; 1:143–155.
135. Flannigan B, Kursunoglu-Brahme S, Snyder S, et al. MR arthrography of the shoulder: Comparison with conventional MR imaging. *AJR.* 1990;155:829–832.
136. Plamer WE, Brown JH, Rosenthal DI. Rotator cuff: Evaluation with fat-suppressed MR arthrography. *Radiology.* 1993;188: 683–687.
137. Winalski CS, Aliabadi P, Wright RJ, et al. Enhancement of joint fluid with intravenously administered gadopentetate dimeglumine: Technique, rationale and implications. *Radiology.* 1993; 187:179–185.
138. Munk PL, Vellet AD, Levin MF. Intravenous adminstration of Gadolinium in the evaluation of rheumatoid arthritis of the shoulder. *Canad Assoc Radiol J* 1993;44:99–106.
139. Seeger LL, Lubowitz J, Thomas BJ. Case report 815. *Skeletal Radiol.* 1993;22:615–617.

Chapter 7

Classification of Rotator Cuff Tears

Michael D. Ciepiela and Wayne Z. Burkhead, Jr.

For many years the goal has been to compare apples to apples and oranges to oranges. The next generation of shoulder surgeons will need to compare Granny Smith's apples to Granny Smith's apples and mandarin oranges to mandarin oranges.

Wayne Z. Burkhead, Jr.

Classification schemes are used for the purposes of identification, diagnoses, treatment, and prognosis in a clinical setting. From a scientific point of view, they are requisite for the meaningful comparison of the results of various modes of treatment. Obviously, the ideal system would allow for the integration of all of these functions. Rotator cuff tears have been organized in a variety of ways. No single method to date appears to have satisfied all surgeons' criteria. Most likely, in the future, the best part of each method will be meshed into an organized, integrated whole.

Codman was the first to attempt classification of rotator cuff tears as observed from a series of 400 painful shoulders.[1] His chart of four common causes of painful shoulders included complete rupture of supraspinatus, partial rupture of supraspinatus, calcified deposits, and tendinitis (frozen shoulder). He classified rotator cuff lesions as follows: (1) an incomplete rupture in the sense that it does not involve the whole thickness of the cuff; (2) a complete rupture, the whole thickness of the rotator cuff and capsule are torn, resulting in direct communication between the subdeltoid bursa and the joint cavity; and (3) a pure transverse rupture was considered an uncommon lesion, pure vertical rents or longitudinal splits paralleling the direction of the cuff fibers. Such a tear was most frequently found in young persons whose tendinous cuff was thick and strong enough to withstand transverse rupture, and invariably, had been situated in the aponeurosis between the subscapularis and supraspinatus with a portion of the cuff "aptly" described by Jones as the coracocapsular ligament, which we now refer to more commonly as the rotator interval.

INCOMPLETE TEARS

Degree or Depth of Tear

Rotator cuff tears have been described according to the amount of tendon material damaged. Partial-thickness tears involve some portion of the tendon, with the remainder intact. These tears are further divided into subgroups, according to whether the tear is adjacent to the articular surface or the bursal surface, or insubstance. Fukuda found a 13% incidence of partial rotator cuff tears in 149 cadaveric left shoulders. Of these tears, 3% were on the bursal side, 3% on the articular side, and 7% were intertendinous.[2]

Ellman separates partial-thickness tears into three grades depending on the depth of the tear.[3] Grade 1 tears have a depth less than 3 mm, which is less than one-fourth of the thickness of the cuff. Only the capsule or superficial fibers are involved. Grade 2 tears are less than 6-mm thick, which is less than one-half of the cuff thickness. Grade 3 tears involve more than one-half the cuff thickness and are subdivided into articular (A) or bursal (B) side tears (Fig. 7–1).

Matsen refers to all partial tears as Grade 1A tears regardless of the depth of tearing.[4]

Shape

Wolfgang, in his classic 1974 article, classified rotator cuff tears according to the pattern they assumed (Table 7–1).[5] He observed small tears to be transverse in nature.

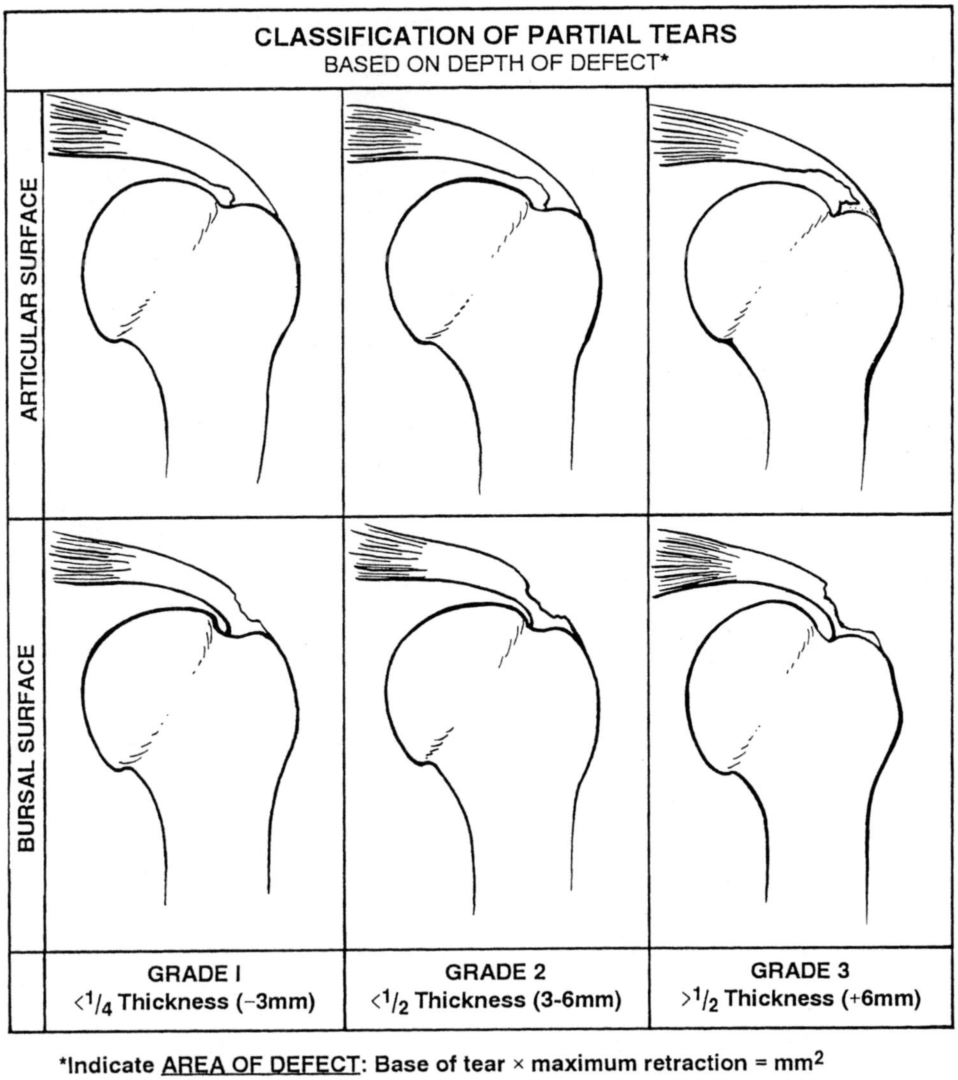

Fig. 7–1. Classification of partial tears offered by Ellman is related to the depth of the defect, as well as the area of the defect. (From Ellman H. Rotator cuff disorders. In: Ellman H, Gartsman GM, eds. *Arthroscopic Shoulder Surgery and Related Disorders.* Philadelphia: Lea & Febiger; 1993:98–119.)

Table 7–1. Wolfgang's Classification of Rotator Cuff Tears

Transverse
Triangular or crescentic
Massive

As these tears enlarged, they assumed a triangular or crescentic configuration. Massive tears resulted from an enlarging of one of the above patterns, either progressively or from severe trauma. A teleological component may be inherent in this classification system, by virtue of the time dependent retraction patterns of the muscles acting on the tear (Fig. 7–2).

A more elaborate classification system, based on shape or configuration of the tear that is dependent on both the size and location of the tear, has been offered by Ellman (Table 7–2).[3] This scheme includes the rare full-thickness vertical tear, as well as the more common transverse linear tear involving the supraspinatus at its insertion (Fig. 7–3). A crescent-shaped tear (Fig. 7–4) is an extension of a transverse linear tear by pull of the infraspinatus and supraspinatus muscles. What were previously referred to generically as triangular-shaped tears are the L-shaped and reverse L-shaped tears (Fig. 7–5). The L-shaped tear is a transverse linear tear with extension into the interval between the infraspinatus and supraspinatus. Conversely, a reverse L tear (Fig. 7–6) has its extension in the rotator interval, between the supraspinatus and subscapularis muscles. The L and reverse L classifications are helpful in determining arm position at the time of repair. A trapezoidal tear (Fig. 7–7), if large enough, involves the insertions of both the infraspinatus and supraspinatus. A massive tear is defined as having extension into the teres minor or anterior subscapularis.

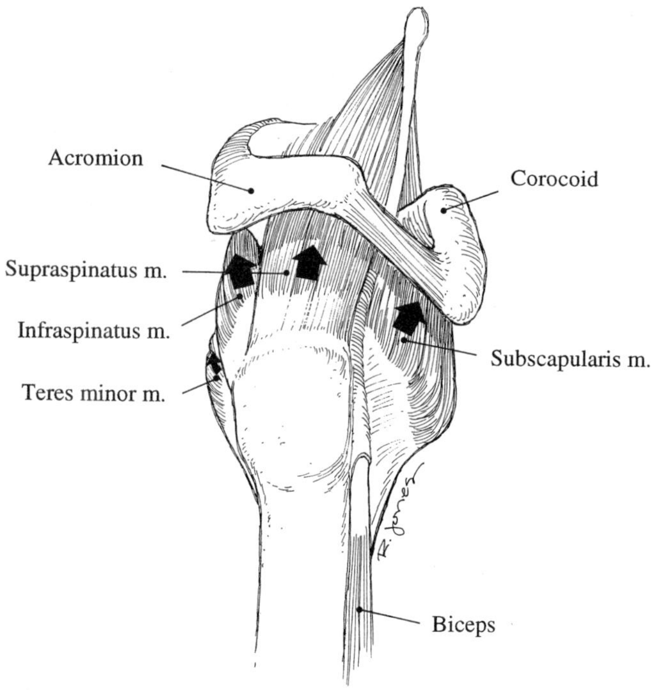

Fig. 7–2. The forces acting on tears are related to the direction and force of the muscles as illustrated. (After Hengst.)

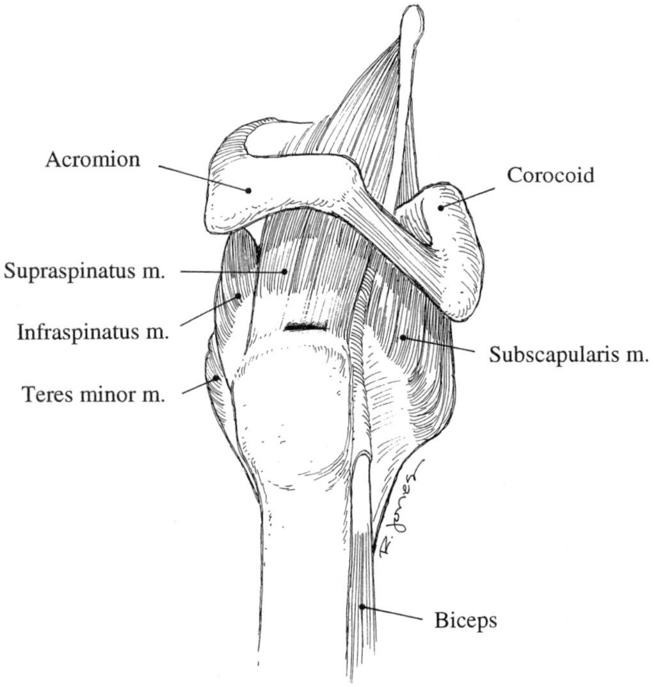

Fig. 7–3. The more common transverse tear at the level of the greater tuberosity. (After Hengst.)

Table 7–2. Pattern of Rupture

Shape	*Location*
Transverse linear	Supraspinatus at insertion.
Crescent	A transverse tear deformed by the pull of infraspinatus and subscapularis.
L-shaped	Extension between infraspinatus and supraspinatus.
Reverse L	Extension into rotator interval.
Trapezoidal	Insertions of infraspinatus and supraspinatus.
Massive	Extension into teres or anterior subscapularis.

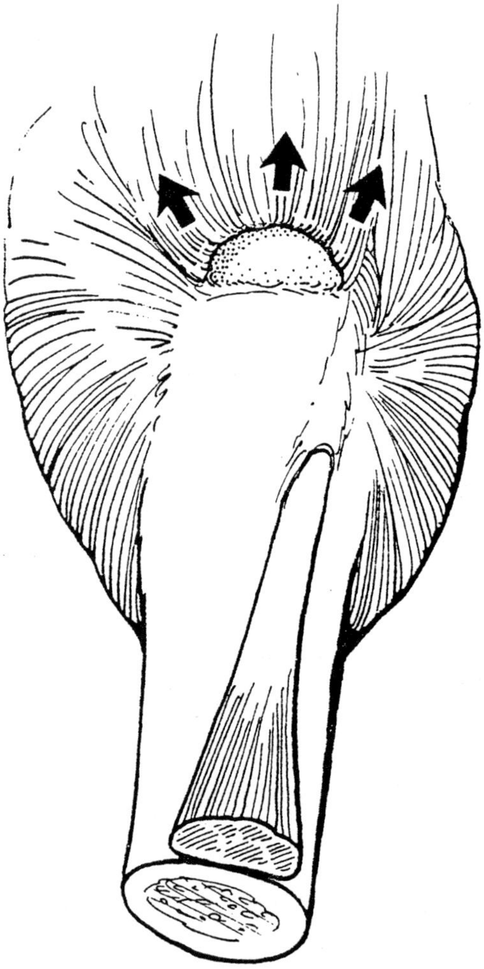

Fig. 7–4. A small crescent-shaped tear. Note deforming forces. (After Hengst.)

Etiology

Neer classified tears by etiology (Table 7–3).[6] He felt that 95% of tears he observed were "impingement tears," occurring in patients older than 40 years of age. He subclassed the predictable size of tears from this group according to duration of the tears, subsequent trauma, and the directional forces of the supraspinatus, infraspinatus, and subscapularis. His second group was termed "traumatic tears." He felt these occurred in pa-

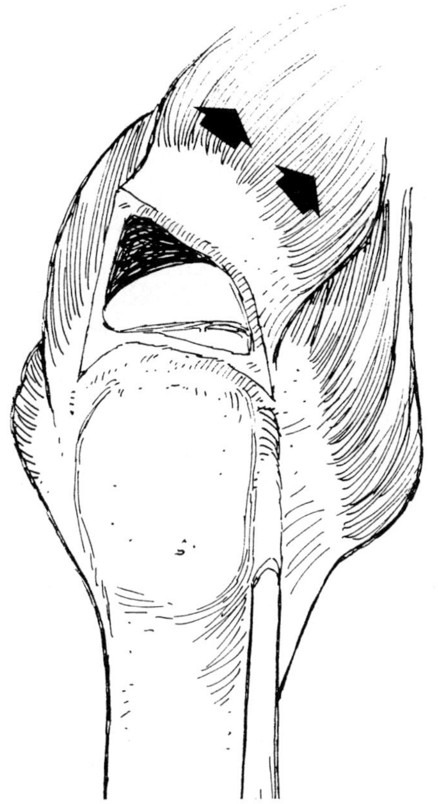

Fig. 7–5. The L-shaped tear is an extension of the transverse linear tear into the interval between the infraspinatus and supraspinatus. (After Hengst.)

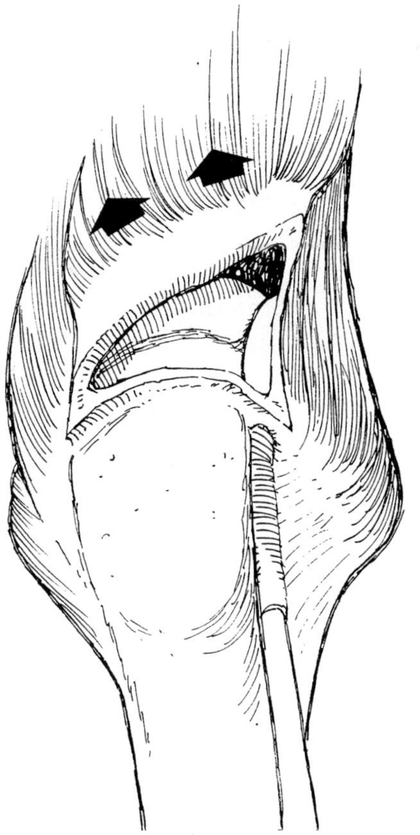

Fig. 7–6. A reverse L-shaped tear extends into the rotator interval which, like the L-shaped tear, creates a triangular-shaped defect. (After Hengst.)

tients less than 40 years old and comprised less than 5% of tears observed. He further subgrouped traumatic tears into those that occurred because of a single injury, repetitive microtrauma, or severe violence. His third classification was "rotator interval tears due to multidirectional dislocation." This type of tear also occurred in patients less than 40 years of age and was found in less than 5% of tears observed. The final group was "acute glenohumeral dislocations after age 40," which were less than 5% of tears observed. Neer used his classification system to develop an algorithm incorporating pathology, prognosis, and treatment. Those that do not follow the impingement theory classify tears as traumatic or degenerative.[7]

Size

Other classification systems define tears by their size only, which is measured at the widest point of retraction after minimal debridement of 1 to 2 mm (Table 7–4). Small tears measure less than 1 cm, medium tears less than 3 cm, large tears 3 to 5 cm, and massive tears greater than 5 cm.[8] Some investigators prefer small tears to be defined as less than 2 cm and massive tears as greater than 4 cm.[9]

Ellman points out that the length of the tear does not always correspond to the difficulty of repair. He proposes the *area* of the tear be measured in centimeters squared.[9] This is calculated using the base of the tear along the former insertion site times the depth of muscle retraction. This approach seems logical, however, because of the individual variation in humeral head size and insertion widths; therefore, an absolute area of the tear may not allow accurate comparison or project the relative difficulty of repair.

Age

Rotator cuff tears have also been classified according to the age of the tear (Table 7–5). An acute tear has been defined as less than 6 weeks old, a subacute tear as 6 weeks to 6 months old, a chronic tear as 6 months to 1 year, and an old tear as greater than 1 year in duration.[9]

Number of Tendons

Matsen's classification is based on the extent to which the musculotendinous insertion of the rotator cuff has failed.[4] Stage 1B tears are full-thickness defects isolated

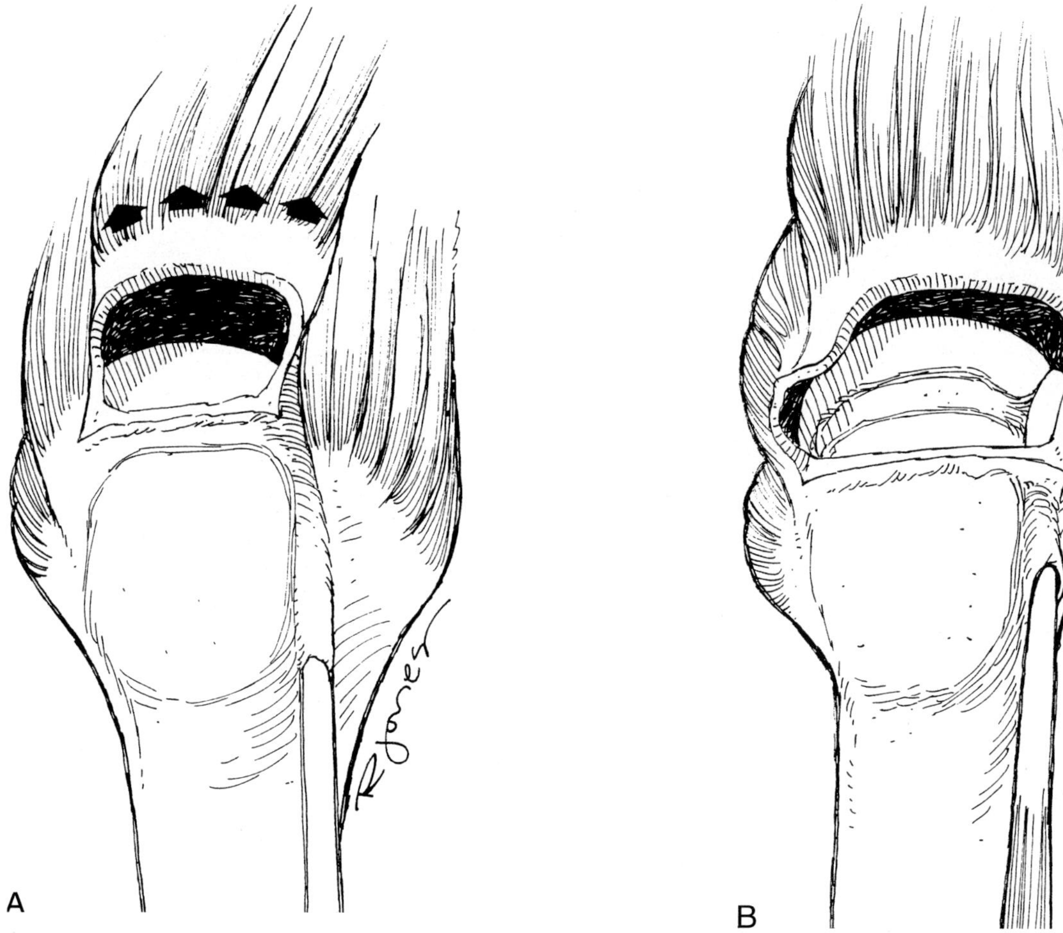

Fig. 7–7. ***A and B,*** **Small and large trapezoidal-shaped tears. (After Hengst.)**

Table 7–3. Neer's Classification of Rotator Cuff Tears

Mechanism	*% of All Tears*	*Age of Patient (Years)*	*Pathology*	*Prognosis*	*Treatment*
"Impingement tears" due to outlet impingement; no injury in 50%	95	Over 40	Centered on the supraspinatus; may be suddenly enlarged by a trivial injury ("acute extension")	Tend to progress slowly unless "acute extension"	Anterior acromioplasty and cuff repair
Traumatic tears	Under 5	Under 40	Usually incomplete supraspinatus tears	Tend to heal	Conservative
Single injury	Rare (without fractures)				
Repetitive microtrauma	Example, baseball pitchers	Under 40	Usually incomplete supraspinatus tears	Tend to heal	Rest; later change style or use
Supreme violence	Traction or "superior dislocation"	Any age	Massive cuff avulsion, often with nerve injuries	Guarded	Early recognition and surgical repair
"Rotator interval tears," enlarged rotator interval of acquired multidirectional dislocations	Under 5	Under 40	"Cleft" Enlargement with instability; arthrogram usually shows ballooning rather than leak	Recurrent dislocations Chronic disability	Repair interval and repair instability, e.g. inferior capsular shift
Acute glenohumeral dislocations after age 40 years		Over 40	Interval and subscapularis tendon torn	May heal	Observe initially

Table 7–4. Size Measured at Widest Point of Retraction

Size	*Width*
Small	Less than 1 cm
Medium	1–3 cm
Large	3–5 cm
Massive	>5 cm
(Ellman)	–measure area of tear in cm^2 –base of tear along former insertion × depth of retraction

Table 7–5. Duration

	Age of Tear
Acute	<6 weeks old
Subacute	6 weeks–6 months
Chronic	6 months–1 year
Old	>1 year

to the supraspinatus. Stage 2 tears involve the supraspinatus and at least a portion of the infraspinatus. Stage 3 tears are full-thickness tears involving supraspinatus, infraspinatus, and subscapularis. Stage 4 tears represent rotator cuff arthropathy.

Topography and Trophicity

Patte developed an elaborate classification system based on anatomic and pathologic considerations (Table 7–6).[10] He first defined the extent of the tear in the sagittal plane. Group I is defined as partial or full thickness and less than 1 cm. This is subgrouped into deep partial, superficial partial, or small full-thickness tears. Group II is defined as a full-thickness tear involving the entire supraspinatus tendon. Group III is a full-thickness tear involving more than one tendon. Group IV is a massive tear with concomitant osteoarthritis.

The next element Patte defined was a topography of the tear in the sagittal plane (Fig. 7–9). He divided the sagittal plane into six segments: segment 1 contains the subscapularis; segment 2 contains the coracohumeral ligament; segment 3 contains the supraspinatus only; segment 4 contains the supraspinatus and the upper one-half of the infraspinatus; segment 5, the supraspinatus and the entire infraspinatus; and segment 6 contains the subscapularis, supraspinatus, and infraspinatus. Patte correlated rotator cuff tears to the defined segments as follows: anterosuperior tears involve segments 1, 2, and 3; superior tears involve segments 2 and 3; posterosuperior tears involve segments 4 and 5; and total cuff tears involve segment 6.

The next portion of Patte's scheme divides the topography of the tear in the frontal plane into three stages (Fig. 7–10). Stage I occurs when the proximal tendon stump is close to its bony insertion. Lesions in which the

Table 7–6. Anatomic-Pathologic Classification

Extent of Tear	
Group I	Partial- or full-thickness <1 cm sagittal Deep partial Superficial Small full-thickness
Group II	Full-thickness entire supraspinatus
Group III	Full-thickness more than 1 tendon
Group IV	Massive tear with osteoarthritis
Topography of Tear in Sagittal Plane Divides Into Six Segments	
Segment 1	Subscapularis
Segment 2	Coracohumeral ligament
Segment 3	Supraspinatus only
Segment 4	Supraspinatus and upper 1/2 infraspinatus
Segment 5	Supraspinatus and entire infraspinatus
Segment 6	Subscapularis, supraspinatus, and infraspinatus
(Then Correlated as Follows)	
Anterosuperior tears	Segments 1, 2, 3
Superior tears	Segments 2, 3
Posterosuperior tears	Segments 4, 5
Total cuff tears	Segment 6
Topography of Tear in Frontal Plane, Three Stages	
Stage 1	Proximal tendon stump close to bony insertion
Stage 2	Tendon stump at level of humeral head
Stage 3	Tendon stump at level of glenoid
Trophic Quality of Muscle, Four Stages–Based on Fatty Degeneration of Muscle as Seen on CT	
1. Fat streaks minimal	
2. Fat streaks less than dark streaks (muscle)	
3. Fat streaks equal to dark streaks (muscle)	
4. Fat streaks greater than dark streaks (muscle)	
State of Long Head of Biceps Correlate to Extent of Tear in Sagittal Plane	
Intact	
Torn	
Dislocated	
For anterosuperior tear, no functional adversity. For Group III—may have superior migration of humeral head.	

tendon stump is at the level of the humeral head are referred to as Stage II. Stage III is defined by the tendon stump being at the level of the glenoid.

Patte attempted to define a trophic quality of muscle as observed on CT. He felt this portion of the schematic to be evolving; however, he divided his observations into four stages. These stages are based on the amount of fat (light streaks) compared to muscle (dark streaks). The stages progress from minimal light streaks, light streaks less than dark, light streaks equal to dark, and light streaks greater than dark streaks.

Patte thought that the state of the long head of the biceps, as it correlates to the extent of the tear in the sagittal plane, to be important. He divided this observation into intact, torn, or dislocated long head of the biceps. Clinically, he stated that for an anterosuperior tear, the condition of the long head of the biceps offers no functional adversity. For Group III tears, however, in his opinion, the long head's absence accelerates superior migration of the humeral head and has a detrimental effect on outcome.

Patte's classification system was designed to provide prognostic and diagnostic data for both operative and nonoperative patients. His goal was to provide clinical studies with the ability to predict the sequelae of tears, although this data has not been accumulated. The various components of this system are useful, but it is not apparent how the components correlate with each other. Neer has provided an algorithm that offers prognosis and treatment plans for his categories of tears. However, the completeness in classifying tears might be inadequate.

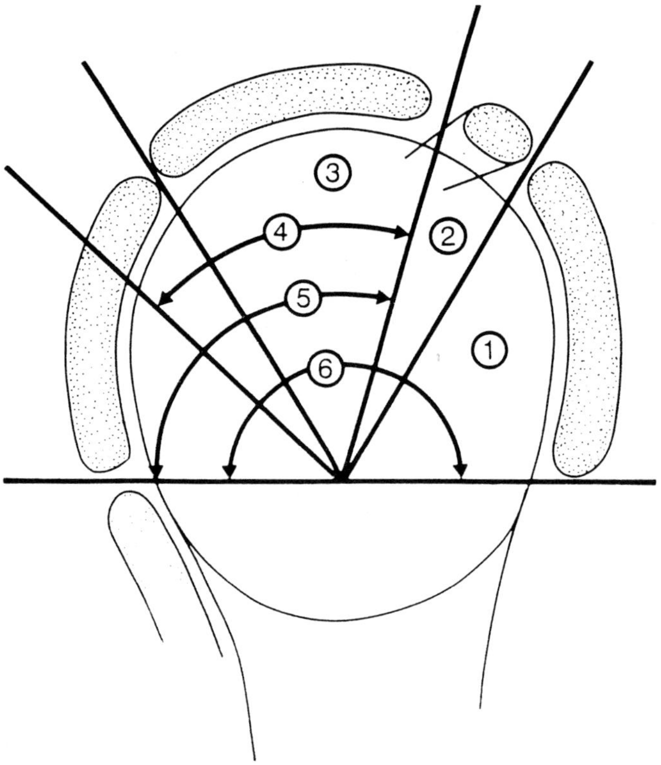

Fig. 7–8. Topography of tears in the sagittal plane. Location of extent of tears determine their division into segments; Anterosuperior lesions: segments 1, 2, and 3; superior lesions: segments 2 and 3; posterior-superior lesions: segments 4 and 5; and total cuff lesions: segment 6.

TOWARDS A UNIFIED CLASSIFICATION SYSTEM

The more traditional classification systems of defining the size or configuration of the tear also lack completeness. However, the familiarity of these methods throughout the literature lends some assistance in preoperative planning as one selects the type of repair necessary. A system that integrates these methods with the methods of Patte seems appropriate, as clearly the trophicity of the muscle and, therefore, it's ability to be rehabilitated is important in the postoperative result. A potential equation exists combining some of the aspects of all the previous classifications with one important (I think) addition for comparing tendon tears: (duration of tear in weeks) × (extent of tear, cm) × (degree of retraction, cm) × (trophicity) divided by the (humeral head diameter). This equation would then provide, with the denominator being the patient's head diameter, an anthropomorphic constant that would allow comparisons of cuff tears in subjects with a large humeral head diameter in whom a 2-cm tear may represent a relatively small area (of the supraspinatus) with subjects who have small diameter humeral heads in whom a 2-cm tear would be relatively larger (involving more than one tendon). The specific tendons involved could then be simply stated. This system would then allow comparisons between subjects with similar tears to evaluate different methods of treatment, and as well, a comparison between subjects with different tears to evaluate the outcome of treatment or nontreatment of different lesions. The value of any classification scheme can be weighed only after its inter and intra observer reliability are tested. Furthermore, even if reliable, classifications that do not alter treatment or prognosis seem superfluous. However, the adoption of a standardized classification would allow us to compare apples to apples and would aid us in perfecting Codman's "end result idea."

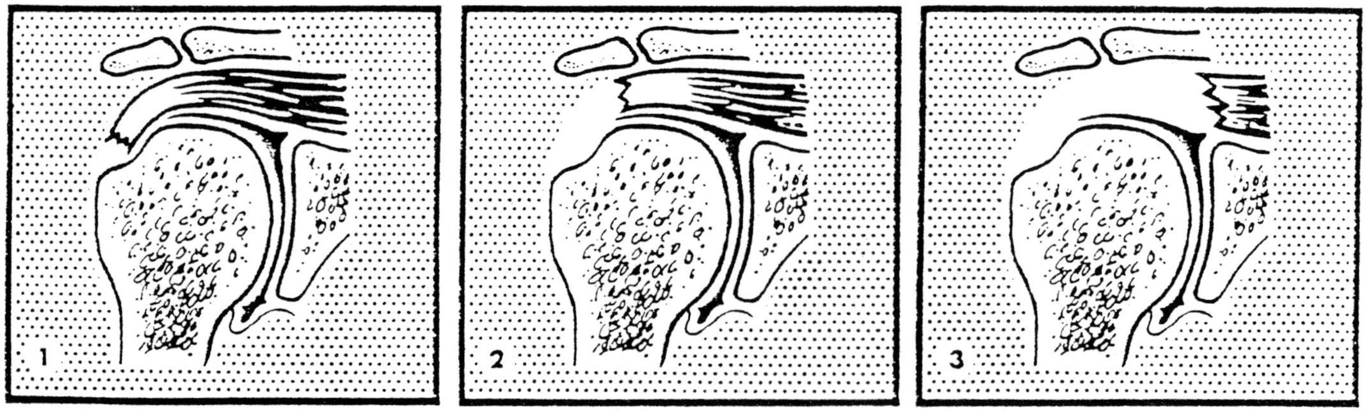

Fig. 7–9. Topography of the tear in the frontal plane. (From Patte D. Classification of rotator cuff lesions. *Clin Orthop.* 1990;254:81–86.) *A,* Stage I: the tendon stump is close to its bony insertion. *B,* Stage II: the tendon stump is at the level of the humeral head. *C,* Stage III: the tendon stump is at the level of the glenoid.

REFERENCES

1. Codman EA. *The Shoulder.* Malabar, FL: RE Krieger; 1934:123–224.
2. Fukuda H, Mikassa M, Ogawa K. The partial thickness tear of the rotator cuff. *Orthop Trans.* 1983;7:137.
3. Ellman H. Rotator cuff disorders. In: Ellman H, Gartsman GM, eds. *Arthroscopic Shoulder Surgery and Related Disorders.* Philadelphia: Lea & Febiger; 1993:98–119.
4. Harryman DT, Mack LA, Wang K, Jackins SE, Richardson ML, Matsen FA. Repairs of the rotator cuff. Correlation of functional results with integrity of the cuff. *J Bone Joint Surg Am.* 1991;73:982–989.
5. Wolfgang GL. Surgical repairs of tears of the rotator cuff of the shoulder. *J Bone Joint Surg Am.* 1974;56:14–26.
6. Neer CS II. Cuff tears, biceps lesions, and impingement. In: Neer CS II, ed. *Shoulder Reconstruction.* Philadelphia: WB Saunders; 1990:63–70.
7. Uhthoff HK, Sarkar K. Classification and definition of tendinopathies. In: Watson MS, ed. *Surgical Disorders of the Shoulder.* Edinburgh: Churchill Livingstone; 1991:259–270.
8. Cofield RH, Lanzer WL. Pathology of rotator cuff tearing in methods of tendon repair (abstract). *Orthop Trans.* 1985;9:42.
9. Ellman H. Surgical treatment of rotator cuff rupture. In: Watson M, ed. *Surgical Disorders of the Shoulder.* 1991: 283–284.
10. Patte D. Classification of rotator cuff lesions. *Clin Orthop.* 1990; 254:81–86.

Section 4

Clinical Disorders

Chapter 8

The Coracoacromial Arch Impingement Syndromes

James A. Shankwiler, Michael D. Ciepiela, and Wayne Z. Burkhead, Jr.

Necessity's sharp pinch.

Shakespeare, King Lear

Webster's dictionary defines impingement thusly: **impinge** (im-pinj) *vb* (L *impingere,* fr. *int pangere,* to strike; see Fang) **1**: to strike, hit or dash (on or upon something), **2**: to touch (on or upon); have an effect.[1] Regardless of the newer theories and nomenclature for the events that take place in the coracoacromial arch, there is no doubt that impingement, even if only in its tertiary definition (i.e., to have an effect) is a valid descriptive term for these syndromes. The fact that it derives from the word fang makes Rockwood's analogy of a "shark's tooth" acromion all the more accurate.

HISTORY

A recent expansion has occurred in the study, understanding, and treatment of impingement syndrome and its related conditions. In fact, interest in this area has existed for quite some time. In 1867 Jarjavey gave what is credited as the first description of subacromial bursitis.[2] Subsequently, in 1872 Duplay described his findings regarding autopsy specimens of post-traumatic shoulders with stiffness and pain.[3] He surmised that injury to the subacromial and/or subdeltoid bursa led to a clinical condition of pain and stiffness that he termed "periarthritis humeroscapularis." Duplay's findings were contested at the time as being attributable to rheumatic or other etiologic factors. In 1931 Meyer identified the importance of the undersurface of the acromion in the etiology of rotator cuff tears.[4] Codman was the first to associate significant changes in the supraspinatus tendon with the changes in the subacromial bursa noted in humeroscapular periarthritis. He stressed the importance of rotator cuff tendinopathy and tearing in shoulder pathology.[5] Subsequently, other investigators including McLaughlin,[6] Smith-Peterson,[7] and Watson-Jones[8] recognized the importance of subacromial impingement in shoulder morbidity. Early surgical reports discussed the performance of complete or lateral acromionectomy for the treatment of this condition. These procedures were complicated by weakness and late detachment of the deltoid, sinuses, scarring, and, in the case of lateral acromionectomy, persistent impingement symptomatology. In 1972 Neer described his results of dissection of 100 scapulae and coined the term "impingement syndrome." [9] He related the importance of the anterior-inferior acromion to mechanical attrition of the supraspinatus tendon and the rationale behind performance of anterior acromioplasty. Since that time, advances in diagnostic and surgical techniques have paralleled an increased understanding of the pathomechanics and treatment of this condition. Despite these advances, controversy still remains concerning the etiology and ultimate management of these lesions.

Anatomy

An understanding of the anatomy of the shoulder girdle is essential for elucidation of the pathomechanics of

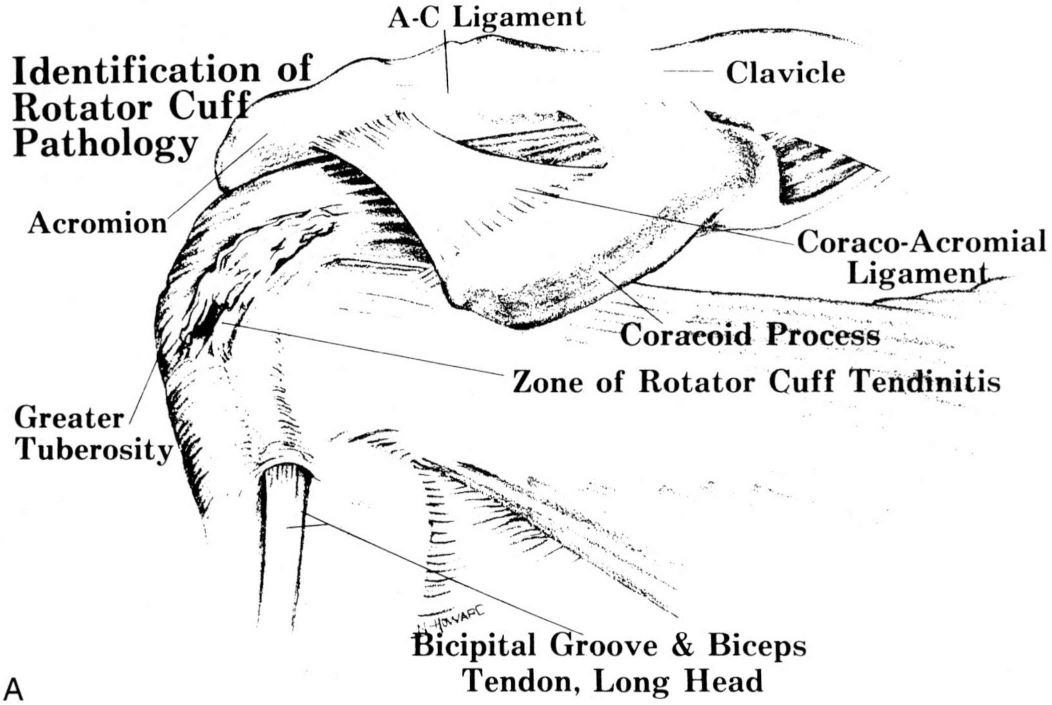

A

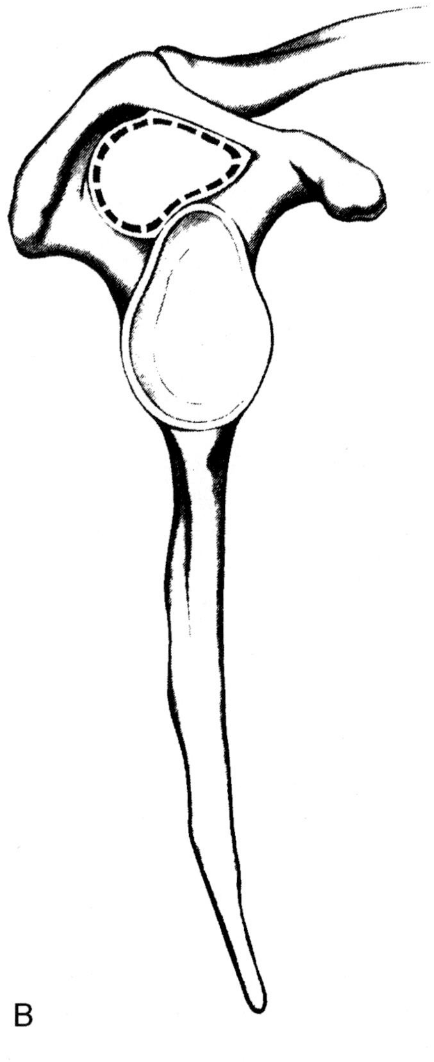

B

Fig. 8–1. *A,* The anatomy of the shoulder is demonstrated here in reference to the coracoacromial arch with the presence of an associated rotator cuff. *B,* The bony and ligamentous anatomy of the coracoacromial arch creates a passage through which the supraspinatus tendon traverses to its insertion on the proximal humerus.

impingement. The scapula has three bony processes: the acromion, the coracoid, and the spine (Fig. 8–1). The acromion is formed from three separate ossification centers: the preacromion, mesoacromion, and meta-acromion (Fig. 8–2). These fuse to form the acromion, usually by the age of 22.[10] The failure of one of these centers to unite creates an os acromiale, with the most common region being between the mesoacromion and meta-acromion. The reported frequency of os acromiale in the population has been quoted as ranging from 2.7 to 6%.[11,12]

Acromial shape has been noted to have an impact on impingement and the incidence of rotator cuff tears. Bigliani et al. evaluated 71 cadavers for acromial morphology.[13] They subsequently described three types: Type I or flat acromions (17%), Type II or curved acromions (43%), and Type III or hooked acromions (40%) (Fig. 8–3). Rotator cuff tears were seen most frequently with Type III acromions (73%), followed by Type II (24%) acromions, with the least number being seen with Type I (3%).

The length of the acromion plays an important role in the development of degenerative changes and associated cuff problems, as illustrated in a recent article by Edelson and Taitz.[14] The investigators also found that rather than the shape of the acromion, the absolute length as well as the slope of the acromion was more important in the production of these degenerative changes (Fig. 8–4). The investigators also point out the importance of exposing the anterolateral corner of the acromion by showing that degenerative changes occurred not only on the acromial facet of the AC joint, but also on the anterolateral aspect of the acromion itself. The overall length was, in turn, related to the shape in the coronal plane. The longest specimens were "cobra-shaped" (Fig. 8–5). A mean length of 6.2 cm (5 to 7.75 cm) was found in 33% of the specimens. The shortest specimens (22%) from disease were square-tipped, with a mean length of 5.2 cm; degenerative changes were found in only 11% of these

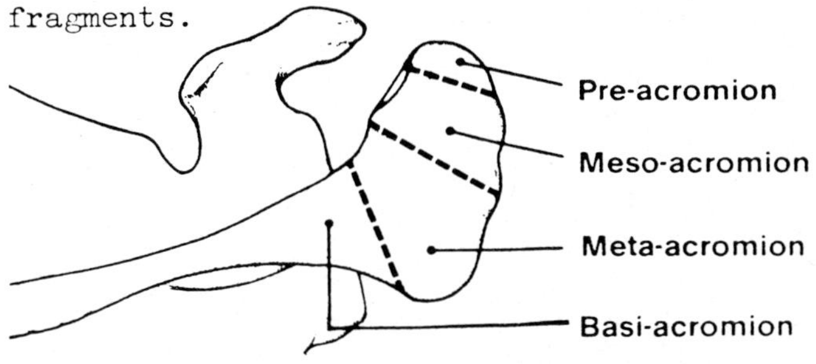

Fig. 8–2. The acromion is formed from the fusion of three separate ossific nuclei: The preacromion, mesoacromion, and meta-acromion. Failure to fuse results in the formation of an os acromiale, with the most common region being between the mesoacromion and meta-acromion.

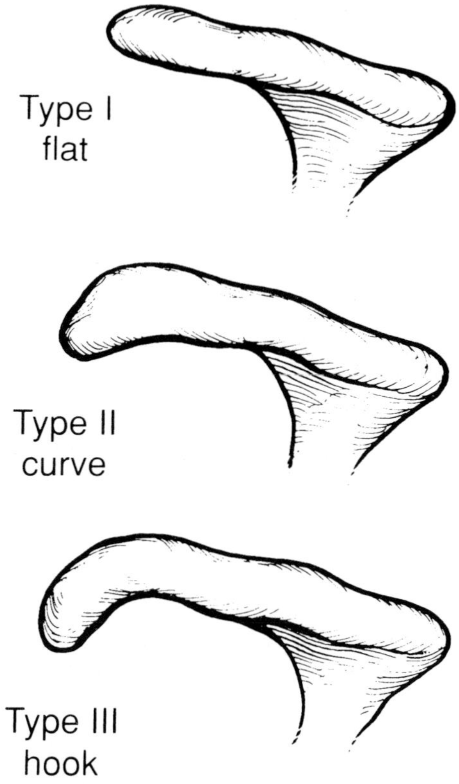

Fig. 8–3. Acromial morphology has been classified into three distinct shapes: Type I or flat (17%), Type II or curved (43%), and Type III or hooked (40%). A higher incidence of rotator cuff tears is associated with Type II and Type III acromial processes. (From Rockwood CA Jr. Shoulder impingement syndrome: Diagnosis, radiographic evaluation, and treatment with a modified Neer acromioplasty. *J Bone Joint Surg Am.* 1993;75:409–423.)

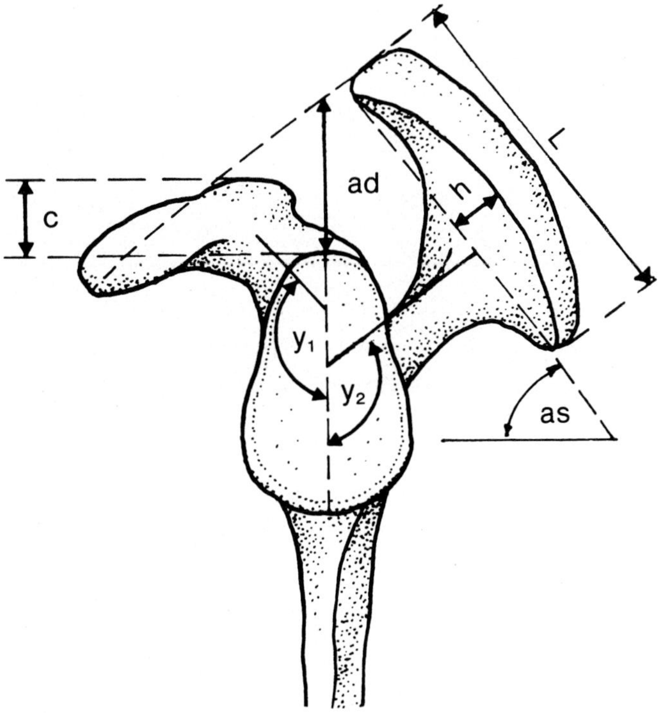

Fig. 8–4. Outlet view to determine the slope of the acromion (AS). As AS increases the greater the acromial slope and the smaller the supraspinatus outlet becomes. (From Edelson JG, Taitz C. Anatomy of the coraco-acromial arch. Relation to degeneration of the acromion. *J Bone Joint Surg Br.* 1992;72:589–594.)

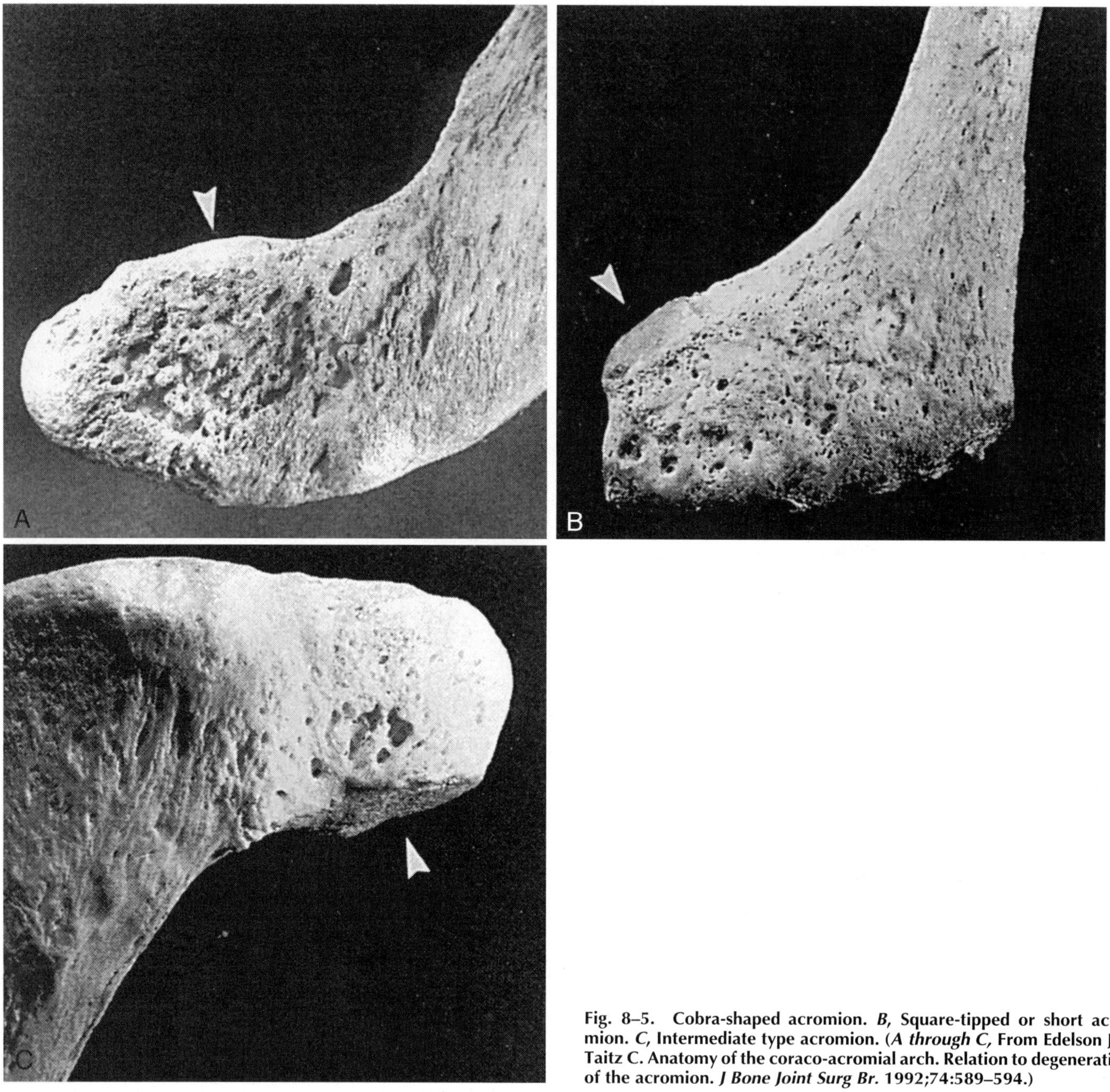

Fig. 8–5. **Cobra-shaped acromion.** ***B,*** **Square-tipped or short acromion.** ***C,*** **Intermediate type acromion. (*A through C,* From Edelson JG, Taitz C. Anatomy of the coraco-acromial arch. Relation to degeneration of the acromion. *J Bone Joint Surg Br.* 1992;74:589–594.)**

specimens. The remainder (45%) were of an intermediate type, with a mean length of 5.8 cm (5 to 7.75 cm); degenerative changes were found in 19% of these cases.

The acromion and the coracoid processes, with their interconnecting coracoacromial ligament, form the coracoacromial arch. It is underneath this arch that the proximal humerus lies and through which the rotator cuff tendons pass to insert on the humeral tuberosities. The rotator cuff consists of four separate muscles with their associated tendons: the supraspinatus, subscapularis, infraspinatus, and teres minor. Clark and Harryman[15] have shown that the rotator cuff tendon is composed of five distinct surgical layers. Between these layers exist many interdigitations, which create a confluent arc of tendon that inserts on the greater and lesser tuberosities and transverse ligament. For a complete description of the anatomy of the rotator cuff see Chapter 2. The tendon of the long head of the biceps runs in the bicipital groove, which is formed between the greater and lesser tuberosities, to insert on the superior labrum and supraglenoid tubercle. In its course it passes intra-articularly underneath the coracohumeral ligament, which lies between and strengthens the interval between the subscapularis and supraspinatus. The subscapularis and supraspinatus tendons in turn form a sheath-like canal, which the biceps traverses. The biceps tendon serves as a weak static head depressor in the normal shoulder.[16] In rotator cuff tears, the tendon may hypertrophy as the head-depressor responsibility of the biceps increases.[17,18]

The subacromial and subdeltoid bursa exist in the area between the acromion and rotator cuff tendons. They are composed at two serosal surfaces in approximation to one another, with a small amount of interposed synovial fluid. The region between the two serosal layers exists as a potential space in the normal, uninflammed shoulder. The bursae act to allow a fluid gliding motion of the rotator cuff underneath the arch. However, inflammation of the bursa and the subsequent formation of fibrous adhesions can limit motion, with associated pain and crepitus.

The subacromial and subdeltoid bursae may play an even greater role in impingement symptomatology. des Marchais et al. believe that a fibrotic thickening of the subacromial bursa in the region of the anterolateral portion of the greater tuberosity produces increased inflammation and pain with elevation of the arm as the tuberosity glides under the acromion. Subsequent bursal thickening alters the normal gliding mechanism with increased pain. They also noted the formation of an anterolateral bursal ulcer averaging 2 cm in diameter in 66% of their cases. Because these observations occurred lateral to the supraspinatus tendon, they concluded that the rotator cuff itself is not the primary source of impingement pathology, but rather the bursal fibrosis and thickening acting on the acromion is.[19]

The vascular supply to the rotator cuff tendons arises from the anterior humeral circumflex, the suprascapular, and the subscapular arteries. Lindblom hypothesized the existence of a "critical zone" of hypovascularity at the insertion of the supraspinatus at the greater tuberosity.[20] Subsequently, Rathbun and Macnab performed injection studies to examine the vascular supply of the supraspinatus.[21] They discovered that humeral adduction led to tension and subsequent decreased blood flow in the region of the critical zone. They proposed that positioning of the arm in adduction caused the blood to be "wrung out." However, microangiographic studies by Moseley and Goldie found no evidence of decreased blood flow to the region.[22] Ianotti et al., using laser Doppler studies, have also shown no evidence of decreased vascular flow.[23]

The muscles of the shoulder girdle interact to generate specific force couples to help balance the humeral head in the glenoid with active motion. Inman noted that during elevation of the arm, the deltoid and rotator cuff tended to act synchronously as a force couple to allow for balanced motion across the joint.[24] The deltoid's origin lies above and external to the glenohumeral articulation, with its insertion being distal into the humeral shaft. As a result, the overall forces produced at the initiation of abduction and the initial 45° of elevation are primarily vertical in nature, creating significant upward shear (Fig. 8–6).[25] The rotator cuff muscle force patterns contrast those of the deltoid. The supraspinatus, being horizontally oriented, primarily generates a compressive force at the joint. This helps centralize the humeral head

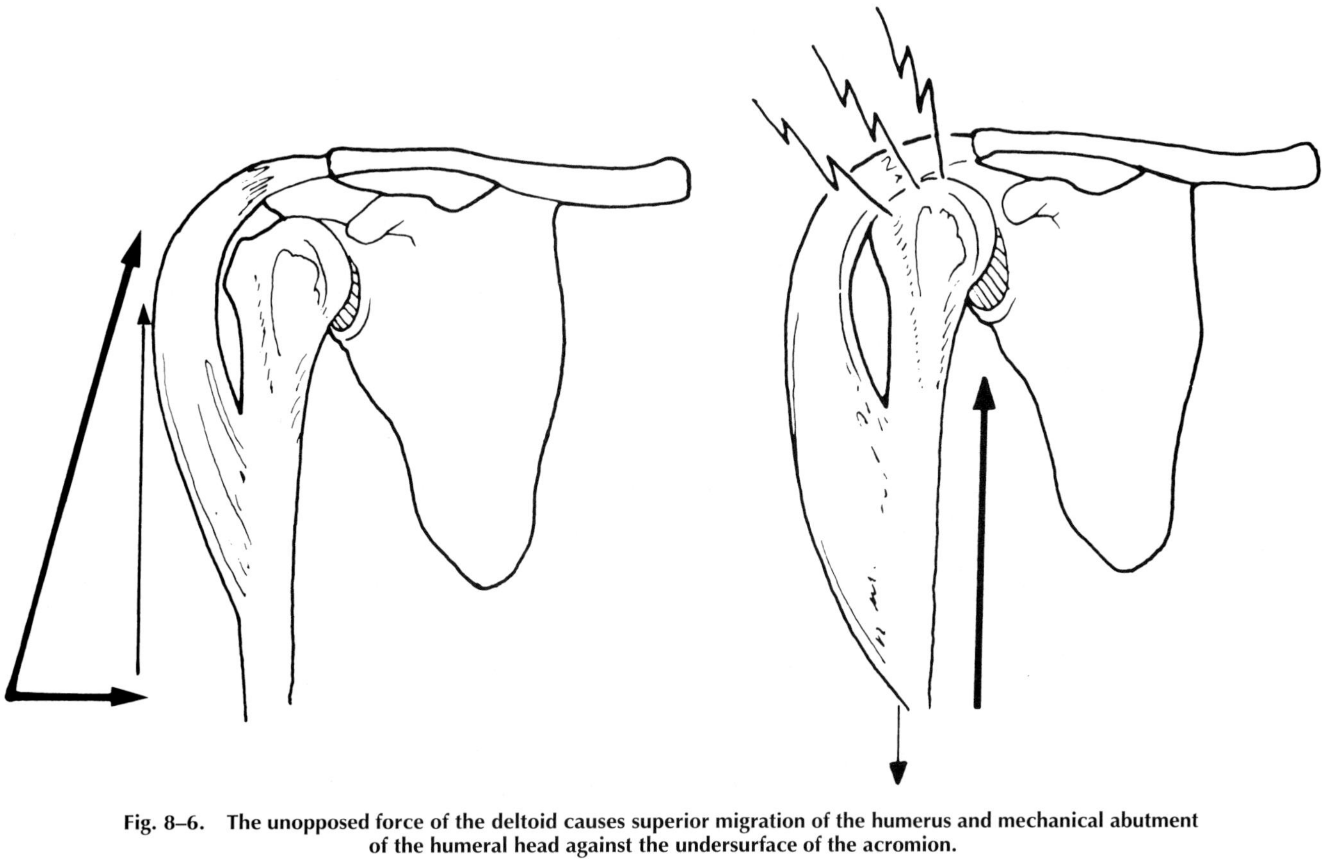

Fig. 8–6. The unopposed force of the deltoid causes superior migration of the humerus and mechanical abutment of the humeral head against the undersurface of the acromion.

in the glenoid during elevation and counteracts the superior migration force of the deltoid. However, the combined action of the subscapularis, infraspinatus, and teres minor is in a primarily downward projection. This generates an opposing inferior or head depressing shear to the upward force of the deltoid (Fig. 8–7). The upward rotation of the scapula also is an important component of elevation. Inman discovered that the upper portion of the trapezius, levator scapulae, serratus anterior, and rhomboids were all active during abduction and flexion.[24] The force couple of the levator scapulae and serratus anterior (flexion and abduction) and upper and lower trapezius (primarily abduction) were essential for proper rotation of the scapula, with elevation of the acromion away from the humeral head (Fig. 8–8). Weakness in any of the muscles of the shoulder girdle can therefore disrupt the normal scapular rhythm and balance and lead to abnormal motion and or impingement.

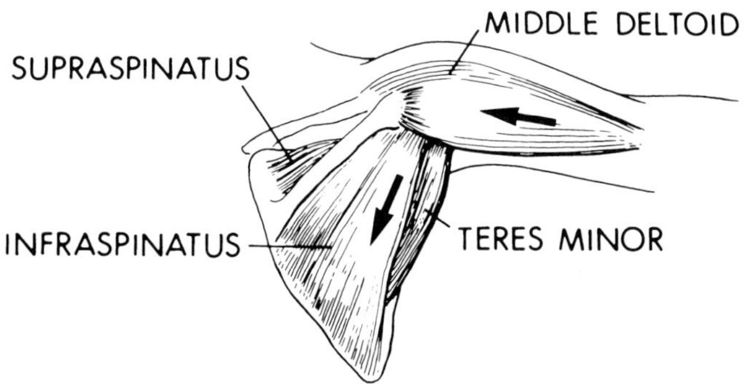

Fig. 8–7. The combined action of the rotator cuff generates a head depressing and stabilizing force which counteracts the force of the deltoid.

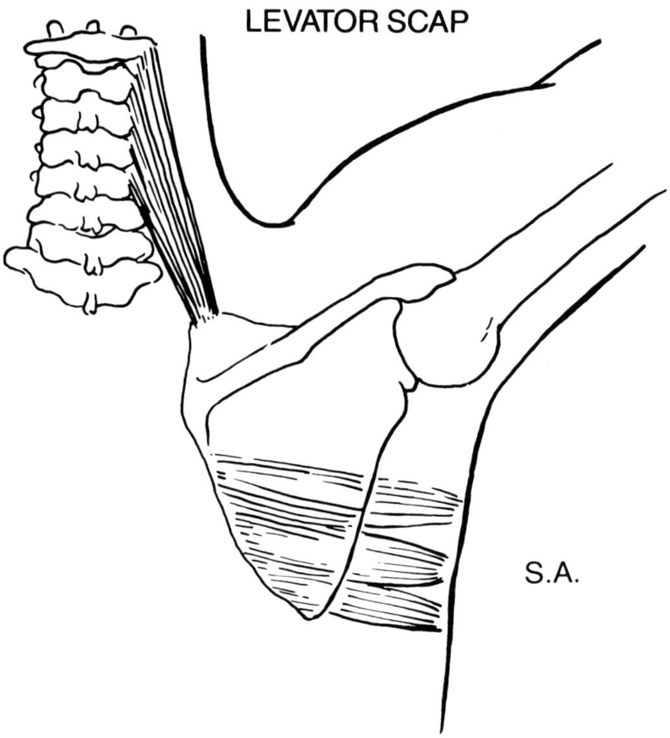

Fig. 8–8. The force couple of the serratus anterior and levator scapula muscles, as well as the upper and lower trapezius, are important for proper rotation of the scapula to prevent mechanical impingement with elevation of the arm. Alteration of this force couple can result in "non-outlet" impingement. (From Perry J. Biomechanics of the shoulder. In: CR Rowe, ed. *The Shoulder.* New York: Churchill-Livingstone; 1988:13.)

Matsen and Harryman described the presence of posterior capsular stiffness in association with impingement syndrome.[26] This would tend to force the humeral head superiorly against the undersurface of the anterior acromion, exacerbating the impingement when the shoulder is flexed. He states that the humeral head rolls up on the tightened posterior capsule similar to the mechanism of a yo-yo on a string. This action, coupled with disuse atrophy, tendinitis, muscle weakness, and subacromial bursal thickening, leads to a self-perpetuating process.

PATHOMECHANICS

Extrinsic

Theories regarding the etiology and development of impingement syndrome can be divided into intrinsic and extrinsic factors (Fig. 8–9). Extrinsic factors are those that act outside of the rotator cuff with subsequent secondary changes. The category of extrinsic causes can be further subdivided into primary and secondary. Primary extrinsic causes occur as a result of mechanical impingement of the rotator cuff against the anterior-inferior aspect of the acromion with subsequent attritional changes. This has traditionally been considered to be the primary mechanism in the etiology of impingement based on Neer's original anatomic study. Neer attributed 95% of all rotator cuff tears to mechanical impingement.[27] Acromial morphology and its relationship to the

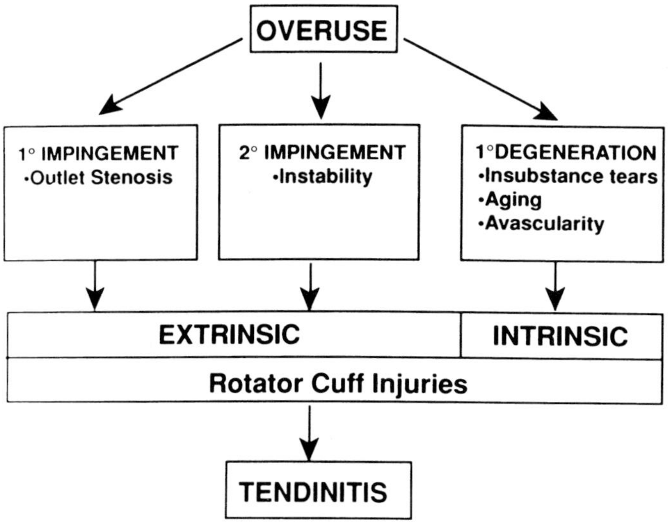

Fig. 8–9. A diagrammatic representation of the intrinsic and extrinsic causes of impingement syndrome. (From Fu F, Harner CD, Klein AH. Shoulder impingement syndrome. *Clin Orthop.* 1991;269:162–173.)

presence of cuff disease has been previously discussed.

Secondary extrinsic causes occur as a result of relative narrowing of the supraspinatus outlet with subsequent mechanical impingement. A primary example of this category is seen in relation to glenohumeral instability. Hawkins,[28] Jobe and Kvitne,[29,30] and Nirschl[31] have reported on the association of instability and secondary impingement syndrome. This is more commonly seen in the younger, athletic patient population, especially in swimmers and throwers. For a more thorough discussion see Chapter 11.

Intrinsic

Included in this group of factors are internal anatomic impingement, functional overload, and intrinsic tendinopathy. Intrinsic factors have been hypothesized to be the inciting etiologic events in the production of impingement syndrome. Codman stated that a critical zone exists at the region of the supraspinatus tendon's insertion.[5] Subsequent studies by Lindblom[20] and Rathbun and Macnab[21] demonstrated an area of relative hypovascularity to exist in this region. Nirschl has proposed that angiofibroblastic changes occur within the tendon as the initial etiologic event[31] (Fig. 8–10). This leads to secondary weakness of the rotator cuff with subsequent superior migration of the humeral head, impingement, and exacerbation of the primary degenerative changes. This mechanism has also been put forth by Ozaki[32] and Ogata and Uhthoff.[33] Ozaki et al. evaluated 200 anatomic specimens and noted that the typical changes associated with mechanical impingement usually were seen only in association with full-thickness rotator cuff tears.[32] Ogata and Uhthoff radiologically and histologically evaluated the undersurface of 76 cadaveric acromions. They noted no correlation between degenerative changes on the undersurface of the acromion and rotator cuff tears and concluded that rotator cuff tears likely are unrelated to mechanical impingement, and, rather, they stem from an intrinsic degenerative tendinopathy.[33] Fukuda et al. performed histologic sections of 12 en-bloc surgical specimens, consisting of the bony insertion, tendon, and musculotendinous junction in patients with bursal side rotator cuff tears. On inspection, he found evidence of both degenerative and mechanical attribution and hypothesized that aging, precarious vascularity, repetitive injury, and mechanical impingement interact in the pathogenesis of bursal side rotator cuff tears.[34] For a more thorough discussion of partial-thickness tears see Chapter 12.

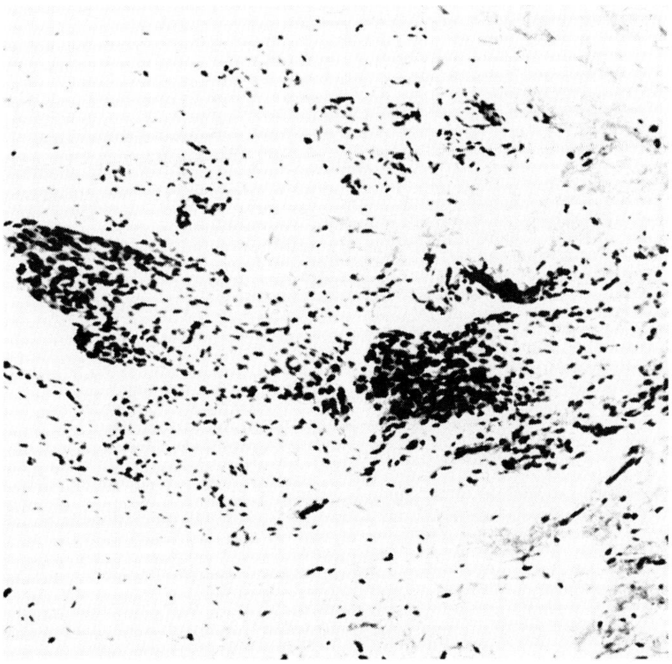

Fig. 8–10. Photomicrograph of primary angiofibroblastic changes within the substance of the rotator cuff tendon at low power (×100).

Probably both intrinsic and extrinsic factors work in concert to create the complex of impingement. Repetitive microtrauma, in association with inflammatory and degenerative changes in the rotator cuff, interact to create a vicious self-propagating cycle with subsequent permanent changes. Persistence of the inciting trauma does not allow for significant healing with progression of the damage, and irreversible changes ultimately leading to complete tearing of the rotator cuff tendon.

CLASSIFICATION

Neer originally divided impingement lesions into three clinical stages. This classification has remained effective in describing the pathology as well as organizing treatment rationales[27,35] (Fig. 8–11). In stage I lesions, overuse of the arm above the horizontal causes edema and hemorrhage. This lesion was felt to be more commonly seen in individuals less than 25 years of age and was reversible with rest and avoidance of the offending mechanism. A single traumatic event, wherein the humerus is impacted into the undersurface of the acromion, also can present in a similar fashion. Neer termed this type of lesion "acute traumatic subacromial bursitis." Again, this condition tends to respond to rest and conservative care.[35]

During stage II, repetition of the insulting events results in thickening and fibrosis of the subacromial bursa and the associated tendinitis. Typically, patients in this group are between 25 and 40 years of age. Neer again felt that the majority of these patients tended to improve with rest and conservative measures. However, persistent pain and disability after several months and failure of conservative care were felt to warrant surgical treatment with anterior acromioplasty and division of the coracoacromial ligament.

Stage III lesions represent partial or complete tearing of the rotator cuff tear, with possible biceps tendon rupture and associated bony changes. This was felt to occur in individuals more than 40 years of age. Neer felt that these patients could be improved after acromioplasty, bursectomy, and rotator cuff repair were performed as indicated.

Neer also has classified impingement with regard to its

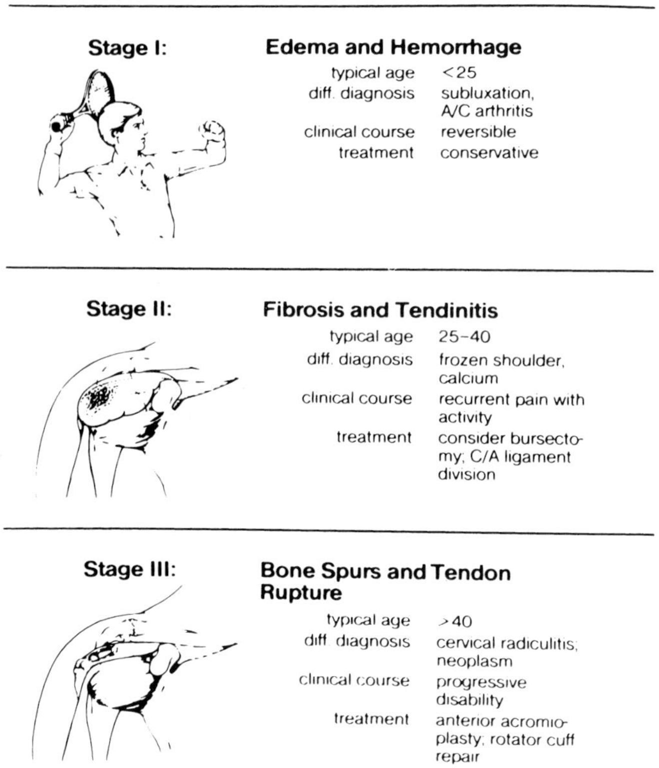

Fig. 8–11. Neer's classification of the three stages of impingement. (From Neer CS II. Impingement lesions. *Clin Orthop.* 1983;173:70.)

etiology into two broad categories: outlet impingement and nonoutlet impingement.[35] Outlet impingement refers to primary anatomic conditions that lead to absolute narrowing of the supraspinatus outlet. Neer felt that this was by far the most frequent cause of impingement. As stated earlier, the shape of the acromion can significantly impact on the rotator cuff and the production of impingement syndrome.[13,14] An acromial process with an acute slope also may encroach on the supraspinatus outlet. Anterior acromial spurs and marginal osteophytes at the AC joint also may narrow the outlet, with subsequent exacerbation of impingement. Os acromiale also may cause direct narrowing of the supraspinatus outlet and is in our opinion best classified with outlet impingement.

Nonoutlet impingement occurs when there is relative narrowing of the supraspinatus outlet with subsequent secondary impingement. Anatomic variations, such as prominence of the greater tuberosity, whether congenital or secondary to previous fracture, may lead to nonoutlet impingement. Relative prominence of the greater tuberosity also may occur with low placement of humeral components in shoulder arthroplasty. In addition, disruption of the normal glenohumeral mechanics, such as in instability, may lead to relative narrowing of the outlet and secondary impingement. Muscular imbalance and scapulothoracic dysfunction as in paraplegia, Erb's palsy, and third-degree AC separation may cause subsequent narrowing of the outlet and impingement. The importance of differentiating between outlet and nonoutlet impingement cannot be overstressed, because the treatment between the two categories often is vastly different. Outlet impingement normally responds to the treatment for classical mechanical impingement of acromioplasty and or distal clavicle excision. Nonoutlet impingement commonly requires specific treatment in regards to the underlying primary pathology rather than the secondary impingement. In this instance, subacromial decompression alone often does not address the etiology of the impingement and fails to treat the problem. The one exception to this is the patient with the minimally malunited greater tuberosity fracture that in the senior author's experience responds well to acromioplasty alone.

CLINICAL PRESENTATION

There is seldom a standard presentation or rigid set of symptoms with which patients invariably appear. For this reason, care must always be taken to perform a thorough evaluation and to look for underlying and/or unexpected etiologies for a given condition. Impingement syndrome is no different in this regard from other medical conditions. A careful, concise history and examination are necessary because masked and/or associated conditions may present in a similar fashion. Typically, patients with impingement syndrome will present with a complaint of pain. They usually do not present acutely, hoping that symptoms will resolve. Frequently, patients complain of specific functional limitations, such as difficulty with dressing, inability to lift objects off shelves, or other activities of daily living requiring use of the arm in elevation and rotation.

Physical inspection may demonstrate atrophy of the deltoid or spinati. Palpation in the region of the subacromial bursa at the lateral aspect of the acromion often may elicit pain. Crepitus secondary to hypertrophy and scarring of the subacromial bursa and/or tearing of the rotator cuff also may be palpable in the subacromial region as the shoulder is moved through a gentle range of motion. Tenderness can often be seen on palpation over the region of the AC joint, especially anteriorly, if significant arthritic change exists. The region of the bicipital groove also may be tender and should alert the examiner to the possibility of associated bicipital tendinitis. Active range of motion is often limited compared with the uninvolved extremity, especially in forward flexion and abduction because of pain and especially above the level of the horizontal. Scapular dysrhythmia may be present with loss of the normal fluid arc of motion normally seen in the involved shoulder. Compared to passive elevation, active elevation of the arm usually is more uncomfortable than passive, because of the presence of associated rotator cuff tendinitis.

Neer described the impingement sign in the evaluation of patients with impingement syndrome (Fig. 8–12).[9] The maneuver is performed by elevation of the humerus as the acromial process is depressed with the examiner's opposite hand. This movement effectively com-

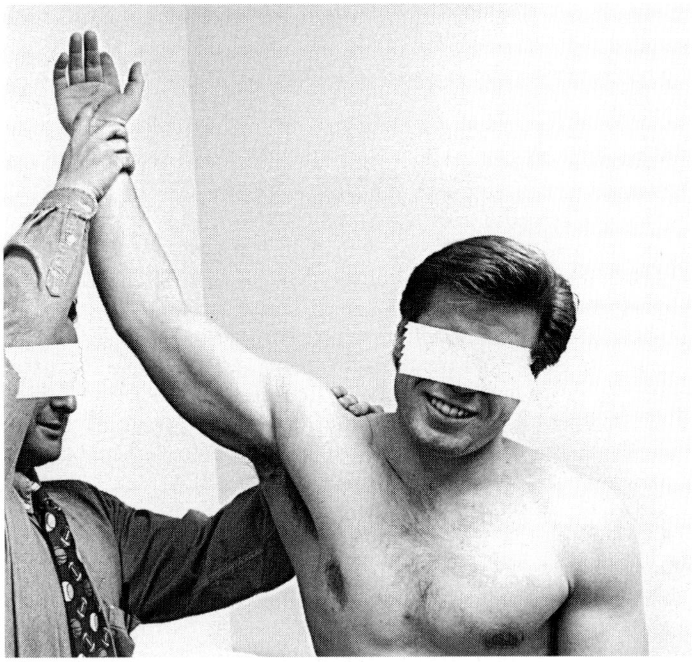

Fig. 8–12. **The impingement "sign" is performed by forward flexion of the arm by the examiner with concurrent downward pressure applied to the superior aspect of the acromion.**

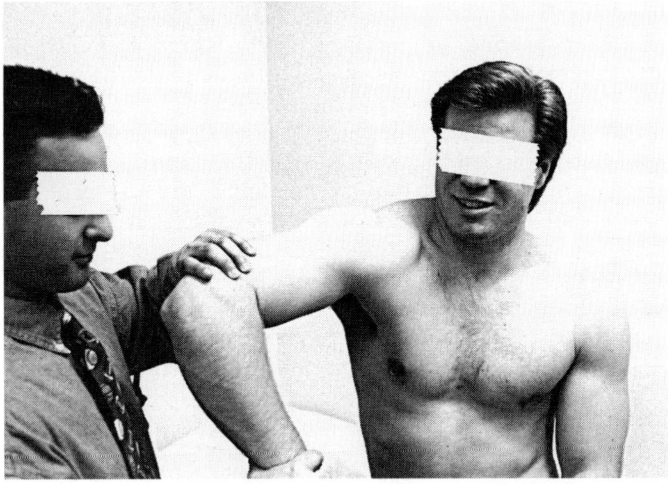

Fig. 8–13. **The impingement reinforcement test is elicited by forward flexion of the arm 90° with subsequent internal rotation of the arm.**

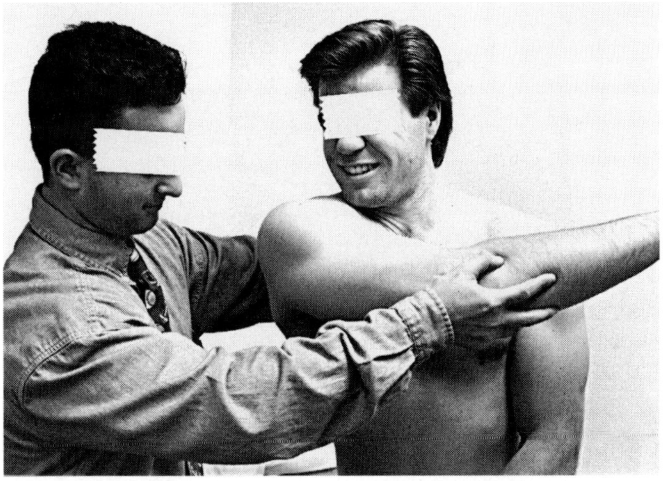

Fig. 8–14. **The horizontal adduction test is performed by forward flexion of the arm 90° with subsequent crossbody adduction, with pain localized to the region of the AC joint. It is important for the patient to localize the pain, with pain over the AC joint indicating AC joint origin and pain over the posterior capsule indicating impingement with a tight posterior capsule. Patients with coracoid impingement will also have pain with this maneuver.**

presses the greater tuberosity against the anterior acromion. Complaint of pain by the patient is considered a positive provocative examination. An additional examination is the impingement reinforcement test or ''Hawkins' sign''(Fig. 8–13).[28] This is done with the shoulder flexed forward 90° with subsequent internal rotation of the arm by the examiner. This effectively drives the greater tuberosity further under the coracoacromial arch with elicitation of pain. Although this test has been used as a diagnostic examination for impingement syndrome, we note that the compression of the AC joint increases with this maneuver.

AC joint arthritis is commonly associated with impingement syndrome and can be evaluated by performance of the horizontal adduction test (Fig. 8–14). The shoulder is brought into 90° of forward flexion and then adducted across the body. The patient should be asked to localize his pain during performance of the test. Pain in the region of the AC joint is considered positive for the presence of AC arthritis. Often posterior shoulder pain also may be elicited by this maneuver, which is caused by the presence of posterior capsular tightness in association with impingement. The hug test (Fig. 8–15) is perhaps more accurate for isolated AC arthralgia. Tenderness at the bicipital groove should alert the examiner to the presence of coexisting bicipital tendinitis. The bicipital groove is best localized with the arm in approximately 10° of internal rotation, because this places it directly anterior. A simple confirmatory examination for bicipital tendinitis is de Anquin's test (Fig. 8–16).[36] In this instance, the arm is rotated while pressure is placed with the examiner's fingers in the region of the biceps tendon. A positive test occurs when the incidence of pain correlates with the moment the tendon is brought under the examiner's fingers. In addition to de Anquin's test, the presence of bicipital tendinitis also can be evaluated by performance of Speed's test[37] and Yergason's sign.[38] In Speed's test, the patient flexes the shoulder against resistance while the elbow is extended and the forearm supinated (Fig. 8–17). A test is positive when pain is localized to the region of the bicipital groove. Yergason's sign requires the patient to forcibly supinate the forearm against resistance while the elbow is flexed with pain in the area of the biceps tendon (Fig. 8–18). Evaluation of muscular tone and strength is an integral part of the examination of patients who have impingement. As stated earlier, atrophy and dysymmetry should be noted by the examiner on initial inspection of the patient. The supraspinatus is tested by placing the arm in internal rotation and abduction in the plane of the scapula, with a downward force being applied to the forearm (Fig. 8–19). Pain and/or weakness on examination may be caused by the presence of tendinitis, partial or complete rotator cuff tears, and/or possible nerve injuries. The strength of the infraspinatus and teres minor can be evaluated by placing the arm at the patient's side with the elbow flexed at 90°, with resistance being applied while the patient attempts to externally rotate the arm (Fig. 8–20). The subscapularis may be tested for tendinitis and tearing using the lift-off test. In this test, the arm is internally rotated and placed against the patient's back, with forceful internal rotation used to elevate the arm against resistance (Fig. 8–21). Pain and weakness with this maneuver are consistent with injury in the subscapularis according to Gerber.[39]

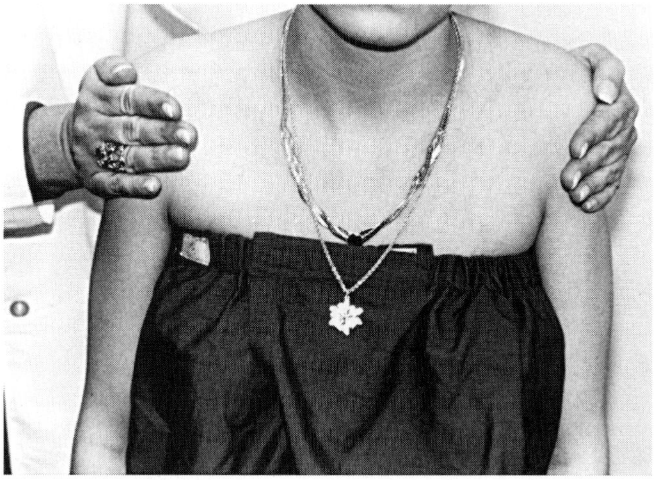

Fig. 8–15. Compression over the lateral shoulder girdle region or "hug test" for AC joint arthritis.

The presence of underlying instability should be strongly suspected in the young athletic patient who presents with impingement symptomatology. The anterior apprehension and relocation tests as described by Jobe can be employed to evaluate for this condition.[29] The patient is placed supine on the table and the arm abducted 90° and, subsequently, externally rotated (Fig. 8–22). The presence of anterior instability is verified by associated pain and apprehension. The second portion of the examination in Jobe's relocation test is performed by repetition of the anterior apprehension maneuver with a posteriorly directed force being applied to the arm,

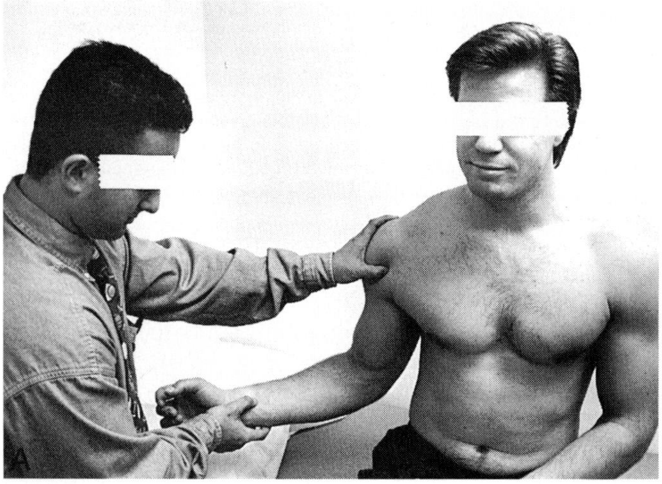

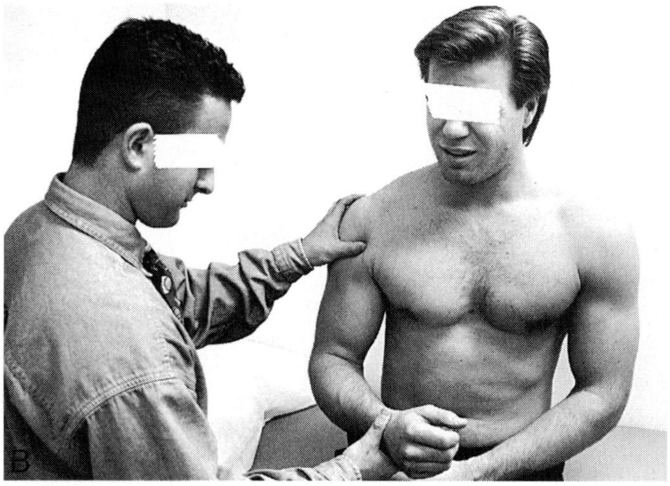

Fig. 8–16. de Anquin's test evaluates for the presence of bicipital tendinitis. *A,* The examiner places pressure over the anterior aspect of the shoulder with the arm being internally and externally rotated. *B,* Pain that occurs with rotation of the biceps tendon underneath the examiner's fingers is considered a positive test.

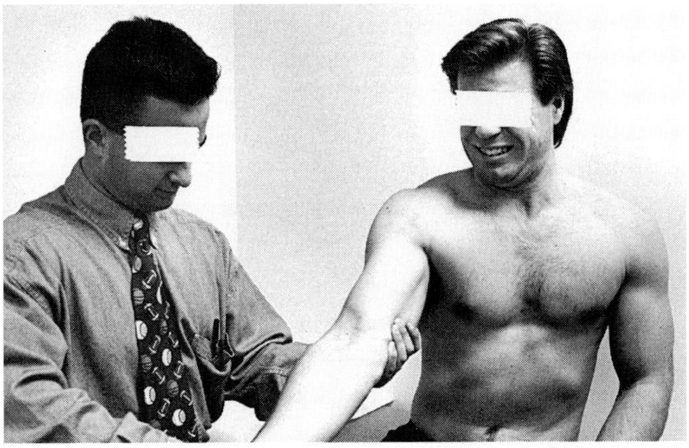

Fig. 8–17. Speed's test is performed by forward flexion of the arm with the forearm in full supination against resistance applied by the examiner. Pain is again localized in the region of the bicipital groove and anterior shoulder with a positive test result.

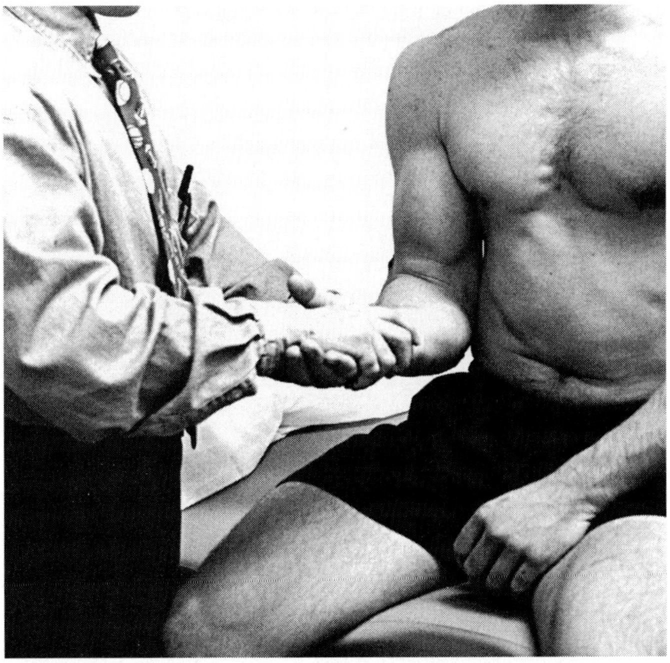

Fig. 8–18. Yergason's test requires the patient to actively supinate against resistance applied by the examiner with pain being elicited over the bicipital groove being considered indicative of biceps tendinitis.

thus preventing anterior subluxation of the humeral head (Fig. 8–23). If pain and apprehension are relieved with the relocation maneuver, an underlying primary etiology of instability should be strongly suspected. For a more thorough discussion of instability and its relationship to rotator cuff disease, see Chapter 11. Neer also described the impingement test for evaluation of patients with potential impingement syndrome[9] (Fig. 8–24). Injection of lidocaine into the subacromial bursa with subsequent relief of the patient pain symptomatology is considered a positive impingement test. Additional selective injections with local anesthetic in the AC joint and bicipital groove can be useful when pain relief is not complete after infiltration of the bursa; pathology is suspected in these areas on examination. After each subsequent injection, the patient should be asked to range the shoulder

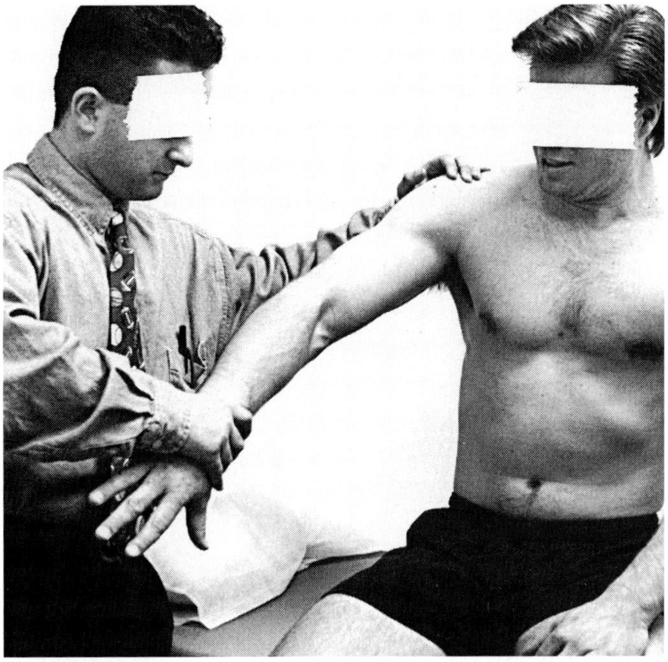

Fig. 8–19. The supraspinatus test is performed by abducting the arm in the plane of the scapula with the forearm pronated against resistance with pain and weakness being present with associated rotator cuff tendinitis.

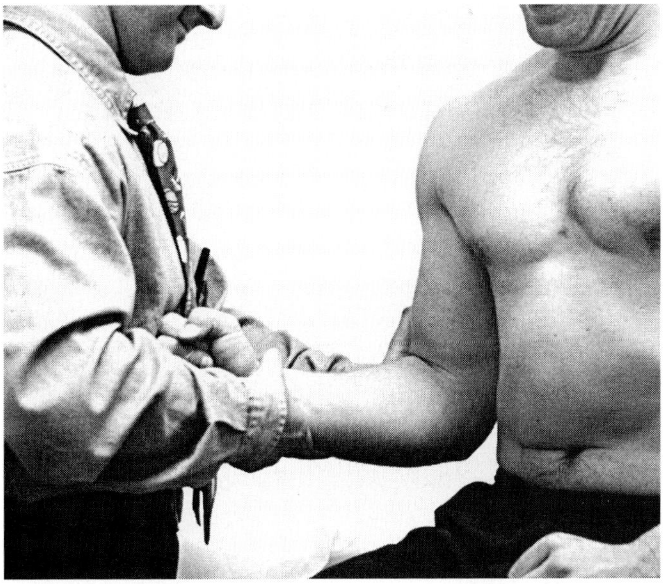

Fig. 8–20. The infraspinatus and teres minor muscles are tested by the patient externally rotating the arm against resistance while holding the elbow firmly at the side. Weakness and pain are consistent with tendinitis and/or tearing of these tendons.

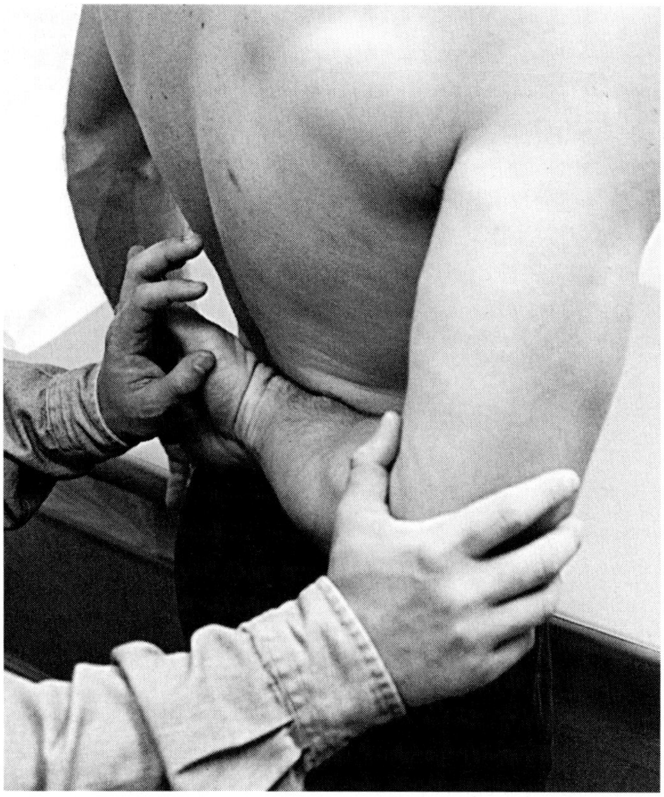

Fig. 8–21. The subscapular lift-off test is performed by the patient internally rotating the shoulder and placing the hand against his back. The arm is stabilized at the elbow by the examiner with the patient asked to internally rotate at the shoulder in order to bring his hand away from his back against resistance. Subscapular tendinopathy will cause associated discomfort and weakness with the maneuver.

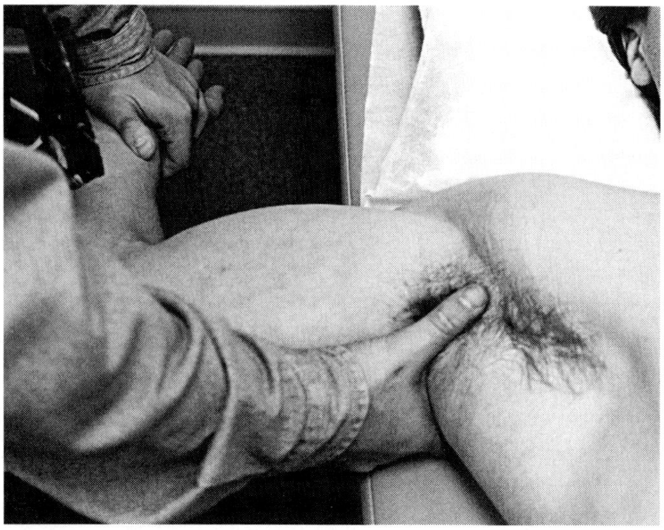

Fig. 8–22. The apprehension maneuver tests for anterior shoulder instability. It is best performed with the patient supine with the arm brought into 90° of abduction and external rotation. Subsequent pain and apprehension of impending dislocation are associated with underlying instability.

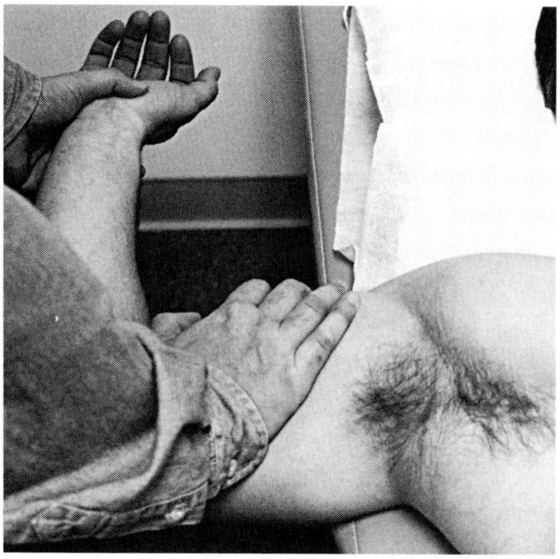

Fig. 8–23. The relocation test is performed in similar fashion to that of the apprehension test except with a posterior directed force being applied by the examiner to the proximal humerus to prevent anterior translation of the humeral head. Relief of discomfort and/or apprehension further confirms the presence of underlying anterior instability.

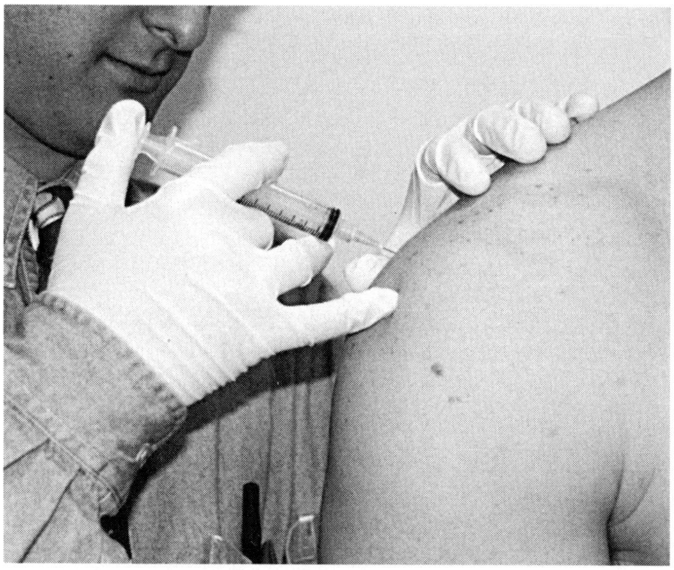

Fig. 8–24. Neer described the impingement "test" wherein local anesthetic is injected into the subacromial region with subsequent re-examination of the shoulder. Relief of previous pain and discomfort with provocative maneuvers for impingement is considered a positive test result.

and report on the degree of remaining pain. The results should be documented carefully by the examiner.

If pain only occurs with specific activities or provocative maneuvers, a selective injection of bupivacaine hydrochloride (Marcaine) 0.25% can be given into the subacromial bursa of the patient. The patient is then asked to perform the activity and report back later that day or the following day. Significant pain relief is confirmatory for impingement.

DIFFERENTIAL DIAGNOSIS OF OTHER INTRINSIC SHOULDER LESIONS THAT CAN MIMIC IMPINGEMENT

AC Joint Derangement

Again, pain often can be elicited on examination by palpation over the anterior superior aspects of the AC joint, with a positive horizontal adduction test or a positive hug test as described earlier in the chapter. Occasionally, patients with isolated AC arthritis will present with shoulder pain without associated impingement or rotator cuff tendinopathy. This is commonly seen in individuals who perform repetitive or powerful overhead activities, such as in weightlifters and some manual laborers, because this routinely places increased stress across the joint. Special radiographs, such as the Zanca view can be obtained to specifically evaluate the AC joint (see Chapter 6). Additional selective injection into the AC joint after first infiltrating the subacromial bursa may help objectively quantify its contribution in association with impingement to the patient's pain symptomatology. No change in pain with subacromial injection, with obliteration of pain with AC joint injection, confirms this diagnosis.

Biceps Tendinitis

Bicipital tendinitis is another commonly seen lesion that occurs with impingement and should also be examined as a possible contributing source of pain. Biceps tendinitis may occur in isolation; however, it is often associated with underlying impingement and rotator cuff tendinopathy.[40] Patients will often present with pain over the anterior region of the shoulder, which is exacerbated with overhead and lifting activities and is often improved with rest. There may not be any associated night pain or specific discomfort noted with lying on the involved shoulder in contrast to that of impingement. Limitation in motion often exists in abduction and forward flexion secondary to pain. Tenderness in the region of the bicipital groove can be elicited by palpation in the region and with performance of Speed's, de Anquin's, and Yergason's provocative maneuvers as described previously. A selective injection of lidocaine (Xylocaine) can also be used in concert with the impingement test to evaluate for the presence of bicipital tendinitis. Standard AP and lateral radiographs seldom show specific changes of isolated biceps tendinitis. The Fisk view can be obtained to better visualize the region of the bicipital groove and biceps tendon (see Chapter 6).

Glenohumeral Arthritis

Glenohumeral arthritis may present with symptomatology similar to rotator cuff tendinopathy. Primary osteoarthritis of the shoulder is less common than that in the knee, hip, or spine, because of the decreased axial loading through the shoulder. The greater mobility of the shoulder predisposes it to repetitive microtrauma with subsequent development of osteoarthritic changes. Heavy laborers and athletes are more likely to develop primary osteoarthritis of the shoulder, because of the increased mechanical demands and stress they place across the joint. Patients who present with complaints of night pain and difficulty lying on the involved shoulder, like impingement syndrome, may confuse the differential diagnosis. Pain, limitation of motion, and crepitation on motion are considered the cardinal signs associated with the presence of arthritic change. Plain radiographs will often show inferior humeral and/or glenoid osteophytes, narrowing of the joint space, calcific loose bodies, and/or cystic and irregular changes at the articular margin. Rotator cuff tears, however, are not commonly associated with osteoarthritis. Rheumatoid arthritis may also involve the shoulder. It rarely presents as an isolated entity but is characteristically seen in association with symmetrical joint involvement elsewhere, especially the hand and wrist. There is a higher incidence of rotator cuff tearing associated with rheumatoid arthritis versus osteoarthritis.[35] Other arthritides may present with pain similar to rotator cuff pathology such as gout, aseptic necrosis, and neuropathic joint disease and, therefore, should be considered in patients with atypical pain patterns, other joint involvement, and the appropriate history and findings.

Calcific Tendinitis

Calcific tendinitis can present with pain similar to that seen with impingement syndrome; however, it usually is of greater intensity and will persist at rest. The diagnosis often may be confirmed by the presence of calcific deposits seen with AP radiographs of the shoulder in internal and external rotation. Frozen shoulder also may present with symptoms like those of impingement in its initial phase. However, it may be differentiated by the rigid limitation present with passive range of motion as well as by selective injection.

Multidirectional Instability

Subtle instability, as stated earlier, can present with symptoms of a secondary impingement syndrome. Young athletic patients, especially swimmers and throwers, need to be evaluated specifically for the presence of this condition in the etiology of their pain.

Adhesive Capsulitis

Adhesive capsulitis may also mimic impingement syndrome. The exact etiology of this condition is still uncertain. It is associated with such conditions as diabetes mellitus, Parkinsonism, thyroid disorders, and cardiovascular disease. Women who have recently undergone breast surgery may also present with this condition. A diffuse inflammatory synovitis occurs with subsequent adherence of the capsule with loss of the normal axillary pouch.

These patients are typically women, within their fourth or fifth decade. A history of diffuse, dull aching pain about the shoulder with weakness and loss of motion over a period of the last few months is often given by the patient. Incidence of night pain with inability to sleep on the involved shoulder may be noted and is similar to that of impingement syndrome. For a full discussion on adhesive capsulitis, see Chapter 17.

Coracoid Impingement

Coracoid impingement must be considered in the differential diagnosis for impingement syndrome and is discussed in detail later in this chapter.

Scapulothoracic Dysfunction

Snapping scapula may also present with pain that may mimic impingement or rotator cuff pathology. In this condition however, the pain and snapping is usually localized over the region of the vertebral border of the scapula with associated snapping noise noted with elevation of the arm. Scapular lateral radiographs and CT scanning may occasionally show the presence of an underlying osteochondroma or other osseous irregularity of the scapula or ribs in relation to the pathology.

Slap Lesions

In association with recent arthroscopic and imaging advances has come an increased interest in the relationship of labral pathology as the basis of intrinsic shoulder pain. In this regard Snyder has described the superior labral anterior to posterior (SLAP) lesion with regard to shoulder pain and disability (see Chapter 10). In this condition, an associated dull aching pain in the shoulder may occur with motion. Discomfort is often noted on lifting and with biceps active motions, because the long head of the biceps often inserts in a portion of the superior labrum. Discomfort with Speed's and/or Yergason's test may be noted on examination, however, without associated tenderness in the region of the bicipital groove on palpation.

The presence of paresthesias and persistent sensory or motor changes should alert the examiner to the possible presence of nerve compression syndromes in the patient. Cervical radiculitis may have referred pain to the shoulder girdle, especially with involvement of the C5–6 disc. Pain with neck motion that is greater than shoulder motion should alert the examiner to evaluate for this condition. Discomfort with Lhermitte's phenomenon may be noted with performance of cervical compression and/or Spurling's tests. Thoracic outlet and peripheral compression neuropathies also may present with a large component of shoulder pain. The location of sensory changes, paresthesias, and responses to provocative maneuvers should be carefully noted by the examiner. Thoracic outlet often will present with anterior shoulder pain and paresthesias into the lunar two digits (distribution of the lower trunk of the plexus). Performance of Wright's maneuver, Adson's test, and/or Roos' overhead grip test may be performed to evaluate for its presence. Suprascapular neuropathy can be associated with pain over the scapula, with significant weakness noted on resistance testing of the supraspinatus and infraspinatus. Viral infections of the brachial plexus (syndrome of Parsonage and Turner) may also present with extreme shoulder pain after a history of previous flu-like symptoms preceding its onset. Neurologic findings are varied with evidence of numbness, weakness, or both. Peripheral compression neuropathies, such as carpal and cubital tunnel syndromes, also may present with a component of shoulder pain and should be considered in the patient with associated paresthesias. Neoplasms of the proximal humerus and scapula also may present with pain complaints similar to that of impingement. Any previous history of carcinoma, especially those with a tendency to metastasize to bone, should alert the examiner to evaluate for this. Finally, visceral complaints, such as cholecystitis, aortic aneurysm, coronary insufficiency, and Pancoast tumors, often present with referred pain to the shoulder girdle. The examiner should be alerted to this possibility when atypical pain patterns and persistence of pain with a negative examination for impingement is present.

RADIOGRAPHIC EVALUATION

Despite the recent expansion in diagnostic imaging techniques, plain radiographs are still considered the best modality in the initial evaluation of patients with shoulder pain. Typically, the basic series of radiographs should include AP, scapular lateral, and axillary views. The AP radiograph may show the presence of a sclerotic rim at the undersurface of the acromion or "sourcil" (eyebrow) caused by increased mechanical loading of the region. The presence of an os acromiale, Hill-Sachs lesion, or subtle glenoid deformity may be demonstrated on axillary radiographs. Two additional views are extremely useful in elucidating the pathology associated with impingement and should be included in the routine initial evaluation: the scapular outlet and 30° caudal tilt views. The scapular outlet view is obtained by placing the patient in the same position as for a true scapular lateral view with the beam angled 10° caudally. This view allows for more definitive visualization of the region through which the supraspinatus passes. The acromial morphology, presence of deformities of the anterior-inferior acromion, and inferiorly directed bony spurs at the AC joint can be discerned with this view. The caudal tilt view is obtained by positioning the patient as for a routine AP radiograph of the shoulder but with the tube angled 30° caudad. This view is extremely helpful in imaging anterior acromial spurs as well as the AC joint. Other conditions such as AC arthritis, calcific tendinitis, prominence of the greater tuberosity, and glenohumeral arthritis also can be readily seen with plain radiographs and should be noted by the examiner. The efficacy of using ultrasonography to image the rotator cuff for the presence of tears has recently been explored. Although ultrasonography offers the benefits of ease and noninvasiveness, it is limited in its ability to adequately visualize tears less than 1 cm in size. Results also tend to be somewhat dependent on the examiner with this modality.[41] Arthrography remains highly sensitive in the evaluation of full-thickness rotator cuff tears and has some facility in demonstrating deep surface partial tears. Both single-contrast (dye only) or double-contrast (air and dye) techniques may be employed. Arthrography may be combined with CT scanning of the shoulder for elucidation of labral lesions or other intra-articular pathology and is especially useful in patients with suspected underlying instability. The advent of MRI has ushered in a new era of imaging techniques that continue to find greater application in regard to orthopaedic injuries. MRI has been shown to be highly sensitive in the evaluation of rotator cuff tears, tendinitis, and labral and capsular lesions of the shoulder.[42,43] However, it remains costly and, therefore, limited as a routine screening procedure. Other imaging modalities, such as technetium bone scanning and CT scans, may be used to evaluate for pathologic entities including neoplasms and intra-articular and/or difficult fracture patterns if present or suspected.

CONSERVATIVE TREATMENT

Neer has stressed the importance of nonoperative treatment in the initial care of patients with rotator cuff tendinitis and partial-thickness tears.[9,27,35] He stressed the importance of rest and avoidance of the offending mechanism, with an early maintenance program for range of motion followed by strengthening only after symptoms had completely resolved. Other investigators, Hawkins and Kennedy,[28,44] Nirschl,[31] Cofield and Simonet,[45] and Jobe and Richardson[46,47] also have stressed the importance of the initial nonoperative management of the lesions.

The initial component of any conservative treatment program is relative rest and restriction from repetition of the insulting event. In association with this, a gentle, passive range-of-motion program should be started to help prevent stiffness and maintain range of motion. Stretching exercises for the anterior, inferior, and posterior shoulder should be performed by the patient as part of the motion program as illustrated (Figs. 8–25 through 8–27). Anterior capsular stretching should not be performed in patients having suspected underlying instability, because this may exacerbate the underlying condition. Pendulum or Codman's exercises are performed easily and are well tolerated by the patient; they should be done as an adjunct to the passive motion program (Fig. 8–28). These exercises are performed by flexing 90° at the waist with the involved arm held dependent and with gentle circular motions in a clockwise and counter clockwise direction. These exercises allow for passive enlargement of the subacromial space by depressing the humeral head with the weight of the arm during motion. Pulley and internal and external rotation exercises can be performed concurrently with Codman's exercises and should be performed 2 to 3 times daily for 5- to 10-minute intervals as tolerated (Figs. 8–29 and 8–30). Additionally, the use of nonsteroidal medications, hot and cold packs, and ultrasound can be instituted during this initial period for symptomatic treatment, if effective. Patients with

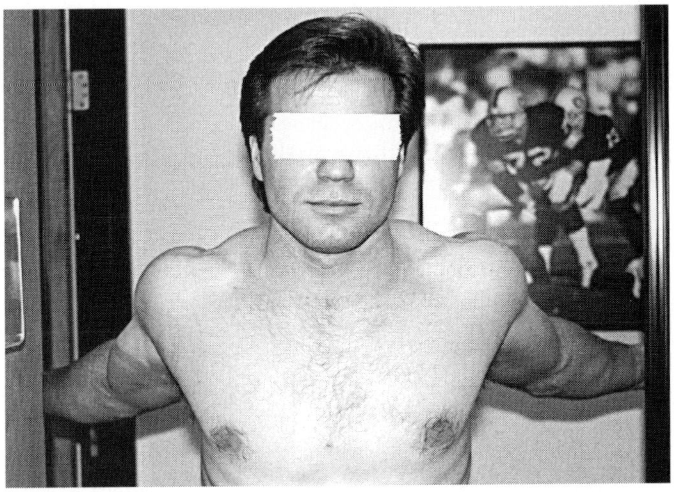

Fig. 8–25. Anterior capsular stretching is best performed in a doorway with the shoulders and arms being brought backwards into extension against the weight of the body. Care must be taken to avoid this maneuver in the presence of underlying anterior instability since it will exacerbate the condition.

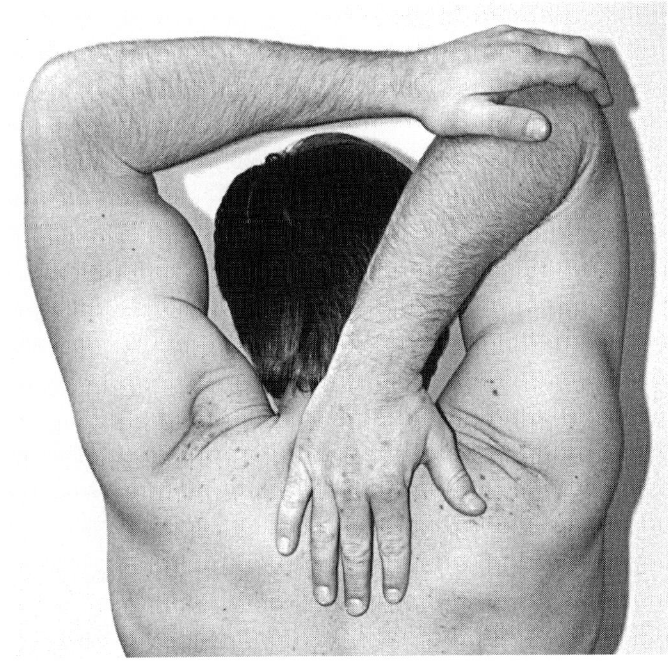

Fig. 8–26. Inferior capsular stretching can be done by the patient by placing the arm in full forward flexion with the opposite hand used to further the flexion of the arm and help maintain appropriate position of the arm for stretching.

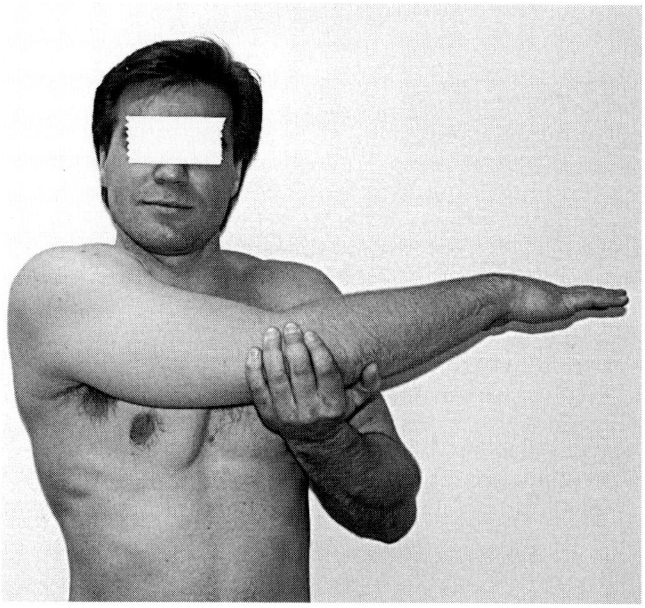

Fig. 8–27. Posterior capsular stretching can be performed by the patient flexing the arm to 90° with subsequent crossbody adduction which is aided by the opposite hand.

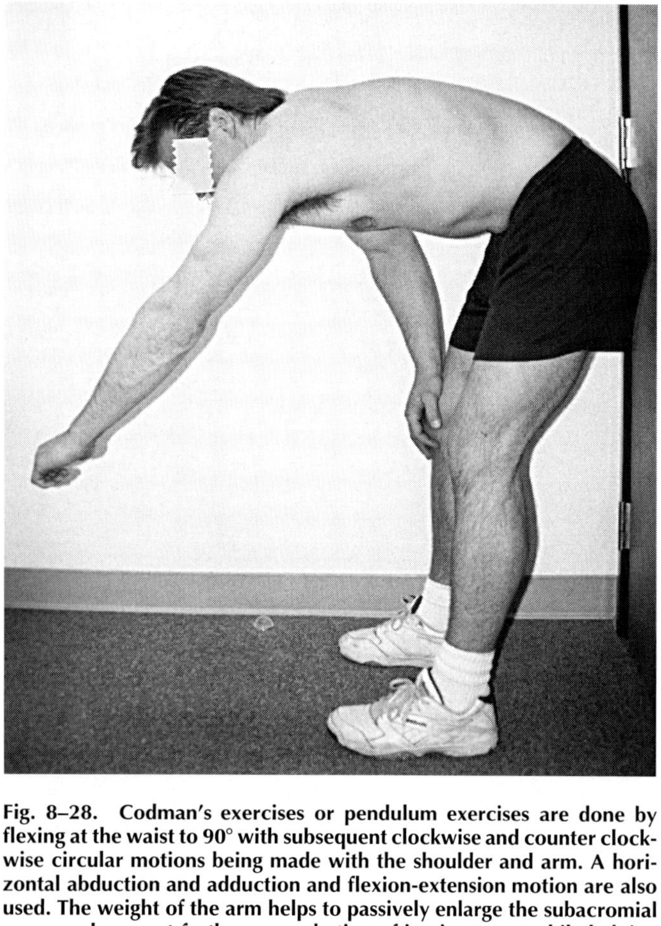

Fig. 8–28. Codman's exercises or pendulum exercises are done by flexing at the waist to 90° with subsequent clockwise and counter clockwise circular motions being made with the shoulder and arm. A horizontal abduction and adduction and flexion-extension motion are also used. The weight of the arm helps to passively enlarge the subacromial space and prevent further exacerbation of impingement while helping maintain range of motion.

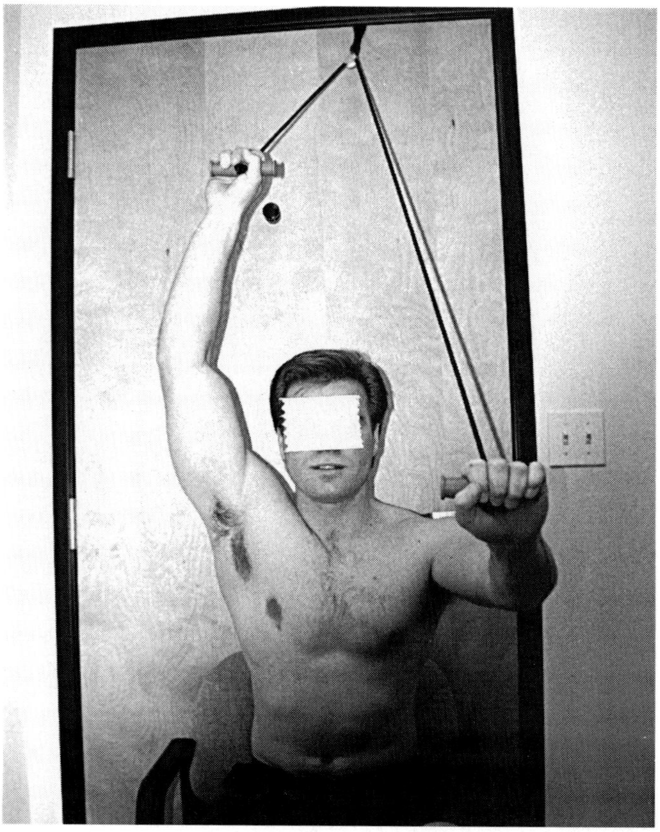

Fig. 8–29. Pulley exercises are an important adjunct to any rehabilitation program to help the return of a normal painless range of motion in flexion and external rotation.

significant limitations in motion or difficulty in performance of passive motion exercises may benefit from a monitored program with a physical therapist using the principles of proprioceptive neuromuscular facilitation (PNF).[48] PNF focuses on the agonist/antagonist muscle couple in response to stretch reflexes and allows for progressive increase in motion by fatigue of the antagonistic muscle group.

The use of steroid injections has been discussed by some investigators in the initial treatment of impingement.[46,49] These injections are given as a mixture of local anesthetic and steroid in the region of the subacromial bursa. Proper technique demands avoidance of direct injection into the rotator cuff tendon. Studies have shown that significant weakness of the tendon can exist for a minimum of 14 days following local injection of steroids.[44] Therefore, associated strengthening programs should be avoided after injection for at least 2 weeks to prevent additional injury. A maximum of three injections are recommended with each spaced at least 6 weeks apart.

After a full, painless range of motion is achieved, the patient may be advanced to a gentle strengthening program for the shoulder. The strengthening program first addresses the internal and external rotators, specifically the infraspinatus, teres minor, and subscapularis mus-

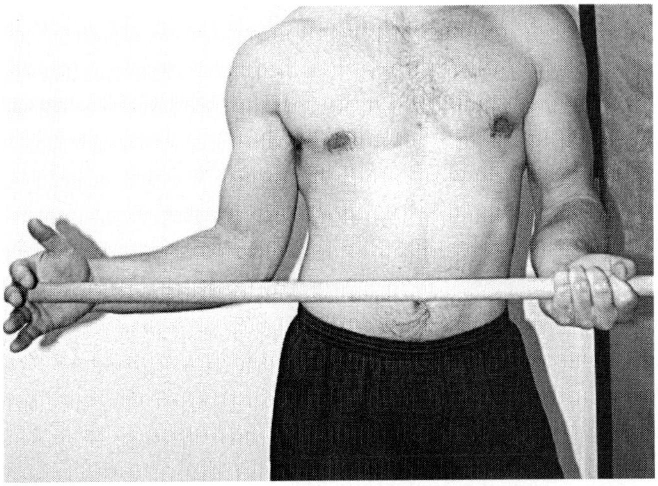

Fig. 8–30. External rotation with a stick. Most patients want to abduct the arm with this maneuver. They should be instructed to keep the elbow tightly applied to the side.

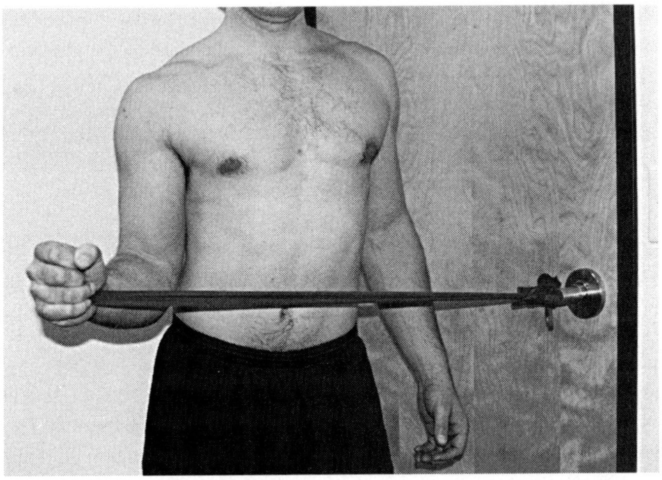

Fig. 8–31. Gentle strengthening exercises can be instituted after a full painless range of motion has been obtained. Strengthening should first focus on the infraspinatus, teres minor, and subscapularis muscles by gentle internal and external strengthening exercises.

cles. These muscles act to generate a head-depressing force and to stabilize the glenohumeral joint as well. A gentle, progressive resistance program using Theraband, rubber tubing, or sheet rubber can be performed easily by the patient on a regular basis. Strengthening should start with internal and external rotation below the horizontal (Fig. 8–31). After strengthening has progressed with the internal and external rotation exercises, abduction and forward flexion exercises can be added (Fig. 8–32). When normal range of motion and near normal strength are obtained, additional exercises for strengthening and generalized conditioning can be employed to prepare the patient for return to work and return to their prior level of activity. Specific training and conditioning relating to the prevention of reinjury to the region

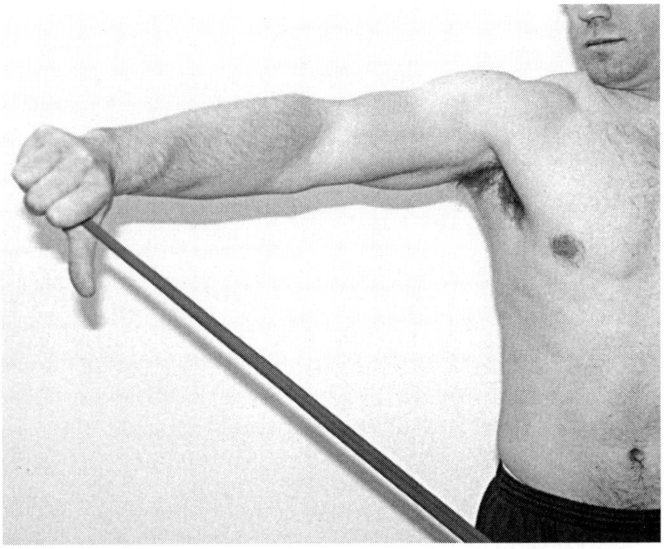

Fig. 8–32. How not to do supraspinatus strengthening: supraspinatus exercise in the thumb down position must be done through a shorter arc than illustrated. This particular exercise is often taught through an even greater range of abduction than shown here. Many patients can be cured by simply stopping them from doing this exercise through an aggressive arc.

should also be employed. This may require work-hardening programs for the laborer, stressing proper techniques involving lifting and the avoidance of repetitive overhead maneuvers. Athletic patients should undergo a gentle, graded return to their sports activity prior to returning to competition. A detailed study of the results of conservative treatment of impingement is found in Chapter 18.

SURGICAL TREATMENT

The surgical treatment of impingement lesions has undergone a steady evolution over the past 50 years. Early theories of the etiology of impingement stressed the importance of the lateral acromion in its production rather than the anterior portion. As a result, complete and lateral acromionectomy was considered the surgical technique of choice. These procedures, however, led to weakening of the deltoid, wound complications, and often persistent symptoms and limitation in function.[9,50] In 1972 Neer described the rationale behind anterior acromioplasty in the treatment of impingement syndrome.[9] Neer's indications for anterior acromioplasty were: (1) pain over 1 year and negative arthrogram with positive impingement injection test, (2) occasional stage II impingement lesions with demonstrable bony prominences at the undersurface of the anterior acromion or AC joint, (3) when repairing a rotator cuff tear, and (4) in association with other procedures for nonoutlet impingement lesions (biceps rupture, malunited greater tuberosity fractures, etc.). He cautions the use of anterior acromioplasty in the patient under 40 years of age, because the acromion often does not fuse until at least 25 years of age, and the majority of changes are transient and respond to conservative measures in this age group.[9,25,33]

His technique, which is described in detail in Chapter 23 makes use of an incision based in Langer's lines that extends from the anterio-lateral aspect of the acromion to just lateral to the coracoid. Subsequent mobilization of the subcutaneous tissue is performed with the deltoid musculature being split in line with the AC joint downward for a maximal distance of 5 cm. The importance of not extending beyond this 5-cm limit cannot be over stressed, because injury to the axillary nerve with subsequent denervation of the anterior deltoid is possible. The tendinous insertion of the anterior deltoid is elevated away from the AC joint and the anterior acromion and is preserved for later repair. An osteotomy is then performed, resecting a triangular wedge of bone that is 0.9-mm thick and approximately 2.0-cm long. The fragment and the attached coracoacromial ligament are then resected. Neer's indications for performance of distal clavicle resection were (1) preoperative assessment revealing painful arthritic change to be present and, (2) if more exposure of the supraspinatus is required, intraoperative assessment.[9] If either or both of these criteria were met, Neer recommended the excision of the distal 2.5 cm of the clavicle. The deltoid is repaired to the acromion and trapezius at the end of the case. Using this technique, Neer originally reported on 16 patients with diagnosis of chronic bursitis or partial tears of the supraspinatus, with 15 of these achieving satisfactory results with normal range of motion and deltoid strength.[9] Thorling et al. studied 51 patients who underwent Neer acromioplasty, with 33 reporting good to excellent results.[51] Sahlstrand evaluated the results of Neer's anterior acromioplasty in 52 patients with impingement, with 40 achieving good or excellent results.[52] Rockwood's modified Neer's acromioplasty technique is described in Chapter 23. His procedure includes removal of the anterior process of the acromion that extends beyond the anterior border of the clavicle in addition to the inferior prominence.[53] He states that this portion of the acromion continues to irritate the subacromial bursa and rotator cuff, thus producing impingement symptoms after removal of the inferior prominence alone. His acromioplasty technique is performed in two steps: first, the portion of the acromion that projects beyond the anterior border of the clavicle is resected vertically with a traditional anterior-inferior acromioplasty afterwards. The second step is a horizontal resection parallel to the posterior acromial border. In his study of 71 patients that underwent a modified Neer acromioplasty, 63 patients reported good or excellent results. In addition to performance of an acromioplasty, additional procedures such as distal clavicle excision and biceps tenodesis can be performed for treatment of other related pathology.[53] Neviaser et al. have described the "four in one" arthroplasty, in which tenodesis of the biceps at the time of acromioplasty and excision of the distal clavicle are performed for treatment of the painful arc syndrome.[54]

Arthroscopic decompression of the rotator cuff has been popularized in the treatment of impingement lesions in the past 10 years. Its technique can be demanding, with an associated learning curve even for experienced arthroscopists. Gartsman reported on a series of 165 patients with impingement treated with arthroscopic acromioplasty.[55] He divided the population into three groups based on the presence of rotator cuff tears. Group 1 consisted of 100 patients who had stage II impingement without evidence of rotator cuff tears; group 2 consisted of 40 patients with partial tears; and group 3 consisted of 25 patients with full-thickness tears of the rotator cuff. In group 1, 86 patients were followed for an average of 2 years, with 81 reporting marked improvement in pain and function. In group 2, 33 of 40 patients reported major improvement at an average of 28.9 months. In group 3, 14 satisfactory and 11 unsatisfactory results were seen at an average follow-up of 30.8 months, with 7 patients eventually requiring open procedure and repair of the rotator cuff. Gartsman concluded that arthroscopic treatment was most effective in stage II impingement and those with partial tearing of the rotator cuff, with inferior results being obtained in complete tears compared with open procedures. Ellman discussed the results in 60 cases treated with arthroscopic acromioplasty for both stage II and III lesions, with 88% of the patients reporting good or excellent results.[56] Similarly, Esch reported on 102 patients who had undergone arthroscopic acromioplasty for stage II and III lesions, with good or excellent results in 80% of patients at an average follow-up of 3 years.[57] Burkhart evaluated the clinical outcome of arthroscopic acromioplasty and rotator cuff debridement in 10 patients with massive tearing of the rotator cuff.[58] All patients had normal active motion and strength preoperatively, with the goal of surgery being pain relief. All 10 reported significant improvement; however, he stressed the importance of normal function and motion preoperatively as a criterion for this form of treatment. For a more thorough discussion of the technique of arthroscopic acromioplasty see Chapters 20 and 21.

Van Hosbeeck et al. compared the results of 53 patients treated with open subacromial decompression to the results of 53 patients who had received similar arthroscopic treatment.[59] Good or excellent results were found to occur in 81.1% of the open group and in 83.1% of the arthroscopic group at 27.3 months and 20.1 months follow-up, respectively. Overall patient satisfaction was slightly higher in the open group (94.3%) than in the arthroscopic group (88.3%). The current accepted standard for surgical treatment of impingement consists of antero-inferior acromioplasty, resection of the coracoacromial ligament with possible excision of the distal 1.5 to 2.5 cm of the clavicle if significant bony excrescences and or AC arthritis exists. The performance of the procedures by open versus arthroscopic methods remains a matter of debate. A certain level of competence and facility with arthroscopic surgery is required for the performance of these techniques arthroscopically. However, to date the literature has not shown a consistent significant difference in rehabilitation time and/or patient satisfaction between the two groups for impingement lesions without associated rotator cuff tearing. Arthroscopic surgery is still viewed as inferior to open techniques for treatment of impingement with associated rotator cuff tears.

Surgical failures with impingement surgery may arise from many sources. Care must be taken during the preoperative evaluation of the patient to rule out associated pathology, such as AC arthritis and/or biceps tendinitis, which may be addressed easily during the index procedures. In addition, care must be taken to establish definitively the existence of impingement syndrome prior to proceeding with surgery. As discussed earlier, many unrelated conditions may present with symptoms that mimic impingement, such as cervical radiculopathy, subtle glenohumeral instability, and glenohumeral arthritis. Hawkins et al. evaluated 51 patients with failed anterior acromioplasty, with 34 of the patients having a diagnosis other than impingement.[60] Surgical technique obviously has profound impact on the postoperative course of the patient. Care should be performed during the acromioplasty to ensure the appropriate amount of bone resection. Over-resection of bone will lead to weakness and predispose to detachment and scarring of the deltoid to the rotator cuff; under-resection will predispose the patient to residual impingement. Meticulous care should also be exercised with repair of the deltoid to its origin, because its detachment will lead to weakness, scarring, and pain.[61] Adherence to an appropriate postoperative rehabilitation program also is necessary and should emphasize initial rest for resolution of residual inflammation in the region, with maintenance of range of motion followed by a gradual strengthening and return of activities after all discomfort has subsided. Finally, appropriate patient selection with realistic expectations of goals being discussed with the patient prior to proceeding with surgery is necessary, because patient occupation and expectations heavily impact on surgical outcome. Hawkins et al.[60] and Saddemi[62] discussed the higher rates of failure and persistence of pain in patients treated with arthroscopic and open acromioplasty for impingement secondary to work-related injuries. Adequate evaluation and treatment require a period of conservative care and observation prior to proceeding with surgical intervention, especially in patients with a higher risk for poor surgical outcome.

Coracoid Impingement

Coracoid impingement results from the encroachment of the coracohumeral space with subsequent abutment of the lesser tuberosity against the coracoid process and may also mimic symptoms of subacromial impingement syndrome.[39,63] Goldthwait first described a clinical entity in patients. Pain from the subcoracoid bursa was referred pain in the upper arm and forearm, and reproduced by rotation of an abducted humerus.[64] This early observation proved accurate, as these patients often present with complaints of dull aching pain in the anterior aspect of the shoulder with radiation into the proximal brachium. Bennett described a cause of anterior shoulder pain as inflammation of the coracoid bursa.[65] He felt lesions in the coracoid region were produced by direct trauma of the humeral head on the coracoid process. He based his observations on his patient population of professional side-arm baseball pitchers.

An underlying history of anterior instability may exist, causing secondary narrowing of the coracohumeral interval, and should be considered in the evaluation of these patients. A previous history of shoulder surgery for instability with the use of bone blocks (i.e., Trillat or Bristow procedures) and/or osteotomy procedures may exist, which would predispose the patient to this condition. Previous fracture of the lesser tuberosity and calcification within the subscapularis tendon have also been reported in the etiology of coracoid impingement.[63] Tenderness may often be noted on palpation in the region of the coracoid. Typically, pain is exacerbated with the motions of forward flexion, adduction, and internal rotation (Fig. 8–33). This may often be accompanied by an audible and palpable snap and pain as the lesser tuberosity rides under the coracoid. Standard plain radiographs may show an elongated and/or overhanging coracoid process. Gerber evaluated patients with CT scans and noted a normal coracohumeral distance of 8.6 mm to be decreased in these patients to 6.7 mm.[39] Dines and colleagues have developed the coracoid index on CT scan.[63] This is a measurement of the projection of the coracoid beyond the line of the glenoid as measured on a CT scan. The

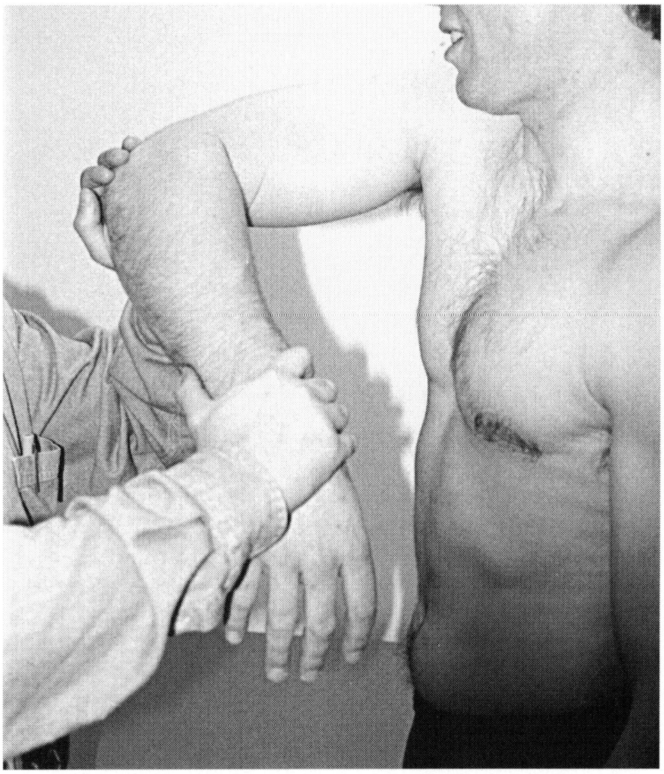

Fig. 8–33. The presence of coracoid impingement can be evaluated by forward flexing the arm to 90°, with subsequent adduction and internal rotation of the arm. An associated snapping may be noted with the maneuver as the lesser tuberosity slides under the coracoid process. Pain is localized by the patient in the region of the coracoid process.

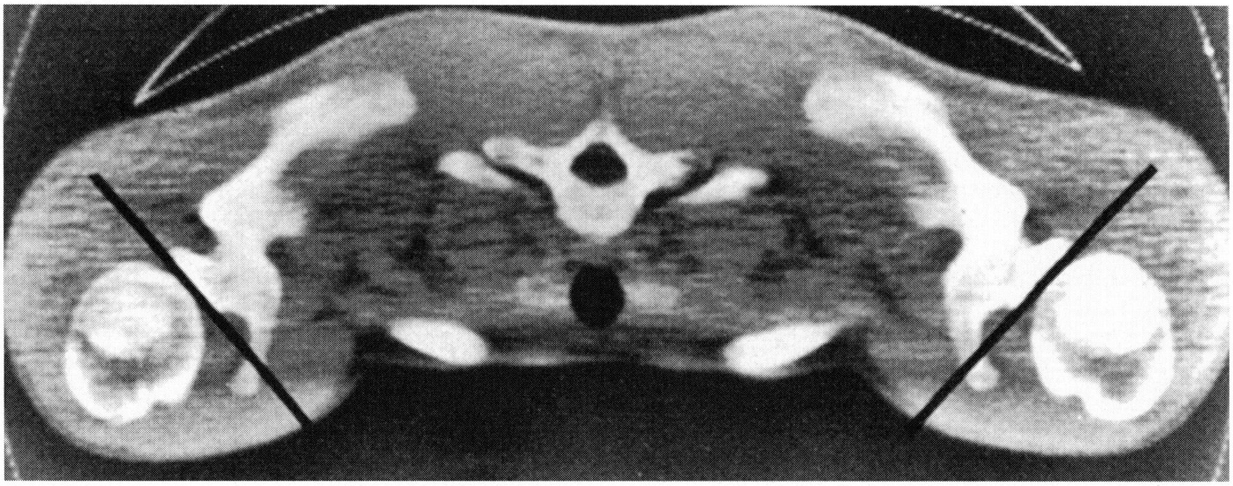

Fig. 8–34. The coracoid index is measured as the distance the coracoid process projection beyond the line from the glenoid rim. The CT scan can also demonstrate medial overgrowth, calcification, or spurring of the coracoid. (From Dines DM, Warren AF, Inglis AE, Pavlov H. The coracoid impingement syndrome. *J Bone Joint Surg Br.* 1990;72:314–316.)

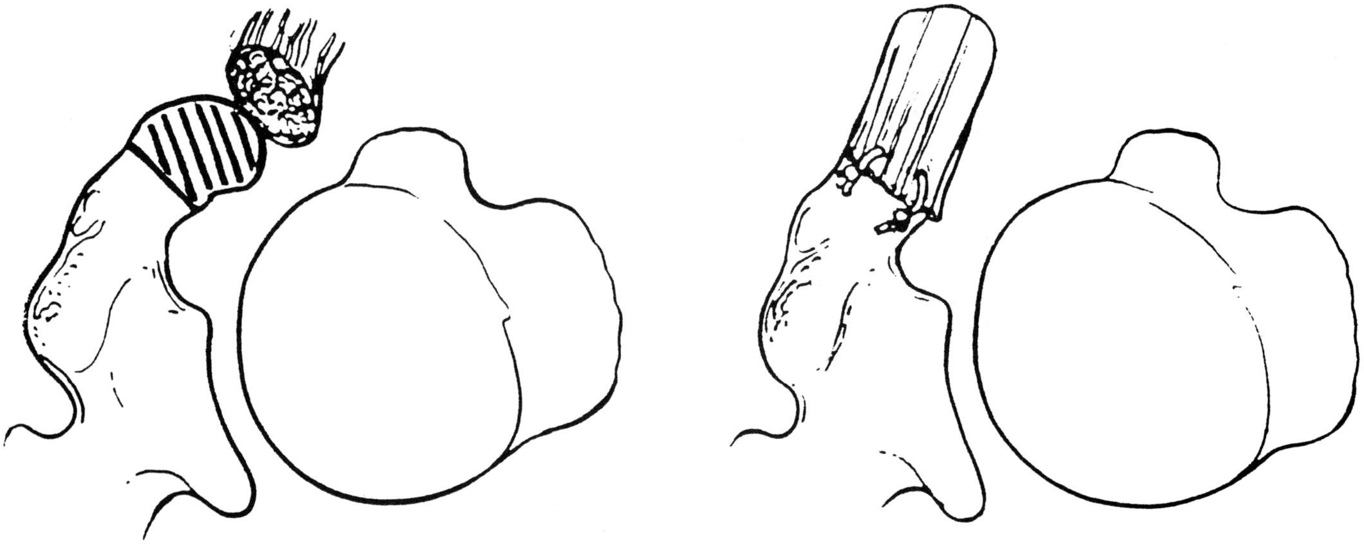

Fig. 8–35. Surgical removal of the distal portion of the coracoid process with reattachment of the conjoint tendon. (From Dines DM, Warren AF, Inglis AE, Pavlov H. The coracoid impingement syndrome. *J Bone Joint Surg Br.* 1990;72:314–316.)

average value in normal patients was 8.2 mm. The one patient measured preoperatively had an index of 3.5 mm (Fig. 8–34).

Friedman has discussed the diagnostic roles of cine MRI in active motion studies in coracoid impingement. However, this remains a purely investigational technique at this time.[66] The diagnosis often may be confirmed by selective injection into the subcoracoid region with local anesthetic with alleviation of the patient's discomfort. Some patients may respond to injections with steroid solution immediately adjacent to the coracoid combined with a strengthening program directed at the external rotators if subtle anterior instability is present. Surgical treatment for these lesions has recently been well defined and is presented later in this chapter.

Gerber et al. classified coracoid impingement into three categories: idiopathic, iatrogenic, and traumatic. Their observation was that the main symptom that the patient presented with was dull pain in the front of the shoulder. Most patients had referred pain to the front of the upper arm with occasional radiation into the forearm. They observed the patients to be most painful with flexion between 80 and 130°. They also observed that patients were most uncomfortable while driving a car, drawing on a blackboard, or during the follow-through phase of throwing. Those patients with iatrogenic coracoid impingement had undergone a bony block type procedure or posterior glenoid neck osteotomy. These procedures alter the normal anatomic relationship between the coracoid and the humeral head. They also felt that traumatic etiologies of coracoid impingement, such as lesser tuberosity fracture or coracoid fracture, altered the normal anatomic relationship between the humerus and the coracoid. They also felt that the cases of idiopathic subcoracoid impingement had some anatomic variant, such as a calcification at the tip of the coracoid, an elongated coracoid, or were soft tissue in nature.[39]

Surgical treatment of patients who have coracoid impingement requires decompression of the coracohumeral region by osteotomy of the coracoid process. This technique has recently been well described in the literature.[63] An incision based in Langer's lines, in line with the axillary fold, can be made with a subsequent deltopectoral approach similar to that used for anterior instability procedures. The clavipectoral fascia then is identified and carefully divided at the lateral aspect of the muscle of the conjoint tendon. The tendon and a portion of the coracoacromial ligament are excised from the tip of the coracoid process, revealing the underlying bone. The coracoid is osteotomized at the neck, with excision of the distal 1.5 cm of the process (Fig. 8–35). The conjoined tendon subsequently is reattached to the remaining coracoid base through drill holes. Dines et al. presented a review of 8 patients treated surgically for coracoid impingement. All claimed significant pain relief postoperatively with complete relief obtained in 6 patients at an average follow-up of 3 years.[63] The senior author has also performed a lateral partial corocoidectomy for this condition.

CONCLUSION

Significant advances have occurred in the understanding and treatment of impingement syndrome and related conditions of the shoulder. Debate still exists as to the exact etiology of impingement, whether it is a primary intrinsic, degenerative event within the tendon or a purely mechanical attrition of the tendon against the acromion. Appropriate diagnosis requires attention to the history and physical examination of the patient with shoulder pain, because many unrelated conditions may mimic impingement and/or coexist with it. Further disparity exists in the ultimate surgical treatment of impingement lesions that fail conservative therapy. The recent advent and expansion of arthroscopic surgery has afforded the practitioner new techniques in the management of impingement. However, like all new modalities, its ultimate role is still being actively determined.

REFERENCES

1. *Webster's Dictionary.* Springfield, IL: Merriam-Webster.
2. Jarjavey JF. Luxation du tendon du biceps humeral et des tendons des peroniers lateraux. *Gaz hebd de med.* Paris 1867;4:325–327, 357–359, 387–391.
3. Duplay. *Arch gen de med.* 1872;2:513.
4. Meyer AW. The minute anatomy of attrition lesions. *J Bone Joint Surg Am.* 1931;13:341.
5. Codman EA. Rupture of the supraspinatus tendon. In: *The Shoulder: Rupture of the Supraspinatus Tendon and Other Lesions in or about the Subacromial Bursa.* Malabar, FL: RE Krieger; 1984:(supplement edition)123–177.
6. McLaughlin HL. Lesions of the musculotendinous cuff of the shoulder. I. The exposure and treatment of tears with retraction. *J Bone Joint Surg Am.* 1944;26:31–51.
7. Smith-Petersen MN, Aufranc OE, Larson CB. Useful surgical procedures for rheumatoid arthritis involving joints of the upper extremity. *Arch Surg.* 1943;46:764–770.
8. Watson-Jones R. *Fractures and Joint Injuries.* 4th ed. Baltimore: Williams & Wilkins; 1960:449–451.
9. Neer CS II. Anterior acromioplasty for the chronic impingement syndrome in the shoulder: A preliminary report. *J Bone Joint Surg Am.* 1972;54:41–50.
10. Chung SMK, Nissenbaum, MM. Congenital and developmental defects of the shoulder. *Orthop Clin North Am.* 1975; 6:382.
11. Liberson, F. Os acromiale—a contested abnormality. *J Bone Joint Surg Am.* 1937;19:683–689.
12. Mudge MK, Wood VE, Frykman GK. Rotator cuff tears associated with os acromiale. *J Bone Joint Surg Am.* 1984;66:427–429.
13. Bigliani LU, Morrison D, April EW. The morphology of the acromion and its relationship to rotator cuff tears. *Orthop Trans.* 1986; 10:228.
14. Edelson JG, Taitz C. Anatomy of the coraco-acromial arch. Relation to degeneration of the acromion. *J Bone Joint Surg Br.* 1992;74:589–594, 1992.
15. Clark JM, Harryman DT II. Tendons, ligaments, and capsule of the rotator cuff: Gross and microscopic anatomy. *J Bone Joint Surg Am.* 1992;74:713–725.
16. Habermeyer P, Kaiser E, Knappe M, et al. Functional anatomy and biomechanics of the long biceps tendon. *Unfallchirurg.* 1987;90: 319–329.
17. Rowe CR (ed). *The Shoulder.* New York: Churchill Livingstone; 1988:145.
18. Ting A, Jobe FW, Barto P, et al. *An EMG analysis of the lateral biceps in shoulders with rotator cuff tears.* Presented at 3rd Open Meeting of the Society of American Shoulder and Elbow Surgeons, California, 1987.
19. des Marchais JE, Mehran RJ, Vezina JN. The etiology of chronic impingement syndrome re-evaluated. In: Takagishi N, ed. *The Shoulder.* Tokyo, Japan: Postgraduate Services; 1987:177–178.
20. Lindblom K. On pathogenesis of ruptures of the tendon aponeurosis of the shoulder joint. *Acta Radiol.* 1939; 20:563.
21. Rathbun JB, Macnab I. The microvascular pattern of the rotator cuff. *J Bone Joint Surg Br.* 1970;52:540.
22. Moseley HF, Goldie I. The arterial pattern of the rotator cuff of the shoulder. *J Bone Joint Surg Br.* 1963;45:780.
23. Ianotti JP, Swiotkowski M, Esterhafi J, Boulas HJ. *Intraoperative assessment of rotator cuff vascularity using laser Doppler flowmetry.* Abstract presented at AAOS Meeting, Las Vegas, 1989.
24. Inman VT, Saunders JB, De CM, Abbott LC. Observations on the function of the shoulder joint. *J Bone Joint Surg.* 1944;42:1.
25. Perry J. Biomechanics of the shoulder. In: Rowe CR, ed. *The Shoulder.* New York: Churchill Livingstone; 1988:13.
26. Matsen FA, Arntz, CT. Subacromial Impingement. In: Rockwood CA, Matsen FA, eds. *The Shoulder.* Philadelphia: WB Saunders; 1990: 628.
27. Neer CS II. Impingement lesions. *Clin Orthop.* 1983;173:70–77.
28. Hawkins RJ, Kennedy JC. Impingement syndrome in athletes. *Am J Sports Med.* 1980;8:151–158.
29. Jobe FW, Kvitne RS. Shoulder pain in the overhand or throwing athlete: The relationship of anterior instability and rotator cuff impingement. *Orthop Rev.* 1989;18:963–975.
30. Jobe FW. Impingement problems in the athlete. *Instr Course Lect.* 1989; 205–209.
31. Nirschl RP. Rotator cuff tendinitis: Basic concepts of pathoetiology. *Instr Course Lect.* 1989;439–445.
32. Ozaki J, Fujimoto S, Nakagawa Y, Masuhara K, Tamai S. Tears of the rotator cuff of the shoulder associated with pathological changes in the acromion: A study in cadaver. *J Bone Joint Surg Am.* 1988;70:1224.
33. Ogata S, Uhthoff HK. Acromial enthesopathy and rotator cuff tear: A radiologic and histologic postmortem investigation of the coracoacromial arch. *Clin Orthop.* 1990;254:39–48.

34. Fukuda H, Hamada K, Yamanaka K. Pathology and pathogenesis of bursal-side rotator cuff tears viewed from en bloc histologic sections. *Clin Orthop.* 1990;254:75–80.
35. Neer CS II. *Shoulder Reconstruction.* Philadelphia: WB Saunders; 1990.
36. Steindler A. Interpretation of pain in the shoulder. *AAOS Instructional Course Lecture.* Ann Arbor: JW Edwards; 1958: 159.
37. Gilcreest EL, Albi P. Unusual lesions of muscles and tendons of the shoulder girdle and upper arm. *Surg Gynecol Obstet.* 1939; 68:903–917.
38. Yergason RM. Rupture of the biceps. *J Bone Joint Surg Am.* 1931; 13:160.
39. Gerber C, Terrier F, Ganz R. The role of the coracoid process in the chronic impingement syndrome. *J Bone Joint Surg Br.* 1985; 67:703–708.
40. Burkhead WZ. The biceps tendon. In: Rockwood CA, Matsen FA, eds. *The Shoulder.* Philadelphia: WB Saunders; 1990;2:791–836.
41. Mack LA, Matsen FA III, Kilconyne RF, et al. Ultrasound: US evaluation of the rotator cuff. *Radiology.* 1985;157:205–209.
42. Seeger LL, Gold RH, Bassett LW, Ellman H. Shoulder impingement syndrome: MR findings in 53 shoulders. *AJR.* 1988;150:343–347.
43. Ianotti JP, Zlatkin MB, Esterhai JL, et al. Magnetic resonance imaging of the shoulder. *J Bone Joint Surg Am.* 73:17–28, 1991.
44. Kennedy JC, Willis RB. The effects of local steroid injections on tendons: A biomechanical and microscopic correlative study. *Am J Sports Med.* 1976;4:11–21.
45. Cofield RH, Simonet WT: Symposium on sports medicine: Part 2, the shoulder in sports. *Mayo Clin Proc.* 1984;59:157–164.
46. Richardson AB, Jobe FW, Collins HR: The shoulder in competitive swimming. *Am J Sports Med.* 1980;8:159–163.
47. Jobe FW. Symposium: Shoulder problems in overhead-overuse sports: Thrower problems. *Am J Sports Med.* 1979; 7:139–140.
48. Fu F, Harner CD, Klein AH. Shoulder impingement syndrome. *Clin Orthop.* 1991;269:162–173.
49. Cofield RH. Current concepts review: Rotator cuff disease of the shoulder. *J Bone Joint Surg Am.* 1985;67:974–979.
50. Neer CS II, Marberry TA. On the disadvantages of radical acromionectomy. *J Bone Joint Surg Am.* 1981;63:416–419.
51. Thorling J, Bjerneld H, Hallin G, et al. Acromioplasty for impingement syndrome. *Orthop Scand.* 1985;56:147–148.
52. Sahlstrand T. Operations for impingement of the shoulder: Early results in 52 patients. *Orthop Scand.* 1989;60:45–48.
53. Rockwood CA Jr. Shoulder impingement syndrome: Diagnosis, radiographic evaluation, and treatment with a modified Neer acromioplasty. *J Bone Joint Surg Am.* 1993;75:409–423.
54. Neviaser TJ, Neviaser RJ, Neviaser JS. The four-in-one arthroplasty for the painful arc syndrome. *Clin Orthop.* 1982;163:107–112.
55. Gartsman GM. Arthroscopic acromioplasty for lesions of the rotator cuff. *J Bone Joint Surg Am.* 1990;72:169–180.
56. Ellman H. Arthroscopic subacromial decompression: Analysis of one to three year results. *J Arthroscopic Rel Surg.* 1987; 3:173–181.
57. Esch JC. Arthroscopic update: Arthroscopic subacromial decompression: Surgical technique. *Orthop Rev.* 1989; 6:738–742.
58. Burkhart SS. Arthroscopic treatment of massive rotator cuff tears: Clinical results and biomechanical rationale. *Clin Orthop.* 1991; 267:45–46.
59. Van Hosbeeck E, Derycke J, Declerq G, et al. Subacromial impingement: Open versus arthroscopic decompression. *Arthroscopy.* 1992; 8:173–178.
60. Hawkins RJ, Chris T, Bokor D, Kiefer G. Failed anterior acromioplasty: A review of 51 cases. *Clin Orthop.* 1989; 243:106–111.
61. Post M. Complications of rotator cuff surgery. *Clin Orthop.* 1990; 254:97–104.
62. Saddemi S, Hawkins R, Moor J, Hawkins J. *Arthroscopic subacromial decompression: Two to four year follow-up study.* Presented at 9th open Meeting of American Shoulder and Elbow Surgeons. San Francisco, CA, February 21, 1993.
63. Dines DM, Warren AF, Inglis AE, Pavlov H. The coracoid impingement syndrome. *J Bone Joint Surg Br.* 72:314–316, 1990.
64. Goldthwait JE. An anatomic and mechanical study of the shoulder-joint, explaining many of the cases of painful shoulder, many of the recurrent dislocation, and many of the cases of brachial neuralgias or neuritis. *Am J Ortho Surg.* 1909;6:579–606.
65. Bennett GE. Shoulder and elbow lesions of the professional baseball pitcher. *J Am Med Assoc.* 1941;117:58–514.
66. Friedman RJ, Bonutti P, Genez B, Norfray J. *Cine MRI of subcoracoid impingement.* Presented at the 9th Open Meeting of the American Shoulder and Elbow Society. San Francisco, CA, February 21, 1993.

Chapter 9

The Acromioclavicular Joint and its Relationship to Rotator Cuff Disease

Michael Watson

The recognition that impingement leads to painful degeneration of the rotator cuff became generally accepted with Neer's paper in 1972.[1] It was Neer's contention that the rotator cuff impinges on the anterior acromion during elevation, leading to the attritional wear and resulting in symptoms and signs described in Chapter 10. The success of anterior acromioplasty in relieving these symptoms attests to the soundness of the observation.[2,3]

A proportion of patients with impingement have symptoms and radiographic signs of AC abnormality. It is accepted practice to excise the joint when performing anterior acromioplasty for impingement in these patients. In many patients, the hypertrophic new bone on either side of the AC joint seems to encroach on the supraspinatus outlet and the surgeon is left to wonder how much of the patient's symptoms are caused by his subacromial impingement, and how much are caused by his AC disorder.[4]

FREQUENCY OF AC DISORDERS IN IMPINGEMENT

The frequency with which AC abnormalities are reported in the impingement syndrome is variable.[5,6] This variation depends on the population served and on the diagnostic criteria. Plainly, in many patients with impingement and radiologically abnormal AC joints, the association is purely coincidental, because we know that many people have asymptomatic though radiologically abnormal AC joints. However, some patients with undoubted impingement have no other radiologically demonstrable lesion, and it must be assumed that the symptoms are caused by impingement involving the radiologically abnormal AC joint.

WIDE POST-TRAUMATIC AC SEPARATIONS

Severe post-traumatic displacement and instability of the AC joint may cause symptoms. Many of the symptoms arise from the disorganized joint itself, but cases exist in which the rotator cuff is distorted and compressed during elevation by post-traumatic scar tissue, new bone, and displaced local structures, such as the lateral clavicle and the anterior acromion.

MRI scanning differentiates these patients into those where the involvement is localized to the AC joint and those where the rotator cuff is involved. Should symptoms justify it, surgical debridement and stabilization of the damaged AC joint is helpful in the former cases. In those cases in which the rotator cuff is involved, such stabilization ought to be combined with subacromial decompression of all the affected structures in order to allow the rotator cuff to heal to its full potential.

LATE AC DISLOCATIONS

The effect of third-degree AC separations in the context of nonoutlet impingement is discussed in Chapter 8.

ANATOMY OF THE AC JOINT

The articular surfaces are virtually planar and normally partially separated by a fibrous meniscus. The two articular surfaces are roughly oval, flattened from above. The articulation is usually approximately sagittal, but a proportion of the population have a degree of lateral inclination, so that the joint space slopes laterally as it rises (Fig. 9–1).[7] Others have a more coronal orientation, the clavicle lying more in front of the acromion. The size of the contact area of the articulation varies from almost a pin-point to the whole medial aspect of the acromion.

The articulation is rarely truly congruous, for horizontal scans reveal that most joints are open anteriorly, with contact between articular surfaces in the posterior part only. Usually the anterior margin of the clavicle coincides with the anterior margin of the acromion but, in some, the acromion projects forward from the line of the clavicle (Fig. 9–2). This depends to a certain degree on the

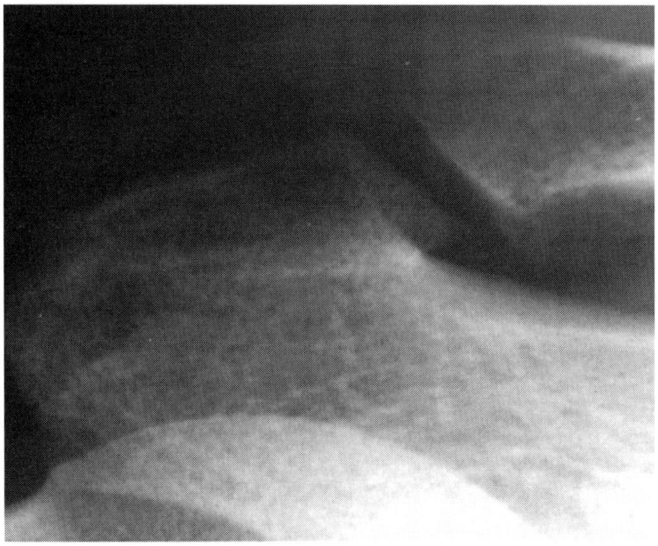

Fig. 9–1. A radiograph of a patient with impingement and a laterally sloping AC joint.

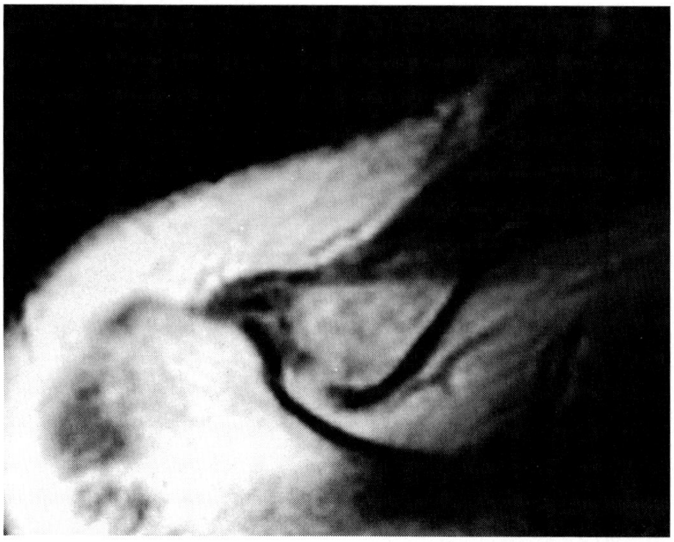

Fig. 9–2. Horizontal MRI scan showing the AC joint. The joint is open anteriorly and the contact area between the two surfaces is incongruous.

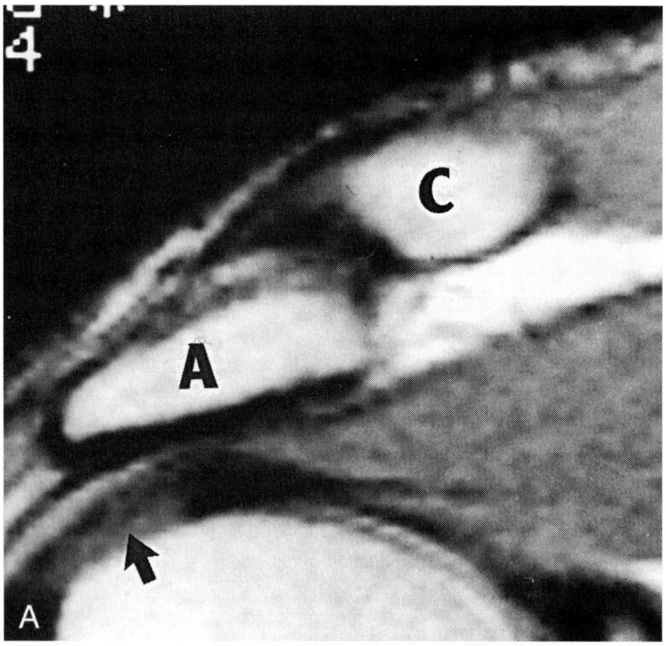

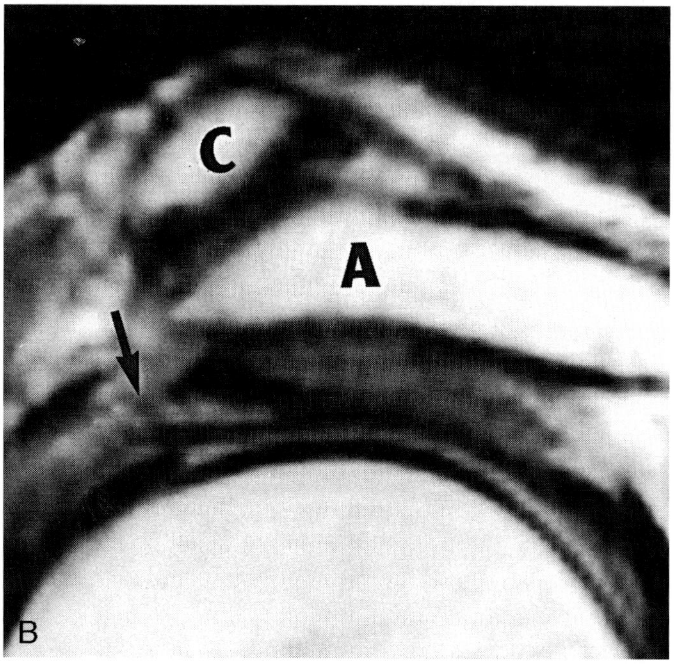

Fig. 9–3. MRI scans through a subluxed degenerated AC joint in a patient with impingement. Note the changes in the insertion of the supraspinatus tendon with irregularity, swelling, and increased hydration; *A*, coronal; *B*, sagittal.

competency of the coracoclavicular ligaments, as well as on the position of the patient's scapula at the time of the examination.

The radiographic appearance of the AC joint is variable; a degree of subluxation of the joint is often seen, with the clavicle overriding the acromion to a variable extent (Fig. 9–3). Irregularity and narrowing of the joint space is also often seen (Fig. 9–4). This is beam angle dependent on plain film radiology.

Movement at the articulation is extremely variable. A degree of passive movement is often demonstrable in the anatomical position in all three planes. In elevation of the arm the variability is again seen; in some patients the joint behaves as though it were almost fused, while in others the clavicle rides over the acromion (Fig. 9–5); in others, the acromion flexes on the lateral clavicle causing a rotatory subluxation.

The joint is bound by a tough capsule. Serial sectioning

has shown that stability depends chiefly on the inferior AC ligament and the coracoclavicular ligaments.[8] The coracoacromial ligament, inserted predominantly into the anteroinferior acromion, is also inserted into and blends with the inferior AC ligament (arrow symbol) (Fig. 9–6).

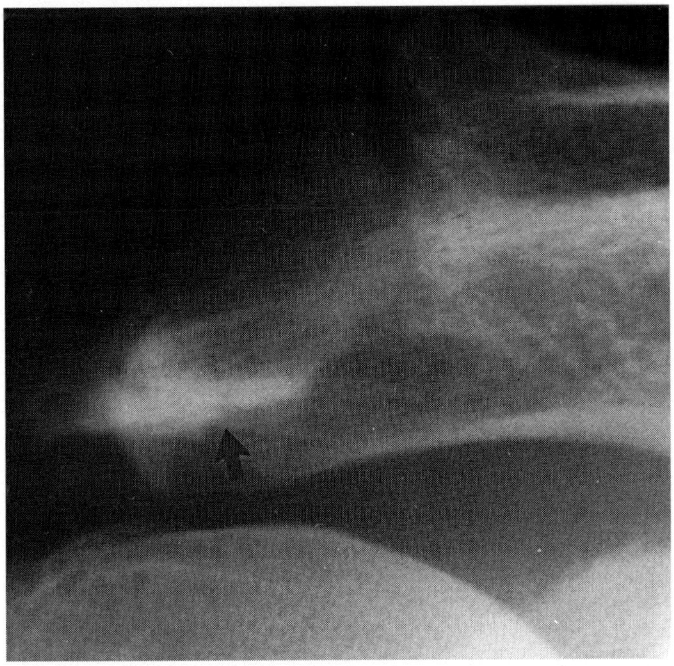

Fig. 9–4. Radiograph showing hypertrophic degeneration of the AC joint, with associated ossification in the insertion of the coracoacromial ligament in a patient with impingement.

CLINICAL DIAGNOSIS

The clinical diagnosis of patients with symptomatic AC joint derangement include a high painful arc (Fig. 9–7) and local tenderness at the AC joint line. This line includes not only the superior joint line but also the anterior joint line as well, which can be easily confused with coracoid tenderness to the less observant or less experienced examiner. Tenderness with crossbody adduction localized to the AC joint, in the absence of positive impingement signs and normal painless strength examination of the supraspinatus, is the sine qua non of isolated AC joint disease. When combined with positive impingement signs and variable degrees of pain and weakness with supraspinatus testing, one most query the role of the AC joint arthritis in the production of the attritional wear in the rotator cuff. An AC joint grind test (Fig. 9–8) measures stability in the horizontal plane and reproduces pain in arthrosis.

In summary then, local swelling and tenderness of a stable AC joint suggests that the impingement is caused by encroachment into the supraspinatus outlet. An unquestionably normal AC joint suggests that the patient has impingement by structures other than this joint.

PLAIN RADIOGRAPHY

Plain radiographs reveal the extent of the osteophytes on the deep surface of the AC joint, as well as a configuration of the acromion in the subacromial space. For a more detailed discussion and radiographic evaluation of the AC joint, refer to Chapter 6.

Patients with shoulder pain who have radiologically abnormal AC joints may be further investigated by MRI.

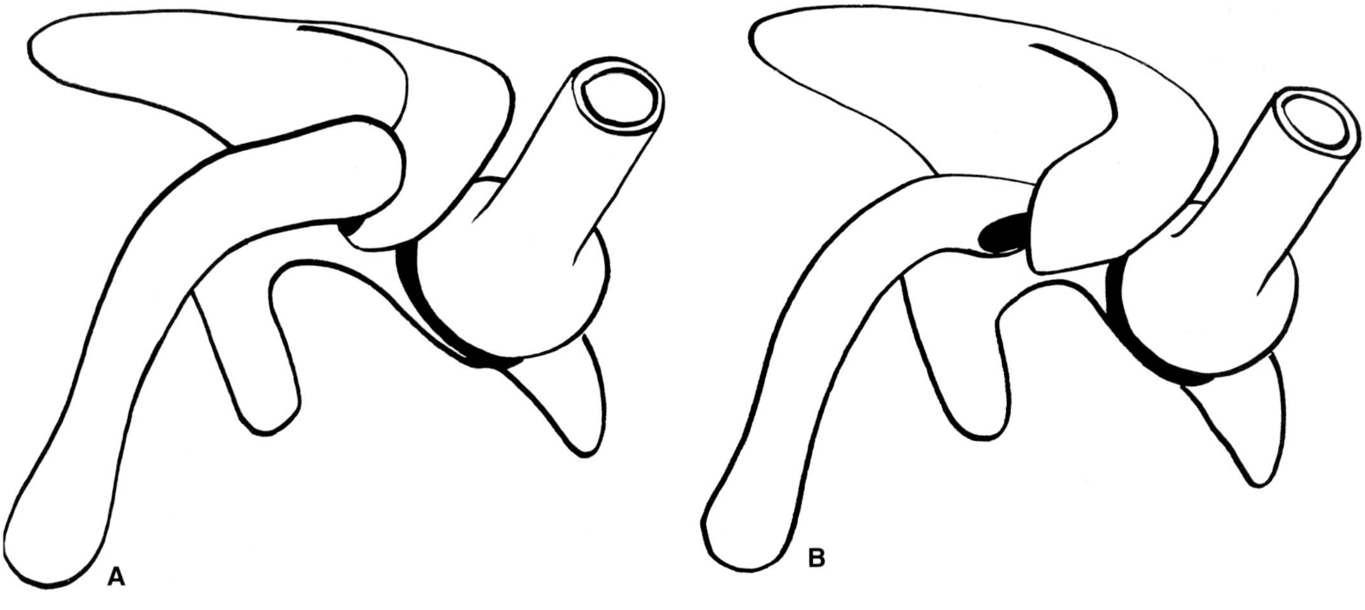

Fig. 9–5. Drawings to show (A) subluxation and (B) rotation at the AC joint during elevation.

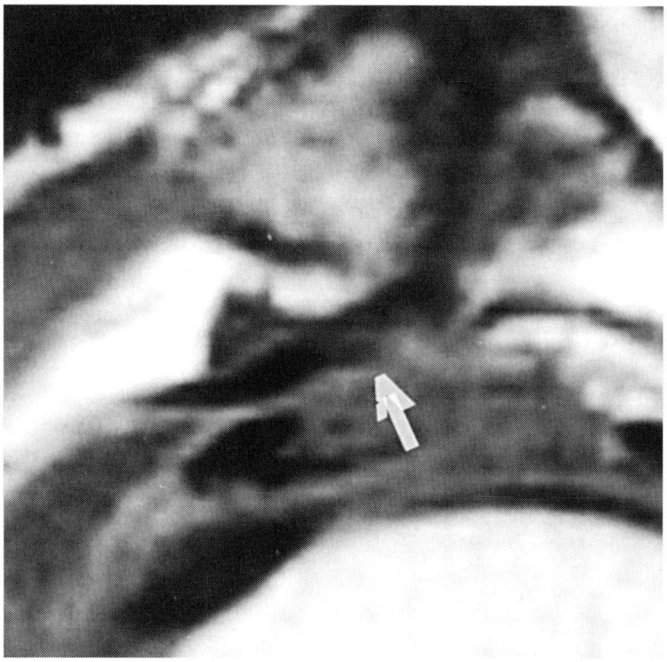

Fig. 9–6. Sagittal MRI to show the coracoacromial ligament inserting into the inferior capsule of the AC joint.

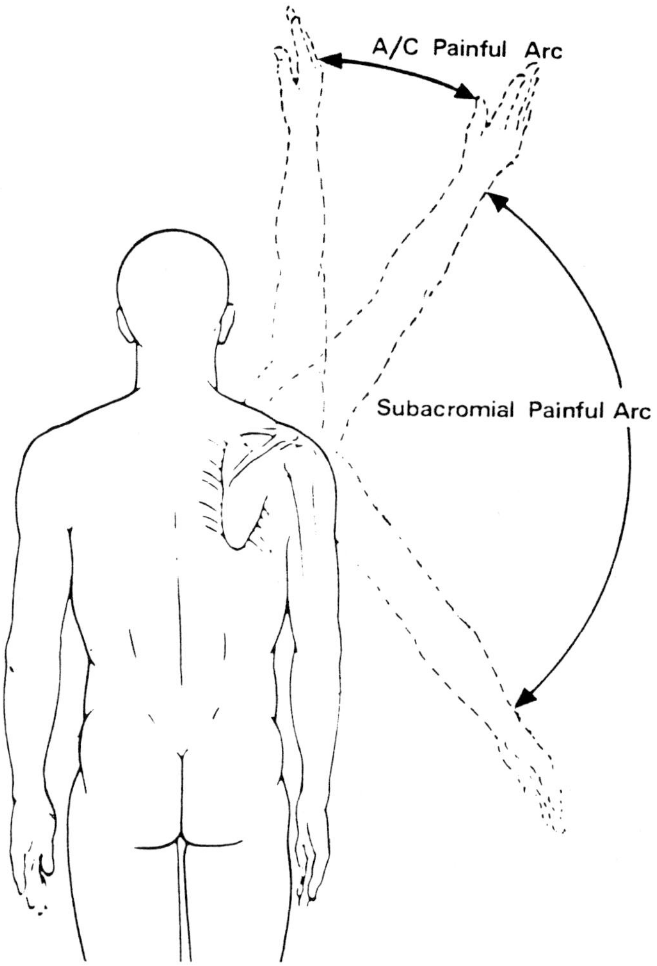

Fig. 9–7. The high painful arc seen in AC joint disease. (From Kessel L, Watson M. The painful arc syndrome. Clinical classification as a guide to management. *J Bone Joint Surg Br.* 1977;59:166–172.)

Other imaging techniques, ultrasound and computerized axial tomography (CAT), do not give an accurate picture of the soft-tissue contribution to the joints or their relationship with the rotator cuff. MRI scans in the anatomical position reveal the true extent of the thickening of the soft tissues on the deep aspect of the joint, and similar scans (taken in forward elevation) show the nature of the impingement. These same scans also give the surgeon a good measure of the nature of the rotator cuff lesion.

I have not found the endoscope helpful in investigating the AC joint, because the presence of the endoscope distorts the very structures under scrutiny.

In the anatomical position, a group of those patients with impingement with radiologically abnormal AC joints show thickening of the inferior AC ligament on MRI (Fig. 9–9). Others show distortion of the adjacent soft tissue by osteophytic new bone on either side of the joint (Fig. 9–10). It is reasonable to assume that a portion of these patient's symptoms are caused by contact and attritional wear of the rotator cuff tendons against these deep swellings on the joint. However, this is impossible to prove for impingement occurs in elevation, not the anatomical position. In the anatomical position, the AC joint overlies the belly of the supraspinatus muscle, not its tendon, where degenerative changes are seen in the impingement syndrome.

BONE SCANNING

Bone scanning generally reveals some increased uptake as well (see Chapter 6).

MRI SCANNING

In elevation, the AC capsule bulges inferiorly, compressing the tendon (Fig. 9–11). In some, the tendon impinges against osteophytes on the deep surface of the joint, the thickened AC joint capsule intervening (Fig. 9–12). At the extremes of elevation, MRI has revealed buckling of the tendon against the superior glenoid (see Chapter 14 for a thorough discussion of the role of posterosuperior impingement).

In some patients with impingement, the nature of the condition cannot be identified until the rotator cuff is exposed surgically. Most patients in this group have hypermobile AC joints, and the clavicle subluxes upwards on the acromion in elevation. This distorts the capsule of the joint, taking with it that part of the insertion of the coracoacromial ligament that blends with the inferior AC ligament. Passive movement of the arm then reveals buckling and snapping of the supraspinatus tendon beneath the tightened coracoacromial ligament in a large number of patients.

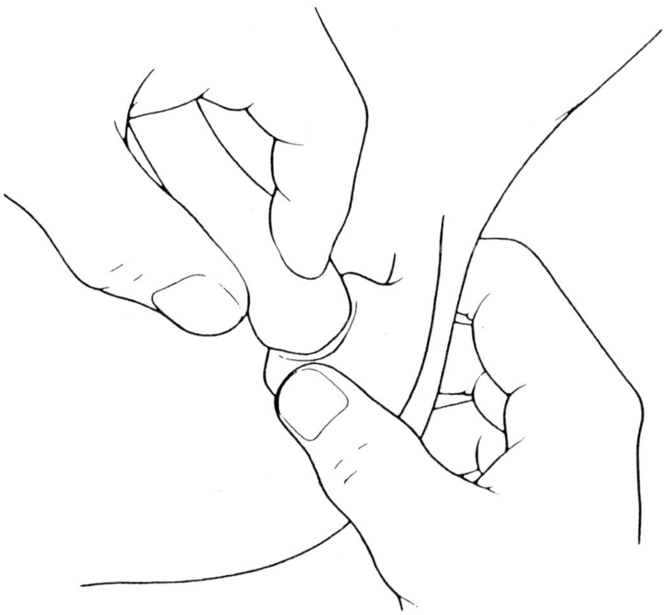

Fig. 9–8. An AC grind test. This test for instability of the AC joint in the horizontal plane and as well is positive in patients with AC joint arthrosis. (From Watson M: Examination of the shoulder: Signs and approaches. In: Watson M, ed. *Surgical Disorders of the Shoulder.* London: Churchill Livingstone; 1991;29–38.)

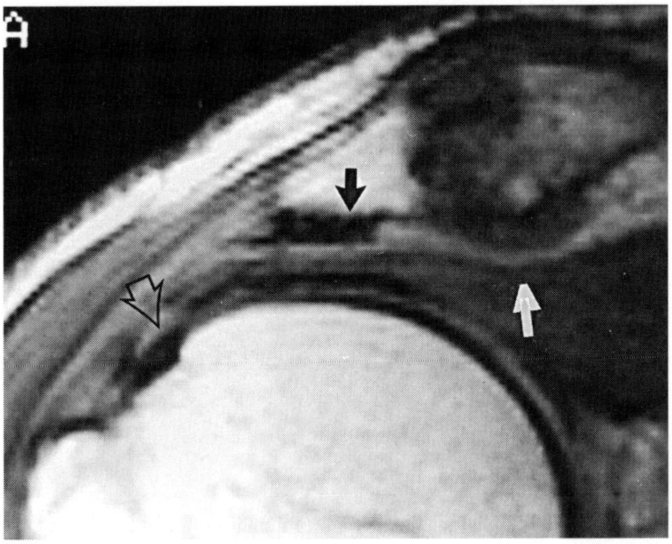

Fig. 9–9. MRI showing thickened inferior AC ligament distorting the belly of the supraspinatus tendon in a patient with impingement (white arrow). Note the irregular edema in the supraspinatus tendon insertion (open arrow) in this view with the arm at the side. Also note the thickened insertion of the coracoacromial ligament (black arrow).

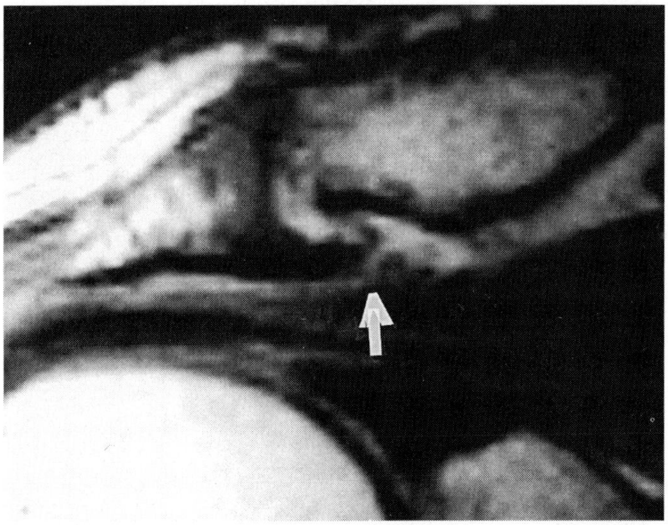

Fig. 9–10. MRI to show distortion of the supraspinatus belly by hypertrophic new bone projecting inferiorly from the acromial side of the AC joint (white) in a patient with impingement. Note the irregular edema in the insertion of the supraspinatus tendon.

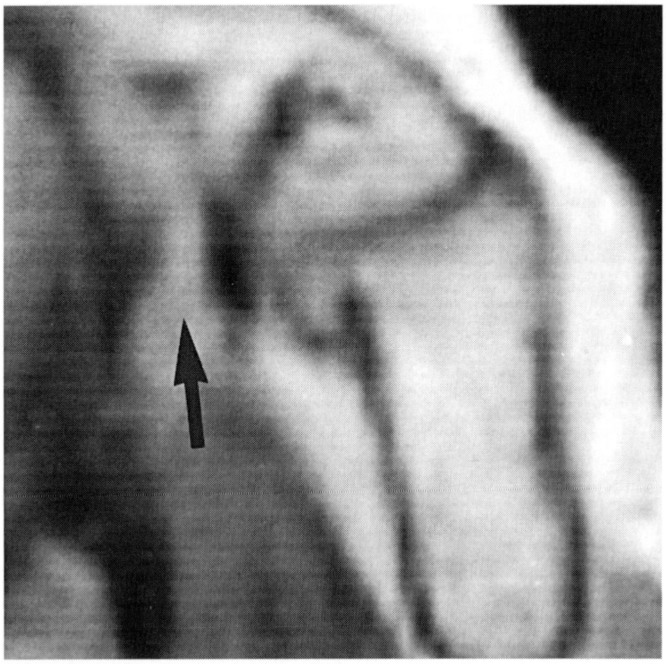

Fig. 9–11. Coronal MRI in elevation in a patient with impingement. Deep to the AC joint the capsule bulges, compressing the underlying supraspinatus tendon which is irregularly edematous in this area (black arrow).

POST-TRAUMATIC CHANGES

The AC joint may be rendered incongruous by injury. Hypertrophic degeneration then leads to enlargement of the joint, as well as stiffness and pain. In such patients, the symptoms are often caused by cuff impingement, in addition to the AC arthropathy, because MRI reveals degenerative changes in the rotator cuff. These areas of increased hydration are often in the deep part of the insertion of the supraspinatus tendon (Fig. 9–13). On occasions the same tissue ruptures, causing a deep surface partial-thickness rupture, Codman's rim rent (Fig. 9–14).[9] In most of these patients, MRI shows that the area

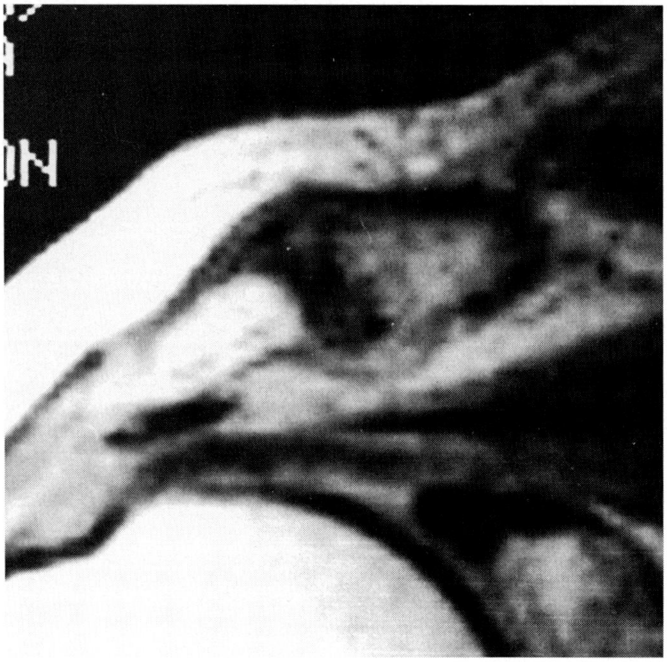

Fig. 9–12. Coronal MRI in the anatomical position showing the combined effects of capsular bulging and osteophytic enlargement of the AC joint in a patient with impingement.

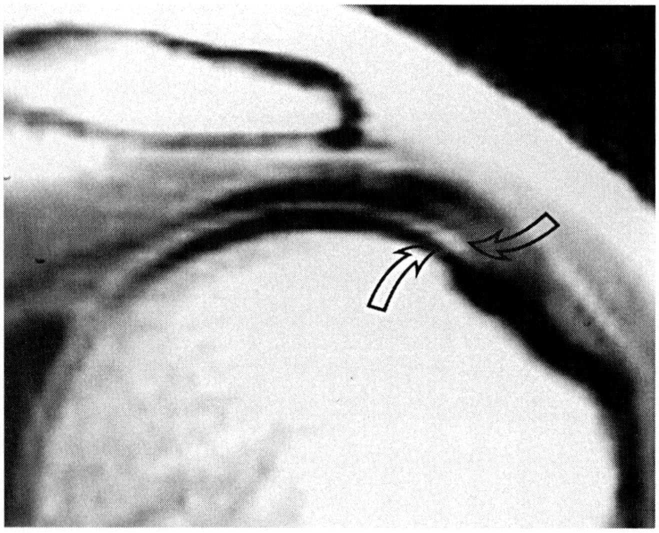

Fig. 9–13. Coronal MRI of the shoulder showing edema in the deep part of the insertion of the supraspinatus tendon (open arrow).

of increased hydration and rupture impinges on the thickened insertion of the coracoacromial ligament in elevation (Fig. 9–15).

Post-traumatic instability of the AC joint may cause symptoms similar to those of impingement; clinically, the two are very similar, with demonstrable laxity of the AC joint and pain during elevation. The impingement test, local anaesthetic in the subacromial bursa, often allows a distinction to be made. MRI also helps, because degenerative changes in the rotator cuff are highly suggestive of impingement. The mechanism of impingement in

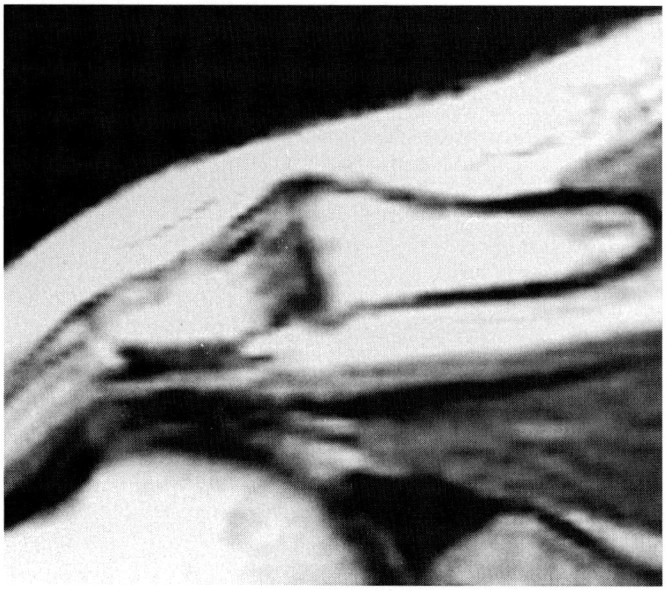

Fig. 9–14. Coronal MRI of the shoulder showing a deep surface partial-thickness rupture, Codman's rim rent associated with mild subluxation of the gently sloping AC joint and thickening of the insertion of the coracoacromial ligament.

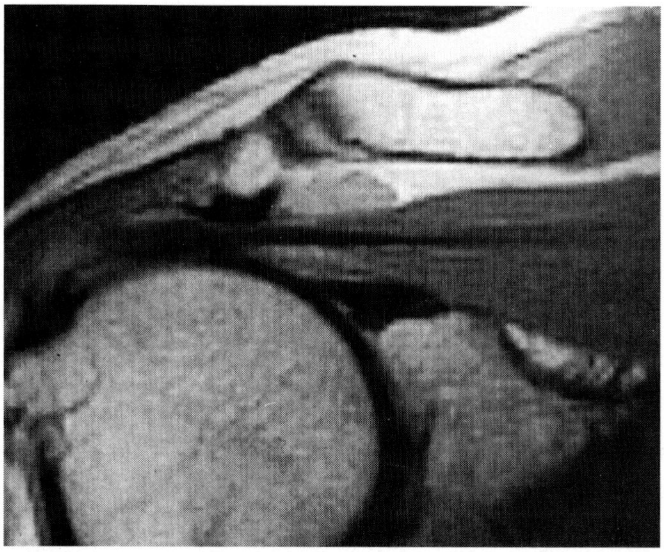

Fig. 9–15. Coronal MRI of the shoulder showing distortion of the supraspinatus musculotendinous junction by thickening in the coracoacromial ligament insertion and edema of the supraspinatus tendon insertion. In elevation the edematous region impinges on the insertion into the AC ligament.

these patients is not necessarily caused by hypertrophy of the AC joint and adjacent soft tissues, because these may not be present. Indeed the condition may be seen after surgical removal of the outer end of the clavicle for post-traumatic arthropathy. In patients with impingement with AC instability, exploration has shown that many have pathological thickening of the coracoacromial ligament. This is distorted via its connection with the AC joint during elevation in a manner very similar to that seen in patients with constitutional laxity of the AC joint, causing supraspinatus tendon impingement.

ROTATOR CUFF

In impingement associated with AC disorders, the rotator cuff changes may be extremely subtle, with very little to be seen endoscopically or radiologically. In these patients, MRI is the best evidence of disease. Areas of increased hydration are seen, almost always near the insertion of the supraspinatus insertion. The affected area is usually the deep part of the tendon. The insertion itself is often healthy; the abnormal area lies just medial to it (Fig. 9–16). In more advances cases there is a deep partial-thickness defect in the supraspinatus tendon in this region, a rim rent (Fig. 9–17). The same region may also house a midsubstance cleavage. This is best seen on MRI (Fig. 9–18), though adroit arthroscopy may demonstrate such cleavage via a rim rent.

Full-thickness cuff tears may be seen too. These can be demonstrated by arthrography and by arthroscopy. The center of the defect is usually near the insertion of the supraspinatus tendon. MRI reveals the extent of the defect and permits preoperative planning. Full-thickness cuff rupture associated with destruction of the inferior joint capsule in degenerative arthropathy of the AC joint may exhibit the "geyser sign," when contrast medium used in arthrography leaks into the AC joint via the cuff defect.

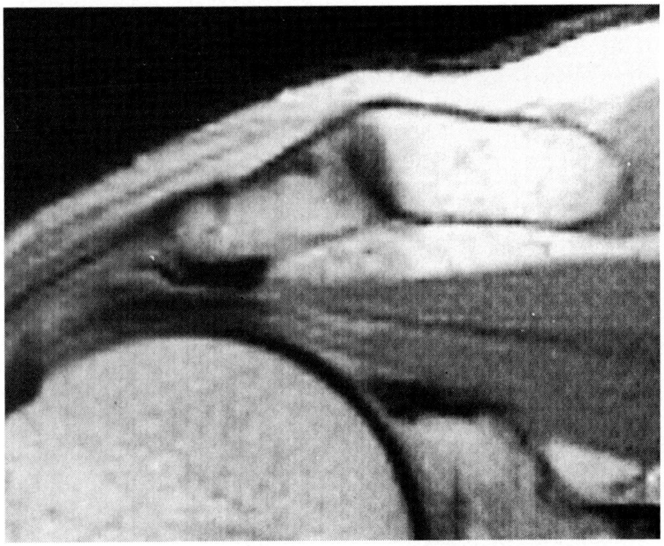

Fig. 9–16. Coronal MRI of the shoulder. The supraspinatus tendon just medial to its insertion is edematous. This is associated with a sloping AC joint and a thickened coracoacromial ligament insertion.

SURGICAL TREATMENT

Severe refractory symptoms justify surgical treatment. The surgeon should satisfy himself that he has identified the source of the impingement, its mechanism, and site. Approximately half the patients in my practice with impingement have AC joint affection.

Examination must include tests for glenohumeral instability. The degree and direction of AC laxity should be assessed too. This can be done usually on the conscious patient, but a preoperative examination under anaesthetic may be required. Overriding of the acromion by the lateral clavicle in elevation suggests that the coracoacromial ligament is the culprit, distorting as a result of AC subluxation in elevation and strangling the buckled supraspinatus tendon.

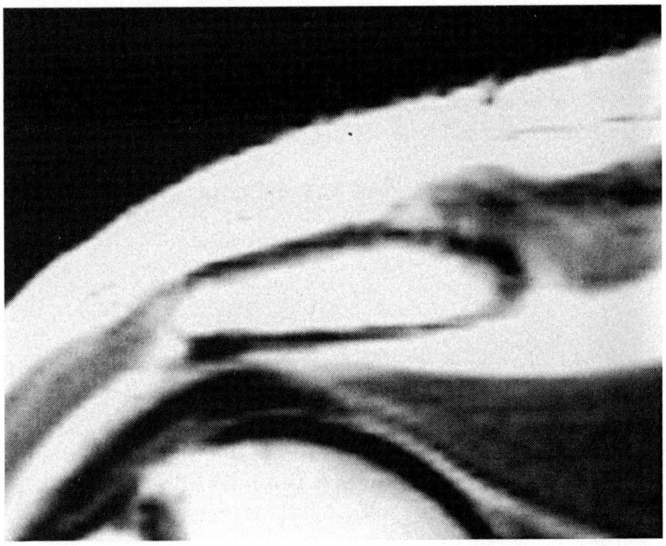

Fig. 9–17. Coronal MRI of the shoulder. A deep-surface, partial-thickness defect near the insertion of the supraspinatus tendon propagates medially within the substance of the tendon, a rim rent.

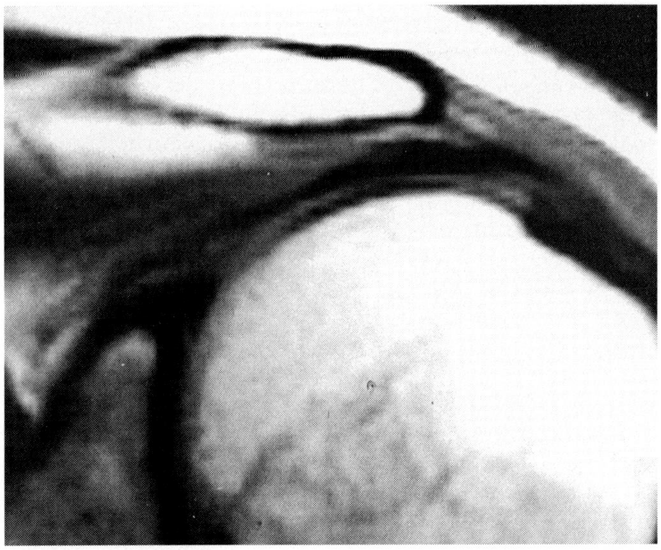

Fig. 9–18. Coronal MRI of the shoulder. A midsubstance cleavage lesion lies within the supraspinatus tendon insertion.

Decompression for impingement and cuff degeneration caused by AC disorders may be done arthroscopically or open. The principle of the procedure is to reduce the swelling on the deep surface of the joint, to divide the coracoacromial ligament, and to widen the supraspinatus outlet. Arthroscopic techniques allow this to be done reliably in expert hands.[10] The occasional arthroscopist is advised to perform an open operation, because it is easy either to overdo or underdo the decompression unless a good deal of training and practice has been put into mastering the arthroscopic technique.

OPEN DECOMPRESSION

Unless the shoulder is mobile and strong, a short period of preoperative mobilization and strengthening under the care and supervision of a trained therapist is worthwhile, because such treatment hastens postoperative recovery. Of course, the preoperative symptoms may prevent any but the gentlest treatment, and in this case the procedure should not be delayed.[11]

After induction of the anaesthetic, the shoulder is prepared and draped to allow generous access. Some elevation of the torso and the scapula is helpful. The AC joint is examined for stability; in all but the most obese patients, this can be done by grasping the acromion with the fingers of one hand and the lateral clavicle with those of the other. Pushing and pulling will then demonstrate the excursion available in all three planes. The joint should then be palpated while the arm is passively elevated to test for subluxation of the clavicle over the acromion in elevation.

Through a skin cleavage line over the acromion, the AC joint and the acromion are exposed. Careful diathermy dissection allows the deltoid origin from the lateral clavicle and the anterior acromion to be peeled off the bone as a single sheet, which includes the anterior part of the capsule of the AC joint. Care should be taken to preserve the fibrous tendon of origin to which sutures are tied during closure.

The capsule of the AC joint is then peeled off the lateral clavicle, preserving the capsular sleeve's attachment to the periosteum of the clavicle. An excision arthroplasty of the joint is then effected by nibbling back the articular surface of the lateral clavicle. Surgeons commonly fail to nibble back the posterior part of the articular surface adequately and leave a point-to-point articulation that is rather painful postoperatively. Therefore, palpate the joint to ensure that the excision has been done completely. Swellings on the deep surface of the lateral clavicle should be felt for and removed by nibbling. It is important to preserve the deep part of the capsule when doing this, for symptomatic postoperative instability may be caused otherwise. Ensure that the articular surfaces do not make contact in elevation of the shoulder too. More bone needs to be nibbled from the lateral clavicle if they do.

The acromion is usually abnormal if the AC joint is abnormal. Commonly the anteromedial aspect is enlarged by mirror-osteophytes reflecting the enlargement of the lateral clavicle. The subacromial space is further narrowed by thickening and, sometimes, even ossification of the insertion of the coracoacromial ligament into the anteroinferior acromion. An osteotome directed posteroinferiorly is used to raise the roof of the subacromial space by removing the anteroinferior acromial projections. The acromial tip projecting beyond the anterior margin of the AC joint is removed together with the anteroinferior hook. The osteotomy necessarily includes the insertion of the coracoacromial ligament. The fragment is removed by section of the ligament, in which care should be taken to preserve the inferior AC ligament, with which the coracoacromial ligament blends in order to preserve as much AC stability as possible. The deep surface of the acromion should be palpated at this stage to identify any residual projections or ligament remnants; these should be removed if found. The lateral margin of the coracoacromial ligament frequently extends laterally behind the acromion and also blends with the coracohumeral ligament medially. Any such extension should be divided under direct vision. It may be necessary to extend the incision in the deltoid laterally by splitting its fibers to achieve this. This decompression allows sufficient access for any repair of the rotator cuff that is required.

The closure must ensure stability of the AC articulation and security of the deltoid origin. The thick tough flaps of AC capsule are closed with interrupted sutures. The articulation should be tested after this; too tight a repair prevents full excursion of the shoulder; too loose a repair and the AC articulation is hypermobile. Strong sutures are then used to repair the deltoid origin back onto fibrous aponeurosis over the acromion; the tough fibrous tendon of origin and the aponeurosis take sutures well, but earlier careless raising of the deltoid origin may necessitate the boring of holes into the acromion to take the sutures. Shoulder excursion should be tested again after this to ensure adequacy of the repair.

The postoperative regime is dictated by the rotator cuff. If it is sound, then early gentle passive mobilization should commence as soon as postoperative symptoms allow. If an insecure repair has been done, then cuff healing dictates the rate of mobilization.

EDITOR'S NOTE

I have been impressed with the frequency with which radiographically abnormal, but seemingly symptom-free AC joints, become painful after surgery for impingement and after total shoulder arthroplasty. The etiology of this, I feel, is two-fold: (1) the patient's shoulder prior to surgery may be so painful from his/her cuff tear or arthritis, that he/she do not move their shoulder enough to insight the AC joint; and/or (2) the relative immobilization of the shoulder postoperatively increases the arthrofibrosis and may accelerate the onset of pain from otherwise silent AC joint arthritis.[10] Over the last 7 years, I have been very liberal in removing the AC joint without regret.

REFERENCES

1. Neer CS II. Anterior acromioplasty for the acromic impingement syndrome in the shoulder. A preliminary report. *J Bone Joint Surg Br.* 1977;59:166–172.
2. Watson M. The refractory painful arc syndrome. *J Bone Joint Surg Br.* 1978;60:544–546.
3. Neer CS II. Impingement lesions. *Clin Orthop.* 1983;173:70–77.
4. Kessel L, Watson M. The painful arc syndrome. Clinical classification as a guide to management. *J Bone Joint Surg Br.* 1977;59:166–172.
5. Taylor GM, Tooke M. Degeneration of the acromioclavicular joint as a cause of shoulder pain. *J Bone Joint Surg Br.* 1977;59:507.
6. Watson M. The impingement syndrome in sportsmen. In: Bateman JE, Welsh RP, Decker BC, eds. *Surgery of the Shoulder.* New York: Churchill Livingstone; 1984:140–142.
7. De Palma AF. *Surgery of the Shoulder.* 2nd ed. Philadelphia: JB Lippincott; 1973.
8. Fukuda K, Craig EV, An K-N, Cofield RH, Chao EUS. Biomechanical study of the ligamentous system of the acromioclavicular joint. *J Bone Joint Surg Am.* 1986;68:434–440.
9. Codman EA. *The Shoulder.* Boston: Thomas Todd, 1934.
10. Gartsman GM. Arthroscopic acromioplasty for lesions of the rotator cuff. *J Bone Joint Surg Am.* 1990;72:169–180.
11. Watson M. Major rupture of the rotator cuff: The results of surgical repair in 80 patients. *J Bone Joint Surg Br.* 1985; 67:618–624.

Chapter 10

The Biceps Tendon and Rotator Cuff Disease

Peter Habermeyer and Gilles Walch

Except in primates, the biceps brachii muscle has but a single origin on the scapula. The horse, for example, which lacks a deltoid muscle, has a strong and "one-headed" biceps muscle that works together with a powerful supraspinatus muscle to antevert the humerus. However, in primates the biceps muscle arises by two heads.[1] The long biceps tendon has migrated away from the scapular level through the phylogenetic rotation of the humeral shaft. This makes it more difficult to understand the way in which the muscle works.

Gradually, new diagnostic techniques and, especially, arthroscopy have shed new light on the pathophysiology of the long biceps tendon. Our knowledge has been greatly enhanced by the routine exposure of the long biceps tendon during open surgery on the rotator cuff, which was introduced by the French surgeon Patte. Routine surgical exposures and diagnostic arthroscopy have provided fundamental new insights into shoulder pathology, which in turn have yielded important implications for the treatment of lesions of the long biceps tendon.

ANATOMY

The long head of the biceps brachii is attached to the posterior superior aspect of the glenoid labrum in about 50% of the population. It attaches to the supraglenoid tubercle in about 20% of cases. In about 30% of cases the long head of the biceps originates in both regions, and sometimes it appears bifurcated.[2] A study of the relationship between the tendon of the long head of the biceps brachii and the glenoid labrum showed that in 70% of the specimens examined, the biceps tendon was blended with the posterosuperior portion of the labrum. Only a small part of the tendon was attached to the supraglenoid tubercle. However, in 25% of the specimens the major portion of the long biceps tendon was attached to the supraglenoid tubercle.[3] A close association between the glenoid labrum and biceps tendon was consistently observed, both grossly and histologically. A primary attachment of the tendon to the superior part of the labrum before its insertion into the supraglenoid tubercle was noted. The collagenous fibers of the labrum and biceps tendon were found to be intimately blended in that area.[4] The cross-sectional characteristics of the long head of the biceps vary during its course: 8.5 × 2.8 mm at the origin, 4.7 × 2.6 mm in the area of strongest demand (the entrance to the bicipital groove), and 4.5 × 2.8 mm at a point 1.5 cm above the musculotendinous junction.[2]

The long head of the biceps muscle receives its blood supply from the brachial artery. The anterior circumflex artery in particular supplies the biceps tendon at the intertubercular groove. The groove portion of the tendon, which is the most susceptible to rupture, possesses an arterial supply in all individuals. The blood supply at that level at least far surpasses the supply to the intra-articular portion of the tendon, where ruptures seldom occur. The vascular factor appears to play a minor role in the pathogenesis of biceps tendon ruptures.[5]

The 9-cm long biceps tendon runs obliquely over the top of the humeral head into the bicipital (intertubercular) groove. It continues down the ventral portion of the humerus, becoming musculotendinous near the insertion of the pectoralis major muscle.

The biceps tendon is intra-articular but extrasynovial. The proximal layer of the synovial sheath reflects back upon itself to form a visceral sheath (vagina synovialis intertubercularis), which extends 4.5 cm past the distal end of the bicipital groove. The extra-articular component of the biceps begins distal to the synovial sheath. The long synovial sheath permits the humeral head to glide up and down on the biceps tendon. The portion of the long head of the biceps tendon inside the bicipital groove possesses a mesotendineum that arises from the posterolateral groove.

The bicipital groove has an average width of 6.2 mm at its central, narrowest portion. The groove is 9.6 mm wide at its entrance and 7.3 mm wide at its exit. The depth of the groove averages 2.2 mm at the entrance, 5 mm at the center, and 2.4 mm at the exit. These figures are based on measurements in 50 specimens.[2]

The medial wall of the bicipital groove is formed by the lesser tuberosity of the humerus. The medial wall angle has shown a high degree of variability in previous studies,[2,6,7] with a mean value of approximately 60°. The correlation between a lower medial wall angle and subluxation or dislocation of the biceps tendon remains unclear.[8,9]

Capsuloligamentous structures play a major role in retaining and stabilizing the long biceps tendon in the intertubercular groove. The subscapularis and supraspinatus tendons fuse to form a sheath that surrounds the biceps tendon at the proximal end of the groove. The roof of the sheath is formed by extensions of the supraspinatus tendon, and the superior part of the subscapularis tendon passes below the biceps tendon to join with fibers from the supraspinatus tendon to form the floor of the sheath. The deep portion of the sheath runs adjacent to the bone and forms a fibrocartilaginous lining for the groove that extends approximately 7 mm.[10]

The rotator cuff is perforated anterosuperiorly by the coracoid process, which separates the anterior border of the supraspinatus tendon from the superior border of the subscapularis tendon, creating the triangular rotator interval. The base of the interval is the coracoid process, from which the coracohumeral ligament originates. The coracohumeral ligament has a broad, thin origin, 1 to 2 cm in width, near the base of the coracoid process along its lateral border. The coracohumeral ligament divides into two main bands, one of which inserts into the tendinous anterior edge of the supraspinatus and the greater tuberosity and the other into the superior border of the subscapularis, the transverse humeral ligament, and the lesser tuberosity of the humerus (Fig. 10–1).[8]

Clark et al.,[10] in a histologic study of the fibrous anatomy of the rotator cuff, found that the collagenous extensions of the coracohumeral ligament envelop the cuff tendons and blend into superficial and deep layers of the supraspinatus and subscapularis and into the articular capsule. This relationship reinforces the capsule at the interval and the borders of the tendon cuff. The coracohumeral ligament is superficial to the shoulder capsule and overlies the biceps tendon, while its superficial and deep branches envelop the anterior part of the supraspinatus tendon.

The superior glenohumeral ligament (SGHL) consistently arises from the labrum adjacent to the supraglenoid tubercle and crosses the floor of the rotator interval.[11] The superior glenohumeral ligament inserts on the superior lateral portion of the lesser tuberosity and is united to the medial aspect of the coracohumeral ligament. The coracohumeral ligament is the superficial portion that covers the long head of the biceps, and the SGHL is the deep part that inserts over the humerus, thus forming a reflection pulley for the biceps tendon. This pulley is also in direct contact with the insertion of the subscapularis situated on its internal border.[10]

The superior glenohumeral ligament and the coracohumeral ligament blend together above the entrance to the bicipital groove, forming a circular sleeve, comparable to a ringband of a finger flexor tendon, that restrains against medial dislocation of the long biceps tendon.[12] The connection of both ligaments at the entrance to the groove has considerable pathogenic importance (Figs. 10–2 and 10–3).

In this respect the superior glenohumeral ligament, previously regarded as insignificant, makes an important contribution to the stability of the intraarticular part of the long head of the biceps tendon.

Traditionally, it was taught that the biceps tendon is retained in the groove by the transverse humeral ligament. Meyer[13] disputed this, finding that this structure was either too weak or entirely absent. The principal structure containing the tendon with the groove below the top of the tuberosity is the falsiform ligament, a ten-

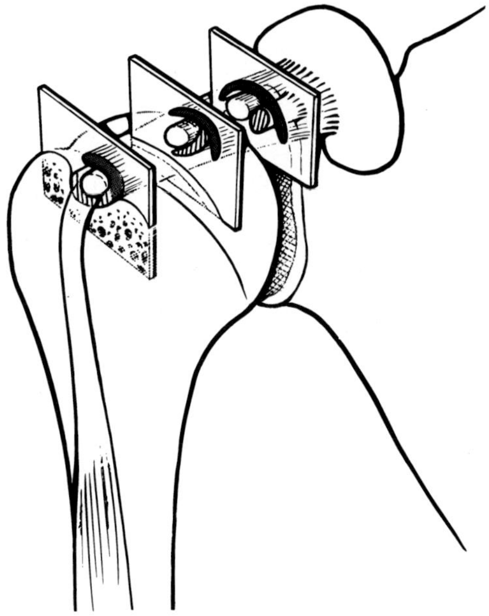

Fig. 10–1. Schematic diagram showing the interelationship of the coracohumeral ligament, superior glenohumeral ligament, and long biceps tendon at several planes in the rotator interval. The long biceps tendon (white) is positioned centrally. The coracohumeral ligament (black) forms a crescent-shaped roof above it and the superior glenohumeral ligament ("hatched area") forms a U-shaped trough.

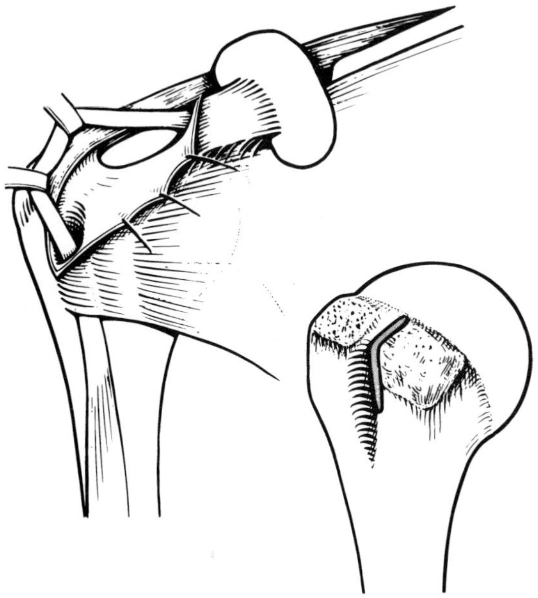

Fig. 10–2. The rotator interval has been opened to demonstrate the common attachment of the coracohumeral ligament and superior glenohumeral ligament on the humeral head.

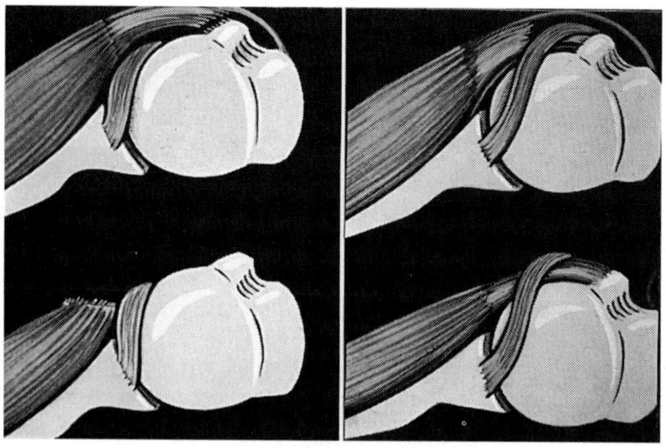

Fig. 10–3. Various patterns of dislocation of the long biceps tendon. Upper right: dislocation of the long biceps tendon over the lesser tuberosity. The deep layers of the subscapularis tendon are intact. Upper left: complete intra-articular dislocation of the long biceps tendon with a rupture of the subscapularis tendon. The anterior fascia is still intact. Lower left: complete intra-articular dislocation of the long biceps tendon with a complete rupture of the subscapularis tendon and the anterior fascia. Lower right: dislocation of the long biceps tendon before an intact subscapularis tendon.

dinous expansion from the insertion of the sternocostal portion of the pectoralis major muscle.

FUNCTIONAL ANATOMY AND BIOMECHANICS OF THE LONG HEAD OF THE BICEPS

Basmajian and Latif[14] characterize the biceps brachii muscle as a flexor of the elbow joint when the forearm is supinated or in a neutral position under strain. The biceps muscle does not contribute significantly to flexion of the pronated forearm. An important function of the biceps muscle at the elbow is in deceleration of the rapidly moving forearm.[15]

The long biceps tendon performs a joint-stabilizing function for up to 90° of abduction and acquires a positive lever arm past 90° of elevation as illustrated in Figures 10–4 and 10–5. The net force vector exerted by the muscle contributes to elevation of the arm in the frontal plane. The biceps is also actively involved in flexion of the arm. The passage of the long head of the biceps tendon around the humeral head simultaneously generates a net force that compresses the humerus against the glenoid and stabilizes the glenohumeral joint. The biceps muscle is active in external but not internal rotation of the upper arm.

The EMG activity pattern of the biceps muscle is marked by a higher primary loading of the tendon in external rotation than in internal rotation. The high passive tension of the long biceps tendon in external rotation thus produces a joint-stabilizing effect (Fig. 10–6). There is not an active contribution from the biceps muscle in external rotation.[16]

Perry[17] did not ascribe particular importance to the biceps muscle during abduction, because the muscle reaches only 36% of its maximum capacity. In our own examinations, however, we have found that the biceps

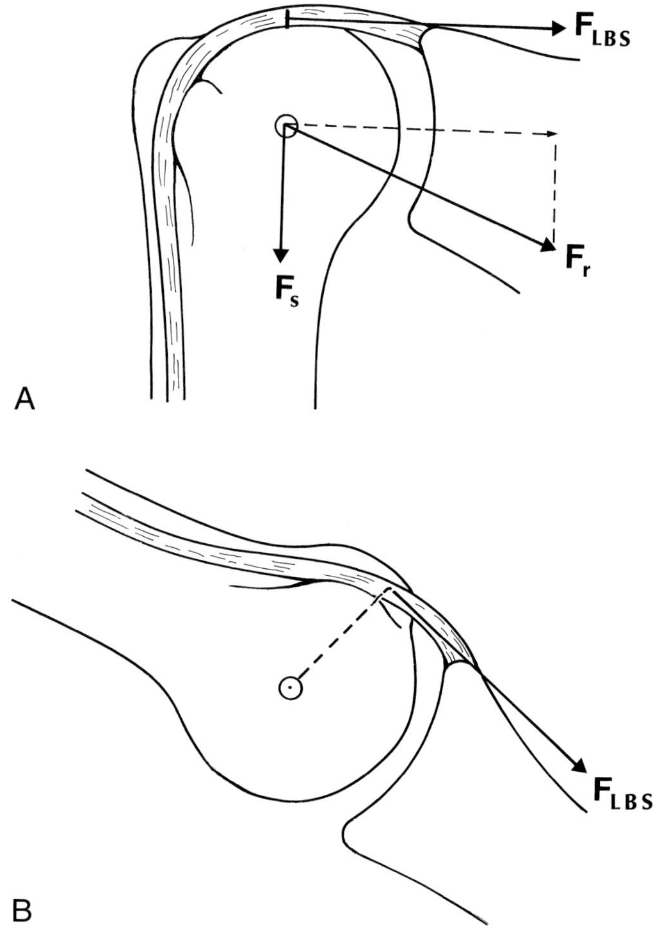

Fig. 10–4. Vector representation of the force parallelogram of the long head of the biceps brachii (LBT). *A,* With the arm in an adducted position, the long biceps tendon winds over the humeral head in such a way that the force vector of the long biceps tendon (F_{LBT}) combines with that of the arm weight (F_S) to create a resultant force (F_r) that stabilizes the glenohumeral joint. *B,* Past 90° of abduction, an effective moment arm is established, and the long head of the biceps actively participates in elevation of the arm.

muscle reached 56% of its maximum capacity during abduction under isokinetic conditions. We were able to prove that the long head of the biceps muscle is active during abduction of the arm in a neutral position. Rupture of the long biceps tendon reduces the abducting force of the arm for 20% (i.e., resulting in 80%).[18]

The long head and short head of the biceps brachii perform a similar function. They are anterior stabilizers of the glenohumeral joint with the arm in abduction and in external rotation. Both heads of the biceps have been shown to perform a stabilizing function in resisting anterior displacement of the humeral head.[9]

PATHOLOGY OF THE LONG BICEPS TENDON AT ITS ORIGIN (ORIGIN LESIONS)

As noted earlier, the long head of the biceps brachii originates at the supraglenoid tubercle and glenoid labrum in the superiormost portion of the glenoid. The

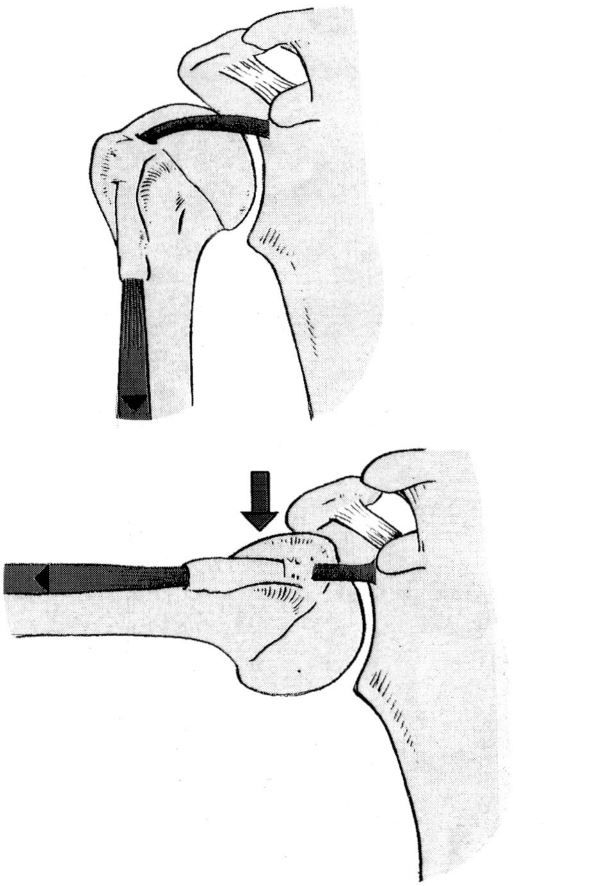

Fig. 10–5. Illustration of the depressor action of the long biceps tendon on the humeral head.

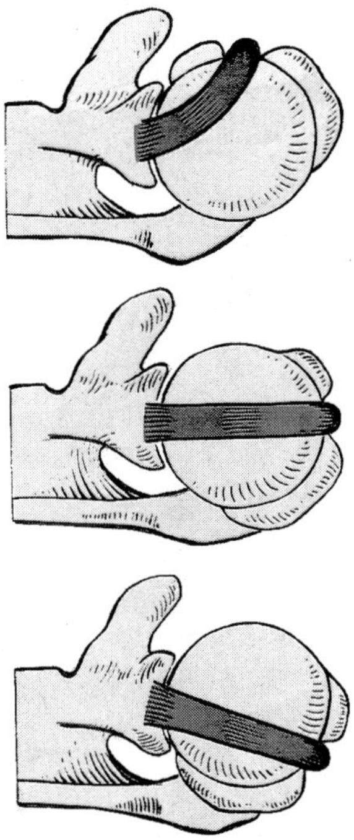

Fig. 10–6. Schematic axial views of the glenohumeral joint showing the change in the position of the long biceps tendon from internal rotation to external rotation. The long biceps tendon has its longest horizontal intra-articular course in external rotation, where a maximum primary stress is exerted on the tendon.[52] A smaller primary stress is exerted in internal and neutral rotation.

major portion of the tendon is blended with the posterosuperior aspect of the labrum.

Damage to the labral-biceps anchor at the glenoid can occur in many different ways. Origin lesions of the biceps are defined as tearing of the biceps-labrum junction at the superior rim of the glenoid.

Andrews[15] describes lesions of the anterosuperior labrum in throwing athletes. These tears are secondary to traction of the biceps tendon. The associated pathology includes biceps tendon tears (10%).[15]

Observations during biceps muscle stimulation have shown the long biceps tendon lifting the labrum off the glenoid near its attachment to the anterosuperior glenoid rim. This is consistent with biomechanical data indicating that the strain in the labrum from the working biceps is greatest when the arm is in overhead abduction.[19] Deceleration trauma is another cause of labrum-biceps injuries.

Three-dimensional, high-speed cinematography with computer analysis has shown that the moment acting about the elbow to extend the joint through an arc of about 50° is greater than 600 in/lbs. The extremely high velocity of elbow extension that is generated must be decelerated through the final 30° of extension. Of the brachial muscles that assist in deceleration of the rapidly extending elbow in the follow-through phase of throwing, only the biceps brachii traverses both the elbow joint and the shoulder joint. Additional forces are generated at the biceps tendon in connection with its function as a "shunt muscle" to stabilize the glenohumeral joint during the act of throwing.[15]

Snyder and colleagues[20] introduced the term "SLAP lesion" in 1990 to denote a pattern of injury involving the long biceps tendon and the superior portion of the glenoid labrum. In a type I SLAP lesion, the superior labrum is markedly frayed but its edges remain firmly attached to the glenoid. A type II lesion also has frayed labral margins, and, additionally, the superior labral-biceps complex is stripped from the underlying glenoid so that the labral-biceps anchor is unstable. Type III lesions show a bucket-handle tear of the superior labrum, and in type IV lesions the bucket-handle tear of the labrum extends into the biceps tendon. As a variation, SLAP lesions have been described in association with complete ruptures of the long biceps tendon.[21,22]

The most common mechanism of a SLAP injury is a fall onto the outstretched arm with the shoulder in abduction and slight forward flexion at the time of impact.[20] SLAP lesions can also result from acute traction on the arm and from an abduction-external rotation mechanism.[22]

The patients complain clinically of shoulder pain that tends to increase with overhead activities. They may report a painful "catching" or "popping" sensation with overhead activities. The most useful diagnostic tests on physical examination are the palm-up test (resisted shoulder flexion with the elbow extended and forearm supinated) and the joint compression-rotation test.[20] Imaging procedures such as radiography, sonography, CT, and MRI have not been very helpful in diagnosing SLAP lesions, but shoulder arthroscopy is extremely valuable for diagnosis and treatment.[19]

PATHOLOGY OF THE LONG BICEPS TENDON AT THE ROTATOR INTERVAL (INTERVAL LESIONS)

An interval lesion is defined as a lesion of the intra-articular portion of the long biceps tendon between its insertion at the supraglenoid tubercle and the entrance to the bicipital groove with no associated rotator cuff pathology. The diversity of pathologic findings has led to confusing descriptions in the literature. The most detailed review of the literature is presented by Burkhead.[23]

Biceps Tendinitis

Tendinitis of the long head of the biceps is characterized clinically by chronic shoulder pain, with tenderness over the bicipital groove and a positive palm-up test. Following these criteria alone, 90% of all painful shoulders would be considered to be caused by tendinitis of the long head of the biceps. However, chronic shoulder pain caused by inflammation of a degenerative or microtraumatic lesion of the long biceps tendon is found in fewer than 5% of cases.[12] Isolated tendinitis of the long head of the biceps can be diagnosed only by arthroscopy. In most cases we find a synovitis of the long head of the biceps accompanied by synovitis of the surrounding capsule and, especially, of the superior glenohumeral ligament. A similar arthroscopic presentation with vascular reaction around the long head of the biceps and the bicipital groove is observed in frozen shoulders.[24]

A true isolated biceps tendinitis may be diagnosed only if the shoulder has a free range of passive mobility. For example, tendinitis of the long head of the biceps is often found in a frozen shoulder. In most cases, however, biceps tendinitis is not an isolated entity but coexists with associated lesions. The early stage of a lesion is frequently marked by an inflammatory reaction commencing at the long head of the biceps and involving the surrounding structures. The senior author, for example, noted biceps tendinitis in 100% of an arthroscopic series of 39 patients who had isolated subluxation or dislocation of the long biceps tendon.

Osteophytes in the area of the bicipital groove can occasionally cause bicipital tendinitis, as a result of mechanical friction. Similar mechanical irritation can result from a fracture of the greater or lesser tuberosity, causing stenosis of the intertubercular groove. This attrition syndrome can be diagnosed by CT, CT arthrography, or MRI. Associated synovial effusion can sometimes be demonstrated by ultrasound or MRI.[25–29]

Isolated Ruptures of the Long Biceps Tendon

Neer[30] estimates that 60 to 70% of long biceps tendon ruptures are accompanied by a lesion of the supraspinatus tendon. Based on clinical criteria alone, "isolated" ruptures of the long biceps tendon had an incidence of 25%. However, when CT arthrography is performed to assess the integrity of the rotator cuff, the incidence of isolated biceps tendon ruptures decreases to only 6% of cases.[31] In an arthroscopically controlled series of 74 patients with intact rotator cuffs, the coauthor found only a 2.2% incidence of isolated biceps tendon ruptures. Given these findings, it must be asked whether an "isolated" rupture of the long biceps tendon can truly exist as a pathologic entity. At the least, every "clinically isolated" biceps rupture should be evaluated by CT arthrography, MRI, or ultrasound to confirm or exclude a concomitant lesion of the rotator cuff.

Meyer,[32] Hitchcock,[7] Paavolainen,[33] and Cone[6] described osseous changes in the bicipital groove as a cause of ruptures of the long biceps tendon. However, CT studies have shown that the depth and width of the bicipital groove do not have pathognomonic significance.[31] Degenerative bone changes in the groove area with cystic deformation, osteophytosis, and irregularities are interpreted as secondary effects of a synovitic process about the bony canal. The chronic tenosynovitis caused by microtrauma and the secondary osseous changes resulting from the synovitis lead, ultimately, to rupture of the biceps tendon. The inflammation is most commonly found at the entrance to the groove, where the biceps tendon is subjected to the greatest mechanical stresses and where biceps tendon ruptures most commonly occur.

Degenerative bone changes were noted in 80% of a series of long biceps ruptures examined in Lyon.[31] However, 20% of the patients did not exhibit these bony features. The patients were predominantly men (91%), 62% were manual laborers with an average age of 53 years, and the dominant side was affected in 80%. The patients had experienced shoulder pain on the affected side for several months before the rupture occurred. The rupture either occurred atraumatically or was precipitated by a trivial trauma, and the rupture site was intra-articular. The etiology obviously relates to chronic overuse.

Besides tenosynovitis and microtrauma, a true adequate gross trauma may be a rare cause of biceps tendon rupture in younger patients. The rupture site may be intra-articular at the entrance to the groove or may involve the tendon origin and coexist with a SLAP lesion.[21,22]

Neer[34] believes that ruptures of the long biceps tendon are a secondary result of subacromial impingement. But *isolated ruptures* of the long biceps tendon do not fit with Neer's theory. If mechanical impingement was the sole cause of the biceps rupture, there should be an associated partial or complete rupture of the supraspinatus tendon.

The intra-articular remnant of the long biceps tendon can lead to significant, painful secondary pathology. Entrapment of the stump can produce chondral lesions of the glenoid or humeral head. In all cases, the rupture is associated with severe synovitis of the articular capsule.

Many spontaneous biceps tendon ruptures take an almost painless course. This occurs when the biceps tendon tears near the base and then disappears in the bicipital groove as a result of muscular traction. The only clinical complaint in these cases is spasmodic discomfort in the area of the biceps muscle.

Subluxation of the Long Biceps Tendon

The terminology and definition of instability of the long biceps tendon are poorly standardized and highly controversial. Dines[35] and Mariani[36] define instability in terms of a subluxation or dislocation of the long biceps tendon, while O'Donoghue[37] refers only to subluxation. Peterson,[38] Paavolainen,[33] and Mayer[32] draw a distinction between subluxation and dislocation. None of these investigators have established criteria for the various definitions.

Walch[12] defines subluxation of the long biceps tendon as a partial and/or transient incomplete loss of contact between the tendon and its bony groove.

We recognize three different types of biceps tendon subluxation.

SUPERIOR SUBLUXATION (TYPE I)

The circular sling of the superior glenohumeral and coracohumeral ligaments (i.e., rotator interval sling) is partially or completely torn, resulting in loss of restraint of the long biceps tendon above the entrance to the groove. The subscapularis tendon, which attaches to the lesser tubercle just below the superior glenohumeral ligament, is largely intact; otherwise a true dislocation is present. The lesion above the entrance to the groove is sometimes marked by an accompanying partial lesion of the supraspinatus tendon on the articular side, directly at the lateral groove entrance, where it forms the roof for the biceps tendon. The pathologic substrate of the type I subluxation is a discontinuity in the tendo-ligamentous rotator interval sling surrounding the long biceps tendon (i.e., lesions of the coracohumeral and superior glenohumeral ligament and a partial rupture of the supraspinatus and/or subscapularis tendon above the entrance to the groove) (Fig. 10–7).

SUBLUXATION AT THE GROOVE (TYPE II)

The lesion responsible for the subluxation is located below the entrance to the bony groove. With this type of lesion, the tendon slips over the medial rim of the bony groove and ''rides'' on the border of the lesser tuberosity. The causal lesion is a detachment of the outermost fibers of the subscapularis tendon. Tearing of the superficial (outer) portions that line the floor of the groove and help anchor the long biceps tendon[10] allows the tendon to displace to a medially subluxated position. The principal criterion for a type II biceps tendon subluxation is a partial rupture of the outer, superficial tendinous portions of the subscapularis muscle, allowing the biceps tendon to ride over the bone of the lesser tuberosity.[39] The type II lesion may be confined to the superior half of the groove or may involve its entire length.

MALUNION AND NONUNION OF THE LESSER TUBEROSITY (TYPE III)

A fracture-dislocation of the lesser tuberosity can progress to a malunion or nonunion that compromises the medial bony restraint of the long biceps tendon, allowing the tendon to subluxate. The patient complains of painful internal rotation of the humerus.

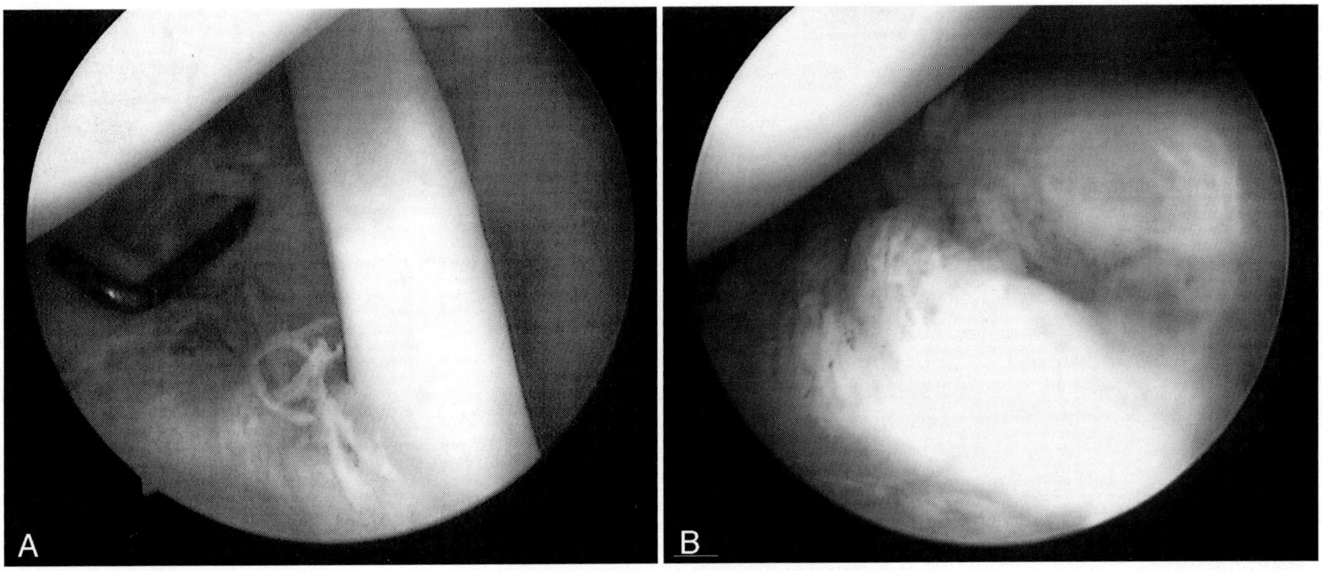

Fig. 10–7. Arthroscopic appearance of a subluxated long biceps tendon. *A*, With the arm in neutral rotation, the long biceps tendon exhibits an apparently normal intra-articular course. *B*, With the arm in internal rotaton, the long biceps tendon subluxates medially against the glenoid labrum.

Lesions Associated with Subluxation of the Long Biceps Tendon

The most common associated lesions, almost invariably present, are biceps tendinitis and capsular synovitis in the area of the rotator interval. Erosion of the deep, medial aspect of the biceps tendon is very common and, if persistent, will lead to partial rupture of the tendon. Partial ruptures secondary to tendon subluxation can also be responsible for "isolated" ruptures of the long biceps tendon. Because of chronic subluxation of the biceps tendon, shearing forces lead to an attrition of the chondral layer on the humeral head.

The subluxation leads to increased mechanical stresses at the tendon attachment, which are transmitted to the anterosuperior portion of the labrum. At arthroscopy, we found that 50% of all tendon subluxations were associated with degenerative changes in the anterosuperior aspect of the labrum.

Pathogenesis of Biceps Tendon Subluxations

External rotation of the adducted arm places a maximal stress on the long biceps tendon at the entrance to the bicipital groove.[16] The tendoligamentous sleeve above the groove entrance and the groove itself create a 90° angle between the horizontal, intra-articular portion of the tendon and the vertical, groove portion. The peak of the lesser tuberosity at the groove entrance represents the junction between the perpendicular segments. During active internal rotation, contraction of the muscle forces the tendon to undergo an "internal subluxation."[12] Passive external rotation of the adducted (hanging) upper arm causes an increased load to be exerted on the tendoligamentous restraint of the tendon in the groove area. In this situation microtrauma or occasionally gross trauma can produce a pathologically increased pressure in the medial groove area, resulting in subluxation of the biceps tendon (Fig. 10–8).

A partial rupture of the supraspinatus tendon on the articular side is associated with concomitant lesions of the coracohumeral ligament, with consequent damage to the roof of the rotator interval (Fig. 10–9). This can have causal significance in a type I subluxation of the long biceps tendon. Clark[10] noted that the interweaving of the supraspinatus tendon and coracohumeral ligament makes an important contribution to the soft-tissue restraint of the long biceps tendon. Once a subluxation has occurred, it perpetuates and aggravates the pathologic stresses in the rotator interval, thereby compounding the damage to the tendoligamentous sling.

The anatomic complex of the tendoligamentous sling formed by the coracohumeral ligament, superior glenohumeral ligament, and the supraspinatus and subscapularis tendon is of central importance for the stability of the long biceps tendon. We call this complex the "rotator interval sling." Partial lesions of the rotator interval sling (Risling lesions) inevitably lead to "subluxation" of the long head of the biceps. The integrity of the rotator interval sling is absolutely essential for biceps stability. (Fig. 10–10) shows a rare example of a stable long head of biceps, with an intact rotator interval sling in the presence of a massive rotator cuff tear. We agree with Cone[6] that changes in the groove area or a low medial wall angle of the groove do not contribute materially to the pathogenesis of subluxation of the long biceps tendon.

The precise cause of a tendoligamentous interval lesion in the absence of a complete rotator cuff tear remains unclear. We do not feel that mechanical outlet impingement[40] or coracoid impingement[35,41] needs to be present. The lesion may be a primary intrinsic lesion of the rotator interval sling caused by trauma or chronic overuse.

Diagnosis

Scarcely any lesion of the shoulder is more difficult to detect clinically than subluxation of the long biceps tendon. The patient notices a painful "snapping" in the

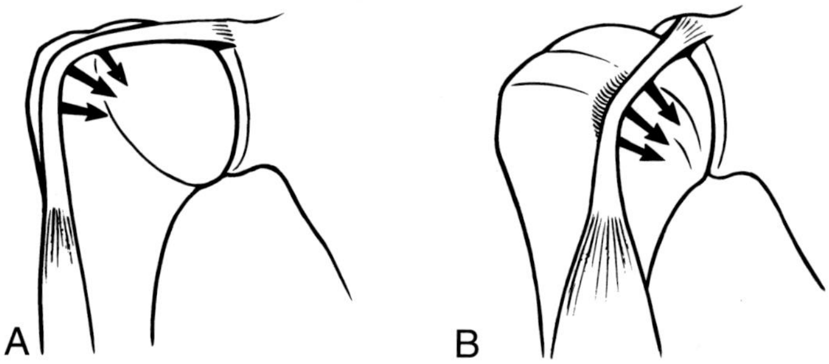

Fig. 10–8. Force vectors acting on the long biceps tendon. Subluxating forces on the long biceps tendon are increased by passive external rotation (*A*) and internal rotation of the arm with active flexion of the elbow and contraction of the LHB tendon (*B*).

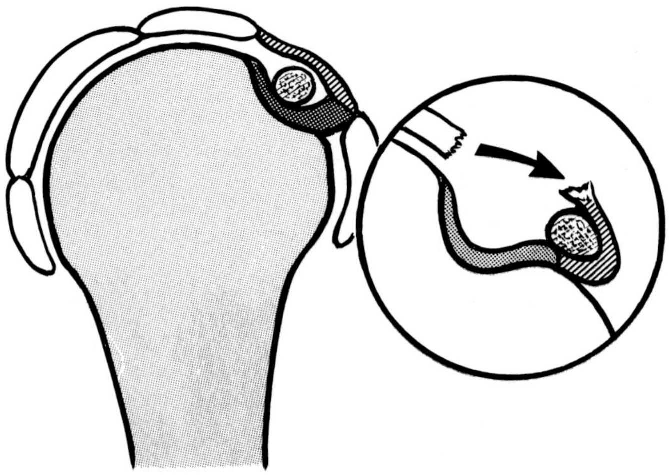

Fig. 10–9. Rupture of the supraspinatus tendon causes detachment of the lateral limb of the coracohumeral ligament, provoking eventually subluxation of the long biceps tendon.

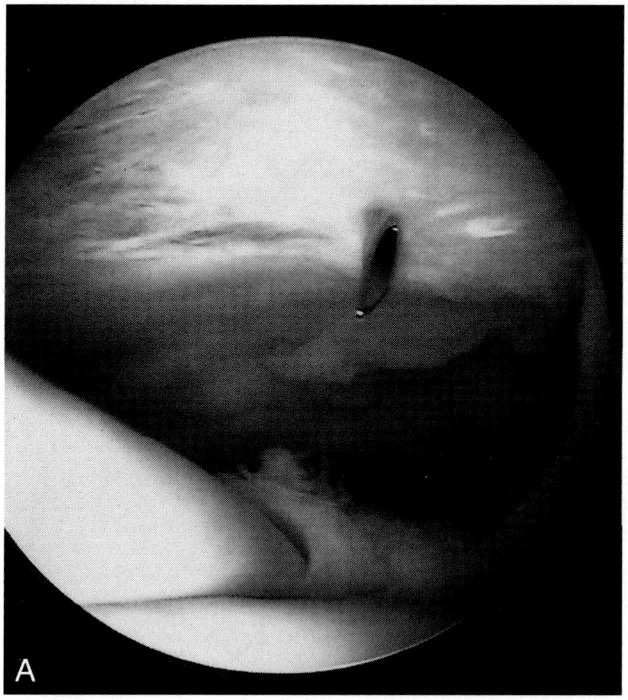

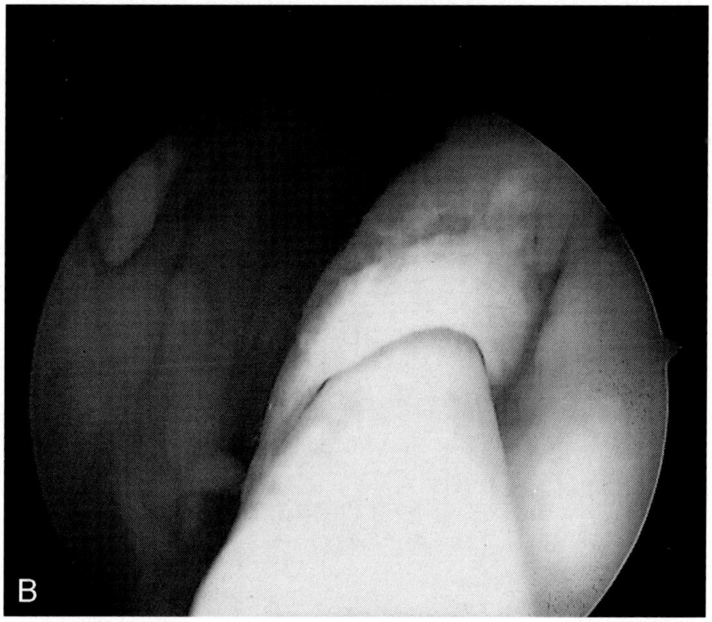

Fig. 10–10. Arthroscopic appearance of the rotator interval sling with a massive rotator cuff tear. *A,* View of the rotator interval sling from the subacromial space. The needle marks the anterolateral border of the acromion. There is a complete avulsion of the rotator cuff. The rotator interval sling is still intact and continues to hold the long biceps tendon in the groove. *B,* Close-up view of the intact rotator interval sling. Remnants of the coracohumeral ligament, subscapularis tendon, and supraspinatus tendon form a "sleeve" that retains the long biceps tendon in the groove.

area of the bicipital groove, which he interprets as a subluxation or dislocation. In reality, however, the gliding mechanism of the tendon in the groove is impaired, and this is manifested as a painful "jump" or "snap." Normally the bicipital groove glides beneath the fixed, taut biceps tendon during elevation of the arm. Standard plain radiographic views are useful for demonstrating a malunion or nonunion of the lesser tuberosity. Contrast arthrography can exclude a complete rotator cuff tear. This is essential before one can assign a diagnosis of biceps tendon subluxation.

CT arthrography is the most reliable technique for the diagnosis of subluxations. Typically the arthrogram shows contrast extravasation at the medial entrance to the bicipital groove and in the proximal portions of the lesser tuberosity. The long biceps tendon "rides" on the medial wall of the groove and remains there during rotation of the arm (Fig. 10–11). These findings are also demonstrable by MRI and by ultrasound imaging in the hands of an experienced sonographer.

A common feature of all three types of lesion is that they are easily missed during open surgery because they are obscured by the clavipectoral fascia and by the coracohumeral ligament. Only a systematic exploration of the rotator interval along the anterior border of the supraspinatus and over the lateral margin of the groove can disclose these lesions. Arthroscopy provides a classic diagnosis of type I superior subluxations (Fig. 10–12; see also Fig. 10–7). Subluxations at the groove (type II) cannot be directly demonstrated by arthroscopy because of the intact ligamentous sleeve at the groove entrance, but the lesion can be indirectly identified by noting descent or medialization of the long biceps tendon. If examination with a probing hook additionally reveals bicipital tendinitis, the arthroscopic diagnosis is considered to be confirmed.

BICEPS TENDON PATHOLOGY ASSOCIATED WITH ROTATOR CUFF TEARS

Whereas origin lesions and rotator interval lesions are rare, isolated conditions, combined lesions of the rotator cuff and long biceps tendon are quite common. In a series of 438 rotator cuff tears operatively treated in Lyon between 1984 and 1991, the long biceps tendon was involved in 45%.

Various forms of biceps tendon pathology may be encountered in the presence of a rotator cuff tear:

Biceps Tendinitis

Biceps tendinitis in this sense refers to the associated tendinitis of a long biceps tendon that is not subluxated or dislocated. Of course, biceps tendinitis is almost always

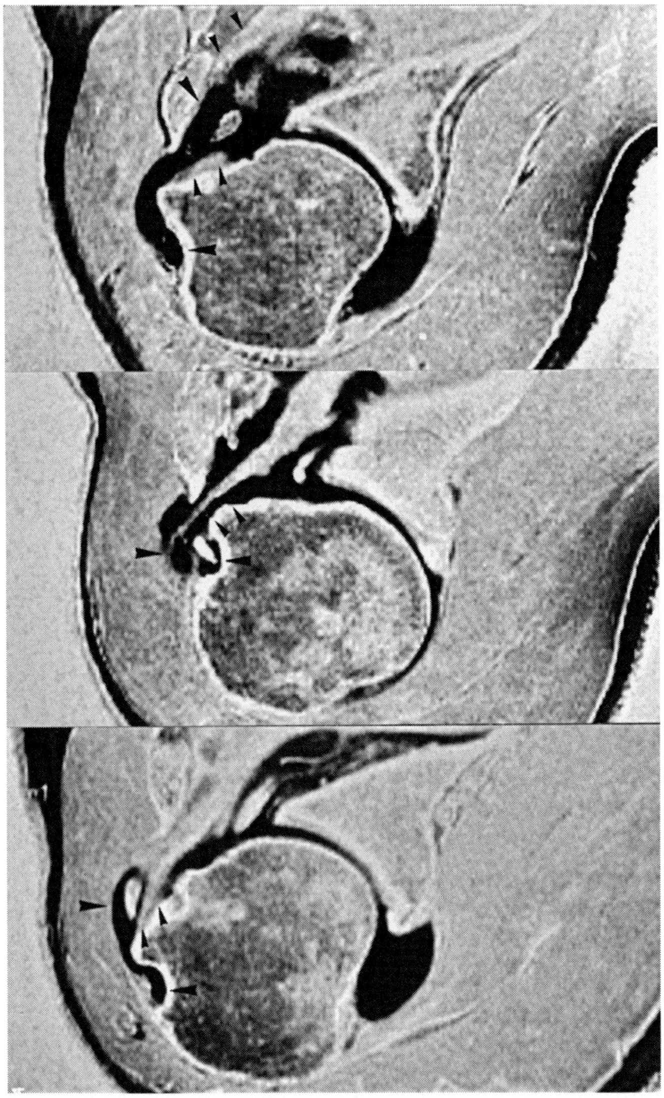

Fig. 10–11. MR images of the long biceps tendon and subscapularis muscle. The scans illustrate a dislocation of the long biceps tendon with and without a subscapularis lesion, and a subscapularis tear associated with a normally positioned biceps tendon. (Courtesy of Beat R. Simmen, MD, Schulthess Clinic, Zurich, Switzerland.)

present as an associated feature of a rotator cuff tear. The reddened appearance of the tendon is caused by inflammation of the tendon sheath, because the tendon itself is initially intact and presents a normal diameter. As the inflammation progresses, there is a superficial erosion of the outer tendon fibers, with inflammation spreading to involve the entire tendon, which still exhibits a normal size.

We also recognize an atrophic form of tendinitis, considered an antecedent of prerupture, in which the tendon fibers are thinned and inflamed. In hypertrophic tendinitis, the tendon may enlarge to the diameter of a finger. These forms of tendinitis may occur in association with all types of rotator cuff tear. Arthroscopy reveals an accompanying synovitis in the rotator interval that also involves the superior glenohumeral ligament. The coracohumeral ligament coursing in the rotator interval clearly serves an important protective function for the biceps tendon. A lesion in that area rapidly exposes the biceps tendon to frictional loading from the coracoacromial ligament and acromion in the subacromial space.

Subacromial impingement secondary to a rotator cuff tear can account for the tendinitis but is not the only factor. The rotator cuff tear compromises the centering of the humeral head in the glenoid, resulting in increased mechanical loading of the long biceps tendon that incites a hypertrophic tendinitis. Chemical alterations in the synovial fluid can also contribute to initiating and sustaining the tendinitis. Rotator cuff tears consistently lead to increased synovial fluid production and may be associated with a change in its chemical composition.[42]

Dislocation of the Long Biceps Tendon

Dislocation of the long head of the biceps is always combined with a lesion of the subscapularis tendon and requires differentiation from the various types of subluxation. The rotator interval sling is destroyed in a dislocation of the long biceps tendon, and there are accompanying subtotal lesions of the subscapularis tendon.

A complete dislocation of the long biceps tendon is defined as a complete displacement of the tendon out of its bony canal. The tendon cannot be continuously reduced by internal or external rotation maneuvers and remains outside the bicipital groove.

Dislocations of the long biceps tendon have been described for many years. Meyer[32] described six cases of biceps tendon dislocation over the intact subscapularis tendon. Petersson[38] in 1986 first described a type of dislocation involving displacement of the biceps tendon below the subscapularis tendon. Collier[43] reported on two posttraumatic cases of intra-articular biceps tendon dislocation. Thus, varying descriptions have been presented on the pathomorphology of the biceps dislocation.

Walch[12] has proposed a classification based upon the pathomorphologic features of the biceps tendon dislocation. This classification system follows.

EXTRA-ARTICULAR DISLOCATION COMBINED WITH A PARTIAL TEAR OF THE SUBSCAPULARIS TENDON (TYPE I)

In this type the long biceps tendon is completely dislocated to a point over the lesser tuberosity. The deeper portions of the subscapularis tendon still insert into the lesser tuberosity, separating the biceps tendon from the joint space. Invariably there is a rupture of the common attachment of the superior glenohumeral ligament and coracohumeral ligament. The biceps tendon, then, is displaced over the anterior wall of the groove and slips or glides medially over the torn fibers of the subscapularis tendon. The clavipectoral fascia covers this lesion externally, and this might give the impression that the subscapularis tendon is intact over its full thickness. It has been shown,[39] however, that the outer attachment of the subscapularis tendon is always torn. This type of dislo-

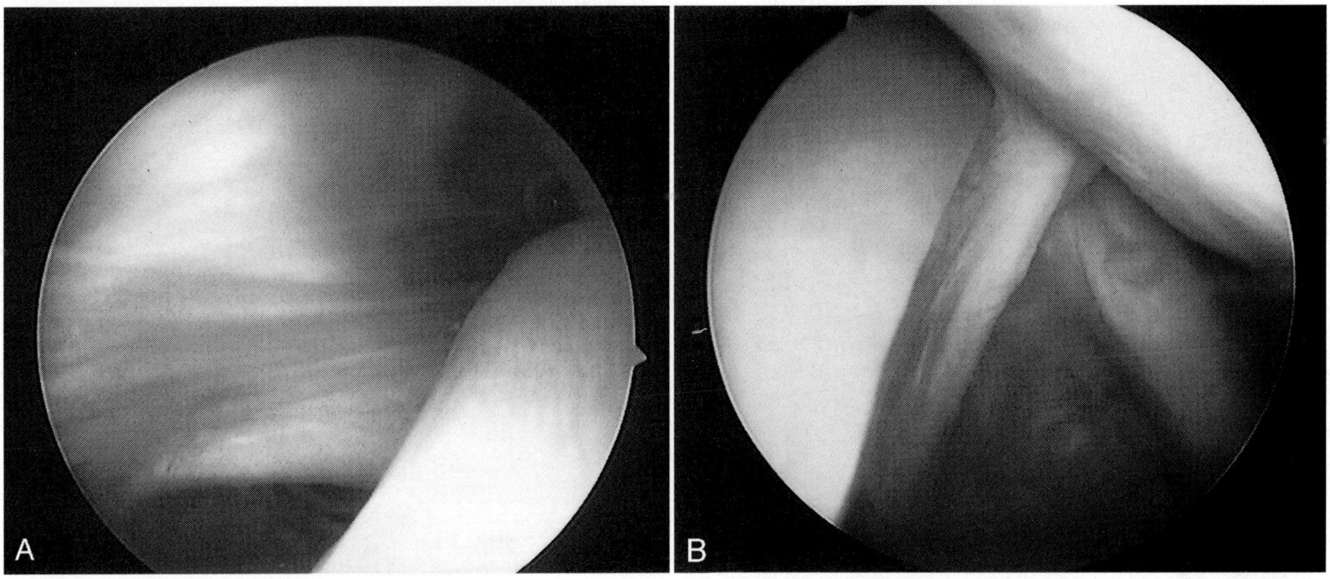

Fig. 10–12. Arthroscopic view of a healthy long biceps tendon at the entrance to the bicipital groove (right shoulder). *A,* Cranial view of the entrance to the groove, demonstrating an intact rotator interval sling. *B,* Long biceps tendon from the laterocaudal aspect. The superior glenohumeral ligament, the principal stabilizer of the long biceps tendon at the groove entrance runs below the long biceps tendon and over the tendon of the subscapularis muscle.

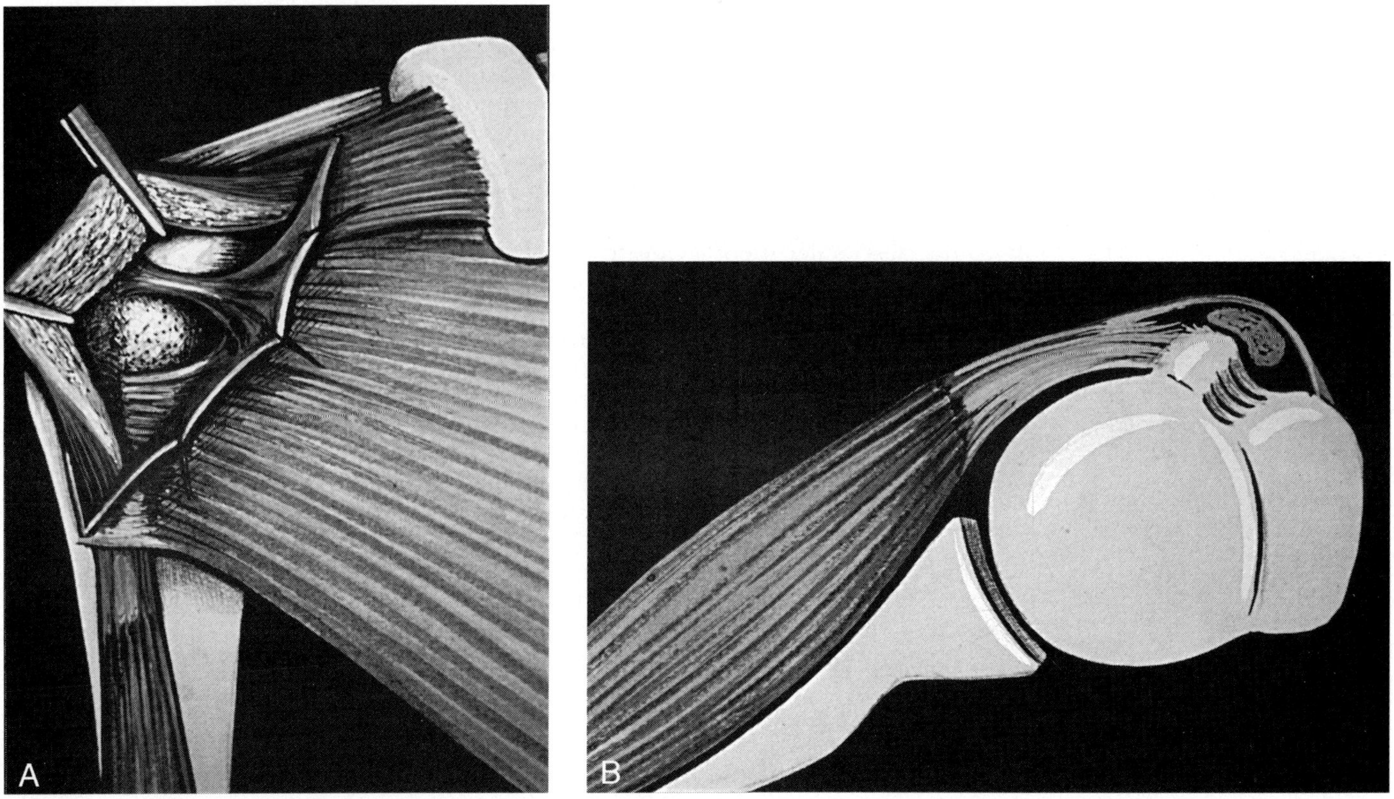

Fig. 10–13. Subluxation of the proximal portion of the biceps tendon at the groove entrance. *A,* In transverse section the long biceps tendon rides on the medial rim of the bony groove. These lesions are hidden by an intact anterior fascia. *B,* Opening the rotator interval exposes the injury of the rotator sling and the lateral fibers of the subscapularis tendon.

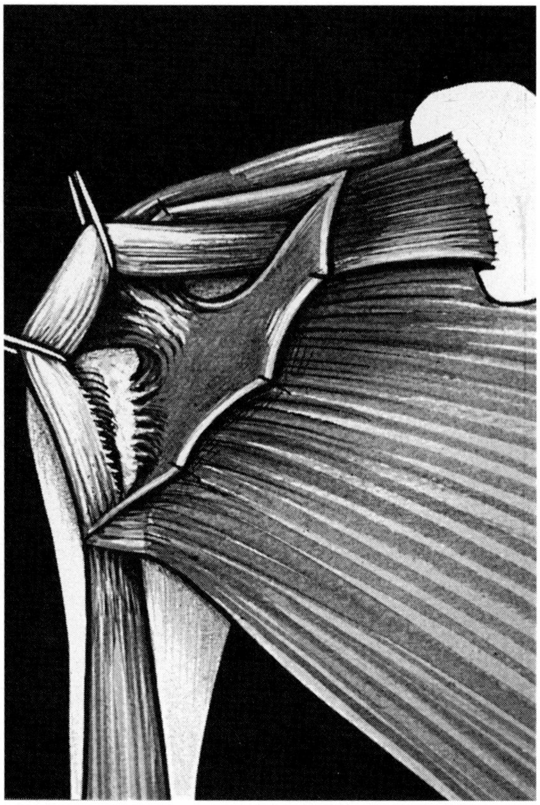

Fig. 10–14. Subluxation of the long biceps tendon with a partial rupture of the lateral fibers of the subscapularis tendon. This lesion spares the rotator sling. It extends over the entire medial rim of the groove.

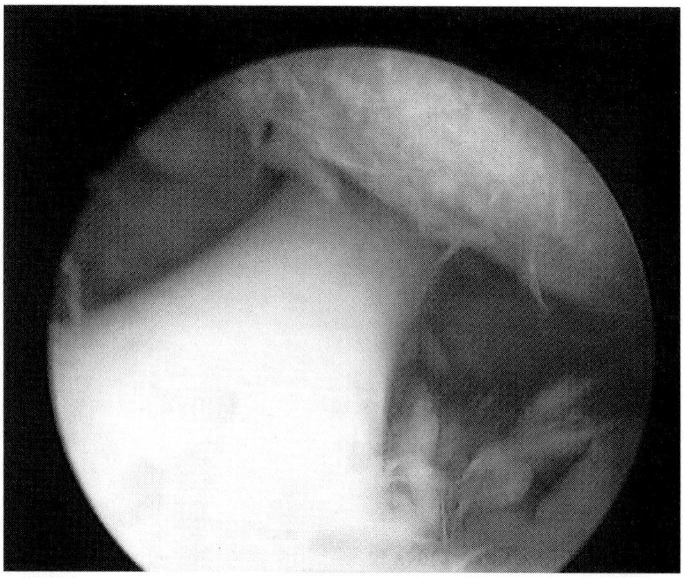

Fig. 10–15. Chondral defect on the humeral head secondary to subluxation of the long biceps tendon. Chronic subluxation of the biceps tendon over the humeral head during internal rotation of the arm can cause mechanical damage to the cartilage covering the humerus.

cation corresponds in its evolution to a type II subluxation but represents a more advanced stage (Figs. 10–13 and 10–14).

Besides the superficial lesion of the subscapularis tendon, there is frequently an associated tear of the rotator cuff. Only systematic exploration of the rotator cuff interval can ensure that the dislocation of the long biceps tendon is not missed.

EXTRA-ARTICULAR DISLOCATION WITH AN INTACT SUBSCAPULARIS TENDON

Dislocation of the long biceps tendon over a completely intact subscapularis tendon is very rare. In a series of 70 patients with subluxations and dislocations of the long biceps tendon, only 2 patients (3%) were found to manifest this condition.[39]

INTRA-ARTICULAR DISLOCATION OF THE LONG BICEPS TENDON COMBINED WITH A COMPLETE TEAR OF THE SUBSCAPULARIS TENDON (TYPE II)

The biceps tendon is widened and flattened as a result of its contact with the lesser tuberosity. It shows a diversity of substance lesions, ranging from erosion to prerupture. The subscapularis tendon is torn from its attachment on the lesser tuberosity, and the long biceps tendon is interposed into the joint space and displaced inferomedially (Fig. 10–15). On the articular side, the biceps tendon is apposed to the glenoid labrum. Entrapment of the tendon in the anterior joint space occurs with each internal rotational movement of the humerus. Usually the proximal two-thirds of the subscapularis tendon is ruptured; rarely is the distal, purely muscular insertion of the subscapularis tendon torn as well. We credit Gerber[44] with drawing attention to the problem of an isolated rupture of the subscapularis tendon and its consequences.

The intra-articular dislocation is often associated with extensive tearing of the rotator cuff. Approximately half of these dislocations have a traumatic etiology.[39]

Associated Lesions

The common insertion of the superior glenohumeral ligament and coracohumeral ligament is always ruptured in the presence of a long biceps tendon dislocation. This is an important sign in arthroscopic examinations. As in subluxations, it is very common to find associated degenerative lesions of the anterosuperior labrum that are believed to result from unphysiologic mechanical loads. In some subluxations and dislocations of the long biceps tendon, we noted chondromalacia of the anterosuperior portion of the humeral head. This results from mechanical friction of the humeral head against the subluxated or dislocated biceps tendon during internal rotation. An example of mechanical friction is demonstrated in Figure 10–15.

Epidemiology

Dislocations of the long biceps tendon predominantly affect men (80%) and tend to involve the dominant side

(83%). The average age of occurrence is 59 years of age.[39] The cause of the dislocation is traumatic in about 63% of cases. The mechanism of the injury may be forced abduction and internal rotation, (e.g., frontal impact of the extended arm against a steering wheel) or a direct fall onto the shoulder.

Diagnosis

The dislocation of the biceps tendon is obscured by the torn rotator cuff, and the clinical presentation matches that of a rotator cuff tear. There are no clinically significant diagnostic tests that can reliably confirm dislocation of the long biceps tendon in the presence of a rotator cuff tear. Typically the pain is exacerbated by movement, especially flexion and internal rotation of the arm, and tends to be worse at night. A history of pseudoparalysis of the arm for several months should raise suspicion of a biceps tendon dislocation combined with an extensive rotator cuff tear.[39]

Standard radiographic views of the shoulder demonstrate the typical features of a rotator cuff tear. In 95% of cases the dislocation of the long biceps tendon is accompanied by a superior migration of the humeral head, reducing the acromiohumeral distance to 7 mm.[39] CT arthrography and MRI can provide an accurate diagnosis of biceps tendon dislocation and can plainly demonstrate the position of the tendon outside the groove. The subscapularis tendon should also be evaluated for injury. Contrast medium that reaches or envelops the lesser tuberosity confirms the presence of a subscapularis rupture.

Arthroscopy is a reliable technique for identifying a dislocation of the long biceps tendon. The pathologic intra-articular course of the biceps tendon and the consistent avulsion of the rotator interval sling are typical of a complete dislocation. Arthroscopy can also disclose the extra-articular type of dislocation in which the articular portions of the subscapularis tendon are still intact. It is again emphasized that whenever arthroscopy is performed to evaluate a rotator cuff tear, the possibility of a subluxation or dislocation of the long biceps tendon should always be considered.

Subluxation of the Long Biceps Tendon Combined with Rotator Cuff Tears

The rotator cuff tear is the predominant lesion in cases of this kind. A subluxation of the long biceps tendon is merely the result of a concomitant rotator interval lesion. Subluxation of the long biceps tendon is generally associated with an isolated rupture of the supraspinatus tendon (Fig. 10–16).[53] In this case the lesion of the supraspinatus tendon is the predominant lesion from a functional standpoint, and the subluxation has very little significance compared with the supraspinatus rupture. It is important only because it may progress to a complete dislocation. Usually this will be an extra-articular dislocation with a partial, superficial tear of the subscapularis

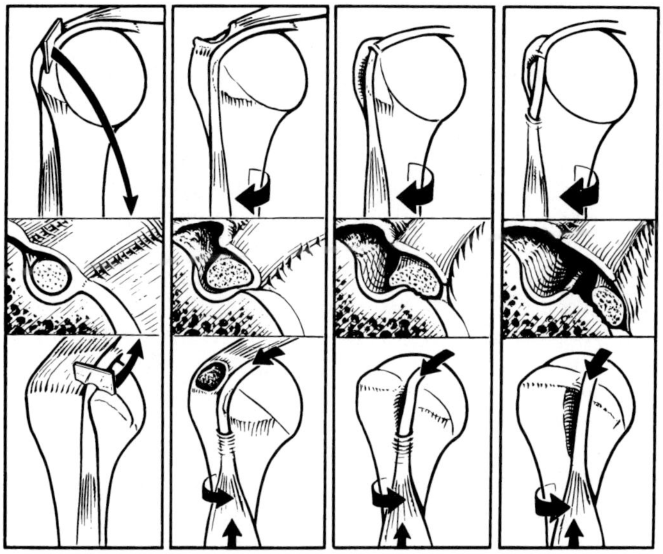

Fig. 10–16. A possible effect of rupture of the supra spinatus tendon on the stability of the LHB: (1) intact supraspinatus; (2) rupture of the supraspinatus allows the coracohumeral ligament to be released, and the LHB has a tendency to be displaced medially; (3) subluxation of the long head of the biceps with a attenuation of the "rotator interval sling;" and (4) complete dislocation of the LHB is a possible evolution. The tendency of medial displacement of the long head of biceps is increased in passive external rotation (above) and in internal rotation with active flexion of the elbow (below).

tendon (type I). We ascribe greater pathognomonic importance to true isolated subluxations of the long biceps tendon, which we described earlier as rotator interval lesions. Thus, because a subluxation of the long biceps tendon is of minor concern in the presence of a rotator cuff tear, we need not discuss it further. It should be stressed, however, that whenever a supraspinatus tendon rupture is identified, the possibility of a coexisting subluxation of the long biceps tendon should be considered.

In summary, we may say that isolated biceps tendon subluxations with an intact rotator cuff are a rare but painful condition that warrants serious attention. By contrast, subluxations that are accompanied by a rotator cuff tear are of less clinical and pathomorphologic concern than the associated rotator cuff tear.

RUPTURES OF THE LONG BICEPS TENDON COMBINED WITH ROTATOR CUFF TEARS

While isolated ruptures of the long biceps tendon are quite rare when the rotator cuff is intact, ruptures of the long biceps tendon are very common when there is a coexisting rotator cuff tear. A series of 196 ruptures of the long biceps tendon combined with rotator cuff tears were diagnosed in Lyon from 1985 to 1992.[45] In 10% of these cases the biceps tendon rupture was associated with a concomitant rupture of the supraspinatus, infraspinatus, and subscapularis. In 9% of the biceps tendon ruptures there was an isolated lesion of the subscapularis, and in 8% of these cases the biceps rupture was combined with a rupture of the supraspinatus. In 7% of cases the biceps tendon rupture was combined with ruptures of the supraspinatus and infraspinatus, and in 6% there was a partial rupture of the supraspinatus on the articular side. Although Neer's impingement theory[34] has gained wide acceptance in the literature, we do not believe that subacromial impingement is the primary factor responsible for combined ruptures of the long biceps tendon and rotator cuff. An epidemiologic study in Lyon[45] showed that the majority of these combined lesions occurred in males on the dominant side. Moreover, the extent of the rotator cuff defect tended to become more severe with increasing age. Neer was never able to demonstrate that the cause of the mechanical outlet syndrome correlated with gender, dominant side, or the severity of rotator cuff pathology.

One must be careful in attributing pathology to a single causal factor, but it is evident that the lesion can originate from intrinsic changes in the rotator cuff. Onset of the rupture is followed by an upward decentering of the humeral head, leading to increased frictional loading of the long biceps tendon in the narrowed subacromial space. The superior migration of the humeral head, coupled with the mechanical loading by the acromion, creates a two-prong mechanism that promotes rupture of the long biceps tendon. The impingement lesion, then, is in our opinion a secondary effect.

The effects of a combined rotator cuff tear and biceps tendon rupture on arm strength are substantial. Dynamometric measurements have shown that an isolated biceps tendon rupture with an intact rotator cuff leads to a strength loss of 15% relative to the unaffected side. An isolated rupture of the supraspinatus tendon was found to be associated with an average strength loss of 42%. The strength loss increased to 51% when both the supraspinatus tendon and long biceps tendon were ruptured.[12] Biceps tendon ruptures occur in some patients who report no prior history of pain; the shoulder was completely asymptomatic until the occurrence of the rupture. The patient usually notices the biceps tendon rupture himself, prompting him to seek medical attention. Ecchymosis and sagging of the muscle belly in the upper arm are usually present as obvious clinical signs. As noted earlier, an effort should be made to exclude an associated rotator cuff tear whenever an "isolated" biceps tendon rupture is identified. A biceps tendon avulsion may be missed in elderly patients who have atrophied shoulder and arm muscles and generally weak muscular tonus.

In some patients, rupture of the biceps tendon is preceded by painful shoulder symptoms that prompt a diagnosis of impingement syndrome. Sometimes the pain disappears when the tendon ruptures, giving rise to the term "saving rupture" (rupture salvatrice). If the shoulder pain persists, however, it is reasonable to assume that a concomitant rotator cuff lesion is present. Neither the initial symptoms experienced by the patient nor the causal circumstances of the biceps tendon rupture (direct or indirect trauma, lifting a heavy load) have any prognostic significance in terms of identifying the pattern of the coexisting rotator cuff tear.[12]

TREATMENT OF LESIONS OF THE BICEPS TENDON AND ROTATOR CUFF

Treatment of Lesions of the Long Biceps Tendon With an Intact Rotator Cuff

ORIGIN LESIONS

A number of arthroscopic surgical techniques have been developed for the treatment of Andrews lesions and SLAP lesions, ranging from simple shaving[19] to various suturing techniques.[22,46] If the SLAP lesion is accompanied by a full-thickness tear of the supraspinatus, the supraspinatus rupture must be treated concurrently with repair of the SLAP lesion. It is our practice to add arthroscopic repair of the supraspinatus tendon if the lesion is a complete rupture.[47] For an incomplete supraspinatus tear on the articular side, we limit the treatment to arthroscopic debridement of the articular side and perform a suturing repair of the SLAP lesion.[22]

ROTATOR INTERVAL LESIONS

Isolated tendinitis of the long biceps tendon with an intact rotator cuff is exclusively an arthroscopic diagnosis. It also may be combined with a mechanical supraspinatus outlet syndrome. Differentiation is required from a frozen shoulder, which is always associated with a limitation of passive joint motion.

The primary treatment for tendinitis of the long biceps tendon is conservative. We recommend the single intra-articular injection of a noncrystalloid cortisone preparation and the oral administration of anti-inflammatory drugs. In the acute stage, a brief period of immobilization and local ice pack therapy afford rapid improvement. A key component of the conservative regimen is physical therapy, which includes isometric and isokinetic strengthening of the rotator cuff to achieve better muscular balance between the rotator cuff and deltoid muscle. We advocate arthroscopic subacromial decompression for chronic bicipital tendinitis combined with a subacromial impingement syndrome.

With an isolated rupture of the long biceps tendon, there is little rationale for advocating surgical treatment. It is important to note that an isolated intra-articular rupture of the long biceps tendon may coexist with a SLAP lesion.[21,22] As stated above, a rotator cuff tear must be excluded in all patients who have a painful isolated rupture of the long biceps tendon. If shoulder discomfort persists despite the exclusion of a rotator cuff tear, we recommend diagnostic arthroscopy to evaluate for intra-articular pathology involving the stump of the long biceps tendon and the glenoid labrum.

We feel that tenodesis of the long biceps tendon in the groove is appropriate only in young patients and in athletes under 40 years of age. Transfer of the long biceps tendon to the short biceps tendon as described by De Palma[48] tends to provoke or exacerbate subacromial impingement. We prefer the technique of Post,[49] which is elegant and simple to perform even when the distal

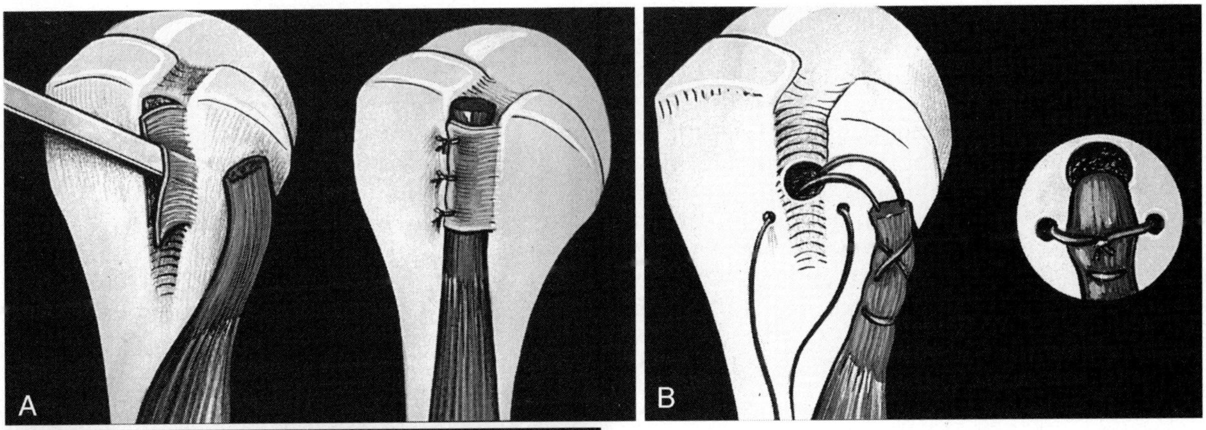

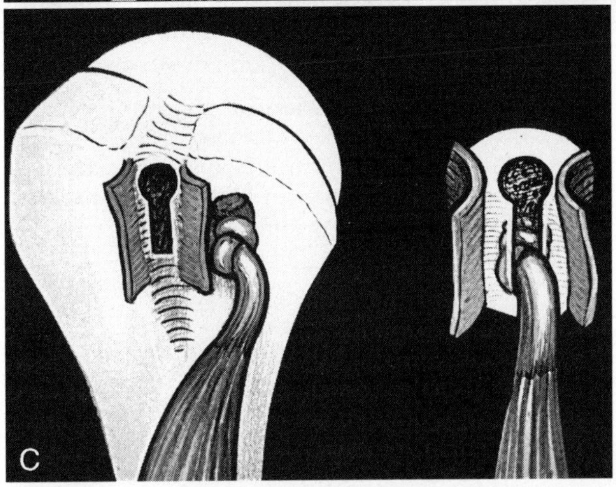

Fig. 10–17. Schematic diagrams of various techniques for tenodesis of the long biceps tendon: *A*, Hitchcock technique (upper left); *B*, Post technique (upper right); *C*, Froimson keyhole technique; *D*, Lipman technique; and *E*, DePalma technique.

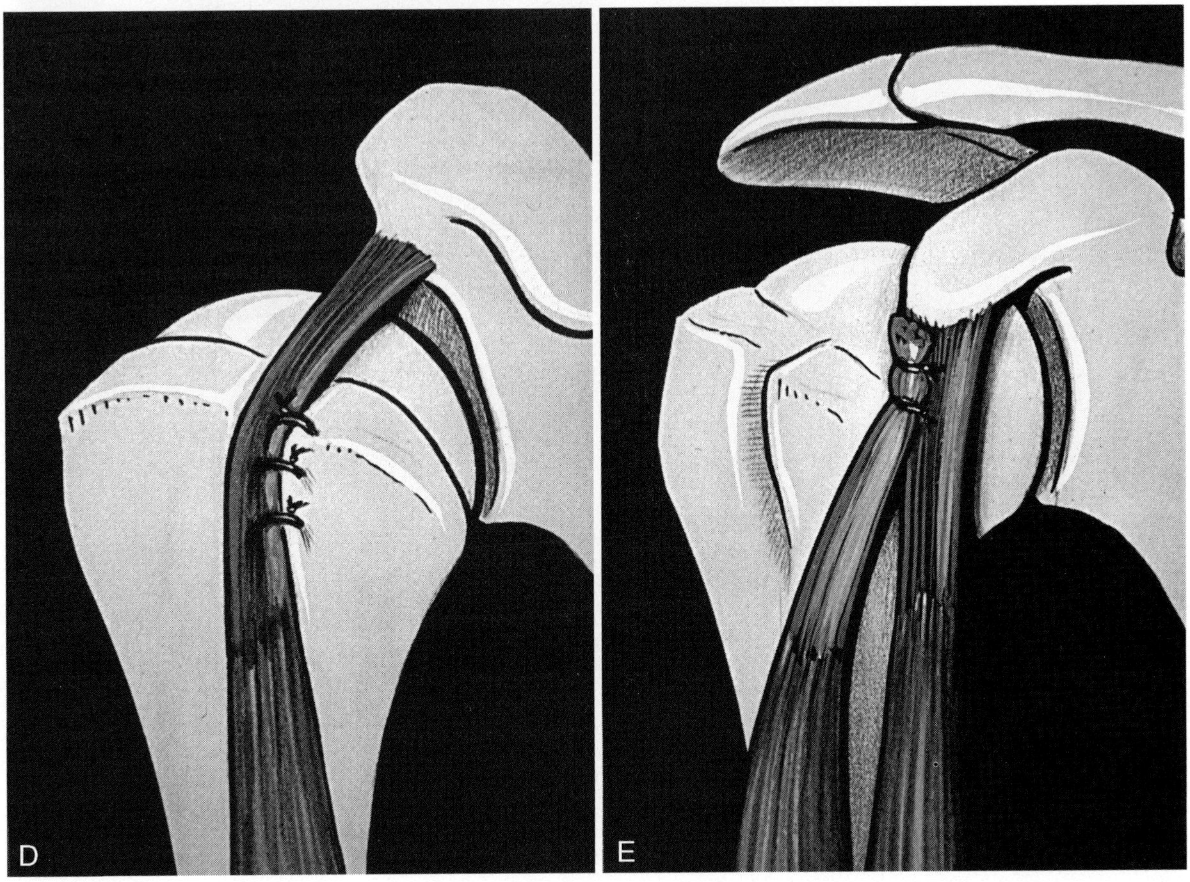

stump of the biceps tendon is very short (Figs. 10–17 and 10–18). Arthroscopic tenodesis of the long biceps tendon in the groove is still in the trial stage and cannot yet be generally recommended.

Arthroscopic and open techniques are available for the surgical management of biceps tendon subluxation. Arthroscopic resection of the long biceps tendon is justified only if the subluxation has severely compromised the quality of the tendon and in the older patient who has concomitant subacromial impingement syndrome. In this case we add arthroscopic subacromial decompression.

The following open operative techniques are available:

1. Internal reconstruction: In this method the subscapularis tendon is reattached to the lesser tuberosity along with the overlying clavipectoral fascia. Various types of suture anchors can be used for this purpose. Particular emphasis is placed on reconstruction of the rotator interval sling. The superior glenohumeral ligament and coracohumeral ligament must be reattached, together with the extensions of the supraspinatus and subscapularis tendons, to form a sling or lasso around the entrance to the bicipital groove for restabilizing the biceps tendon.
2. Recentering of the long biceps tendon: With a very recent biceps tendon subluxation, fibrous tissue and osteophytes have not yet filled the bicipital groove, and the tendon is still thin. In this situation a simple suture repair is adequate for restoring the tendon to the center of the groove. However, if the biceps tendon is widened, thickened, and torn, two options are available: (1) tenodesis in the groove (e.g., using the technique of Post,[50] Hitchcock[7] or Froimson[50]) (see Fig. 10–9) or (2) the Walch tubularization technique[12] (see Fig.10–19), in which the widened and damaged tendon is curled into a tube and fixed with a running suture, and the floor of the groove is deepened with an impactor.

In the case of a malunion or nonunion of the lesser tuberosity, the fracture surfaces are freshened and the fragments reduced and immobilized by internal fixation with screws or staples. This can be supplemented by a tenodesis of the long biceps tendon.

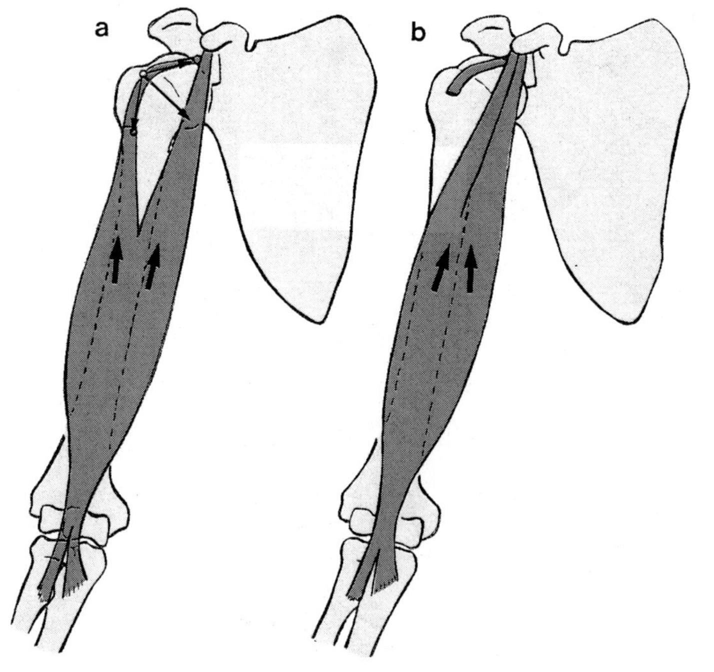

Fig. 10–18. **Vector analysis of the forces exerted on the glenohumeral joint by an intact long biceps tendon, *A*. The DePalma tenodesis results in increased proximalization of the humeral head, *B*.**

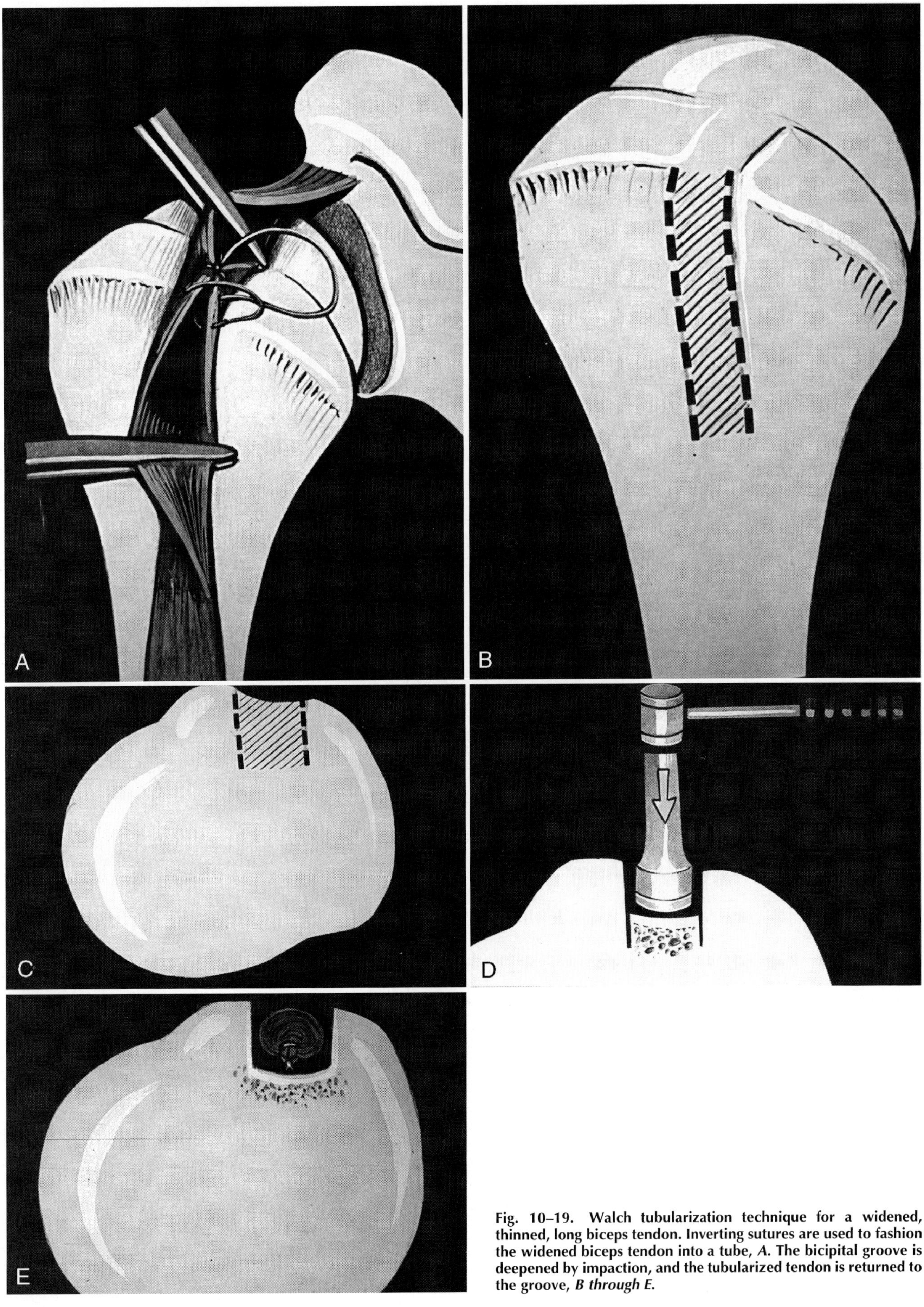

Fig. 10–19. Walch tubularization technique for a widened, thinned, long biceps tendon. Inverting sutures are used to fashion the widened biceps tendon into a tube, *A*. The bicipital groove is deepened by impaction, and the tubularized tendon is returned to the groove, *B through E*.

Treatment of Lesions of the Long Biceps Tendon Combined with Complete Rotator Cuff Tears

TENDINITIS

If the rotator cuff tear is reparable, the goal should be to preserve the long biceps tendon if at all possible, provided the tendon shows moderate tendinitis and only superficial erosive lesions. But if severe atrophic changes are noted during repair of the rotator cuff, biceps tenodesis is the most elegant solution, as it forestalls rupture and provides a quasi-functional reconstruction. We also tenodese a tendon that exhibits hypertrophic tendinitis. In this case it is difficult to recenter the thickened tendon, which no longer fits comfortably in the groove, so tenodesis provides the most favorable solution.

With a massive rotator cuff tear that is no longer reparable (acromiohumeral distance less than 7 mm), the remaining long biceps tendon is very often responsible for the pain, because it serves as the final restraint to proximal migration of the humeral head and becomes entrapped between the humeral head and acromion. We[12] have had good results with arthroscopic tenotomy of the biceps tendon at the base. The rationale for this isolated tenotomy, performed without subacromial decompression, is that a gradually progressive subacromial stenosis is not painful for the patient, and remarkably good active mobility is maintained. Following arthroscopic division of the long biceps tendon, there is no immediate slippage or descent of the biceps muscle, as the tendon is usually wedged within the groove. The sagging effect is considerably delayed, and patients are subjectively satisfied with the cosmetic result. A further upward migration of the humeral head has not been seen after resection of the long head of the biceps.

If dislocation of the long biceps tendon is noted during the open repair of a rotator cuff tear, and if the quality of the tendon appears good, we perform a biceps tenodesis. Of course we add an anterior acromioplasty to the cuff repair and tenodesis, and for extensive ruptures we perform an extended acromioplasty that includes resection of the lateral end of the clavicle. Neer[40] even suggests lateralization of the long biceps tendon to achieve better closure of the cuff.

The tenodesis should be performed close to the groove entrance, rather than at a more proximal level. If the biceps tendon if fixed to the supraspinatus tendon at a higher level in its intra-articular course, this will create potentially damaging opposing forces between the supraspinatus tendon and long biceps tendon.

RUPTURE OF THE LONG BICEPS TENDON

If there is already a rupture of the long biceps tendon with a concomitant rotator cuff tear, the biceps rupture does not require special therapeutic attention. However, one should check the intra-articular segment of the long biceps tendon to assess the potential for entrapment and to determine the extent of associated labrum pathology. If the biceps tendon stump becomes displaced into the joint space and entrapped there, it should be arthroscopically resected.

CONCLUSION

As the fifth tendon of the rotator cuff, the long biceps tendon not only functions as a flexor of the forearm but also contributes to flexion and abduction of the arm and exerts a joint-stabilizing effect during rotation. Thus, it is an important stabilizer of the shoulder joint.

The long biceps tendon is divisible into an intra-articular portion, a groove (canalicular) portion, and an extracanalicular portion in its course over the humeral head. Pathologic changes develop at the origin of the tendon, in its intra-articular portion at the rotator interval, and within the groove. The stability of the tendoligamentous structures at the entrance to the groove (rotator interval sling) and the restraint of the tendon in the groove have major pathologic significance. The pathogenesis of bicipital tendinitis and subluxation has its origin at these locations. The various types of dislocation are necessarily associated with lesions of the subscapularis tendon and supraspinatus tendon. Rotator cuff tears correlate with the occurrence of lesions of the long biceps tendon.

The long biceps tendon and rotator cuff also comprise a unit in terms of clinical diagnosis. One can never diagnose a rotator cuff tear without also considering a lesion of the long biceps tendon. At the same time, rotator cuff pathology frequently commences with pathology of the long biceps tendon.

Isolated lesions of the long biceps tendon with an intact rotator cuff pose a therapeutic challenge to the surgeon. The younger the patient and the less severe the rotator cuff pathology, the greater the need is for an anatomic repair. Conversely, resection takes precedence over repair in older patients and in patients with more extensive rotator cuff tears.

REFERENCES

1. Inman VT, Saunders M, Abbot LC. Observations on the function of the shoulder joint. *J Bone Joint Surg.* 1944;1–30.
2. Habermeyer P, Kaiser E, Knappe M, Kreusser T, Wiedemann E. Zur funktionellen Anatomie und Biomechanik der langen Bizepssehne. *Unfallchirurg.* 1987; 90:319–329.
3. Pal GP, Bhatt RH, Patel VS. Relationship between the tendon of the long head of biceps brachii and the glenoidal labrum in humans. *Anat Rec.* 1991;229:278–280.
4. Cooper DE, Arnoczky SP, O'Brien SJ, Warren RF, DiCarlo E, Allen AA. Anatomy, histology and vascularity of the glenoid labrum. An anatomical study. *J Bone Joint Surg Am.* 1992;74:46–52.
5. Hermann B, Steiner D. Arterial supply of the human long biceps tendon. *Acta Anat Basel.* 1990;137:129–131.
6. Cone RO, Danzig L, Resnick D, Goldman AB. The bicipital groove: Radiographic, anatomic and pathologic study. *AJR.* 1983;41: 781–788.
7. Hitchcock HH, Bechtol CO. Painful shoulder: Observations on role of tendon of long head of biceps brachii in it's causation. *J Bone Joint Surg Am.* 1948;30:263–273.
8. Harryman DT, Sidles JA, Harris SC, Matsen III FA. The role of the rotator interval capsule in passive motion and stability of the shoulder. *J Bone Joint Surg Am.* 1992;74:53–66.
9. Itoi E, Kuechle DK, Newman SR, Morrey BF, AN KN. Stabilizing function of the biceps in stable and unstable shoulders. *J Bone Joint Surg Br.* 1993;75:546–550.
10. Clark JM, Harrymann DT. Tendons, ligaments and capsule of the rotator cuff. *J Bone Joint Surg Am.* 1992;74:713–725.

11. O'Brien SJ, Arnoczky SP, Warren RF, Rozbruch RS. Developmental anatomy of the shoulder and anatomy of the glenohumeral joint. In: Rockwood CA, Matsen FA III, eds. *The Shoulder.* Philadelphia: WB Saunders; 1990;1:16–17.
12. Walch G. *La pathologie de la longue portion du biceps.* Conference d'enseignement de la SOFCOT, Paris 1993.
13. Meyer AW. Spolia anatomica. Absence of the tendon of the long head of biceps. *J Anat.* 1913;48:133–135.
14. Basmajian JV, Latif V. Integrated actions and functions of the chief flexors of the elbow. A detailed electromyographic analysis. *J Bone Joint Surg Am.* 1957;39:1106–1118.
15. Andrews J, Carson W, McLeod W. Glenoid labrum tears related to the long head of the biceps. *Am J Sports Med.* 1985;13:337–341.
16. Habermeyer P. Isokinetische Kräfte am Glenohumeralgelenk. *Hefte zur Unfallheilkunde.* Berlin: Springer;1989:1–114.
17. Perry J. Biomechanics of the shoulder. In: Rowe CR, ed. *The Shoulder.* New York, Edinburgh: Churchhill Livingstone; 1988;1–15.
18. Lucas DB. Biomechanics of the shoulder joint. *Arch Surg.* 1973; 107:425–432.
19. Grauer JD, Paulos LE, Smutz WP. Biceps tendon and superior labral injuries. *Arthroscopy.* 1992;8:488–497.
20. Snyder SJ, Karzel RP, Del Pizzo W, Ferkel RD, Freidman MJ. SLAP lesions of the shoulder. *Arthroscopy.* 1990;6:274–279.
21. Burkhart SS, Fox DL. SLAP lesions in association with complete tears of the long head of the biceps tendon: A report of two cases. *Arthroscopy.* 1992;8:31–35.
22. Habermeyer P, Brunner U, Treptow U, Wiedemann E. Arthroskopische Over-the top-Naht zur Behandlung von S.L.A.P. Läsionen der Schulter. *Arthroskopie.* 1993:6:263–271.
23. Burkhead WZ Jr. The biceps tendon. In: Rockwood CA Jr, Matsen III FA, eds. *The Shoulder.* Vol 2. Philadelphia: WB Saunders; 1990:791–836.
24. Wiley AM. Arthroscopic appearance of frozen shoulder. *Arthroscopy.* 1991;7:138–143.
25. Ahovuo J, Paavolainen P, Slatis P. Diagnostic value of sonography in lesions of the biceps tendon. *Clin Orthop.* 1986;202:184–188.
26. Carrillon Y, Tavernier, Tran-Minh VA, Bochu M. *Etude comparitive prospective de trois methodes d'imagerie dans la pathologie de la coiffe des rotateurs.* Échographie, arthrographie associëe au scanner et imagerie par rësonance magëtique. Lyon, France, 1993.
27. Chan TW, Dalinka MK, Kneeland JB, Chervot A. Biceps tendon dislocation: Evaluation with MR imaging. *Radiology.* 1991;179: 645–652.
28. Middleton WD, Reinus WR, Totty WG. Ultrasonographic evaluation of the rotator cuff and biceps tendon. *J Bone Joint Surg Am.* 1986; 68:440–450.
29. Tavernier T, Lapra C, Bochu M. *IRM dans la pathologie de la coiffe rotateurs.* Lyon, France, 1993.
30. Neer CS, Bigliani NU, Hawkins RJ. Rupture of the long head of the biceps related to subacromial impingement. *Orthop Trans.* 1977; 1:111.
31. Dejour D, Tayot O. La rupture isolëe de la longue portion du biceps. *Journëes Lyonnaise de l'Epaule.* Lyon, France; 1993.
32. Meyer AW. Spontaneous dislocation and destruction of tendon of long head of biceps brachii. *Arch Surg.* 1928;17:493–506.
33. Paavolainen P, Slatis P, Aalto K. Surgical pathology in chronic shoulder pain. In: Bateman J, Welsh P, eds. *Surgery of the Shoulder.* Philadelphia: BC Decker; 1984:313–318.
34. Neer CS. Impingement lesions. *Clin Orthop.* 1983;173:70–77.
35. Dines D, Warren RF, Inglis AE. Surgical treatment of lesions of the long head of the biceps. *Clin Orthop.* 1982;164:165–171.
36. Mariani EM, Cofield RA. The tendon of the long head of the biceps brachii: Instability, tendinitis and rupture. *Advances in Orthopaedic Surgery.* Baltimore: Williams & Wilkins; 1988: 262–268.
37. O'Donoghue DH. Subluxing biceps tendon in the athletes. *Clin Orthop.* 1982;164:26–30.
38. Peterson CJ. Spontaneous medical dislocation of the tendon of the long biceps brachii. *Clin Orthop.* 1986;211:224–227.
39. Nové-Josserand L. Subluxation et luxation du tendon du long biceps. *Journëes Lyonnaise de l'Epaule.* Lyon, France; 1993.
40. Neer CS. *Shoulder Reconstruction.* 1st Ed. Philadelphia: WB Saunders; 1990.
41. Gerber C, Terrier F, Zehnder R, Ganz R. The subcoracoid space. An anatomic study. *Clin Orthop.* 1987;215:132–138.
42. Neer CS, Craig EV, Fukuda H. Cuff tear arthropathy. *J Bone Joint Surg Am.* 65:1232–1244.
43. Collier SG, Wynn-Jones CH. Displacement of the biceps with subscapularis avulsion. *J Bone Joint Surg.* 1990;72:145.
44. Gerber C, Krushell R. Isolated rupture of the tendon of the subscapularis muscle. *J Bone Joint Surg Br.* 1991;73:389–394.
45. Walch G. Synthëse sur l'epidemiologie et l'ethiologie des ruptures de la coiffe des rotateurs. *Journëes Lyonnaise de l'Epaule.* Lyon, France; 1993.
46. Snyder SJ. *Repair of type II SLAP lesion using suture anchors and permanent mattress sutures.* Ninth Annual San Diego Shoulder Meeting, San Diego, CA; 1992.
47. Wiedemann E, Habermeyer P. Neue arthroskopische Technik zur Naht von Rotatorenmanschettenrupturen. In: Hofer H, Hertel P, eds. *Arthroskopie und Chirurgie der Schulter. Fortschritte Arthroskopie.* Vol 8. Stuttgart: Enke; 1992:74–77.
48. De Palma AF. *Surgery of the Shoulder.* 3rd ed. Philadelphia: JB Lippincott; 1983;266–276.
49. Post M, Benca P. Primary tendinitis of the long head of biceps. *Clin Orthop.* 1989;246:117–125.
50. Froimson Al. Keyhole tenodesis of biceps origin at the shoulder. *Clin Orthop.* 1974;112:245–249.
51. Kapandji IA. *Funktionelle Anatomie der Gelenke.* Vol 1. Stuttgart: Enke; 1984:28.

Chapter 11

Anterior Instability and its Relationship to Cuff Disease in Throwing Athletes

Patrick A. Ruwe, Ronald S. Kvitne, and Frank W. Jobe

The traditional concept of "shoulder impingement" and rotator cuff dysfunction has evolved considerably over the past 20 years.[1,2] Impingement problems in the older nonathletic population can be attributed to degenerative causes, characterized by proliferative processes along the subacromial arch, which lead to compromise of the subacromial outlet, vascular insufficiency, and rotator cuff injury. Until recently, overhand athletes presenting with chronic shoulder symptoms and impingement signs were also felt to have primary dysfunction of the rotator cuff.[3] However, the proposed mechanism of subacromial impingement and compressive cuff wear is generally not seen in the young overhand athlete. Although undersurface rotator cuff fraying and labral wear is often seen arthroscopically, there is usually a relatively normal appearance within the subacromial space. In addition, recent cadaveric studies have shown that impingement symptoms produced during provocative testing, such as that described by Neer (forward flexion and internal humeral rotation), are not the result of impingement of the supraspinatus tendon beneath the coracoacromial arch. Rather, they appear to be the result of impingement between the undersurface of the supraspinatus and infraspinatus portions of the rotator cuff and the posterior-superior labrum.[4–6]

A critical review of the results from surgical treatment has also led to a better overall understanding of shoulder impingement. Given the excellent results obtained by Neer and other investigators with anterior acromioplasty, athletes who did not respond to conservative measures were previously treated surgically with a subacromial decompression. Tibone et al.[7,8] reported their results using an open acromioplasty for treatment of overhand athletes with rotator cuff dysfunction secondary to impingement. Unfortunately, only 27% of skilled collegiate and professional pitchers were able to return to their same competitive level without pain.[8] The results of arthroscopic subacromial decompression have also revealed that although athletes using overhand motions obtained good pain relief, their return to high level competitive overhand sports remained unpredictable.[9]

What has emerged from these and other studies is an evolution of the concepts concerning shoulder instability, impingement, and rotator cuff tears in the throwing athlete.[10–19] The chronic repetitive stresses associated with the overhead throwing motion can progress along a continuum of cumulative microtrauma, progressive instability, glenohumeral subluxation, "internal" impingement, and finally rotator cuff tears.[2,20–31]

An accurate diagnosis and treatment of any patient who presents at any point along this continuum requires a thorough understanding of the pertinent shoulder anatomy, the basic biomechanics of the throwing motion, and the complex interrelationship of mobility and stability of the shoulder joint.

SHOULDER ANATOMY

A complex array of static and dynamic stabilizers around the shoulder joint provide the necessary balance between functional mobility and stability.[32–36] In addition, negative intra-articular pressure of −4 mm Hg contributes to stability. In the cadaveric model, simple venting of the capsule results in an average 52% increase in humeral head translation.[37]

Although the glenohumeral contact area is relatively small, recent evidence has shown that the concavity of the glenoid provides significant stability to the humeral head when combined with a compressive force. The concavity-compression model holds that as the shoulder girdle muscles generate compressive forces across the glenohumeral joint, they provide stabilization of the joint.[38] The glenoid labrum (fibrocartilaginous rim) increases the surface area and concavity of the glenoid fossa, further improving stability without impeding joint mobility.

The most important static shoulder constraints are the capsuloligamentous structures. The joint capsule, although redundant, affords some degree of stability through selective tightening of the anterior and inferior portions of the capsule during humeral abduction and external rotation. The capsule is further reinforced via the glenohumeral ligaments.[28,39–41] The superior glenohumeral ligament, present in approximately 90% of shoulders, arises from the glenoid tubercle, anterior to the long head of the biceps tendon. It runs inferior and laterally to insert on the proximal aspect of the lesser tuberosity. Its primary role is in resisting inferior translation with the arm adducted to the side, together with an equal contribution from the inferior glenohumeral ligament.[42]

The middle glenohumeral ligament, present in approximately 70% of shoulders, arises from the labrum below the superior glenohumeral ligament and inserts just medial to the lesser tuberosity under the subscapularis tendon to which it adheres.[43] The middle glenohumeral ligament's contribution to stability is variable. However, cordlike middle glenohumeral ligaments serve as an important secondary restraint to anterior translation.[44]

The inferior glenohumeral ligament complex, present in approximately 90% of shoulders, is the main static stabilizer of the abducted shoulder. It consists of an anterior and posterior band with an axillary pouch, or hammock-like sling, draped in between.[45] It takes origin from most of the anterior glenoid labrum and inserts into the anatomic neck of the humerus.[43]

In the throwing position (90° humeral abduction and maximum external rotation) the inferior glenohumeral ligament and the anterior inferior glenoid labrum are the most significant structures providing passive restraint at the anterior glenoid margin.[43] In this position, the anterior band of the inferior glenohumeral ligament fans out to support the head, and the posterior band becomes cordlike. The converse is seen with internal rotation.[46]

Dynamic stability is achieved through the synchronous firing of the rotator cuff and scapular rotator musculature. The rotator cuff muscles (supraspinatus, infraspinatus, teres minor, and subscapularis) originate from the body of the scapula and insert onto the greater and lesser tuberosities of the humerus. These muscles provide stability by centering and compressing the humeral head within the glenoid fossa. The scapular rotators (trapezius, serratus anterior, rhomboids, and levator scapulae) position the scapula (glenoid) for optimum stability throughout the entire overhead throwing motion.

BIOMECHANICS

A brief review of the basic biomechanics of throwing will illustrate the delicate balance between functional mobility and glenohumeral stability. The sequence of shoulder motion among throwers in different sports is relatively constant. A preparatory phase positions the arm, which is then cocked for acceleration. The acceleration phase culminates with ball release followed by deceleration and follow-through.[47] The pitching motion has been studied in the most detail and, therefore, will be presented here.[48–56] The overhand throwing motion has been divided into five stages (Fig. 11–1): windup (stage 1) ends as the ball leaves the nondominant glove hand; early cocking (stage II) proceeds as the ball is released from the glove hand, the shoulder abducts, and externally rotates and terminates as the forward foot contacts the ground; late cocking (stage III) continues as the dominant shoulder achieves maximum external rotation; acceleration (stage IV) begins with internal humeral rotation and ends with ball release; deceleration (stage V) begins after ball release and comprises 30% of the time required to dissipate the excess kinetic energy of the throwing motion; and follow-through (stage VI) completes the remaining 70% of this time frame and ends when all motion is complete.

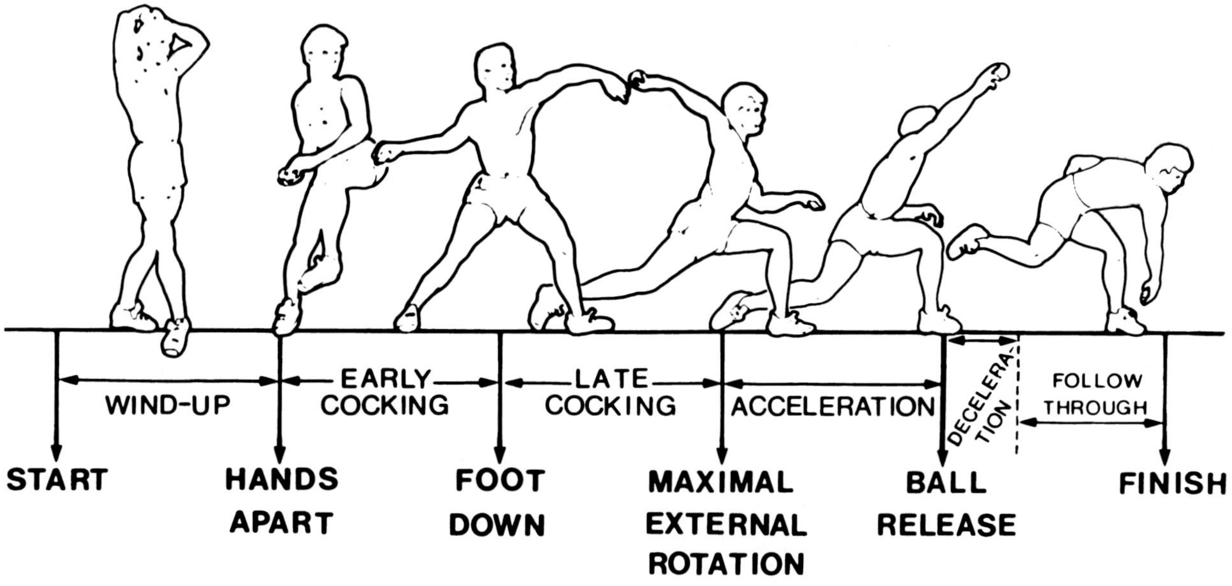

Fig. 11–1. Five stages of the overhand throwing motion: stage I, windup; stage II, early cocking; stage III, late cocking; stage IV, acceleration; and stage V, follow-through.

An athlete must depend on an extremely complex, synchronous firing pattern of the muscles about the shoulder, elbow, trunk, and lower extremities in order to generate the momentum necessary to throw a baseball. During the windup and early cocking phases of throwing, the deltoid muscle abducts the dominant arm. Throughout late cocking, the infraspinatus and teres minor muscles externally rotate the humerus, the biceps maintains elbow flexion at 90°, and the subscapularis decelerates the externally rotating humerus. The pectoralis major, latissimus dorsi, and triceps muscles provide the forward propulsive force during the acceleration phase. In the deceleration phase eccentric muscle contractions of the teres minor, as well as increased activity of the trapezius, serratus anterior, and rhomboids, control the deceleration of the extremity.

Activity of the rotator cuff and scapular rotators (dynamic stabilizers) is necessary throughout the entire throwing motion to help maintain glenohumeral congruency. A small deficiency of either the dynamic or static stabilizers can have a cumulative effect in compromising shoulder function.

Early fatigue of the dynamic anterior shoulder stabilizers initiates a cascade of changes in the throwing mechanism, including scapulohumeral dysynchrony, scapular winging, dropped elbow, and increased lumbar lordosis. These changes may lead to inconsistency or early fatigue. When recognized early, most athletes respond to a combined strengthening, power, and endurance program directed toward the rotator cuff, scapular rotators, and trunk stabilizers. Continued fatigue allows transfer of the repetitive stresses associated with throwing to the anterior static stabilizers and subsequent anterior translation of the humeral head secondary to attenuation of the static restraints. With progressive forward translation, the posterosuperior undersurface of the rotator cuff impinges upon the posterior glenoid labrum leading to secondary internal impingement. Thus, shoulder pathology in this setting can progress along a continuum from mild laxity, to anterior subluxation, secondary internal impingement, and eventual rotator cuff tearing. This injury pattern has been identified as the "instability-complex."

DIAGNOSIS

The successful treatment of shoulder problems in athletes requires an accurate diagnosis that begins with a thorough history and physical exam. Adjuvant tests such as arthrogram, CT scan, and MRI are obtained only after a working diagnosis has been established and should serve the physician as a tool for confirmation rather than enlightenment.

Symptoms of instability are often vague and the physical findings are often subtle. Pain is the most common complaint in throwing athletes with shoulder problems and can assist greatly in making the proper diagnosis when its spatial relationship with athletic activity is properly delineated. Pain that is associated with a specific phase of the throwing motion (i.e., late cocking or acceleration) is most likely caused by mild anterior instability. Shoulder pain that is exacerbated with progressive activity is usually associated with rotator cuff tendinitis and/or subacromial bursitis. Pain at rest or pain that occurs during the night can be the result of a partial or complete rotator cuff tear. As predicted, a rotator cuff tear in a throwing athlete is especially disabling and can be a career-threatening injury.

Before initiating the shoulder exam, it is important to remember that the shoulder is often a site of referred pain, most commonly from neurovascular problems or from the cervical spine. These potential problems should be routinely evaluated and excluded.

Examination of the shoulder itself begins with inspection, both static and dynamic. Static examination is directed toward evidence of muscle wasting. Deltoid wasting is characterized by squaring off of the shoulder or prominence of the acromion and indicates a possible axillary nerve lesion. A more selective wasting of the anterior deltoid is often seen in throwers with significant shoulder pain secondary to instability or impingement. A prominent scapular spine is a result of supraspinatus and infraspinatus wasting, generally secondary to a rotator cuff tear, but may represent suprascapular nerve entrapment that is often seen in overhand athletes such as volleyball, baseball, and water polo players.

Dynamic inspection is directed toward evaluating asynchrony of scapulohumeral motion. Elevation and/or upward rotation of the scapula before humeral abduction may be a subtle and an early sign of rotator cuff dysfunction.

Next, all four joints of the shoulder (glenohumeral, scapulothoracic, sternoclavicular, and acromioclavicular) should be palpated. The entire clavicle, the acromion, the scapular body, and the spine should be assessed for tenderness, crepitation, deformity, and temperature. Asymmetry, muscle atrophy, bony deformity, decreased range of motion, crepitus, and areas of localized swelling or tenderness should be documented. Careful palpation about the shoulder not only provides additional clues to the diagnosis, but may direct therapeutic modalities to areas of injury or inflammation. Various conditions associated with palpable tenderness include AC joint tenderness, which may indicate AC synovitis or perhaps osteoarthritis; subacromial space tenderness, which might indicate subacromial bursitis, rotator cuff impingement, or a rotator cuff tear; and intertubercular tenderness, which may be a sign of biceps tendinitis or subluxation.

Range of motion, both active and passive, should be assessed with the patient seated to minimize compensatory actions of the spine and pelvis that may mislead the examiner. Diminished shoulder range of motion following an acute injury may be caused by pain as a sequelae of an AC joint separation, glenohumeral joint dislocation, or a fracture about the shoulder girdle. Lost shoulder range of motion in the absence of recent trauma may be the result of chronic subacromial bursitis, rotator cuff tendinitis, cuff tearing, adhesive capsulitis, or osteoarthritis. Audible or palpable crepitus about the shoulder girdle associated with passive or active range of motion may represent scarring within the subacromial soft tissues or scapulothoracic bursa, osteoarthritis of the AC or glenohumeral joint, a tear of the glenoid labrum, or loose bodies within the joint itself.

Muscle strength testing allows the physician to evaluate the integrity of the musculotendinous unit while also assessing neurologic function. Muscle asymmetry or weakness identified with manual muscle testing may represent deficiencies in strength of certain muscles. Observed weakness noted on selective testing of the biceps muscle, rotator cuff, or scapular rotators may be an indication of underlying tendinitis, muscle strain, tear, or even nerve impairment. Recognition of muscle weakness serves as a reminder to strengthen these weakened muscles during rehabilitation. Strength measurements obtained isokinetically (Cybex, Lido, or Biodex systems) can also provide an objective estimation of weakness. This information, when used as a baseline, can provide a reference for subsequent strength gains achieved during rehabilitation.

Of crucial importance in the throwing athlete is the association of impingement with shoulder instability. However, a distinction must be made between instability and laxity. Shoulder laxity may be defined as excessive translation of the humeral head on the glenoid in the absence of clinical symptoms or pathological changes. Normal shoulders may exhibit laxity without being unstable. Instability is then defined as asymmetrical laxity associated with clinical symptoms on pathologic changes. In unstable shoulders, laxity is not obliterated by humeral rotation with secondary capsular tightening.

Glenohumeral instability can be described in terms of etiology, frequency, degree, direction, and volition.[57] Etiology may be atraumatic or traumatic. Traumatic instability may be subdivided into macrotrauma (single traumatic event), which is common in football players and weightlifters, or microtrauma (recurrent or cumulative), which is common in overhand athletes.

Frequency may be acute, chronic, or recurrent. Degree is divided into dislocation and subluxation. The degree of subluxation can be graded according to Cofield to allow standardization for comparison. Grade 1 involves translation less than 50% of the humeral head. Grade 2 describes translation greater than 50%. Grade 3 involves translation to the glenoid rim or perched, and grade 4 describes subluxation over the glenoid rim.

The direction may be unidirectional (anterior, or posterior, inferior) or multidirectional antero-inferiorly, postero-inferiorly, or global. Finally, instability may be voluntary or involuntary. Voluntary instability is not commonly seen among competitive athletes and generally is not associated with psychiatric disorders.

Unfortunately, information gathered during classic stability testing may be confusing. Although impingement signs and apprehension signs are relatively straightforward, signs of mild instability (subluxation) are often subtle and must not be overlooked. The examination begins with the normal shoulder. This decreases the patient's anxiety and establishes a baseline for comparison. Patients without evidence of instability on the affected side with contralateral laxity should be suspected of guarding. Before any test of glenohumeral stability is performed, the humeral head should be compressed into the glenoid fossa to ensure concentric reduction. The most sensitive means of eliciting occult anterior glenohumeral instability is achieved through the use of the "classic" apprehension sign followed by the "relocation test."[26] These maneuvers are best performed with the patient relaxed and lying supine. The arm to be tested is positioned off the edge of the examining table in 90° abduction and 90° external rotation. In this position, the apprehension test is performed by gently applying an anteriorly directed force to the posterior aspect of the humeral head (Fig. 11–2). Marked apprehension (or apprehension and pain) in this setting indicates gross instability, as seen with recurrent dislocations. The sensation of pain without apprehension may denote primary subacromial impingement or mild anterior instability (subluxation), with secondary internal impingement between the undersurface of the supraspinatus and infraspinatus portions of the rotator cuff and the posterior superior glenoid rim (Fig. 11–3). To differentiate primary subacromial impingement from primary instability (subluxation) with secondary internal impingement, the relocation test is performed. This is again accomplished with the shoulder abducted 90° and externally rotated 90°. However, gentle pressure is applied to the anterior aspect of the humeral head and this force is directed posteriorly (Fig. 11–4). Patients who have no change in their perception of pain will likely have primary subacromial impingement. Whereas, those patients whose pain is relieved most likely have primary mild anterior instability (subluxation) and secondary internal impingement, as they can now tolerate further external humeral

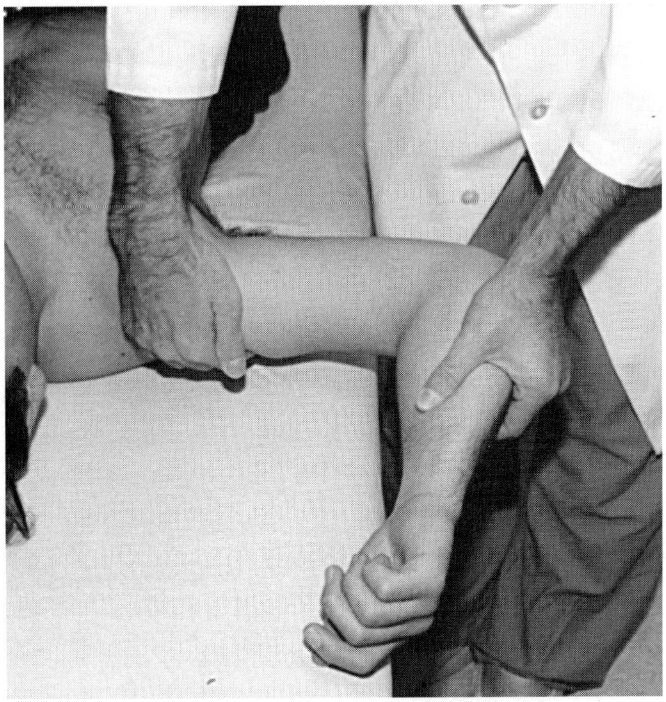

Fig. 11–2. Apprehension test: with the shoulder held in 90° abduction and maximum external rotation, an anteriorly directed force is applied with gentle fingertip pressure to the posterior humeral head.

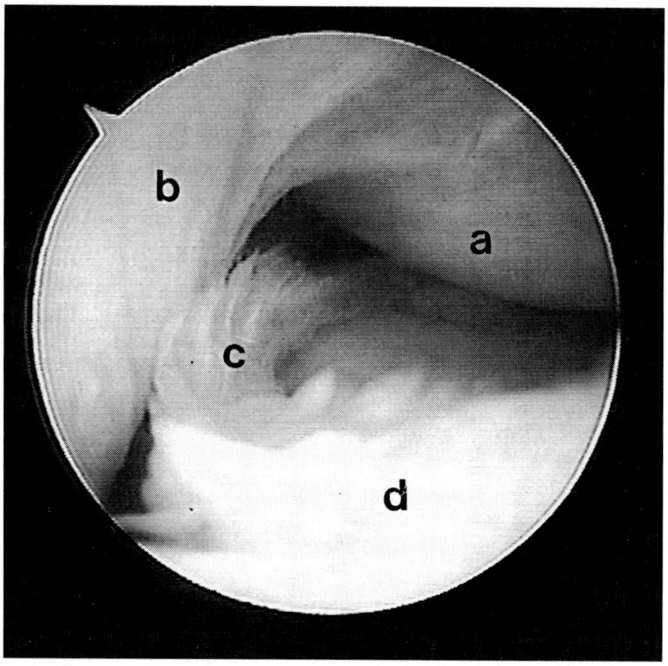

Fig. 11–3. Posterior glenoid impingement: *A,* anteriorly translated humeral head; *B,* undersurface rotator cuff fraying; *C,* site of impingement along posterior glenoid rim; and *D,* glenoid fossa.

rotation while the humeral head is maintained in a reduced position (Fig. 11–5).

Glenohumeral translation is further assessed with the patient supine by the load and shift test. The patient's arm is grasped and placed in a position of approximately 20° of abduction and forward flexion. The humerus is then loaded in an axial direction and anterior stresses are applied to the humeral head, noting the degree of anterior translation.

The load and shift test measures translation in the range of glenohumeral motion when the capsular restraints are lax. The apprehension test measures laxity at extremes of motion when the specific capsular ligaments are under tension. By performing the load and shift test in varying degrees of internal and external rotation on both the affected and contralateral shoulders, the examiner is able to assess the competency of the glenohumeral complex and uncover subtle laxity patterns as well.

An evaluation would not be complete without radiographic analysis. Unfortunately, standard radiographs supply little diagnostic information for a throwing athlete. They must, however, be included in the investigation of persistent shoulder pain to rule out infection, fracture, or an unsuspected neoplasm. Patients with chronic recurrent instability or an acute traumatic glenohumeral dislocation may exhibit a bony defect within the posterior aspect of the humeral head (Hill-Sachs deformity) or a deficiency of the anterior, inferior glenoid rim (Bankart lesion). Additional diagnostic procedures including arthrography, CT arthrography, or MRI have not been proven effective to date. For those patients with suspected occult instability, an examination under anesthesia and diagnostic arthroscopy has been most helpful

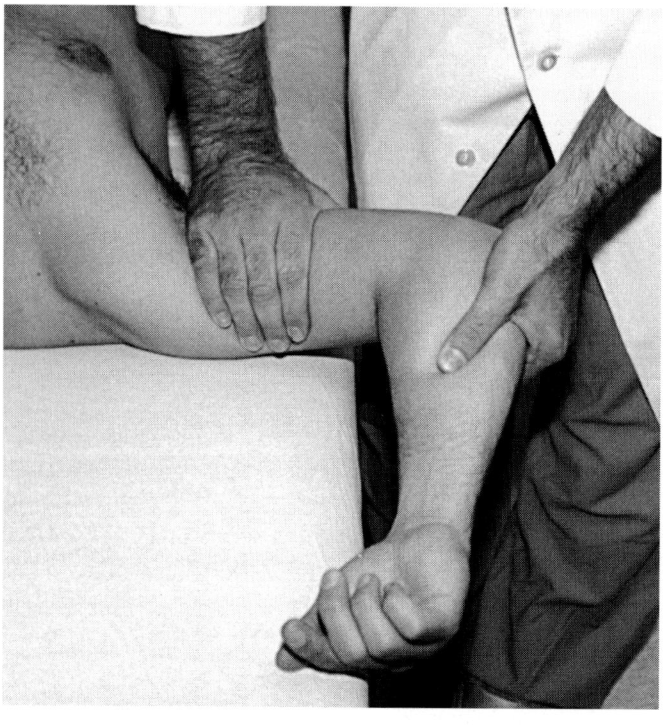

Fig. 11–4. Relocations test: with gentle pressure applied to the anterior humeral head (maintaining the head in a reduced position), further external humeral rotation is achieved.

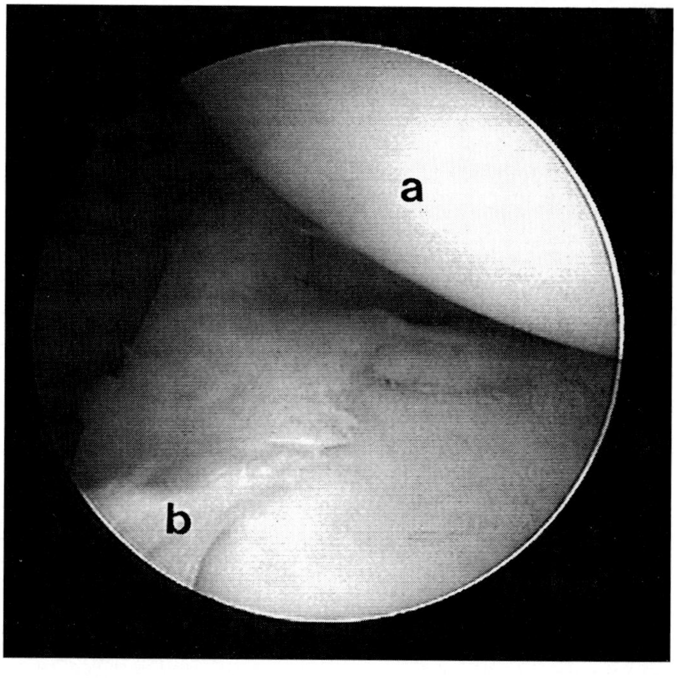

Fig. 11–5. Reduced position of glenohumeral joint: *A,* humeral head "reduced" and *B,* glenoid rim with fraying.

in confirming the diagnosis.[58,59] Findings on diagnostic arthroscopy consistent with subtle anterior instability include an enlarged bare area, articular impression lesions on the posterior humeral head, posterosuperior undersurface fraying of the rotator cuff, and evidence of undersurface internal rotator cuff impingement along the posterosuperior aspect of the glenoid rim when the arm is placed in the throwing position.

CLASSIFICATION

Based upon the information obtained through a detailed history, physical examination and preliminary diagnostic arthroscopy, most throwing athletes with refractory anterior shoulder pain can be classified into one of four groups (Table 11–1).[26]

Group I

These athletes have shoulder pain associated with pure primary subacromial impingement but no shoulder instability. Impingement testing elicits pain, whereas instability tests are negative. On occasion, athletes with severe impingement have experienced pain with apprehension testing. However, because their shoulder is stable, this pain is not relieved with relocation testing. Examination under anesthesia also reveals a stable joint. Arthroscopic findings may include undersurface fraying or partial-thickness tearing of the rotator cuff, but the glenoid labrum and glenohumeral ligaments are usually normal. The subacromial space, however, is often obscured because of fibrosis and scarring of the subacromial bursa. The acromion process may have an inferior osteophyte that, together with the coracoacromial ligament, can be seen impinging upon the superior surface of the rotator cuff. In our experience, this group includes a relatively small number of athletes, most of whom are over the age of 35.

Group II

As a result of repetitive throwing and chronic microtrauma to the capsule and glenoid labrum, these athletes have developed primary instability (subluxation) and secondary internal impingement. As expected, these athletes have pain with impingement testing. By virtue of their underlying mild primary instability, these athletes also have pain or discomfort (but not apprehension) with apprehension testing. When the relocation test is then added, the pain is relieved, as the humeral head is held in a reduced position, and the pinching of the rotator cuff is relieved. Unfortunately, examination under anesthesia is not very helpful, as their primary instability is often so subtle that it goes undetected. Arthroscopically, these athletes demonstrate undersurface rotator cuff fraying, anterior glenoid labral damage, posterior-superior glenoid labral damage, attenuation of the inferior glenohumeral ligament, and anterior translation (subluxation) of the humeral head.[4,6,58] Occasionally, posterior labral damage and chondral defects in the posterior humeral head have been seen.

Table 11–1. Classification of Shoulder Injury

Group I	Pure Impingement No instability
Group II	Primary instability caused by chronic labral microtrauma Secondary impingement
Group III	Primary instability caused by generalized ligamentous hyperelasticity Secondary impingement
Group IV	Pure instability No impingement

Group III

These athletes have generalized ligamentous hyperelasticity and, as a result, have also developed primary shoulder instability with secondary internal impingement. Because of their generalized ligamentous laxity, these patients often exhibit hyperextension of the elbow, knee, or metacarpal-phalangeal joints and the ability to place the abducted thumb on the forearm.[60] As noted in Group II, these athletes have pain with impingement testing, and pain (but not apprehension) with apprehension testing. Performance of the relocation test again relieves the pain associated with apprehension testing, as the humeral head is prevented from subluxating anteriorly. Examination under anesthesia often demonstrates bilateral shoulder laxity. Arthroscopic findings may include undersurface rotator cuff fraying. Typically, there is also attenuation or hypoplasia of the inferior glenohumeral ligament and marked laxity of the anterior joint capsule allowing easy glenohumeral subluxation with gentle manipulation but without associated glenoid labral damage or humeral head chondromalacia.

Group IV

This last group of athletes have pure primary instability without impingement. There usually is a history of a single traumatic event that has produced an anterior glenohumeral joint subluxation or dislocation. This trauma may be as trivial as a forceful slide into a base or associated with a more violent collision with another player. These athletes do not usually have impingement findings. However, they exhibit pain, apprehension, or both with apprehension testing and relief of these symptoms with relocation testing. Under anesthesia they will have gross anterior instability. Characteristic arthroscopic findings include a normal rotator cuff, anterior glenoid labral damage (Bankart lesion), posterior humeral head defects (Hill-Sachs lesion), and a dislocatable humeral head. By classifying these athletes according to their particular pathological process, a more rational and standardized treatment program can be instituted with hopefully improved results.

TREATMENT

Most shoulder injuries in the throwing athlete are the result of chronic repetitive microtrauma. Consequently, an initial period of relative rest (avoidance of throwing) is indicated. Oral nonsteroidal anti-inflammatory medication is recommended in order to reduce inflammation about the shoulder. The judicious use of cortisone preparations, when injected about the shoulder, bathe the inflamed tissues and promote healing. However, the reader is cautioned against using more than three injections over a 3- to 6-month period of time for any condition. Various physical therapy modalities including cryotherapy, contrast baths, phonophoresis, iontophoresis, and electrical stimulation can also be employed. These techniques create an environment about the inflamed tissues that will reduce swelling and facilitate the body's own healing response.

As pain and swelling subside, a supervised muscle strengthening program is undertaken to reestablish muscle synchrony about the shoulder. Special emphasis is made to regain flexibility as well as strength, power, and endurance of the rotator cuff muscles, deltoid, scapular rotators and stabilizers, pectoralis major, coracobrachialis, biceps, and triceps. Strengthening begins with isometric exercises and moves toward progressive resistive exercises, isotonic exercises, and finally isokinetic training. Those patients with underlying glenohumeral joint instability must be protected from further injury by avoiding shoulder hyperextension or abduction and external rotation. This precaution should be applied throughout the rehabilitation regardless of the exercise being performed. An aggressive conservative rehabilitation program is continued for 3 to 6 months. If symptoms persist and the athlete is unable to return to throwing, consideration must be given for surgical intervention.

Examination under anesthesia and preliminary diagnostic arthroscopy allows confirmation of the presumptive diagnosis and helps to direct surgical treatment. For patients with classic subacromial impingement and those rare overhead athletes under 35 with refractory primary subacromial impingement without instability (group I) a subacromial decompression, either open or arthroscopic, is required.[1,8,15] It is essential that underlying instability be ruled out prior to decompressing a young throwing athlete with pain. A proper decompression, when undertaken, must include an anteroinferior acromioplasty and resection of the subacromial bursa and coracoacromial ligament. Distal inferior clavicular osteophytes, if present, must also be resected. In the absence of instability, a frayed or partially torn rotator cuff indicates primary subacromial impingement, which responds favorably to decompression. Those athletes with a complete rotator cuff tear, however, will require a rotator cuff repair. This can be accomplished using either an open or arthroscopically assisted technique.[7]

Those athletes in groups II and III have underlying primary instability with secondary internal impingement. Arthroscopic subacromial decompression in these individuals does not address their underlying instability. With time, recurrence of the impingement syndrome is expected. These athletes, as well as those in Group IV (pure instability without impingement), require glenohumeral joint stabilization in order to eliminate the instability and

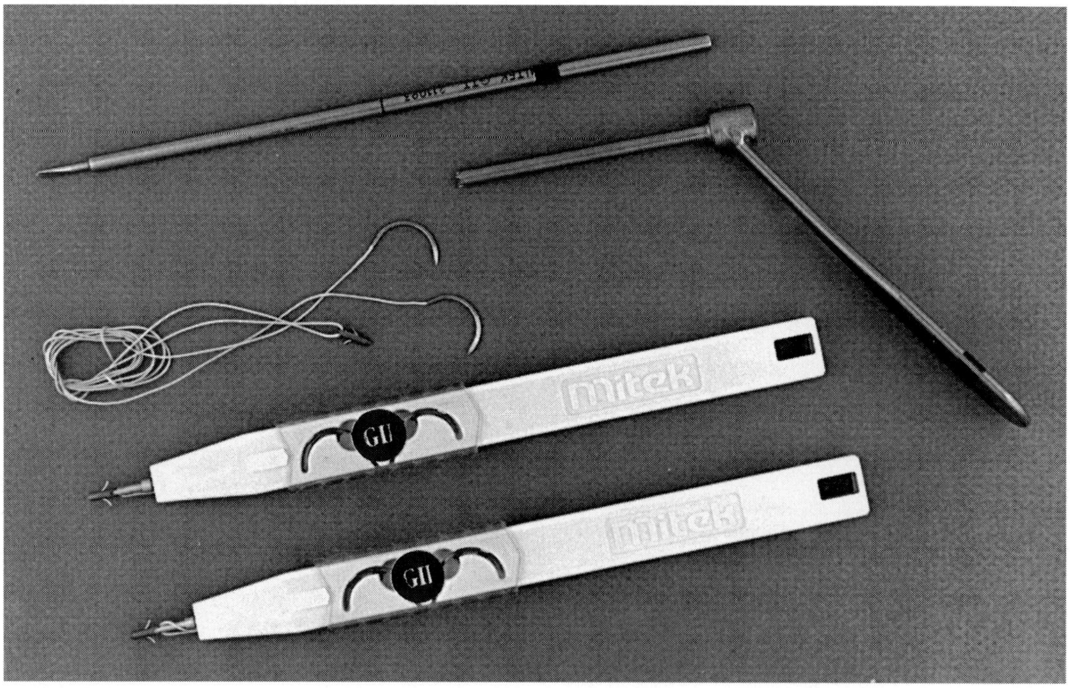

Fig. 11–6. Mitek instrumentation: preloaded G-2 Mitek anchors with No. 1 Ethibond sutures.

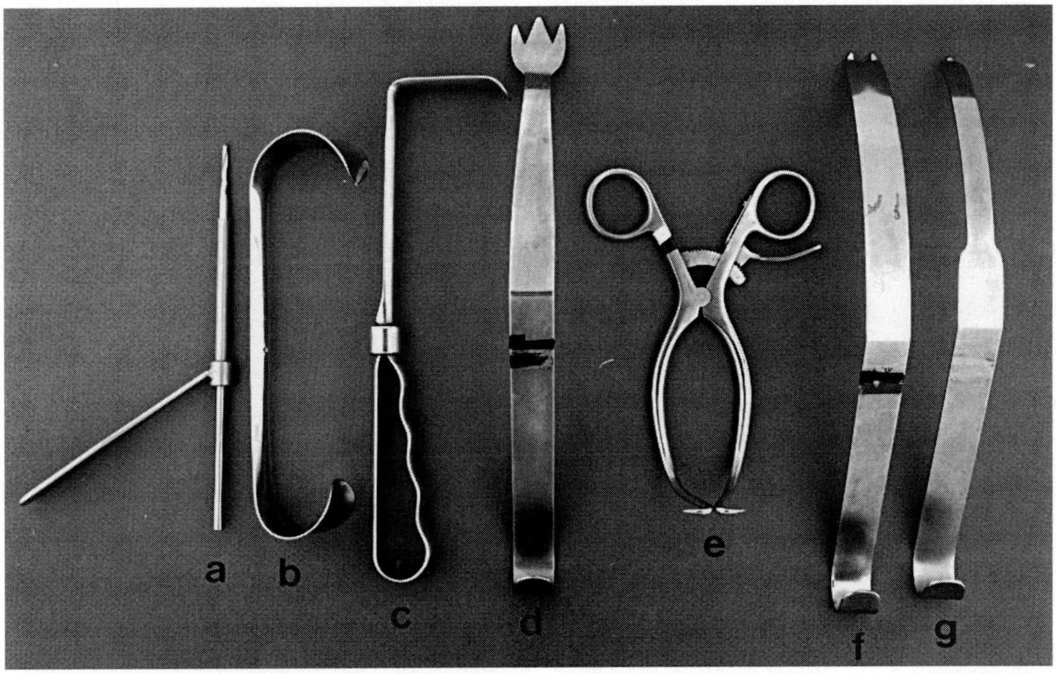

Fig. 11–7. **Anspach shoulder instruments: *A,* Mitek drill and drill guide; *B,* modified Goulet retractor; *C,* long narrow Richardson retractor; *D,* pitchfork retractor; *E,* modified Gelpi retractor; *F,* double-pronged humeral head retractor; and *G,* single-pronged humeral head retractor (narrow).**

their symptoms. Recently, this has been accomplished using an Anterior Capsulolabral Reconstruction (ACLR),[22,61–63] which is a modification of the procedure originally described by Bankart[64] and Rowe.[65] The capsular shift, which is fashioned on the glenoid side of the joint, tightens the attenuated or redundant capsule at the precise site of instability. Our most recent modification of this procedure now uses the Mitek instrumentation system (Fig. 11–6) to anchor the capsular flaps securely to the anterior neck of the scapula, adjacent to the glenoid margin. Numerous surgical techniques used in athletes have been previously described to address anterior glenohumeral instability.[66–69] However, we believe that the ACLR technique follows the four essential principles that will most successfully allow a throwing athlete a full and timely return to their former level of competition. First, all muscle attachments and their proprioceptive fibers must not be violated. Second, the glenohumeral joint capsule must not be excessively shortened, as this would limit postoperative shoulder mobility and thereby interfere with function and ultimate performance. Third, the anterior glenoid labrum and capsule must be reinforced at the exact point of instability. Finally, full range of shoulder motion must be regained quickly through proper postoperative abduction splinting and a specific rehabilitation program.

SURGICAL TECHNIQUE

Minor modifications of existing surgical instruments (Anspach Shoulder Instruments, Lake Park, FL) (Fig. 11–7) facilitate the operative technique by providing improved surgical exposure, limiting local soft tissue trauma, and reducing the need for additional surgical assistants.

After preliminary diagnostic arthroscopy, the patient is positioned supine with the involved extremity supported by a Parker arm board. Two folded surgical towels placed beneath the body of the scapula provide additional stability for the shoulder girdle and allow for posterior retraction of the humeral head. Through an anterior axillary skin incision, the deltopectoral interval is divided, retracting the cephalic vein laterally with the deltoid muscle (Fig. 11–8). Modified Goulet retractors maintain patency of the deltopectoral interval (Fig. 11–9), allowing exposure of the underlying conjoined tendon. The conjoined tendon is then dissected from the underlying subscapularis muscle and retracted (together with the pectoralis major muscle) medially using a long narrow Richardson retractor (Fig. 11–10). The arm is now externally rotated to provide improved exposure of the subscapularis muscle and to position the long head of the biceps laterally "out of harm's way." Needle-point electrocautery is used to split the subscapularis horizontally along the direction of its fibers at the junction of the upper two thirds and lower one third (Fig. 11–11). Blunt dissection beginning medially and progressing laterally is used to develop the interval between the overlying subscapularis and the closely adherent underlying joint capsule. A modified Gelpi retractor is then inserted to maintain this interval. Next, a blunt-tipped, three-pronged "pitchfork" retractor is carefully positioned along the anterior scapular neck just medial to the glenoid rim to allow wide exposure of the glenohumeral joint capsule (Fig. 11–12).

At this point, the capsule is incised horizontally in line with the subscapularis division (Fig. 11–13). With manual distraction of the glenohumeral joint, a narrow single- or double-pronged humeral head retractor is placed across the joint to the posterior glenoid rim to retract the humeral head laterally. This allows better visualization of the joint and anterior glenoid rim. Stay sutures placed in the superior and inferior capsular flaps at the level of the glenoid rim allow improved handling of these capsular tissues. With sharp dissection, the capsule and periosteum are elevated from the anterior scapular neck. The inferior flap must be dissected inferiorly to the 6-o'clock position to allow sufficient superior advancement (shift) in order to completely eliminate the redundant inferior capsular pouch. If the labrum is intact and the capsule merely redundant (group III), the capsulotomy, when carried out medially, must avoid cutting the intact labrum. If a Bankart lesion is encountered (groups II and IV), the damaged labrum is incised and elevated along with the capsular flaps and incorporated into the capsular reconstruction.

Using the No. 2 Mitek drill bit, drill sleeve, and power

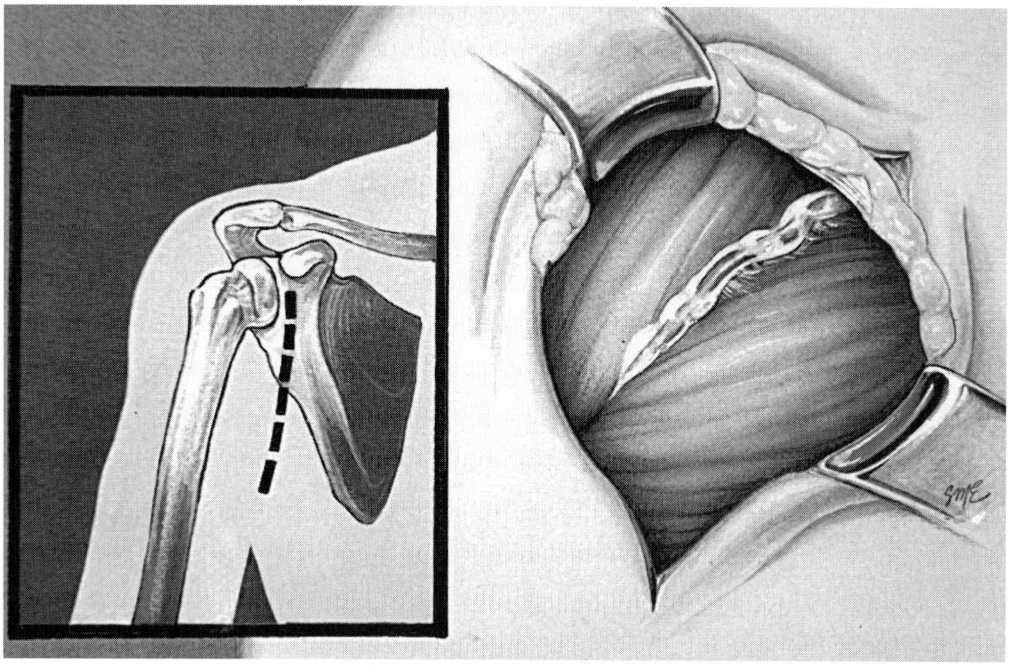

Fig. 11–8. Anterior axillary skin incision and deltopectoral groove.

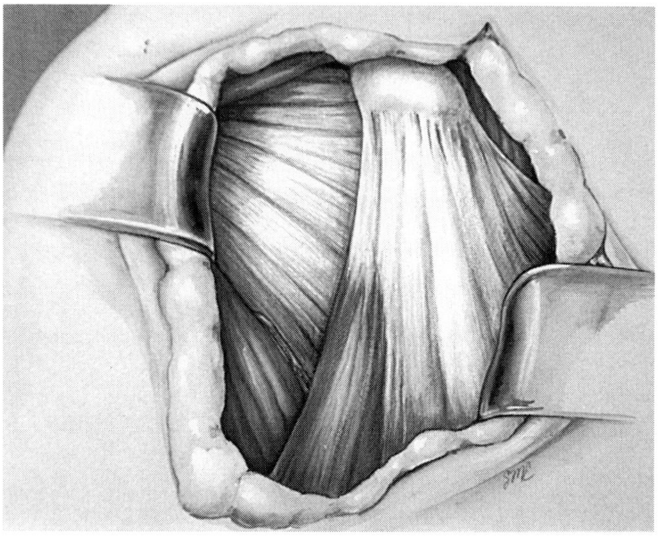

Fig. 11–9. Exposure of conjoined tendon.

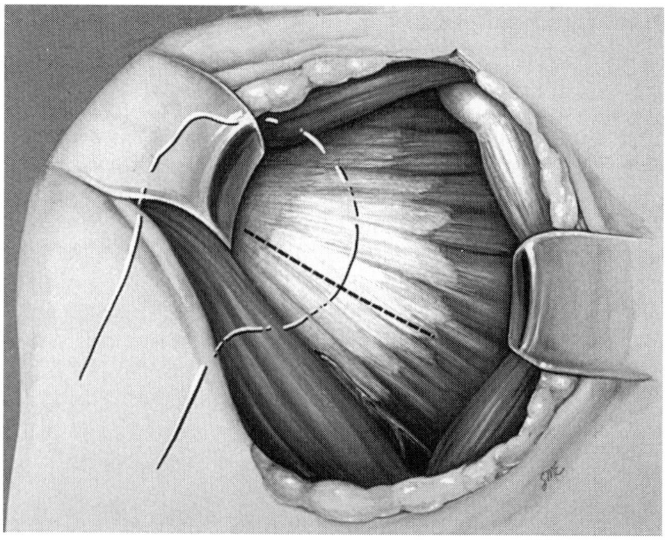

Fig. 11–10. Exposure of subscapularis muscle.

drill, three drill holes are created along the anterior glenoid rim 2 to 3 mm medial to the articular margin (Fig. 11–14). These drill holes will be located at the 2-, 4- and 5-o'clock positions for the right shoulder and 10-, 8- and 7-o'clock positions for the left shoulder (Fig. 11–15). The Mitek drill bit is marked to indicate the correct tunnel depth to accommodate the Mitek GII anchor and its attached suture. These are then inserted sequentially into each drill hole.

By applying tension along the inferior stay suture, the inferior capsular flap is advanced superiorly and secured into position using the double stranded No. 1 Ethibond sutures (Fig. 11–16). It is essential that each anchoring suture be placed within the capsule at the level of the glenoid margin, as marked by the stay suture. Placement of sutures laterally will excessively tighten the capsule when these sutures are tied and potentially limit postoperative range of motion. The superior capsular flap is then shifted inferiorly over the inferior capsular flap and secured into position using the same double-limbed sutures (Fig. 11–17). The humeral head retractor may be removed to relieve undue tension on the capsular flaps before tying these sutures. The arm is now positioned in 90° abduction and 75 to 85° of external rotation, as nonabsorbable sutures are used to closed the remaining capsulotomy in a ''pants-over-vest'' fashion (Fig. 11–18). The

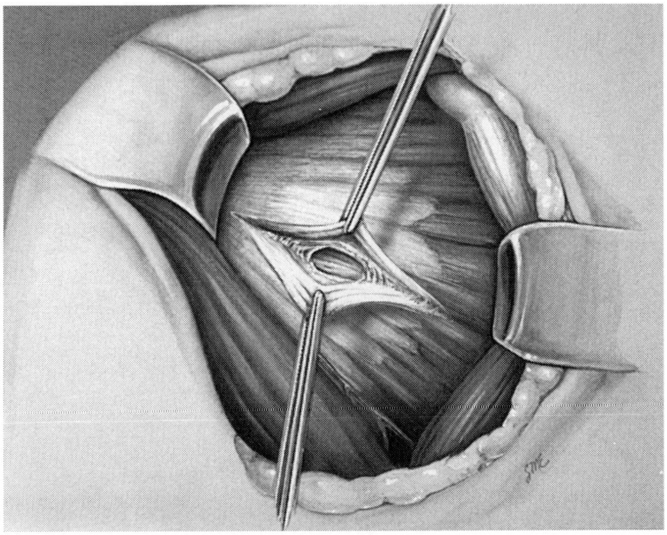

Fig. 11–11. Subscapularis muscle split at junction of upper two thirds and lower one third.

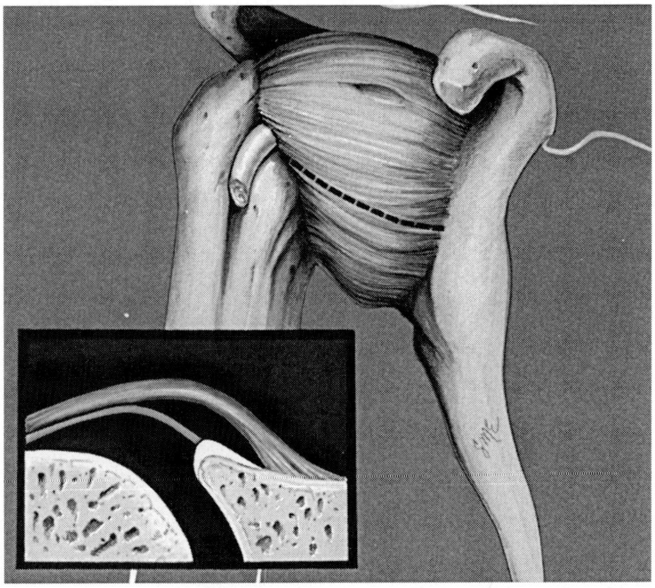

Fig. 11–13. Capsular incision located at junction of upper two thirds and lower one third. Inset: redundant anterior capsule with underlying synovial lining and intact glenoid labrum.

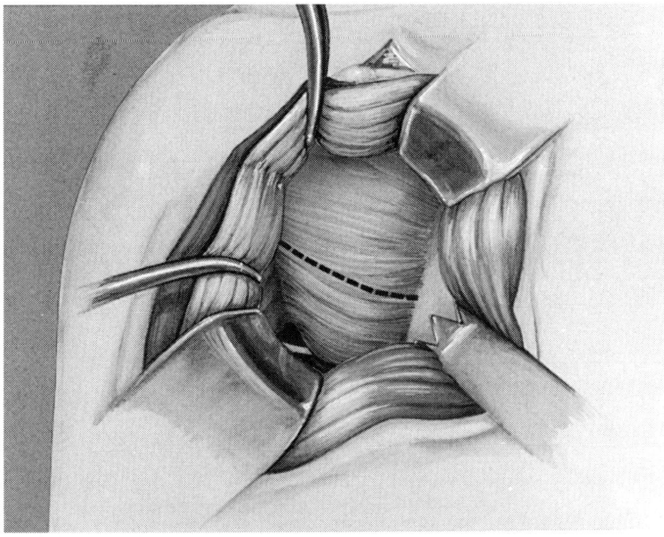

Fig. 11–12. Glenohumeral joint capsule exposure. Dotted line indicates sight of capsulotomy.

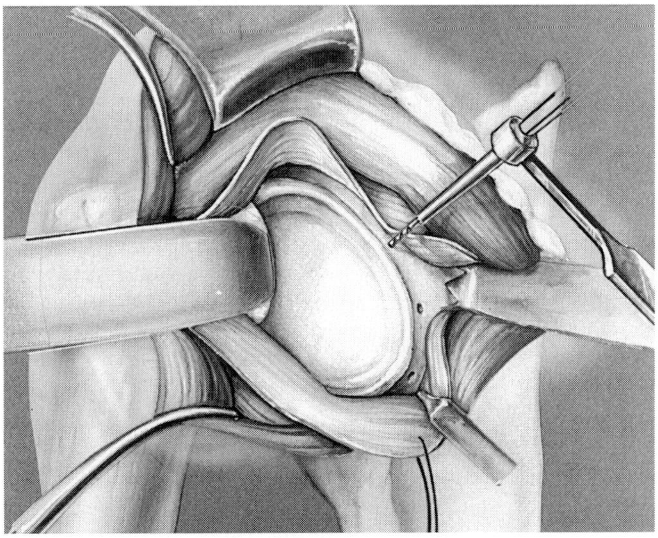

Fig. 11–14. Mitek system used to drill anchoring holes for Mitek sutures.

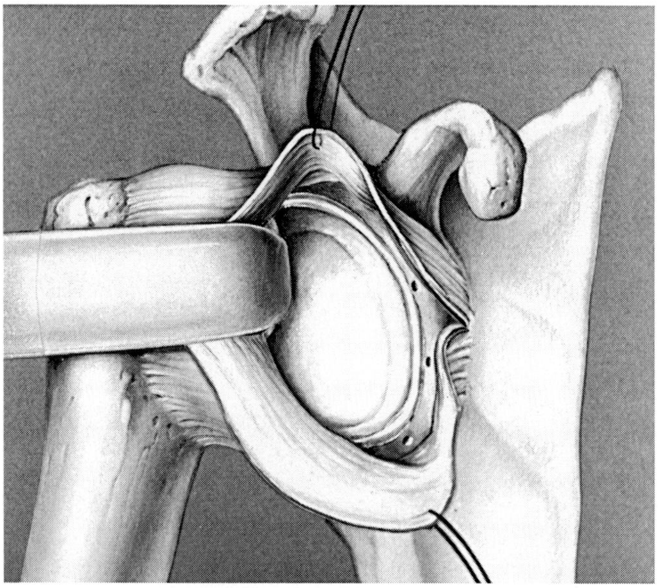

Fig. 11–15. Drill holes located along anterior glenoid rim.

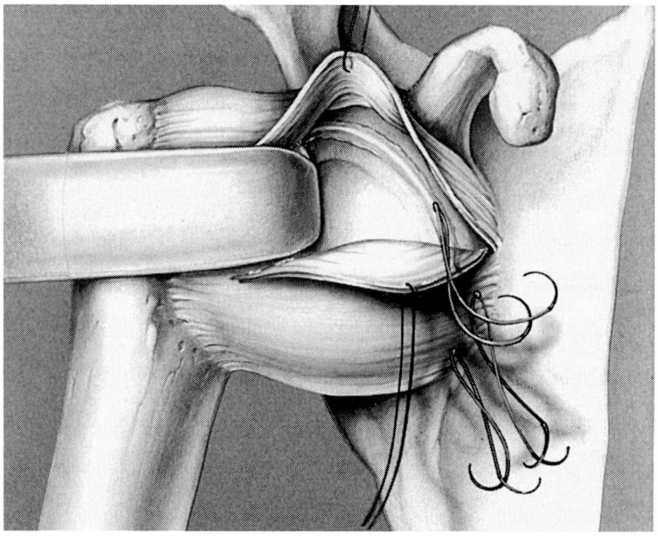

Fig. 11–16. Inferior capsular flap shifted superiorly and "anchored" into position.

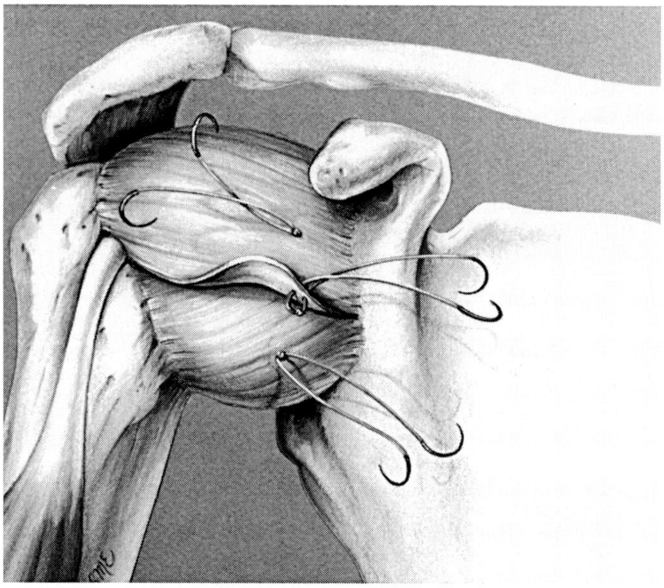

Fig. 11–17. Superior capsular flap shifted inferiorly, overlying the inferior flap.

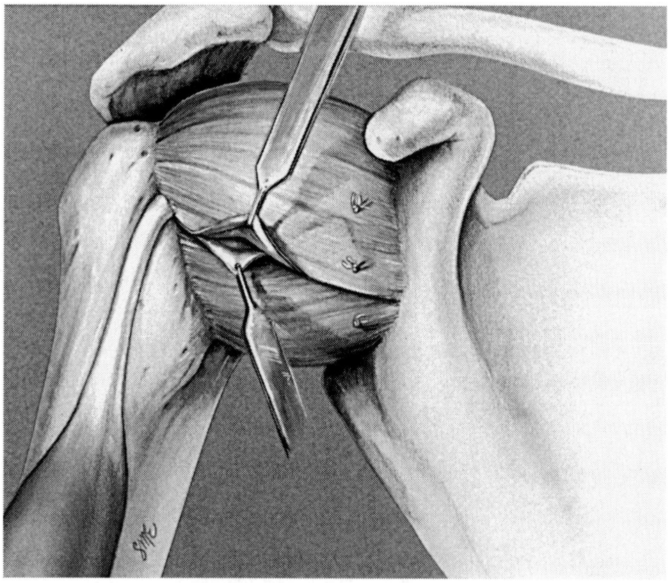

Fig. 11–18. Closure of capsulotomy in "pants-over-vest" fashion.

subscapularis is reapproximated and routine wound closure is performed (Fig. 11–19). This capsular shift procedure eliminates the capsular redundancy, reinforces the glenohumeral joint at the site of previous instability, and provides secure fixation of these tissues to the anterior glenoid rim. The throwing patient is then placed in a shoulder-arm-system postoperative orthosis (Zinco Industries, Pasadena, CA), which maintains the arm in 90° humeral abduction, 45° external rotation, and 30° forward flexion. This position allows for capsular healing in a position of function, facilitates rehabilitation, and allows for an earlier return to full range of shoulder motion. The splint is worn at all times except during rehabilitative exercises and is discontinued when the patient can actively abduct and forward flex the arm to 90° (usually within 2 weeks).

REHABILITATION

The rehabilitation program begins on the first postoperative day and continues for approximately 6 to 12 months. Each session lasts approximately 45 minutes to 1 hour. The patient is assigned ball-squeezing exercises and is encouraged to perform wrist flexion and extension exercises. The shoulder is passively ranged in abduction, flexion, and external rotation as tolerated. This is done in the scapular plane with no forced motion. Active, as-

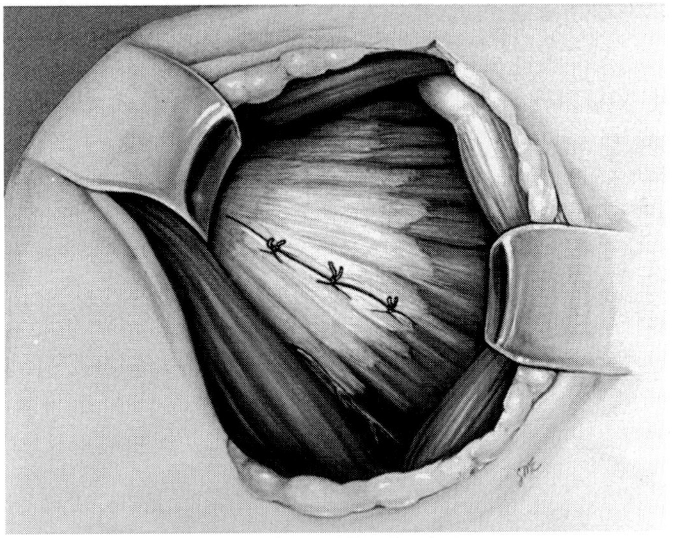

Fig. 11–19. Closure of subscapularis muscle.

sisted shoulder range of motion, as well as isometric abduction strengthening exercises, are continued.

Within 2 weeks most patients can actively abduct the arm from 0 to 90°. Active internal rotation exercises, with the arm at the side along with external rotation to neutral, are begun with the use of rubber tubing to provide gentle resistance. As the patient progresses, shoulder extension exercises in the prone position and external rotation to tolerance in the side-lying position are added. Shoulder shrugs and active shoulder abduction exercises to 90° are also carried out.

For the first 2 months following surgery, strengthening exercises are continued with emphasis on the rotator cuff muscles. Strengthening exercises in horizontal abduction and shoulder flexion are added, and upper body endurance training with an ergometer at low resistance is begun. Within 8 to 12 weeks most patients have achieved full forward flexion and abduction, with some minor restriction in regard to full external rotation. Early in the rehabilitation period, this is acceptable in order to protect the anterior capsule from being stretched too vigorously until all soft-tissue healing is complete. As all pain resolves, a vigorous strengthening program is undertaken using isokinetic training machines using three different speeds to increase the strength, power, and endurance of the rotator cuff muscles. Strengthening of the scapular rotators, biceps, triceps, pectoralis, and deltoid muscles are added and continued for a minimum of 1 year.

After 6 months an isokinetic strength and endurance test can be performed to evaluate internal and external rotation, flexion/extension, and abduction/adduction. If the patient has at least 80% strength of the contralateral shoulder, a progressive throwing program is begun. By 9 months postsurgery these patients are throwing for 30 minutes each day, while continuing a total body conditioning program. Within 8 to 12 months most patients reach a point where strength, power, and endurance is restored, muscle synchrony returns to normal, and performance is maximized. At this time, the athlete is allowed to return to all activities but is encouraged to maintain an ongoing home maintenance program of shoulder flexibility and strengthening exercises.

RESULTS

From December 1989 through July 1990, 35 consecutive athletes (including 18 baseball players, 13 of whom were pitchers) with shoulder pain secondary to anterior glenohumeral instability, which had failed to improve with conservative therapy, underwent an anterior capsulolabral reconstruction.[70] There were 12 professional, 11 collegiate, and 8 recreational athletes. At a minimum follow-up of 24 months, the results were graded as excellent in 24 patients (71%), good in 9 patients (26%), and poor in 1 patient (3%). Overall, 25 (74%) of the 34 athletes returned to their prior competitive level and competed in their sport for at least one complete season. Five (15%) of the 34 patients returned to the same sport but at a lower level of competition and 4 (11%) did not return to their sport. Twelve (67%) of the 18 baseball players, including 9 (69%) of 13 baseball pitchers, and 6 (86%) of 7 professional baseball pitchers returned to their prior level of competition. Athletes required an average of 12 months to return to full competition. Pitchers were initially restricted from pitching at full speed for a minimum of 6 months; however, we have now extended this restriction to 1 year to allow additional time for rehabilitation.

The one poor result was a 20-year-old competitive college swimmer who sustained a traumatic anterior shoulder dislocation while playing hockey 21 months after his initial shoulder reconstruction. Although considered a failure of surgery, he was treated conservatively and has returned to his previous level of competitive swimming.

Four of the 34 patients (12%) have undergone additional surgery following their index operation. One professional outfielder lost 25° of external humeral rotation and required an anterior capsular release. Although his range of motion returned to normal, he did not return to professional baseball. Three baseball pitchers underwent arthroscopic debridement for posterior shoulder pain. The two professional pitchers returned to their same level of competition. The remaining patient, a college-level pitcher, lost velocity on his pitches and ultimately changed positions (becoming a catcher).

The average loss of postoperative range of motion was 2°. There were no intraoperative or postoperative complications in patients involved in this study. Radiographs obtained at follow-up also demonstrated that all Mitek anchors had remained well seated within the glenoid neck in all patients.

SUMMARY

In the overhead or throwing athlete, the shoulder is extremely vulnerable to injury because of repetitive, high-energy forces. When these stresses are applied at a rate that exceeds the rate of tissue repair, progressive damage to the shoulder's stabilizing structures can occur. With continued throwing, the static restraints become progressively attenuated, allowing anterior glenohumeral subluxation. Initially, the dynamic stabilizers can compensate for this mild instability with increased muscle activity. However, prolonged activity may lead to fatigue. Over time, these compensatory mechanisms can become overloaded. The humeral head may then subluxate anteriorly allowing the undersurface of the rotator cuff to impinge along the posterior superior glenoid rim, causing pain and possibly limiting function.

Fortunately, conservative management is effective in most chronic overuse injuries and includes an initial period of relative rest (avoidance of throwing), oral nonsteroidal anti-inflammatory medication, a physical therapy program structured to provide local modalities to reduce inflammation, and a strengthening program for the rotator cuff and scapular rotators. For those athletes with continued symptoms, surgical intervention may become necessary. The appropriate surgical treatment will depend on the diagnosis. In the young throwing athlete with shoulder pain, it is essential to recognize that instability or occult subluxation, rather than impingement, is the primary underlying pathology.

The anterior capsulolabral reconstruction addresses the problem of instability by correcting the capsular redundancy and/or labral damage. When performed in the manner described, muscle attachments and proprioceptive muscle fibers are not disturbed and full shoulder range of motion can quickly be achieved. We believe this most recent surgical technique and postoperative rehabilitation program has resulted in a significant improvement in our ability to correct instability in those athletes who have failed a prolonged course of conservative care. Prevention of these injuries may hopefully be attained through continued research into the basic biomechanics and the pathoanatomy associated with overhand sports. In addition, further modifications of existing surgical techniques and refinement of rehabilitation programs may continue to more predictably and successfully return these athletes to their prior competitive level.

REFERENCES

1. Neer CS. Anterior acromioplasty for the chronic impingement. *J Bone Joint Surg Am.* 54:41–50.
2. Neer CS. Impingement lesions. *Clin Orthop.* 1983;173:70–77.
3. Jobe FW, Glousman RE. Rotator cuff dysfunction and associated glenohumeral instability in the throwing athlete. In: Paulos, Tibone, eds. *Operative Techniques in Shoulder Surgery.* Rockville, MD: Aspen Systems; 1991:127–133.
4. Jobe CM, Sidles J. *Evidence for a superior glenoid impingement upon the rotator cuff.* Presented at the 5th International Conference on Surgery of the Shoulder. Paris, France, July 1992.
5. Walch G, Bioleau P, Noel E, Donnell, ST. Impingement of the deep surface of the supraspinatus tendon on the posterosuperior glenoid rim: An arthroscopic study. *J Shoulder Elbow Surg.* 1:238–245, 1992.
6. Walch G, Liotard JP, Bioleau P, Noel E. *Posterosuperior impingement in the throwing athlete.* Presented at the 5th International Conference on Surgery of the Shoulder. Paris, France, July 1992.
7. Tibone JE, Elrod B, Jobe FW, et al. Surgical treatment of tears of the rotator cuff in athletes. *J Bone Joint Surg Am.* 1986;68:887–891.
8. Tibone JE, Jobe FW, et al. Shoulder impingement syndrome in athletes treated by anterior acromioplasty. *Clin Orthop.* 1985;198:134–140.
9. Fly WR, Tibone JE, Glousman RE. *Arthroscopic subacromial decompression in athletes less than 40 years old.* Presented American Shoulder and Elbow Surgeons 6th Open Meeting. New Orleans, LA, February 1990.
10. Anderson T, Bergfeld J. Common throwing injuries of the shoulder. *Mediguide to Orthop.* 1983;4:1–5.
11. Barnes D, Tullos HS. An analysis of 100 symptomatic baseball players. *Am J Sports Med.* 1978;6:62–67.
12. Blazina ME, Saltzman JS. Recurrent anterior subluxation of the shoulder in athletes: A district entity. *J Bone Joint Surg Am.* 1969; 51:1037–1038.
13. Jobe FW. Impingement problems in the athlete. *Instr Course Lect.* 1989;38:205–209.
14. Jobe FW. Painful athletic injuries of the shoulder. *Clin Orthop.* 1983; 173:117–124.
15. Jobe FW. *Rotator cuff problems in the athlete.* AAOS Specialty Day, AOSSM. February 7, 1988.
16. Jobe FW, Jobe CM. Painful athletic injuries of the shoulder. *Clin Orthop.* 173:117–124, 1983.
17. Neer CS, Welsh RP. The shoulder in sports. *Orthop Clin North Am.* 1977;8:583–591.
18. Norwood LA, Del Pizzo W, Jobe FW. Anterior shoulder pain in baseball pitchers. *Am J Sports Med.* 1978;6:103–106.
19. Tullos HS, Erwin WD, Wood GW, et al. Unusual lesions of the pitching arm. *Clin Orthop.* 1982;169–182.
20. Garth WP, Allman FL, Armstrong WS, et al. Occult anterior subluxation of the shoulder. *Am J Sports Med.* 1988;15:579–585.
21. Hawkins RJ, Kennedy JC. Impingement syndromes in athletes. *Am J Sports Med.* 1980;8:151–158.
22. Jobe FW, Bradley JP. *Anterior capsulolabral reconstruction.* Videotape Library of the American Academy of Orthopaedic Surgeons. 1987, V.T. No. 21–041.
23. Jobe FW, Bradley JP. The diagnosis and non-operative treatment of shoulder injuries in athletes. *Clin Sports Med.* 1989;8:419–438.
24. Jobe FW, Bradley, JP. Rotator cuff injuries in baseball: Prevention and rehabilitation. *Sports Med.* 1988;6:378–387.
25. Jobe FW, Bradley JP, Pink M. Impingement syndrome in overhand athletes, Part II. *Surgical Rounds in Orthop.* 1990;4:39–41.
26. Jobe FW, Kvitne RS, Giangarra CE. Shoulder pain in the overhand or throwing athlete: The relationship of anterior stability and rotator cuff impingement. *Orthop Rev.* 1989;18:963–975.
27. O'Brien SJ, Warren RF, Schwartz E. Anterior shoulder instability. *Orthop Clin North Am.* 1987;19:395–408.
28. O'Connell P, Nuber G, Mileski R, Lauteenschlager E. The contribution of the glenohumeral ligaments to anterior stability of the shoulder joint. AAOS Specialty Day, AOSSM. February 11, 1990.
29. Rockwood CA. Subluxation of the shoulder: The classification, diagnosis and treatment. *Orthop Trans.* 1979;4:306.
30. Rowe CR. Recurrent transient anterior subluxation of the shoulder: The "Dead-arm Syndrome." *Clin Orthop.* 1987;223:11–19.
31. Rowe CR, Zarins B. Recurrent transient subluxation of the shoulder. *J Bone Joint Surg Am.* 1981;63:863–872.
32. Cain PR, Mutschler TA, Fu FH, Lee SK. Anterior stability of the glenohumeral joint: A dynamic model. *Am J Sports Med.* 1987; 15:144–148.
33. D'Alessandro DF, Jobe FW, Perry J, Glousman RE, Pink M. *Dynamic stabilizers of the glenohumeral joint: An anatomic and electromyographic analysis.* AAOS Specialty Day, American Shoulder and Elbow Society. February 11, 1990.
34. Glousman RE, Jobe FW, Tibone JE, et al. Dynamic EMG analysis of the throwing shoulder with glenohumeral instability. *J Bone Joint Surg.* 1988;70:220–226.
35. Gowan ID, Jobe FW, Tibone JE, Perry J, Moynes DR. A comparative electromyographic analysis of the shoulder during pitching: Professional versus amateur pitchers. *Am J Sports Med.* 1987; 15:586–590.
36. Jobe FW, Moynes DR, Tibone JE, Perry J. An EMG analysis of the shoulder in pitching–A second report. *Am J Sports Med.* 1986; 12:218–220.

37. Wulken N, Spervescage C, Brene F. *The contribution of capsule and arthroscopic pressure to glenohumeral joint stability. A biomechanical study.* Presented at the 5th International Conference on Surgery of the Shoulder. Paris, France, 1993.
38. Bowen MK, Warner SJP, Deng XH, Warren RF, Torzilli PA. *The effect of joint compression on stability of the glenohumeral joint.* Presented by the 5th International Conference on Surgery of the Shoulder. Paris, France, 1993.
39. Moseley HF, Overgaard B. The anterior capsular mechanism in recurrent anterior dislocation of the shoulder: Morphological and clinical studies with special reference to the glenoid labrum and the glenohumeral ligaments. *J Bone Joint Surg Br.* 1962;44:913.
40. O'Brien SJ, Neves MC, Rozbruck SR, et al. *The anatomy and histology of the glenohumeral ligament complex of the shoulder.* AAOS Specialty Day, AOSSM. February 11, 1990.
41. Pollack RG, Bigliani LU, Flatow EL, Soslowsky LJ, Mow VC. *The mechanical properties of the inferior glenohumeral ligament.* AAOS Specialty Day, American Shoulder and Elbow Society. February 11, 1990.
42. Motzkin N, Ito E, Morrey BF, An KN. *Role of capsular structures in inferior shoulder stability.* Presented at the 5th International Conference on Surgery of the shoulder. Paris, France, 1992.
43. Turkel SJ, Panio MW, Marshall JL, Girgis FG. Stabilizing mechanisms preventing anterior dislocation of the glenohumeral joint. *J Bone Joint Surg Am.* 1981;63:1208–1217.
44. Morgan CD, Snyder SJ, et al. *Arthroscopic anatomy and variations of capsular ligaments based on 102 cadaver dissections.* AAOS Annual Meeting, Washington D.C., 1992.
45. O'Brein SJ, Neves ML, Arnoczky SP, et al. The anatomy and histology of the inferior glenohumeral ligament complex of the shoulder. *Am J Sports Med.* 1990;19:449–456.
46. O'Brein SJ, Arnozcky SP, Warren RF, Rozbruch SR. Developmental anatomy of the shoulder and anatomy of the glenohumeral joint. In: Rockwood CA, Matsen F, eds. *The Shoulder.* Philadelphia: WB Saunders; 1990:1–33.
47. Jobe FW, VanderWilde RS. Chronic shoulder problems in Athletes. In preparation for Orthopaedic Knowledge Update V. American Academy of Orthopaedic Surgeons.
48. Albright JA, Jokl P, Shaw R, et al. Clinical study of baseball pitchers: Correlation of injury to the throwing arm with method delivery. *Am J Sports Med.* 1978;6:15–21.
49. Atwater AE. Biomechanics of overarm throwing movements of throwing injuries. *Exer Sport Sci Rev.* 1979;7:43–85.
50. DiGiovine NM, Jobe FW, Pink M, Perry J. An electromyographic analysis of the upper extremity in pitching. *J Shoulder Elbow Surg.* 1992;1:15–25.
51. Gainor BJ, Piotrowski G, Puhl J, et al. The throw: Biomechanics and acute injury. *Am J Sports Med.* 1980;8:114–118.
52. Nuber GW, Gowan ID, Jobe FW, et al. EMG analysis of classical shoulder motion. *Trans Orthop Res Soc.* 1986;11:11.
53. Perry J. Anatomy and biomechanics of the shoulder in throwing, swimming, gymnastics and tennis. Symposium on injuries of the shoulder in the athlete. *Clin Sports Med.* 1983;2:247–270.
54. Perry J, Glousman RE. Biomechanics of the athletic arm. In: Nicholas JA, Hershman EB, eds. *The Upper Extremity in Sports Med.* St. Louis: CV Mosby; 1990:727–751.
55. Poppen NK, Walker PS. Normal and abnormal motion of the shoulder. *J Bone Joint Surg Am.* 1976;58:195–201.
56. Tullos HS, King JW. Throwing mechanism in sports. *Orthop Clin North Am.* 1973;4:709–720.
57. Cofield RH, Irving JF. Evaluation and classification of shoulder instability with special references to exam under anesthesia. *Clin Orthop.* 1987;223:32–43.
58. McGlynn FJ, Caspari RB. Arthroscopic findings in the subluxating shoulder. *Clin Orthop.* 1974;183:173–178.
59. Mizuno K, Hirohata K. Diagnosis of recurrent traumatic anterior subluxation of the shoulder. *Clin Orthop.* 1983;179:160–167.
60. Durkan JA, Wynne GF, Haggerty JF. Extra-articular reconstruction of the anterior cruciate ligament deficient knee. *Am J Sports Med.* 1989;17:112–117.
61. Jobe FW, Giangarra CE, Kvitne RS, Glousman RE. Anterior capsulolabral reconstruction of the shoulder in athletes in overhand sports. *Am J Sports Med.* 1991;19:428–434.
62. Jobe FW, Glousman RE. Anterior capsulolabral reconstruction. *Tech Orthop.* 1989;3:29–35.
63. Kvitne RS, Jobe FW. The diagnosis and treatment of anterior instability in the throwing athlete. *Clin Orthop.* 1993;291:107–123.
64. Bankart SAB. The pathology and treatment of recurrent dislocations of the shoulder joint. *Br J Surg.* 1938;26:23–29.
65. Rowe CR, Patel D, Southmayd WW. The Bankart procedure: A long-term end-result study. *J Bone Joint Surg Am.* 1978;60:1–16.
66. Aamoth GM, O'Phelan EH. Recurrent anterior dislocation of the shoulder: A review of 40 athletes treated by subscapularis transfer. *Am J Sports Med.* 1977;5:188–190.
67. Bigliani LU, Kurzweil PR, Schwartzbach CC, Flatow EL, Wolfe, I. *Inferior capsular shift procedure of anterior inferior shoulder instability in athletes.* AAOS Specialty Day, AOSSM. February 12, 1989.
68. Lombardo SJ, Kerlan RK, Jobe FW, et al. The modified Bristow procedure for recurrent dislocation of the shoulder. *J Bone Joint Surg Am.* 1976;58:256–261.
69. Neer CS, Foster CR. Inferior capsular shift for involuntary inferior and multidirectional instability of the shoulder: A preliminary report. *J Bone Joint Surg Am.* 1980;62:897–908.
70. Montgomery III WH, Jobe FW. Functional outcomes in athletes following a modified anterior capsulolabral reconstruction. Submitted *Am J Sports Med.* 1993.

Chapter 12

Partial-Thickness Cuff Tears

Hiroaki Fukuda, Edward V. Craig, Kaoru Yamanaka, and Kazutoshi Hamada

In the large spectrum of rotator cuff tendon pathology, the rotator cuff diseases include strain, inflammation, fibrosis, partial-thickness and full-thickness tears of the cuff, and ultimately cuff-tear arthropathy. After the introduction of shoulder arthrography, the diagnosis of full-thickness cuff tears became both accurate and objective. We have gradually accumulated knowledge of rotator cuff diseases since then. However, the diagnosis of partial-thickness cuff tears is still problematical in spite of the introduction of arthroscopy, ultrasonography, and MRI. It is unfortunate to observe, even today, that many patients with partial-thickness cuff tears are being treated under the diagnosis of "R bursitis" or "frozen shoulder," not infrequently for years. Furthermore, even after the correct diagnosis is reached, patients have been under-treated in many instances because of the term "partial" in partial-thickness tears. In reality, however, the surgical treatment of the extensive intratendinous lamination, for example, can be as difficult as treatment of the massive cuff tear.

By definition, a partial-thickness tear of the supraspinatus tendon is one of the three subtypes of tear with no communication between the glenohumeral joint and the subacromial bursa: (1) the bursal-side tear, in which the tear is only on the bursal side of the tendon; (2) the intratendinous tear, in which the tear is only in the tendon, without any communication with either the subacromial bursa or the shoulder joint; or (3) the joint-side tear, in which the tear is only on the joint side of the tendon (Fig. 12–1). The extent of tearing is at least one-third of the tendon thickness.

Partial-thickness tears, as a component of rotator cuff disease, are now considered to play a more significant role than previously recognized in contributing to the patient's disability and should, therefore, receive more attention. In this chapter the pertinent anatomy and histology, clinical features, diagnosis, pathology, treatment, and results of partial-thickness cuff tears are described. All of the information is based on our experiences with 39 surgically proven cases and the histological studies of 249 cadaveric supraspinatus tendons.

PERTINENT ANATOMY AND HISTOLOGY

The rotator cuff consists of four muscles: the subscapularis, the supraspinatus, the infraspinatus, and the teres minor muscles. They all arise from the scapula and are inserted into the tuberosities of the humerus. The vascular anatomy of the rotator cuff has been described by many investigators. In particular, the supraspinatus tendon receives its blood supply from the muscle belly through branches of both subscapular and suprascapular arteries and from bone through branches of the anterior circumflex humeral artery. The critical portion defined by Codman, which is located just proximal to the supraspinatus insertion and where most of the pathology occurs, is the area of anastomosis or watershed of these blood vessels and is known to be hypovascular. Within the tendon the blood vessels are more abundant in the bursal part than in the articular part.[1]

In normal aging of the supraspinatus tendon, Wilson[2] reported that loss of the regular wavy appearance of the tendon was an initial sign of degeneration. Further changes of the tendon were described as becoming granular, homogenous, and fibrillar. Yamanaka and Fukuda[1] demonstrated evidence of hyperplasia of the intima in the arterioles of the tendon with age (Fig. 12–2). This is further evidence, in addition to the reported results of microangiographic studies, of increasing hypovascularity in the critical portion of the supraspinatus tendon. The tenocytes in the articular part of the tendon adapt themselves to the low oxygen tension and transform into chondrocytes through metaplasia. The numbers of arterioles on the articular part are fewer than any other portions of the tendon. Therefore, the degeneration caused by hypovascularity with age is most conspicuous in the articular part of the tendon.

At the supraspinatus insertion the regular transitional four layers become more irregular and local disruption of the four layers appears more frequently as age increases (Fig. 12–3). The disruption appears to be a reparative process of the tendon insertion and the area involved is considered less resistant to mechanical stress.

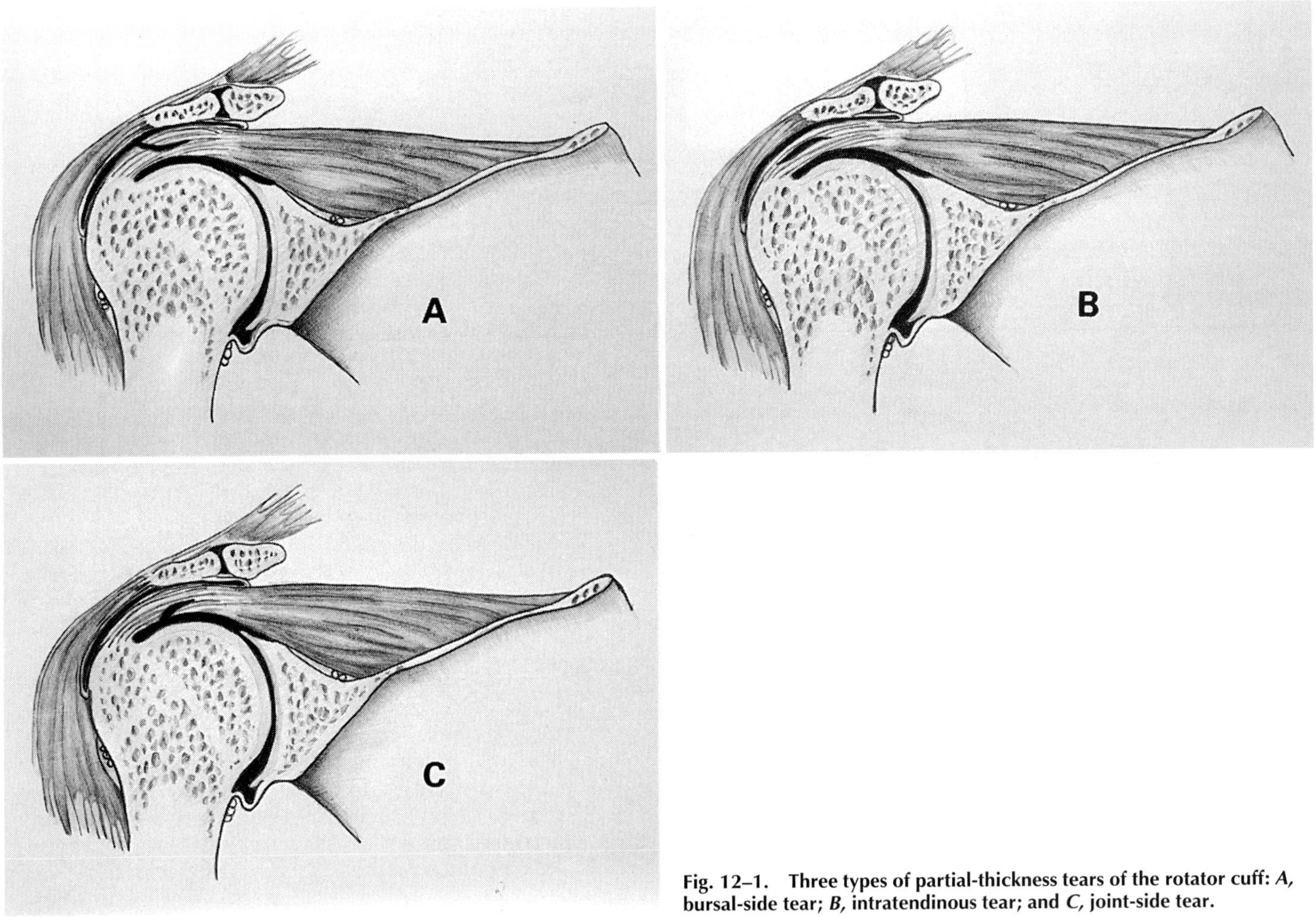

Fig. 12–1. Three types of partial-thickness tears of the rotator cuff: *A*, bursal-side tear; *B*, intratendinous tear; and *C*, joint-side tear.

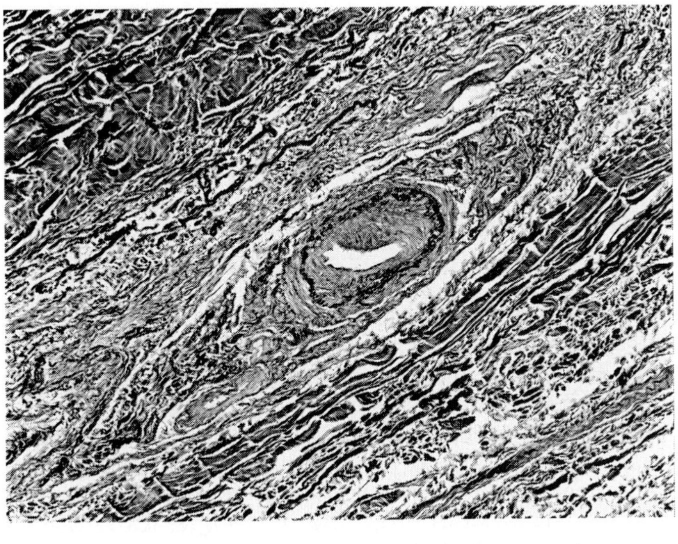

Fig. 12–2. An expression of changes of aging in the supraspinatus tendon. Intimal hyperplasia in an arteriole in the critical portion (E-v-G, original magnification ×96).

Rotator cuff tears are common after the age of 40. The incidence of rotator cuff tears in cadavers has been variously reported with a range of 6 to 19% for full-thickness tears and 6 to 33% for partial-thickness tears. Partial-thickness tears appear to be about twice as common. Yamanaka and Fukuda[1] reported on 249 cadaver shoulders (average age = 57.5 years) in which they found a 7% incidence of full-thickness tears. The incidence of partial-thickness tears was 13%; 2.4% were on the bursal-side, 7.2% were intratendinous, and 3.6% were on the joint-side (Table 12–1).

PATIENTS

The series consisted of 19 patients with bursal-side tears, 4 with intratendinous tears, and 16 with joint-side tears. There were 30 men and 9 women included. The average age was 45.9 years. The right side was involved in 21 patients and the left side in 18 patients. Twenty-two patients remembered definite trauma. The duration of symptoms averaged 13.3 months before surgery. The average follow-up was 34 months.

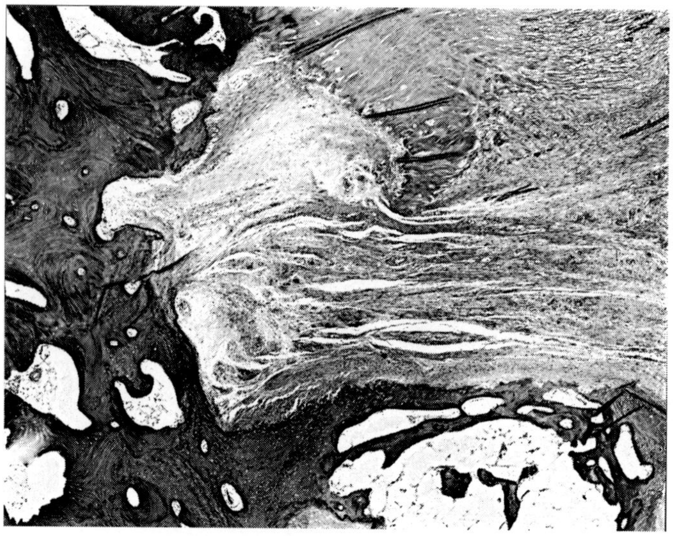

Fig. 12–3. Changes at the supraspinatus insertion. Destruction of the normal four layers of the tendon insertion, accompanied by proliferation of fibers and new capillaries (azan, original magnification ×37).

Table 12–1. Incidence of Rotator Cuff Tears in Cadaveric Specimens (n=249)

Type of Tear	*Specimens*		*Percentage*
Full-thickness tears		18	(7)
Partial-thickness tears			
Bursal-side tears	6		
Intratendinous tears	18	33	(13)
Joint-side tears	9		

CLINICAL FEATURES

The age of the patient is important in rotator cuff disease. Subacromial impingement may afflict patients at any age, but cuff tears are extremely rare below age 40 years and are common after age 50 years. Athletic patients in their second and third decades are not included in this study. Since Codman's original description, a history of trauma has been considered important for the diagnosis of a cuff tear. However, trauma has probably been over-emphasized. Recent studies have shown a lower incidence of trauma in patients with full-thickness tears (e.g., approximately 50% of the patients in Neer's series).[3] According to Neer, this kind of tear is referred to as an "acute extension" of a tear, which prior to the injury may have been a partial-thickness tear.[3a] The incidence of trauma in our series of 39 partial-thickness cuff tears was rather high at 56%.

The physical signs and symptoms of rotator cuff disease are multi-various and essentially nonspecific. However, they may be categorized into two groups: (1) those caused by inflammation, such as subacromial bursitis and rotator cuff tendinitis (designated here as category A), and (2) those caused by the torn tendon per se (designated here as category B). There is no clear delineation in symptomatology between partial-thickness and full-thickness cuff tears. Some of the commonly observed signs are as follows:

1. Pain: spontaneous pain and motion pain are almost always present in all stages. Night pain is the most annoying type of spontaneous pain. The bursal-side tear presents the severest pain among the three subtypes of partial-thickness tears. However, concomitant subacromial bursitis is almost always noted in both intratendinous and joint-side tears based on our surgical and pathological findings. The degree of pain may not be proportional to the size of the tear but proportional to the degree of inflammation.
2. Fluid sign: this sign was described by Codman[4] as indicating the accumulation of fluid in the subacromial bursa. The fluid sign is often seen in chronic full-thickness tears and less frequently in bursal-side partial-thickness tears.
3. Arc of pain: the pain in the arc between 70 to 120° of active elevation of the arm on the involved side. This test may become more pronounced when internal rotation is added by increasing the impingement.
4. "Distraction test:" this test was described by Fukuda[5] and is done to reconfirm the presence of an impingement lesion after the positive arc of pain. The arc of pain may disappear on passive elevation of the arm with a longitudinal traction against the patient's axilla because of distraction of the subacromial space.
5. Impingement sign: this sign was described by Neer in 1983. According to Neer, "to elicit the impingement sign, the humerus is elevated as the scapula is depressed with the opposite hand so that the greater tuberosity is compressed against the anterior acromion. This almost invariably produces pain if an impingement lesion is present. This maneuver also produces pain when other conditions are present, such as frozen shoulder, gleno-humeral instability, acromioclavicular arthritis . . ."[3]
6. Impingement injection test: this injection test has been known as Brown's procaine test and was popularized by Neer[3] with his concept of subacromial impingement. Complete temporary relief of pain by the injection of 10 mL of lidocaine (Xylocaine) into the subacromial space is positive. Although assessment is subjective, this is the most reliable test to prove the presence of an impingement lesion. Failure to relieve the pain indicates a cause other than impingement.
7. Drop arm sign: the sign is positive when the passively elevated arm cannot be held there and drops with gravity. The sign may be negative when the cuff tear is confined to the supraspinatus tendon but may appear in a large tear in which the infraspinatus tendon is also involved. It is also positive in paralysis of the C5 nerve root or if the pain is extreme.
8. Crepitus: crepitus is more marked in stage III lesions, especially when there is a full-thickness cuff

Table 12–2. Analysis of Signs and Symptoms of Rotator Cuff Tears

Those Caused by the Inflammation (category A)	*Those Caused by the Torn Tendon Per Se (category B)*
Pain	Drop arm sign
Fluid sign	Crepitus
Arc of pain	Muscle weakness
Distraction test	Spinati atrophy
Impingement sign	
Impingement injection test	
Contracture	

tear. However, it is also audible in the early stages of impingement.

9. Muscle weakness: weakness of abduction and external rotation is subtle and may not be appreciated until the cuff tear becomes massive involving the infraspinatus tendon. Testing muscle strength is also influenced by pain.
10. Atrophy of supraspinatus and infraspinatus: atrophy of the spinati appears in 2 to 3 weeks after an acute tear of the rotator cuff and also in chronic tears.
11. Contracture: Codman[4] described preservation of passive motion and the absence of contracture as characteristic of full-thickness cuff tears. It is true in general. Those patients with partial-thickness tears, however, tend to develop contracture. The reason for this difference is not clear, but the inflammatory process may be involved. In the presence of contracture, those tests listed here as numbers 3, 4, 5 and 7 are not valid.

Those symptoms, signs, or tests above described from 1 to 6 and possibly 11 are considered to belong mainly to category A, while those from 7 to 10 belong to category B. Thus, the signs and symptoms of rotator cuff tears have been rather arbitrarily categorized (Table 12–2). As the vicious cycle of subacromial impingement continues, the rotator cuff tear progresses from a partial-thickness tear to a full-thickness tear. When the relative balance of components between categories A and B is considered in a given patient, the former predominates in the early stages of impingement and the latter in stage III. This categorization of signs will have some implications for the treatment of rotator cuff tears.

DIAGNOSIS

Plain Radiographs

Plain radiographs are usually normal in the early stages of impingement and in partial-thickness or small cuff tears.

Shoulder Arthrography

Shoulder arthrography can demonstrate a partial-thickness cuff tear involving only the articular side of the cuff. The diagnosis was made by arthrography in 12 of 16 joint-side tears in the authors' series. However, shoulder arthrography is unable to demonstrate partial-thickness cuff tears involving only the bursal side. This bursal-side tear constitutes an important but often overlooked pathology of the rotator cuff after middle age.

Subacromial Bursography

Subacromial bursography was first performed by Lindblom[6] in 1939 and was advanced by Mikasa[7] in 1979 to evaluate the superficial surface of the rotator cuff. Fukuda and associates[8] reported 6 cases of bursal-side partial-thickness tears diagnosed by subacromial bursography. There was pooling of the injected contrast medium in the cuff tissue (Fig. 12–4), which was reconfirmed at surgery (Fig. 12–5). They recommend bursography following a negative shoulder arthrography for those patients with a persistent symptom complex of subacromial impingement. Interpretation of the bursogram, however, can be subtle and often difficult. The correlation between bursographic and operative findings was accurate in 6 of 9 cases in their experience. Subacromial bursography was performed in 13 cases of this series and was revealed as positive in 6 cases. The accuracy of bursography for the diagnosis of the bursal-side tear has not reached the point that arthrography has in the diagnosis of the full-thickness tear. Nevertheless, the value of the positive bursogram cannot be overstressed.

Shoulder Ultrasonography

Matsen and coworkers[9] first introduced shoulder ultrasonography to aid the diagnosis of rotator cuff lesions in 1984. The technique is noninvasive and, therefore, can be applied to the contralateral shoulder for comparison. The cuff defects are revealed as absence of the normal tissue echoes and failure of the tissue to move synchronously with the humeral head environments. Ultrasonography was performed in 16 shoulders in this series in which 15 were interpreted as abnormal. Two of four intratendinous tears were diagnosed by this method (Fig. 12–6). In a larger series of 141 patients from the University of Washington Shoulder Clinic, ultrasonography showed a specificity of 98% and a sensitivity of 91% when compared with surgical findings.[10] However, ultrasonic differentiation of scarring, partial-thickness, and small full-thickness cuff tears remains difficult. Even with experienced ultrasonographers, cuff tears smaller than 1 cm are often missed. With improvement in technology and the technique of ultrasonography, resolution may improve and demonstrate small partial-thickness tears, especially intratendinous tears.

Magnetic Resonance Imaging

MRI of the rotator cuff has been increasingly used. The criteria for diagnosing full-thickness tears have been

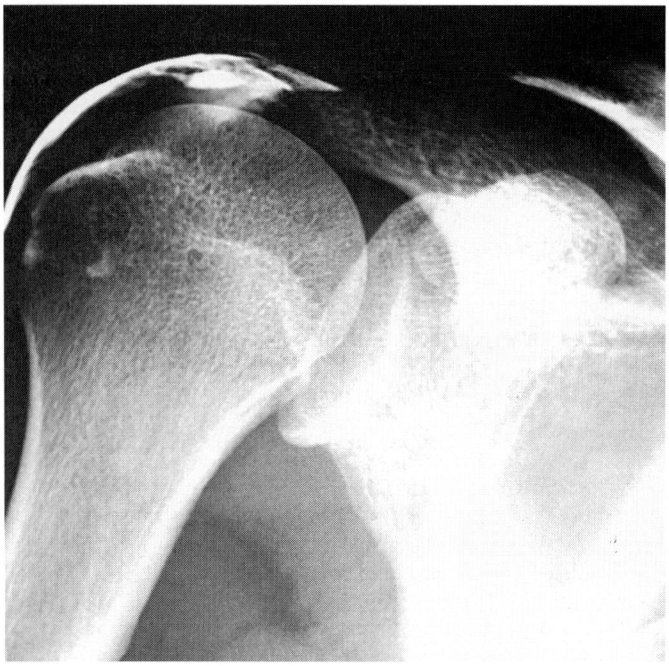

Fig. 12–4. Subacromial bursogram showing a localized pooling of the contrast medium in the cuff tissue.

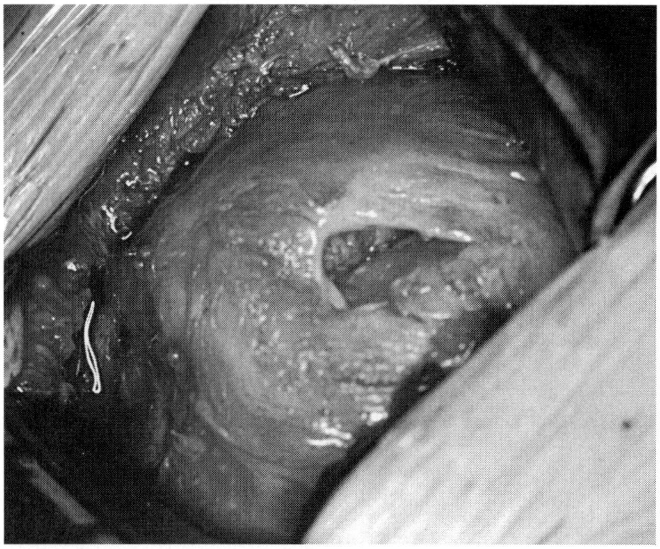

Fig. 12–5. A bursal-side partial-thickness tear was noted at surgery in the critical portion of the supraspinatus tendon.

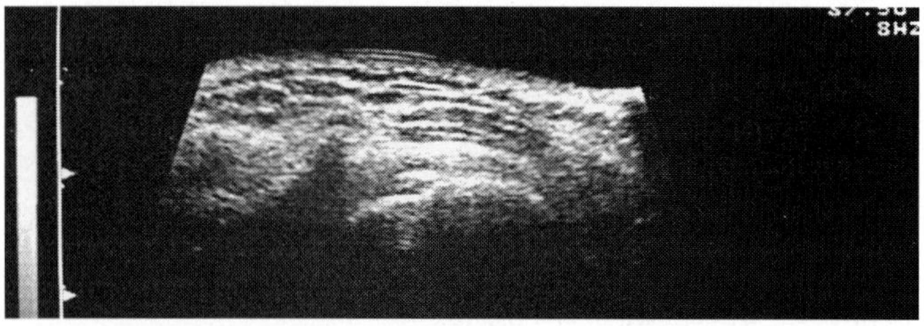

Fig. 12–6. Ultrasonogram showing a hyperechoic band in the supraspinatus tendon which was found to be an intratendinous tear at surgery.

fairly well established: a discontinuity of the tendon on T1-weighted images that reveals as fluid signal on T2-weighted images.[11] The use of MRI for diagnosing partial-thickness cuff tears has been attempted, but the criteria have yet to be defined, especially in the reoperated cases. MRI was not used in this series.

Shoulder Arthroscopy

The arthroscope can identify joint-side partial-thickness tears in the glenohumeral joint and bursal-side partial-thickness tears in the subacromial bursa, as well as the quality of the cuff tendon. In addition to the diagnosis, some surgeons perform arthroscopic decompression of the undersurface of the acromion without repairing the cuff defect. Arthroscopy was not used for diagnosis or treatment in this series.

Exploration

Six of 19 bursal-side tears and 2 of 4 intratendinous tears were diagnosed only after exploration. Incising along the supraspinatus tendon fibers to find intratendinous tears underneath did not do any harm even after negative explorations.

The Color Test

The joint-side rotator cuff tear and its extension are usually diagnosed by arthrography. However, it is not always possible at surgery to determine the exact site and extension of the tear when one is viewing the apparently intact bursal floor. "The color test,"[12] an intraoperative staining test with indigo carmine solution or methylene blue solution, was devised and was helpful in 7 of 14 joint-side tears. The tendon sheath for the long head of biceps brachii muscle and the rotator interval are two sites that are normally stained. They should serve for surgical orientation.

TREATMENT AND RESULTS

Treatment Option Based On Pathology

Treatment for rotator cuff disease varies according to the pathology. Most surgeons agree with this principle. However, for the rotator cuff tear, being either full-thickness or partial-thickness, we still do not know the answers to the following questions: Is spontaneous and anatomical healing possible? If it is possible, under what condition? How often does it occur? How long does it take? Codman[4] stated concerning partial-thickness tears that spontaneous healing occurred as a rule, but it was not substantiated by histologic evidence. We studied histologic sections from 12 en bloc surgical specimens of bursal-side cuff tears.[13] In most histologic sections examined, the proximal stumps showed chondrometaplasia of tendon tissue and were covered with thin layers of fibrinoid material. No active reparative process was observed in any portion examined, except in the distal stumps and at the insertions. It appears that healing is prevented by separation between the stumps, avascularity of the proximal stump (Figs. 12–7 and 12–8), and subacromial impingement. Therefore, it was concluded that most bursal-side cuff tears gradually progress through a vicious cycle and that the possibility of spontaneous healing is extremely low.

The same tendency was observed in two intratendinous tears (Fig. 12–9) and eight intratendinous tears associated with joint-side tears (Fig. 12–10). The intratendinous tearing was located in the midlayer of the tendon, and its axis is parallel to tendon fibers. The inner surface of the intratendinous tears appeared smooth in most of the specimens (Fig. 12–11), which suggested the presence of shear within the tendon. No active repair was noted in and adjacent to the intratendinous tearing.[13a]

On the other hand, we have experienced many "cures" in arthrographically verified full-thickness tears with conservative treatment. What is the explanation for this apparent contradiction? It may be explained as follows: in the total picture of the rotator cuff tear, if those signs and symptoms caused by inflammation (designated earlier as category A) are alleviated, and if those caused by the torn cuff per se (designated earlier as category B)

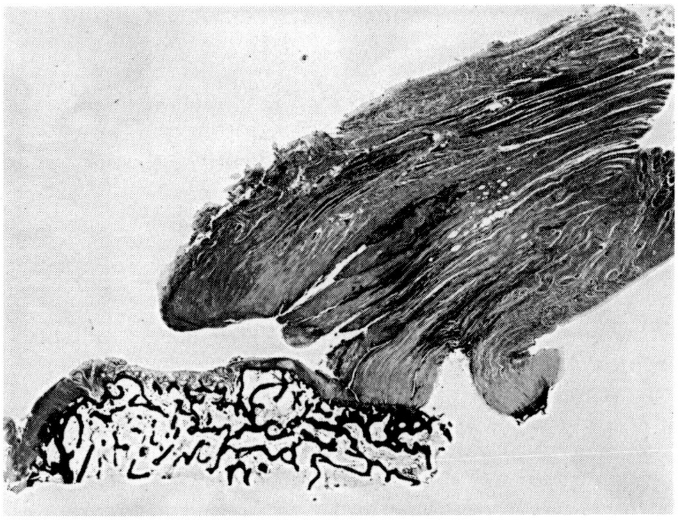

Fig. 12–7. A photomicrograph of a bursal-side partial-thickness cuff tear involving more than one-half thickness of the tendon in a 57-year-old man (azan, original magnification ×1).

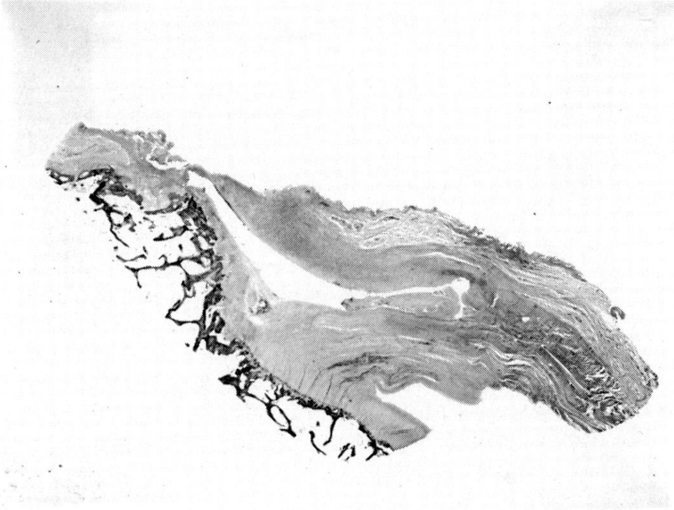

Fig. 12–9. A photomicrograph of an intratendinous tear of the supraspinatus tendon in a 42-year-old man, the distal end of which is close to the bursal floor (hematoxylin-eosin, original magnification ×1).

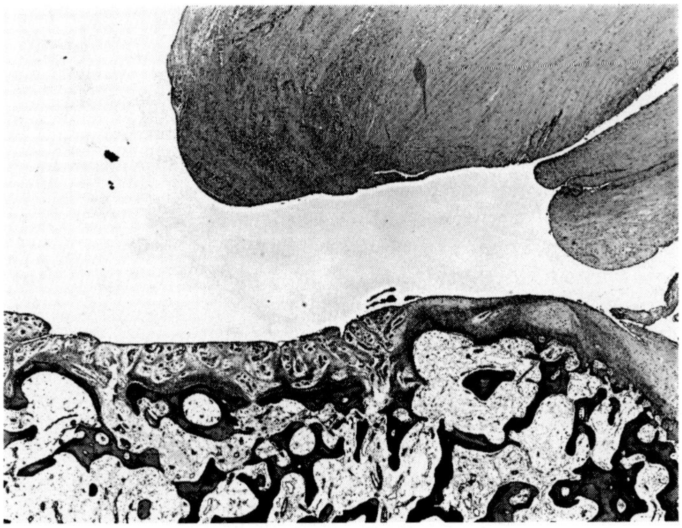

Fig. 12–8. A higher magnification reveals the proximal stump to be avascular with chondrometaplasia, while the distal stump to be well vascularized. There is no apparent evidence of successful repair (azan, original magnification ×15).

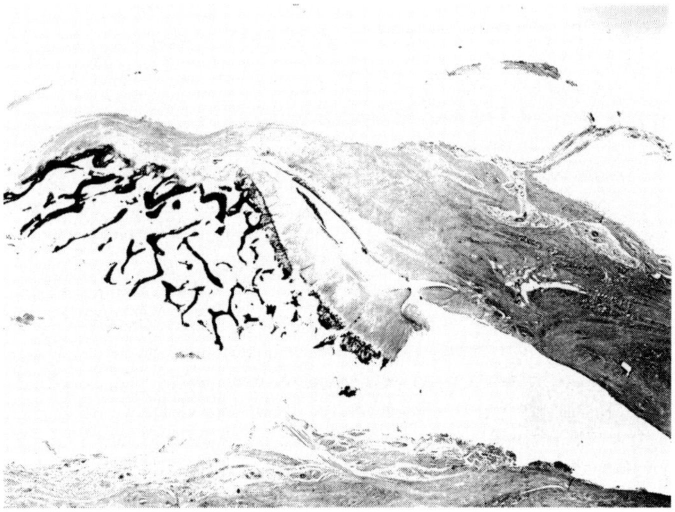

Fig. 12–10. A photomicrograph of a joint-side tear in a 67-year-old man that reaches almost four-fifths of the tendon thickness (hematoxylin-eosin, original magnification ×1).

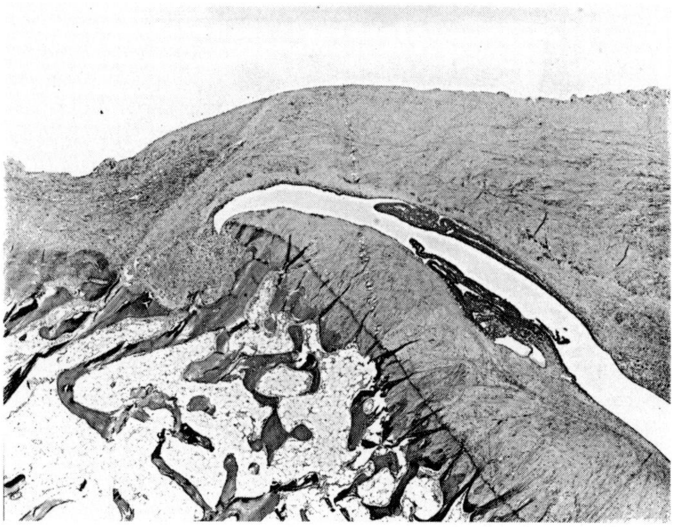

Fig. 12–11. A higher magnification showing the tearing in the midlayer of the tendon and its axis as being parallel to tendon fibers. The inner surface of the intratendinous tear is smooth and is covered by fibrinoid material suggesting the presence of shear within the tendon. No evidence of active repair is noted (hematoxylin-eosin, original magnification ×38).

settle either by the spontaneous healing of the torn tendon (which is unlikely) or by compensation of the residual cuff muscles, prime movers, and other extrinsic shoulder muscles, then a clinical cure may be obtained. Thus, conservative and surgical treatments are both possible therapeutic options. Conservative treatment is first adopted to relieve category A. If reasonable pain relief is accomplished within a certain period of time, muscle strengthening exercises are then prescribed to obtain a new scapulo-humeral rhythm. However, if pain relief cannot be obtained or category B continues to give patients much disability, surgical treatment is indicated. The length of time for conservative treatment varies from 2 weeks to 3 to 4 months, depending on the stages and the surgeon.

Conservative Treatment and Results

Conservative treatment is primarily indicated for tendon or bursal inflammation. Time, local rest, cold or heat, massage, acupuncture, nonsteroidal anti-inflammatory medication, modification of activities, gentle exercises for maintaining and increasing range of motion, and later muscle-strengthening are methods of treatment. The judicious use of no more than three to four steroid injections into the subacromial space or around the biceps tendon can also be helpful. If these conservative treatments fail to provide a response within 12 weeks, Neer[3] recommends arthrography to detect the presence of a full-thickness cuff tear. According to Cofield's review[14] of the literature in 1985, several investigators have observed patients with full-thickness cuff tears doing well with conservative treatment. The incidence of such satisfactory results was reported variously as 33%, 44%, and 59%. In the 90% of good results reported by Brown in 1949, stage I and stage II impingement must have been included. Because of uncertain diagnosis for both bursal-side and intratendinous tears, follow-up studies with conservative treatment for those categories are not available in a large series. Our results of conservative treatment for joint-side tears are satisfactory in approximately 40% of the cases.

Most bursal-side tears respond poorly to conservative treatment. Once the vicious cycle of subacromial impingement has been established and/or the tear is deep, conservative treatment is rarely helpful. We therefore operate early when a bursal-side tear is suspected from severe clinical manifestations and a positive bursogram. Conservative treatment is extended 3 to 6 months when it is suspected from physical signs alone.

In summary, conservative treatment for the rotator cuff diseases is effective in relieving inflammation in all stages. However, once a cuff is torn, whether it is a partial or a full tear, satisfactory results can be expected in only approximately 50% or less of such patients with conservative treatment. Spontaneous healing of the torn cuff tendon has not been substantiated.

Surgical Treatment and Results

Surgery for the partial-thickness cuff tear is indicated when conservative treatment fails, especially in order to relieve persistent pain. Different treatments have been employed, such as arthroscopic debridement, complete excision of the damaged area with tendon repair as an open procedure, subacromial decompression (both arthroscopic and open methods), or some combinations of the above procedures. We adopted open decompression (anterior acromioplasty) with excision of the involved tendon and repair in all 39 shoulders after an average period of 4.6 months of conservative treatment. AC arthroplasty was added in nine of the shoulders. Gross acromial spurring was noted in two shoulders. Nineteen bursal-side tears, 4 intratendinous tears, and 16 joint-side tears were noted in the critical portion of the supraspinatus tendon. The tear involved at least one-third of the tendon thickness in all patients.

Under general anesthesia an anterosuperior approach is used because of its excellent exposure of the supraspinatus and its environs with minimum deltoid detachment. The tendon repair is preceded by anterior acromioplasty. Bursal-side tears are now identified, but synovial proliferation may mask the small cuff defect. In order to detect both intratendinous and joint-side tears, the critical portion of the supraspinatus tendon and the adjacent area should be carefully palpated for a thinned area. "Puckering" may be seen when milking the tendon digitally or with a probe. Injecting color dye into the glenohumeral joint (the color test)[12] or incising the tendon along its fibers may be necessary to locate the undersurface tear site. The torn portion of the tendon is then excised in an elliptical or isosceles fashion until the healthier tissue is met and oversewn side to side or to a trough in the greater tuberosity.

Postoperative rehabilitation should be surgeon-oriented and individualized, because only the surgeon can tell the quality of both the tendon and the repair. The recent trend is to gain a full range of motion of the shoulder by early passive motion exercises (the second to third postoperative day) and to gain strength later. Approximately 5 to 6 weeks are necessary for the strong reattachment of the deltoid before active elevation of the arm is allowed. Six to 12 months are needed for the return of full use of the arm after successful repair of the cuff tear.

The results were assessed according to Neer's criteria.[15] Thirty-six of the 39 shoulders were rated satisfactory with an average follow-up of 34 months. Two patients continued having pain in overhead activity. One patient was lost to follow-up. We recommend this combined procedure for the following reasons: (1) the pathology is usually localized, (2) the diseased portion has low potential for tissue repair, (3) the progression of tearing can be prevented, (4) subacromial decompression is doubly ensured by both anterior acromioplasty and tenorrhaphy after the excision of the diseased portion of the tendon, and (5) tendon excision can be readily done in the same anterior acromioplasty exposure.

In 1972 Neer[15] treated partial-thickness cuff tears with anterior acromioplasty alone unless the tendon was thin, threatening complete tear, in which case repair was indicated. In a recent large series of Neer and associates, all 30 partial-thickness tears were treated with anterior acromioplasty; however, 20 of these tears were large enough to require tendon repair in addition.

Ellman[17] developed the technique of arthroscopic subacromial decompression (ASD) in 1985. He reported that among 20 partial-thickness tears, 15 had a satisfactory result using ASD, but 5 required additional surgery. Gartsman[18] demonstrated that arthroscopic acromioplasty is effective for chronic tendinitis and partial-thickness tears obtaining excellent to good results in 83% of 40 patients with an average follow-up of 29 months. Ogilvie-Harris and associates[19] treated 57 partial tears with arthroscopic debridement alone and found that only half achieved satisfactory results.

It is difficult to compare different treatments at this point because most series are small with short follow-ups. Furthermore, as requested by Ellman,[20] quantitative recording of the extent of partial-thickness tears should be available for the meaningful comparison of various reports.

CONCLUSIONS

Partial-thickness tears of the rotator cuff, consisting of the three subtypes the bursal-side tear, the intratendinous tear, and the joint-side tear, are not rare and have been up to this time a cause of nondocumented shoulder disability. However, these tears are now recognized as an important entity in the spectrum of subacromial impingement syndrome. The clinical diagnosis of partial-thickness tears is notably difficult and has often been mistaken for periarthritis, bursitis, tendinitis, bicipital tenosynovitis, or frozen shoulder. In addition to arthrography and arthroscopy, bursography, ultrasonography and MRI have been added to our armamentarium for more accurate diagnosis, especially of bursal-side and intratendinous tears. Surgery is indicated for those partial-thickness tears refractory to conservative treatment for 3 to 6 months. We recommend a combined procedure of anterior acromioplasty and subsequent tenorrhaphy after excision of the torn portion of the tendon. We have performed this type of surgery in 39 patients in whom 19 bursal-side tears, 4 intratendinous tears and 16 joint-side tears were identified. Satisfactory results were obtained in 36 of 39 (92%) shoulders with an average follow-up of 34 months.

REFERENCES

1. Yamanaka K, Fukuda H. Ageing process of the supraspinatus tendon with reference to the rotator cuff tears. In: Watson MS, ed. *Surgical Disorders of the Shoulder.* Edinburgh: Churchill Livingstone; 1991:247–258.
2. Wilson CL. Lesions of the supraspinatus tendon. *Arch Surg.* 1943; 46:307–325.
3. Neer CS II. Impingement lesions. *Clin Orthop.* 1983;173:70–77.

3a. Neer CS II. *Shoulder Reconstruction.* Philadelphia: WB Saunders; 1990:59.

4. Codman EA. *The Shoulder. Rupture of the Supraspinatus Tendon and Other Lesions in or About the Subacromial bursa.* Boston: Thomas Todd; 1934.
5. Fukuda H. Therapeutic regimen for periarthritis scapulohumeralis and rotator cuff tear. *Seikeigeka.* 1984; 35:83–90 (in Japanese).
6. Lindblom K. Arthrography and roentgenography in ruptures of the tendons of the shoulder joint. *Acta Radiol.* 1939;20:548–562.
7. Mikasa M. Subacromial bursography. *J Jpn Orthop Assoc.* 1979;53: 225–231.
8. Fukuda H, Mikasa M, Yamanaka K. Incomplete thickness rotator cuff tears diagnosed by subacromial bursography. *Clin Orthop.* 1987;223:51–58.
9. Matsen FA III, Kilcoyne RF. Sonographic evaluation of the rotator cuff. *Orthop Trans.* 1984;8:42.
10. Mack LA, Nyberg DA, Kilcoyne RF, et al. Sonography of the postoperative shoulder. *AJR.* 1988;150:1089–1094.
11. Iannotti JP, Zlatkin MB, Esterhai JL, et al. Magnetic resonance imaging of the shoulder: Sensitivity, specificity and predictive value. *J Bone Joint Surg Am.* 1991;73:17–29.
12. Fukuda H, Mikasa M, Ogawa K, et al. "The color test": An intraoperative staining test for joint-side rotator cuff tearing and its extension. *J Shoulder Elbow Surg.* 1992;1:86–90.
13. Fukuda H, Hamada K, Yamanaka K. Pathology and pathogenesis of bursal-side rotator cuff tears viewed from en bloc histologic sections. *Clin Orthop.* 1990;254:75–80.

13a. Fukuda, Hamanaka K, Nakajima T, et al. Pathology and pathogenesis of the intratendinous tearing of the rotator cuff viewed from en bloc histologic sections. *Clin Orthop.* 1994;304:60–67.

14. Cofield RH. Current concept review. Rotator cuff disease of the shoulder. *J Bone Joint Surg Am.* 1985;67:974–979.
15. Neer CS II. Anterior acromioplasty for the chronic impingement syndrome in the shoulder. *J Bone Joint Surg Am.* 1972;54:41–50.
16. Neer CS II, Flatow EL, Lech O. *Tears of the rotator cuff: Long-term results of anterior acromioplasty and repair.* Presented at the Fourth Open Meeting of the American Shoulder and Elbow Surgeons. Atlanta, GA, February 1988.
17. Ellman H. Arthroscopic subacromial decompression: A preliminary report. *Orthop Trans.* 1985;9:49.
18. Gartsman GM. Arthroscopic acromioplasty for lesions of the rotator cuff. *J Bone Joint Surg Am.* 1990;72:169–180.
19. Ogilvie-Harris DJ, Wiley AM. Arthroscopic surgery of the shoulder: A general appraisal. *J Bone Joint Surg Br.* 1986;68:201–207.
20. Ellman H. Diagnosis and treatment of incomplete rotator cuff tears. *Clin Orthop.* 1990;254:64–74.

Chapter 13

The Rotator Interval Lesion

Katsuya Nobuhara

In some patients with painful unstable shoulders the clinical picture does not fall into one of the routinely recognized disease states. For example, these patients may at times appear to have shoulder instability and at other times may seem to have impingement problems. However, routine radiologic examinations do not disclose a rotator cuff tear or a traumatically induced unstable shoulder.

The purpose of this chapter is to report a new clinical entity of the shoulder that is painful and oftentimes associated with anteroinferior instability. It is caused by an abnormality in the rotator interval and for the purpose of this chapter is referred to as the rotator interval lesion.

My interest in this entity dates to 1970 when a 33-year-old woman presented complaining of pain and stiffness in her shoulder to such an extent that she could not hold a newspaper open. This condition had interfered with her activities of daily living for 13 years. At approximately 18 years of age she had participated in strenuous sports, but she had no history of trauma. Clinical evaluation revealed acute tenderness of the lateral side of the coracoid process, pain when lifting the arm, and instability. All conservative treatments had been ineffective. Because injury to the rotator cuff was suspected, arthrography was performed; however, no definite signs of a rotator cuff tear were seen. At first, we could not arrive at a diagnosis, but a re-examination of the video recording of dynamic arthrography revealed leakage of the contrast medium into the rotator interval. We therefore considered that there might be a relation between the patient's symptoms as described and an abnormality in the rotator interval region. Without these findings, this patient would have been treated under a diagnosis of tendinitis, impingement syndrome, subluxation, or instability of the shoulder.[1] However, because of these findings the patient was taken to the operating room and her rotator interval was explored and repaired by the technique described in detail later in this chapter. Her almost 25-year follow-up forms the epilogue of this chapter.

ANATOMY AND PATHOPHYSIOLOGY

The space between the superior border of the subscapularis and the adjacent supraspinatus is termed the "rotator interval" (RI). It is formed by thin elastic, membranous tissue. The coracohumeral and the superior glenohumeral ligaments, as well as the capsule, help strengthen the tissue in the RI (Fig. 13–1).[2]

Observations made during shoulder operations in patients with a normal RI show that the tension of the structures constituting the interval space is constant during downward traction of the upper extremity whether the humerus is held in internal or external rotation. Moreover, the tissues constituting the RI normally do not become depressed or collapse inward during this maneuver. The RI forms a straight line in external rotation and becomes loose in internal rotation of the shoulder. It acts like a sleeve, changing its shape in each position to make shoulder motion smooth.

In patients with an abnormal RI, downward traction of the upper extremity in an internally rotated position causes the humeral head to subluxate inferiorly because of the untethered pull of the subscapularis (Fig. 13–2); this is not present in otherwise healthy joints in which the coracohumeral ligament resists this downward force. When the arm is placed in the dependent position and downward traction is applied, the humeral head sublux-

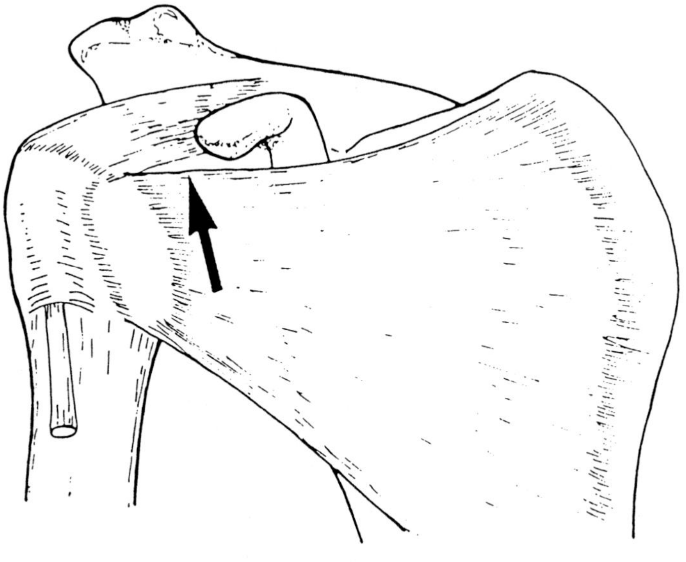

Fig. 13–1. The rotator interval (arrow).

ates inferiorly as if it were loose. This distinctive feature disappears when the coracohumeral ligament becomes taut during external rotation. In an elevated position, the humeral head may slip inferiorly and posteriorly, suggesting a posteroinferior instability.

CLASSIFICATION

Two clinical entities emerge as the result of RI injury. Type I, the contracted state, occurs when the RI is damaged, the subacromial bursa and the coracohumeral ligament become inflamed, and adhesions occur about the structures. This can result in contracture of the soft tissues, especially in older individuals. With more force and greater involvement of the surrounding tissues, instability may occur; this usually occurs in younger patients. Thus, disorders of the RI are classified as type I (contracted state) when associated with inflammatory changes of the more superficial tissues and as type II (unstable state) when associated with greater involvement of the deeper tissues (Fig. 13–3).

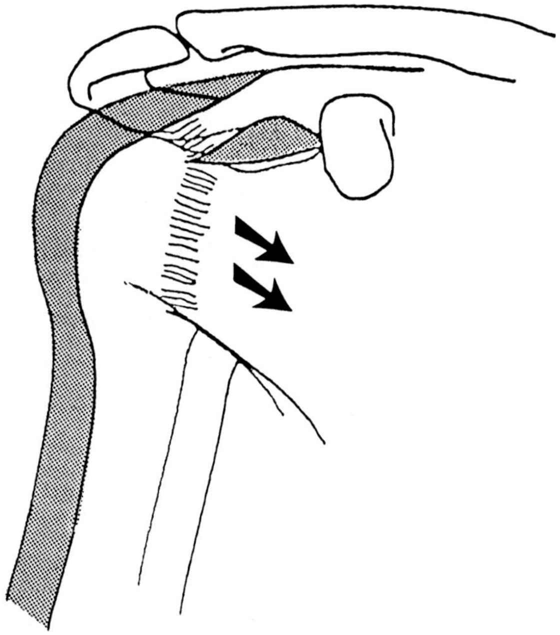

Fig. 13–2. An anteroinferior instability (arrow) with RI lesion.

DIAGNOSIS

The average age of patients with type I (contracted) RI lesions was 42 years of age; in contrast, the average age of patients with type II (unstable) RI lesions was 24 years of age. Both types of lesions consistently manifest pain. In the majority of type II patients, there is loosening or some degree of instability; no such findings are present in type I patients. Similarly, there is no anteroposterior instability in type I patients, while a significant number of patients with type II RI lesions have anteroposterior instability.

All patients complain of persistent soreness in the shoulder that is unresponsive to conservative treatment. Pain is most severe during abduction and external rotation. Slipping of the humeral head occurs in type II patients in varying degrees while in the elevated position. The normal rounded contour of the lateral aspect of the shoulder is lost as the deltoid flattens when the humeral head subluxates anteroinferiorly during the application of downward traction to the dependent upper extremity. This does not occur when downward traction is applied during external rotation of the arm, because the coracohumeral ligament becomes taut.

RADIOGRAPHIC FINDINGS

Plain radiographs clearly demonstrate an anteroinferior subluxation when downward traction is applied to the dependent upper extremity. This finding is not observed in radiographs taken with the shoulder in external rotation. Posteroinferior instability can be detected in the anteroposterior film taken during active elevation. During these active movements, symptoms of pain and discomfort arise as synchronous motion is lost. Even in the type I lesion, there is also a dysfunction of the shoulder motion.

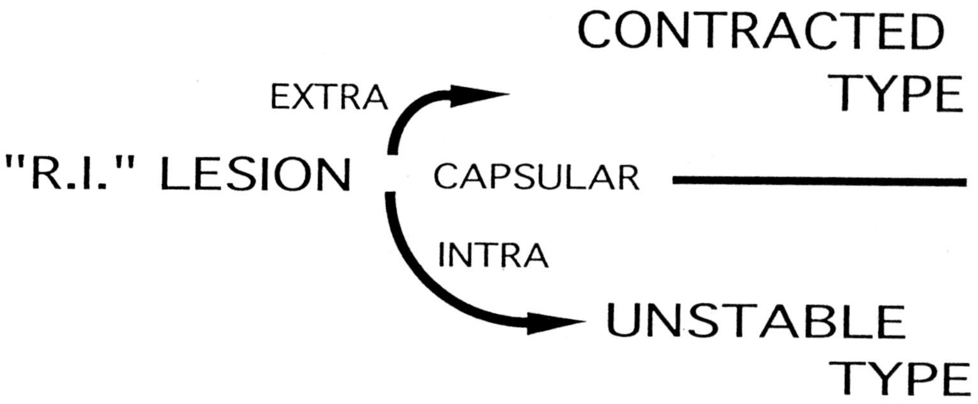

Fig. 13–3. Two types of RI lesions.

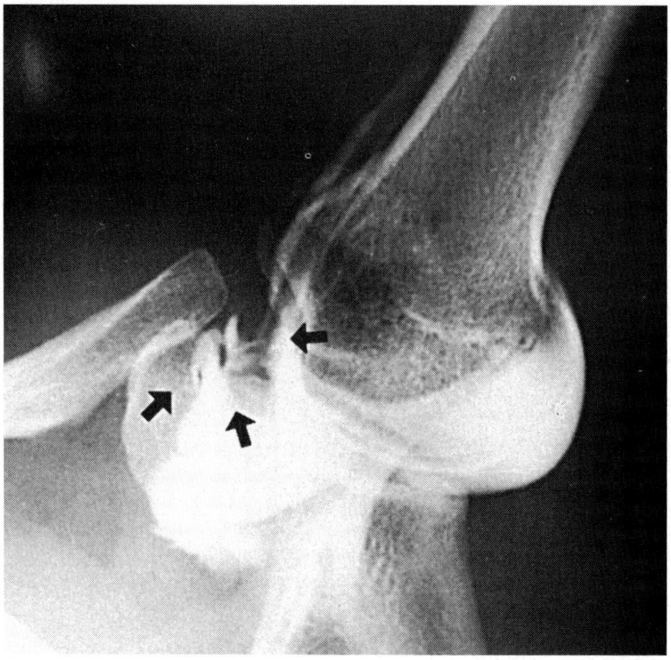

Fig. 13–4. An arthrogram showing contrast medium pouting the RI space (arrow) in a type II lesion.

Standard arthrographic films usually are interpreted as normal until the arm is actively elevated and externally rotated into the overhead position; the contrast medium is then seen pouting into the RI space (Fig. 13–4). This finding can easily be observed during dynamic cineradio-arthrography as the upper extremity is actively elevated and externally rotated. This phenomenon is always present in type II lesions but almost always absent in type I RI lesions. Obliteration of the subscapularis bursa was observed in 100% of type I and 25.8% of type II RI lesions.

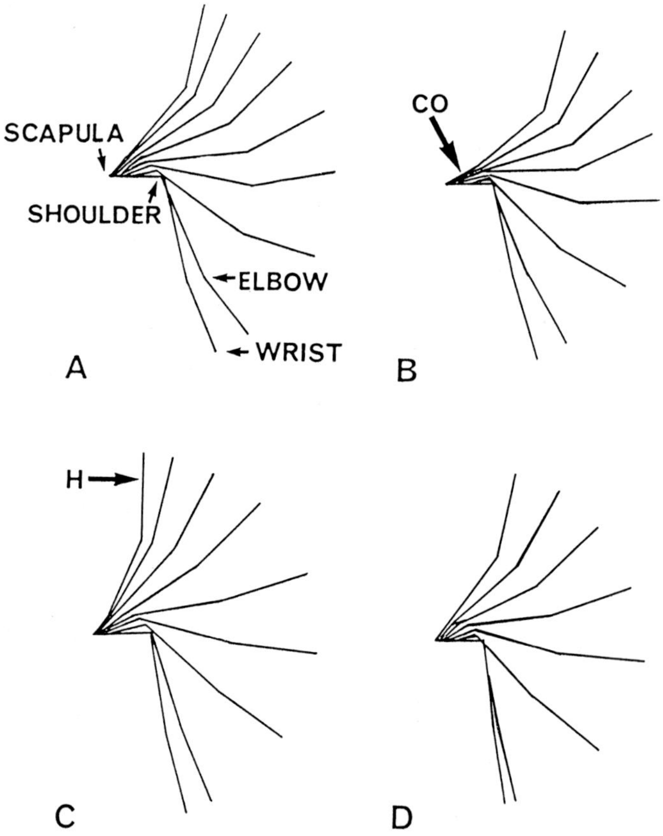

Fig. 13–5. The stick to stick diagram of shoulder movement. In a Nac Selgraph 2D system, 4 LEDs were placed on the medial border of the scapular spine, on the angle of the acromion, on the epicondyle of the humerus, and over the wrist joint. *A,* In normal shoulders. *B,* Preoperative diagrams in a type I RI lesion (arrow CO indicates a limited scapular movement). *C,* Preoperative diagram in a type II (arrow H indicates a hypermobility of the shoulder motion). *D,* Postoperative diagram in a type II RI lesion.

MOTION ANALYSIS

Using a computerized motion analyzer (Nac Selgraph 2D system, Nac Corporation, Japan), hypermobility and abnormal motion of the scapula in a patient with a RI lesion is easily demonstrated (Fig. 13–5). In the early stage of shoulder motion, downward adduction motion of the scapula decreases and upward rotation motion starts early. A pattern of the scapulohumeral rhythm precedes about 20° as compared to normal shoulder motion.

MEASUREMENT OF INTRACAPSULAR PRESSURE

The intracapsular pressure pattern is not remarkably different from the pressure in the normal shoulder. Because of pain produced in the elevated externally rotated position in patients with a RI lesion, the intracapsular pressure may continue to rise even when the arm is returned to the side of the body (Fig. 13–6).

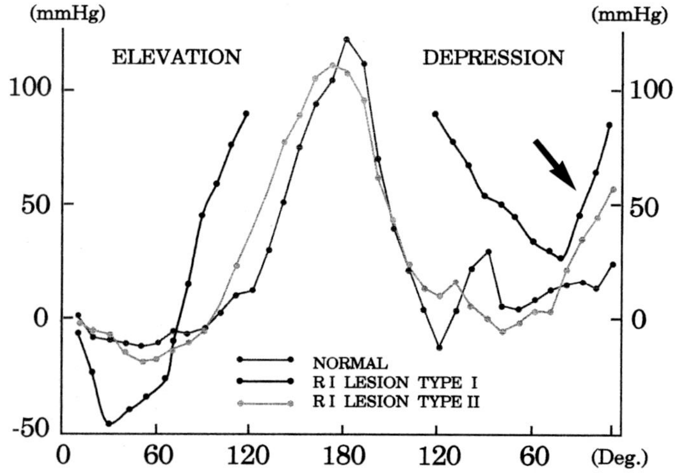

Fig. 13–6. Diagram of the intracapsular pressures. Comparison of normal to the two types of RI lesions. Arrow indicates the intracapsular pressure may continue to rise even when the arm is returned to the side of the body.

ARTHROSCOPIC FINDINGS

The articular surface of the tissues in the RI appear inflamed. In severe cases, granulation tissue may extend to the undersurface of the subscapularis and may also appear over the surface of the long head of the biceps.

ELECTROMYOGRAPHIC FINDINGS

With dynamic EMG, an increased integration value moving time average of all muscles around the shoulder is observed in a patient with a RI lesion. This finding is seen clearly in the upper fibers of the trapezius and in the middle and anterior fibers of the deltoid. The upper segment of the trapezius participates in the movement throughout all phases of shoulder motion.

TREATMENT

Conservative Treatment

In the early stage of a RI lesion, no harm is done even if the RI lesion is mistaken for sprain or contusion, because conservative treatment (such as a sling and rest) usually is sufficient in 90% of all cases. However, clinicians should be aware of the presence of the RI lesion, because the remaining 10% do not improve with conservative treatment alone; complaints, all referable to the shoulder joint, will persist.

After 3 weeks of various conservative treatment, dynamic arthrography should be performed if the patient still complains of pain on motion and instability of the shoulder. However, the decision for surgery should not be made immediately, even when there is the pouting of a contrast medium in the RI space, because there is still a possibility of improving the condition by means of joint distention with the infusion of a mixture of 10 mL of 0.5% lidocaine (Xylocaine) and 10 mL of Isovist into the joint or by forced elevation and rotation motion. Extravasation of contrast medium into the subscapularis bursa may reduce the intracapsular pressure, thereby relieving the patient from pain and discomfort. In the contracted state or type I RI lesion that is unresponsive to distention, the anterior path is recommended for rehabilitation because of the inability to externally rotate the arm. The anterior pathway is achieved in internal rotation of the shoulder and elbow flexion. From this position, the shoulder is elevated gradually (Fig. 13–7).[3]

Operative Treatment

Under general anesthesia, an anterolateral incision is made one finger-breadth lateral to the coracoid process. The deltoid muscle fibers are separated, and the subacromial bursa is incised but not resected. Adhesion of the subacromial bursa exists in all type I lesions and in 80% of type II RI lesions.

Stay sutures are placed through each cut edge of the bursa, while a suture is placed beneath the coracohumeral ligament to act as a traction suture to identify the RI lesion (Fig. 13–8). Another suture is placed through the superior border of the subscapularis and also is used as a traction suture, thereby making the RI lesion more visible. The edges of the supraspinatus and adjacent subscapularis are roughened and closed with interrupted nonabsorbable sutures while the shoulder is held in the externally rotated position. The coracohumeral ligament is then pulled over the repaired RI and sutured in place. The bursal incision is repaired with absorbable interrupted sutures. In patients with severe RI lesion, a thin membranous tissue may be the only remnant left of the

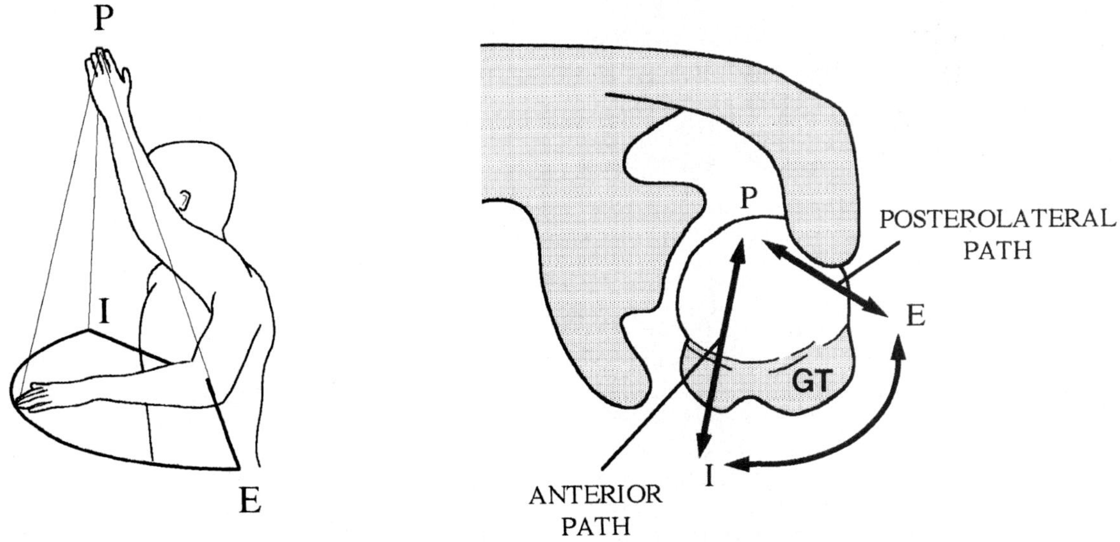

Fig. 13–7. Illustrates the pathways of the greater tuberosity in shoulder motion. Right: top view of the shoulder joint, showing the two pathways of the greater tuberosity, the anterior path and the posterolateral path. GT, greater tuberosity; P, pivotal position; I and E, internal and external rotation position.

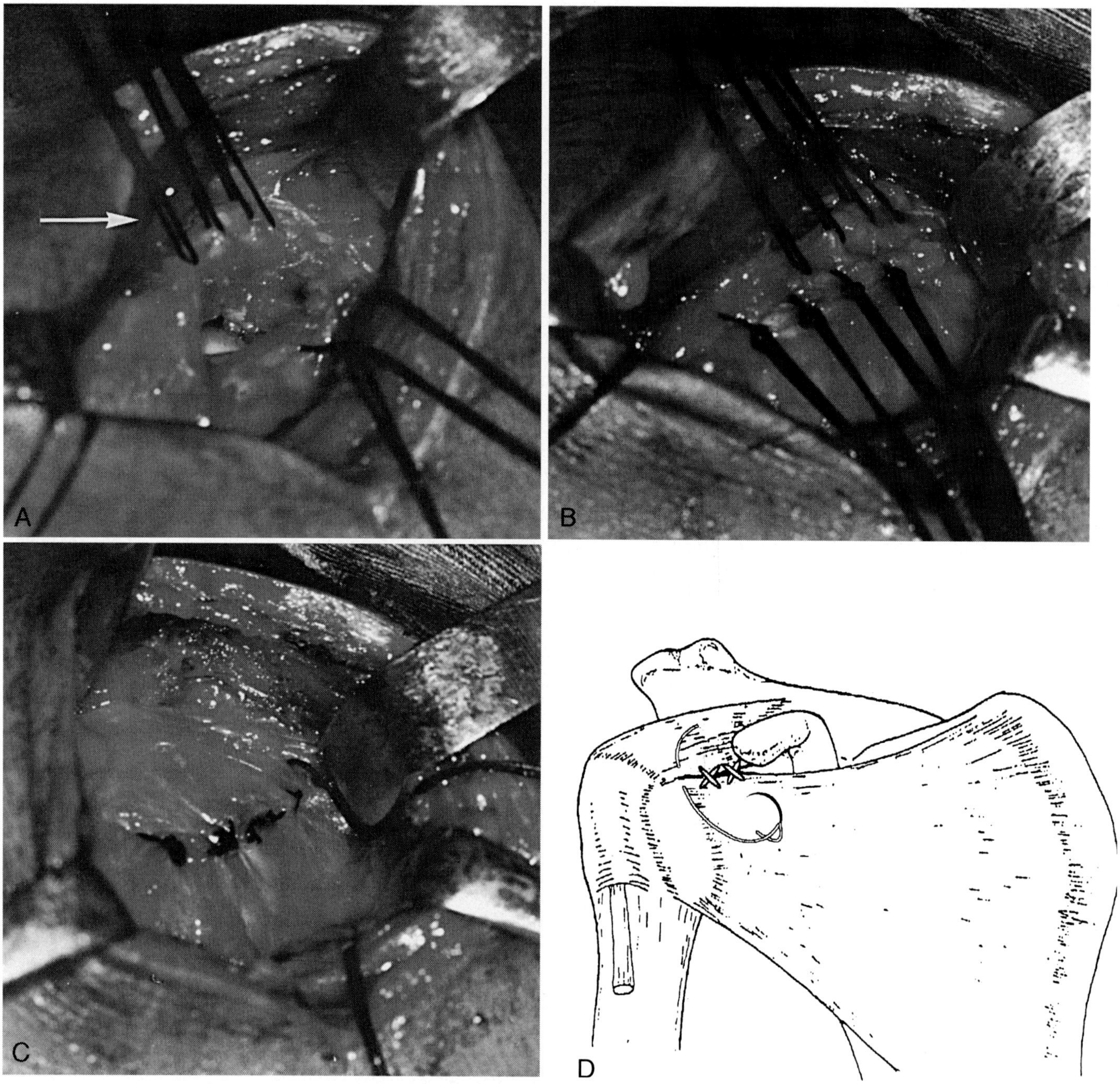

Fig. 13–8. ***A,*** **How to repair the RI lesions. The white arrow indicates the coracohumeral ligament with stay sutures.** ***B,*** **Repaired RI lesion.** ***C,*** **Repaired RI lesion augmented with coracohumeral ligament.** ***D,*** **Illustration of repaired RI lesion.**

original tissues. In this event, the attenuated thin membranous tissue should be resected before the repair is made.

The coracohumeral ligament usually is resected in type II patients to prevent adhesions and to make early exercises of the shoulder possible. The arthroplasty of the second joint of the shoulder (resection and release of the coracoacromial ligament, removal of adhesions, and acromioplasty) should be done for all type I patients.

During the operation, a variety of findings may be observed. Abnormal laxity caused by atony and a dell or indentation of the RI are easily appreciated in type II RI lesions (Fig. 13–9). A complete "open-mouthed" RI is often seen in type I RI lesions (Fig. 13–10). In chronic cases with subsequent and repeated minor traumas, several irregular layers of adhesive tissues around the RI may be noted (Fig. 13–11). This finding explains the persistence of pain, limited range of motion, and contracture associated with this condition.

Inflamed synovium bordering the tendons may be found in 18% of patients; hypertrophy and elongation of the middle glenohumeral ligament may be observed in 14% of cases. A slight inflammation and elongation of the anteroinferior margin of the labrum may be noted

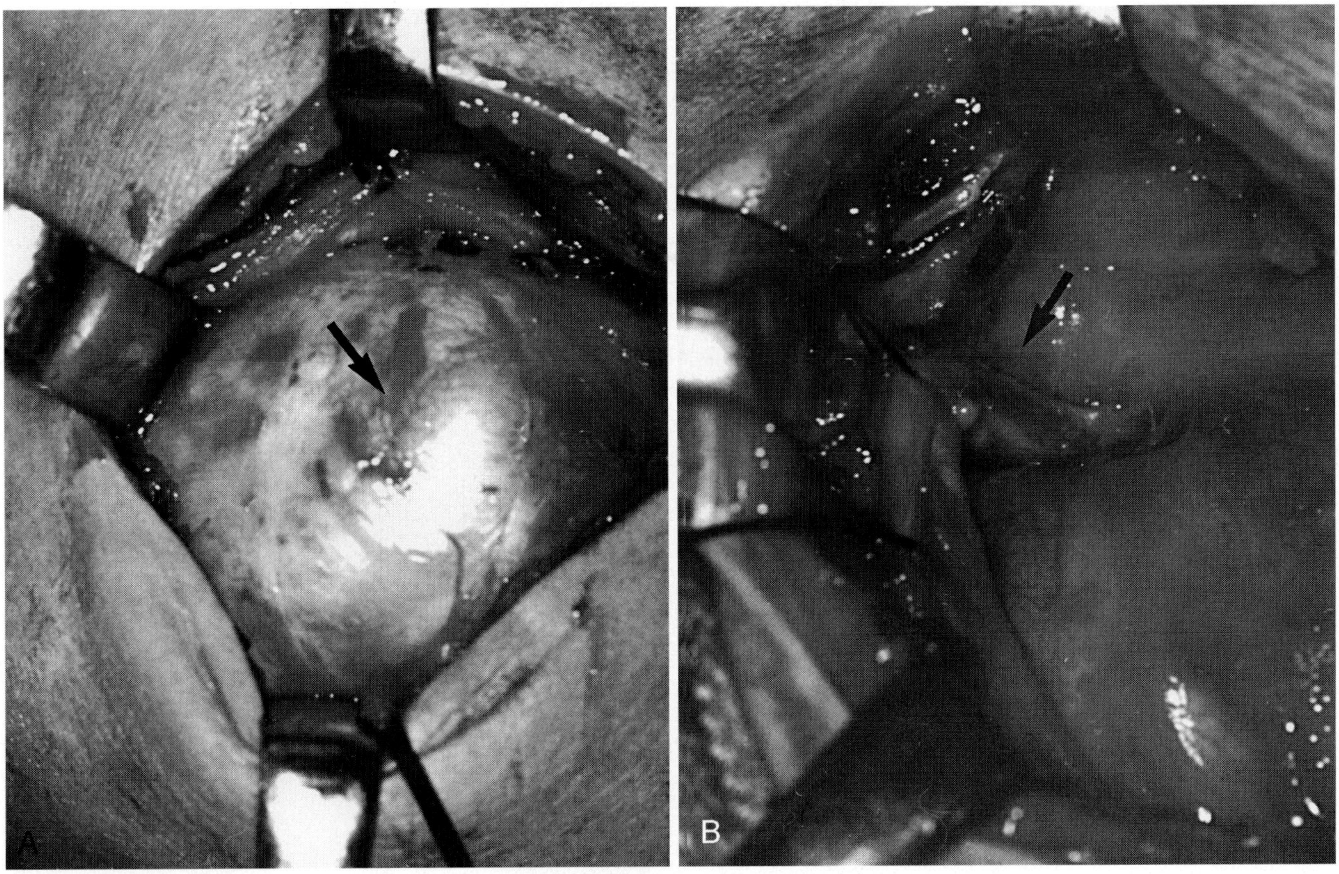

Fig. 13–9. *A,* An abnormal slackness (arrow) of the RI. *B,* A dell (arrow) of the RI.

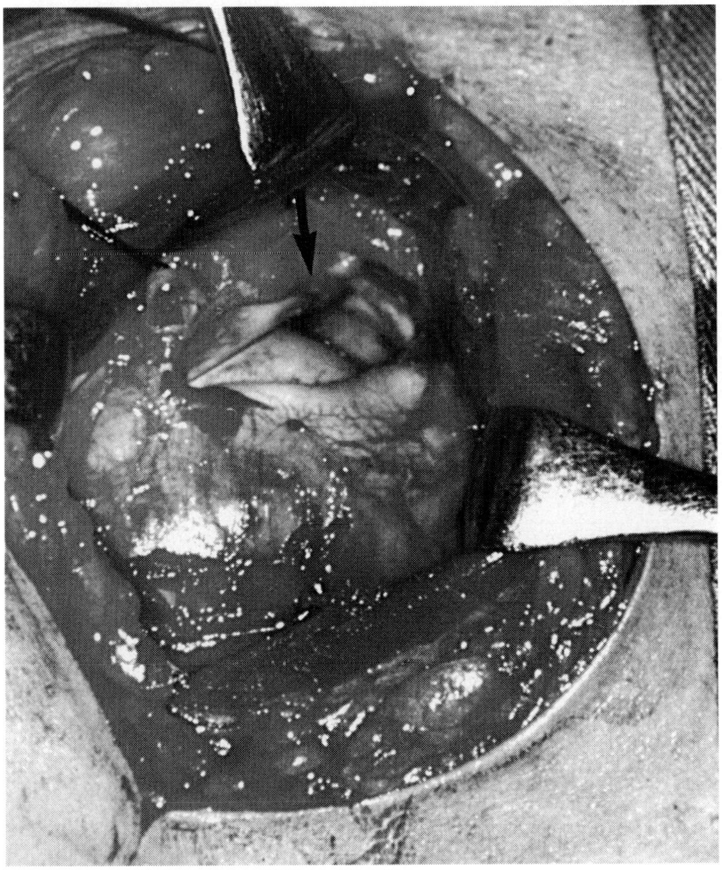

Fig. 13–10. A complete "open-mouthed" (arrow) RI.

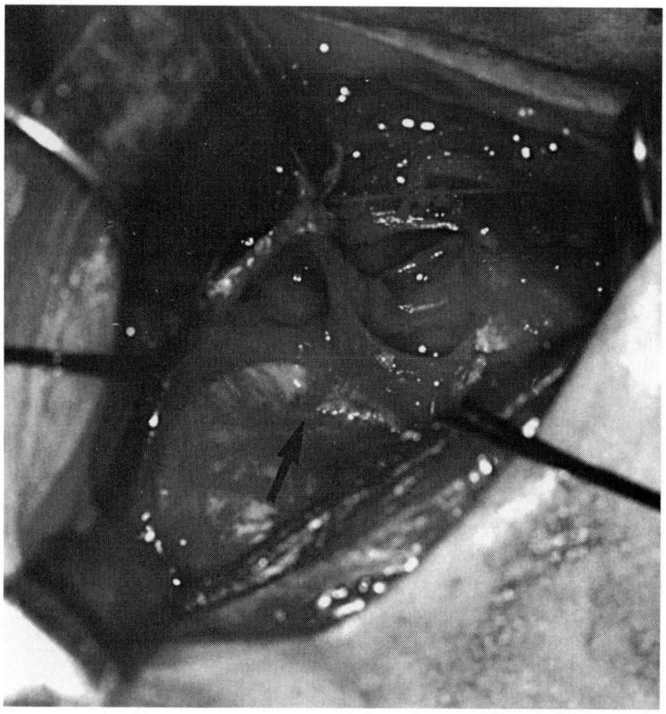

Fig. 13–11. Several irregular layers of adhesive tissues (arrow) around the RI.

in 35% of patients. Granulation tissue on the long head of the biceps may be seen in 54% of cases and was present on the undersurface of the superior aspect of the subscapularis in 28% of cases. Lastly, degenerative changes may be noted in the glenoid.

Postoperative Care

Postoperatively, a skin traction with the arm in the elevated position is applied for 3 to 5 days. The patient is then placed in a shoulder spica cast in Zero position, about 130° of elevation in the scapular plane with the arm in neutral position, for a period of 16 to 18 days (Fig. 13–12). On the third day in the cast, the upper part of the cast is bivalved, and elevation exercises, including exercises of the long head of the biceps, are performed vigorously. Thereafter, the arm is lowered and the patient is enrolled in a gentle active and passive motion exercise program.[4]

MATERIALS AND METHODS

Two hundred and thirty-three patients with 240 RI lesions were treated surgically from 1970 through 1992. The age ranged from 11 to 68 years, with an average age of 26.5 years. There were 170 male and 63 female patients. The ratio of left to right shoulders was 72:168. Seven cases were bilateral. In general, laborers and athletes had a greater frequency of type II RI lesion, as compared with the overall population of patients who were included in this series.

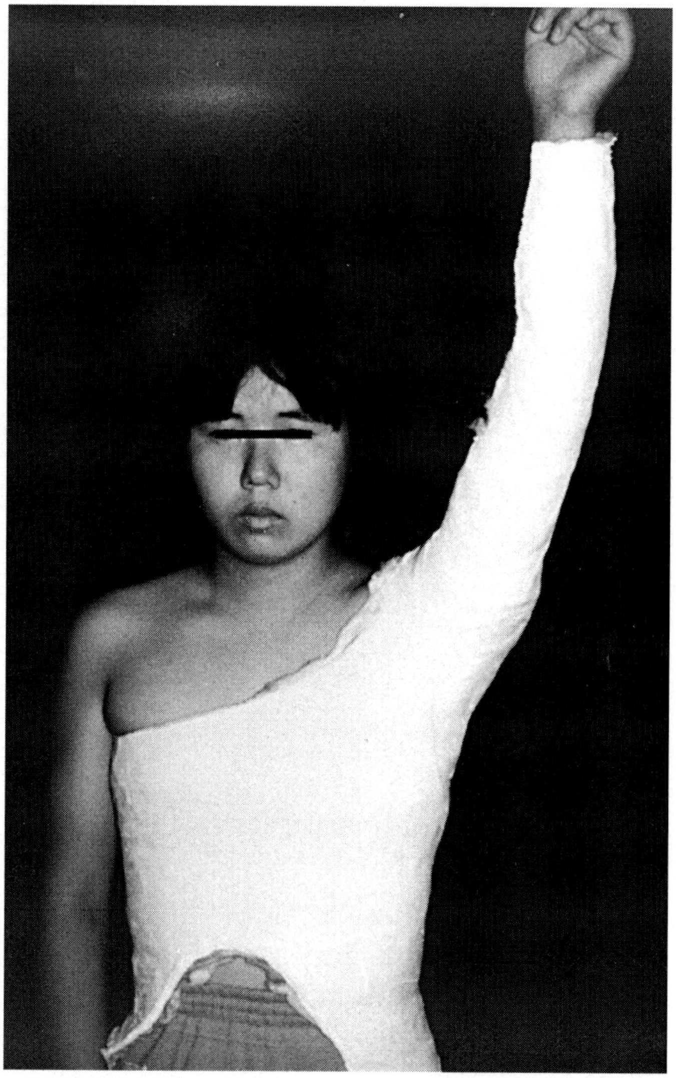

Fig. 13–12. A shoulder spica case in Zero position.

Ninety-eight shoulders (40.8%) had history of trauma, whereas 109 shoulders (45.4%) had no history of trauma but were involved in strenuous sports activities. The remaining 33 cases (13.8%) had no known history of physical problems involving the shoulder. The average time between the traumatic incident and the onset of pain at the time of diagnosis was 27 months. The maximum time that had elapsed before operation was 13 years.

The unstable (type II) group included 199 cases (85%) or 205 shoulders. The male-to-female ratio was 150:49; the left-to-right ratio was 50:155. Type II lesions occurred more frequently in the right side of young athletes, with an average age of 24 years. The presenting symptom was pain in 99% of the 205 shoulders. Tenderness existed at the lateral portion of the coracoid process just above the RI. Pain on motion occurred with the arm in the elevated and externally rotated position. Anteroinferior instability was noted in 90% and slipping phenomenon was observed in 75%, but the facioscapulohumeral angle remained at a range of 80 to 85°. Anteroposterior instability was noted in 47%. Unexpectedly, dysfunction was rela-

Table 13–1. Clinical Features

Type and Number	*Contracted Type 34 cases (%)*	*Unstable Type 199 cases (%)*
Pain	96	96
Anteroinferior instability	0	90
Anteroposterior instability	0	47
Slipping	0	75
Languidness	40	53
Dysfunction	96	99

tively infrequent (19%). Languidness or limp (dead arm) sensation was experienced in 53%, and tingling sensation in 23%.

The contracted state (type I) group included 34 patients (15%), or 35 shoulders. The male-to-female ratio was 20:14, and the average age of 42 years was high compared with that of the type II group. The left-to-right ratio was 13:22. The chief complaint was pain (96%). Dysfunction was observed in 96% of the shoulders (Table 13–1). Within the rotator cuff tear category, incomplete tear, complete tear, and RI lesion each constituted approximately a third of the cases. However, the ratio of each group treated surgically was 4:2:3 (Fig. 13–13).

As for the relationship between age and injury, RI lesions are more common among younger patients (78%), whereas massive tears are more frequent in the older age group (with an average of 60 years) (Fig. 13–14). Following surgical repair of the RI lesion, the scapulohumeral rhythm is almost (but not completely) restored to normal.

RESULTS

Two hundred and twenty-two shoulders were evaluated in the follow-up study. The follow-up period lasted from 6 months to 23 years, with an average of 7.3 years.

Pain

One hundred and twenty-three shoulders (55%) were completely relieved of pain. Eighty-eight shoulders (40%) were improved but had some pain with the overexertion of the shoulder or with strenuous activities, while 11 shoulders (5%) were unchanged and continued to have pain with any motion of the shoulder, as before the operation. Thus, good to excellent results were seen in 95% of all the cases undergoing operation.

Range of Motion

Ninety percent of the shoulders regained full range of motion except for slight limitation of internal rotation. Among the 34 cases of type I (contracted) in which range of motion could not reach 150° of elevation before surgery, 29 had significant improvement with only a slight limitation of motion. Only 5 shoulders had no appreciable improvement postoperatively.

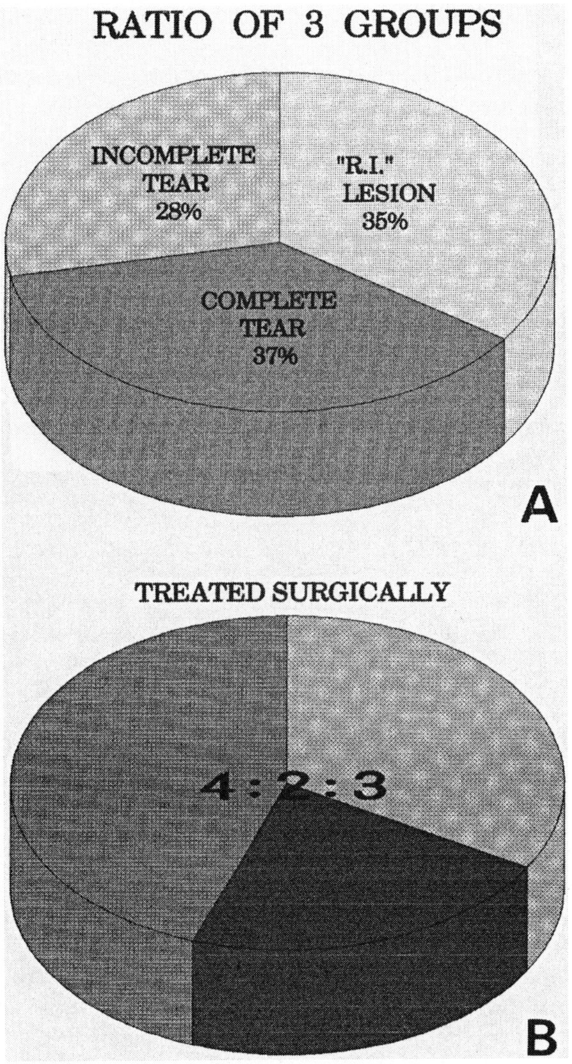

Fig. 13–13. Diagrams of the ratio of three groups (incomplete rotator cuff tears, complete rotator cuff tears, and the RI lesion). *A,* Ratio of cases treated conservatively. *B,* Ratio of cases treated surgically.

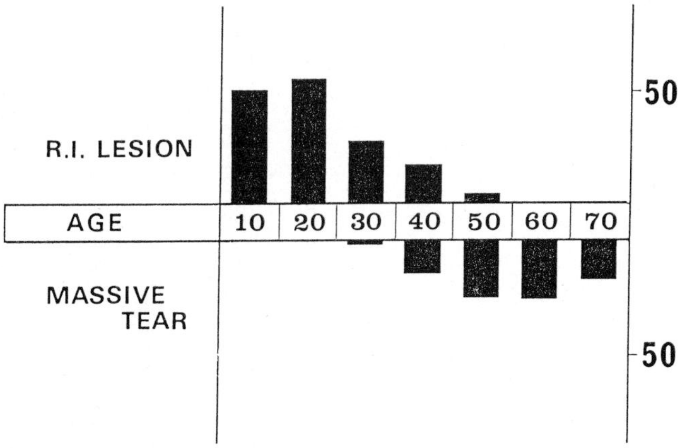

Fig. 13–14. Diagram of relationship of the age and the frequency in the RI lesions and massive tears of the rotator cuff.

Muscle Strength

One hundred and sixty-two shoulders (72%) regained normal muscle strength postoperatively. However, a slight decrease of muscle power was noted in 62 shoulders (28%). Many of these patients no longer had to restrict strenuous sports activities.

Stability

One hundred and fifty-five shoulders (70%) had good shoulder stability, while 60 shoulders (27%) improved significantly but had a slight and persistent instability. Seven shoulders continued to have poor glenohumeral stability postoperatively.

Activities of Daily Living

One hundred and eighty-nine shoulders (85%) achieved normal activities of daily living, while 22 shoulders (10%) were improved but still had below-normal activities of sports and labor. Short-term follow-up within 1 year revealed that the rate of patient satisfaction was comparatively low (70%) at the beginning but improved with time and reached 85% at the time of this study (Table 13–2).

DISCUSSION

The RI lesion is a new disease entity that often resembles the findings of a rotator cuff tear or traumatic recurring subluxation of the shoulder. It occurs more often in younger people, as compared with a massive rotator cuff tear that is typically observed in older individuals. Two types of disease states have been described. In type II the lesion can be diagnosed easily when anteroinferior instability is elicited upon application of downward traction to the upper extremity during internal rotation motion. Instability does not occur when downward traction is applied in external rotation. In type II loosening and instability usually are seen among younger patients. Moreover, in the elevated externally rotated position of the upper extremity, a painful posteroinferior instability may result. This disease entity can be documented clearly if dynamic cineradio-arthrographs are taken when the upper extremity is exercised in the overhead and externally rotated position, because leakage of the contrast medium to the RI space may be observed as a result of increased intracapsular pressure.

Included in this series were athletes who were able to return to their previous level of activities, including professional baseball players, volleyball players on the Japan Olympic Team, a professional golfer who became the All-Japan Tournament Champion, and a high school judo champion. We believe without doubt that all practicing orthopedic surgeons have encountered patients with similar complaints.

Table 13–2. Follow-up Study* (222 shoulders)

	Cases	%
Pain:		
Complete relief	123	55
With overuse	88	40
No change	11	5
ROM		
Full range	200	90
Slight limitation	17	7
Limited	5	2
MMT		
Normal	162	72
Weak	60	27
Stability		
Excellent	155	70
Good	60	27
Poor	7	3
ADL		
Normal	189	85
Improved	22	10
No improvement	11	5

*Note. Follow-up period 23 to 0.5 years (average = 7.3 years).

Relationship with Sports

The tissues of the RI have a flexible structure; however, they are easily damaged by violent force and are easily inflamed with frequent use of the shoulder. Our data indicate that more than 45% of the RI lesions resulted from overexertion of the shoulder in competitive sporting activities.

In a throwing motion, the shoulder performs two functions: (1) it serves as a platform of the upper extremity and (2) it acts as a fulcrum of the upper arm lever. One can achieve the optimum efficiency through a propeller motion with the speed and the power accumulated with the balance between the upper arm and the lower limb. Immediately following the "windup" of the upper and lower extremities on the ipsilateral side, the fulcrum is shifted to the foot on the contralateral side. At this point, the ball on one hand and the fulcrum of the opposite foot form the longest lever.[5]

In the acceleration phase the body first moves forward, followed by the shoulder; the elbow comes last along with the hand while being forced to form a big arc. Early in this phase, the anterior shoulder muscles are in a state of high stress, because they are maximally stretched. When they contract from the stretched external rotation to the internal rotation position, more stress is applied to the anteroposterior muscle unit of the shoulder. The humeral head locates anteriorly to the glenoid in early phase and shifts posteriorly in the late phase. The infraspinatus tendon that is contracting eccentrically acts as the brake. The acceleration phase is the shortest phase in the entire throwing motion and takes only 0.12 seconds, according to our data.

Since 1988 we have treated 37 athletes whose shoulders have both an RI lesion and a tear of the infraspinatus. The subjects in this series included 33 baseball players (including 23 professional players) and 4 professional volleyball players. The age ranged from 11 to 36 years, with an average age of 22 years. The length of time they engaged in sports activities ranged from 3 to 15 years, with an average of 9.7 years. The male-to-female ratio was 33:4, and the ratio of dominant arm to nondominant arm was 33:4.

The symptoms included severe tenderness at the RI and at the insertion of the infraspinatus and pain on motion with the arm in the horizontal plane or in the elevated position. Arthrography shows leakage of the contrast medium into the RI and to the subacromial bursa through the perforated infraspinatus tendon. Patients have normal muscle strength but hardly can throw because of severe pain. Pain on motion occurs mainly in acceleration phase. Comparing the pain with rotation to pain with elevation, the ratio is 81:19. This finding suggests that an anterior instability as a result of the RI lesion may be caused by the posterior shift of the humeral head to the glenoid during throwing motion (Fig. 13–15), re-

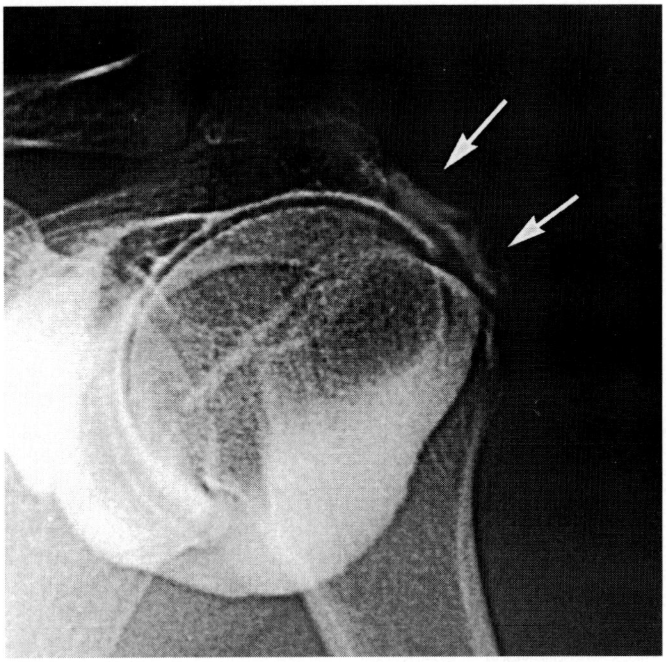

Fig. 13–16. A leakage of contrast medium from the infraspinatus tendon (arrow).

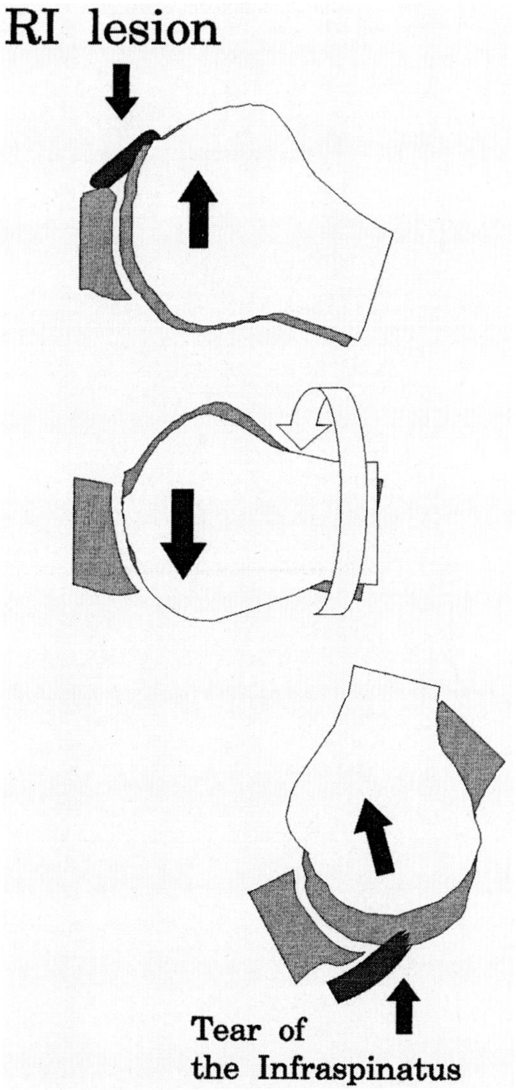

Fig. 13–15. Diagram showing the mechanism by which the RI lesion may cause tears to the infraspinatus.

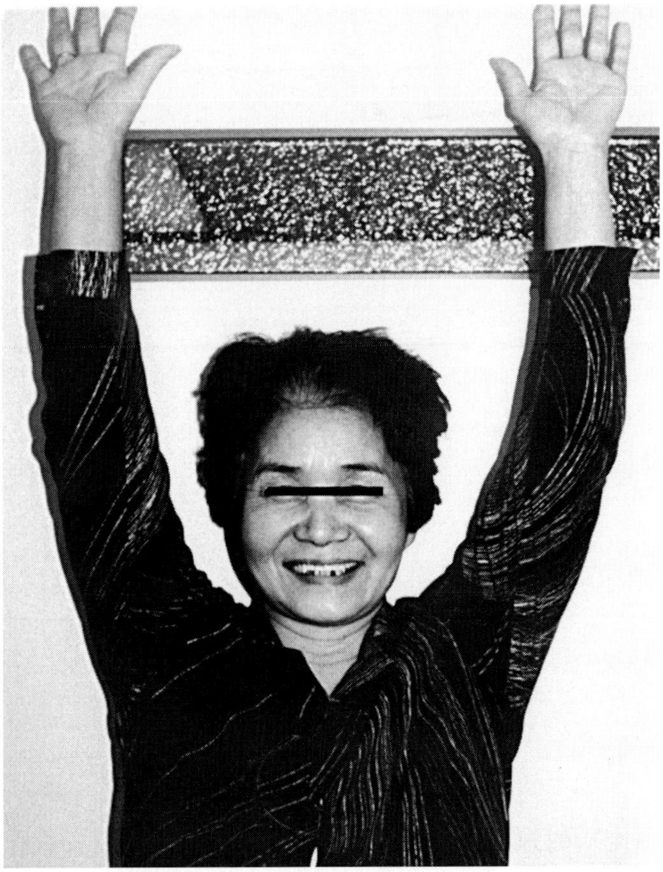

Fig. 13–17. Fifty-five-year-old woman who has normal range of motion of the operated shoulder with RI lesion.

sulting in injury to the posterior musculature and tearing of the infraspinatus tendon (Fig. 13–16).

Conservative treatment such as a sling and a swathe, rest, no throwing, and joint distention during arthrography was effective. Thirty patients healed within 3 months with conservative treatment. Seven patients underwent surgery because of continued pain and dysfunction.

Based on our data, anterior instability of the shoulder in this group of patients may be caused by injury of the posterior musculature of the shoulder.

EPILOGUE

In late 1992 the patient described in the beginning of the chapter came back to our hospital for follow-up. Physical examination revealed normal range of motion of the operated shoulder with RI lesion. This patient is now 55 years old. She no longer experiences any night pain or pain on motion of the shoulder (Fig. 13–17).

CONCLUSION

Based on our data, we conclude that the RI lesion is a new disease entity that differs from tendinitis, subluxation, or impingement syndrome. This lesion is seldom diagnosed by the practicing general orthopedic surgeon. This disease entity, however, responds promisingly to conservative treatment; only approximately 10% of patients needed surgery. Of the 10% treated with surgery, 95% had good to excellent results.

REFERENCES

1. Nobuhara K, Ikeda H. Rotator interval lesion. *Clin Orthop.* 1987; 223:44–50.
2. Rowe CR. *The Shoulder.* New York: Churchill Livingstone; 1988:237–244.
3. Sohier R. *Kinesitherapy of the Shoulder.* Bristol: John Wright & Sons; 1967:6–19.
4. Saha AK. *Theory of Shoulder Mechanism.* Springfield: Charles C. Thomas; 1961:54–55.
5. Malone TR. *Throwing Injuries* Baltimore: Williams & Wilkins; 1989:6–24.

Chapter 14

Posterosuperior Glenoid Impingement

Gilles Walch

Shoulder pain frequently occurs in athletes who practice throwing sports and has been the subject of numerous publications.[1–6] The typical pain in throwers lies posteriorly and is produced by the cocking maneuver (i.e., 90° of abduction and full external rotation). There are three theories as to the origin of the pain and its pathogenesis: (1) the subacromial impingement syndrome,[1–3] (2) instability with secondary impingement,[4] and (3) excessive traction on the tendons and capsuloligamentous structures during exercise.[5,6] Any intra-articular lesion can be analyzed arthroscopically.[7] Based on arthroscopic observations, a further explanation is proposed, which is impingement between the deep surface of the rotator cuff and the posterosuperior border of the glenoid.

PATIENTS AND METHODS

Between December 1, 1989 and June 30, 1991, 17 athletes without clinical evidence of anterior instability were examined arthroscopically for pain in the shoulder specifically related to the throwing position.[7] Table 14–1 summarizes the sports practiced. All but one of the athletes were throwers. There were 11 men and 6 women, with a mean age at arthroscopy of 25 years (range = 15 to 30 years). The dominant arm was affected in all of the throwers; the nondominant arm was affected only in a bodybuilder.

All of the patients had chronic shoulder pain that worsened progressively when they practiced their sports. In some of the patients, the pain was prolonged into the night and into the day following competitions. The mean duration from the onset of symptoms to presentation was 27 months (range = 12 to 60 months). All had received nonoperative therapy to some extent, including nonsteroidal anti-inflammatory drugs, physiotherapy, rest, and local injections.

Table 14–1. Main Sport Practiced by the Patient

Sport	*No. of Patients*
Tennis*	6
Volleyball*	5
Handball	4
Javelin	2
Bodybuilding	1

*One patient played both tennis and volleyball competitively.

All of the patients had a radiographic workup consisting of anteroposterior plain radiographs in neutral, external, and internal rotation, a lateral view of the glenoid (as described by Bernageau et al.[8]), and a single contrast arthrogram followed by computed tomography. One patient had a MRI scan and an ultrasound scan instead of CT arthrography.

Arthroscopy was performed on all patients under general anesthesia. The patients were placed in the lateral decubitus position with the arm in vertical and horizontal double traction (as described by Gross and Fitzgibbons[9]). The arthroscope was introduced through a routine posterior portal. A probe introduced through an anterior portal confirmed the absence of a Bankart lesion (pathognomonic of anterior instability). After routine diagnostic arthroscopy, the traction was removed and the arm was placed in full external rotation and examined in varying degrees of abduction. All cases showed impingement between the posterosuperior part of the glenoid rim and the insertion of the supraspinatus and infraspinatus at the level of greater tuberosity (Fig. 14–1).

RESULTS

Symptoms

All of the patients complained of diffuse shoulder pain that was worse in the posterior part of the shoulder. In 10 patients, the pain disappeared when the sports activity was stopped but returned each time the sport was resumed. The pain became permanent in seven patients, preventing sleep and affecting everyday activities. None of the patients presented with dislocation, subluxation, or the sensation of instability in the shoulder.

Clinical Examination

The data for the clinical examination are outlined in Table 14–2. Examination typically reproduced pain when

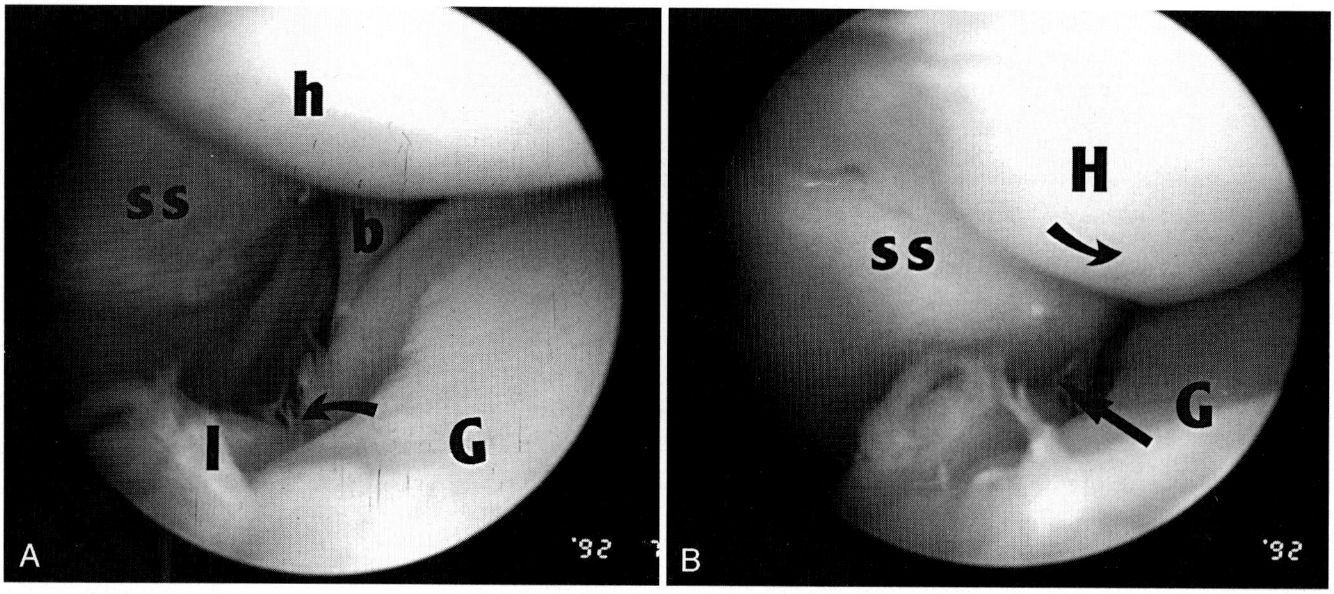

Fig. 14–1. *A,* **Arthroscopic evaluation of the patient with posterosuperior impingement showing posterior superior labral tear (arrow). This midposition view shows the relationship of the supraspinatus (SS), biceps (B), humeral head (H), labrum (L), and glenoid at this point.** *B,* **Progressive abduction and external rotation (curved arrow) of the humerus allows arthroscopic visualization of the impingement between the supraspinatus (SS) and the glenoid rim (arrow).**

Table 14–2. Clinical Findings with Posterosuperior Impingement

Test	*Result*	*No. of Cases*
Active flexion	Normal	17
Passive external rotation	Equal	13
	Increased	4
Impingement sign (Neer)	Positive	17
Modified impingment sign (Hawkins)	Positive	17
Supraspinatus strength (Jobe)	Normal but painful	5
	Decreased	12
Infraspinatus strength in 90° of abduction	Normal	11
	Normal but painful	6
Apprehension test	Painful	17
Relocation test (Jobe)	Positive	17

Table 14–3. Radiological Examination

Radiological Examination	*Findings*	*No. of Cases*
Plain radiographs	Posterosuperior humeral head geode	8
	Sclerosis or microcysts of the tuberosity	8
	Abnormal posterior border of glenoid	1
	Normal	3
Contrast arthrography	Rupture deep surface supraspinatus	8
	Normal	9
CT arthrogram	Abnormality of posterosuperior glenoid edge	10
	Mean humeral retrotorsion (range)	10° (0 to 26°)

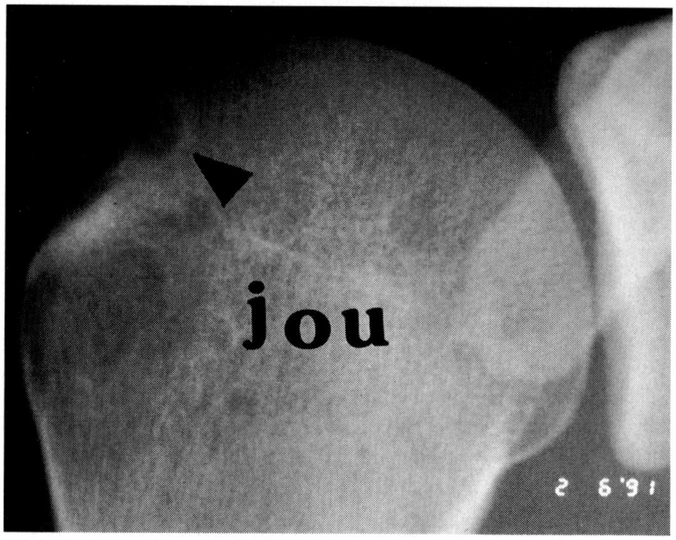

Fig. 14–2. Plain radiograph showing geode in tuberosity.

the arm was held in full external rotation and then moved between 90 and 150° abduction. Evidence of rotator cuff problems usually was present, notably at the supraspinatus.

External rotation at 90° abduction had a mean value of 104° (range = 92 to 115°). In four patients, external rotation averaged 15° more compared to the normal opposite side. Atrophy of the supraspinatus and infraspinatus fossae was never found. Two patients demonstrated a positive sulcus sign bilaterally but no evidence of instability.

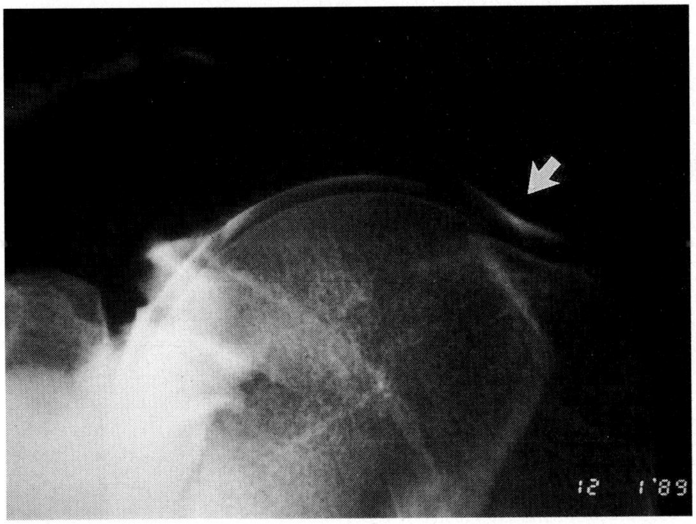

Fig. 14–3. Arthrogram showing partial rupture of the undersurface of supraspinatus.

IMAGING STUDIES

Table 14–3 outlines the results of the imaging studies. Conventional radiography showed an abnormality in 14 cases. In five cases, the greater tuberosity had geodes (Fig. 14–2) or sclerosis with microcysts, as found with degenerative rotator cuff tears. In one case, on the lateral glenoid view, an osteophyte was noted on the posterior border of the glenoid fossa. The plain radiographs were completely normal in only three cases.

Preoperative contrast radiography is performed routinely in those cases with signs of supraspinatus damage. The arthrogram was positive in eight cases, showing broaching of the deep surface of the supraspinatus tendon, with leakage of contrast into its substance shaped either like a flame or a cloud (Fig. 14–3). There was never communication with the subacromial bursa. There was no significant difference in age between patients with (26 years) and without (24 years) a partial rupture.

The CT scan that immediately followed the arthrogram was done to (1) check the integrity of the labrum-inferior glenohumeral ligament complex, (2) analyze the posterior border of the glenoid, and (3) measure humeral retrotorsion by viewing supracondylar cuts.

None of the patients had an anterior lesion; however, 10 patients had bony changes at the posterosuperior part of the glenoid. Obvious small osteophytes were seen occasionally, but differences usually were revealed by comparison with the normal contralateral shoulder, slight sclerosis or rounding of the rim, or wearing down of the posterosuperior labrum (Fig. 14–4).

Humeral retrotorsion was measured from the periphery of the articular cartilage that forms the anatomical neck. Using this landmark, the normal value lies between 25 and 35°.[10] The mean angle in this series was 10° (range = −5 to 30°), clearly much lower than normal.

Arthroscopic Findings

The arthroscopic findings were recorded on videotape and are presented in Table 14–4. None of the patients had a Bankart lesion. When the arm was placed in the throwing position, all patients demonstrated impingement between the posterosuperior edge of the glenoid and the insertion of the rotator cuff (Figs. 14–5 and 14–6). All cases showed that, at the end of the throwing movement, the posterior labrum separated from the glenoid, allowing the latter's sharp edge to come into contact with the undersurface of the cuff. Contact occurred between 90 and 150° abduction, in the area between 9 o'clock and 11 o'clock on the posterior edge of the glenoid. The labral lesions appeared similar to degenerative types, with irregular scuffing and small flap tears that could lie within the joint. In two cases, the lesion extended toward the superior labrum but never in front of the insertion of the biceps.

In eight cases, there was an osteochondral lesion of the humeral head that was situated higher than the classic Hill-Sachs lesion and was adjacent to the posterior sulcus or more distal and separated by a strip of normal cartilage. The osteochondral lesion was always less than 1 cm in size and only a few millimeters in depth and could

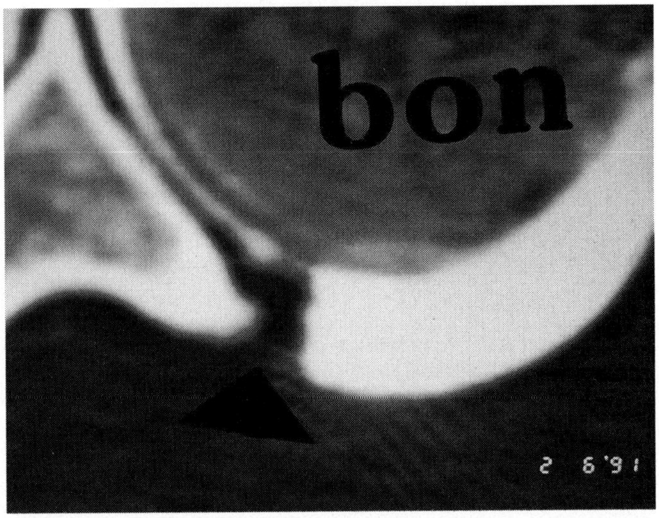

Fig. 14–4. Modification of the posterior glenoid rim on CT arthrogram.

Table 14–4. Arthroscopic Findings

Findings		*No. of Cases*
Posterosuperior glenoid impingement of rotator cuff, arm in throwing position		17
Posterosuperior labral lesion		12
Osteochondral fracture of humeral head		8
Cuff lesions (Ellman classification)		
Supraspinatus:	grade I	2
	grade II/III	7
Infraspinatus:	grade I	2
	grade II/III	1

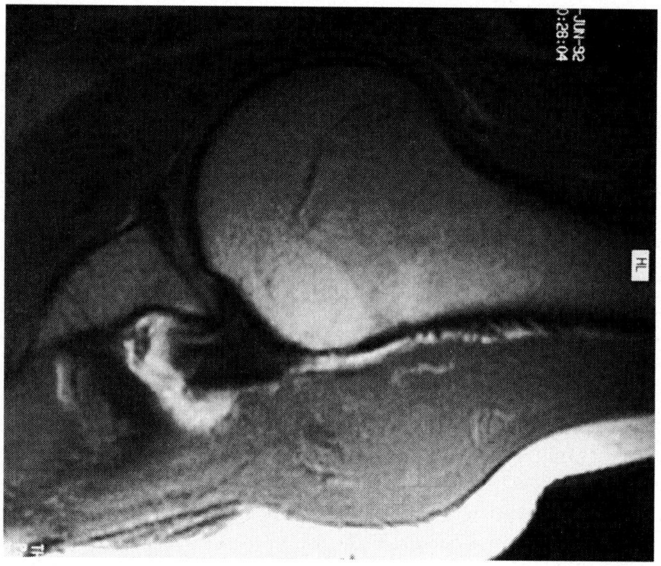

Fig. 14–5. MRI imaging of posterosuperior glenoid impingement between the posterior edge of the glenoid and the deep surface of the supraspinatus and infraspinatus tendons.

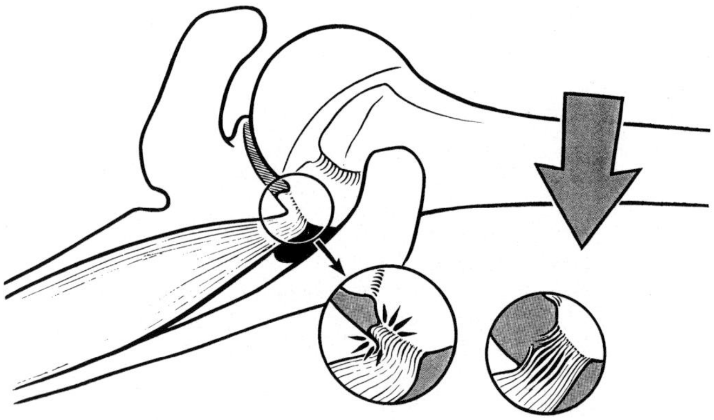

Fig. 14–6. Line drawing illustrating posterior superior glenoid impingement and subsequent injury.

correspond to humeral impaction on the posterosuperior part of the glenoid. However, it was never possible to demonstrate this impact at arthroscopy.

The majority of cuff lesions affected the supraspinatus. Four cases were difficult to differentiate, as some tears extended into the depth of the tendon, dissecting it into two layers.

DISCUSSION

This study has described arthroscopically confirmed impingement of the deep surface of the rotator cuff and the posterosuperior border of the glenoid while the arm was placed in the position of abduction and external rotation. Perry[11] stressed that this could occur during the "cocking" phase, but she did not indicate whether the contact was physiological or pathological or whether it could give rise to lesions. More recently, in a study of frozen cadaveric shoulders, Jobe[12] showed that the tendinous insertion of the rotator cuff became jammed between the humeral head and the glenoid when the arm was placed in the throwing position. We have seen this arthroscopically in patients without cuff symptoms or pathology and in patients who were not throwing athletes. It seems probable that the contact is, in fact, physiological and can be found to varying degrees in normal subjects. Excessive external rotation does not appear to be an important etiological factor, as it was found to be increased in only four patients when compared to the other side; this is a normal finding in throwers. Only 2 of 17 patients had evidence of hyperlaxity by having a positive sulcus sign.

Measurement of humeral retrotorsion is still the subject of much discussion. The upper humeral landmark can be the line of insertion of the capsule on the humeral neck[13] or the articular margin[10], as chosen here. There is no doubt that the average angle in this series was abnormally low and therefore could be an etiological factor in impingement. However, two of our patients had normal angles but were still symptomatic.

Etiology of the Cuff Lesions

Radiography must be performed by a radiologist familiar with the technique for cuff lesions. Two of our patients had normal initial arthrograms, but their shoulders had not been manipulated after injection of contrast. Cuff lesions were demonstrated on a second arthrogram that was performed correctly. After injection, the shoulder must be actively mobilized through abduction and adduction; traction then must be applied in the axis of the arm. Leakage of contrast into the supraspinatus may be minimal and must be sought at the level of the greater tuberosity. Eight of our patients had contrast running into the substance of the supraspinatus tendon on arthrography. Five had a localized disruption of the capsule, exposing the undersurface of the fibers to a depth of 3 mm, which was not demonstrable arthrographically. Four patients had only fraying of the capsule. We agree with Ellman[14] that simple capsular tears do not constitute a true cuff rupture, because they frequently are found in patients older than 50 years of age. However, they are much rarer in young subjects, and, as Snyder et al.[15] suggest, are clearly traumatic and not degenerative in origin.

Rotator cuff lesions have been described as either tendinitis (Neer grade II) or partial/total ruptures (Neer grade III). Many investigators cite subacromial impingement as the reason these lesions occur,[1,12,14,16–18] even if the superficial bursal fibers of the tendon are intact. The standard treatment is then anterior acromioplasty or division of the coracoacromial ligament. However, Tibone et al.[3] found this release insufficient, as only 22% of their throwing athletes returned to the same sporting level afterwards. This is similar to our experience, in which we found that throwing athletes are improved by an anterior acromioplasty but are never cured of pain when throwing; this lesion may explain why these athletes fail to return to performing at the highest level.

Because of this, Jobe et al.[4] proposed the theory that in throwing athletes the impingement is secondary to anterior instability. The cuff lesions are said to occur when the anteriorly subluxed humeral head compromises the tendons under the acromial arch while the arm is cocked. Because none of our patients had evidence of anterior instability, the mechanism cannot apply to our patients. Furthermore, in the throwing position, the greater tuberosity lies posterior to the acromial arch; it is impossible for the cuff tendons to become trapped when the head is subluxed anteriorly. In fact, the anterior structures have to be normal for impingement to occur posteriorly. The positive relocation sign found in all our patients can be explained by the fact that pushing the humeral head posteriorly stops it from impinging on the posterior part of the glenoid.

Andrews et al.[5] felt that the lesions occur from excessive traction, repeated thousands of times on the rotator cuff. This hypothesis is very plausible, except that it does not explain why the subscapularis, which is in exactly the same mechanical environment, is involved so rarely.

Uhthoff et al.[19] and Yamanaka and Fukuda[20] thought that progressive degeneration of the tendinous fibers on the deep surface causes partial rupture at this site. This theory was based on histological studies that apparently were performed on adults older than 50 years of age. This mechanism cannot explain the cause of the tears in athletes younger than 30 years.

We hypothesize that the lesions on the undersurface of the cuff are caused by impingement on the posterior edge of the glenoid when the arm is in the throwing position. This impingement probably is physiological, but in throwing athletes the repetitive nature of their sport on their dominant arm leads to mechanical damage and the lesions that are observed.

Etiology of the Posterior Labral and Glenoidal Lesions

In 1977, Lombardo et al.[21] reported four cases of posterior glenoidal lesions in professional pitchers who needed surgical debridement of the posterior part of the joint. They suggested that the lesions were caused by excessive traction on the posterior capsule during the final phase of throwing. In 1978, Barnes and Tullos[22] also described posterior glenoidal lesions (named "Bennett's lesions" after the radiologist who first described them) in eight baseball players. The lesions were posteroinferior glenoidal subperiosteal osteophytes, often associated with a tear of the glenoidal labrum. Barnes and Tullos thought that these lesions were a sequela of capsular tears or a result of previously undetected posterior humeral subluxation. It seems that the lesions seen on CT arthrography in this study are a combination of those described by Lombardo et al.[21] and Barnes and Tullos.[22]

More recently, Snyder et al.[23] have reported posterior labral lesions associated with lesions of the humeral head. They attributed these lesions to a single violent traumatic event that caused "a combination of compression force on the superior joint surface and a proximal subluxation force on the humeral head." None of our patients had suffered a clear traumatic event, and none had labral lesions of the SLAP 1 (superior labral anterior posterior) type extending anterosuperiorly in front of the insertion of the long head of biceps. However, the lesions produced from trauma between the humeral head and the glenoid, as reported by Snyder et al.,[23] look similar to those seen arthroscopically in this series. It is possible that some SLAP lesions may be caused by posterosuperior impingement.

TREATMENT

Conservative treatment with rest, nonsteroidal anti-inflammatory medications, and physical therapy affords rapid clinical improvement in many patients. While a leisure athlete can stop throwing, the high-level competitive athlete finds difficulty with such a drastic alteration. In these individuals one must try to change the shoulder motion during throwing to avoid the horizontal retropulsion associated with this lesion. Unfortunately, in some patients, the change in body mechanics leads to loss of a level of competition. Older athletes, especially those with partial tears of the supraspinatus, find it difficult if not impossible to change their throwing motions at age 27 or 28. The next step in regard to aggressiveness and treatment of this includes arthroscopic debridement of the supraspinatus lesion and the posterior-superior labrum. My experience has been that this gives transitory improvement; however, the impingement and the pain recur, oftentimes immediately upon resumption of throwing activities.

Recently, in patients whose retrotorsion is less than 10°, a rotational humeral osteotomy of 20° with shortening of the subscapularis was proposed, as described previously by Weber.[24] This technique avoids the impingement in external rotation as illustrated in Figure 14–7. This technique, which avoids the impingement in external rotation, has been performed 15 times to date. Ten cases have greater than 1-year follow-up. Six athletes have had a complete recovery and have resumed their sports at the same level, while three athletes are better but still experience pain during full intensive sporting activity. There was one nonunion, which healed after a second operation; however, this patient is unable to return to her sport. What emerges from the early study is that if there is already a deep, partial-thickness tear of the supraspinatus with dissection into the tendon, this procedure does not seem to relieve their pain or allow them to return to sport. On the other hand, if the supraspinatus tendon is not yet damaged, results are good. Still, our follow-up is short and our clinical experience is insufficient to recommend this operation routinely.

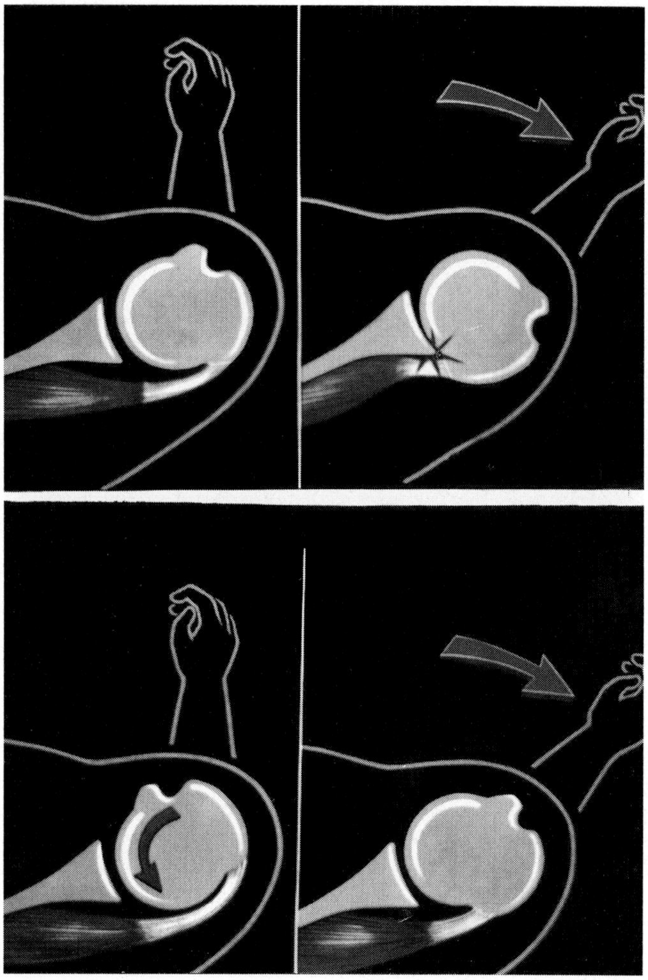

Fig. 14–7. ***A and B,*** **For humeral osteotomy and full external rotation, posterior superior impingement occurs with the damage to the posterior glenoid labrum, posterior humeral head, and supraspinatus tendon.** ***C and D,*** **After humeral osteotomy and Putti-Platt procedure (Weber procedure) with the same degree of external rotation, there is no further impingement.**

CONCLUSION

Dynamic arthroscopic visualization of the shoulder in full external rotation and varying degrees of abduction has suggested new ideas as to the cause of well-known lesions of the rotator cuff and posterior border of the glenoid in throwing athletes. Further clinical and radiological studies are needed to define the role of humeral retrotorsion in the etiology of this condition. Possibly, some of these athletes may require a humeral rotation osteotomy to control their symptoms and return to high-level sports.

REFERENCES

1. Neer CS, Welsh RP. The shoulder in sports. *Orthop Clin North Am.* 1977;8:583–591.
2. Hawkins RJ, Kennedy JC. Impingement syndrome in athletes. *Am J Sports Med.* 1980;8:151–158.
3. Tibone JE, Jobe FW, Kerlan RK, Carter VS. Shoulder impingement syndrome in athletes treated by anterior acromioplasty. *Clin Orthop.* 1985;198:134.
4. Jobe FW, Tibone JE, Jobe CM, Kvitne RS. The shoulder in sports. In: Rockwood CA, Matsen FA, eds. *The Shoulder.* Philadelphia: WB Saunders; 1990;2:961–990.
5. Andrews JR, Broussard TS, Carson WG. Arthroscopy of the shoulder in the management of partial tears of the rotator cuff: A preliminary report. *Arthroscopy.* 1985;1:117–122.
6. Olgilvie-Harris DJ, Wiley AM. Arthroscopic surgery of the shoulder: A general appraisal. *J Bone Joint Surg.* 1986; 68:201–207.
7. Walch G, Liotard JP, Boileau P, Noel E. Un autre conflit de l'épaule: "le conflit glénoïdien postero-superieur." *Rev Chir Orthop.* 1991; 77:571–574.
8. Bernageau J, Debeyre J, Ferrane J. Intérêt du profil glénoïdien dans les luxations récidivantes de l'épaule. *Rev Chir Orthop.* 1976; 62(suppl 2):142–147.
9. Gross RM, Fitzgibbons TC. Shoulder arthroscopy: A modified approach. *Arthroscopy.* 1985;1:156–159.
10. Kronberg M, Brostrom LA, Soderlund V. Retroversion of the humeral head in the normal shoulder and its relationship to normal range of motion. *Clin Orthop.* 1990;253:113–117.
11. Perry J. Anatomy and biomechanics of the shoulder in throwing, swimming, gymnastics, and tennis. *Clin Sports Med.* 1983; 2:247–270.
12. Jobe CM. Evidence for superior glenoid impingement of the rotator cuff. Personal communication at the 4th Congress of the European Society of Shoulder and Elbow Surgery. Milan, Italy, October 1990.
13. Laumann U, Kramps HA. Computer tomography in recurrent shoulder dislocation. In: Bateman JE, Welch RP, eds. *Surgery of the Shoulder.* Philadelphia: BC Decker; 1984:84–85.
14. Ellman H. Diagnosis and treatment of incomplete rotator cuff tears. *Clin Orthop.* 1990;254:64–80.
15. Snyder SJ, Pachelli AF, Del Pizzo W, Friedman MJ, Ferkel RD, Pattee G. Partial thickness rotator cuff tears: Results of arthroscopic treatment. *Arthroscopy.* 1991;7:1–7.
16. Gartsman GM. Arthroscopic acromioplasty for lesions of the rotator cuff. *J Bone Joint Surg Am.* 1990;72:169–180.
17. Neer CS. Anterior acromioplasty for the chronic impingement syndrome in the shoulder: A preliminary report. *J Bone Joint Surg Am.* 1972;50:41–49.
18. Penny JN, Welsh RP. Shoulder impingement syndromes in athletes and their surgical management. *Am J Sports Med.* 1981;9:11–15.
19. Uhthoff HK, Lohr J, Sarkar K. The pathogenesis of rotator cuff tears. In: Takagishi N, ed. *The Shoulder.* Tokyo, Professional Postgraduate Services; 1990:211–212.
20. Yamanaka K, Fukuda H. Pathological studies of the supraspinatus tendon with reference to incomplete thickness tears. In: Takagishi N, ed. *The Shoulder.* Tokyo, Professional Postgraduate Services; 1990:220–224.
21. Lombardo SJ, Jobe FW, Kerlan RK. Posterior shoulder lesions in throwing athletes. *Am J Sports Med.* 1977;5:106–110.
22. Barnes DA, Tullos HS. An analysis of 100 symptomatic baseball players. *Am J Sports Med.* 1978;6:62–67.
23. Snyder SJ, Karzel RP, Del Pizzo W, Ferkel RD, Friedman MJ. SLAP lesions of the shoulder. *Arthroscopy.* 1990;6:274–279.
24. Weber BG, Simpson LA, Hardegger F. Rotational humeral osteotomy for recurrent anterior dislocation of the shoulder associated with a large Hill-Sachs lesion. *J Bone Joint Surg.* 1984; 66:1443–1450.

Chapter 15

Disruption of the Subscapularis

William F. Tucker, Jr. and James F. Silliman

The discussion of injuries to the musculotendinous units of the rotator cuff in the past has focused primarily on the superior components of the cuff, namely the supraspinatus and infraspinatus. Few reports of injury to the subscapularis are available for review. This chapter will address both the historical and recent concepts of trauma to the subscapularis, its diagnosis, treatment, and significance.

Most early reports of subscapularis injury were in association with recurrent anterior shoulder dislocations. Subscapularis laxity has long been postulated as a predisposing factor to recurrent anterior instability of the shoulder.[1] This is the underlying basis for reconstructive procedures, such as the Putti-Platt and Magnuson-Stack operations.[1–4] Descriptions in the English language literature of actual disruption of the subscapularis date back to at least 1834, when Smith described tears of the subscapularis tendon from the lesser tubercle in seven shoulders examined at autopsy.[5] Hauser detailed two case reports of subscapularis avulsions associated with anterior dislocation and recurrent anterior instability in 1954.[6]

Isolated case reports of tendinous avulsion in adults without antecedent history of dislocation or instability have also appeared.[7–12] The mechanisms of injury in these reports have varied from typical abduction-external rotation injuries to direct trauma associated with aggravated assaults. Several reports also exist of lesser tuberosity avulsions occurring in adolescents.[13–16] The injury in these patients was an apophyseal avulsion of the lesser tuberosity. These avulsions tended to be less displaced than those encountered in adults and were more often responsive to conservative treatment.

Recently, two articles detailing findings in larger groups of patients with similar histories and injuries have appeared. Neviaser et al. described 31 patients, all over the age of 35, with concurrent rupture of the rotator cuff and anterior dislocation of the shoulder.[17] In eight of these patients the subscapularis was found to be ruptured from the lesser tuberosity, along with a portion of anterior capsule. These were the only patients in the cohort who developed recurrent instability (three had recurrent dislocation, while five developed persistent subluxation.) Their symptoms of anterior instability, as well as night pain, all resolved following repair of the subscapularis and associated anterior capsular lesion.

Gerber and Krushell detailed 16 patients with isolated rupture of the subscapularis who had no prior history of dislocation or symptoms of recurrent instability.[18] The chief complaints of these patients were shoulder pain and weakness, particularly in internal rotation. Again, these symptoms were relieved following successful repair of the isolated lesion.

ANATOMY

The subscapularis arises from the entire medial two thirds of the anterior scapula, with the exception of the areas adjacent to the superior and inferior angles which allow attachment of the serratus magnus.[19] The muscle then courses anterolaterally beneath the scapular neck and is focused into a broad tendon at the level of the glenoid rim. The tendinous portion continues laterally towards its insertion on the lesser tubercle, with the fibers intermingling with those of the glenohumeral joint capsule, particularly in the lateral 2 cm. Additionally, there exists in many shoulders a further more muscular insertion onto the humerus over the 2 to 3 cm just distal to the lesser tubercle.[1,2] Innervation of the subscapularis is derived from the upper and lower subscapular nerves, from primary rami C5 and C6 of the brachial plexus.

Classically, the subscapularis was described as an internal rotator of the glenohumeral joint, which also acted to draw the head of the humerus anteriorly and inferiorly.[19] More recently, attention has focused on the role of the rotator cuff musculature as a dynamic stabilizer of the shoulder.[1,20,21] All cuff musculature adds to glenohumeral joint stability by seating the humeral head within the gleno-labral socket.[20,21] In the midportion of shoulder range of motion, the rotator cuff is the primary, dynamic stabilizer against anterior, posterior, and inferior translation of the humeral head. It is only at the relative extremes of joint excursion, or when the cuff musculature is not functioning properly, that the capsulo-ligamentous structures come under excessive tension.[21]

The subscapularis balances the action of the external rotators (the supraspinatus, infraspinatus, and teres minor), preventing anterior displacement of the humeral head.[1,22,23] Cadaveric studies estimating the force generating capacities of the individual cuff muscles reveal the strength of the subscapularis to slightly exceed that of the supraspinatus, infraspinatus, and teres minor combined.[22] The relative absence or weakness of the subscapularis has been associated with an increased probability of recurrent anterior dislocation and was considered by some early investigators to represent the *sine qua non* of recurrent dislocation.[1,2]

In the normal shoulder, a complex interaction of static and dynamic restraints is required to maintain normal joint integrity. Selective, serial-cutting experiments on cadavers have shown the subscapularis to be a primary stabilizer with the shoulder held in 0° of abduction.[23] As the shoulder moves through an arc of abduction, the middle glenohumeral ligament shares with the anterior-superior fibers of the inferior glenohumeral ligament and the subscapularis in preventing anterior instability at 45° of abduction.[20,23,24]

Clearly, there is no single restraint to anterior dislocation in the normal shoulder. Rather, a complex interaction of static and dynamic structures act in concert to prevent anterior instability. As this concept is studied further, a greater understanding of each individual component's role in both normal and high demand situations will undoubtedly evolve.

MECHANISMS OF INJURY

The majority of patients with subscapular injury present with a history of anterior shoulder dislocation. The most common mechanism for dislocation is forceful abduction and external rotation. The humeral head is levered against the anterior stabilizers, finding the path of least resistance as it travels out of the confines of the glenohumeral joint.

In 13 patients who had no previous shoulder surgery and whose symptoms developed without initial dislocation, Gerber and Krushell described "violent external rotation of the adducted arm" as the mechanism of injury in seven patients, while six patients were described as having "hyperextension" injuries.[18] Other isolated case reports of subscapular disruption without a history of dislocation describe mechanisms of injury including external rotation-abduction, direct trauma, and iatrogenically induced seizures as the inciting etiology.[7–12]

In patients without previous surgery, the injury tends to appear after the age of 40. Studies in cadavers revealed subscapular tensile strength to vary considerably from patient to patient but overall to wane significantly with age.[25] This reduction in strength was secondary to a decrease in cross-sectional area and an increase in areas of ectopic calcification, which presumably act as stress risers in the tendon under stress.[25] It is postulated that the probability of subscapular injury increases with age in a given patient.

In contrast to subscapular rupture, lesser tuberosity avulsion is not limited to patients older than 40 years of age. A total of six cases exist in the literature of patients with open physes who suffered lesser tuberosity avulsions.[13–16] None of these injuries were in association with dislocation or persistent instability. The most common mechanism of injury reported was forceful external rotation with the arm in approximately 60° of abduction. This is the position that places the subscapularis under maximal tension.[9] In the skeletally immature patient, the injury occurs as an apophyseal avulsion.

Lesser tuberosity avulsion injuries also occur in adults.[8–12] Again, forced abduction/external rotation is the most common etiology of injury. Isolated reports of injuries associated with direct trauma and one case of medicinally induced seizures leading to lesser tuberosity avulsion also exist.[8,9,11,12] One gymnast is also reported to have had an insidious onset of symptoms without acute injury.[10]

PATHOLOGY

Gerber and Krushell did not find evidence of injury to the inferior glenohumeral ligament in any of their 16 patients with subscapular rupture not associated with anterior dislocation.[18] It is interesting to note that ruptures reported without initial dislocation have not been associated with the development of recurrent instability. Indeed, in selective cutting experiments, isolated transection of the subscapularis lead to an increase in external rotation but did not allow dislocation of the shoulder.[20,23]

In contrast, in 31 shoulders with initial dislocation, all 8 patients who had documented subscapular rupture went on to develop recurrent instability as a complaint (3 with recurrent dislocation and 5 with recurrent subluxation).[17] All of these patients did have disruption of the associated anterior capsule, but none of them suffered a Bankart lesion.[26] Isolated repair of their subscapularis and anterior capsular lesions alleviated all symptoms of instability.

From the data available, it appears that isolated injury, even rupture, of the subscapularis is not associated with recurrent instability, while subscapularis disruption with a history of dislocation (and therefore concomitant capsular injury) does predispose to instability. These data suggest it is not the labral injury seen in the Bankart lesion but, rather, the associated damage to the anterior capsulo-ligamentous structures, specifically the inferior glenohumeral ligament, which produces recurrent instability of the shoulder in these patients.[20,23,24]

DIAGNOSIS

Symptoms associated with rupture of the subscapularis should be divided into two categories, patients with and those without previous history of dislocation. In patients with previous dislocation, especially those over 40 years of age, subscapular injury should be suspected with a history of recurrent instability following reduction. The great majority of patients in this age group do not experience recurrent instability.[17] Care should be taken not to attribute loss of internal rotation strength to an associated axillary nerve injury, as was the case in 29 of 31 patients with rotator cuff rupture associated with anterior

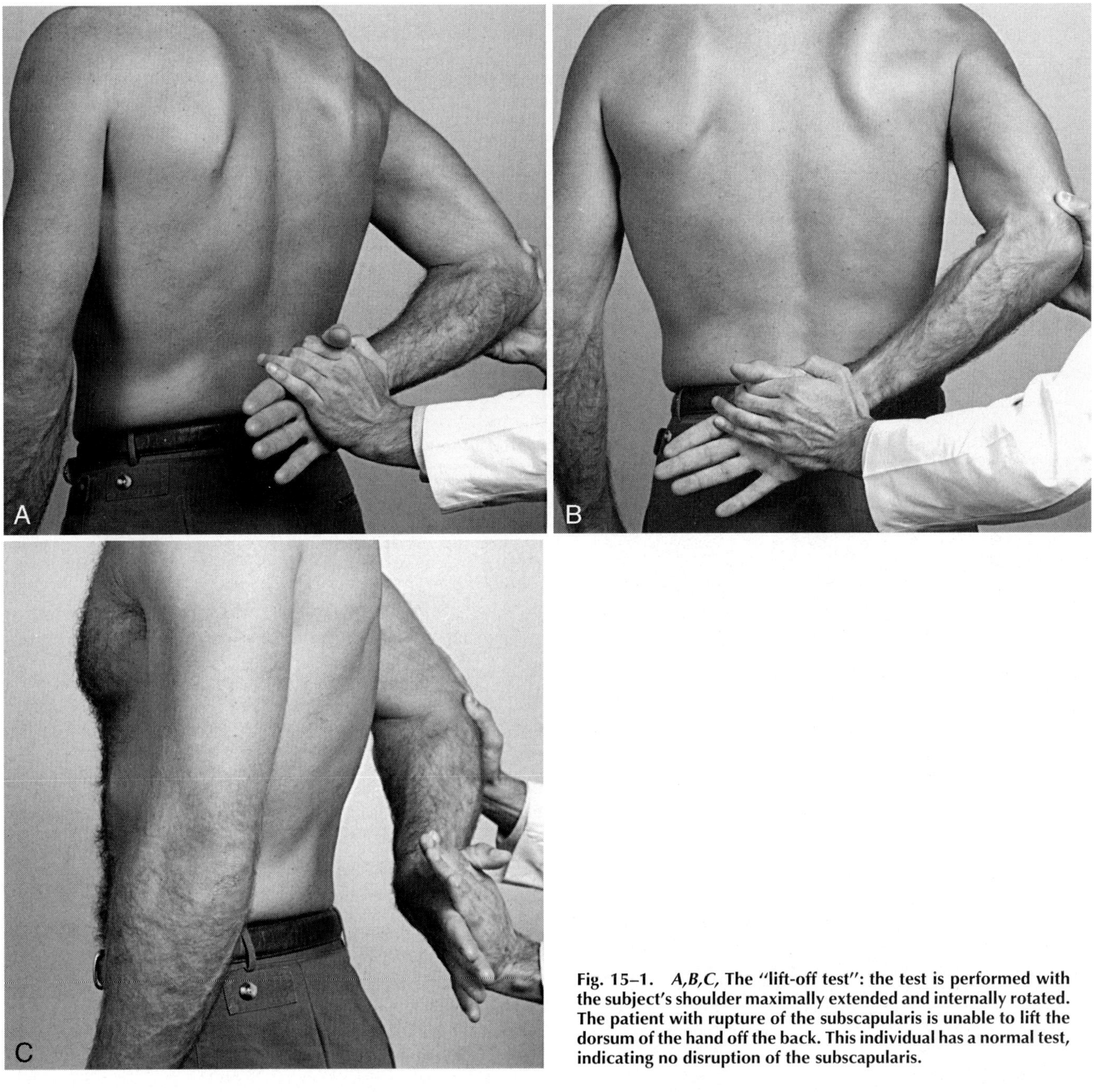

Fig. 15–1. *A,B,C,* **The "lift-off test": the test is performed with the subject's shoulder maximally extended and internally rotated. The patient with rupture of the subscapularis is unable to lift the dorsum of the hand off the back. This individual has a normal test, indicating no disruption of the subscapularis.**

dislocation in the group of patients of Neviaser et al. Pain, especially at night, is the other common complaint of patients with subscapular injury associated with previous dislocation.

The symptom complex may be more subtle in patients without a history of dislocation and, therefore, no associated instability. In Gerber and Krushell's series, all patients could remember an acute, painful injury, and all were treated initially for a "muscle strain."[18] Once again these patients will note a loss of strength in the shoulder, most notably in internal rotation. Pain was also noted with active use both above and below the level of the shoulder. This is in distinction to patients with tears of other cuff muscles, who typically note a lessening of symptoms with use of the arm below shoulder level.[18]

Gerber and Krushell described a clinical diagnostic test for use with rupture of the subscapularis.[18] The "lift-off test" was considered pathological in 12 of 13 patients with isolated rupture of the subscapularis. The test is performed with the patient's shoulder maximally extended and internally rotated (Fig. 15–1). The dorsum of the hand rests on the lumbar region. The patient with an intact subscapularis should be able to lift the dorsum of the hand off the back against resistance. The patient with rupture of the subscapularis is unable to lift the dorsum of the hand off the back. It is required that the patient have full passive internal rotation for the test to be considered valid. To confirm the validity of this test, it was performed on 162 other patients with and without shoulder pathology.[18] The test was normal in all patients without associated subscapular rupture and was considered "pathological" in 8 of 9 patients with documented full thickness tears of the rotator cuff involving the subscapularis. The test was also noted to revert to normal following successful repair of the subscapular injury. This test may also be useful in diagnosis of postsurgical disruption or dehiscence of subscapularis repairs following anterior approaches to the shoulder, whether or not the initial pathology included subscapular injury.

Clinically, patients with subscapular rupture were also noted to have an increase in passive external rotation, with a poor end-point relative to the contralateral side. Pain is associated with passive external rotation and patients report this pain to improve with abduction of the externally rotated extremity.[18]

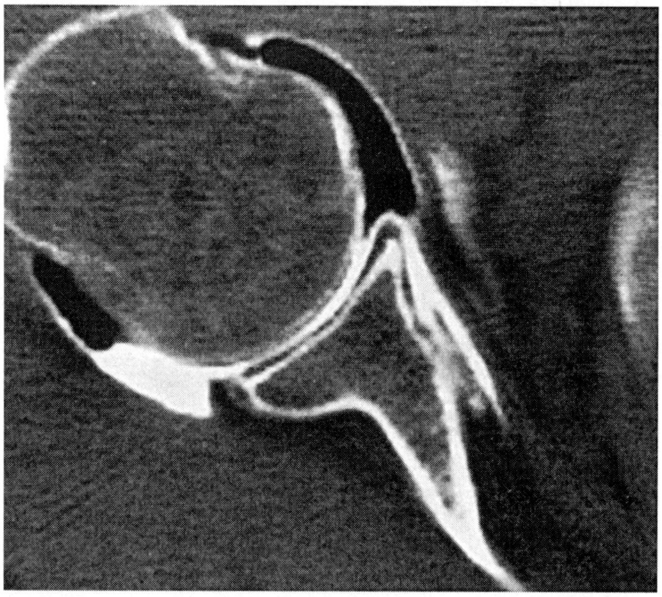

Fig. 15–2. CT arthrography shows a crescent of injected air extending without interruption into the bicipital groove. This is proof that the subscapularis tendon has been separated from the lesser tuberosity. Note that the anterior labrum is normal. (From Gerber C. Isolated disruption of the tendon of the subscapularis muscle. *J Bone Joint Surg Br.* 1991;73:389–394.)

DIAGNOSTIC STUDIES

Radiography

Plain film radiographs provide no information in rupture of the subscapularis without associated fracture; they may be useful in cases of lesser tuberosity avulsion with resultant disruption of the insertion of the subscapularis. Axillary views and images with the humerus in maximal internal rotation will best delineate the avulsed lesser tuberosity.[10,11,14] Typically, the fragment is visualized off the anterior-inferior border of the glenoid. Care should be taken to avoid the pitfall of diagnosing "calcific tendonitis" of the long head of the triceps or subscapularis, as is frequently the case.[8] These are unusual sites for radiologically identifiable calcific tendonitis and a history of such a diagnosis should lead to suspicion of lesser tuberosity avulsion.

Arthrography

Arthrography is often diagnostic in the face of subscapularis rupture. AP views will sometimes demonstrate medial dislocation of the tendon of the biceps into the

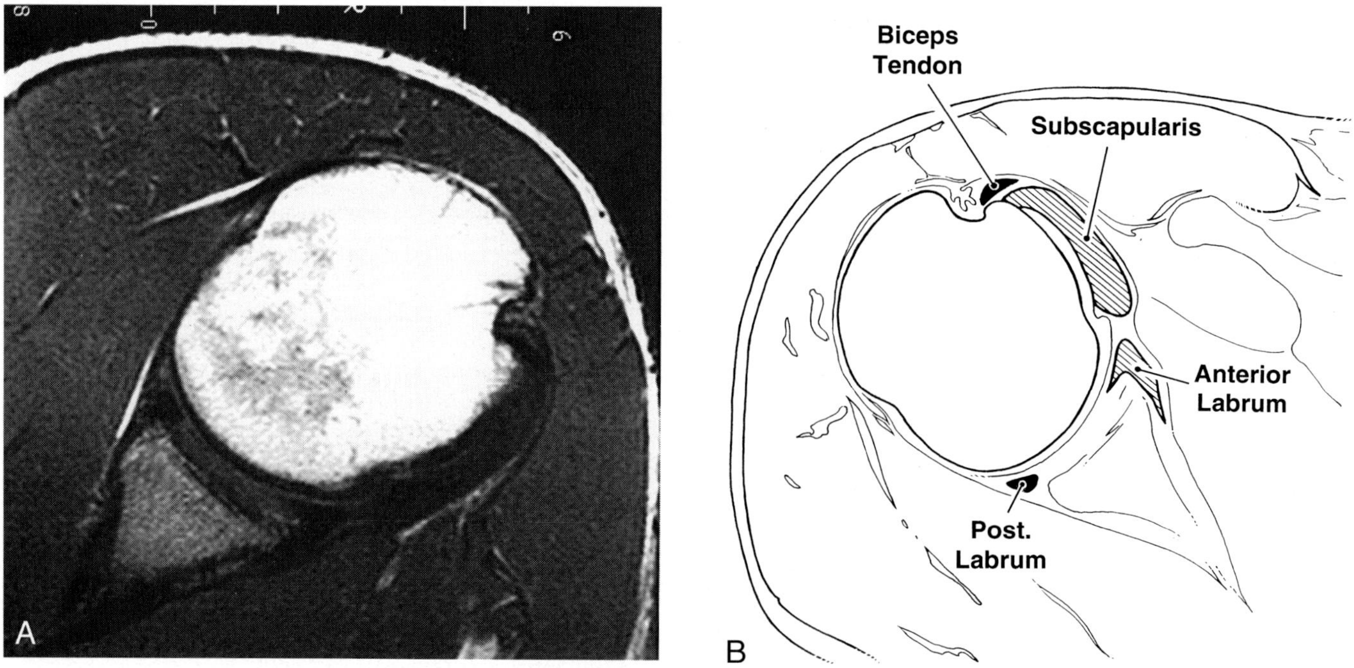

Fig. 15–3. MRI image *(A)* and line drawing *(B)* of an uninjured shoulder demonstrating normal anatomy of the subscapularis and biceps tendons. (Courtesy of Paul Weatherall, MD)

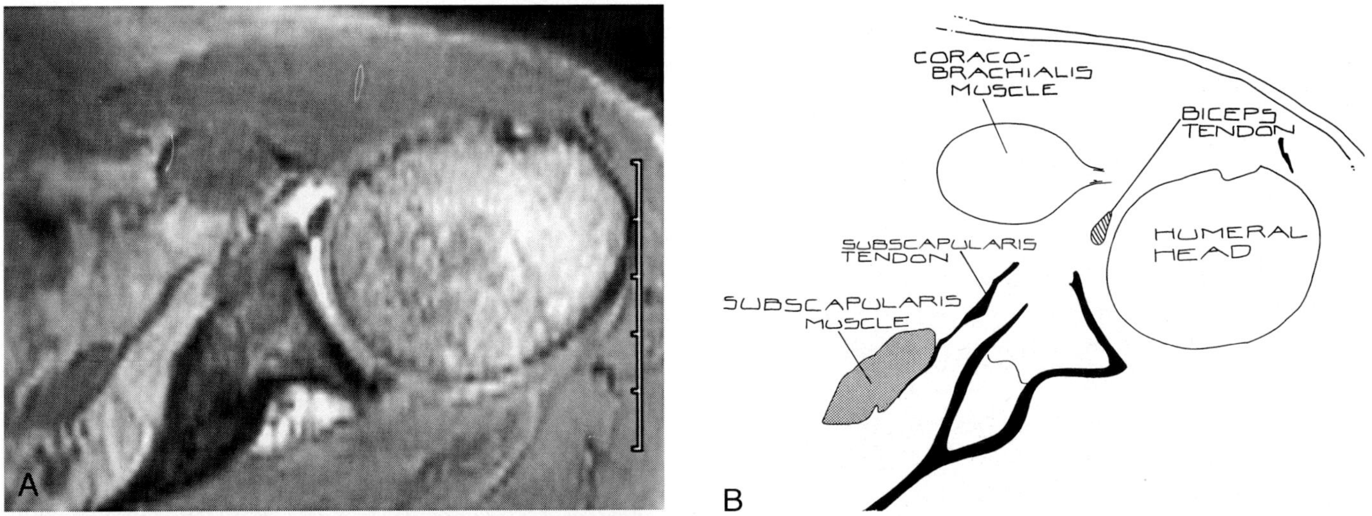

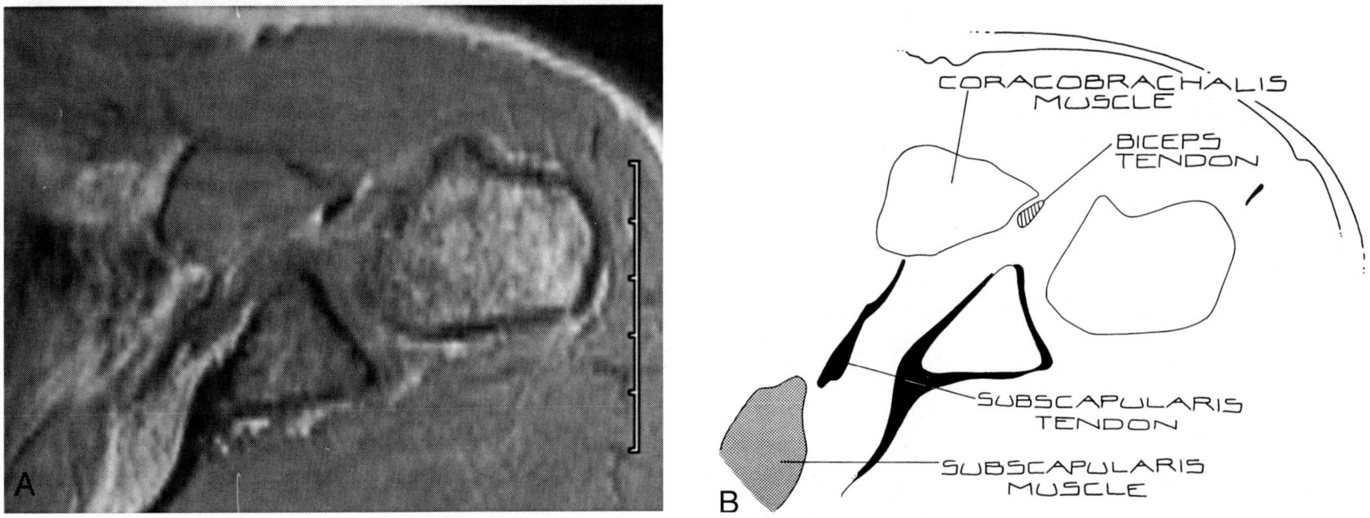

Figs. 15–4 and 15–5. Subscapularis tendon rupture: ***these serial axial MRI images (A)*** **and line drawings** ***(B)*** **demonstrate the dislocated biceps tendon, as well as the subscapularis (anteromedial to the glenoid).**

shoulder. This is pathognomonic of subscapular rupture.[18,27] Lateral views reveal a ventral defect in the capsule and an intact supraspinatus.[18]

Postarthrography CT scans often document continuity of the dye column in the shoulder with the bicipital groove (Fig. 15–2).[18] CT scans can also assess the degree of atrophy of the subscapularis muscle.

Ultrasonography

Ultrasonography reveals loss of the subscapularis echogenic line at its insertion into the lesser tuberosity.[18]

MRI

MRI, when available, is the diagnostic procedure of choice, as it best defines the overall anatomy of the shoulder, ruling out other injuries and better delineating the tissue quality associated with the subscapular injury. Its only significant drawbacks are cost and availability.

Axial images in the uninjured shoulder demonstrate the subscapularis inserting onto the lesser tuberosity and the biceps tendon located in the bicipital groove (Fig. 15–3). Axial images in the shoulder with subscapularis disruption reveal fascia in direct apposition to the lesser tuberosity without interposing subscapularis tendon.[18,27] The line of low signal intensity representing the subscapularis tendon is often visualized anteromedial to the anterior edge of the glenoid (Figs. 15–4 and 15–5). In cases of lesser tuberosity avulsion, the avulsed fragment can also be visualized, with or without associated biceps tendon dislocation (Figs. 15–6 through 15–9). Coronal images may also reveal dislocation of the long head of the biceps tendon into the shoulder, with disruption of the subscapular insertion (Fig. 15–10).[28–30]

Arthroscopy

Arthroscopic examination can also diagnose subscapularis rupture (Fig. 15–11). However, if the capsule and

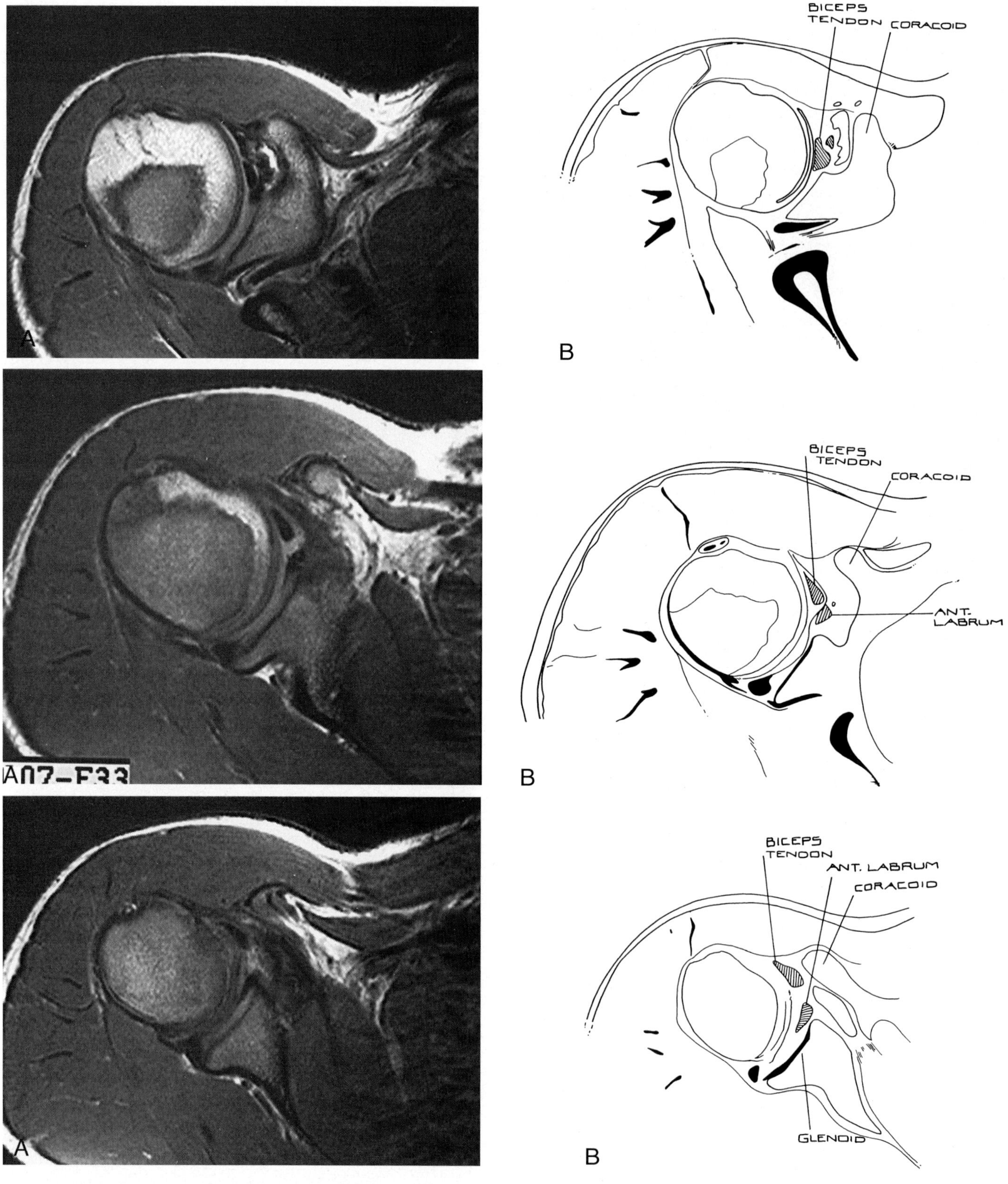

Figs. 15–6 through 15–9. Lesser tuberosity avulsion: these serial axial MRI images *(A)* and corresponding line drawings *(B)* delineate the MRI findings associated with lesser tuberosity avulsion. (Courtesy of Paul Weatherall, MD.)

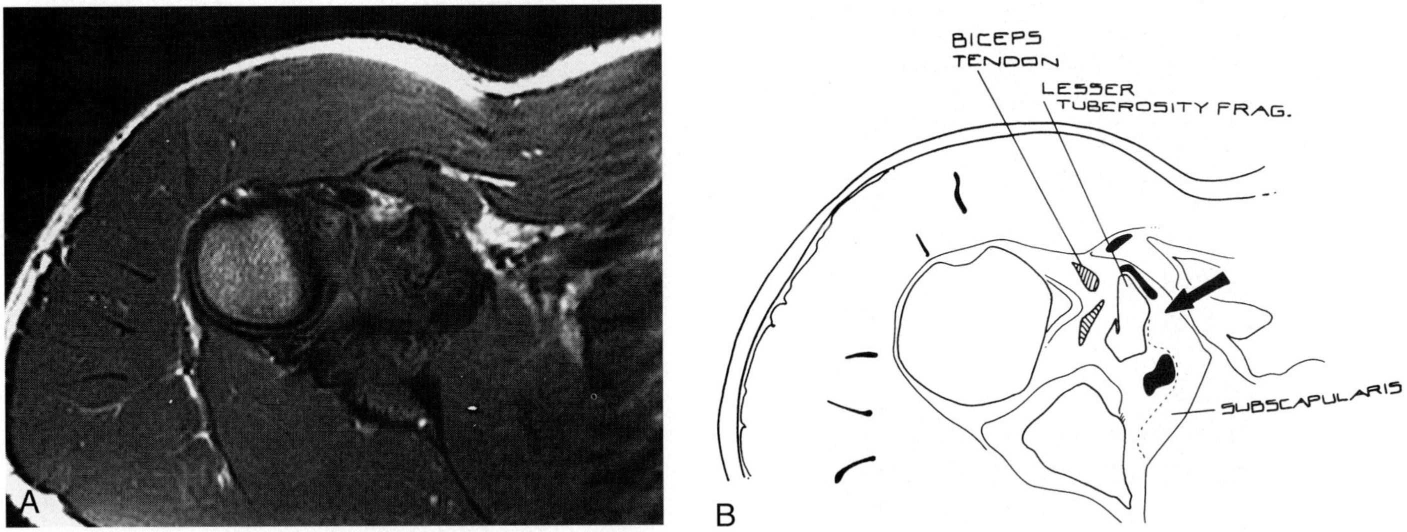

Figs. 15–6 through 15–9.—*Continued*

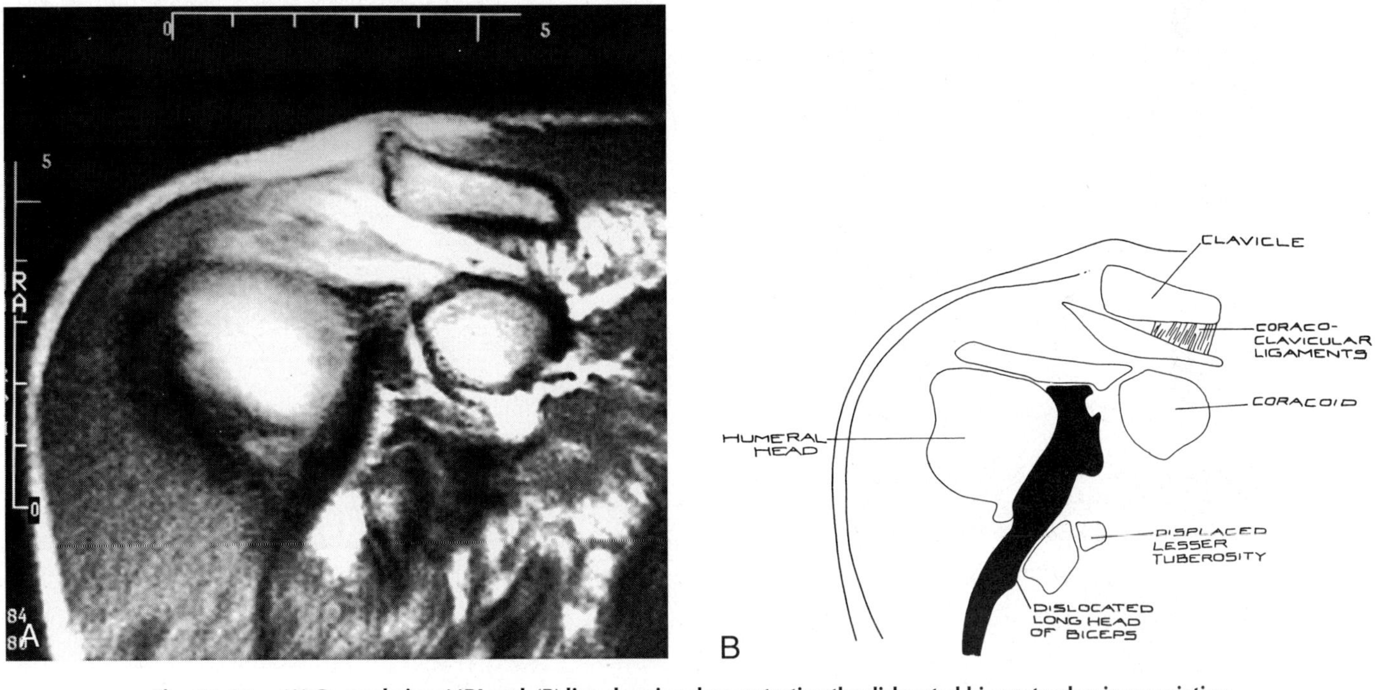

Fig. 15–10. ***(A)*** **Coronal view MRI and** ***(B)*** **line drawing demonstrating the dislocated biceps tendon in association with a lesser tuberosity avulsion injury.**

the superior band of the subscapularis tendon are intact, the diagnosis of a significant tear can be missed.

TREATMENT

The key to treatment of subscapular disruption lies in its diagnosis. In cases both with and without dislocation, diagnosis is often delayed, thereby allowing progressive scarring around the subscapularis tendon and brachial plexus, as well as retraction of the tendon stump. A heightened level of suspicion is warranted particularly in the older, at-risk patient.

Surgical repair of the disrupted tendon is recommended through an anterior delto-pectoral approach, which affords access to both the lesser tuberosity and the retracted tendon stump (Figs. 15–12 and 15–13). Care must be taken to avoid injury to the juxtaposed brachial plexus, particularly in delayed repairs. In most cases, reanastomosis with a trough in bone technique provides a very satisfactory repair. Heavy, nonabsorbable sutures passed through drill holes in the bone, or used with su-

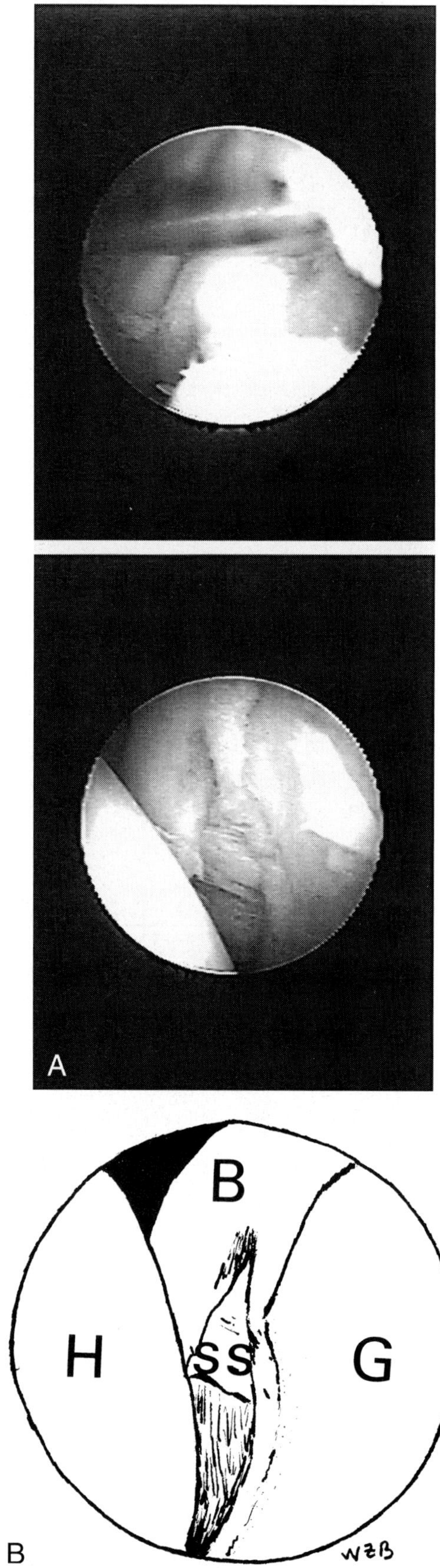

Fig. 15–11. *(A)* Arthroscopic image and *(B)* line drawing demonstrating findings of subscapularis rupture. The subscapularis (ss) is avulsed. The biceps (B) takes a more inferior and medial course through the joint.

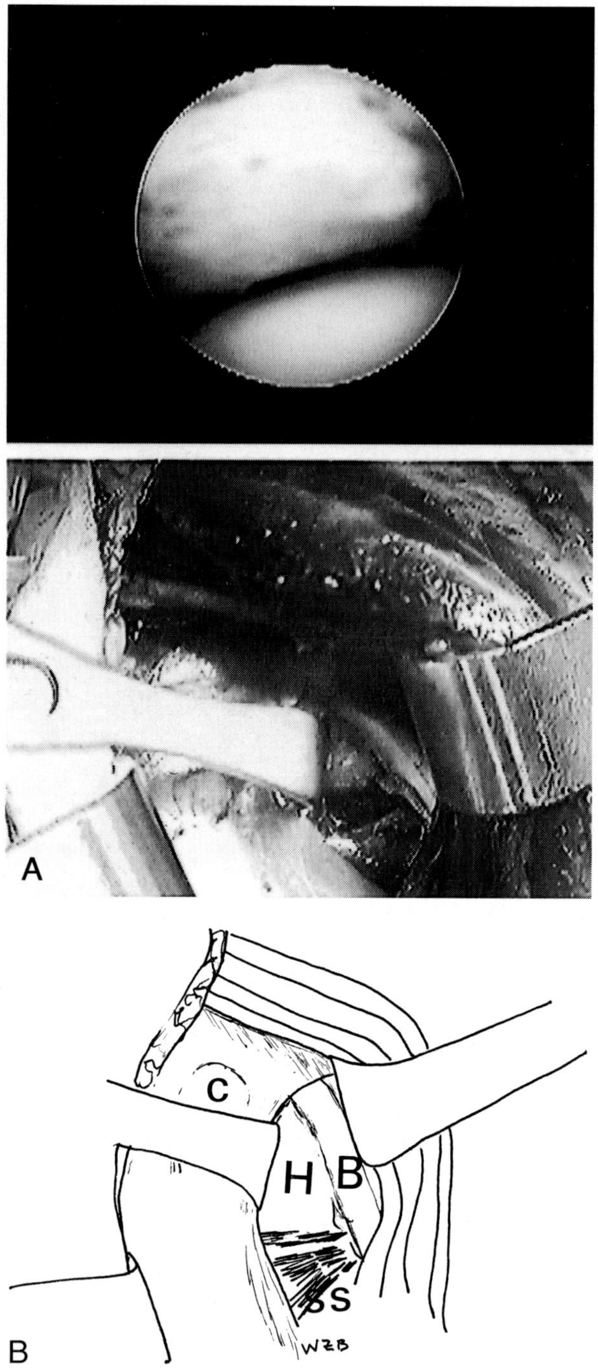

Fig. 15–12. *(A)* Intraoperative photograph and *(B)* corresponding line drawing of delto-pectoral approach for subscapularis injury. Labels: H–humeral head, B–biceps tendon, SS–subscapularis, C–conjoined tendon.

ture anchors, are recommended. Given the shallow depth of the lesser tuberosity, using suture anchors to attach the tendon to an area of freshened bone is often technically easier than formation of a formal trough with drill holes for suture placement. In the instance an unsuspected subscapular injury is encountered during repair of other shoulder pathology through a more superior approach, suture anchors can greatly facilitate subscapular reattachment in the distal portion of the exposure. If displaced, the biceps tendon should be replaced in the bicipital groove (Fig. 15–14).[30]

In adult patients with displaced lesser tuberosity avulsion, surgical repair with suture has been successful.[8,9,11] Earwaker reported on two patients who underwent excision of the avulsed lesser tuberosity fragment with primary repair of the subscapularis tendon to bone.[8] One patient did well, while the other continued to suffer from instability and pain.

Adolescents with lesser tuberosity avulsion seem less likely to sustain displaced fractures.[14,15] Nondisplaced lesser tuberosity avulsions may be treated conservatively, with early immobilization for 4 to 6 weeks, followed by progressive increases in range of motion. Successful results have been reported with this protocol, despite failure to demonstrate osseous union in two of three cases reported.[14,15] Individuals with displaced fractures should undergo surgical restoration of their normal anatomy, even if this requires osteotomy of the malunited lesser tuberosity fragment.[13]

PROGNOSIS

In isolated tears at early follow-up (6 months), Gerber noted 9 of 12 patients with primary ruptures of the subscapularis that were repaired had regained "normal passive internal rotation."[18] All repaired patients also reversed their pathological "lift-off test." At this early follow-up, no patients had yet regained full strength of internal rotation.

In a separate study of patients with other rotator cuff pathology, Gerber found that shoulders with massive tears and an irreparable subscapularis tear had an age-adjusted 48% functional value compared to 82% in shoulders with a functioning subscapularis following rotator cuff repair.[31] Obviously, repair is indicated wherever possible to return a more functional shoulder.

In Neviaser's report of reattachment of the subscapularis to the lesser tuberosity in patients with previous dislocation, all patients had good relief of nocturnal pain and full return of abduction.[17] Muscle strength about the

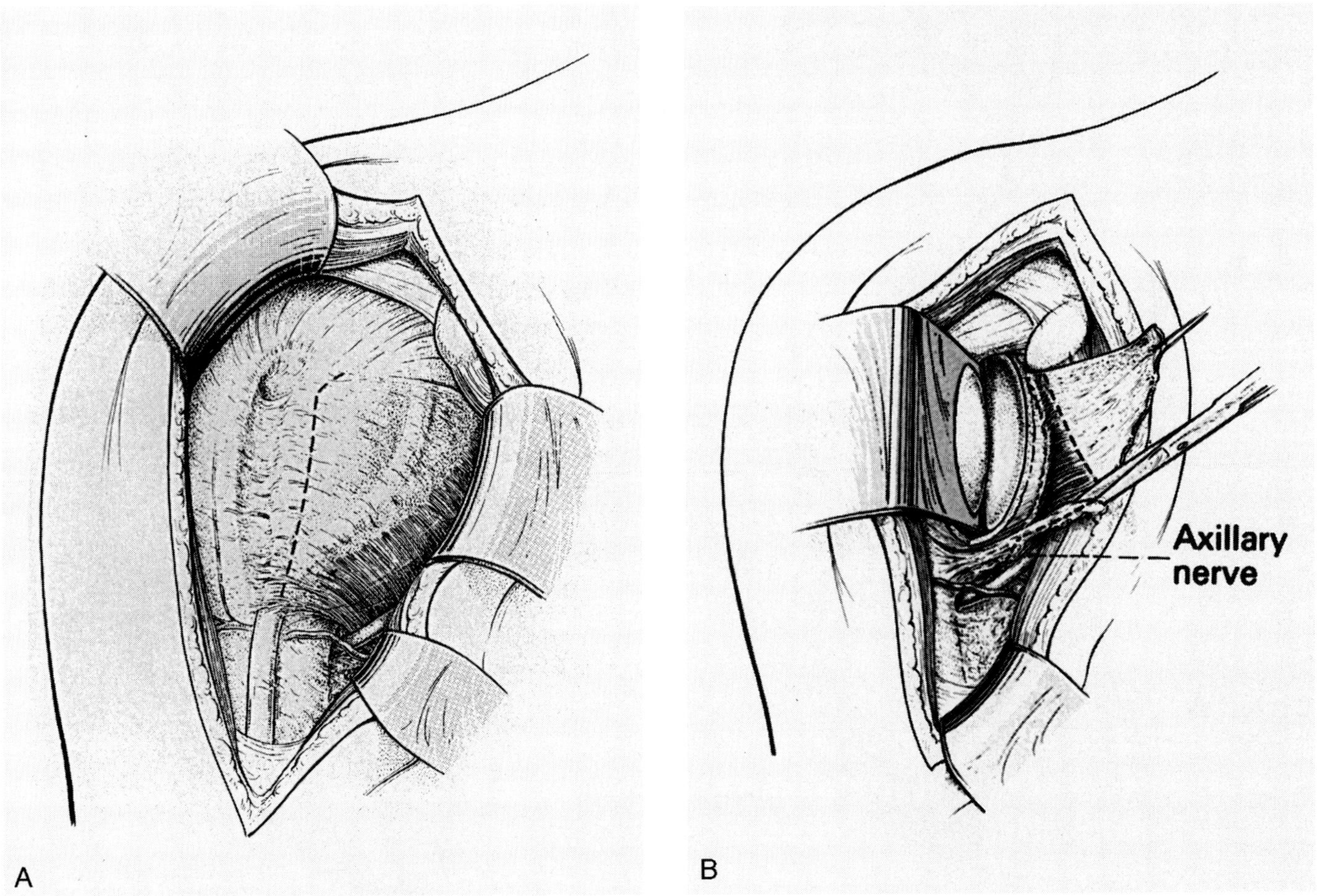

Fig. 15–13. Diagrams of a right shoulder with a ruptured subscapularis tendon. *A,* The humeral head is covered with thin scar tissue that can be mistaken for intact tendon. The biceps tendon may be dislocated medially into the joint. The scar which has replaced the subscapularis tendon is incised vertically (dotted line). *B,* The lesser tuberosity is found to be bald. Scar tissue is excised to reveal the tendon (dotted line), the axillary nerve being carefully protected. *C,* The subscapularis tendon is transfixed with heavy sutures and the musculotendinous unit is prepared for reinsertion. (From Gerber C. Isolated rupture of the tendon of the subscapularis muscle. *J Bone Joint Surg Br.* 1991;73:389–394.)

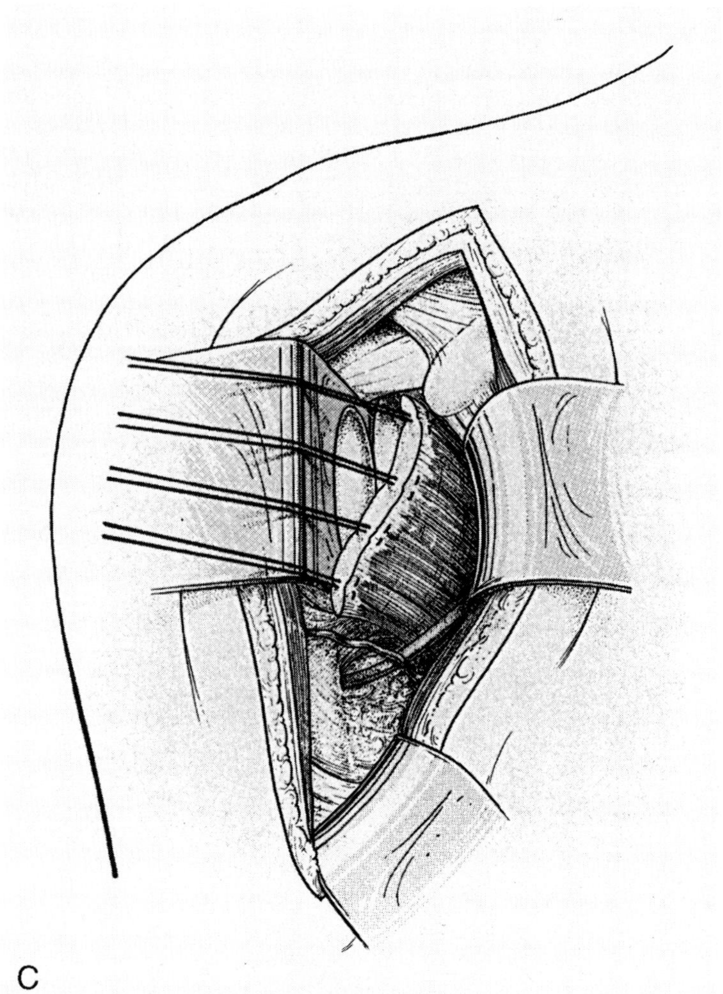

Fig 15–13—*continued*

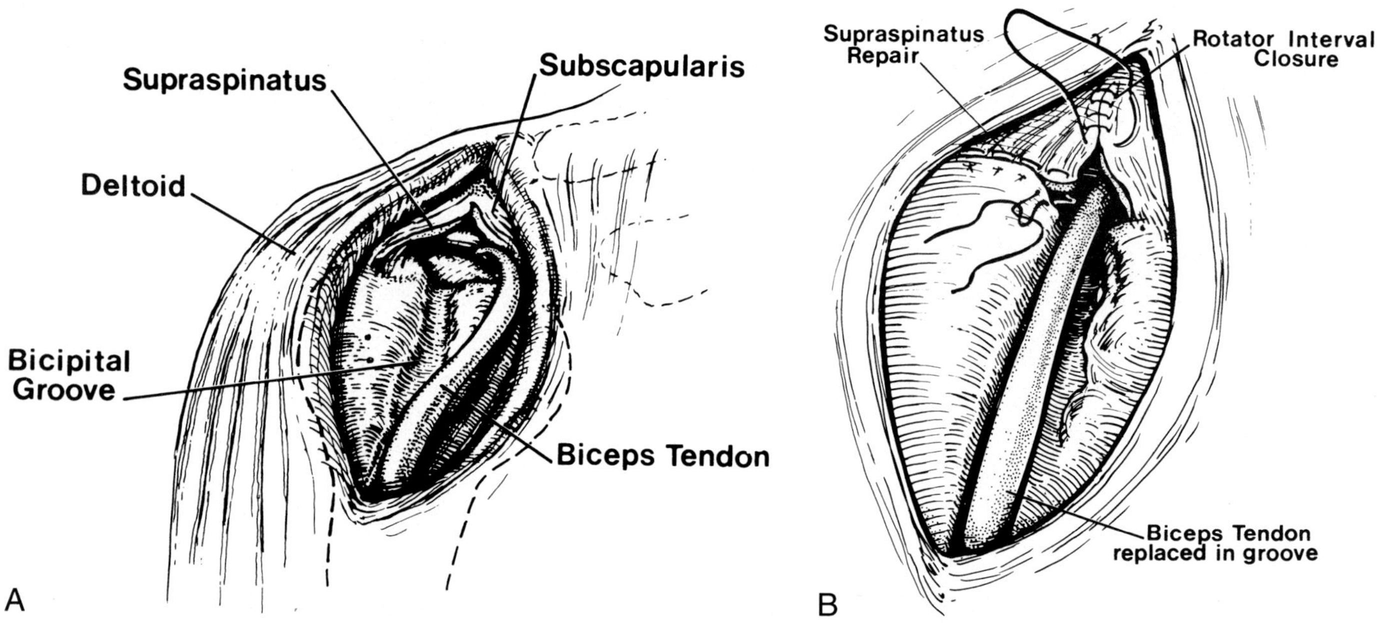

Fig. 15–14. ***A,*** **Rotator cuff tear and dislocated biceps tendon.** ***B,*** **The rotator cuff has been repaired and the rotator interval closed with the biceps tendon replaced in the bicipital groove. (From Rockwood CA, Matsen FA, eds.** ***The Shoulder.*** **Philadelphia: WB Saunders; 1990.)**

shoulder was described as 4 to 4+ in all shoulders. At 2 years following surgery, they reported no incidence of recurrent instability.

Similarly, adult and adolescent patients with preserved or restored anatomic alignment of the lesser tuberosity fragment following avulsion injury did well overall.[8,9,11,14,15] Every effort should be made to restore normal anatomy following these injuries, as patients without satisfactory repair did not do well in long-term follow-up.[8,13]

CONCLUSIONS

While isolated subscapularis disruption does not predispose to recurrent anterior instability of the shoulder, it is associated with significant morbidity. Patients typically complain of weakness in internal rotation and pain with passive external rotation. Subscapularis injury in association with a history of dislocation, and therefore concomitant disruption of the anterior capsulo-ligamentous restraints of the shoulder, results in the additional complication of recurrent instability.

The key to early diagnosis of subscapularis disruption is a high index of suspicion from the history and the appropriate physical exam. Subscapularis disruption must be included in the differential diagnosis of patients with shoulder pathology. It should be suspected particularly in the patient over the age of 40 who presents with weakness and pain in the shoulder, with or without a history of dislocation. Physical exam of patients with suspected subscapularis disruption should emphasize testing of internal rotation strength, passive external rotation, and assessment of the "lift-off test" as described by Gerber and Krushell.[18] Confirmation of the diagnosis and ruling out of other associated pathology is accomplished with ancillary diagnostic studies, preferably MRI if available.

Primary repair is indicated in patients with subscapular disruption associated with pain, weakness or recurrent instability. Early diagnosis of the condition allows repair prior to subscapular stump retraction and prevents fibrosis between the tendon stump and adjacent brachial plexus.

We recommend repair with a trough in bone technique or with implantable suture anchors to an area of freshened bone through a delto-pectoral approach, which allows excellent access to both the lesser tuberosity and retracted tendon stump. Most reports to date indicate that patients with primary repair do quite well and are relieved of symptoms of pain and recurrent instability.

REFERENCES

1. DePalma AF, Cooke AJ, Probhakar M. The role of the subscapularis in recurrent anterior dislocations of the shoulder. *Clin Orthop.* 1967; 54:35–49.
2. Symeonides PP. The significance of the subscapularis muscle in the pathogenesis of recurrent anterior dislocations of the shoulder. *J Bone Joint Surg Br.* 1972;54:476–483.
3. Karadimas J, Rentis G, Varouchas G. Repair of recurrent anterior dislocation of the shoulder using transfer of the subscapularis tendon. *J Bone Joint Surg Am.* 1980;62:1147–1149.
4. Hovelius I, Thorling J, Fredin H. Recurrent anterior dislocation of the shoulder: Results after the Bankart and Putti-Platt operations. *J Bone Joint Surg Am.* 1979;61:566–569.
5. Smith JG. Pathological appearances of seven cases of injury of the shoulder joints, with remarks (Abstract from The Medical Gazette, May 1834). *Am J Med Sciences.* 1835;16:219–224.
6. Hauser EDW. Avulsion of the tendon of the subscapularis muscle. *J Bone Joint Surg Am.* 1954;36:139–141.
7. Collier SG, Wynn-Jones CH. Displacement of the biceps with subscapular avulsion. *J Bone Joint Surg Br.* 1990;72:145.
8. Earwaker J. Isolated avulsion fracture of the lesser tuberosity of the humerus. *Skeletal Radiology.* 1990;19:121–125.
9. Haas SL. Fracture of the lesser tuberosity of the humerus. *Am J Surg.* 1944;63:253–256.
10. Labriola JH, Mohaghegh HA. Isolated avulsion fracture of the lesser tuberosity of the humerus: A case report and review of the literature. *J Bone Joint Surg Am.* 1975;57:1101.
11. McAuliffe TB, Dowd GS. Avulsion of the subscapularis tendon: A case report. *J Bone Joint Surg Am.* 1987;69:1454–1455.
12. McGuinness JP. Isolated avulsion fracture of the lesser tuberosity of the humerus. *Lancet.* 1939;1:508.
13. Paschal SO, Hutton K. Isolated avulsion fracture of the lesser tuberosity in adolescents: A report of two cases and review of the literature. Unpublished, 1993.
14. Ross GJ, Love MB. Isolated avulsion fracture of the lesser tuberosity of the humerus: Report of two cases. *Radiology.* 1989;172:833–834.
15. Shibuya S, Ogawa K. Isolated avulsion fracture of the lesser tuberosity of the humerus: A case report. *Clin Orthop.* 1986;1:215–218.
16. White GM, Riley LH. Isolated avulsion of the subscapularis insertion in a child: A case report. *J Bone Joint Surg Am.* 1985;67:635–636.
17. Neviaser RJ, Neviaser TJ, Neviaser JS. Concurrent rupture of the rotator cuff and anterior dislocation of the shoulder in the older patient. *J Bone Joint Surg Am.* 1988;70:1308–1311.
18. Gerber C, Krushell RJ. Isolated rupture of the tendon of the subscapularis: Clinical features in 16 cases. *J Bone Joint Surg Br.* 1991; 73:389–394.
19. Gray HG. In: Dick TP, Howden R, eds. *Gray's Anatomy: The Classic Collectors Edition.* London: Crown Publishers; 1977:383–384.
20. Bowen MK, Warren RF. Ligamentous control of shoulder stability based on selective cutting and static translation experiments. *Clin Sports Med.* 1991;10:757–782.
21. Harryman DT, Sidles JA, Matsen FA. Mechanisms of shoulder stability. Individual Orthopaedic Instruction Videotape VT-2314 at American Academy of Orthopaedic Surgeons 58th Annual Meeting. February 1993.
22. Keating JF, Waterworth P, Shaw-Dunn J, Crossan J. The relative strengths of the rotator cuff muscles: A cadaver study. *J Bone Joint Surg Br.* 1993;75:137–140.
23. Turkel SJ, Panio MW, Marshall JL, Girgis FG. Stabilizing mechanisms preventing anterior dislocation of the gleno-humeral joint. *J Bone Joint Surg Am.* 1981;63:1208–1217.
24. O'Brien SJ, Neves MC, Arnoczky SP, et. al. The anatomy and histology of the inferior gleno-humeral ligament complex of the shoulder. *Am J Sports Med.* 1990;18:449–456.
25. Reeves B. Experiments on the tensile strength of the anterior capsular structures of the shoulder in man. *J Bone Joint Surg Br.* 1968; 50:858–865.
26. Neviaser RJ. Personal communication, March 1993.
27. Crues JV, Fareed DO. Magnetic resonance imaging of shoulder impingement. *Techniques Orthop.* 1992;7:39–49.
28. Chan TW, Dalinka MK, Kneeland JB, Chervrot A. Biceps tendon dislocation: Evaluation with MR imaging. *Radiology.* 1991;179:649–652.
29. Petersson CL. Spontaneous medial dislocation of the tendon of the long biceps brachii. *Clin Orthop.* 1986;211:224–227.
30. Burkhead WZ. In: Rockwood CA, Matsen FA, eds. *The Shoulder.* Philadelphia: WB Saunders; 1990:829.
31. Gerber C. Latissimus dorsi transfer for the treatment of irreparable tears of the rotator cuff. *Clin Orthop.* 1992;275:152–160.

Chapter 16

Calcifying Tendinitis

Hans K. Uhthoff and K. Sarkar

Calcifying tendinitis is a relatively common disorder of a tendon characterized by multifocal calcific deposits, which in the course of time disappear either after spontaneous resorption or after surgical removal. The disappearance of the calcium deposit is followed by complete functional, and probably anatomical, restitution of the tendon. Thus, the process of calcification in calcifying tendinitis may be considered as the reactive type in which calcification occurs in an apparently viable soft tissue, as opposed to the dystrophic type where calcium mineral deposits at a site of nonviable soft tissue. Although the disorder is most often observed in the rotator cuff tendons of the shoulder, it is also described at other sites adjacent to the hip, elbow, and wrist.

TERMINOLOGY

Soft-tissue disorders of the shoulder have always presented a diagnostic problem and challenge. Although various imaging techniques have improved our diagnostic capabilities, a reliable interpretation of the variations in images is lacking, because the benign nature of these lesions often precludes surgical procedures, at least a biopsy.

Since the early description of Duplay (1872), the subacromial bursa has been blamed as the major source of shoulder pain. It was Duplay[1] who coined the term "periarthritis humero-scapularis," which is a nonspecific diagnosis covering all soft-tissue disorders except tears. This term is still in use for want of a more specific term. The advent of radiography enabled the identification of calcification in soft tissues. Painter (1907),[2] Bergemann and Stieda (1908),[3] and Stieda (1908)[4] believed that the subacromial bursa was the primary site of calcification; hence, the disorder was called calcified bursitis. However, Codman (1934)[5] rightly stated that the deposits did not arise in the bursa but in the underlying tendon. In 1912 the first histologic description was published by Wrede,[6] demonstrating that chondroid changes preceded calcium deposition and, consequently, the process took place in living tissue.

Although the intratendinous localization of calcium deposits was subsequently confirmed by many investigators,[7–9] inaccurate terms such as peritendinitis calcarea,[8] and calcified peritendinitis[10] continued to be in use even as late as 1979. In the English literature, intratendinous calcification is commonly referred to as calcific or calcified tendinitis. However, the term calcifying tendinitis, which first appeared in the English literature in 1952,[10a] seems to reflect better the dynamic nature of the disease that undergoes three consecutive events: (1) formation of multifocal calcium deposits, (2) spontaneous resorption of those deposits, and (3) finally, reconstitution of the tendon. In giving preference to this term we agree with the terminology of de Sèze and Welfling[11] who called the disorder "tendinite calcifiante." Because the clinical stages of the disease are at times accompanied by acute pain and the pathological process characterized by granulation tissue, the term tendinitis seems more appropriate than tendinosis.

INCIDENCE

During a round table discussion at an international symposium on the rotator cuff disorders held in Ottawa, Canada, in May, 1993, North American shoulder surgeons maintained that the overall incidence of calcifying tendinitis is decreasing, while surgeons from Japan and Europe were not able to confirm such a trend.[12] In the literature, the incidence of calcifying tendinitis shows a wide variation. It seems to depend not only on the available clinical material and diagnostic techniques, but also on the country under study. The classical study of Bosworth[13,14] in the United States reported an incidence of 2.7% among 6,061 office workers who had no symptoms. In Switzerland, Rüttimann[15] reported an incidence of 20% among 100 asymptomatic individuals. In France, Welfling and his collaborators[16] found a 7.5% incidence of calcification in 200 shoulders of asymptomatic persons. However, when they examined radiographs of 925 symptomatic shoulders, the incidence of calcification was 6.8%. The lower incidence among the symptomatic group was believed to be caused by a difference in age distribution. Patients with calcification were generally younger than those without calcification.

With respect to the preferred site of calcification, Plenk[17] noted that 82% of the deposits occurred in the supraspinatus tendon. In the same tendon, De Palma and Kruper[18] found an incidence of 74% and Bosworth[13] found an incidence of 51%.

Females are affected by calcification more often than males, with the incidence varying between 76.7 and 57%.[13,14,16,18–20] The age distribution is quite characteristic. De Palma and Kruper[18] reported that 36% of the patients were between 40 and 50 years of age. In our series, 42% were in this age range.[20] In the series reported by Welfling and his colleagues,[16] the highest incidence was seen in patients between 31 and 40 years of age. Not one of their patients was over the age of 71. The lack of calcific deposits in old persons was also observed by McLaughlin[21] in a postmortem study of approximately 1000 cadavers.

The right shoulder appears to be involved somewhat more often than the left shoulder.[18,20] The incidence of bilateral involvement seems to increase with the length of the follow-up. Bilateral involvement was found in 24.3% in Welfling and his collaborators' study,[16] 13% among De Palma and Kruper's patients,[18] and 17% in our series.[20] Welfling and his associates[16] also radiographed the hips of the patients with calcifying tendinitis of the shoulder and found 62.5% incidence of calcification, whereas in the control group incidence of calcification was only 4%. Despite this observation, the investigators concluded that no generalized disease process was responsible for calcifying tendinitis, and that constituted a disease entity of its own.

In De Palma and Kruper's study,[18] 41% of the patients were housewives and 27% included salespersons, executives, and professionals. In our study,[20] 43% of the patients were housewives and 44% performed clerical work. Persons doing heavy manual labor seem to suffer less from calcifying tendinitis. Any relation between calcifying tendinitis and trauma has been denied by most investigators.

ETIOLOGY AND PATHOGENESIS

The etiology of calcifying tendinitis remains unknown. Because the disease is not associated with abnormalities of calcium or phosphorus metabolism, local changes within the cuff tendon preceding calcification have been the subject of much speculation. Codman[5] believed that degeneration of the tendon is the prime factor leading to calcification through a dystrophic process. This concept has gained widespread acceptance. McLaughlin[21] described the earliest lesion as focal hyalinization and fibrillation of tendon fibers that become detached from the surrounding normal tendon. Continued motion of the tendon grind the detached, curled fibers into a "wen-like substance" consisting of necrotic tissue that eventually calcifies. Steinbrocker[22] postulated that the disorder begins with necrosis and fraying of the tendon fibers, which are then replaced by a fibrinoid mass surrounded by leukocytes and histiocytes. Calcium is deposited on this mass by an unknown mechanism. According to Macnab,[23] the cuff tendons suffer from reduced vascularity because of pressure from the prominent humeral head that wrings out the vessels in the tendon. The resulting hypoxia induces separation and fragmentation of collagen fibers, cell death, and ultimately calcification.

Our concept of the pathogenetic mechanism of calcifying tendinitis is entirely to the contrary. We believe that neither degeneration nor necrosis of the tendon fibers is the initiating event and that the process of calcification is actively mediated by cells in a viable environment.[20,24,25] However, because of the anatomical position of the cuff tendons as they bend over the humeral head, there may be bouts of hypoxia in the area compromising tissue viability that becomes susceptible to calcification.

By clinicopathological correlations, we envisage the pathogenesis of calcifying tendinitis evolving through three distinct stages: (1) precalcific, (2) calcific, and (3) postcalcific (Fig. 16–1). In the precalcific stage, the site for future calcification, approximately 1.5 to 2 cm from the bony insertion and in the tendon proper, undergoes fibrocartilaginous transformation. In the ensuing calcific stage, calcium salts are deposited in this area. For the convenience of description, we have used the term "formative phase" to denote the initial period of the calcific stage. Following a variable period of inactivity, the spontaneous resorption of the calcific deposits begins, mediated by macrophages brought into the area by proliferating blood vessels. This is the latter phase of the calcific stage, which we have termed the "resorptive phase". As the calcium crystals are removed, the space that had been taken up by the deposit is occupied by granulation tissue and the postcalcific stage begins. The granulation tissue progresses to a mature scar, which undergoes remodeling and reconstitutes the tendon with the recovery of function.[20,24,25]

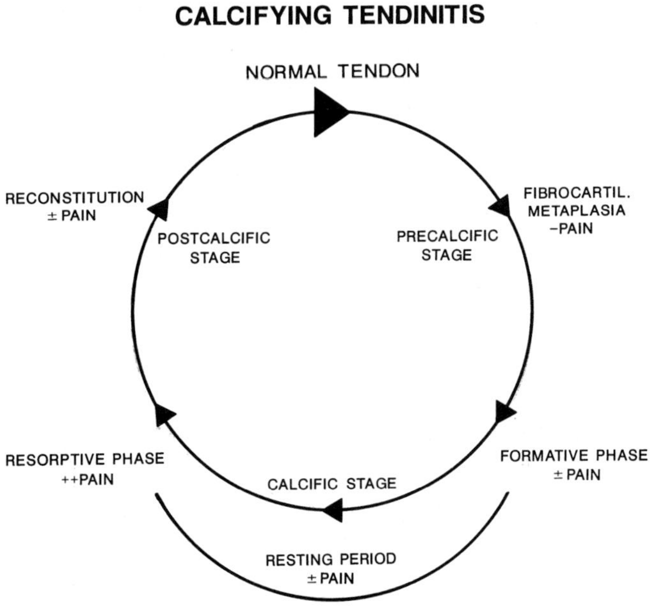

Fig. 16–1. Evolution of calcifying tendinitis. A schematic representation of our hypothesis.

CLINICAL PRESENTATION

The understanding of the pathogenetic mechanism of calcifying tendinitis is a prerequisite for a proper clinical evaluation and management. The usual clinical perception is that in any disease acute symptoms represent the initial stage and subsiding or chronic symptoms indicate the recovery stage. However, in calcifying tendinitis it is entirely the opposite. The formative phase of calcification is usually accompanied by minimal symptoms, or the deposit is discovered accidentally. Thus, the disease seems to begin with symptoms characteristic of a chronic state. Larger deposit may lead to the impingement syndrome, a fact already observed during surgery by Baer in 1907.[26]

It is during the ensuing phase of resorption of calcium deposits when acute symptoms appear, because of cellular and vascular proliferation together with edema that raise the intratendinous pressure. The pain may be further exacerbated by impingement secondarily to the increased volume of the tendon in the unyielding subacromial space. Symptoms may become chronic after the resorption of calcium while the tendon is in the process of reconstitution.

The subclinical nature of the formative phase has been reported by many investigators. Codman[5] noted that "the usual history is not acute pain in the beginning." Wilson[27] observed that many patients know about the presence of a calcium deposit for months or years prior to an acute attack. Pinals and Short[28] stated that "calcium deposition precedes rather than follows the development of an acute attack of calcific periarthritis, and the attack is accompanied by a disintegration and gradual disappearance of the deposit." Gschwend and coworkers[29] noted that the calcification is often symptomless at the beginning but its disappearance is very painful.

These reports clearly indicate that we are not dealing with two unrelated disease processes, namely acute and chronic calcific tendinitis, but with two phases of the same disease. Lippmann[19] warned that the failure to recognize the proper phase might result in attributing "magical healing powers" to "useless therapeutic measures" and "to the performance of needless surgical procedures."

According to Simon,[30] a relationship exists between the intensity of symptoms and duration. Acute symptoms may last up to 2 weeks; subacute symptoms may last 3 to 8 weeks; chronic symptoms may persist for 3 months or more. The briefness of acute symptoms was also noted by Pendergrass and Hodes[31] even in the absence of treatment. Wrede[6] and other investigators observed that clinical symptoms are often absent.

An increase in pain during the night is not uncommon. The patient cannot sleep on the affected shoulder. The range of motion is usually decreased by pain. Kessel and Watson[32] described the painful arc between 70 and 110° of abduction. Patients often complain of a sensation of catching when going through the arc of motion. We believe that this is caused by localized impingement. Such an impingement between the calcium deposit and the coracoacromial arch were mentioned by Baer[26] and Wrede.[6] In the presence of long-standing symptoms, an atrophy of both spinati muscles may be present. During the acute phase, patients refuse to move the shoulder because of excruciating pain. Any attempt to mobilize the glenohumeral joint is resisted. Typically, patients hold their arm close to the body in internal rotation.

The involvement of the subacromial bursa in different phases of calcifying tendinitis has not been documented in detail. There is no doubt that in the chronic state the subacromial bursa is not significantly involved. Any reaction tends to be limited to the site of the impingement where hyperemia can be seen. Carnett[33] noted that bursitis forms a minor and infrequent feature in calcifying tendinitis. The bursa has been alleged to be the major source of pain during the acute stage. Yet, during surgery, the bursal reaction is so minimal that the calcific deposit can be seen through the bursal wall. Litchman and his colleagues[34] have also noted the absence of bursal inflammation. It is probable that as deposits rupture into the bursa, a crystalline bursitis may develop, causing pain. We have shown evidence of phagocytic resorption of deposits that ruptured into the bursa.[35] In Welfling's study,[16] of the 12 patients in whom the deposit ruptured into the bursa, only 8 patients showed symptoms.

RADIOLOGY

Radiographs should be taken in all patients suspected of having calcifying tendinitis. Once diagnosed, radiologic follow-up is absolutely necessary. This follow-up allows an assessment of changes occurring in density and extent of the deposit.[36] The initial radiographs should include an anteroposterior view in neutral, external, and internal rotation. Films taken in internal rotation will reveal deposits in the infraspinatus and teres minor tendons, whereas those taken in external rotation will reveal deposits in the subscapularis tendon. The latter site of calcification is a rare occurrence. In calcifying tendinitis, the calcium deposits are localized inside the tendon proper 1.5 to 2.0 cm away from the insertion of the tendon into bone. Thus, they are easily distinguishable from stippled calcifications that may occur at tendon insertions. Should a rupture into the bursa occur, a crescent-like shadow overlying the actual calcification is seen extending over the greater tuberosity.

Bosworth[13] has proposed a classification of calcifying tendinitis into three categories based on the size of the deposits: (1) small, measuring up to 0.5 mm in diameter; (2) medium, measuring from 0.5 to 1.5 mm; and (3) large being greater than 1.5 mm. He concluded that small deposits were of little clinical significance, whereas the larger deposits could give rise to pain. Patte and Goutallier[37] proposed another classification by distinguishing between localized and diffuse forms of calcification. The localized form was round or oval, homogeneously dense, and situated close to the bursal wall. These deposits were believed to heal spontaneously. On the other hand, the diffuse form was situated much deeper, close to the bony insertion and with a heterogenous appearance on radiographs. This type produced more symptoms and took longer to disappear. In our experience, both classifications are of little clinical value.

Radiographs, in addition to confirming the presence or absence of calcification and localization of the deposit, also help to indicate the phase of the deposits. De Palma and Kruper[18] described two types of calcification. According to their results, type I showed a fluffy, fleecy appearance and its periphery was poorly outlined. This type was usually seen in patients with acute pain. The type II deposit was more or less discrete, with a uniform density and well-defined outline. Patients with this type of calcification had subacute or chronic pain. De Sèze and Welfling[11] also reported that patients with deposits that were less dense with ill-defined margins had acute pain. On the other hand, calcification in patients with chronic pain was dense with well-defined margins. These investigators described the following radiologic sequence in acute cases: (1) first, a fluffy, ill-defined intratendinous deposit, (2) followed by calcific material in the bursa, and (3) finally, the disappearance of calcium.

Our own observations are generally in accordance with those of De Palma and Kruper[18] and De Sèze and Welfling.[11] During the formative phase deposits are homogeneously dense and well defined (Fig. 16–2). On the other hand, during the resorptive phase deposits are fluffy, cloud-like and ill-defined (Fig. 16–3). Moreover, the density is irregular. In some cases, during the resorptive phase it may be difficult to identify the deposit in ordinary radiograms. In that situation, a xerogram may be helpful. Ruptures into the bursa are seen only in the resorptive phase. However, we feel that rupture into the bursa does not occur in all cases. The resorption of the residual material in the tendon takes far longer than in the bursa. Calcifying tendinitis and full substance tears can coexist.[37a]

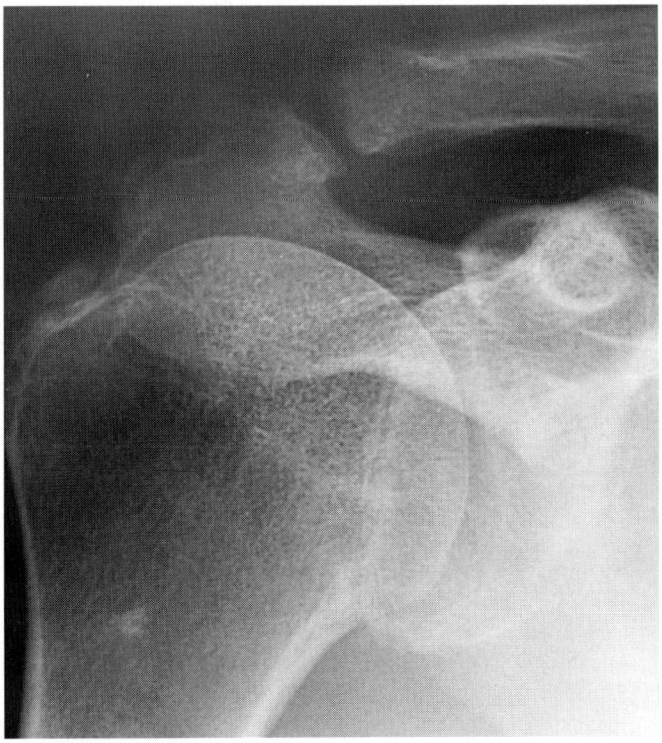

Fig. 16–2. Radiograph demonstrating the calcium deposit in the formative phase.

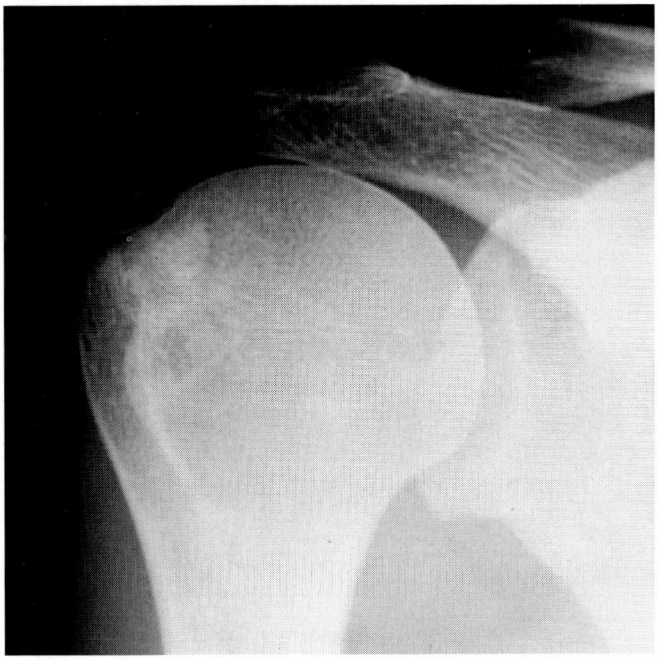

Fig. 16–3. Radiograph demonstrating the deposit in the resorptive phase.

We have attempted to correlate clinical symptoms with radiologic signs and the consistency of deposits in 41 patients undergoing surgery.[38] In 24 out of 31 patients with chronic symptoms, the radiologic signs were compatible with the formative phase, while the consistency of the calcific material during surgery was chalk-like in 29 out of 31 patients. Of 10 patients with acute symptoms, 8 had radiographic features characteristic of the resorptive phase, and 9 had toothpaste-like consistency of the deposit at surgery.

In our hospital, bursograms have not proven to be of value. Arthrograms, on the other hand, will show a clear separation between the deposit and the joint cavity. However, arthrograms are indicated only in certain circumstances, especially when a tear is suspected. The absence of degenerative joint diseases has been noted by most investigators. In only three of our patients did we find evidence of acromioclavicular osteophytes. All three patients were aged in their sixth decade.

PATHOLOGY

In biopsy specimens obtained during surgery of the tendinous tissue containing calcium, the deposits under the scanning electron microscope appear as irregularly ovoid masses disrupting and fragmenting the collagen fibers (Fig. 16–4). Microscopically, the deposits are mul-

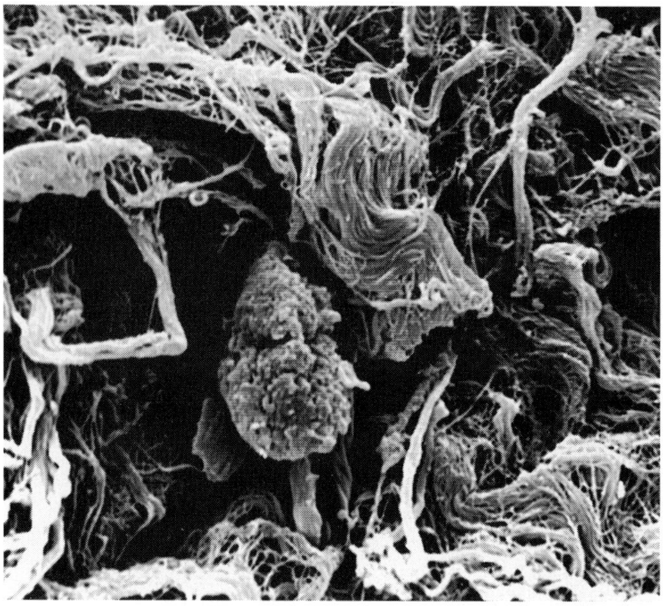

Fig. 16–4. Scanning electron micrograph showing an ovoid calcific deposit in the center surrounded by fibrillated and fragmented bands of collagen fibers (×2.600).

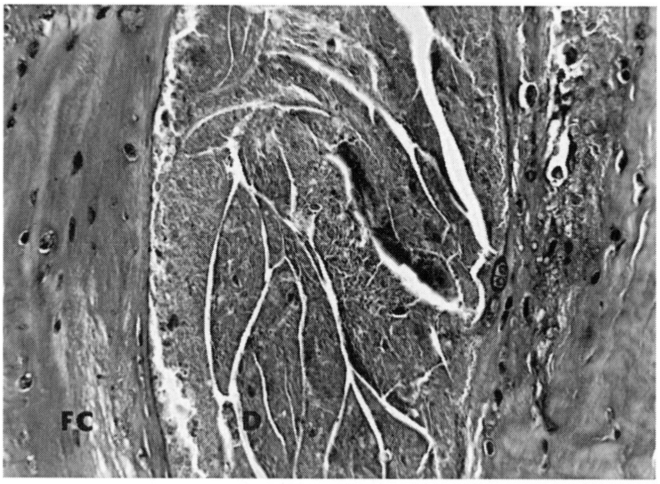

Fig. 16–5. Section showing fibrocartilaginous tissue (FC) on either side of a calcific deposit (D), characterizing the formative phase (hematoxylin-eosin, ×60).

tifocal, interrupted by strands of connective tissue (Fig. 16–5). The size and shape of the deposits are quite irregular, and the contents are granular or in clumps. The surrounding connective tissue may present a variegated appearance. Some deposits are adjacent to areas of fibrocartilage, containing chondrocytes and a metachromatic matrix that show no signs of degeneration or necrosis (Fig. 16–6). We believe that the fibrocartilage is the result of a metaplastic transformation of the collagenous fascicles in the tendon proper that occurs as the initial step before calcification. The fibrocartilaginous tissue then persists during the formative phase of the calcific stage, because it contains the chondrocytes that mediate the appearance of calcium crystals, which begin mainly in matrix vesicles (Fig. 16–7). Interestingly, Archer and colleagues[38a] were able to detect collagen type II in the fibrocartilage. The crystal-containing vesicles tend to coalesce with each other, thus producing large deposits. This area, then, represents the formative phase of the calcific stage.

In some other areas, the deposits abut against relatively avascular areas of tendinous tissue with tenocytes and fibers with minimal wavy configuration (Fig. 16–8). These areas could represent the deposits in resting phase when no addition to the mass is occurring nor is it being resorbed.

What is considered to be the characteristic lesion of calcifying tendinitis is called the "calcium granuloma."[39] In this lesion, the calcific deposit is surrounded and infiltrated by cells consisting mainly of phagocytosing

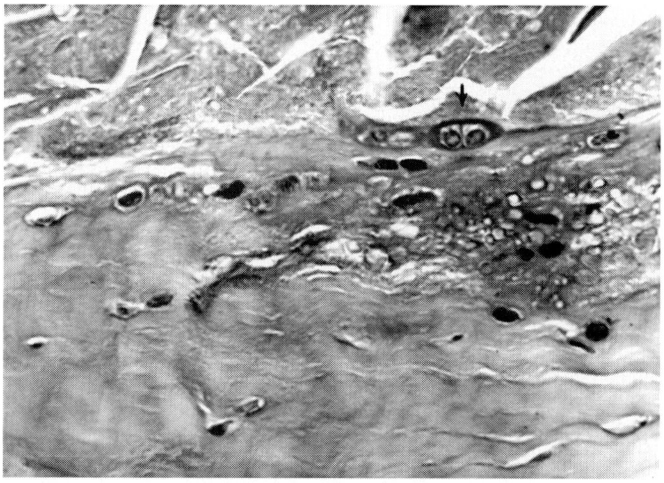

Fig. 16–6. Higher magnification of the same section showing viable chondrocytes (arrow) next to the calcific deposit (hematoxylin-eosin, ×120).

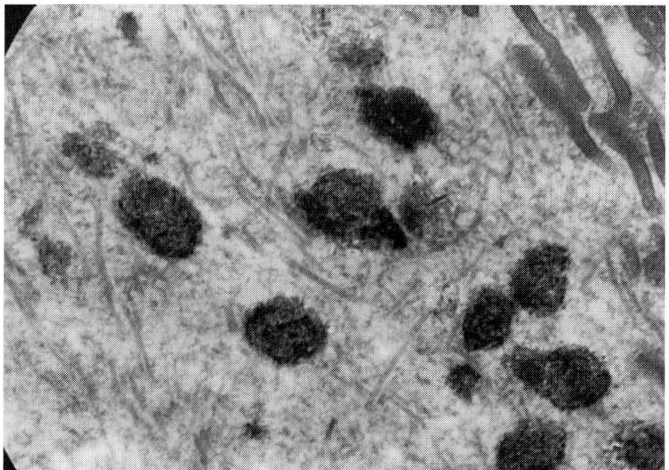

Fig. 16–7. Transmission electron micrograph showing matrix vesicle-like structures containing crystalline material suggesting hydroxyapatite (uranyl acetate and lead citrate, ×54,000).

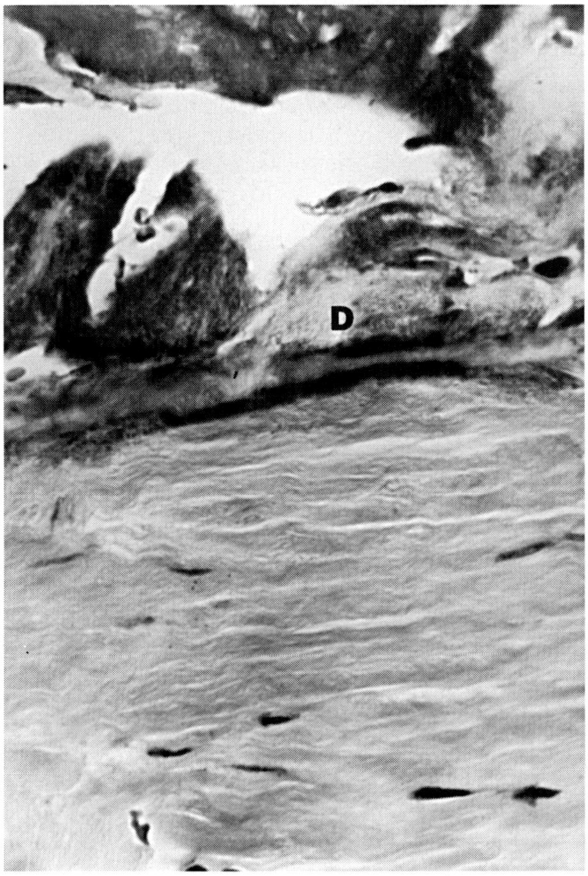

Fig. 16–8. Section showing collagenous bands of the tendon proper bordering calcific deposit (D), representing the resting phase (hematoxylin-eosin, ×120).

macrophages and multinucleated giant cells (Fig. 16–9), some fibroblasts, and infrequently a small to moderate number of polymorphonuclear leukocytes. In the immediate vicinity, there is an abundant number of hyperemic vessels. With the electron microscope, numerous phagosomes containing densely staining calcific substance are seen in the macrophages (Fig. 16–10). "Calcium granuloma" represents the resorptive phase of the calcific stage. It appears likely that cellular and vascular proliferation raises the intratendinous pressure to such

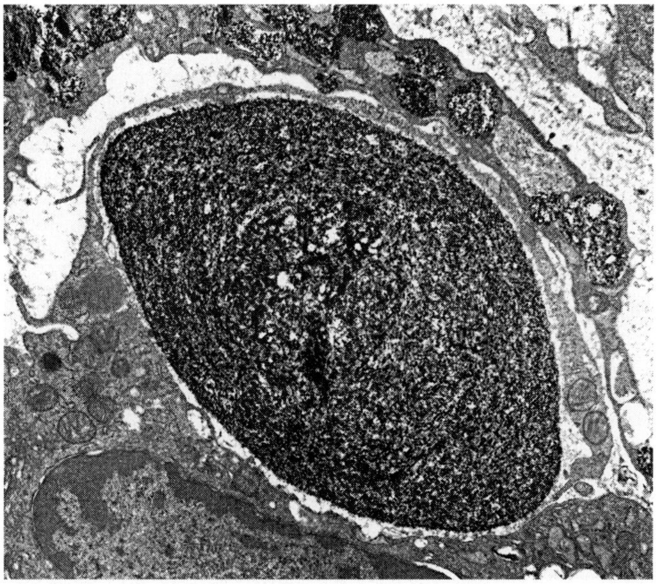

Fig. 16–10. Transmission electron micrograph showing a macrophage engulfing a portion of calcific deposit. Similar deposits are seen in phagosomes of the cytoplasm of another macrophage (Uranyl acetate and lead citrate, ×18,000).

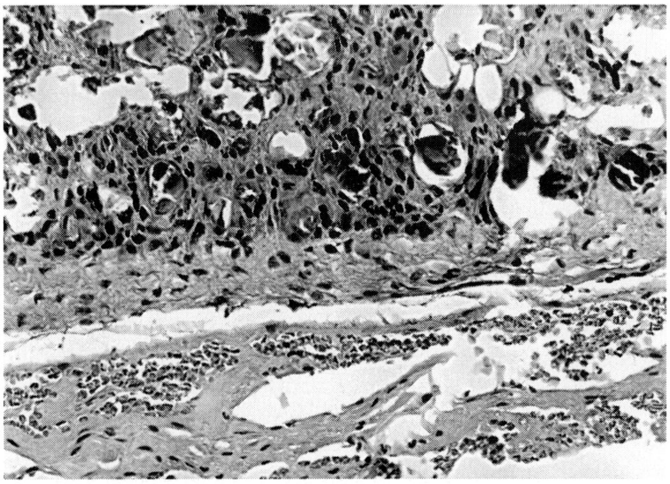

Fig. 16–9. Section showing a "calcium granuloma" with macrophages and multinucleated giant cells in the process of phagocytosing calcific deposit, indicating the resorptive phase. Congested vascular channels are seen at the periphery (hematoxylin-eosin, ×60).

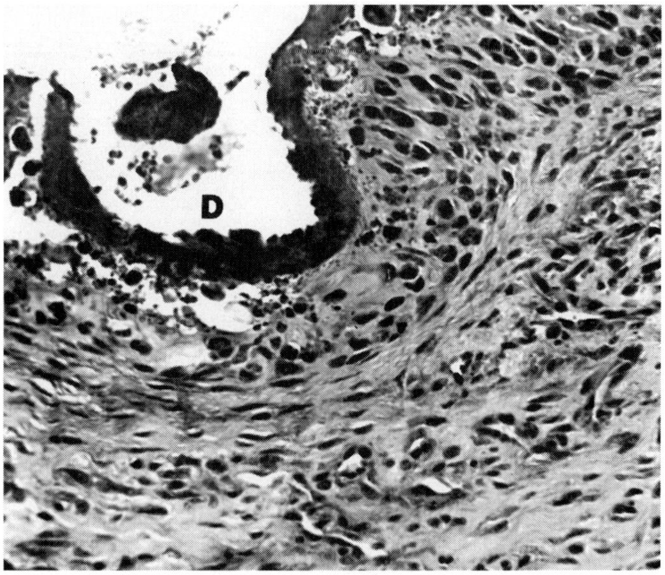

Fig. 16–11. Section showing proliferation of fibroblastic cells in the area of the disappearing deposit (D) (hematoxylin-eosin, ×60).

an extent that acute symptoms are induced with intense pain and impaired mobility of the joint.

Resorption of calcium and proliferation of fibrovascular tissue forming scar proceed simultaneously (Fig. 16–11), so that the space once occupied by the calcific deposit is now replaced by fibroblastic cells producing collagen fibers and numerous thin-walled capillaries (Fig. 16–12). At sites of collagen synthesis the formation of collagen type III predominates, as can be shown by monoclonal antibody staining. With the removal of calcium, the intensity of cellular reaction consisting of macrophagic activity disappears, and the vessels become nonhyperemic. This decreases the intratendinous pressure and seems responsible for the subsidence of the symptoms. The postcalcific stage begins with return of function, and remodeling of the scar tissue that replaces the calcific deposit (Fig. 16–13).

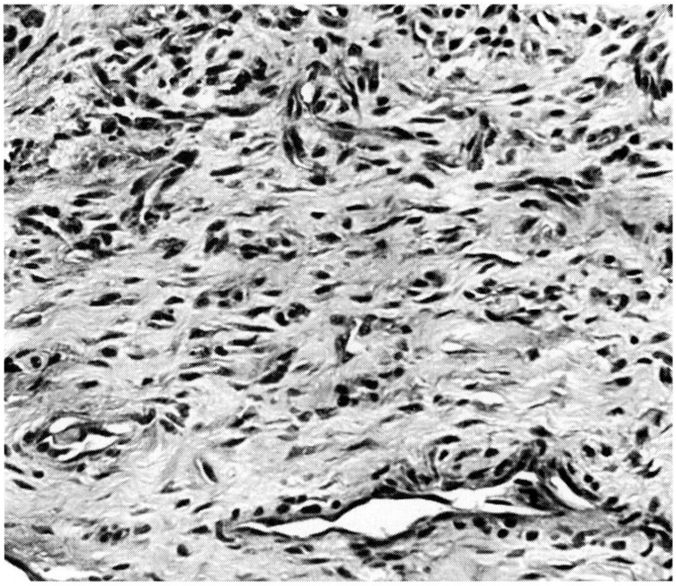

Fig. 16–12. Higher magnification of the same section showing numerous vascular channels (hematoxylin-eosin, ×120).

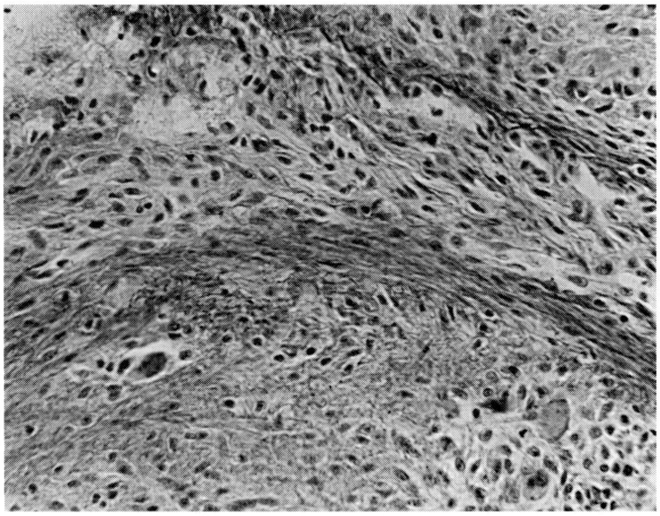

Fig. 16–13. Section of an area of scar showing axial alignment of cells and fibers suggesting remodeling (hematoxylin-eosin, ×60).

It is to be emphasized that, because of the multifocal nature of the deposit, one focus may exhibit the histology of the resting phase while an adjacent one may be in the resorptive phase. The predominant type of the lesion, however, can be predicted by the clinical symptoms, radiologic aspect of the deposit, or even the gross appearance and consistency of the deposit when observed during surgery.

LABORATORY INVESTIGATIONS

No abnormalities in calcium and phosphorus metabolism were identified, and serum values including alkaline phosphatase were within normal limits. We performed tissue typing in 50 patients with calcifying tendinitis and 36 patients who had a tear of the rotator cuff. The results were compared with 982 controls. HLA-A1 was present in 50% of the patients with calcifying tendinitis and in 27.8% of the patients with tear compared to 26.7% in controls.[40] There was a statistically significant difference between patients suffering from calcifying tendinitis and those having a tear ($p = 0.025$).

DIFFERENTIAL DIAGNOSIS

Not all calcifications in the rotator cuff tendons should be diagnosed as calcifying tendinitis. Radiographs showing stippled calcification overlying the greater tuberosity are evidence of dystrophic calcification. These deposits occur in the fibrocartilaginous portion of the tendon at its insertion and are much closer to the bone than the deposits in calcifying tendinitis that occur in the tendon proper. Histologically, the dystrophic deposits in the fibrocartilage of the enthesis appear as exophytes from the tidemark, and they tend to increase with age. They clearly are an expression of degenerative changes and may give rise to symptoms pertaining to enthesopathy. An accompanying degenerative change in the bone and/or the joint is often present.

Calcification of the dystrophic type in relation to the torn margins of the rotator cuff have also been reported. Wolfgang[41] found radiologic evidence of calcification in as high as 23% of patients with the cuff tear prior to surgery. This is not the general experience. However, infrequent calcification in complete tears, whether identified radiologically or histologically, has been reported by McLaughlin and Asherman[42] and in our own studies.[43]

Massive calcification is a component of the Milwaukee shoulder syndrome[44] and cuff tear arthropathy.[45] There are significant changes in the glenohumeral joint in both of these conditions that do not occur in calcifying tendinitis. Calcifying tendinitis may mimic a bone tumor, a fact well documented by Toriyama and collaborators.[45]

TREATMENT

There is no apparent uniformity of treatment for calcifying tendinitis, and it seems to be greatly influenced by the training and expertise of the physician involved. Therefore, it is not surprising to find rheumatologists generally favoring a conservative approach, while the surgeons tend to proceed with an operative procedure after a reasonable period of conservative treatment. Because the duration of the resorptive (acute) phase usually does not exceed a few weeks and because conservative treatment should last at least 2 to 3 months, it happens that surgery is mostly performed during the formative or the resting phase.

Conservative

The vast majority of patients will undergo conservative treatment initially. Gschwend and his collaborators[29] believe that conservative care is successful in 90% of the patients. In a series of patients followed by Litchman and his colleagues,[34] only 1 out of 100 patients required surgery. There is common agreement as to the need for adequate physiotherapy, which involves range-of-motion and pendulum exercises. This should then be followed by a program of muscle strengthening. In acute cases, attempts at gentle mobilization may be preceded by local application of ice. In patients with chronic pain, however, local heat, especially in the form of infrared treatment, seems preferable. Although ultrasonography is said to be able to break up calcium deposits, there is no randomized study proving the value of this treatment. The relief of pain observed by Griffin and Karselis[46] was thought to be caused by a physiological rise in tissue temperature. We believe that the main aim of physiotherapy should be to decrease muscle spasm, to improve local blood flow, and to prevent stiffness. We also recommend placing the arm in abduction on a pillow to relieve pain, particularly in acute cases. This will also improve the blood supply to that part of the tendon which is the site of the calcium deposition.

Patterson and Darrach[47] and Lapidus[48] recommend needling and injection of local anesthetics in patients with acute symptoms. The repeated perforations decrease the intratendinous pressure. An added lavage may help to remove part of the deposit, which at this stage is in a cream-like state. The needle is inserted at the site of maximum tenderness and its exact localization is confirmed by radiogram. Among 400 patients, Harmon[49] obtained excellent results in 78.9%. De Palma and Kruper[18] were less successful: good results were obtained in only 61%, fair results in 22%, and no response in 17%.

During the acute stage, some investigators have suggested adding corticosteroid to the local anesthetic. Gschwend and his collaborators[29] feel that the action is short and the effect exclusively directed at symptoms. However, corticosteroids inhibit vascular proliferation, local hyperemia, and macrophage activity. Therefore, it is not surprising that Lippmann[19] warns that corticosteroids might abort the activity that produces the disruption and eventual resorption of the deposit. In Harmon's opinion,[49] the addition of corticosteroid does not accelerate the process of resorption but could reduce muscle spasm. Murnaghan and McIntosh[50] injected 27 patients with lidocaine and 24 with hydrocortisone locally without finding a difference in results. During the acute phase, analgesics are administered to reduce the excruciating pain. Nonsteroidal anti-inflammatory drugs are also given, but their value remains undetermined.

X-radiation was used in the past as a treatment modality for calcifying tendinitis but now remains of historical interest only.[51,52] In an informative study, Plenk[17] submitted 38 patients to radiation; a lead shield was interposed between the source of radiation and the shoulder in 17 patients, but 21 patients received direct radiation. The calcium deposit disappeared in 67% of the shielded patients but disappeared in only 44% of those directly radiated. In this context, the opinion of Gschwend and his collaborators[29] is instructive: "Therapy cannot hinder success."

Surgical

We believe that surgery is indicated either in the formative phase or in patients where the deposit fails to resorb. Litchman and his colleagues[34] felt that prolonged waiting with chronic symptoms could lead to shoulder stiffness. This view, however, is not commonly shared. Gschwend and his collaborators[29] have proposed three criteria that should be met before surgery is performed: (1) progression of symptoms, (2) constant pain interfering with activities of daily living, and (3) absence of improvement of symptoms after conservative therapy. Moseley[53] recommended restricting the indication for surgery to patients having a large deposit in the mechanical (chronic) phase. He, like other investigators, suggests a conservative approach for patients in the acute phase. In summary, restricting management solely to surgical methods is currently considered too aggressive. This contradicts the advice of Bosworth,[13] who maintains that the quickest and the most dependable way to rid the patient of pain would be surgery.

SURGICAL TECHNIQUE

In order to lower the risk of postoperative infection, we recommend waiting at least 4 weeks after the last intrabursal or intra-articular injection before proceeding with surgery. The removal of the deposit is done under general anesthesia using an approach recommended by Neer,[54] starting at the anterior aspect of the acromion and ending at the coracoid process. The fibers of the deltoid are bluntly separated.[29] We do not detach the origin of the deltoid from the acromion. The opening of the bursa is followed by an inspection of the bursal cavity, in particular, the floor of the bursa. Free draping of the arm allows internal and external rotation as well as abduction and adduction. The site of bursal reaction is noted. With longitudinal traction of the arm, the surgeon's small finger is introduced into the space between the coracoacromial arch and the rotator cuff to determine the constraints of this interval. If it is too tight, the coracoacromial ligament is partially resected. This partial resection is replaced by an anterior acromioplasty if an acromial beak or spur exists. It is noteworthy that Vebostad[55] could find no improvement in results with routine anterior acromioplasty following the evacuation of the deposit. Goutallier and Du Parc[56] have recently recommended an anterior acromioplasty without removal of the deposit. Although they reported favorable results, we wonder whether such a procedure will find general acceptance.

In general the bursal reaction is minimal, allowing for an easy localization of the deposit. In some instances, a localized bursal reaction is present at the site of the deposit. The tendon is now incised longitudinally over the deposit which is then curetted. Following a copious lavage, we only close the tendon incision when both edges do not fall together spontaneously. Early in the postoperative stage, gentle passive range-of-motion exercises are started in the recovery room by a physiotherapist. We recommend positioning of the arm in abduction whenever possible, but do not use an abduction pillow. Postoperative corticosteroid injections should be avoided. Complete disappearance of symptoms after surgery can take several months.[57]

Increasingly, arthroscopic surgery is being performed to evacuate the calcium deposits. It is obvious, however, that this procedure is accomplished more easily during the acute phase when the consistency of the deposit is creamy or pus-like. Evacuation during the chronic phase, when the consistency is chalk-like, is more difficult to perform, and we doubt whether a complete removal is possible, even when using a burr or a resector. Ellman[58] has reported his technique and results of removing the deposit through a bursoscopy. From his description one gains the impression that the procedure is done during the resorptive phase; the content of the deposit empties spontaneously into the bursa after incision of the cuff.

Re and Karzel[59] have described a technique that is somewhat different. During arthroscopy, the deposit is localized (a hyperemic area on the articular surface of the tendon may reveal its presence). An absorbable suture is then put through the tendon. It helps to find the exact site during the subsequent bursoscopy. If the consistency of the deposit is hard and dry, a resector is used for a more aggressive debridement.[59]

CONCLUDING REMARKS

In calcifying tendinitis, as in any other disease process, a thorough understanding of the pathogenesis is a prerequisite for proper treatment. Calcifying tendinitis is a self-healing disease going through successive stages in which the formation of the deposit is followed by its resorption. Whereas surgery may be indicated during the phase of formation or during the resting phase, it is never indicated during the resorption phase where the deposit undergoes phagocytic resorption. Although this latter phase is the most painful, the treatment should be conservative. Following resorption of the deposit, a tendon reconstitution takes place spontaneously.

ACKNOWLEDGEMENT

Work in the authors' laboratory has been supported by the Medical Research Council of Canada. We sincerely thank Dr. J. Wiley for his helpful advice.

REFERENCES

1. Duplay S. De la périarthrite scapulohumerale et des raideurs de l'épaule qui en sont la consequence. *Arch Gen Med.* 1872;513:542.
2. Painter CF. Subdeltoid bursitis. *Boston Med J.* 1970;156:345–349.
3. Bergemann D, Stieda A. Uber die mit Kalkablagerungen einhergehende Entzündung der Schulterschleimbeutel. *Münich Med Wschr.* 1908;52:2699–2702.
4. Stieda A. Zur Pathologie der Schultergelenkschleimbeutel. *Arch Klin Chir.* 1908;85:910–924.
5. Codman EA. *The Shoulder.* Boston: Thomas Todd, 1934.
6. Wrede L. Uber Kalkablagerungen in der Umgebung des Schultergelenkes und ihre Beziehungen zur Periarthritis humeroscapularis. *Langenbecks Arch Klin Chir.* 1912;99:259–272.
7. Sandstrom C. Peritendinitis calcarea: Common disease of middle life: Its diagnosis, pathology and treatment. *AJR.* 1938;40:1–21.
8. Sandstrom C, Wahlgren F. Beitrag zur Kenntnis der "Peritendinitis calcarea" (sog. "Bursitis calculosa") speziell vom pathologisch-histologischen Gesichtspunkt. *Acta Radiol. (Stockh)* 1937; 18:263–296.
9. Schaer H. Die Periarthritis humeroscapularis. *Ergebn Chir Orthop.* 1936;29:211–309.
10. Dieppe P. Crystal deposition disease and the soft tissues. *Clin Rheum Dis.* 1979;5:807–822.
10a. Plenk HP. Calcifying tendinitis of the shoulder. *Radiology.* 1952; 59:384–389.
11. De Sèze S, Welfling J. Tendinites calcifiantes. *Rhumatologie.* 1970; 22:5–14.
12. *The rotator cuff of the shoulder.* An International Symposium. May 20–22, 1993, Ottawa, Canada.
13. Bosworth BM. Calcium deposits in the shoulder and subacromial bursitis: A survey of 12,122 shoulders. *JAMA.* 1941; 116:2477–2482.
14. Bosworth BM. Examination of the shoulder for calcium deposits. *J Bone Joint Surg.* 1941;23:567–577.
15. Ruttimann G. *Über die Häufigkeit röntgenologischer Veränderungen bei Patienten mit typischer Periarthritis humeroscapularis und Schultergesunden.* Inaugural dissertation, Zurich 1959.
16. Welfling J, Kahn MF, Desroy M, et al. Les calcifications de l'épaule. II. La maladie des calcifications tendineuses multiples. *Rev Rhum Ed Fr.* 1965;32:325–334.
17. Plenk HP. Calcifying tendinitis of the shoulder. *Radiology.* 1952; 59:384–389.
18. DePalma AF, Kruper JS. Long term study of shoulder joints afflicted with and treated for calcific tendinitis. *Clin Orthop.* 1961; 20:61–72.
19. Lippmann RK. Observations concerning the calcific cuff deposits. *Clin Orthop.* 1961;20:49–60.
20. Uhthoff HK, Sarkar K. Tendopathia calcificans. *Beitr Orthop Traumat.* 1981;28:269–277.
21. McLaughlin HL. Lesions of the musculotendinous cuff of the shoulder. III. Observations on the pathology, course and treatment of calcific deposits. *Ann Surg.* 1946;124:354–362.
22. Steinbrocker O. The painful shoulder. In: Hollander JE, ed. *Arthritis and Allied Conditions.* 8th ed. Philadelphia: Lea & Febiger,

1972.
23. Macnab I. Rotator cuff tendinitis. *Ann R Coll Surg Engl.* 1973; 53:271–287.
24. Uhthoff HK. Calcifying tendinitis, an active cell-mediated calcification. *Virchows Arch A Pathol Anat Histopathol.* 1975;366:51–58.
25. Uhthoff HK, Sarkar K, Maynard JA. Calcifying tendinitis. *Clin Orthop.* 1976;118:164–168.
26. Baer WS. The operative treatment of subdeltoid bursitis. *Johns Hopkins Hosp Bull.* 1907;18:282–284.
27. Wilson CL. Lesions of the supraspinatus tendon. Degeneration, rupture and calcification. *Arch Surg.* 1943;46:307–325.
28. Pinals RS, Short CL. Calcific periarthritis involving multiple sites. *Arthritis Rheum.* 1966;9:566–574.
29. Gschwend N, Patte D, Zippel J. Die Therapie der Tendinitis calcarea des Schultergelenkes. *Arch Orthop Unfallchir.* 1972;73:120–135.
30. Simon WH. Soft tissue disorders of the shoulder. Frozen shoulder, calcific tendinitis, and bicipital tendinitis. *Orthop Clin North Am.* 1975;6:521–539.
31. Pendergrass EP, Hodes PJ. Roentgen irradiation in treatment of inflammations. *AJR.* 1941;45:74–106.
32. Kessel L, Watson M. The painful arc syndrome. *J Bone Joint Surg Br.* 1977;59:166–172.
33. Carnett JB. The calcareous deposits of so-called calcifying subacromial bursitis. *Surg Gynecol Obstet.* 1925;41:404–421.
34. Litchman HM, Silver CM, Simon SD, Eshragi A. The surgical management of calcific tendinitis of the shoulder. *Int Surg.* 1968; 50:474–482.
35. Uhthoff HK, Sarkar K, Hammond DI. The subacromial bursa: A clinicopathological study. In: Bateman JE, Welsh RP, eds. *Surgery of the Shoulder.* Philadelphia, Toronto: BC Decker; 1984:121–125.
36. Uhthoff HK, Sarkar K, Hammond I. Die Bedeutung der Dichte und der Schürfe der Abgrenzung des Kalkschattens bei der Tendinopathia calcificans. *Radiologe.* 1982;22:170–174.
37. Patte D, Goutallier D. Calcifications. *Rev Chir Orthop Reparatrice Appar Mot.* 1988;74:277–278.
37a. Hsu HC, Wu JJ, Jim YF, Chang CY, Lo WH, Yang DJ. Calcific tendinitis and rotator cuff tearing: A clinical and radiographic study. *J Shoulder Elbow Surg.* 1994;3:159–164.
38. Uhthoff HK, Sarkar K. Calcifying tendinitis. In: Rockwood CA, Matsen FA, eds. *The Shoulder.* Philadelphia: WB Saunders; 1990: 774–790.
38a. Archer RS, Bayley JI, Archer CW, Ali SY. Cell and matrix changes associated with pathological calcification of the human rotator cuff tendons. *J Anat.* 1993;182:1–11.
39. Pedersen HE, Key JA. Pathology of calcareous tendinitis and subdeltoid bursitis. *Arch Surg.* 1951;62:50–63.
40. Sengar DPS, McKendry RJ, Uhthoff HK. Increased frequency of HLA-A1 in calcifying tendinitis. *Tissue Antigens.* 1987;29: 173–174.
41. Wolfgang GL. Surgical repairs of the rotator cuff of the shoulder. *J Bone Joint Surg Am.* 1974;56:14–26.
42. McLaughlin HL, Asherman EG. Lesions of the musculotendinous cuff of the shoulder. *J Bone Joint Surg Am.* 1951;33:76–86.
43. Earnshaw P, Desjardins D, Sarkar K, Uhthoff HK. Rotator cuff tears: The role of surgery. *Can J Surg.* 1982;25:60–63.
44. Halverson PB, McCarty DJ, Cheung HS, Ryan LM. Milwaukee shoulder syndrome. *Ann Rheum Dis.* 1984;43:734–741.
45. Neer CS II, Craig EV, Fukuda H. Cuff-tear arthropathy. *J Bone Joint Surg Am.* 1983;65:1232–1244.
45a. Toriyama K, Fukuda H, Hamada K, Noguchi T. Calcifying tendinitis of the infraspinatus tendon stimulating a bone tumor. *J Shoulder Elbow Surg.* 1994;3:165–168.
46. Griffin EJ, Karselis TC. Physical agents for physical therapists. In: *Ultrasonic Energy.* 2nd ed. Springfield, IL: Charles C Thomas; 1982.
47. Patterson RL, Darrach W. Treatment of acute bursitis by needle irrigation. *J Bone Joint Surg.* 1937;19:993–1002.
48. Lapidus PW. Infiltration therapy of acute tendinitis with calcification. *Surg Gynecol Obstet.* 1943;76:715–725.
49. Harmon HP. Methods and results in the treatment of 2580 painful shoulders. With special reference to calcific tendinitis and the frozen shoulder. *Am J Surg.* 1958;95:527–544.
50. Murnaghan GF, McIntosh D. Hydrocortisone in painful shoulder. Controlled trial. *Lancet.* 1955;21:798–800.
51. Baird LW. Roentgen irradiation of calcareous deposits about the shoulder. *Radiology.* 1941;37:316–324.
52. Brenckmann E, Nadaud P. Le traitement des calcifications périarticulaires de l'épaule par radio thérapie. *Arch D'Electric Med.* 1932; 40:27–29.
53. Moseley HF. The results of nonoperative and operative treatment of calcified deposits. *Surg Clin North Am.* 1963;43:1505–1506.
54. Neer CS II. Impingement lesions. *Clin Orthop.* 1983;173:70–77.
55. Vebostad A. Calcific tendinitis in the shoulder region. A review of 43 operated shoulders. *Acta Orthop Scand.* 1975;46:205–210.
56. Goutallier D, Duparc F. *Surgical treatment of calcifying tendinitis by decompression without removal of the deposit- A 4-year follow-up. The rotator cuff of the shoulder.* An International Symposium. May 20–22, 1993, Ottawa, Canada.
57. McKendry RJR, Uhthoff HK, Sarkar K, St George-Hyslop P. Calcifying tendinitis of the shoulder: Prognostic value of clinical, histologic and radiologic features in 57 surgically treated cases. *Rheumatology.* 1982;9:75–80.
58. Ellman H. *The Controversy of arthroscopic vs. open approaches to shoulder instability and rotator cuff disease.* Fourth Open Meeting of the American Society of Shoulder and Elbow Surgeons. American Academy of Orthopedic Surgeons. Atlanta, Georgia, 1988 Symposium.
59. Re LP, Karzel RP. Management of rotator cuff calcifications. *Orthop Clin North Am.* 1993;24:125–132.

Chapter 17

Frozen Shoulder Syndrome: Frozen Shoulder, Idiopathic Chronic Adhesive Capsulitis, Post-Traumatic Stiff Shoulder, and Painful Stiff Shoulder

Wayne Z. Burkhead, Jr.

What's in a name? That which we call a rose by any other name would smell as sweet.

William Shakespeare, Romeo and Juliet

When I see a patient with frozen shoulder syndrome (idiopathic adhesive capsulitis), I am frequently reminded of a definition I heard of the term "idiopathic" given by Mercer-Rang at the Texas Orthopaedic Association in 1987. Idiopathic: the doctor is an idiot and the patient is pathetic. I hope you will agree, after reading this chapter, that most cases of "idiopathic chronic adhesive capsulitis," whether it be mild unforgotten trauma in the predisposed individual, early osteoarthritis, partial-thickness rotator cuff tears that escape radiographic diagnosis, or a previously undiagnosed systemic illness, do have an etiology. Furthermore, it's of paramount importance to understand that this symptom complex or syndrome represents a response of individuals to a condition, local or remote, which depending on when the patient presents in the course of their illness may have a different clinical picture, diagnostic tests, and response to treatment. If one does not realize this from the outset and performs an acromioplasty or manipulation in the early stages of this process, then you the surgeon will look like an idiot and the patient will be pathetic. On the other hand, if you make an accurate diagnosis of a resectable tumor or unrecognized diabetes, then you can look like a hero.

TERMINOLOGY

Every generation of physicians since the late 1800s who have faced the patient with a painful stiff shoulder have coined a term to describe this puzzling condition. Duplay used the term "periarthrite scapulo-humerale."[1–4] Putnam anglicized the term in 1882 in his description of the treatment of a form of painful periarthritis of the shoulder.[5] In using these terms, both Duplay and Putnam displayed their recognition of the global tenderness around the shoulder girdle in these patients, which is not necessarily limited to the glenohumeral joint. Codman was the first to use the term "frozen shoulder," and I would think that many would still agree with his remarks that, "This is a class of cases that I find difficult to define, difficult to treat, and difficult to explain from the point of view of pathology."[6] J.S. Neviaser, who in 1945 coined the term "adhesive capsulitis" to better describe the adhesion of the inflamed thickened and contracted capsule to the humeral head, also discussed the typical arthrographic findings.[7–11] Moseley recognized that there were a variety of causes of frozen shoulder and he felt, as Codman had several years before him, that the term periarthritis would eventually be replaced by more specific diagnoses, allowing more individualization of care.[12] The biceps tendon as the etiology for adhesive capsulitis was introduced by Pasteur when he coined the term "teno bursite."[13] Lippmann and DePalma also associated pathology in the biceps with frozen shoulder and recommended tenodesis for it's treatment.[14,15] Steinbrocker coined the term "shoulder-hand syndrome" to describe the combination of a painful stiff shoulder with swelling and pain in the hand associated with ongoing stiffness and progressive trophic changes.[16]

Since 1945 investigators have used range of motion, arthrography, historical data, or a combination of all three to classify these patients. Quigley used the term "the checkrein shoulder" to distinguish a subgroup of patients with "frozen shoulder" who had a definite audible and palpable pop followed by improved range of motion at the time of manipulation.[17] These patients, who generally had been symptomatic for a shorter time, had better results than the other group who had frozen shoulders. Reeves used the term "post-traumatic stiff shoulder" to describe patients who at arthrography had a decreased joint volume but whose subscapularis recess was still open and the biceps tendon sheath was normal. He distinguished these patients from a second group of patients in his series who had a more restricted arthrogram, including absence of filling of the subscapularis bursa and biceps tendon sheath in addition to an obliterated inferior recess.[18] Lundberg separated primary frozen shoulder and secondary frozen shoulder based on historical evidence of trauma.[19] Kay used the term "early capsulitis" to designate patients who had shoulder abduction of greater than 90°.[20] He used the term "frozen shoulder" for patients with less than 90° shoulder abduction. Withers based his classification on examination under anesthesia.[21] Patients with "irritative capsulitis" had a normal examination under anesthesia, whereas patients with "adhesive capsulitis" had no change in their preanesthetic motion. R.J. Neviaser used both arthrographic and clinical criteria to classify patients with frozen shoulders. Patients who had shoulder abduction greater than 90° and a joint volume that was restricted to 10 to 12 mL were designated as having painful stiff shoulders. Patients who had abduction less than 90° and whose arthrograms revealed an even more restricted joint volume (5 to 10 mL) were deemed as having adhesive capsulitis.[22] De Seze and Welfling referred to this condition as "L'epaule Bloquee" and discussed the capsular contracture in postmortem specimens.[23–25]

Regardless of what this has been called over the years, the patients have in common varying degrees of restriction, shrinkage if you will, of their joint volume. In trying to explain this concept to patients over the years I have called this the "shrink wrap shoulder," frequently using the analogy of shrink-wrapping or the cellophane that is placed tightly around perishable items at the grocery store to hold them to a plastic tray. If the cellophane wrap is loose, the food can slide around and rotate on the tray. If the wrapping is tight, as is the capsule in frozen shoulder, no motion can occur between the tray and the food.

Irrespective of the label the most important distinction to make is whether this syndrome or symptom complex is secondary to a benign, local, or remote process that will be "self-limited" or secondary to a malignant process that will "limit the self" or be self-eliminating if left untreated. For the purpose of this chapter this "rose," which unlike Shakespeare's rose smells anything but sweet, will be referred to as frozen shoulder syndrome (FSS).

ETIOLOGY

Pain

Pain is the single common denominator in patients with FSS. The inciting event or condition that causes the pain differs from patient to patient. Local or intrinsic inflammatory conditions of the shoulder have long been identified with frozen shoulder syndrome. Duplay believed that the etiology lay in the inflammation of the subacromial bursa. Pathologic processes in the subdeltoid bursa or calcified deposits within the rotator cuff are postulated by a number of investigators to lead to periarthritis.[26–28] Riedel put forward the theory that pathology in the joint capsule rather than the bursa or tendon was responsible for the syndrome.[29] Tenosynovitis of the long head of the biceps was felt by other investigators to be the precipitating event.[13–15] Varying degrees of trauma are associated with FSS. Major skeletal trauma and soft-tissue injury are relatively easy to diagnose with radiographic and imaging techniques. Surgical trauma following mastectomy with and without node dissection or head and neck surgery can result in FSS. Even a minor procedure done in a remote location, such as simple ganglion cyst removal from the hand, can result in FSS in the high risk patient. Although major trauma and events such as surgery are relatively easy to recall, what can be commonly overlooked in these patients is a long forgotten minor trauma or transient overuse.[6,30,31]

Immobilization

DePalma theorized that in addition to a painful process, a period of prolonged muscular inactivity because of the pain was a major etiological factor in frozen shoulder. Confirmation of the immobilization factor in patients with FSS is found in the work of Coventry,[32] Harmon,[33] Johnston,[34] Bruckner and Nye,[35] Lundberg,[19] and Binder.[36]

Personality Factors

Periarthritic personality is a term coined by Coventry to describe a "peculiar constitutional and emotional state," which he felt was one of three factors requisite for developing adhesive capsulitis.[32] An inappropriate response to stress was found commonly in patients with painful stiff shoulders by Lorentz.[37] Bruckner and Nye reported an associated depressive personality as a significant risk factor in developing frozen shoulder.[35] Quigley, on the other hand, felt that many of the patients' unusual personalities were a result of the painful shoulder and their sleep disturbance rather than the cause.[17] Wright and Haq found no evidence of a typical personality disorder,[38] however, these patients with periarthritis tended to worry more and sleep less soundly prior to the onset of pain when compared to a control group. Fleming and colleagues found significantly increased somatic anxiety levels in women when compared to controls.[39]

We know now that pain, depression, and anxiety are closely linked. Whatever underlying personality traits these patients have, I have no doubt that they are magnified by the sleep disturbance that accompanies this condition.

RISK FACTORS

The risk factors and conditions associated with FSS are listed in Table 17–1. Several of the more commonly recognized risk factors are discussed here.

METABOLIC DISORDERS

Diabetes

There is a much higher than normal association between frozen shoulder and diabetes with the incidence of diabetics being 2 to 4 times the rate in the general population.[40–43] The incidence is higher in patients who are Insulin dependent (type I diabetes). These patients have as high as 36% incidence of adhesive capsulitis and are more likely to have bilateral shoulder involvement.[40,44,45]

Table 17–1. Conditions Associated With Adhesive Capsulitis*

Intrathoracic Disorders
Ischemic heart disease, aortic aneurysm, Pancoast tumor, mediastinal tumors, pleural tumor
Abdominal Disorders
Gastric ulcer, cholecystitis, cholelithiasis, **subphrenic abscess, splenic processes, liver tumors,** and **hepatitis**
Metabolic Disorders
Diabetes, hyperthyroidism, hypothyroidism, hyperparathyroidism, and osteomalacia
Bone Disorders
Metastatic tumor, primary bone tumor, malignant and benign, avascular necrosis, and Paget's disease
Cervical Spine Disorders
Cervical spondylosis, cervical disc degeneration, and herniation, **neoplasm,** disc, or **epidural space infection**
Trauma
Fractures of the upper extremity including the shoulder girdle, shoulder dislocation, traumatic bursitis, and rotator cuff tear
Neurogenic Disorders
Suprascapular nerve entrapment, thoracic outlet syndrome, neuralgia amyotrophy—Parsonage and Turner syndrome, cervical radiculitis, carpal tunnel syndrome, ulnar nerve neuritis, radial nerve entrapment, axillary nerve entrapment, and diabetic polyneuropathy
Joint Disorders
Degenerative or traumatic arthritis of AC joint, degenerative or traumatic arthritis of the glenohumeral joint, inflammatory arthritis, septic arthritis, crystalline arthritis, hemophilic arthritis, and osteochondromatosis
Soft-Tissue Disorders About the Shoulder
Impingement syndrome, rotator cuff tendinitis, degeneration, and partial tearing, tendinitis of LHBB, subacromial bursitis, calcific tendinitis, fibrositis, and shoulder-hand syndrome. Fibrositis of soft-tissue tumor including ganglion with a suprascapular nerve entrapment. Soft-tissue tumors of the upper extremity, head, and neck. **MFA, lymphoma,** and **sarcoma.**

*Note. Bold indicates conditions which potentially limit the self.

Cheiroarthropathy, characterized by a "waxy" thickening and induration of the skin and other connective tissues including joint capsules commonly seen in the hands and frequently associated with Dupuytren's contracture, trigger finger, and PIP joint contractures, is not an uncommon sequelae of Insulin dependent diabetes mellitus. In these patients, frozen shoulder can occur bilaterally in as many as 77%.[44] The longer the patient has been diabetic, the more likely it is that they will develop frozen shoulder.

Thyroid Disorders

FSS, or as Duncan referred to it "toxic periarthritis," is associated with hyperthyroidism and frequently resolves when the hyperthyroidism is corrected.[30,38,46–53,] Bowman has reported a definite association between FSS and hypothyroidism.[54] Wohlgethan reviews the possible cause and effect of hyperthyroidism and frozen shoulder:[47] (1) thyroid myopathy may contribute to the limitation of shoulder motion; (2) connective tissue proliferation in thyroid acropachy leads to stiff joints similar to frozen shoulder; and (3) hyperthyroidism leads to activation of the sympathetic nervous system, the mechanism is not known, but thyroid hormones have actions similar to catecholamines or they may alter the number and function of sympathetic cells.[55,56] Many patients in this age group with FSS are on thyroid replacement for hypothyroidism. Therefore, evaluation of these patients should include thyroid testing as both over and under treatment of thyroid deficiency can result in this syndrome.

Other Hormonal Disorders

Other hormonal disorders associated with frozen shoulder include primary and secondary Addison's disease, isolated ACTH deficiency, and hypopituitarism.[56–58]

Intrathoracic Disorders

Of all of the causes of frozen shoulder or painful shoulder in the older patient, none is better described or recognized than the Pancoast tumor: bronchogenic carcinoma in the superior sulcus with invasion of the brachial plexus, shoulder pain, and the development of FSS.[59–65] It must be remembered that a clear apical lordotic chest radiograph does not exclude the possibility that the patient has a malignant process in the chest. Onuigbo stressed the frequency with which patients who have bronchogenic carcinoma in regions of the lung other than the apex present with shoulder pain.[66] Mediastinal lesions causing pressure on the phrenic nerve or small peripheral pleural lesions can be missed on the conventional chest radiograph. For the patient at risk (e.g., the smoker with typical symptoms), chest CT scanning has a much higher yield. Demaziere and Wiley reported on three cases of primary chest wall tumors presenting as FSS. All were diagnosed after the fact.[67] The pain that develops in cases of carcinoma of the lung is generally an intense burning or dull aching pain in and around the region of the scapula; the patients commonly complain of the pain radiating down the arm and there is frequently an associated paresthesia.[68] In a review of 150 cases of upper lobe bronchogenic carcinoma, 14% presented with shoulder and arm pain.[68]

FSS in tuberculosis patients tends to be generally mild, according to Johnston.[34] Saha noted an association between frozen shoulder, emphysema, and chronic bronchitis.[69] Ischemic heart disease has been known to be associated with FSS for many years.[31,70–72] This recognition has led to early gentle range of motion of the shoulder as part of protocols for cardiac rehabilitation.

NEUROGENIC DISORDERS

Cervical Radiculitis

Many investigators have noted a relationship between cervical disc degeneration, cervical radiculitis, and frozen shoulder syndrome.[19,72–77] Recently a case-controlled study by Hargreaves and colleagues confirmed a statistically significant relationship between frozen shoulder and previous neck pain, previous neck trauma, and limitation of range of motion of the cervical spine at the $P < .05$ level.[78] Theories as to the role of cervical nerve root irritation in the production of frozen shoulder include (1) chronic irritation of cervical sympathetic fibers in the anterior cervical nerve roots[77] and (2) referred pain with concomitant reduction in available range of motion.[75] Many times the patients will complain only of neck stiffness and shoulder pain, and the shoulder will be their primary focus because of the severe pain and loss of motion. Frequently, it is only after the FSS has resolved that the patient becomes more focused on their neck symptomatology.

Peripheral Neuropathies

One thing that has struck me over the years is the degree of referred shoulder pain present in patients with peripheral nerve entrapment. Patients with a stiff painful shoulder and associated paresthesias must be carefully evaluated to rule out carpal tunnel, cubital tunnel, or radial tunnel syndromes.

One particularly painful problem around the shoulder is the syndrome of Parsonage and Turner or "neuralgia amyotrophy," as they would have liked it to have been known.[79] This syndrome is characterized by severe pain across the shoulder and upper arm followed by atrophic paralysis in muscles about the shoulder. Neuralgia amyotrophy may follow trauma, surgery, and vaccinations, as well as viral and bacterial infections. While usually self-limited, this condition can lead to FSS in some patients.[80] Patients may continue to suffer from FSS even after their neurogenic focus has resolved, as in the "11th nerve syndrome" in which, following neck dissection, the stiff and painful shoulder can persist despite recovery of the trapezius.[81]

Central Neurologic Conditions

The clinician must be aware that FSS may be the presenting complaint in patients with Parkinsonism in up to 8% of cases,[82] 12.7% of patients with Parkinsonism develop FSS.

The painful stiff shoulder is a well recognized cause of prolongation of rehabilitation in hemiplegic patients. The fact that this is related to FSS and not rotator cuff tears or spasticity was proven arthrographically by Rizk and associates.[83]

FSS AS A "FORME FRUSTE" OF RSD

Many of the features of FSS resemble an isolated reflex sympathetic dystrophy of the shoulder. Yoshida has identified, via a calcitonin gene related peptide labelling technique, sensory fibers of the middle cervical cord and sympathetic nerves from the cervical ganglion distributed in abundance in the shoulder joint capsule and subacromial bursa.[84] This histologic evidence of a neural link to the sympathetic nervous system lends credence to those investigators who, since Steinbrocker's original description of the "shoulder-hand syndrome," have postulated that FSS is a forme fruste of algodystrophy.[16,85–88]

The clinical, radiologic, and cinegraphic behavior of many cases of frozen shoulders is similar to that of RSDS.[86] Recent evidence that frozen shoulder is related to sympathetically maintained pain comes from Jeracitano, who demonstrated significant abnormalities in the mechanisms controlling shoulder skin temperature especially during the re-warming phase following cold stress using thermographic evaluation.[87] Laser flow doppler evaluation has also shown reduced skin blood flow in patients with frozen shoulder.[87,88] Careful evaluation of a patient with FSS will frequently reveal a shiny texture to their skin with marked cutaneous hypersensitivity. This is especially true in the patient with postoperative FSS. A detailed description of reflex sympathetic dystrophy, the theories behind it's production, and it's treatment are beyond the scope of this chapter.

EPIDEMIOLOGY/NATURAL HISTORY

The annual cumulative risk for developing frozen shoulder has been estimated at 2%.[19] The nondominant arms in women are more commonly effected.[19,81] Whites are more commonly affected than blacks.[89] The mean age of onset occurs in the sixth decade, with onset before the age of 40 being rare. Although proposed associations with menopause have been shown to be a consequence of increased age,[19] my experience has been that many of the patients I have seen who are under the age of 40 or in their early 40s have had surgically or medically created menopause. The mean age for men is slightly greater than that of females (55 years versus 52 years).[19] Diabetics tend to develop the condition earlier. Occupation does not appear to play a significant role. A seasonal variation has been suggested by Lundberg.[19] Associated ipsilateral, cervical, and trapezius pain is quite common. In 6 to 17% of patients the contralaterat shoulder develops a similar condition within 5 years.[90] No well-documented case of recurrence of the condition in the same shoulder has been described, although Rowe and Leffert described a patient who appeared to suffer recurrence in the same shoulder.[23] My experience has been that although the exact same condition does not recur in a patient, many patients that are seen in their 70s and 80s with end stage osteoarthritis or rotator cuff tear arthropathy do have a history of a "frozen shoulder" treated successfully with cortisone 20 years before.

Different investigators have used different terms to describe the now well-recognized phases of FSS. Reeves used the terms painful phase, adhesive phase, and resolution phase, which correspond to Rowe's freezing, frozen, and thawing phases (Fig. 17–1).[18,23] Reeves demonstrated that the painful phase lasted approximately 10 to 36 weeks, the adhesive phase 4 to 12 months, and the resolution phase 5 to 26 months. The total duration of symptoms lasted 12 to 42 months, with a mean duration of 30.1 months.[18] These studies, along with a recent study by Shaffer and colleagues, indicate that FSS is a protracted painful condition.[91] Many years later, significant numbers of patients, especially men, have residual clinically detectable limitation of shoulder motion (60%) and a smaller number have residual functional shoulder disability (11%).[91] This differs from the study of Grey, in which the use of simple analgesics, hypnotics, reassurance, and the passage of time of 2 years results in normal shoulders in 24 of 25 patients treated in this manner.[92]

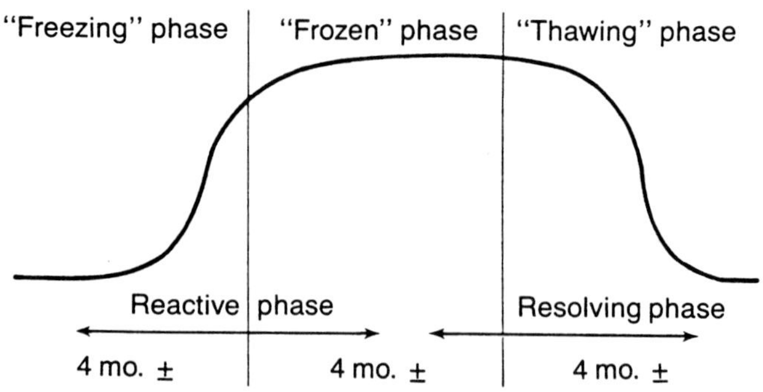

Fig. 17–1. The natural history of idiopathic frozen shoulder is illustrated by Rowe. When left untreated, the syndrome consists of three phases, the average length of which approximates 4 months, but the length may vary. (From Rowe CR, Leffert RD. Idiopathic chronic adhesive capsulitis ("frozen shoulder"). In: Rowe CR, ed. *The Shoulder.* New York: Churchill Livingstone; 1988: 155–163.)

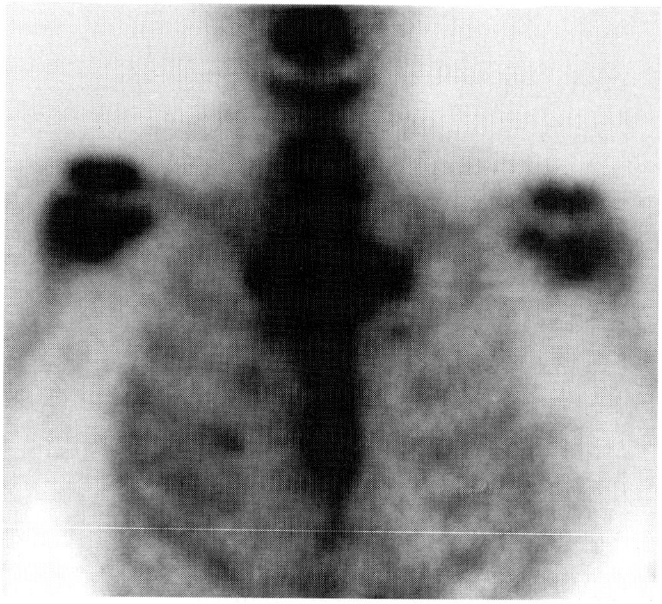

Fig. 17–2. Bone scan showing mild uptake not only in the AC joint and glenohumeral joint, but also in the sternoclavicular joint and coracoid process in the right shoulder (reader's left).

Anatomy

The importance of recognizing that frozen shoulder includes the entire shoulder girdle complex is borne out by bone scanning, which frequently shows uptake not only in the glenohumeral joint, the AC joint, mild uptake in the sternoclavicular joint, and uptake over the coracoid process as well (Fig. 17–2). Patients present with global pain. The trapezius pain and parascapular discomfort seen in these patients is related in some to the increased scapulothoracic motion required for the same degree of arm elevation, placing stress on the rhomboids, trapezius, serratus, and levator scapulae, and in others is related to referred pain from cervical origin.

The prime structure, however, that needs to be understood with regard to pathogenesis and treatment is the glenohumeral joint capsule. The capsule, which attaches around the periphery of the glenoid and spans across to attach to the anatomic neck of the humerus, is normally a loose blousy structure whose surface area is almost twice that of the humeral head.[93] The capsule bridges the gap between the supraspinatus and subscapularis superiorly, the thickening of which in this region is the coracohumeral ligament (see Chapter 2).

Except in the region of the rotator interval above and the inferior recess below, the glenohumeral ligaments and capsule are thickened by the muscular and tendinous attachments of the rotator cuff. The inferior capsule has only the soft muscular portion of the subscapularis present and, in it's most inferior portion, no muscular or tendinous attachments. It is in this region that the redundant fold is normally present while the arm is at the side (Fig. 17–3). This redundant fold, which makes up the axillary pouch of the inferior glenohumeral ligament, disappears as the arm is abducted. The synovial recesses have been well described. Anteriorly be-

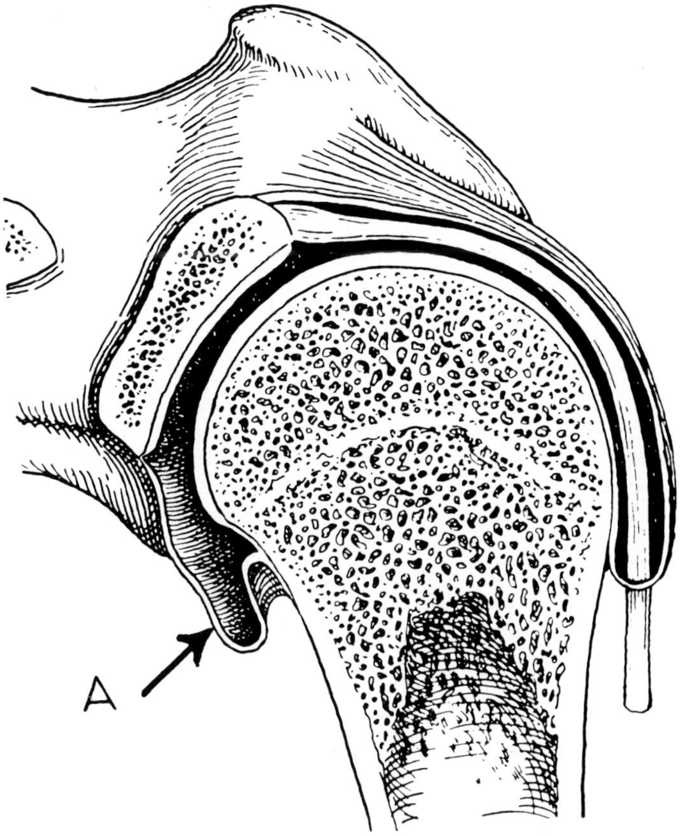

Fig. 17–3. The dependent fold of the axillary recess is normally quite lax and represents a potential space for descent of the humeral head. (From Neviaser JS. Adhesive capsulitis of the shoulder. A study of the pathological findings in periarthritis of the shoulder. *J Bone Joint Surg.* 1945;27:211–222).

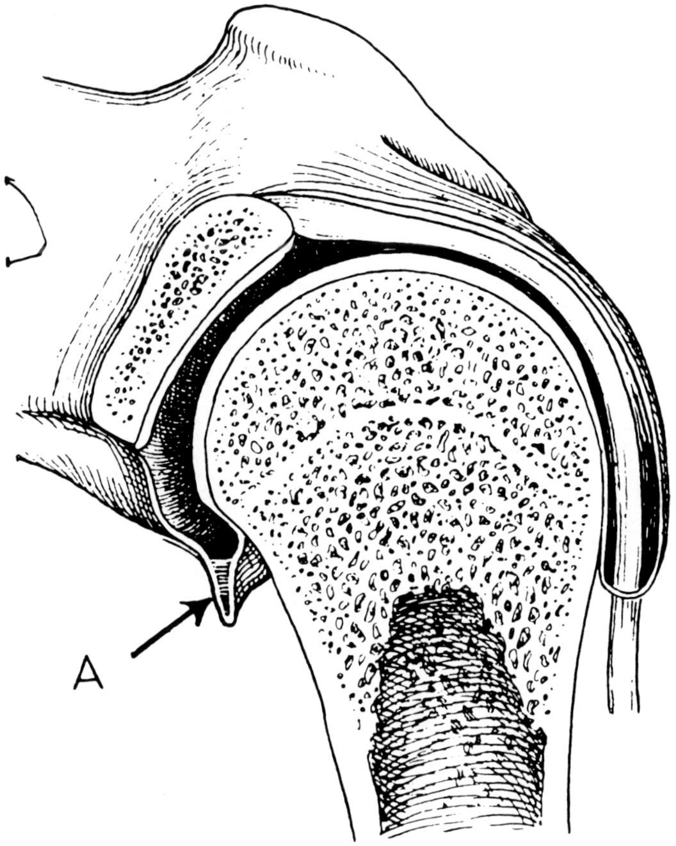

Fig. 17–4. The capsule adheres to the humeral head as well as to itself with obliteration of the axillary fold. (From Neviaser JS. Adhesive capsulitis of the shoulder. A study of the pathological findings in periarthritis of the shoulder. *J Bone Joint Surg.* 1945;27:211–222, 1945.)

tween the superior and middle glenohumeral ligament, the subscapular bursa, as it is known, communicates normally with the glenohumeral joint. The inferior recess is the area of redundant inferior capsule, previously described, and posteriorly an out-pouching deep to the infraspinatus muscle may occur, known as the infraspinatus bursa.[83] The rotator interval, in my opinion, can also be thought of as a recess or potential space in that it is normally quite loose and on arthrography in the lax individual can be seen to expand (see Chapter 13). The synovial membrane lines the capsule and is in continuity with all of the recesses, including the reflection of the capsule that invests the long head of the biceps.

Histologically, the capsule consists of bundles of tightly packed, high-tensile strength type I collagen aligned with the axis of stress.[94] Cells of the synovial membrane covering the inner surface of the capsule are supported by a fibrillar network containing a mixture of types I and III collagen molecules. Because of the smooth muscle of the vasculature, the synovial layer contains type V collagen as well.[95] Electron microscopic examination shows no structural differences between the shoulder capsule and other joint capsules, and like other capsular tissue it's tensile strength decreased with age.[95] There are comparatively few fibrocytes in the glenohumeral capsule in the normal state.[96]

GROSS PATHOLOGICAL CHANGES

Neviaser, who coined the term "adhesive capsulitis," described the gross pathological changes based on operative cases. These included a conspicuous absence of synovial fluid and adherence of the once redundant capsule to itself and to (Fig. 17–4) the humeral head. Under direct observation, when the capsule was sharply separated from the cartilage no bleeding could be detected. This led Neviaser to postulate that the adhesion was not due to vascular bands. Under direct observation during manipulation, he noted that the capsule would separate from the head, similar to an "adhesive plaster" being pulled away from the bare skin. The capsule was thicker than normal and adhesions were discernable at the reflected fold of the capsule, distal to the anatomical neck.[7,9]

Early on, most of the interest in this condition focused on the adhesion of the inferior recess as the source of restricted motion. More recently, DePalma, Nobuhara,

Ozaki, and Neer have commented on the role of the contracted rotator interval and coracohumeral ligament and have recommended it's release at the time of open shoulder manipulation.[15,97–99] It appears that DePalma was the first to comment on the coracohumeral ligament in cases of frozen shoulder. He noted that it was frozen in a shortened position, converted into a tough inelastic band of fibrous tissue spanning the interval between the coracoid and the tuberosities. In it's contracted state, it serves as a forceful checkrein to external rotation, and DePalma incised it at the time of biceps tenodesis to the coracoid.[15] Ozaki has stated that it is the main cause of recalcitrant chronic adhesive capsulitis.

HISTOPATHOLOGY

Neviaser examined microscopic sections of the thickened adherent joint capsule and found changes of chronic inflammation in the subsynovial layer. These cellular changes of chronic inflammation, fibrosis, and perivascular infiltration in the subsynovial layer of the capsule, and not the synovium, were understood to be consistent with a reparative inflammatory process (Fig. 17–5).[7,9]

McLaughlin, in contra-distinction, reported a 10% nonspecific proliferative synovitis at the time of open release.[31] He observed that the capsular folds and pouches were obliterated by adhesion of the adjacent synovial surfaces.

Kay and Slater examined the shoulder capsule tissue from diabetic patients with frozen shoulder and found an appearance identical to that seen in plantar fibromatosis and Dupuytren's disease (i.e., fibroblast and myofibroblast proliferation). The vascular changes suggested diabetic microangiopathy. They felt that a thickened, more dense capsule was responsible for this loss of motion (Fig. 17–6).[100] This differentiation between the histological features of diabetic frozen shoulder and the other types of frozen shoulder may, in the future, have implications for both diagnosis, classification, and treatment.

Lundberg could not demonstrate intra-articular adhesions. Histological evaluation in his series showed that the synovial layer was mostly unchanged. However, there was more compact dense collagen layer in the shoulder capsule with increased fibrous tissue, increased fibroblast numbers, and increased vascularity without an inflammatory cell infiltrate.[19] Again, a similarity in morphology to Dupuytren's was noted. Structural changes were absent in the collagen fibers on electron microscopic examination. Increased levels of glycosominoglycans, particularly dermaten sulfate, and reduced levels of glycoprotein were noted. These changes are suggestive of a repair reaction.[19] Simmonds described a local increase in vascularity in the joint capsule, which is related to a chronic inflammatory reaction in the supraspinatus tendon as the underlying cause.[101] Ozaki found fibrosis, hyalinization in the contracted connective tissue and subsynovial tissue, along with an absence of the synovial cell layer on the joint side of the rotator interval (Fig. 17–7).

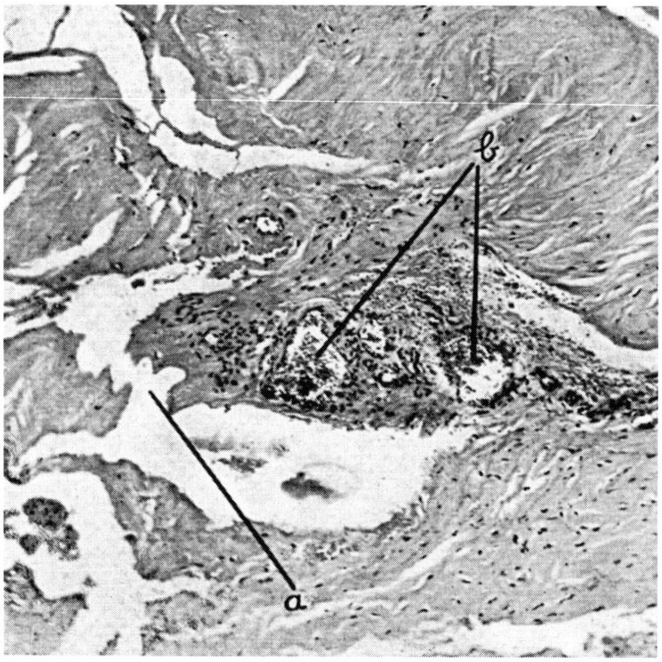

Fig. 17–5. Photomicrograph (× 80) of the capsule shows (*A*) Degeneration of collagen in the subsynovial area; and (*B*) vascular dilatation and perivascular infiltration. (From Neviaser JS. Adhesive capsulitis of the shoulder. A study of the pathological findings in periarthritis of the shoulder. *J Bone Joint Surg.* 1945;27:211–222.)

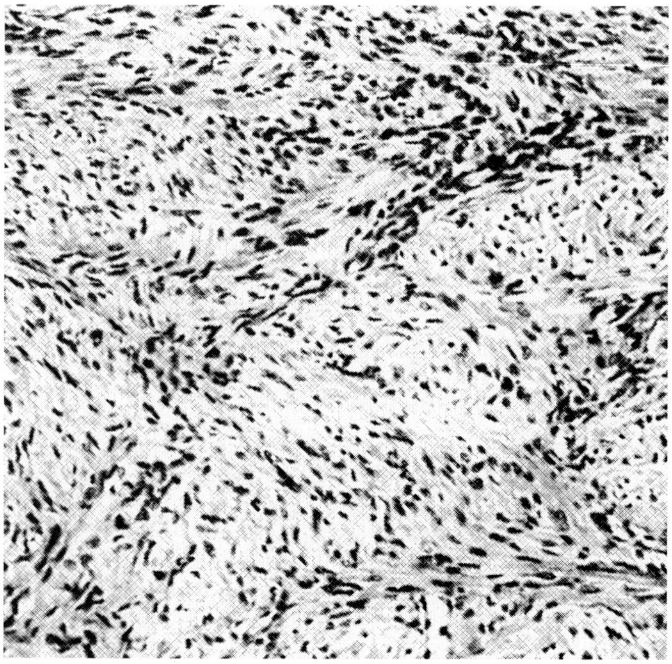

Fig. 17–6. Fibroblast and myofibroblast proliferation seen in the capsule of patient with frozen shoulder secondary to diabetes. (From Kay N, Slater D. Fibromatoses and diabetes mellitus. *Lancet.* 1981;II:303.)

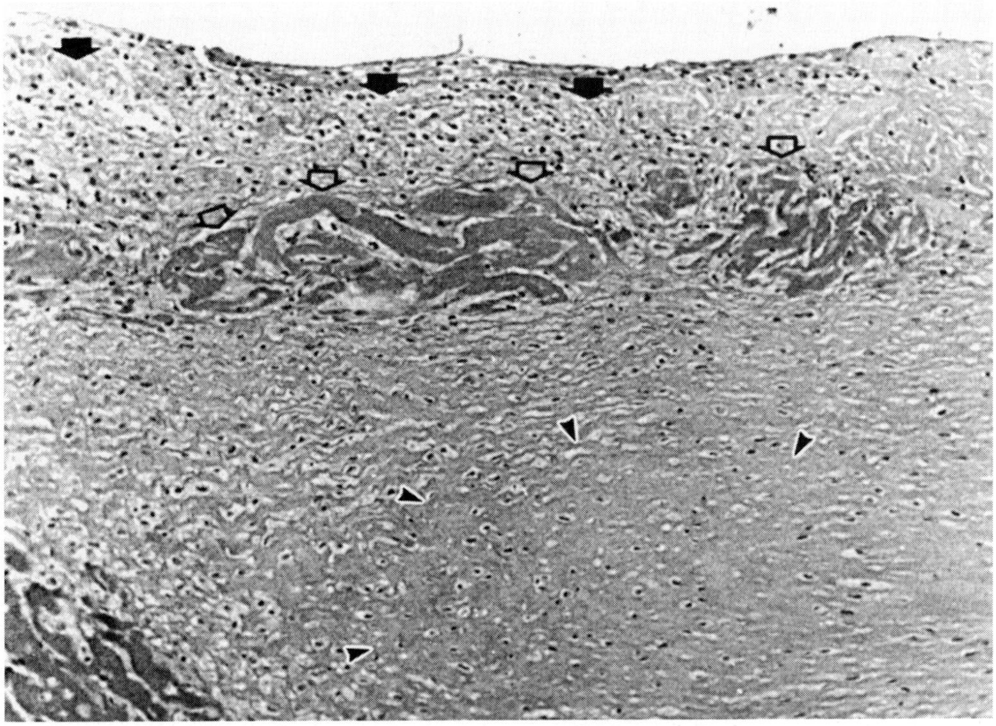

Fig. 17–7. Photomicrograph (× 40) showing the contracted coracohumeral ligament and rotator interval in a patient who had chronic adhesive capsulitis of the shoulder. (From Ozaki J, Nakagawa Y, Sakurai G, Tamai S. Recalcitrant chronic adhesive capsulitis of the shoulder. *J Bone Joint Surg Am.* 1989;71: 1511–1515.)

HISTOCHEMISTRY

MacNab postulated that loss of blood supply in the critical zone could initiate degeneration of collagen and that this localized degeneration of collagen could induce an autoimmune response. Evidence for this, includes a round cell infiltrate and pyroninophilic lymphoid cells found in the capsule.[102,103]

Other investigators have been unable to reproduce consistent evidence for an immunological etiology for adhesive capsulitis.[93,104–106] Acute phase reactants, complement, immunoglobulins (apart from IGA), immune complexes, and autoantibodies to a variety of connective tissues are normal or absent in patients with adhesive capsulitis. High-dose corticosteroids are ineffective in preventing it's development and do not have a marked effect on established disease.

In a controlled series of 25 frozen shoulder patients by Bulgen et al., no significant difference in the presence of rheumatoid, anti-nuclear antibodies, or anti-nuclear factors. Immunoglobulin clonification, immunoelectrophoresis, lymphocyte transformability, and DNA synthesis in response to mitogens are all also nonrevealing. A small depression in serum IGA was noted. The significance of this awaits further evaluation. Kessel et al. screened 50 frozen shoulder patients for autoantibodies to smooth muscle collagen and cartilage, as well as compliment and immune complexes.[107] No immunological disturbance was in evidence.

Four controlled studies have addressed the prevalence of HLA-B27 antigen in patients with FSS. The consensus of all of these studies is that no increase in prevalence is present in this group of patients.[108–110]

In summary, histologic studies fail to consistently show evidence of inflammatory cell infiltrates, granulomas or vasculitis in synovium, capsule, or rotator cuff, and unlike other auto-immune disorders it does not recur. However, because of the nature of this syndrome, the pathologic changes seen in the capsule and synovium may differ with varying timing of obtaining these specimens. A summary of surgical, arthroscopic, and histologic findings are found in Table 17–2.

Clinical Presentation

HISTORY

Although a variety of euphemisms have been used to describe the stages of frozen shoulder, all investigators who have treated this syndrome realize that it does go through characteristic clinical stages. It is important that a thorough history be obtained in terms of the exact duration of the symptoms in order to make this diagnosis and stage the patient.

PHASE ONE—THE PAINFUL OR FREEZING PHASE

Classically, an otherwise healthy patient presents with an insidious onset of generalized aching in the shoulder. The statement, "I just woke up with it," is not uncommon. Frequently the point of maximum pain is the deltoid insertion. The pain is constant and nagging, and it

Table 17–20. Surgical and Arthroscopic Findings

Study	*No. of Patients*	*Duration of Symptoms*	*Findings*
Neviaser (1945)[7]	10		Adhesive capsule to humeral head capsule thickened and tense; axillary fold adhesions; chronic inflammatory changes in capsule with fibrosis; no synovitis.
Lundberg (1969)[19]	20		No adhesions; thickened capsule; periarticular inflammatory changes in rotator cuff.
DePalma (1973)[15]	42	"Long and protracted"	Low grade inflammatory process in capsule and periarticular structures.
Simmonds (1979)[101]	4		Vascular thickened cuff; chronic inflammatory changes, subacromial bursa; no adhesions.
Haéri Maitland (1981)[173]	24	Mean 8 mo.	No adhesions; 1 rotator cuff tear; 2 biceps tendon tear; 5 chronic synovitis; 8 normal axillary fold.
Cofield (1983)[181]	3	3 years	Synovitis, chondromalacia, and capsular scarring.
Ogilvie-Harris Wiley (1986)[174]	81	>6 months	Small joint capacity, mild synovitis, no adhesions—17, partial-rotator cuff tear
Neviaser Neviaser (1987)[122]			Stages 1–4 (as described in text); synovitis and adhesions in varying degrees.

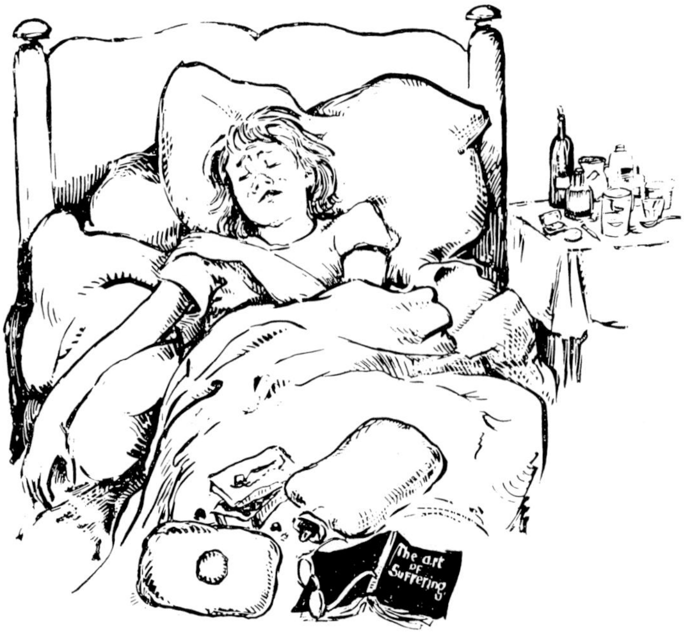

Fig. 17–8. A typical night for a patient with untreated adhesive capsulitis. (From Moseley HF. In: Moseley HF, ed. *Shoulder Lesions.* Edinburgh: Churchill Livingstone; 1972:99–118.)

seems to the patients that there is nothing they can do to get comfortable (Fig. 17–8). If normally a picture is worth 1,000 words, the illustration from Moseley's book is worth 10,000 words in regard to describing the patient during the painful or freezing phase of adhesive capsulitis. The pain is much worse with motion, especially sudden motions. The pain is more severe at night and, as the shoulder is dependent to the heart in the decubitus position, is much worse when the patients lie on their affected shoulder. Typically, nonsteroidal anti-inflammatory medications and over-the-counter analgesics offer little to no relief. The only way the patients feel they can keep their arm comfortable is to keep it close to their side in an internally rotated and adducted position. Frequently, the patients realize that if they don't move their shoulder, they don't have as much discomfort; so they avoid moving their shoulder. They are then led down the primrose path to keep immobilizing their shoulder and avoiding positions that cause pain for several weeks to several months before presenting to the doctor.[18] Careful recording of a patients' histories at the time of their first evaluation may reveal that they did a little more activity than usual shortly before the onset of symptoms or that they did have an episode of pain during a specific activity. A common precipitating event occurs when the arm is placed in an extended internally rotated posture, such as occurs when one reaches into the back seat of a car from the front to lift a briefcase or to take care of a child's needs. This minor type of trauma is often forgotten in the context of a doctor's visit unless specifically queried.

PHASE TWO—ADHESIVE, FROZEN, OR STIFFENING PHASE

The painful phase of frozen shoulder gives way to the adhesive or frozen phase. This phase lasts generally from 4 to 12 months.[18,23] The patient's pain has settled down. Sometimes patients will get through the entire painful phase of their shoulder feeling that "it is something that is going to get well," only to present during the stiffening or frozen phase. Patients in this phase frequently have parascapular symptoms, because of the compensatory motions required to achieve simple elevation and rotation for activities of daily living.

PHASE THREE—RESOLUTION OR THAWING PHASE

The final phase of frozen shoulder may last 5 to 26 months. During this phase the pain eases and limitation of motion slowly improves. Some patients rather dramatically improve. Common statements during the follow-up of patients in this phase include, "it happened overnight" or "in just this last week I have made tremendous progress in my motion," or "I almost canceled this appointment I feel so much better."

PHYSICAL EXAMINATION

An equal loss of passive and active range of motion is the hallmark of established FSS. Range of motion is measured and recorded per the American Shoulder and Elbow Surgeons' Standard, Table 17–3.[91] Physical examination corresponds with the phase during which the patient presents. In the painful stage of freezing, especially in the patient with an early RSD picture, clinical examination is difficult in the office because of severe discomfort. During the early freezing, and later in the thawing phase, varying degrees of motion loss occur. During early freezing when motion is still preserved, or late thawing phase in which motion has almost returned, clinical examination for impingement can be performed. Patients often will have pain with impingement and impingement reinforcement testing; however, subacromial injection incompletely relieves their pain and the loss of passive range of motion persists. Take caution with the female patient with only a few weeks of shoulder symptoms and subtle loss of internal rotation that does not return dramatically with subacromial injection. These patients who are in the early phase of FSS may have a dramatic steroid flare of pain, rapidly lose motion, and frequently blame the doctor and this injection for worsening their condition.

DIAGNOSTIC TESTING

Many patients that I see currently arrive without the benefit of having been seen by a primary care physician. Therefore, because of the severity of some of the associated conditions, an ability to perform a thorough workup is required. It is important to know what to order, when to order it, and why you've ordered it.

Hematologic/Chemistry Evaluation

In order to rule out a remote or metabolic etiology for frozen shoulder, routine blood work is required. A CBC with sedimentation rate, serum chemistry, and thyroid function tests are done as a screening panel. Further blood testing, such as rheumatoid factor, ANA, or serum cortisol levels, is done only if the routine blood work suggests the possibility that the patient may have a diagnosable systemic illness.

Table 17–3. Measurements of Range of Motion of the Shoulder

Measurement	*Plane*
Forward flexion	Sagittal plane, thumb up
Forward elevation	Scapular plane, midway between sagittal plane and coronal plane, thumb up
Abduction	Coronal plane, thumb up
External rotation	Elbow at side, flexed 90°, forearm supinated
Internal rotation	Tip of thumb relative to spinal level

Plain Film Radiology

It is critical to obtain a complete set of shoulder radiographs. This includes five views of the shoulder, an AP in internal and external rotation, an axillary lateral, a caudal tilt view,[111] and an outlet view.[112] A local cause of frozen shoulder is AC joint arthritis, which in general is best viewed with a lighter technique. Therefore, I require that at least one of the radiographs is obtained with the following technique (for the average patient): with the patient standing with their back against a grid and the AC joint centered on the film at a distance of 40 inches, an exposure of 3/20 second, at 62 KV, 200 MA is performed.

Shoulder radiographs are reported usually as normal in patients with frozen shoulder.[113] Mild to moderate osteopenia may be observed, depending on the stage and the patient's premorbid bone density. Minor degenerative changes of the humeral head in the area of the greater tuberosity, as well as narrowing of the subacromial space, in 19 and 12% respectively, have been reported.[113] Erosions of the humeral head can occur with frozen shoulder and must be distinguished from radiographic projectional artifacts but do not alter the prognosis.[114]

In order to obtain a good external rotation view on patients with adhesive capsulitis, the patient must either be in a standing position and turned obliquely, or they must be rolled up onto the affected shoulder. Unfortunately, the patient lying on their affected shoulder will, in many patients, cause a great deal of pain and they will not be able to stay in that position long enough to obtain a radiograph. If adequate external rotation radiographs are performed in the 40- to 50-year-old female patient with this condition, an early osteophyte of osteoarthritis of the glenohumeral joint can frequently be observed (Fig. 17–9).

Radionucleide Scanning

Bone scans with technetium 99-M pertechnetate (Tc99m HDP) consistently show an increased uptake in patients with frozen shoulder, regardless of etiology.[86] The uptake is generally nonfocal, mild to moderate in degree, and involves not only the humeral head but sometimes the coracoid and the AC joint. Wright and colleagues noted a favorable association between a hot bone scan and response to corticosteroid injections.[115] Other investigators have confirmed Wright's findings of increased uptake of Tc99m HDP.[113,116] Binder and associates could not prove that bone scanning predicted the severity of the disease, arthrographic findings, or the eventual recovery.[113]

Although bone scanning does not help in prognostication, it's main goal is to rule out a metastatic deposit, which would give an extremely hot local foci of uptake versus the generalized uptake typical of FSS. Using bone scans Smith et al. identified three patients with lesions of the midshaft of the humerus presenting with classic FSS.[117] Before a surgeon sends a patient out of the office for a several-month period of time to recover gradually from a condition, it is critical that one has ruled out an occult metastasis.

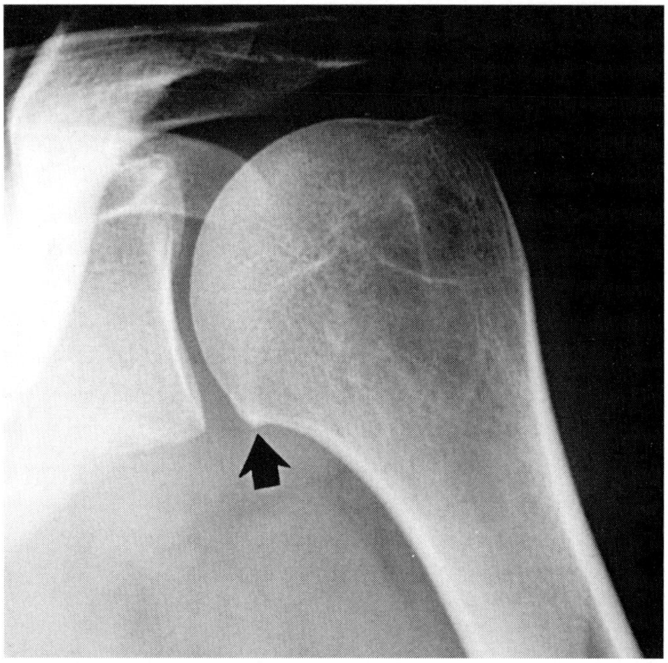

Fig. 17–9. Early osteoarthritis as evidenced by the small humeral osteophyte is seen not uncommonly in 40- to 60-year-old woman who presents with "idiopathic" FSS.

Arthrography

The use of arthrography to make the diagnosis of adhesive capsulitis has been promoted by J.S. Neviaser[9] and Kernwein et al.[118] The criteria for having adhesive capsulitis are decreased joint volume, an irregular joint outline, and variable filling of the bicipital tendon sheath. The subscapularis bursa, axillary fold, infraspinatus recess, and rotator interval are all absent (Fig. 17–10). Several investigators have been able to demonstrate a strong correlation between the severity of the volumetric capsular contraction and the patient's clinical range of motion.[10,18,19,119,120] However, recently Itoi and Tatata failed to document a direct correlation between the severity of the contracture and range of motion. The prognosis for recovery is not directly related to arthrographic findings.[113] Arthrography was used as well to document tearing of the capsule during manipulation under anesthesia.[18,19,121] Lundberg noted that tears in the capsule allowed dye to flow out of the shoulder joint rather than tears in the rotator cuff tendons proper.[19] R.J. Neviaser and T.J. Neviaser used joint volume to separate the painful stiff shoulder with a moderately restricted joint volume (10 to 12 mL) from patients with adhesive capsulitis who had a markedly restricted joint volume (5 to 10 mL).[122] This type of approach confuses matters and does not really help as much with staging of the patient as does the history, because patients both in the freezing and thawing phase will have a restricted volume, but not as restricted as patients in the frozen phase.

Arthrography can be used to rule out a large partial-thickness or a small full-thickness rotator cuff tear with a secondary frozen shoulder. Over the years, many patients

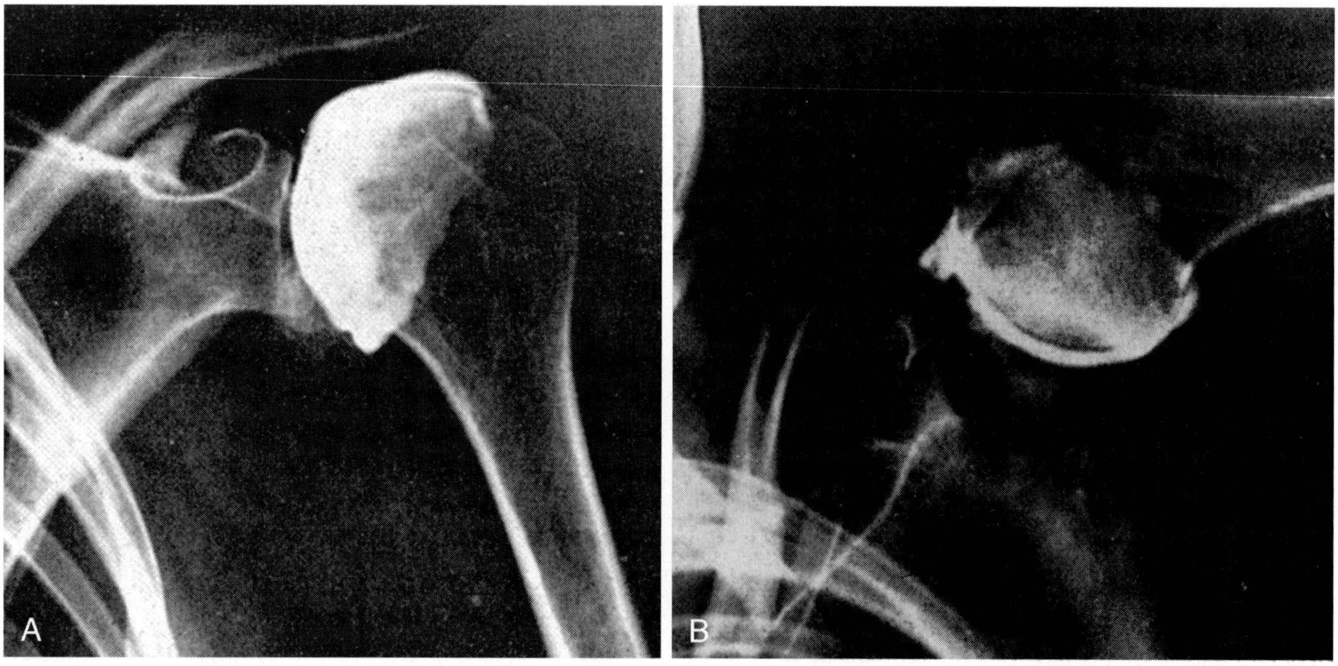

Fig. 17–10. *A*, Arthrogram of a case of adhesive capsulitis. Note the decreased joint capacity and the almost complete obliteration of the axillary fold as well as the subscapularis bursa and biceps sheath. *B*, The arm is in the maximum abducted position. Note the humeral head cannot descend into the contracted axillary recess. (*A and B*, From Neviaser JS. Arthrography of the shoulder joint. *J Bone Joint Surg.* 1962; 44:1321–1330.)

have presented with this diagnostic dilemma: a history of trauma followed by a stiff shoulder. A small full-thickness rotator cuff tear can lead to subacromial bursitis and a full blown FSS clinical picture. The arthrogram is extremely useful in this group of patients to (1) rule out the rotator cuff tear and (2) at the time of the arthrogram, if the joint volume is restricted and there is no rotator cuff tear, the radiologist can then instill corticosteroids and perform gentle distention and effectively treat the patient for their FSS. In the patient without trauma, I seldom, if ever, order an arthrogram. Many of these patients present in the freezing or irritative phase of this syndrome. The arthrogram is in these individuals quite a painful process, and the dye from the arthrogram can exacerbate their synovitis. The volumetric contraction requisite for the diagnosis can be confirmed in the clinic setting at the time of glenohumeral brisement.

MRI Scanning

MRI scanning, like arthrography and bone scanning, is valuable in ruling out a local cause for adhesive capsulitis. The diagnosis of FSS can be made if one pays attention to the inferior capsular fold in patients to see whether it is thickened or contracted (Fig. 17–11). The addition of a gadolinium arthrogram enhances our ability to diagnose this problem with MRI scanning by allowing the joint volume to be depicted; however, it is at this time cost-prohibitive for the bulk of patients with this problem. Like a bone scan, MRI can rule out a metastatic lesion, avascular necrosis, and reveal partial-thickness cuff tears, subacromial fibrosis, or other intrinsic causes of FSS as well.

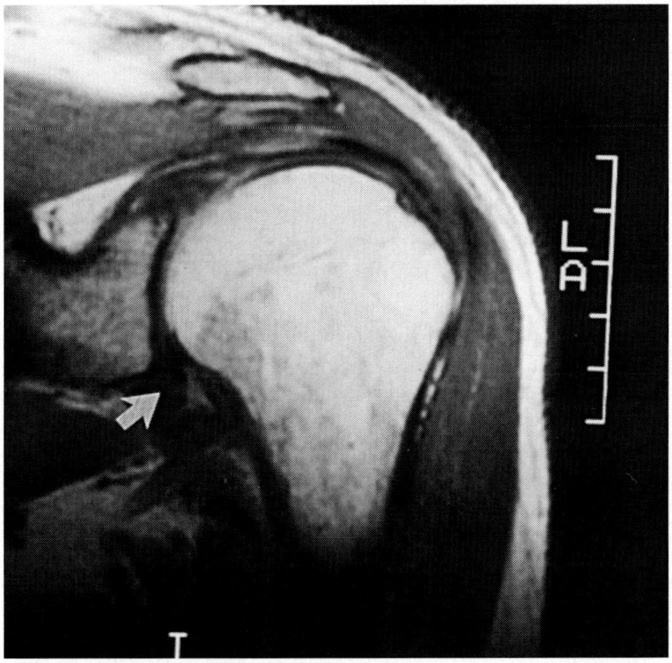

Fig. 17–11. MRI scan of diabetic stiff and painful shoulder. Note thickening of inferior capsule.

Thermography

Thermography has been used successfully as an objective method to assess response to therapy in various inflammatory arthritides.[123] Middleditch and Jarman first investigated frozen shoulder using thermography.[77] Recently, Vecchio and colleagues screened patients with unilateral frozen shoulder and compared them to 86 patients with unilateral rotator cuff lesions.[124] Differences in skin temperature distribution were found in 82% of subjects with frozen shoulder, with nearly three-fourths of these having reduced skin temperature, although there was no consistent pattern of skin temperature found in patients with rotator cuff tendinitis.

BONE DENSOMETRY EVALUATION

Bone densometry studies of the affected humeral head show an average of 50% reduction in bone mineral content compared to the unaffected side. This finding was independent of age, did not increase with extended duration of illness, and did not restore with time.[19] I have no experience with either thermography or bone densometry as diagnostic tools for this condition.

ARTHROSCOPIC EVALUATION OF FROZEN SHOULDER PATIENTS

An arthroscopic staging system has been recommended by T.J. Neviaser. The patients in his series had pathognomonic arthrographic findings and failure to improve with conservative care prior to arthroscopy. His system is as follows:[125]

> Stage I is the preadhesive stage in which there is a patchy, low-lying, fibrinous, erythematous pannus of synovitis about the joint (Fig. 17–12), particularly visible in the dependent axillary fold. This corresponds to the preadhesive painful or frozen phase. Early synovitis has been confirmed arthroscopically by other investigators.[96,126] These patchy nodules of granulation (Fig. 17–13) have been found to represent vasculitis on histologic examination.[126]

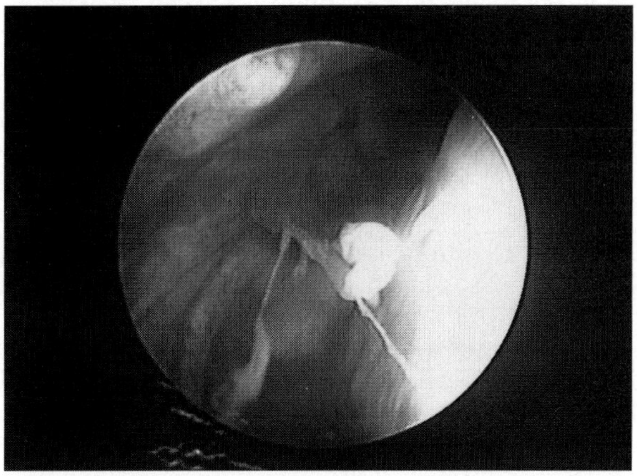

Fig. 17–12. Stage I adhesive capsulitis.

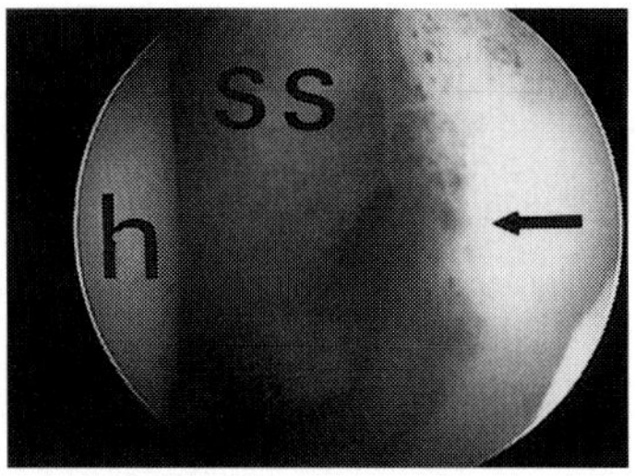

Fig. 17–13. Patchy nodules of granulation tissue which on biopsy are found to be areas of vasculitis.

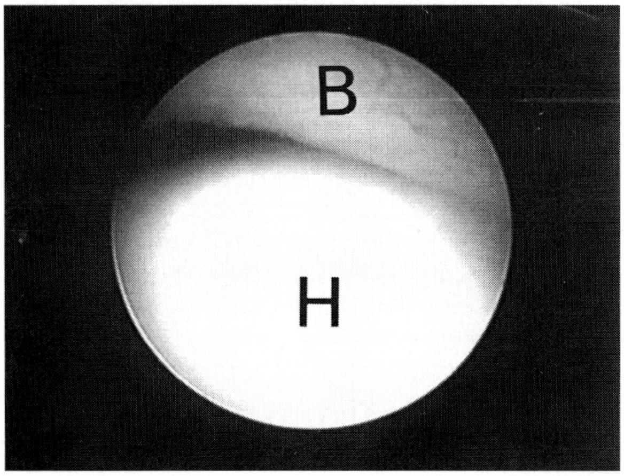

Fig. 17–14. The biceps tendon is seen closely applied to the humeral head in stage II.

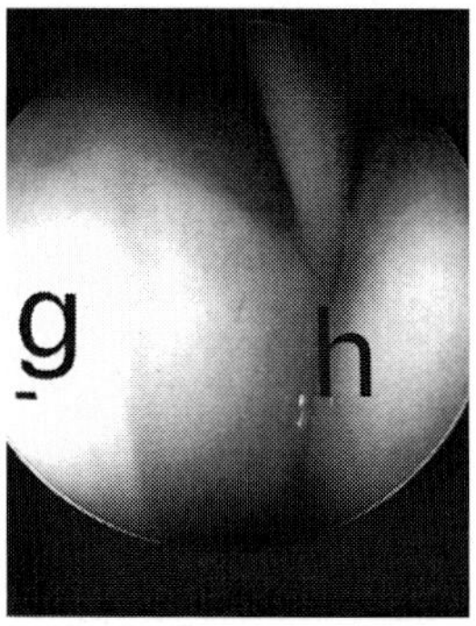

Fig. 17–15. "Fluffy" synovitis characteristic of stage III adhesive capsulitis.

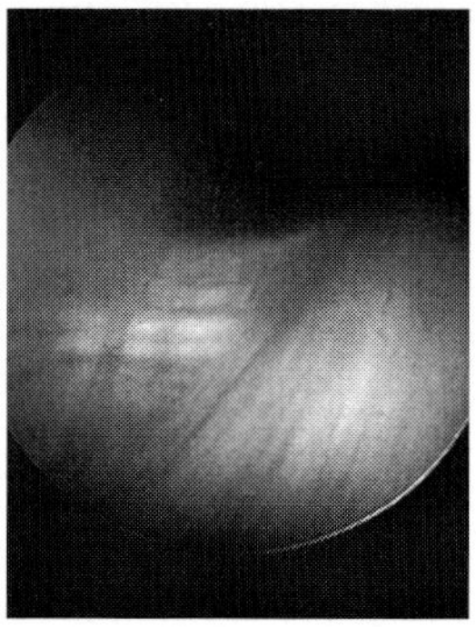

Fig. 17–16. A fibrotic axillary recess in stage IV adhesive capsulitis.

Stage II, according to Neviaser, is the most active and probably the most painful. He maintains that adhesions grow within the joint and restriction of the capsular structures is demonstrated by the loss of the normal space between the humeral head and biceps tendon (Fig. 17–14), as well as between the humeral head and glenoid. In fact, the humeral head cannot be pulled away from the biceps tendon or glenoid, even with traction. It has been my experience that arthroscopy during this stage is quite difficult and may result in a lot of head scuffing unless the shoulder is predistended. In Stage III (Fig. 17–15), the synovitis abates and only residual pink "fluffy synovitis is left." The restriction of motion and loss of humeral head and glenoid space are evident.
In Stage IV, which corresponds to the frozen stage, synovitis is no longer evident, but it is impossible to visualize the dependent fold which "almost disappears once the adhesions have matured" (Fig. 17–16). Wiley found no obliteration by adhesions.[1] It may be that he was looking for the band-like adhesions one associates with bowel surgery and that can occasionally be seen in the bursa.

The clinical manifestations of the stages, according to Neviaser are (1) stage I, the insidious onset of pain or discomfort in the shoulder; (2) stage II, increasing pain, especially at night with loss of motion, with most patients noting loss of internal rotation; (3) stage III, pain is usually of less concern and loss of motion becomes the major concern; and (4) stage IV, the presenting complaint is usually loss of motion with the patient experiencing pain at the extremes of motion. Neviaser recommends manipulation of the shoulder with the patient under general anesthesia as the treatment of choice for the refractory cases of adhesive capsulitis.

Treatment Options in FSS

> We have all had to claim that the idiopathic frozen shoulder is a self-limited condition and that the majority of patients become pain-free with full range of motion within a year or 18 months. Our problem has been: How can we shorten the painful period effectively.
> Rowe, 1984

Once the diagnosis is secure, there are many treatment alternatives for patients with frozen shoulder (Table 17–4). Like any other condition with multiple treatment options, these options should be explored with the patient; in general a course with a high benefit to risk ratio should be taken, and the patient should be encouraged to participate in the choice of treatment.

Analgesia and Hypnotherapy

Pain control, the reassurance of a firm diagnosis, and medication for sleep goes a long way in securing the patient's trust and confidence that they will recover. My experience, as well as the experience of other investigators over the years, has been that nonsteroidal anti-inflammatory medications are less helpful in this condition than other conditions concerning the shoulder.[36] Transcutaneous electrical neural stimulation (TENS), oral narcotic agents, and nonsalicylate analgesics have been found to be effective.[126,127] These patients' sleep disorders must be addressed aggressively. The patient is generally instructed to sleep sitting in a recliner or propped up in bed, if they haven't already learned to do so. Several commercial wedge pillows are available. A recliner is frequently the favorite place to sleep. A moist heating pad at night frequently will be beneficial.

Because these patients may need hypnotic medication for a prolonged period, my drugs of choice for this aspect of their care are nonaddictive. My preference is to use diphenhydramine hydrochloride (Benadryl), 25 to 50 mg, for sleep or a low dosage of dibenzoxepine (Doxepin), 10 mg initially, increasing the dosage by 1 tablet h.s. until a good night's sleep is obtained. My experience has been that a low dosage of dibenzoxepine taken fairly early in the evening, around 7 or 8 pm, is well tolerated and does not cause the patient to be groggy the next day. Amitriptyline in conjunction with lithium hydrochloride or lithium carbonate has been shown by Tyber to improve patients with painful shoulder conditions.[128] If patients are given too much of an antidepressant on their first dosage, it may take them 2 or 3 days to "wake up," and they will never take the medication again. Whereas, if you can slowly and gradually increase the medication to the point where they sleep well, they will be much more tolerant and not risk addiction to diazepam derivative hypnotics or oral narcotic agents.

Table 17–4. Suggested Therapies for the Frozen Shoulder

Analgesics/Hypnotics
Non-steroidal anti-inflammatory drugs
Heat and ultrasound
Physiotherapy and graded exercises
Corticosteroids (oral, intra-articular, intrabursal, local, paired)
Stellate ganglion blockage
Suprascapular nerve block
Calcitonin
Magnetic necklace
Dimethyl sulphoxide (topical)
Arthrographic distension (brisement)
Hydraulic distention (brisement) with and without corticosteroid
Joint irradiation
Manipulation under anesthetic (early/late) with or without injectable or systemic oral corticosteroids

Oral Corticosteroids

Systemic steroids have been recommended for use.[103] Although Binder and associates noted a more rapid initial recovery compared with controls, at a 5-month follow-up there was no distinguishable difference between those who had received steroids and those who had not.[36] In discussing the side effects, especially weight gain in the patient over 40 years old, I find few patients who want to follow this treatment pattern. In some patients who have such severe pain, a short course of oral corticosteroids is warranted. To limit the fluid retention from this medication, hydrochlorothiazide (50 mg) is given on an every other day while on the prednisolone. A summary of results of the use of anti-inflammatory and oral corticosteroids is in Table 17–5.

Table 17–5. Anti-Inflammatory and Oral Corticosteroid Therapy

Study	*No. of Patients*	*Therapy*	*Study Type*	*Outcome*
Blockley et al.[182] (1954)	32	Oral cortisone 2.5 g over 4 weeks and exercise vs. placebo and exercises	Double Blind Placebo Controlled	Improved pain relief and shoulder mobility No improvement in rate of recovery.
Duke et al.[183] (1981)	59	Naproxen vs. Indomethacin	Double Blind	No difference Limited usefulness and gastrointestinal side effects.
Famaey & Ginsberg[184] (1984)	50	Brufen 600 mg. vs. Diclofenac 100 mg. over 2 weeks	Double Blind	Improvement in pain & range of movement. By day 14, 50% good or very good. Equal efficacy. 11 gastrointestinal side effects.
Ward et al.[185] (1986)	26	Diclofenac vs. Paracetamol	Sequential Double Blind	No significant benefit Diclofenac over Paracetamol
Binder et al.[36] (1986)	40	Prednisone 10 mg over 4 weeks, 5 mg × 2 weeks exercise vs. placebo and exercise	Double Blind Placebo Controlled	Reduction in pain No improvemnet in rate of recovery.

Physical Therapy

It is critical that the patient start pendulum exercises early with short periods of exercises, 2 to 3 minutes every 1 to 2 hours having been recommended by Watson-Jones.[129] It must be emphasized on the first visit that no matter what else is done for the shoulder, the exercises are the most important thing for the patient's recovery. The dependent patient must be assured that they can do the exercises on their own better than having someone do the exercises with them. These patients may require more supervision and encouragement but still must be managed with Kessel's philosophy and Cotton's Doctrine, "We cannot cure you. We can show you how to cure yourself."[129,130]

Physical therapy modalities have never been shown to have any benefit on their own.[113] The role of the physical therapist with these patients is instruction and encouragement. My strong feeling is that there is no role for painful passive stretching in the treatment of this condition at any phase, and that this maneuver is not only expensive when applied on a daily basis after ultrasound, infrared, and other modality treatment, but is counterproductive to the goals (i.e., the patient is responsible for his shoulder). The patients frequently experience so much pain between therapy sessions that they cannot do their home exercises gently on their own. I often use the analogy of the piano teacher as the role of the therapist. For some patients who are dependant and not willing to do their exercises on their own, at least they will do them a night or two before they go to therapy so they can at least tell their "teacher" that they have practiced. Rizk et al. found that pulley traction in abduction with TENS was more effective in the short run when compared to Codman's exercise and pulley. However, the patient received a total of 2 hours of traction a day. Physical therapy has been shown to cure or improve, only 50 to 60% of patients after 4 to 5 months[126,131] and 30% of the patients in one study noted an exacerbation of their pain with physiotherapy.[132] I have seen patients with physical therapy bills approaching $10,000 for the treatment of this self-limited condition. No society can afford this.

Stretching Exercises

The regimen and timing of exercises should be taught so that the patient has no excuse not to exercise several times a day. Using a pulley early on the painful stage of adhesive capsulitis is sometimes difficult and as well requires the patient to be at home; however, as their pain settles down, pulley exercises can be instituted for flexion. On the other hand, wall walking exercises both facing the wall (flexion) and standing sideways to it (abduction) can be done anywhere. A tree or truck can be offered as a substitute for the wall when an injured worker who would rather stay home and watch TV rather than stay on the job site in a light duty position states, "I can't do my exercises at work." Stick external rotation exercises and internal rotation passively up the back are reinforced (see Chapter 18). I personally do not recommend abduction exercises at all until full passive external rotation is achieved. Kessel has described exercises in recumbency (Fig. 17–17) and standing (Fig. 17–18), which promote active external rotation in both the adducted and abducted position.[130]

Strengthening Exercises

Murnaghan recommends using the program described by Hughes and Neer for total shoulder arthroplasty.[133,134] Once the pain settles down, an intensive strengthening program with the aim of restoring equal function to both upper extremities is achieved.[33] In my practice, strengthening exercises are not begun until a near full painless range of motion is achieved.

Mobilization Techniques

Many physical therapists recommend scapular mobilization to "teach the patient not to use their scapula as much." Nicholson, in a controlled study, compared patients doing mobilization and found no significant difference in pain scores between two patient groups after 4 weeks of treatment.[135] Therapists need to be reminded that elevating the scapula is the only way the patient *can* elevate the arm during the frozen or adhesive phase.

Intra-Articular Injection

Injection therapy into the inflamed structures around the shoulder is a well-established method for treating many common shoulder problems. A number of injection protocols have been investigated in the treatment of frozen shoulder. In a controlled, blinded multicenter study of 37 patients with frozen shoulder, Richardson found no difference in outcome in regards to pain and range of motion between two groups of patients. One group received both glenohumeral and subacromial prednisolone acetate, 25 mg, on their initial visit and then again 2 weeks later. These patients were compared with controls receiving injections of normal saline. However, it should be noted that when Richardson monitored attempted intra-articular injections by arthrography, he noted an inability of most physicians to successfully enter the glenohumeral joint.[136] Because of the rise in performance of arthroscopy, I do not think this is true of most orthopaedic surgeons. Weiss recommended an arthrogram to better determine the anatomic landmarks to insure glenohumeral injection.[137]

In another study, 55 patients with 60 painful stiff shoulders were treated with paired injections of 20 mg of methylprednisolone acetate into the subacromial bursa weekly, with up to three injections. In this group, in contradistinction to Richardson's patients, 80% of patients had their pain abolished after 2 weeks and 95% were pain-free after 4 weeks. By 8 weeks, 73% achieved 150° of abduction and 53% achieved 45° of external rotation. Only 8% of the patients were considered to be treatment

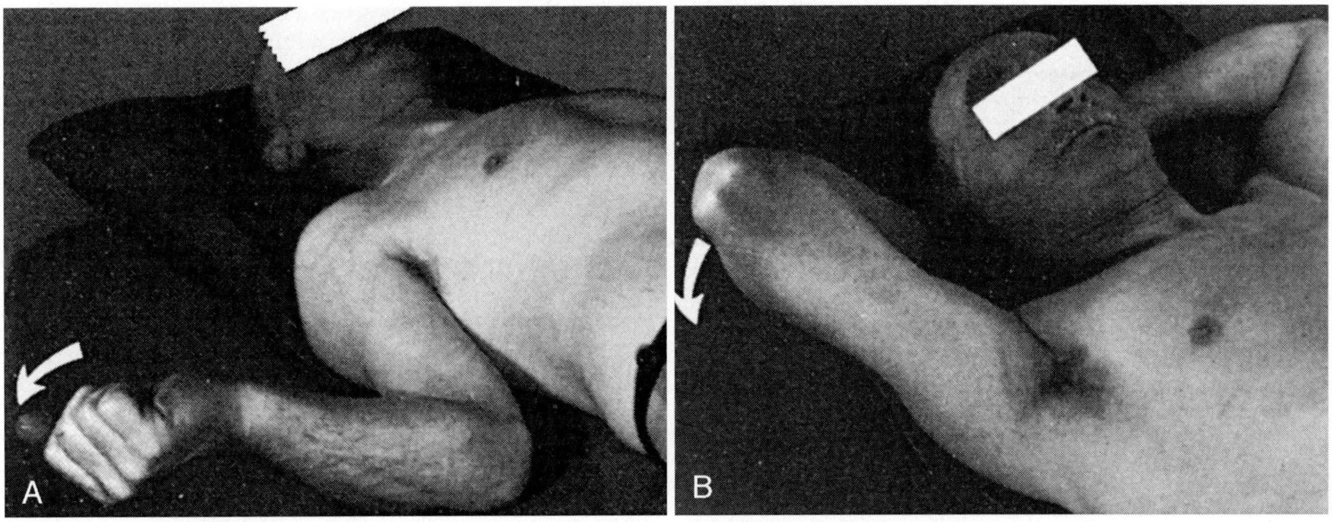

Fig. 17–17. *A and B,* Kessel has recommended exercises in recumbency which promote external rotation in both the adducted and abducted position, as well as standing. Again, these are exercises that can be done anywhere without the use of a therapist. (From Kessel L. Injuries of the shoulder. In: Wilson JN, ed. *Watson-Jones' Fractures and Joint Injuries.* 5th ed. New York: Churchill Livingstone; 1976:522–532.)

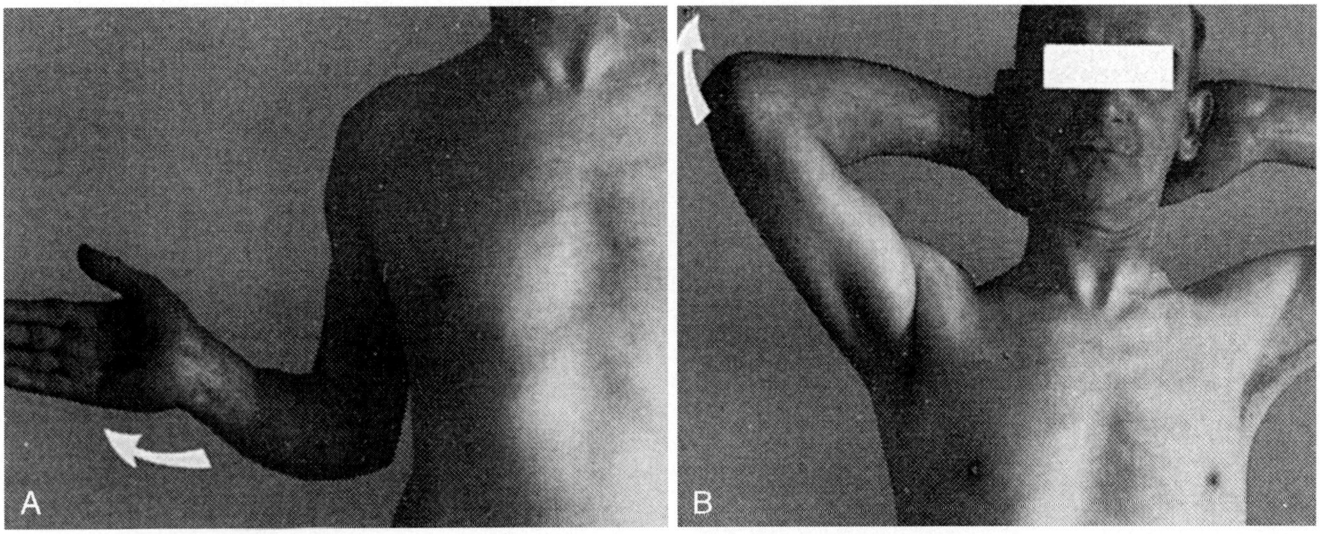

Fig. 17–18. *A,* With the patient standing, the arm is actively externally rotated. *B,* With the patient standing, the arm is placed in a position of abduction/external rotation and active external rotation is encouraged. (*A and B,* From Kessel L. Injuries of the shoulder. In: Wilson JN, ed. *Watson-Jones' Fractures and Joint Injuries.* 5th ed. New York: Churchill Livingstone; 1976: 522–532.)

failures after 8 weeks, because of limited range of motion and continued aching discomfort.[138]

Bulgen et al. found similar results in using 20 mg of methylprednisolone acetate as a paired injection and found no significant difference at 6 month follow-up between a group that was treated with nonsalicylate analgesics, mild sedation, and pendulum exercises.[113] Several studies have reviewed intra-articular injections of corticosteroids.[139–143] Intra-articular injections were shown to be better than trigger-point injections,[142] but not significantly different than stellate ganglion blocks. The use of intra-articular injections alone have some theoretical benefits in the treatment of the patient in the early freezing phase of FSS. Wild et al. combined diagnostic and therapeutic injections in 31 patients using local anesthetic, steroid, and contrast material injected intra-articularly. All patients improved by 8 months, and five rotator cuff tears were identified.[144] On the other hand, the rate of return of shoulder motion was unaffected by intra-articular cortisone according to Quin.[145]

Other Injection Techniques

Murnaghan injected two groups of patients with adhesive capsulitis; injection of the joint capsule with either 25 mg. of hydrocortisone acetate or 2% lidocaine (Xylocaine) was felt to be equally beneficial.[146] Dacre et al. evaluated periarticular triamcinolone, physiotherapy, or both in 62 patients. These investigators found that injection alone was equally beneficial with or without physical therapy and was more cost effective.[147] Rizk et al. studied varying types of injection therapy combined with physical therapy. There was no significant difference in outcome between intrabursal injection and intra-articular injection. In the end result there was no difference between injection of steroid and lidocaine and injection of lidocaine alone.[148]

Steinbroker and Argyros reviewed the results of local injection.[149] Although it is tempting to inject the area of maximum tenderness around the shoulder, my experience has been that this does not commonly relieve the pain or improve motion in patients with FSS, unless they have calcific tendinitis as an intrinsic cause. In fact, frequently these patients have so much "steroid flare" that their motion actually decreases, because they cannot do their exercises because of the severity of the pain. Kraft has recommended trigger-point injections into areas in which light to moderate pressure on specific firm bands of muscle fibers reproduce the patient's pain.[150,151] Intra-articular morphine has been used successfully by Joshi and McCarroll.[152]

Suprascapular Nerve Block

Koppel and Thompson postulated that the suprascapular nerve was the culprit in producing pain in FSS.[153] They injected and later operated on patients with this condition and found a transverse band of compression of the nerve at the level of the transverse ligament. Lee and Khunadorn could not demonstrate slowing of the suprascapular nerve in patients with painful stiff shoulders following hemiplegia.[154] Suprascapular nerve block was used by Wassef for management of frozen shoulder twice weekly, for a total of two to four treatments. This approach proved to be simple, highly successful, and reproducible and is based on the fact that the suprascapular nerve contains a high proportion of sympathetic fibers supplying the shoulder joint.[155]

Calcitonin Injections

In a prospective randomized analysis of 50 cases, a treatment program of early mobilization associated with the administration of subcutaneous calcitonin (Sandoz) for 21 days (100 units). A significant increase in pain control was found as compared to a treatment group in which physical therapy alone was used. There was no significant difference in the speed of recovery between these two groups.[86]

Distention Arthrography or Brisement

The initial description of this maneuver was by Andren and Lundberg in 1965.[121] Subsequently, other investigators have reported on its use.[18,156–160] During this maneuver, increasing volumes of saline are injected, generating intra-articular pressures of 1000 to 1500 mm Hg.[18] Although Reeves noted that the recovery of motion was longer when distention arthrography was compared with manipulation, it clearly has little risk, and my experience, like that of Older,[157] has been that it rather rapidly relieves the patient's pain and makes it much easier for the

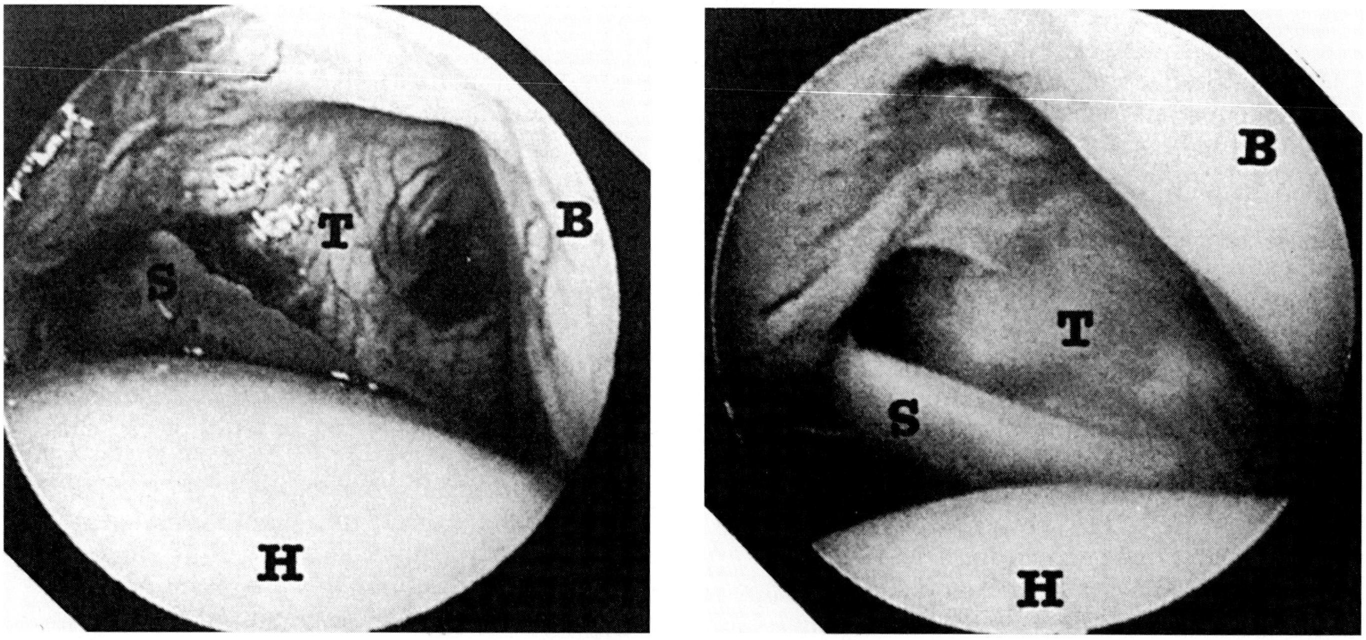

Fig. 17–19. ***A,*** **Hyperemic hypertrophic synovial tissue (T) enveloping the superior margin of the subscapularis tendon (S) and the long head of the biceps tendon (B) at the anterior margin of the glenohumeral joint. (H) humerus.** ***B,*** **Immediately following hydraulic distension of the joint capsule, the hyperemic synovial tissue (T) has receded. The subscapularis (S) and biceps (B) are well defined, demonstrating the intra-articular effect of hydraulic distention. (H) humerus. (From Fareed DO, Gallivan WR. Office management of frozen shoulder syndrome.** ***Clin Orthop.*** **1989;2:177–183.)**

patient to follow their exercise program. Simon reported the technique in patients under a general anesthetic.[110] Fareed and Gallivan treated 20 patients as outpatients under local anesthesia using sequential distention with up to 40 mL of cold saline being instilled in 10 mL increments.[160] The immediate effects of distention have been documented by them at impingement (Fig. 17–19). Jacobs et al. found that combining intra-articular steroids improved the results.[161] It is this technique that I currently employ that is described under the heading in this chapter Author's Preferred Treatment.

Manipulation

The use of manipulation in the treatment of FSS is as controversial as the diagnostic entity itself. Manipulation under anesthesia was first recommended by Duplay.[1–4] Over the years, varying degrees of enthusiasm have existed for this treatment mode. Manipulation under anesthesia, like most of the other treatments described, shortens the frozen phase of the syndrome, although perhaps not affecting the total duration or natural history of it.[19,33,158] McLaughlin pointed out that in addition to the obvious complications of manipulation (i.e., fracture of the humerus, dislocation of the shoulder, and injury to the brachial plexus or it's branches) that in several cases that he opened, the subscapularis tendon was frequently torn from it's insertion. Kessel pointed out that a complication from a manipulation could turn "a nuisance into a disaster." DePalma stated that "manipulation was a dangerous and futile procedure," while Charnley, although not impressed with the technique, considered that the bad reputation of early manipulation is "without foundation."[162] The complication of rapid "refreezing" after performing a manipulation of patients' shoulders who are in the acute or freezing stage of frozen shoulder is well described and controversy also exists on the timing of manipulation, with some investigators finding that the results were better if done within the first 6 months and others being more impressed that waiting a longer period of time for better results.[163] Even in series in which no more aggressive care than analgesics and exercises are employed, manipulation is required in only 25% of patients.[129] Using brisement and an exercise program, I manipulate less than 10% of the patients I see with this condition. If manipulation is to be carried out safely, it must be carried out under a general anesthetic with muscle paralysis and in a setting such as a general hospital in which complications such as fracture, nerve or blood vessel injury, or dislocation can be recognized and treated.

Technique of Manipulation

If one has ruled out old fracture, patients with moderate bone atrophy, and patients who are unable to cooperate with a required post manipulation exercise, and after several months of home exercises, the patient has not improved, then manipulation can be performed. The recommended technique of shoulder manipulation requires a short lever arm (Figs. 17–20 and 17–21); i.e. the surgeon's hands are close to the shoulder to avoid stress (1) across the elbow leading to collateral ligament injuries or (2) across the humerus resulting in spiral fractures

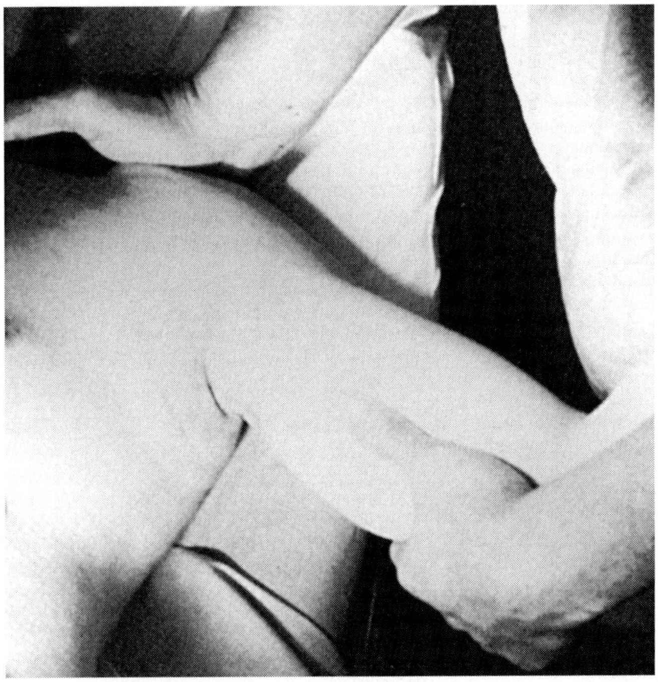

Fig. 17–20. The surgeon's hands are placed close to the shoulder to avoid a spiral fracture of the humerus or ligamentous or bony injury to the elbow during closed manipulation. (From Neviaser TJ. Adhesive capsulitis. *Orthop Clin North Am.* 1987;18:439–443.)

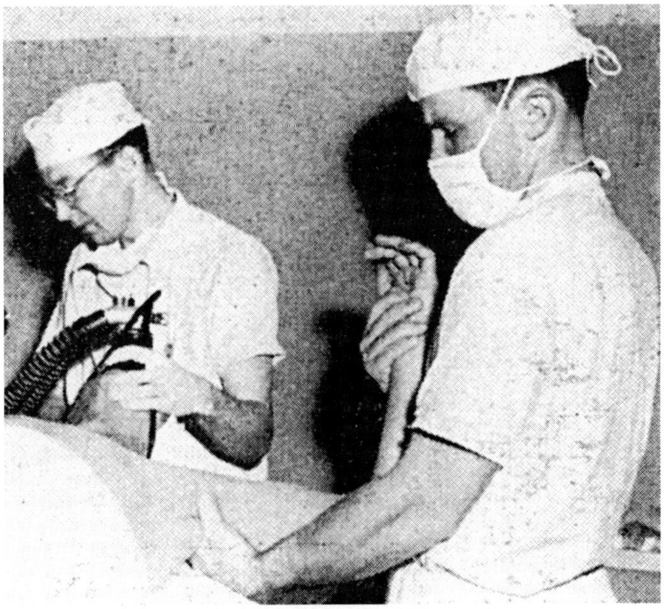

Fig. 17–21. To increase the lever arm, the forearm and humerus can be rotated together, as recommended by Quigley. (From Quigley TB. Checkrein shoulder, a type of frozen shoulder. *N Eng J Med.* 1954; 250:188–192.)

during rotation. Quigley has demonstrated how not to do a shoulder manipulation (Fig. 17–22).[17]

The sequence of events in manipulation varies among investigators. Most investigators prefer to stretch the inferior capsule first, taking care to stabilize the scapula while the arm is abducted. The shoulder can then be moved through internal and external rotation in an effort to obtain the greatest range of motion to the limit of safety. A definite audible and palpable release of resistance that may be experienced on manipulation is thought to be a good prognostic sign.[17,33,73,89,107]

My personal technique is to flex the arm first, the short lever arm technique is used with my hands proximal to the elbow joint. I worry about abducting the arm, which cannot externally rotate, and levering the greater tuberosity against the acromion, which risks a fracture. In my hands, manipulation always follows a diagnostic arthroscopy to rule out an irritative phase and prior to arthroscopy the joint is distended. It seems to me that the palpable release is softer after arthroscopy, perhaps because of the distention or perhaps the hole created in the capsule serves as a stress riser and less force is required to rupture the capsule. Following full flexion, the patient's arm can then be externally rotated at the side, some stress can be gently applied across the elbow after release of the inferior capsule, and then the arm carefully abducted. In a position of 90° of abduction the arm is then internally and externally rotated. I prefer to do manipulations with the patient in the lateral position so that as the final maneuver, the hand can then be brought up the back in extension and internal rotation to a point equal to the opposite side. Leffert has warned against internal rotation during the manipulation, fearing rupture of the teres minor and infraspinatus. However, I have been unable to document a single case in which this has been reported. Using this technique of premanipulation brisement or arthroscopy, 30 shoulders have been manipulated without fracture.

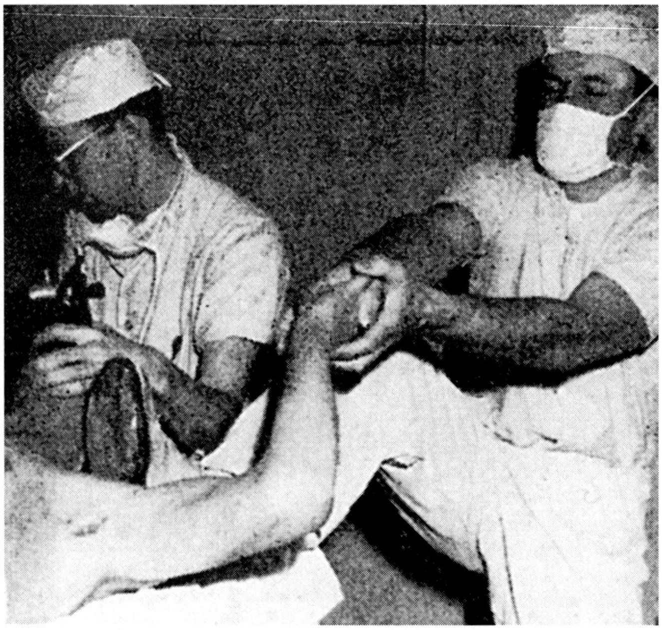

Fig. 17–22. **Quigley also illustrated the absolute wrong way to manipulate the shoulder. (From Quigley TB. Checkrein shoulder, a type of frozen shoulder. *N Eng J Med.* 1954;250:188–192.)**

Postmanipulation care is extremely important. Neviaser described a postmanipulation treatment plan that is cost-prohibitive in this day and age: 3 to 5 days in the hospital after surgery with the arm tied to the bed, in a position of abduction and external rotation, with in-hospital therapy for 5 days. He recommended abduction splinting for 3 weeks postsurgery.[120] It is critical that the patient start exercising their shoulder immediately after manipulation. If this can only be accomplished with parenteral analgesia, then the patient will need to remain hospitalized. However, most patients can go home after a few hours, if their pain is controlled and they understand the importance of and how to do their exercises.

The reports of the results of shoulder manipulation vary, as do the reports of other treatments for this condition, with 26 to 81% of patients significantly improved.[18,33,73,89,119,159] No well-controlled studies substantiate any claims of superiority for this method of treatment over the others previously described.

Although the relationship of duration of symptoms to outcome from manipulation is not reported in most series,[119,159,164] Kessel and colleagues felt that patients with prior symptoms lasting more than 6 months had a much more dramatic response to manipulation than those patients whose symptoms were of less than 6 months duration.[107]

Manipulation and Corticosteroids

Several investigators have reported manipulation in conjunction with either steroid injection or systemic steroids. These investigators report improvement in their patients as well, but again these are not compared to manipulation alone.[17,20,119,142,159,164,165] Parker et al., using Haggart's Classification, (Table 17–6), found excellent results in 68%, good results in 5%, fair results in 2%, and poor results in 0% of the 22 patients following manipulation with corticosteroid injections. Three recurrences, two that were diabetic patients and one that was transient posterior deltoid paralysis, occurred as complications.[158,166,167] Loyd and Loyd and most recently Ekelund and Rydell have used combination treatment for adhesive capsulitis including distention arthrography, intraarticular anesthetic, and steroid combined with manipulation.[168,169] Combination treatment is felt by these in-

Table 17–6. Haggart's Classification for Results From Treatment of FSS[158]

Excellent	Full range of motion with no pain
Good	Occasional discomfort but full range of motion
Fair	Recurrent mild shoulder discomfort with decreased range of motion but able to function
Poor	Decreased range of motion, constant pain, and unable to resume activity

vestigators to be safe and cost-effective and yields immediate results.

Because of the resulting side effects, the use of systemic steroids remains controversial. Bayley believed that steroids did increase the rate of recovery of flexion and external rotation. Angiolini and colleagues felt that systemic steroids were without benefit.[170] I use arthroscopy to determine whether I will use systemic steroids. I almost always use intra-articular injectable steroids at the time of brisement, prior to the closed manipulation. If, on arthroscopy, the capsule is quite erythematous and synovitis is present, IV Decadron is given in the operating room. A short tapering dose of Decadron is then sent home with the patient.

Manipulation Under Local Anesthesia

Manipulation of the shoulder with local anesthesia has been advocated by Galula et al.,[171] Loyd and Loyd, and Wiser; however, when compared to other techniques of manipulation, the results are not as good.[168,172] There was a strong inverse correlation between the degree of disability at the time of the treatment and the outcome from this treatment method.

ARTHROSCOPY AS A TREATMENT MODALITY

Arthroscopic treatment of adhesive capsulitis has become a topic of several recent reports. The main advantage of arthroscopic examination, as previously described as a staging aid as well as a diagnostic tool, especially of unsuspected intra-articular pathology. It does allow joint distention, however, debridement of capsular adhesions and release of a tight contracted capsule operatively remains controversial. Ha'eri and Maitland reviewed the results in patients treated arthroscopically for adhesive capsulitis at an average of 8 months after onset of shoulder pain and stiffness. They were able to enter the joint in all patients but had some difficulty visualizing the intra-articular structures in two cases.[173] In a 10-year review, Ogilvie-Harris and Wiley found that arthroscopy was useful in treating frozen shoulder as well as early osteoarthritis and isolated tears of the labrum and biceps. In the early part of their series, distention via the arthroscope followed by manipulation was used. Later, a "freeing up" procedure with a blunt instrument or in some cases, a progressive incision of the anterior capsule was performed to improve movement in a controlled manner.[174] Thirty-seven patients were reviewed by Wiley.[126] A smaller 3.8-mm arthroscope was occasionally required, because it was impossible to introduce a standard arthroscope into the stiff painful shoulder. Using arthroscopic distention combined with manipulation, all 37 patients eventually recovered, with 20 patients recovering as early as 3 months later and 17 patients requiring a recovery time from 6 months to 2 years. No complications were noted. McGraw and Turba retrospectively reviewed 15 patients treated with arthroscopy combined with manipulation under general anesthesia. Joint distention combined with debridement of capsular adhesions yielded full range of motion and pain relief in all 15 patients in their series from 3 to 6 months postoperatively.[175] In a prospective study, Hsu and Chan found that arthroscopic distention, when compared with manipulation and physical therapy, provided comparable results with respect to pain relief, restoration of motion, and final outcome. Physical therapy alone was significantly less effective. The investigators felt that arthroscopy was more controlled and allowed diagnoses of unsuspected rotator cuff tears in 18% of their patients.[176]

OPEN SURGICAL RELEASE

In patients (i.e., those at risk to develop a fracture with closed manipulation) with marked osteopenia or those with post total shoulder FSS in which the implant may serve as a stress riser, open surgical release and manipulation under direct observation should be considered. McLaughlin recommended open surgical release with excision of the biceps, release of the subscapularis tendon, and release of joint adhesions by blunt dissection.[177] Neviaser recommended open release of the inferior capsule as well (Fig. 17–23). Later, he modified his approach, sparing the biceps and subscapularis (Fig. 17–24). The shoulder could then be manipulated more safely and avoid uncontrolled injury to the bony and ten-

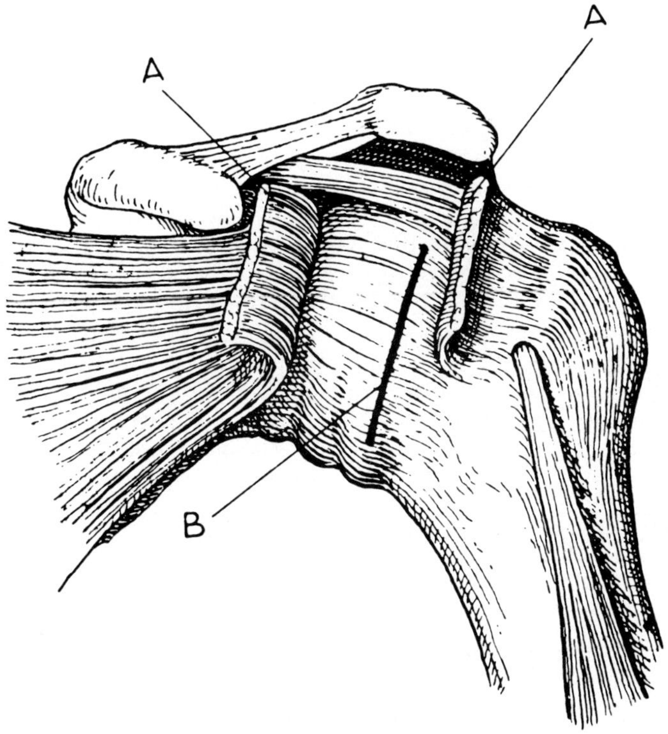

Fig. 17–23. Neviaser's operation for capsular release involved cutting down the subscapularis and cutting the capsule. This procedure evolved into Figure 24, in which only the capsule was cut and the subscapularis preserved. (From Neviaser JS. Adhesive capsulitis of the shoulder. A study of the pathological findings in periarthritis of the shoulder. *J Bone Joint Surg.* 1945;27:211–222.)

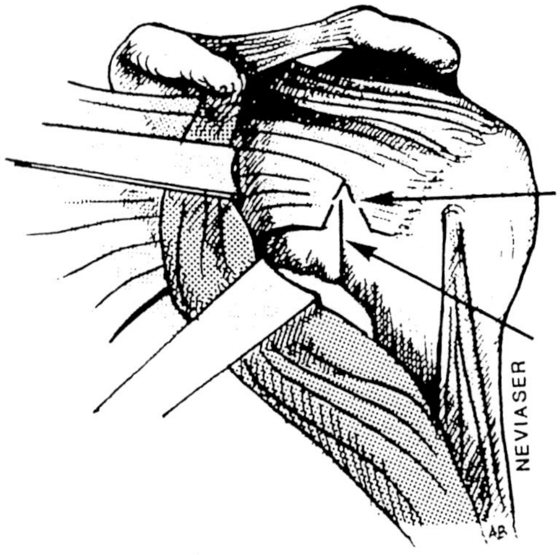

Fig. 17–24. The capsule was cut and the subscapularis preserved. (From Neviaser RJ, Neviaser TJ. The frozen shoulder. Diagnosis and management. *Clin* Orthop. 1987;223:59–64.)

dinous anatomy. Leffert recommends releasing only those structures demonstrable at open operation through a deltopectoral approach to be responsible for the restricted motion.[163] Kieras and Matsen used a deltopectoral approach as well, but they lengthened the subscapularis and incised the anterior inferior joint capsule in conjunction with lysis of subdeltoid adhesions and coracohumeral ligament excision.[178]

Since the days of Codman, an obliterative type of subacromial bursitis with adhesions in the bursa have been described in patients with adhesive capsulitis. Because many of the patients who develop this entity as a secondary condition have underlying partial-thickness cuff tears and AC joint arthritis, and because the coracohumeral ligament is the primary block to external rotation in these patients; many investigators prefer a superior open technique, combined with coracohumeral ligament release, which allows release of the sometimes dense subacromial bursal adhesions.[98,179,180] Ozaki followed 16 patients from 3 to 9.5 years following open coracohumeral ligament release, release of bursal adhesions, and manipulation. A full range of motion was achieved within 3 months and was retained in all but one patient.[98]

Technique of Open Superior Release

A 5- to 6-cm skin incision can be made in Langer's Lines and a delto-trapezial fascial split is used. An acromioplasty is performed and the coracoacromial ligament excised. A thorough subacromial bursectomy is performed. This includes a sweeping motion of the index finger posteriorly along the posterolateral corner of the acromion, removing all bursal adhesions, in the infraspinatus-teres minor area. The coracohumeral ligament is identified as it runs from the base of the coracoid to the lesser and greater tuberosities (Fig. 17–25). The arm is then externally rotated to it's maximum extent. The coracohumeral ligament will become quite prominent, often in neutral external rotation or less. The coracohumeral ligament is then divided at the base of the coracoid. Once the adhesions between the cuff and acromion are released and the coracohumeral ligaments are released, the humeral head can easily be pulled away from the acromion and coracoid. A finger can be placed between the coracoid and the humerus, whereas previously it could not. Following return of external rotation, the shoulder can then be safely manipulated into abduction tearing the inferior capsule. If, during this phase, the subscapularis appears to be at risk of rupturing, then a controlled subscapularis Z-lengthening can be performed. However, after release of the coracohumeral ligament, there is much less tension on the subscapularis tendon during the external rotation phase of manipulation and I have not found this to be necessary.

TREATMENT OF PATIENTS WITH ADHESIVE CAPSULITIS—AUTHOR'S PREFERRED TREATMENT

Management of the patient with adhesive capsulitis should be (1) cost-effective, (2) stage dependent, and (3) individualized to the patient's own needs. It is difficult, sometimes, for the doctor and patient to remember that this is, in most patients, a self-limited condition, which although the patient may have some persistent mild stiffness and discomfort in their shoulder, is not life-threatening or severely disabling. If, on the first or second office visit after a diagnostic work-up, the patient is given a thorough explanation of the condition and treatment options, most will not go from doctor to doctor or shop for a quick cure from chiropractors, laser surgery, or acupuncturists.

In patients who present to my office with atraumatic subacute shoulder pain, stiffness, and negative plain film radiology, a subacromial injection of lidocaine is only performed to determine which component of the pain is emanating from isolated subacromial pathology. If the patient has full resolution of their symptoms with subacromial injection and full return of their range of motion, then the diagnosis of FSS is ruled out at least at this time. The patient who may be predisposed, i.e. the 40- to 60-year-old female patient, should be warned that she may progress to FSS. When subacromial injection of lidocaine does not result in rapid return of a patient's range of motion, I am much more cautious and I do not inject corticosteroid into the subacromial bursa. I have seen numerous patients over the years who have had subacromial injections in a doctor's office in the early freezing stage, only to progress farther into the freezing phase of FSS. Because the injection is temporally associated with an increase in pain and sometimes by a rapid loss of motion, frequently patients blame the injection and the doctor that gave it to them for the worsening of their condition.

In patients in whom subacromial injections do not give significant relief, a glenohumeral joint diagnostic injection is then performed. The landmarks for this injection

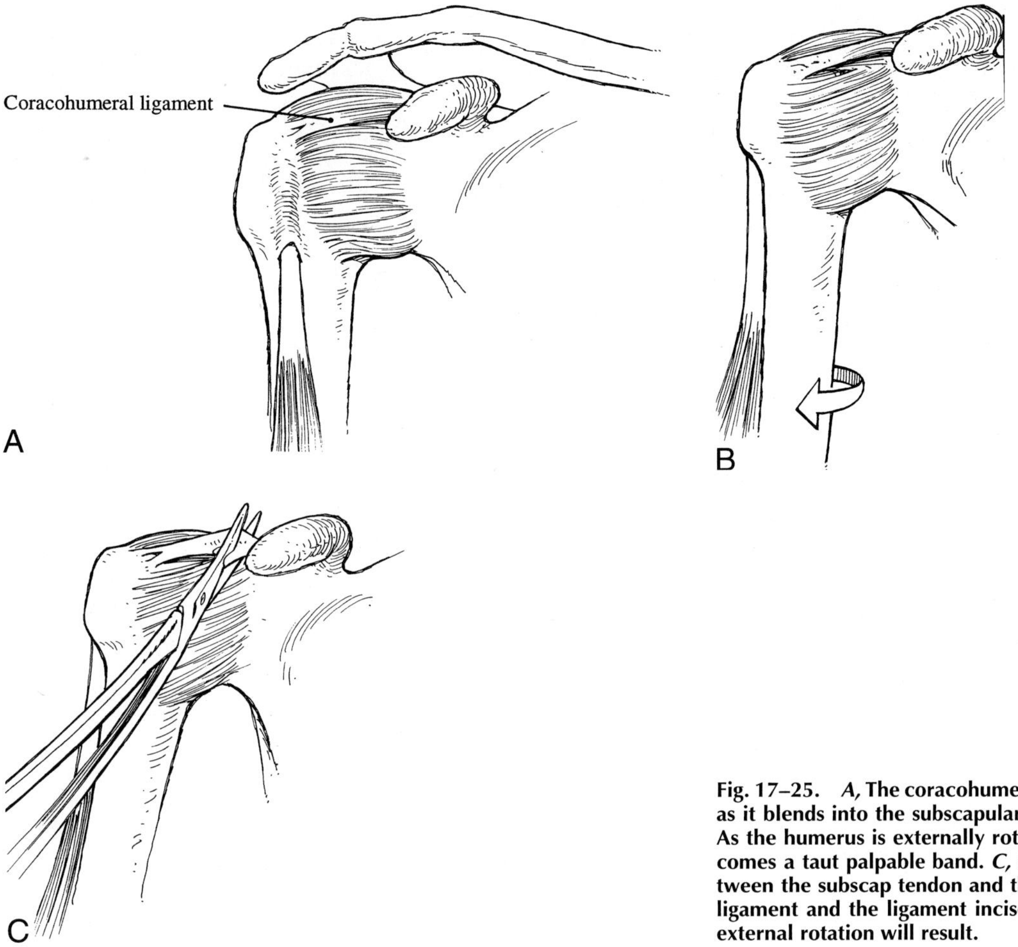

Fig. 17–25. ***A,*** **The coracohumeral ligament is in neutral hard to define as it blends into the subscapularis and supraspinatus tendon edges.** ***B,*** **As the humerus is externally rotated, the coracohumeral ligament becomes a taut palpable band.** ***C,*** **Scissors are placed in the interval between the subscap tendon and the leading edge of the coracohumeral ligament and the ligament incised. Frequently a dramatic increase in external rotation will result.**

are the same as for arthroscopy of the glenohumeral joint (i.e., 2 cm inferior to the posterolateral corner of the acromion and 1 cm medial). A skin wheal is raised with a 0.25-gauge needle and then lidocaine is *slowly* injected, and the 0.25-gauge needle advanced in the direction of the coracoid process until the sudden loss of resistance indicates entry into the glenohumeral joint. In larger patients, a spinal needle is used to anesthetize the posterior capsule and glenohumeral joint.

Lidocaine is slowly injected into the glenohumeral joint once the pressure is released from the syringe. If the lidocaine is injected slowly, the joint can be anesthetized prior to developing the severe intra-articular pressure that can occur in patients with adhesive capsulitis in a short period of time. Should backflow occur with a small volume, (i.e., 5 to 6 mL) then I feel confident that the patient has FSS. This injection does not, however, rule out a remote cause for the syndrome. Once the joint is thoroughly anesthetized with lidocaine, a solution of 7 mL of bupivacaine hydrochloride (Marcaine) with 1 mL of 6 mg per mL. Betamethasone (Celestone) is then instilled. One or 2 minutes are then allowed to pass. Now there is approximately 10 to 12 mL of fluid in the joint. During this procedure, if the pain becomes intolerable, it is important for the surgeon to simply release the syringe, thus lowering the pressure within the joint.

Following the bupivacaine hydrochloride with betamethasone, a 20-mL syringe of saline is connected to the 0.20-gauge spinal needle. Using the hydraulic distention method of Lundberg, we gradually slowly distend the joint capsule to the point of either rupture or patient intolerance. In general, the slow gradual application of pressure with intermittent removal of pressure can result in the patient eventually receiving a full 35 to 40 mL of volume into their glenohumeral joint. A palpable, visible, and sometimes audible rupture frequently occurs in the anterior aspect of the shoulder, in the region of the subscapularis recess or rotator interval. Then the patient is instructed in pendulum exercises. The patient is re-examined approximately 15 minutes after the procedure. Nearly total pain relief with improved but not complete return of motion is the rule after office brisement.

Typically, after the brisement procedure, the patient can at least sleep at night and do their exercises effectively on their own. Furthermore, the patient rapidly loses the hopelessness with which some present. Rest at night is facilitated with low doses of antidepressant medication, doxepin hydrochloride (Sinequan), or diphenhydramine hydrochloride. The chronicity of the problem and the sometimes dependent personality seen in this disorder makes me cautious in recommending diazepam derived sleep medications for fear of habituation. A

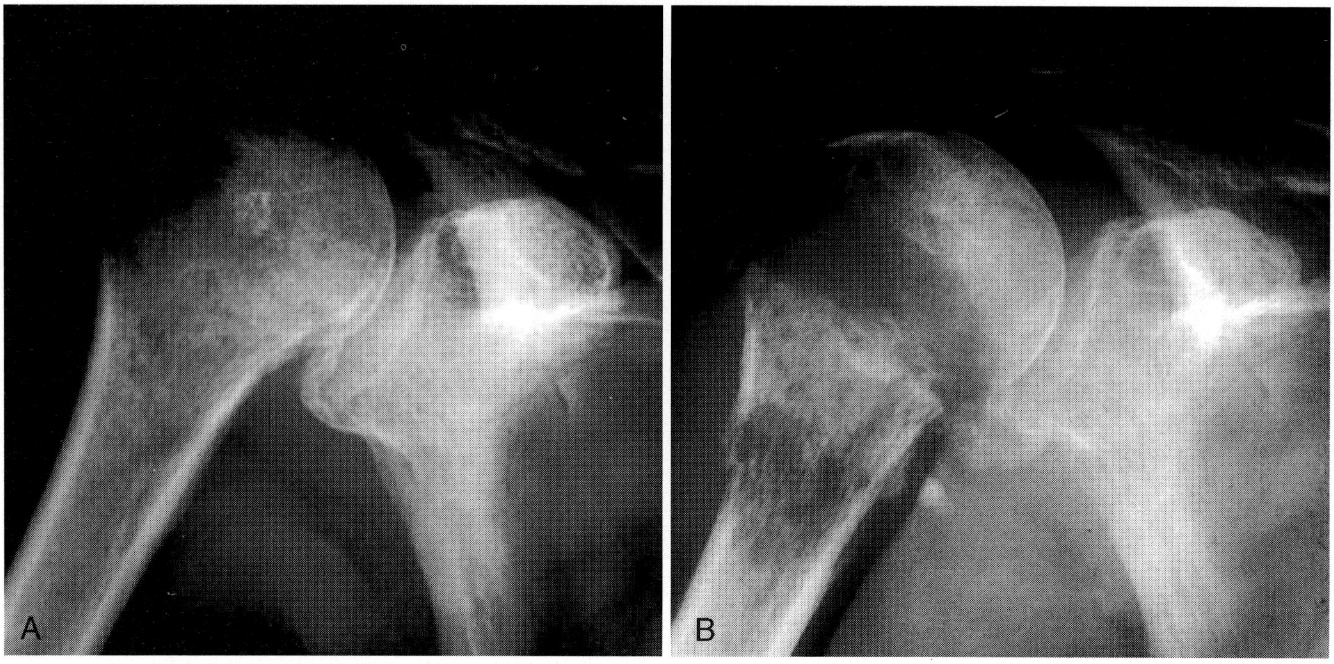

Fig. 17–26. ***A,*** **Radiograph of patient who responded temporarily to corticosteroid injections and was given the diagnosis "idiopathic" adhesive capsulitis.** ***B,*** **Radiograph taken 2 months later of the same patient when she presented with increasing pain. Diagnosis: malignant fibrous histiocytoma.**

methylprednisolone (Medrol) Dosepak, as well as adequate analgesia for 72 hours, is also prescibed. The patients are instructed in pendulum, pulley, internal rotation, and external rotation exercises, and they are not sent for formal physical therapy unless they fail to grasp the exercises.

Patients are then seen again 6 weeks following their initial evaluation. Seldom is a second brisement procedure required, although occasionally if patients continue to have pain at the end range of motion consistent with a persistent subacromial process, a subacromial injection can be performed at this time. Patients at this time are encouraged to continue their exercises and are seen again 6 weeks later. As long as the patients continue to make progress, even if it is slow, surgery is not recommended. Patients who make absolutely no progress and in whom diagnostic work-up has failed to reveal any intrinsic cause of a frozen shoulder syndrome, repeat brisement in conjunction with diagnostic and operative arthroscopy followed by manipulation under general anesthetic is performed. In patients with an intrinsic cause for their FSS (such as rotator cuff tendinopathy, impingement syndrome, or AC joint arthritis) an open acromioplasty, CA ligament release, AC joint excision, and coracohumeral ligament release is performed prior to the manipulation. The manipulation is then performed under direct visualization. In failed acromioplasies, an open release combined with repeat acromioplasty, release of the oftentimes dense subacromial scar, AC joint excision, coracohumeral ligament excision, and manipulation are performed. Subscapularis Z-lengthening has not been required in any of my patients except those with painful stiff shoulders secondary to hemiplegia or with heterotopic ossification from head injury.

SUMMARY

What emerges from the literature is the fact that there are a group of patients, some of whom are hard to define, who possess certain medical, orthopedic, or psychosocial factors (either alone or in combination) that produce a syndrome, the sequelae of which we refer to as FSS. The presence of these factors should alert the physician that he is dealing with a patient who is at risk of developing FSS. At some point in the future, more exacting diagnostic groupings based on the histopathology may aid in treatment.

Whether the pathogenesis involves adhesion of the capsular surfaces or whether fibroblastic proliferation secondary to cytokine production mediates a capsular contracture response, the one single factor that the physician can impact most at this time is the factor of the period of immobility. Binder and colleagues found that half of their patients had received no advice whatsoever about their painful shoulder from their primary care physician. Only 25% of those receiving advice were told to exercise their shoulders, whereas the remaining 75% were told to rest. The importance of not over-immobilizing a minor shoulder injury will need to be emphasized to the primary care physicians who will serve as the "gate keepers" in our new health care systems. Careful identification of and explanation to the patient at risk for developing this condition will hopefully prevent its full blown manifestation. The cost-effectiveness of an ounce of prevention will well be worth a pound of cure for this condition.

Although some of these patients seem neurotic and depressed, many of these patients are just perfectionistic and do not want to do the wrong thing, and because their shoulder hurts when they move it, they just simply do not move it if they are not given instructions to do so. After several months of troubled sleep, these patients are emotionally labile; but like most patients, if treated kindly, they are seldom uncooperative. Reassurance, intra-articular brisement, and a "tincture of time" is all that is required for most to recover. Finally, the importance of a thorough diagnostic workup to avoid confusing a self-limited process with a self-eliminating processes warrants re-emphasis (Fig. 17–26).

REFERENCES

1. Duplay S. *Arch Gen Med.* 1872;2:513–542.
2. Duplay S, Reclus P. *Traite de Chirurgie.* Paris: G. Masson; 1880–1882; 1:825.
3. Duplay S. De la periarthrite scapulo-humerale. *Rev Prat Trav Med.* 1896;53:226–227.
4. Duplay S. On scapulo-humeral periarthritis. (Paris Clinical Lectures.) *Med Presse.* 1900;69:571–573.
5. Putnam JJ. The treatment of a form of painful periarthritis of the shoulder. *Bost Med Surg J.* 1882;107:536.
6. Codman EA. *The Shoulder.* Malabar, FL: RE Kreiger; 1984.
7. Neviaser JS. Adhesive capsulitis of the shoulder. A study of the pathological findings in periarthritis of the shoulder. *J Bone Joint Surg.* 1945;27:211–222.
8. Neviaser JS. Adhesive capsulitis of the shoulder. *AAOS Inst Course Lect.* 1949;6:281–291.
9. Neviaser JS. Arthrography of the shoulder joint. *J Bone Joint* 1962; 44:1321–1330.
10. Neviaser JS. *Arthrography of the Shoulder.* Springfield, IL: Charles C. Thomas; 1975.
11. Neviaser JS. Adhesive capsulitis and the stiff and painful shoulder. *Orthop Clin North Am.* 1980;11:327.
12. Moseley HF. *Shoulder Lesions.* Springfield, IL: Charles C. Thomas; 1945:66.
13. Pasteur F. Les algies de lepaule et la physiotherapie de la teno-bursites bicipitale. *J Radiol Electrol.* 1932;16:419.
14. Lippmann RK. Frozen shoulder, periarthritis, bicipital tenosynovitis. *Arch Surg.* 1943;47:3.
15. DePalma AF. Loss of scapulohumeral motion (frozen shoulder). *Ann Surg.* 1952;135:193.
16. Steinbrocker O. Shoulder-hand syndrome. *Am J Med.* 1947; 3: 402–407.
17. Quigley TB. Checkrein shoulder, a type of frozen shoulder. *N Eng J Med.* 1954;250:188–192.
18. Reeves B. Arthrographic changes in frozen and post traumatic stiff shoulders. *Proc R Soc Med.* 1966;59:827–830.
19. Lundberg BJ. The frozen shoulder. *Acta Orthop Scand.* 1969;119:1–59.
20. Kay N. The clinical diagnosis and management of frozen shoulders. *Practitioner* 1981;25:164–172.
21. Withers RJW. The painful shoulder: Review of one hundred personal cases with remarks on the pathology. *J Bone Joint Surg Am.* 1949;31:414–417.
22. Neviaser RJ. Painful conditions affecting the shoulder. *Clin Orthop.* 1983;173:63–69.
23. Rowe CR, Leffert RD. Idiopathic chronic adhesive capsulitis ("frozen shoulder"). In: Rowe CR, ed. *The Shoulder.* New York: Churchill Livingstone; 1988:155–163.
24. De Seze S, Ryckevaert A, Welfling J, et al. Les lesions anatomiques de l'epaules bloquee. *Rev Rheum.* 1960;27:323–327.
25. De Seze S, Ryckevaert A, Welfling J, et al. L'epaule bloquee et ses lesions. *Rev Rheum.* 1963;30:306–319.
26. Painter CF. Subdeltoid bursitis. *J Med Surg.* 1907;156:345–349.
27. Mumford EB, Martin FJ. Calcified deposits in subdeltoid bursitis. *J Am Med Assoc.* 1931;97:690–694.
28. Baer WS. The operative treatment of subdeltoid bursitis. *Bull Johns Hopkins Hosp.* 1907;18:282–284, 1907.
29. Riedel R. Die versteifung des schultergelenkes durch hangenlassen des armes. *Mnchen Med Wschr.* 1916;63:1397.
30. Dickson JA, Crosby EH. Periarthritis of the shoulder: An analysis of two hundred cases. *J Am Med Assoc.* 1932;99: 2252–2257.
31. McLaughlin HL. On the frozen shoulder. *Bull Hosp Jt Dis.* 1951; 12:383–393.
32. Coventry MB. Problem of the painful shoulder. *J Am Med Assoc.* 1953;151:177–185.
33. Harmon PH. Methods and results in the treatment of 2580 painful shoulders. *Am J Surg.* 1958;95:527–544.
34. Johnston JTH. Frozen shoulder in patients with pulmonary tuberculosis. *J Bone Joint Surg Am.* 1959;41:877–882.
35. Bruckner FE, Nye CJS. A prospective study of adhesive capsulitis of the shoulder in a high risk population. *Q J Med.* 1981;198:191–204.
36. Binder A, Hazleman BL, Parr G, Roberts S. A controlled study of oral prednisolone in frozen shoulder. *Br J Rheum.* 1986; 25:288–292.
37. Lorentz TH, Musser MJ. Life stress emotions and painful stiff shoulders. *Ann Intern Med.* 1952;37:1232–1337.
38. Wright V, Haq AM. Periarthritis of the shoulder I: Aetiological considerations with particular reference to personality factors. *Ann Rheum Dis.* 1976;35:213–219.
39. Fleming A, Dodman S, Beer TC, Crown S. Personality in frozen shoulder. *Ann Rheum Dis.* 1976;35:456–457.
40. Bridgman JF. Periarthritis of the shoulder and diabetes mellitus. *Ann Rheum Dis.* 1972;31:69–71.
41. Lequesne M, Dang N, Bensasson M, Mery C. Increased association of diabetes mellitus with capsulitis of the shoulder and shoulder-hand syndrome. *Scan J Rheum.* 1977;6:53–56.
42. Pal B, Anderson J, Dick WC, Griffiths ID. Limitation of joint mobility and shoulder capsulitis in insulin and non-insulin dependent diabetes mellitus. *Br J Rheum.* 1986;25:147–151.
43. Sattar MA, Luqman WA. Periarthritis: Another duration-related complication of diabetes mellitus. *Diabetes Care.* 1985;8:507–510.
44. Fisher L, Kurtz A, Shipley M. Association between cheiroarthropathy and frozen shoulder in patients with insulin dependent diabetes mellitus. *Br J Rheum.* 1986;25:141–146.
45. Moren-Hybbinette I, Moritz U, Schersten B. The clinical picture of the painful diabetic shoulder: Natural history, social consequences and analysis of concomitant hand syndrome. *Acta Med Scand.* 1987;2:73–82.
46. Meulengracht E, Schwartz M. Course and prognosis of periarthritis humeroscapularis. *Acta Med Scand.* 1952;143: 350–360.
47. Wohlgethan JR. Frozen shoulder in hyperthyroidism. *Arthritis Rheum.* 1987;30:936–939.
48. Oldham BE. Periarthritis of the shoulder associated with thyrotoxicosis. *N Z Med J.* 1959;29:766–770.
49. Bland J, Frymoyer J, Newberg AH, Reeves R. Rheumatic syndromes. *Endocrine Dis.* 1979;9:23–65.
50. Duncan WS. The relationship of hyperthyroidism to joint conditions. *J Am Med Assoc.* 1928;91:1779–1782.
51. Skillern PG. *The association of periarthritis of the shoulder with hyperthyroidism.* Annual Meeting of the American Goiter Association. St. Louis, MO. May 1–3, 1952.
52. Chapman EM, Maloof F. Bizarre clinical manifestations of hyperthyroidism. *N Engl J Med.* 1946;254:1–5.
53. Weiss JJ, Thompson GR, Woodbury D. Hyperthyroidism presenting as acute shoulder pain. *Mich Med.* 1973;72:771–774.
54. Bowman CA, Jeffcoate WJ, Patrick M, Doherty M. Bilateral adhesive capsulitis, oligoarthritis and proximal myopathy as presentation of hypothyroidism. *Br J Rheum.* 1988;27:62–64.
55. Swanson JW, Kelly JT, McConahey WM. Neurologic aspects of thyroid dysfunction. *Mayo Clin Proc.* 1984;56:504–512.
56. Ingbar SH. The thyroid gland. In: Wilson JD, Foster DW, eds. *Wil-*

liams Textbook of Endocrinology. 7th Ed. Philadelphia: WB Saunders; 1985:682–815.
57. Choy EH, Corkill M, Gibson T. Isolated ACTH deficiency presenting with bilateral frozen shoulder. *Br J Rheumatol.* 1991;30:226–227.
58. Calbarese LH, White CS. Musculoskeletal manifestations of Addison's disease. *Arthritis Rheum.* 1979;22:558.
59. Pancoast HK. Superior pulmonary sulcus tumor. *J Am Med Assoc.* 1932;99:1391–1396.
60. Hass LL, Harvey RA, Melchor CF. Radiation management of apical lung tumors. *J Thor Surg.* 1957;33:496–525.
61. Herbut PA, Watson JS. Tumor of the thoracic inlet producing the Pancoast Syndrome. *Arch Path.* 1946;42:88–103.
62. Groves LK. Superior pulmonary sulcus tumor or Pancoast Syndrome. Report of twelve patients treated with surgery and radiation. *Cleve Clin Q.* 1962;29:135–143.
63. Hall WC. The origin of tumors occurring in the apex of the lung. *AJR.* 1940;44:838–847.
64. Shaw RR, Paulson DL, Kee JL. Treatment of the superior sulcus tumor by irradiation followed by resection. *Ann Surg.* 1961;154:29–40.
65. Dee PE, Sauth RG, Gullickson MJ, Ballinger CS. The orthopaedist and apical lung carcinoma. *J Bone Joint Surg. Am.* 1960;42:605–608.
66. Onuigbo WIB. Lung cancer and shoulder pain. *Dis Chest.* 1964; 45:488–491.
67. DeMaziere A, Wiley AM. Primary chest wall tumor appearing as frozen shoulder. *J Rheumatol.* 1991;18:911–9114.
68. Engleman RM. Shoulder pain as a presenting complaint in upper lobe bronchogenic carcinoma: Report of 21 cases. *Conn Med.* 1966; 30:273–276.
69. Saha ND. Painful shoulder in patients with chronic bronchitis and emphysema. *Am Rev Respir Dis.* 1966;94:455–456.
70. Askey JM. The syndrome of painful disability of the shoulder and hand complicating coronary occlusion. *Am Heart J.* 1961;22:1–12.
71. Ernstene AC, Kinell J. Pain in the shoulder as a sequel to myocardial infarction. *Arch Intern Med.* 1940;66:800–806.
72. Wright V, Haq AM: Periarthritis of the shoulder II: Radiological features. *Ann Rheum Dis.* 1976;35:220–226.
73. Quigley TB. Indications for manipulation and corticosteroids in the treatment of stiff shoulders. *Surg Clin North Am.* 1969;43:1715, 1720.
74. Kamieth H. Radiography of the cervical spine in shoulder periarthritis. *Z Orthop.* 1965;100:162–174.
75. Cinquegrana O. Chronic cervical radiculitis and its relationship to chronic bursitis. *Am J Phys Med.* 1968;47:23–30.
76. Kingsley G, Gibson T. Frozen shoulder—a comparative clinical and radiographic study. *Br J Rheum.* 1986;25:58.
77. Middleditch A, Jarman P. An investigation of frozen shoulder using thermography. *Physiotherapy.* 1984;70:433–439.
78. Hargreaves C, Cooper C, Kidd BL, Ellis R, Cawley M. Frozen shoulder and cervical spine disease. *Br J Rheum.* 1989;28:78–79.
79. Parsonage MJ, Turner JWA. Neuralgia amyotrophy. *Lancet.* 1948; 1:973.
80. Mumenthaler M, Narakas A, Gilliott RW. Brachial plexus disorders. In: Dyck PJ, Thomas PK, Griffin JW, Low PA, Poduslo JF, eds. *Peripheral Neuropathy.* Philadelphia: WB Saunders; 1984;1383–1424.
81. Patten C, Hillel A. The 11th nerve syndrome. Accessory nerve palsy or adhesive capsulitis? *Arch Otolaryngol Head Neck Surg.* 1993; 119:215–220.
82. Riley D, Lang AE, Blair RDG, Birnbaum A, Reid B. Frozen shoulder and other shoulder disturbances in Parkinson's disease. *J Neuro Neurosurg Psych.* 1989;52:63–66.
83. Rizk T, Christopher RP, Pinals RS, Salazar JE, Higgins C. Arthrographic studies in painful hemiplegic shoulders. *Arch Phys Med Rehabil.* 1984;65:254–256.
84. Yoshida N, Kikuchi S, Sagiura Y. *Sympathetic and sensory innervation of the shoulder joint.* Presented at Fifth International Conference on Surgery of the Shoulder, Paris, July 14, 1992.
85. Kozin F. Painful shoulder and the reflex sympathetic dystrophy syndrome. In: McCarty DJ, ed. *Arthritis and Allied Conditions.* 9th ed. Philadelphia: Lea & Febiger; 1979:1091–1120.
86. Waldburger M, Meier JL, Gobelet C. The frozen shoulder: Diagnosis and treatment. *Clin Rheum.* 1992;11:364–368.
87. Jeracitano D, Cooper RG, Lyon LJ, Jayson MIV. Abnormal temperature control suggesting sympathetic dysfunction in the shoulder skin of patients with frozen shoulder. *Br J Rheum.* 1992:31:539–542.
88. Mani R, Cooper C, Kidd BL, Cole JD, Cawley MID. Use of laser doppler flowmetry and transcutaneous oxygen tension electrodes to assess local autonomic dysfunction in patients with frozen shoulder. *J Roy Soc Med.* 1989;82:536–538.
89. Connolly J, Regan E, Evans OB. Management of the painful, stiff shoulder. *Clin Orthop.* 1972;84:97–103.
90. Rizk TE, Pinals RS. Frozen shoulder. *Semin Arthritis Rheum.* 1982; 11:440–452.
91. Shaffer B, Tibone JE, Kerlan RK. Frozen shoulder. A long-term follow-up. *J Bone Joint Surg Am.* 1992;74:738–746.
92. Grey RG. The natural history of "idiopathic" frozen shoulder. *J Bone Joint Surg Am.* 1978;60:564.
93. Kessel L. *Clinical Disorders of the Shoulder.* New York: Churchill Livingstone; 1982;82.
94. Gay S, Gay ER, Miller JE. The collagens of the joint. *Arthritis Rheum.* 1980;23:937.
95. Kaltsas DS. Comparative study of the properties of the shoulder joint capsule with those of other joint capsules. *Clin Orthop.* 1983; 173:20–26.
96. Nash P, Hazelman BL. Frozen shoulder. *Balliere's Clin Rheum.* 1989; 3:551–566.
97. Nobuhara K, Sugiyama D, Ikeda H, Makiura M. Contracture of the shoulder. *Clin Orthop.* 1990;254:105–110.
98. Ozaki J, Nakagawa Y, Sakurai G, Tamai S. Recalcitrant chronic adhesive capsulitis of the shoulder. *J Bone Joint Surg Am.* 1989; 71:1511–1515.
99. Neer CS II, Satterlee C, Dalsey R, Flatow E. The anatomy and potential effects of contracture of the coracohumeral ligament. *Clin Orthop.* 1992;280:182–185.
100. Kay N, Slater D. Fibromatoses and diabetes mellitus. *Lancet.* 1981; 2:303.
101. Simmonds FA. Shoulder pain with particular reference to frozen shoulder. *J Bone Joint Surg Br.* 1979;31:426–432.
102. MacNab I. Rotator cuff tendinitis. *Ann R Coll Surg Eng.* 1973; 53:271–287.
103. MacNab I. The painful shoulder due to rotator cuff tendinitis. *RI Med J.* 1971;54:367–374.
104. Bulgen DY, Hazleman BL. Letter. *Lancet.* 1981;2:760.
105. Bulgen DY, Binder A, Hazleman BL, Park JP. Immunological studies in frozen shoulder. *J Rheumatol.* 1982;9:893–898.
106. Young A. Immunological studies in the frozen shoulder. In: Bayley J, Kessel L, eds. *Shoulder Surgery.* Berlin-Heidelberg: Springer-Verlag; 1982:110–113.
107. Kessel L, Bayley I, Young A. The frozen shoulder. *Br J Hosp Med.* 1981;25:334–338.
108. Rizk TE, Pinals RS. Histocompatibility type and racial incidence in frozen shoulder. *Arch Phys Med Rehabil.* 1984;65:33–34.
109. Seignalet J, Sany J, Caillens JP, Lapinski H. Lack of association between HLA-B27 and frozen shoulder. *Tissue Antigens.* 1982; 18:364.
110. Simon WH. Soft tissue disorders of the shoulder. *Orthop Clin North Am.* 1949;6:521–539.
111. Rockwood CA, Szalay EA, Curtis RJ, Young DC, Kay SP. X-ray evaluation of shoulder problems. In: Rockwood CA, Matsen FA, eds. *The Shoulder.* Vol I. Philadelphia: WB Saunders; 1990:178–200.
112. Neer CS II, Poppen NK. Supraspinatus outlet. *Orthop Trans.* 1987; 11:234.
113. Binder AI, Bulgen DY, Hazleman BL, et al. Frozen shoulder: An arthrographic and radionuclear scan assessment. *Ann Rheum Dis.* 1984;43:365–369.
114. Morris IM, Mattingly PC, Thompson AJ. Radiological erosions in frozen shoulder. *Br J Rheumatol.* 1990;29:293–294.
115. Wright MG, Richards AJ, Clarke MB. 99-M pertechnetate scanning in capsulitis. *Lancet.* 1975;2:15.
116. Stodell MA, Nicholson R, Scot J, Sturrock RD. Radioisotope scanning in painful shoulder syndromes. *Ann Rheum Dis.* 1979; 38:496.
117. Smith CR, Binder AI, Paice EW. Lesions of the midshaft of the humerus presenting as shoulder capsulitis. *Br J Rheumatol.* 1990; 29:386–388.
118. Kernwein GA, Roseberg B, Need WA. Arthrographic studies of the shoulder. *J Bone Joint Surg Br.* 1957;39:1267–1279.

119. Helbig B, Wagner P, Dohler R. Mobilization of frozen shoulder under general anesthesia. *Acta Orthop Belg.* 1983;49:267–274.
120. Neviaser TJ. Adhesive capsulitis. *Orthop Clin North Am.* 1987; 18:439–443.
121. Andren L, Lundberg BJ. Treatment of rigid shoulders by joint distention during arthrography. *Acta Orthop Scand.* 1965;36:45–53.
122. Neviaser RJ, Neviaser TJ. The frozen shoulder diagnosis and management. *Clin Orthop.* 1987;223:59–64.
123. Rajapakse C, Grennan DM, Jones C, Wilkinson L, Jayson M. Thermography in the assessment of peripheral joint inflammation—A reevaluation. *Rheum Rehabil.* 1981;20:81–87.
124. Vecchio PC, Adebajo AO, Chard MD. Thermography of frozen shoulder and rotator cuff. *Clin Rheum.* 1992;11:382–384.
125. Neviaser TJ. Intra-articular inflammatory diseases of the shoulder. *Inst Course Lect.* 1989;38:199–204.
126. Wiley AM. Arthroscopic appearance of frozen shoulder. *Arthroscopy.* 1991;7:138–143.
127. Rizk TE, Christopher RP, Pinals RS, Higgins C, Frix R. Adhesive capsulitis (frozen shoulder): A new approach to its management. *Arch Phys Med Rehabil.* 1983;64:29–33.
128. Tyber MA. Treatment of the painful shoulder syndrome with amitriptyline and lithium carbonate. *Can Med Assoc J.* 1974; 111:137–140.
129. Watson-Jones R. Simple treatment of stiff shoulders. *J Bone Joint Surg Br.* 1963;45:207.
130. Kessel L. Injuries of the shoulder. In: Wilson JN, ed. *Watson-Jones' Fractures and Joint Injuries.* 5th Ed. New York: Churchill Livingstone; 1976:522–532.
131. Cotton FJ, Peterson T. Physiotherapy in fracture treatment. *J Bone Joint Surg.* 1934;16:658–662.
132. Hazleman BL. The painful stiff shoulder. *Rheum Rehabil.* 1972; 2:413–421.
133. Murnaghan P. Frozen shoulder. In: Rockwood CA, Matsen FA, eds. *The Shoulder.* Vol. II. Philadelphia: WB Saunders; 1990:837–858.
134. Hughes MA, Neer CS. Glenohumeral joint replacement and postoperative rehabilitation. *Phys Ther.* 1975;55:850–858.
135. Nicholson GG. The effects of passive joint mobilization on pain and hypomobility associated with adhesive capsulitis of the shoulder. *Orthop Sports Phys Ther.* 1985;6:238–246.
136. Richardson AT. The painful shoulder. *Proc R Soc Med.* 1975; 68:731–736.
137. Weiss JJ, Ting YM. Arthrography assisted intra-articular injection of steroids in treatment of adhesive capsulitis. *Arch Phys Med Rehabil.* 1978;59:187–285.
138. Roy S, Oldham R. Management of painful shoulder. *Lancet.* 1976; 1:1322–1324.
139. Lee M, Haq AM, Wright V, Longston E. Periarthritis of the shoulder: A controlled trial of physiotherapy. *Physiotherapy.* 1973; 59:312–315.
140. Lee PN, Lee M, Haq AM, et al. Periarthritis of the shoulder: Trial of treatments investigated by multivariate analysis. *Ann Rheum Dis.* 1974;33:116–119.
141. Williams NE, Seifert MH, Cuddigan JHB, Wise RA. Treatment of capsulitis of the shoulder. *Rheum Rehabil.* 1975;14:236.
142. Hollingworth GR. Comparison of injection techniques for shoulder pain. *Br Med J (Clin Res).* 1983;7:1339–1341.
143. Thomas D, Williams RA, Smith DS. The frozen shoulder: A review of manipulative treatment. *Rheum Rehabil.* 1980;19:173–179.
144. Wild JJ, Fain RH, Tullos HS. Adhesive capsulitis of the shoulder: A conservative management technique. *Orthop Trans.* 1983;7:80.
145. Quin CG. Frozen shoulder: Evaluation of treatment with hydrocortisone injections and exercises. *Ann Phys Med.* 1965; 8:22–29.
146. Murnaghan GF, MacIntosh D. Hydrocortisone in the painful shoulder—a controlled trial. *Lancet.* 1955;2:798.
147. Dacre JE, Beeny N, Scott DL. Injections and physiotherapy for the painful stiff shoulder. *Ann Rheum Dis.* 1989;48:322–325.
148. Rizk TE, Pinals RS, Talaiver AS. Corticosteroid injections in adhesive capsulitis: An investigation of their value and site. *Arch Phys Med Rehab.* 1991;72:20–22.
149. Steinbroker O, Argyros TG. Frozen shoulder: Treatment by local injection of depot corticosteroids. *Arch Phys Med Rehabil.* 1974; 55:209–213.
150. Kraft GH, Johnson EW, Laban MM. The fibrositis syndrome. *Arch Phys Med Rehabil.* 1968;49:155–162.
151. Travell JG, Simmons DG. *Myofascial Pain and Dysfunction: Trigger Point Manual.* Baltimore: Williams & Wilkins; 1983:410–424.
152. Joshi GP, McCarroll SM. Intra-articular morphine for the management of frozen shoulder. *Anes.* 1992;47:627.
153. Koppel H, Thompson W. Pain and the frozen shoulder. *Surg Gynecol Obstet.* 1959;109:92–96.
154. Lee K, Khunadorn F. Painful shoulder in hemiplegic patients. A study of the suprascapular nerve. *Arch Phys Med Rehabil.* 1986; 67:818–820.
155. Wassef MR. Suprascapular nerve block—a new approach for the management of frozen shoulder. *Anes.* 1992;47:120–124.
156. Conti V. Arthroscopy in rehabilitation. *Orthop Clin North Am.* 1979; 10:709–711.
157. Older MWJ. Distention arthrography of the shoulder joint. In: Bayley J, Kessel L, eds. *Shoulder Surgery.* Berlin-Heidelberg: Springer-Verlag; 1982:123–127.
158. Haggart GE, Digman RJ, Sullivan TS. Management of the frozen shoulder. *J Am Med Assoc.* 1956;161:1219–1222.
159. Lloyd-Roberts GC, French PR. Periarthritis of the shoulder, a study of the disease and its treatment. *Br Med J.* 1959;1:1569–1571.
160. Fareed DO, Gallivan WR. Office management of frozen shoulder syndrome. Treatment with hydraulic distention under local anesthesia. *Clin Orthop.* 1989;2:177–183.
161. Jacobs L, Barto M, Wallace W. Intra-articular distention with steroids in the management of frozen shoulder. *Br Med J.* 1991; 302:1498–1501.
162. Charnley J. Periarthritis of the shoulder. *Postgrad Med J.* 1959; 35:384.
163. Leffert RD. The frozen shoulder. *Instr Course Lect.* 1985;34:199–203.
164. Haines JF, Hargadon EJ. Manipulation as the primary treatment of the frozen shoulder. *J R Coll Surg Edinb.* 1982;27:271–275.
165. Hill J, Boqumill H. Manipulation in the treatment of frozen shoulder. *Ortho.* 1988;11:1255.
166. Parker R, Froimson A, Winsberg D, Arsham N. Frozen shoulder. Part I: Chronology, pathogenesis, clinical picture, and treatment. *Orthopedics.* 1989;12:871–873.
167. Parker R, Froimson A, Winsberg D, Arsham N. Frozen shoulder. Part II: Treatment by manipulation under anesthesia. *Orthopedics.* 1989;12:989–990.
168. Loyd JA, Loyd HM. Adhesive capsulitis of the shoulder: Arthrographic diagnosis and treatment. *South Med J.* 1983;76:789.
169. Ekelund A, Rydell N. Combination treatment for adhesive capsulitis of the shoulder. *Clin Orthop.* 1992;2:105–109.
170. Angiolini G, Pasquinelli V, Putti C. La roentgenterapia nella cura della periartrite della spalla. *Minverva Medica.* 1965;56:504–508.
171. Gilula LA, Schoenecker PL, Murphy WA. Shoulder arthrography as a treatment modality. *Am J Roentgenol.* 1978;131:1047–1048.
172. Wiser HI. Painful primary frozen shoulder—mobilization under local anesthesia. *Arch Phys Med Rehabil.* 1977;58:406–408.
173. Ha'eri GB, Maitland A. Arthroscopic findings in the frozen shoulder. *J Rheumatol.* 1981;8:149–152.
174. Ogilvie-Harris DJ, Wiley AM. Arthroscopic surgery of the shoulder. A general appraisal. *J Bone Joint Surg Br.* 1986;68:201–207.
175. McGraw JM, Turba JE. Frozen shoulder—treatment by arthroscopy and manipulation. *Orthop Trans.* 1989;13:661–662.
176. Hsu SY, Chan KM. Arthroscopic distension in the management of frozen shoulder. *Int Orthop.* 1991;15:79–83.
177. McLaughlin HL. The frozen shoulder. *Clin Orthop.* 1961;20:126–131.
178. Kieras DM, Matsen FA. Open release in the management of refractory frozen shoulder. *Orthop Trans.* 1991;15:801–802.
179. De Seze S. Les epaules douloureuses et les epaules bloquees. *Concours Medical.* 1974;96:5329–5357.
180. Neer CS. Less frequent procedures. In: Neer CS II, ed. *Shoulder Reconstruction.* Philadelphia: WB Saunders; 1990:426–427.

Section 5

Conservative Treatment of Cuff Defects and Impingement Syndrome

Chapter 18

Conservative Management of Partial-Thickness Rotator Cuff Lesions

David S. Morrison

The most common shoulder disorders seen by an orthopaedic surgeon relate to injuries of the rotator cuff. However, few of us have an adequate understanding of the etiology of rotator cuff injuries, fewer still have even a passing knowledge of the theory and practice of rotator cuff rehabilitation. It is not an exaggeration to state that approximately 100% of the American population sustains an acute or attritional injury to their rotator cuff at some point in their lifetime. Recent cadaveric studies have shown that up to 39% of individuals over the age of 60 can be expected to have full-thickness rotator cuff tears,[1] and the incidence of partial-thickness rotator cuff injuries is much higher. If all rotator cuff tears were symptomatic, surgical rotator cuff repair would undoubtedly be our primary orthopaedic procedure. This, of course, is not the case. By comparing a number of studies regarding the incidence of rotator cuff tears in a cadaveric population,[3-5] as well as others that have documented the incidence of rotator cuff tears in an asymptomatic group of patients studied by MRI scan,[2] we come to the conclusion that probably only about 25% of patients with full-thickness rotator cuff tears are symptomatic. The question, therefore, is not why only 25% of these patients are symptomatic, but why the remaining majority of patients have little or no symptoms from a full-thickness rotator cuff tear.

An equally perplexing question is why someone with a small partial-thickness rotator cuff tear (Fig. 18-1), comprising only 5 to 10% of the superficial surface of their rotator cuff, can have unrelenting and disabling pain while someone with a small complete thickness rotator cuff tear can be completely asymptomatic and able to participate in reasonably high-caliber athletics without difficulty. Some of this may be explained by the stability biomechanics as discussed in Chapter 28, but this does not explain all of our patients, because patients with apparently stable rotator cuff tears may have severe unrelenting pain, whereas patients with apparently unstable and progressive rotator cuff tears can present mainly with a complaint of weakness and little, if any, pain.

One thing is certain, however, and that is that once a full-thickness rotator cuff tear becomes symptomatic, the vast majority of these rotator cuff tears continue to be symptomatic unless treated surgically. In our experience, once a full-thickness rotator cuff tear has been diagnosed, treatment is surgical. This chapter is limited to a discussion of the nonoperative management of partial-thickness rotator cuff lesions. To date, there are no studies in the literature that document a satisfactory outcome for nonoperative treatment of full-thickness rotator cuff tears when compared to operative management. Several investigators have attempted to perform acromioplasty alone, mainly arthroscopically, with debridement and nonrepair of rotator cuff tears. Their results are inferior to their own controls who underwent repair of their rotator cuff tears and are also inferior to other studies on the outcome from surgical repair of full-thickness rotator cuff tears.[8-11] With that in mind, debridement without repair of rotator cuff tears cannot be recommended. The following discussion relates to the treatment of partial-thickness rotator cuff tears only, because in our experience the response to physical therapy of full-thickness rotator cuff tears is limited at best and quite often results in increasing complaints of pain and weakness. As a matter of fact, one of our indications for an MRI scan of the shoulder is failure to respond to a conservative management program or increasing pain or disability secondary to the performance of the rehabilitation protocol.

In some patients, undoubtedly, there are other underlying problems such as instability, intrinsic tendonopathy, and old fractures that contributed to the patients symptoms. The decision, therefore, as to whether to proceed with conservative management for a rotator cuff lesion relates not only to the extent of that lesion but the etiology of the lesion and the expectations of the individual patient.

ETIOLOGY AND CLASSIFICATIONS OF ROTATOR CUFF INJURIES

The etiology, classification, and historical evolution of our understanding of rotator cuff pathology have been previously presented. An etiologic classification that we

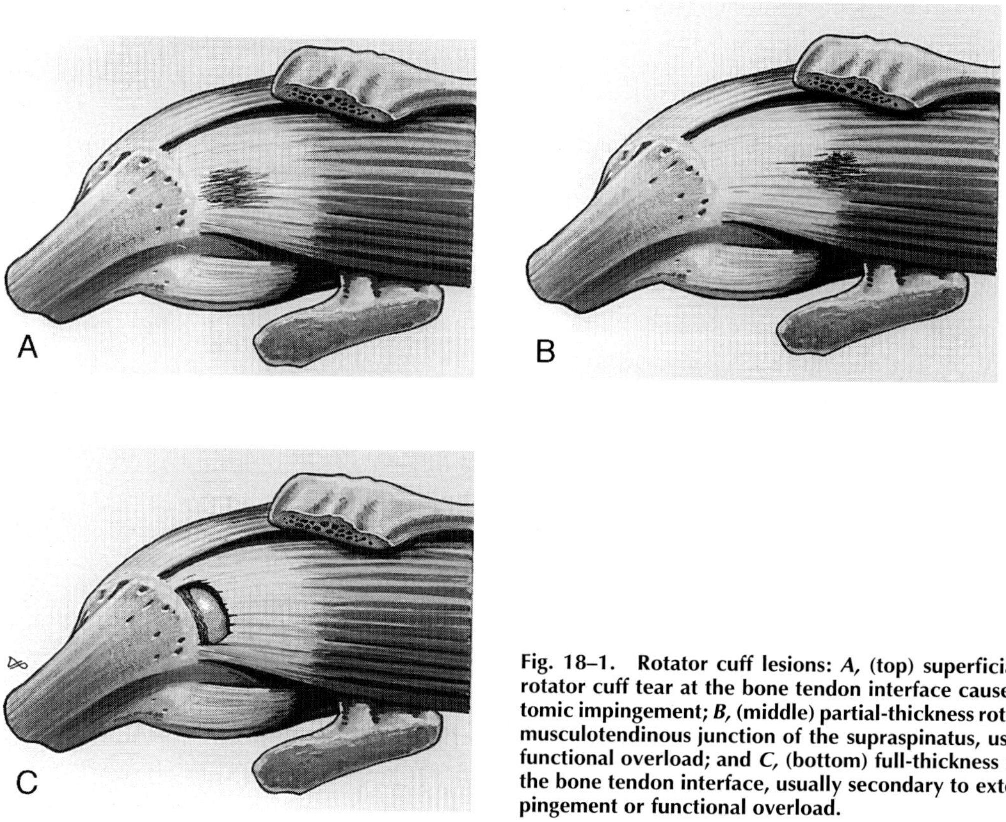

Fig. 18–1. Rotator cuff lesions: *A,* (top) superficial partial-thickness rotator cuff tear at the bone tendon interface caused by external anatomic impingement; *B,* (middle) partial-thickness rotator cuff tear at the musculotendinous junction of the supraspinatus, usually secondary to functional overload; and *C,* (bottom) full-thickness rotator cuff tear at the bone tendon interface, usually secondary to external anatomic impingement or functional overload.

have found useful in decision making in treatment is summarized in Table 18-1.

It is important to emphasize that external anatomic impingement, although responsible for the majority of rotator cuff injuries, particularly in a group over the age of 40, does not account for all rotator cuff pathology. To date, there are no good studies and no solid scientific evidence as to what percentage of rotator cuff injuries are caused by true external anatomic impingement as opposed to these other etiologies. In this author's opinion, approximately 80% of rotator cuff injuries are caused by true external anatomic impingement, 5% are secondary to instability of the glenohumeral joint, 5% caused by intrinsic tendon degeneration, and 5% caused by functional overload of the rotator cuff. However, determining the exact etiology in the individual patient can be exceedingly difficult, because more than one etiology can be at work at any one time.

Take for example the young baseball pitcher who sustains a infraspinatus/teres minor injury early in the season secondary to overuse. These lesions usually occur at the musculotendinous junction rather than in the impingement area. Surgery is almost never indicated and rehabilitation is the treatment of choice. However, if the problem persists for a prolonged period, the patient will develop disuse weakness of his rotator cuff, and thus lose the depressor effect of the oblique rotator cuff muscles. This can then result in minute superior migration of the humeral head and true external anatomic impingement

Table 18–1. Etiologic Classification of Rotator Cuff Injuries

External Anatomic Impingement
Related to acromial morphology
Instability related
Secondary to anatomic abnormalities
AC separation
Ununited anterior acromial epiphysis
Acromial fracture malunion
Displaced greater tuberosity fracture
Internal Anatomic Impingement
SLAP lesion
Deep surface rotator cuff tears
Functional Overload
Strain caused by overuse
Partial thickness tear secondary to overload
Tendon-bone interface
Musculotendinous junction
Complete rotator cuff tear.
Intrinsic Tendonopathy

on the acromion. If the patient presents at this point in time, his symptoms and his physical examination will be entirely consistent with external anatomic impingement, although the true etiology of his problem relates to an original rotator cuff overload injury. The presentation of a patient with intrinsic tendon degeneration is similar. It is possible that there exists a group of patients who undergo true degeneration in the critical zone of the supraspinatus tendon. This results in pain and subsequent disuse weakness of the rotator cuff. This then results in loss of the depressor effect of the rotator cuff muscles and superior migration with secondary external anatomic impingement.

There are numerous other combinations of etiology that could be considered, but the point here is that we probably will never know the true etiology of rotator cuff damage in about 20% of our patients; however, we need to recognize that in the remaining 80% true external anatomic impingement appears to be the primary etiology.

PHILOSOPHY BEHIND THE MANAGEMENT OF ROTATOR CUFF INJURIES

Understanding of the etiologic classification of rotator cuff injuries alone is not sufficient to fully understand the methods and goals of rehabilitation. Review of the basic biomechanics of shoulder elevation in Chapter 4 is recommended.

In the normal individual, the space between the greater tuberosity and the undersurface of the acromion is approximately 6 to 7 mm. The thickness of the rotator cuff tendon in this area is approximately 5 to 6 mm. Therefore, there is little clearance between the rotator cuff and the normal acromion. With adequate function of the rotator cuff, the humeral head does not ride up during arm elevation, and, therefore, impingement does not occur.

As an individual ages, it appears that the massive deltoid muscle retains it strength longer than the relatively small and weak rotator cuff muscles. According to one theory, this allows the deltoid to overpower the rotator cuff during elevation, allowing the humeral head to rise up and causing the anterior acromion to impinge upon the rotator cuff muscles. The treatment of this condition, which has become known as impingement syndrome, therefore is to increase the space between the anterior acromion and the rotator cuff tendons. There are two ways of correcting this problem. One of them is to approach the situation surgically, with an anterior acromioplasty, to remove the undersurface of the anterior third of the acromion and increase the clearance between the acromion and the rotator cuff. However, this procedure is usually not necessary, because the same increase in clearance can often be obtained through another approach. That is, if we can lower the humeral head several millimeters, then we effectively increase the subacromial space in a fashion similar to an acromioplasty and also decompress the rotator cuff muscles. This can be accomplished by physical therapy. The oblique muscles of the rotator cuff, i.e. the inferior half of the infraspinatus and the subscapularis as well as the entire teres minor, attach to the humerus at approximately a 45° angle to the shaft (Fig. 18-2). During the initiation of elevation, these muscles act not only as humeral head stabilizers and rotators, but also as significant humeral head depressors. Therefore, if we can strengthen the inferior portion of the rotator cuff muscles while at the same time either weakening or at least not strengthening the deltoid muscle, we can re-establish the normal balance between the deltoid and the rotator cuff muscles and allow elevation of the humerus without superior migration of the humeral head, thus preventing impingement syndrome. This is the basis of our rehabilitation program for rotator cuff disease.

Although this is admittedly a simplistic look at a rather complex problem, it is quite useful to our basic understanding of impingement syndrome. Obviously, there are additional factors to consider, such as the scapular stabilizers and the accessory muscles of humeral movement, but understanding the basic principles of balance between humeral head elevation and depression is the basis of understanding the theory behind rotator cuff rehabilitation.

Aside from understanding the basic force couple of glenohumeral elevation, it is equally important to under-

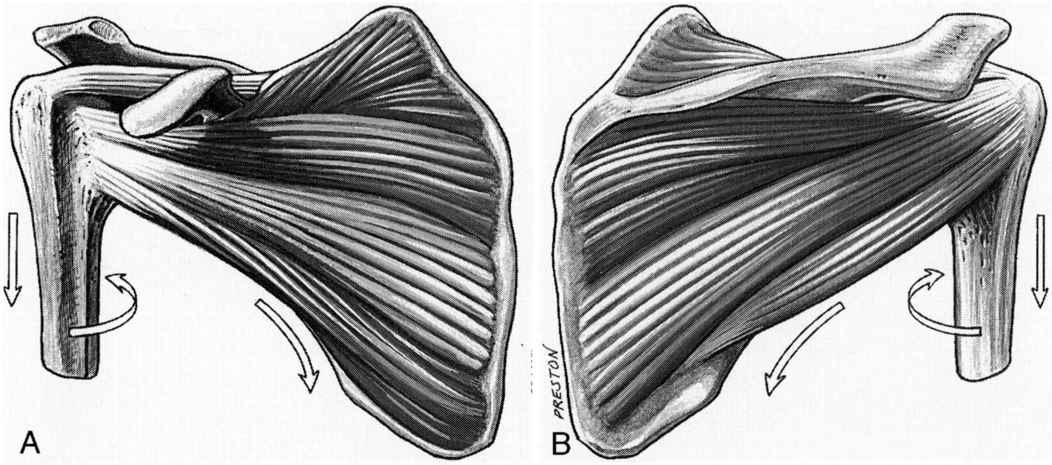

Fig. 18–2. The inferior half of the subscapularis and the infraspinatus as well as the entire teres minor attach at an oblique angle to the shaft of the humerus. In the therapy protocol, these muscles are exercised at the side to enhance their depressor effect upon the humeral head. The deltoid muscle is not exercised, because to do so would negate the benefits gained through strengthening of the oblique rotator cuff muscles.

stand the scapulothoracic force couple. Often rehabilitation fails to address the importance of the scapulothoracic force couple. This is particularly true in patients with impingement syndrome secondary to instability or in cases of AC ligament disruption in which the scapular positioning muscles must work overtime in order to compensate for ligamentous injuries. The glenoid fossa must move in synergy with the humeral head and shaft so that the instant center of humeral rotation is as close as possible to the same position throughout the extremes of functional movement. This concomitant movement of the glenoid and humeral head helps to improve glenohumeral congruency by maintaining the proper length-tension relationships of the muscles that anchor the humerus to the scapula. Likewise, during full elevation or abduction the scapula needs to rotate out of the way of the humerus to prevent impingement of the greater tuberosity on the rotator cuff. This function is controlled by the scapular balancing muscles, that is, the upper and lower trapezius, the serratus anterior, and the rhomboids.

Therefore, complete impingement rehabilitation should place its emphasis upon strengthening three main areas: humeral head depressors (subscapularis, infraspinatus, and teres minor), scapular balancing muscles (upper and lower trapezius, serratus anterior, and rhomboids), and the prime humeral positioners (deltoid, pectoral major, and latissimus dorsi). It is important to understand, however, that in the vast majority of patients, strengthening the humeral head depressors alone is entirely sufficient to control the symptoms of impingement syndrome. It is only in high-demand patients, such as athletes or in those who have concomitant shoulder girdle pathology (e.g., instability), in which we would recommend the full three-phase rehabilitation protocol.

BASIC TREATMENT PROTOCOL

The initial phase of the treatment protocol can be divided into three areas of concentration: decreasing inflammation, soft-tissue stretching, and finally rotator cuff strengthening. Patients that suffer from impingement syndrome need adequate rest from the activities that have inflamed their rotator cuff. Rest is often too short. The length of time may vary from a few days to a few weeks, depending upon the underlying etiology and the degree of inflammation. Nonsteroidal anti-inflammatory medication and a limited number of subacromial steroid injections are useful to decrease inflammation but are mainly symptomatic treatments that do not address the underlying problem. Physical therapy modalities such as phonophoresis, iontophoresis, or ultrasound appear to have little effect on the natural history of rotator cuff problems and would not ordinarily be used. Under normal situations, inflammation can usually be controlled within one or two weeks to the extent that pain has been decreased sufficiently to allow stretching and strengthening exercises. We believe that before any rotator cuff strengthening can be started, the shoulder must have a full normal range of motion. In our experience, a stiff shoulder is a painful shoulder. This not only limits the usefulness of strengthening exercises, but also tends to cause increased pain as the therapy protocol is advanced.

The stretching exercises that we use are passive and active assisted, which are usually performed by the patient at home with only an occasional follow-up in physical therapy. These simple stretching exercises are described extensively in Chapter 8 and need not be discussed here.

Once a full normal range of motion has been obtained, then the strengthening protocol can begin. Isometric exercises directed toward the oblique muscles of the rotator cuff with the arm at the side are the first step. The arm is held in neutral rotation with the elbow bent 90°. Isometric external rotation is performed against the resistance of the patient's opposite hand or an inanimate object such as a wall. Force is exerted for 10 seconds and is followed by 2 seconds of rest. This is repeated for 10 repetitions. Then internal rotation is resisted for another set of 10 repetitions of 10 seconds each. Internal and external rotation exercises are alternated until 3 sets of 10 repetitions of each have been performed. The amount of pressure exerted is determined by the amount of pain that the patient experiences; only minimal transient pain is acceptable. Once forceful isometric exercises are tolerated with minimal pain, light isotonic exercises are introduced using Theraband or surgical tubing. In these exercises, the tubing is tied to a doorknob and the arm is internally or externally rotated against the resistance of the tubing to a position of neutral rotation (Fig. 18-3). The arm is held in the neutral position for 10 seconds and then is rested for 2 or 3 seconds. This is repeated through 10 repetitions, and again, the goal is to perform three sets of 10 repetitions of both internal and external rotation. The resistance should be such that when the patient reaches the tenth repetition in the third set he is unable to hold the position for the full 10 seconds. If the patient finds that he is unable to hold the position for the full 10 seconds halfway through his third set, then the initial resistance during the first two sets has been too severe. If, on the other hand, the patient is able to complete the 3 sets without any problem, then the resistance has been too light. When performed properly this strengthening program should only take about 12 to 15 minutes twice a day. Once the patient has obtained pain relief through these stationary exercises, he can then begin dynamic rotator cuff strengthening at the side. The same exercises are slowly performed through an arc of $-30°$ to $+30°$ of rotation, with an emphasis on the eccentric phase of contraction (3 seconds concentric, 7 seconds eccentric). Again, 3 sets of 10 repetitions of internal and external rotation are used.

It is important that the deltoid be relaxed during these exercises and that all effort be directed toward rotation and not abduction. To assist in eliminating any abduction, effort can be made to hold a magazine between the lateral chest wall and the inner surface of the upper arm. This requires an adduction force and eliminates any deltoid contracture. The patient is advised that cuff reconditioning is at least a 6-week process. This length of time is required to obtain a satisfactory decrease in inflam-

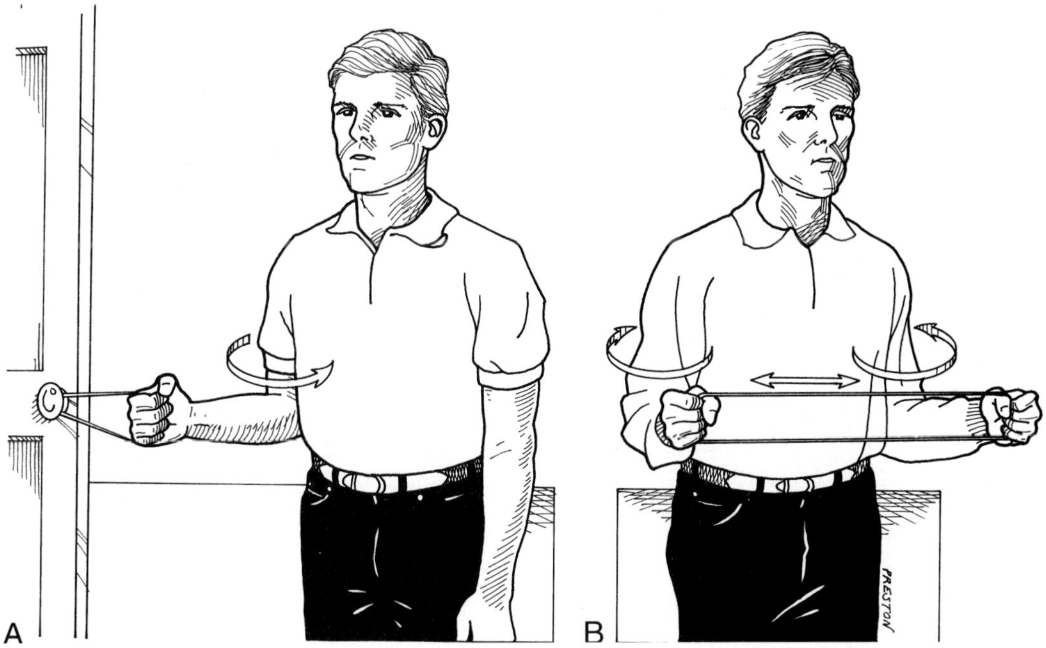

Fig. 18–3. Internal and external rotation exercises are performed at the side using rubber tubing. It is important to keep the upper arm against the chest and to avoid deltoid contracture during the initial phase of rehabilitation.

mation and the necessary strength in the oblique rotator cuff muscles to eliminate pain and prevent further impingement. In our experience patients will begin to experience relief from their symptoms by 4 to 6 weeks on this protocol. If they have no improvement whatsoever by 6 weeks or if the exercises are irritating their shoulder, then it is usually an indication that they are not likely to respond to the exercise protocol, and a longer period of rest is prescribed. It is important not to perform deltoid strengthening exercises during this initial phase of the rehabilitation, because a strong deltoid tends to pull the humeral head up, decreasing the subacromial space and increasing the symptoms of impingement. Therefore, the initial goal is a strong rotator cuff and a relatively weak deltoid.

The patient continues his or her exercises at home and is evaluated about 3 weeks after initiation of the program. Patients who have difficulty complying with a home program can be seen on a regular basis by a physical therapist, but this is not usually necessary. In the majority of patients who are not active athletes, symptoms can be controlled simply through the above protocol. There is a tendency for symptoms to recur in about 17% of patients who have satisfactory initial results, but these patients almost always respond to resumption of their exercises.

In high-caliber athletes, eccentric cuff strengthening is the final stage of cuff rehabilitation prior to scapular stabilization exercises. Eccentric cuff strengthening is particularly important in patients that participate in repetitive overhead activities that require humeral deceleration. Side-lying, eccentric external rotation with a dumbbell is added, with emphasis on low weight and high repetitions. The patient is instructed to avoid overloading these muscles with heavy weight, as the external rotators are relatively weak even in nonpathologic shoulders. Five to 8 pounds would be considered heavy levels of resistance for these exercises. Internal rotators also receive eccentric attention but require heavier poundage during training. Athletes involved in activities that require overhead movements can be progressed to high-speed isokinetics performed in the plane of the scapula. Patients presenting with weakness or decreased control of the scapular positioning muscles should then receive appropriate strengthening exercises. Exercises such as upright or bent-over rowing, shoulder shrugs, latissimus pull-downs, or specific exercises that closely mimic the athlete's functional movements can be added as necessary.

Once the humeral head depressors are strong and scapular balancing has been achieved, strengthening techniques are directed at the prime humeral positioners. These techniques are directed at the glenohumeral muscles and emphasize three component motions, which include shoulder flexion/extension, adduction/abduction, and internal/external rotation. These movements are performed against resistance and combine optimum sequencing of muscle facilitation, allowing muscles to contribute their components of action consistently. This form of manual patterning closely resembles movements used in the patient's sport or overhead work activities.

RESULTS OF BASIC TREATMENT PROTOCOL

We recently completed an extensive review of our results using the described treatment protocol.[7] A group of 770 patients with a diagnosis of impingement syndrome following history, physical examination, and radiographic examination were included in this study. Patients with concomitant adhesive capsulitis, cervical radiculopathy, suprascapular nerve palsy, or full-thickness rotator cuff tears were later excluded from this series, leaving a total of 669 patients; 51 patients were lost to follow-up and two patients died, leaving a final study group of 616 patients and a retrieval rate of 92%. The study group was comprised of 386 men and 230 women. The average age was 42 years (range: 15 to 81 years). We divided the study group into four age categories as follows: (1) under age 20 (33 patients); (2) ages 21 to 40 (253 patients); (3) ages 41 to 60 (252 patients); and (4) over the age of 60 (78 patients). In 406 patients (66%), the dominant shoulder was involved; nondominant involvement was seen in 190 patients (31%), whereas bilateral shoulder involvement was noted in 20 patients (3%). The average duration of symptoms was 16 months, with a range of 1 day to 240 months. We separated the patients into three categories based upon length of symptoms: (1) acute, less than 4 weeks (86 patients, 14%); (2) nonacute, 1 to 6 months (228 patients, 37%); (3) chronic, greater than 6 months (302 patients, 49%). In addition to history and physical examination, radiographs including anteroposterior, axillary, and supraspinatus outlet views were obtained. Using the criteria described by Bigliani and Morrison, we analyzed the acromial morphology in the radiographs of each patient.[6]

An important consideration in this study was our attempt to evaluate the patient's prior treatment history upon presentation to our clinic. Sixty percent of our patients had been seen and treated by a physician prior to their presentation in our clinic. More than half of the treating physicians (55%) were orthopaedic surgeons. Thirty-seven percent of patients stated they had received "physical therapy" for their impingement syndrome prior to transferring treatment to our facility. All of these attempts at therapy had failed to improve the patient's symptoms.

All patients were treated with the basic treatment protocol described above. The high caliber athletes, which comprised only approximately 7% of our patient population, were then progressed to the full three-phase rehabilitation protocol. The vast majority of the patients required only intermittent visits with a physical therapist for follow-up and an occasional refresher course in their exercises, which they performed at home. Follow-up in this study averaged more than 2 years, and all patients were evaluated using the UCLA rating scale.

Overall, 413 patients (67%) had a satisfactory outcome: 186 patients (30%) were rated as demonstrating excellent results and 227 (37%) were rated as demonstrating good results. However, 172 patients (28%) did not improve with conservative treatment and went on to arthroscopic subacromial decompression at an average of 7 months after the initiation of treatment at our facility (average of 23 months after onset of their symptoms); 31 (5%) had unsatisfactory results but declined operative intervention; of these patients, 26 were classified as fair and 5 were classified as having poor results.

It is interesting to note that in the patients with a satisfactory result the majority began to experience resolution of their symptoms within 4 to 6 weeks of the initiation of the treatment protocol. In those patients who did not demonstrate significant improvement by 8 weeks, most went on to fail conservative treatment. Of the 413 patients with satisfactory results, 74 (17%) experienced recurrence of their symptoms during the follow-up period. These recurrent symptoms either resolved spontaneously or with resumption of the exercises in every case. A smaller group of patients responded to their initial exercise program but failed to respond to resumption of exercises when their symptoms recurred. These patients were included among the unsatisfactory results. Sixty-eight percent of the male patients and 65% of the female patients had satisfactory results with conservative treatment; 69% of patients with dominant shoulder involvement had satisfactory results, whereas satisfactory results of 60% were seen with nondominant shoulder involvement.

With regard to acromial morphology, we found no statistical difference in the patients response to conservative management based upon acromial morphology. Of our 120 patients with a diagnosis of concomitant AC arthritis, only 57% had satisfactory results with regard to their rotator cuff pain with conservative management. This could be the result of irritation of the rotator cuff secondary to AC joint osteophyte formation or trapezius muscle spasm secondary to the AC joint arthritis. When we looked at our results with regard to the patients' age at presentation, it was in group 4, those patients over the age of 60, in which we found a significant decrease in their response to the treatment protocol (55% were satisfactory). With regards to the duration of symptoms, the acute patients (symptoms less than 4 weeks) fared best with a 78% achieving satisfactory results. In the nonacute group (symptoms 1 to 6 months), the results were slightly less satisfactory with 63% responding to the protocol. Finally, in the chronic group (symptoms longer than 6 months), 67% of the patients experienced a satisfactory result.

We were careful to eliminate patients with radicular disease and/or limited cervical range of motion from this study group. The treatment of these patients' primary pathology is usually sufficient to correct their shoulder symptoms. Statistically significant less satisfactory results were found in patients over age 60 and in those patients aged 21 to 40. The reasons for this bimodal distribution are unclear. In patients over 60 years of age, poor tendon quality and/or undiagnosed full-thickness rotator cuff tears may account for the poor results. The 21 to 40 age group is an active athletic population and may be involved in more exacerbating activities than the 41 to 60 age group. However, this is speculation. We did not note any significant difference in results with respect to gender.

Two-thirds of all patients in this study had dominant shoulder involvement. These patients had better results than those patients with nondominant or bilateral shoulder involvement. It is interesting to note that patients with type II acromial morphology fared no better than those with type III acromions, which is in contrast to the findings of a relationship between acromial morphology and tears of the rotator cuff. This suggests that patients with Type III acromions have a predisposition to rotator cuff tears but are not at a disadvantage for conservative treatment of rotator cuff tendinitis. A long-term follow-up of these patients has been undertaken in an effort to follow the natural history of their rotator cuff problems.

It should be noted that the results of this study may not be indicative of the results in a general orthopaedic population. Our study group came from a referral practice in which 60% of our patients had previously been seen and treated by another physician, with over half of those treating physicians being orthopaedic surgeons. All of these patients had been treated with rest and anti-inflammatory medication, and nearly 40% of them had been seen and treated with a physical therapy program. It is reasonable to assume that a significant number of patients seen and treated by our referring physicians obtained relief of their symptoms and therefore were not referred to our clinic. Thus, the results of the present study, which shows a 67% response rate to physical therapy, may be significantly lower than that which is possible in a general orthopaedic practice. We believe that a response rate closer to 85% satisfactory results with conservative management would be a reasonable expectation.

TREATMENT BY ETIOLOGY

External Anatomic Impingement

As noted earlier, external anatomic impingement syndrome can be caused by several etiologies. Among these are acromial morphology, instability, and anatomic abnormalities. An attempt must be made to determine the exact etiology of the impingement prior to beginning a conservative management and rehabilitation program. If the primary problem is an anatomic abnormality, such as an AC separation with a drooping scapula, then a reconstruction of the ligaments using a technique such as the Weaver-Dunn repair would be in order. An acromial fracture with impingement on the greater tuberosity or a greater tuberosity fracture with proximal displacement and impingement upon the acromion need to be anatomically reduced for relief of symptoms. The treatment of an ununited anterior acromial epiphysis is dependent on the size of the epiphysis, as well as factors in the patient's age and activity level. Recommending whether it should be excised or repaired is not the purpose of this chapter, but rather recognition of this as an etiology of rotator cuff injury and the possible need for correction prior to rehabilitation is noted. Even after correction of one of these anatomic abnormalities, the rotator cuff injury caused by their presence will often remain. At that point, the routine physical therapy protocol for impingement syndrome is used.

Patients with instability-related impingement present another problem. In these individuals, the lax glenohumeral ligaments allow the humeral head a certain degree of motion in all directions, not just anteriorly inferiorly. This can result in superior migration of the humeral head with impingement of the greater tuberosity and supraspinatus tendon on a relatively normal acromion. Therefore, the treatment in these patients is usually not an acromioplasty but rather involves stabilization of the glenohumeral joint. This stabilization can be obtained surgically when necessary but often can be obtained through conservative means with rotator cuff rehabilitation. The initial protocol used for instability is the same as that for primary impingement syndrome, but once initial relief of symptoms has been obtained, then a general shoulder strengthening and scapular stabilization program is undertaken to control future symptoms in what is usually a highly athletic population.

Once the physician has made the diagnosis of external anatomic impingement syndrome and has ruled out the possibility of any anatomic abnormalities as contributing factors, then a conservative management program can be undertaken.

Internal Anatomic Impingement

Internal anatomic impingement syndrome is a theory put forth independently by two investigators (Christopher Jobe and Gilles Walch) and relates to the etiology of deep surface rotator cuff tears and superior labral detachments (SLAP lesions). In abduction and external rotation in a person with a lax shoulder, the humerus subluxes anteriorly, allowing the greater tuberosity to impinge on the posterior superior aspect of the glenoid. This can result in pinching of the deep surface of the rotator cuff between the greater tuberosity and the glenoid with partial-thickness deep surface disruption. It may also result in shearing off the posterior superior labrum from its glenoid attachment or the creation of a bucket handle tear of the labrum. In addition to this we believe that a fall or a blow to the outstretched arm in a forced elevated position will bring the greater tuberosity into contact with the superior glenoid, also resulting in damage to the deep rotator cuff and possible disruption of the biceps tendon attachment along the superior and anterior superior aspect of the glenoid margin (Fig. 18-4). In the patients with instability, the treatment is a therapy protocol for instability of the shoulder rather than a rotator cuff protocol. If the patient's symptoms are mainly caused by instability and their internal anatomic impingement was simply a secondary problem, a conservative or surgical protocol for instability will usually correct all the patient's symptoms. If however the etiology of the patient's symptoms is not instability but rather is pain related to the superior labral detachment and/or biceps lesions, then surgical management must necessarily include stabilization of the disrupted superior labrum.

Functional Overload

Overuse syndrome is a well recognized problem throughout the body and is particularly apparent in the shoulder. The reason for this is that more than any other athletically active joint the shoulder relies on its musculature for stabilization and protection. Functional over-

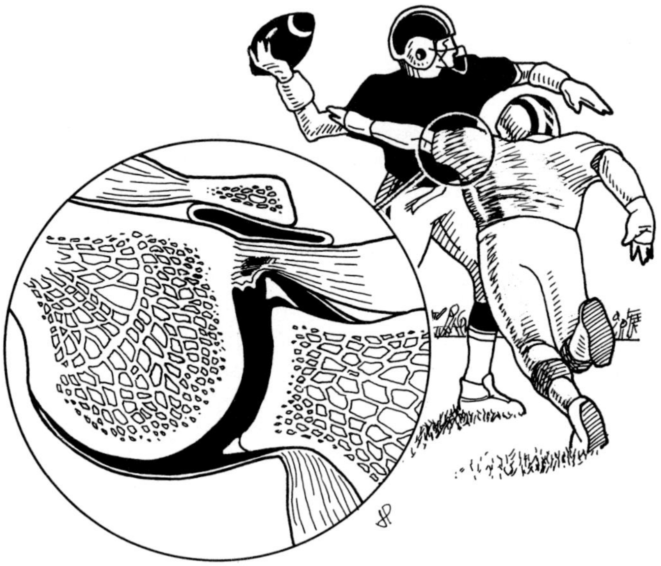

Fig. 18–4. Forceful impact with the arm in the fully elevated position can bring the greater tuberosity to bear upon the superior aspect of the glenoid. This may result in shearing off of the superior glenoid labrum and pinching of the rotator cuff between the greater tuberosity and the glenoid. Unlike the posterior superior impingement described by Jobe, laxity is not a prerequisite for this injury to occur.

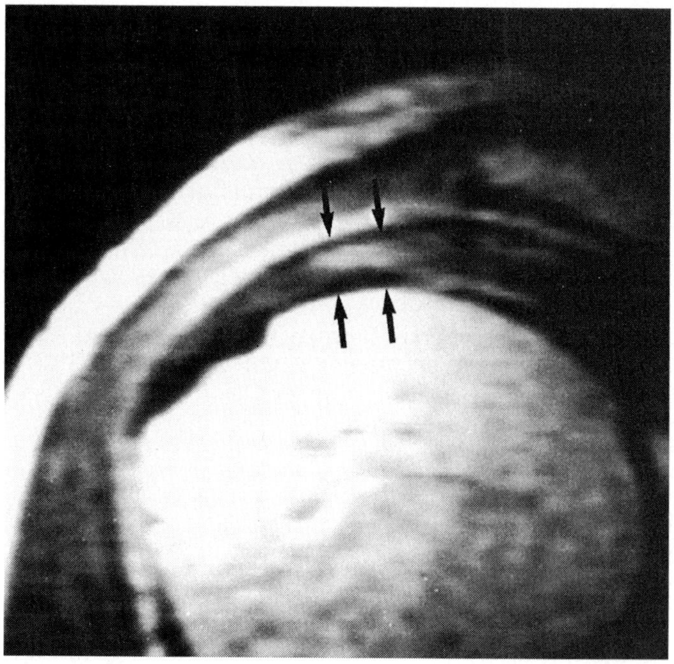

Fig. 18–5. MRI scan of a tear at the musculotendinous junction of the supraspinatus muscle in a 23-year-old professional volleyball player. Note the good quality of the tendon distal to the lesion and the supraspinatus muscle proximal to the lesion.

load of the shoulder is exceptionally common at the beginning of an athletic season or after a prolonged layoff. Simple muscle fatigue and overuse will result in the athlete complaining of a burning type pain in the shoulder often radiating down to the lateral deltoid or in the infraspinatus fossa. They rarely have sharp pains in the shoulder, and although their arm fatigues easily, the pain usually clears quickly after icing down at the completion of the practice session.

These athletes are best treated with the standard rotator cuff protocol described above and the judicious use of anti-inflammatory medications, ice following activity, and a decrease in the intensity of their training. In our experience, it is rarely necessary to completely eliminate the offending activity but rather the use of common sense and modification of the activities is recommended. An example would be a high school baseball pitcher who is also a good hitter. We would decrease the amount of pitching that the athlete performs, but keep him involved in baseball by playing him at first base or as a designated hitter during his rehabilitation. These injuries are often caused by fatigue. As the athlete's arm tires, he begins to drop from a full overhead throwing position to a partial sidearm delivery. This puts excess strain on the elbow and also the altered biomechanics of the pitching motion results in further strain on the rotator cuff. The treatment of these individuals involves having their throwing motion observed from a technical point of view, and when the individual begins to show signs of fatigue or loss of accuracy, the player should be removed from the game before the rotator cuff is reinjured.

The initial treatment of overuse syndrome relates to modification of the athletic activity to decrease irritation as much as possible, anti-inflammatory medications to control the inflammation of the rotator cuff, ice applications following athletics to decrease swelling, and a progressively aggressive rotator cuff strengthening program and general shoulder stabilization program to improve strength and functional stability.

A small number of these athletically active patients develop partial-thickness rotator cuff tears because of overload. This usually occurs from a single massive traumatic event such as an off-balance throw or a fall. These injuries occur in two locations: either at the musculotendinous junction or at the tendon/bone interface. Injuries at the musculotendinous junction will usually heal by themselves with conservative management as discussed above. However, it can take exceptionally long for these to heal completely. It is not unusual for a musculotendinous disruption diagnosed by MRI scan to take 5 to 6 months to heal. It is rarely necessary to operate on these individuals, but if surgery is contemplated, then a good localization of the lesion with MRI or at the time of surgery is absolutely necessary (Fig. 18-5). The treatment in these patients is a limited excision of the damaged portion of the musculotendinous unit with primary repair. An acromioplasty is usually not necessary in these individuals. When the partial-thickness disruption occurs at the tendon/bone interface, however, the results of conservative management are much less predictable. Often, these patients can recover through standard conservative means, but more frequently once the tendon/bone interface has been disrupted, then surgical repair is indicated. It should be noted, however, that such partial-thickness rotator cuff tears secondary to overload in an athletic population are fairly rare. Surgical management of such a lesion would be considered an unusual occurrence.

Full-thickness rotator cuff tears caused by functional overload are also fairly uncommon occurrences. They usually result from a single violent injury, such as being thrown from a dirt bike or falling to the ground in an unusual position during contact athletics. In our experience, there is no conservative management for full-thickness rotator cuff tears of this type, and the treatment is always surgical if medically feasible.

Intrinsic Tendonopathy

If we believe that intrinsic tendonopathy is a major etiology of rotator cuff pain, physical therapy would be expected to have little effect upon the natural history of rotator cuff disorders. If internal rotator cuff tendon degeneration was a normal process of aging, we could expect to give temporary pain relief with anti-inflammatory medications and conservative care, but we would also expect the tendon degeneration to progress with time and result in increasing symptoms and debilitation. Fortunately, this is usually not the case. Even if internal tendon degeneration is a significant etiology of rotator cuff pain, it appears that it may be self-limiting and that a well-reasoned approach to rotator cuff rehabilitation often results in a satisfactory outcome. With this in mind, we treat patients with suspected intrinsic degeneration of the rotator cuff with our standard external anatomic impingement protocol. The difference, however, is that these patients are usually in an older age group than the standard anatomic impingement patients, and therefore they have a tendency to not be as compliant with their rehabilitation protocol. With this in mind, we must often modify the protocol to include more frequent follow-ups with a physical therapist. It is often necessary to continue anti-inflammatory medications on a long-term basis, as opposed to the usual 3 to 6 weeks. In addition, a modification of offending activities is in order in these patients if long-term relief is to be obtained.

CONCLUSION

So, what's the bottom line in shoulder rehabilitation. The vast majority of patients who present to our office having previously undergone "shoulder rehabilitation" have not experienced a therapeutic benefit. Most of these patients are treated (with hot packs, massage, and ultrasound), given a bill, and sent home. It is rare that we see a patient who actually had a functional exercise program prescribed, who understood the etiology of their shoulder pain, and knew the goals of their rehabilitation program. In our study of the conservative management of impingement syndrome, nearly 40% of our patients had been seen and treated elsewhere with physical therapy to no avail. The fact that a patient had failed with a physical therapy protocol elsewhere had no bearing on their response to our protocol. Overall, we had a 70% satisfactory outcome rate with conservative management where previous treatment had apparently failed. The program described is simple, inexpensive, and quick and therefore has a relatively high compliance rate as far as rehabilitation protocols go. If a patient fails to comply with the program, however, the solution is usually not surgery, because if the patient fails to comply with a treatment protocol designed to keep him out of the operating room, he is unlikely to cooperate in a satisfactory rehabilitation protocol after the fact.

REFERENCES

1. Bigliani LU, Morrison DS. Relationship between acromial morphology and rotator cuff tears. *Orthopaedic Transactions.* 1986; 10:216.
2. Sher JS, Uribe JW, Posada A, Murphy BL. Abnormal MRI scans in shoulders of asymptomatic patients. *Orthopaedic Transactions.* 1993; 17:1025.
3. Keyes EL. Observations on rupture of the supraspinatus tendon: Based upon a study of 73 cadavers. *Ann Surg.* 1933;97:849-856.
4. Codman EA, Akerson IB. The pathology associated with rupture of the supraspinatus tendon. *Ann Surg.* 1931;93:348.
5. Cotton RE, Rideout DF. Tears of the humeral rotator cuff. *J Bone Joint Surg Br.* 1964;46:314-328.
6. Morrison DS, Rosen MA. Correlation of acromial morphology and the results of arthroscopic subacromial decompression. In: Post, Morey, Hawkins, eds. *Surgery of the Shoulder.* 1991.
7. Morrison DS, Frogameni A. Conservative management of impingement syndrome. *J Shoulder Elbow Surg.* 1993;2:22-23.
8. Olsewski JM, Depew A. Arthroscopic subacromial decompression and rotator cuff debridement for stage II and stage III impingement. *Arthroscopy.* 1994;10:61-68.
9. Zvijac JE, Lemak LJ, Levy HJ. Arthroscopic subacromial decompression in the treatment of full thickness rotator cuff tears—A three to six year follow up. *J Shoulder Elbow Surg.* 1994;2:13.
10. Kurokawa M, Hirasawa Y. Arthroscopic subacromial decompression for rotator cuff tears. *J Shoulder Elbow Surg.* 1933;2:46.
11. Montgomery TJ, Yerger B, Savoie FH III. Management of rotator cuff tears: A comparison of arthroscopic debridement and surgical repair. *J Shoulder Elbow Surg.* 1994;3:70-71.

Chapter 19

Conservative Management of Rotator Cuff Tears

Dana G. Seltzer, Paolo Kechele, Carl Basamania, and Charles A. Rockwood, Jr.

Although most orthopaedic surgeons recognize the desirability of initially treating shoulder impingement syndrome conservatively, there has been a reluctance to manage rotator cuff defects nonoperatively. There is an abundance of literature describing operative treatment of impingement syndrome and rotator cuff tears, but there is a glaring lack of scientific articles discussing the conservative management of these conditions. To our knowledge, no randomized prospective study comparing conservative treatment of rotator cuff tears to operative management has been published in the English literature.

The purpose of this chapter is to review the literature concerning nonoperative management of rotator cuff tears, describe the philosophy of the senior author (CAR) for the treatment of rotator cuff defects, discuss its rationale, and outline our protocol for the conservative management of rotator cuff tears.

LITERATURE REVIEW

The orthopaedic literature is replete with both data and theories that serve as the foundation for the design rationale of a specific conservative rehabilitation program for the treatment of symptomatic rotator cuff disease. At the same time, this data supports the hypothesis that a conservative treatment program should provide effective treatment of rotator cuff defects in many patients. Several categories of supportive literature can be identified: (1) rotator cuff degeneration is a natural phenomenon of aging that frequently results in the production of rotator cuff defects, many of which are asymptomatic; (2) biomechanical theories may explain why some rotator cuff lesions are symptomatic and others are not; (3) conservative treatment programs have provided satisfactory results for many patients with rotator cuff defects, though reported results are variable; (4) degenerative processes within the glenohumeral joint are not commonly seen despite the prevalence of rotator cuff defects; (5) acromioplasty, in association with rotator cuff debridement, can provide satisfactory results for the treatment of full-thickness rotator cuff defects; and (6) persistent rotator cuff defects are commonly noted after rotator cuff repair.

Neer originally described the shoulder impingement syndrome as a continuum of disease progressing from inflammation and edema to fibrosis, with the final stage being acromial spurring and full-thickness rotator cuff tears.[1,2] He empirically stated that approximately 95% of the rotator cuff tears in his practice could be attributed to chronic impingement syndrome.[3] Ogata and Uhthoff, based upon the analysis of 76 autopsy specimens, disagreed with Neer and stated that rotator cuff tears were more likely the result of an intrinsic degenerative tendinopathy, rather than secondary to chronic impingement.[4] We believe that both tendon degeneration and impingement play significant roles in the development of most rotator cuff tears.

Numerous cadaver studies have documented high incidences of rotator cuff defects in the elderly, with increasing prevalence directly correlated to advancing age.[2,5–15] Reported incidences of full-thickness defects range from 5%[24] to 40%[12] and are largely dependent upon the age group being studied. If partial-thickness defects are included, one report describes rotator cuff lesions in 73% of patients greater than 70 years of age,[12] and another report documents an incidence of nearly 100% in individuals over 70 years of age.[6–8] This suggests that there is a normal degenerative process that occurs naturally with aging, and it implies that many rotator cuff defects remain asymptomatic and never come to the attention of an orthopaedic surgeon. In fact, Pettersson reported arthrographically proven rotator cuff defects in nearly 50% of asymptomatic subjects between the ages of 55 and 85 years.[11]

Theories to account for the numerous asymptomatic tears include the "suspension bridge model" proposed by Burkhart.[16–19] Burkhart has arthroscopically and anatomically described a "rotator crescent" and a "rotator cable" that span the supraspinatus and infraspinatus insertions into the greater tuberosity of the humeral head. He has proposed that the cable acts as a suspension bridge, so that rotator cuff defects occurring within the crescent would not have a tendency to propagate. This theory is based on the assumption that the cable is the support structure upon which rotator cuff function is based, and the premise that balanced force couples in both the coronal (deltoid versus inferior rotator cuff) and transverse (anterior versus posterior rotator cuff) planes allows the shoulder to function asymptomatically despite a rotator cuff defect. Burkhart proposed three kinematic patterns of function: stable, unstable, and fixed fulcrum kinematics. He further proposed that patients presenting with painful shoulders despite good strength and normal range of motion (stable kinematics) be subjected only to subacromial decompression rather than rotator cuff repair to alleviate their pain. We would go further and recommend that these patients be treated with a conservative treatment program, as a similar result is likely to be achieved.[20]

McLaughlin described five reasons for avoidance of early rotator cuff repair, and he advised early repair only for rotator cuff tears associated with grossly displaced tuberosity fractures and massive rotator cuff avulsions where the need for repair was obvious from the initial patient encounter.[21] He pointed out that approximately 25% of cadavers had torn or degenerated rotator cuffs, many of which he felt must have been asymptomatic. He also stated that his clinical experience showed that around 50% of patients with rotator cuff defects would spontaneously recover comfortable and useful shoulder function with time. He also commented that acute defects of the rotator cuff should be considered chronic from the moment they occur, because of the degenerative tendon tissue generally involved in the defect. He mentioned this as the primary reason for late repairs offering similar end results to acute repairs. In addition, he stated that the diagnosis of a rotator cuff lesion could be misleading initially because of the associated pain, and he felt that early surgery carried a higher risk of being an unnecessary operation.

Rowe stated that "the majority of (rotator cuff) lesions should respond satisfactorily to conservative measures consisting of: A) instructing the patient to use his shoulder in a way to avoid repetitious irritation of the rotator cuff tendon, and B) moist heat, pendulum exercises, and occasional subacromial injection of the shoulder with corticosteroids."[22] He mentioned two exceptions to this basic rule: (1) the proven complete avulsion in the young adult and (2) the complete avulsion in the elderly patient associated with disabling pain that does not respond to conservative treatment.

It is clear that rotator cuff defects can be a different entity in young adults, as opposed to elderly patients. Rotator cuff defects may result from violent trauma such as motor vehicle accidents in young or middle-aged adults, and these injuries should not be treated as equivalent to the ruptured degenerative cuff defects that are classically seen in the elderly patient with chronic impingement. However, this is a much less common injury, comprising only 8% of rotator cuff injuries in a large series of patients treated at the Mayo Clinic (Rochester, MN),[23] and Neer stated that less than 5% of rotator cuff tears occur in this younger population.[3]

We do not subscribe to management schemes that promote early treatment of acute defects in the elderly population to prevent "retraction, scarring, tendon edge degeneration, and muscle atrophy,"[24] as we have observed that the restoration of full passive range of motion and subsequent placement on a strengthening program consistently provides these patients with satisfactory results.[20]

Itoi and Tabata retrospectively reported their results for the conservative treatment of 62 arthrographically documented rotator cuff tears in 54 patients treated over a 10-year period and followed for a minimum of 1 year (range = 1 to 9 years).[25] During this same time period, they operated on 196 shoulders in 188 patients with rotator cuff pathology, while treating 124 shoulders in 114 patients conservatively (39%). Their indications for surgical intervention were (1) patients less than 30 years of age, (2) middle-aged patients engaged in physical labor, and (3) middle-aged or elderly patients whose symptoms persisted or were aggravated by a course of conservative treatment. They described their conservative treatment program as "various combinations of rest, anti-inflammatory agents, and local injection of analgesic with or without steroid." Once the symptoms had subsided, active and passive range of motion and strengthening exercises were initiated. The investigators achieved satisfactory results in 82% of their study patients, noting that patients with good range of motion prior to starting treatment had significantly better results than those patients who initially had markedly decreased range of motion and strength. They reported an apparent diminution of results with time, noting that patients followed more than 6 years had significantly worse outcomes at final follow-up when compared to patients with less than 6-year follow-up. In addition, patients experiencing symptoms for less than 1 year prior to treatment fared better than those with more prolonged pretreatment symptoms.

Samilson and Binder reported their short term follow-up results on 194 shoulders in 181 patients treated conservatively, only 41 of whom had reasonable follow-up, and compared these results with 33 shoulders in 33 patients treated operatively.[26] They achieved good or excellent results in 59% of patients treated conservatively compared with the 84% of satisfactory outcomes in patients treated operatively. This study is greatly marred by the deficiency in documentation of rotator cuff tears and the lack of clinical follow-up data.

Nonoperative treatment results reported by other investigators have included success rates ranging from 33%[27] to 92%.[28] Wolfgang reported improvement in only 33% of patients,[27] whereas Takagishi found satisfactory results in 44% of patients with conservative treatment.[29] Brown reported return of full function in 87% of rotator cuff tear patients treated with a conservative program if they initially had full abduction.[30] These cuff defects were not documented, and it seems likely that some of these patients may not have had full-thickness defects. However, even in patients with profound weakness consistent with large rotator cuff defects, Brown achieved satisfactory outcomes in 53%. Tabata and colleagues documented the highest published rate of recovery from conservative management (92%).[28]

In our experience, the presence of massive rotator cuff defects does not necessarily imply eventual progression to "cuff tear arthropathy."[31] We believe that the term "cuff tear arthropathy" describes a disease entity in which the rotator cuff defect is only a small factor in a multifactorial disease process.[32]

This specific rehabilitation program is effective in relieving symptoms of rotator cuff defects caused by chronic impingement for the same reasons it gives satisfactory results in the treatment of stage II shoulder impingement. Maintenance of depressive and compressive forces supplied by the remaining rotator cuff muscles, as well as strengthening of other shoulder girdle muscles with depressive action, is necessary to prevent excessive superior migration of the humeral head during abduction and forward flexion.[33] Posterior capsular stretching and the preservation of a normal passive range of motion are important to diminish static restraints that contribute to the development of impingement symptoms in patients with rotator cuff lesions.[34] The contribution of impaired scapular rotation to impingement symptoms is minimized by strengthening the scapular rotators.[35]

The senior author has reported on his long term follow-up results of patients undergoing debridement of irreparable, degenerative lesions of the rotator cuff.[36] The vast majority of these patients achieved satisfactory results that have not diminished over time. We strongly believe that a good two-stage acromioplasty[37] and the specific rehabilitation protocol outlined here are responsible for the relief of symptoms in these patients. Other investigators have also reported good results for debridement of full-thickness rotator cuff defects,[16,18,38] although one of these investigators reported a decline in results with time.[39] The performance of an adequate subacromial decompression or acromioplasty provides an environment that allows the patient to comfortably complete the specific rehabilitation program, which is primarily responsible for the control of the symptoms of rotator cuff disease. Results will deteriorate with time if patients do not maintain their passive range of motion and/or omit the maintenance strengthening program. However, resumption of the specific program will generally result in resolution of the recurrent symptoms.

Several investigators have reported satisfactory results in patients with persistent or recurrent rotator cuff defects after rotator cuff repair.[40–42] Examination of the postoperative rotator cuff repair reveals that there is no correlation between symptom relief and the integrity of the repair at follow-up. We must infer from these reports that an intact rotator cuff is not necessary for a pain-free, functional shoulder, and we believe that these patients have satisfactory outcomes because an adequate acromioplasty was performed and the patient was placed and maintained on a specific rehabilitation program postoperatively.

The orthopaedic literature, while not providing much direct evidence that a specific conservative rehabilitation program is effective in the treatment of patients with rotator cuff defects, does contain significant evidence to support the hypothesis that a conservative approach should be effective in treating many patients with full-thickness rotator cuff defects. Our clinical results concur with this hypothesis.[20]

CONSERVATIVE TREATMENT PHILOSOPHY AND PROTOCOL

Our basic treatment philosophy is based on the tenet that the majority of rotator cuff defects are the result of a degenerative process within the tendon combined with chronic impingement that can naturally occur with aging. It is for this reason that the senior author has treated his patients with rotator cuff problems and/or the shoulder impingement syndrome with a conservative rehabilitation program.

During the initial visit, the diagnosis of a rotator cuff lesion or shoulder impingement syndrome is established, based upon the patient history, physical examination, and standard AP, axillary, and 30° caudal tilt radiographs. Patients with rotator cuff defects generally have more profound weakness of external rotation, are usually older, and frequently have more limited range of motion. Specific rotator cuff stress radiographs, such as a strap view, can be helpful in differentiating the two conditions if standard radiographs exhibit a normal acromio-humeral distance. In patients with defects in the rotator cuff, active abduction against a strap around the trunk and arms causes superior migration of the humeral head in the rotator cuff deficient shoulder.[45] We do not routinely obtain specialized secondary radiographic studies (arthrogram, ultrasound, CT-arthrogram, or MRI) to confirm or rule out the diagnosis of a rotator cuff tear, because the presence or absence of a tear does not change our treatment plan. Although the differentiation in diagnosis does not change our treatment plan, the course of rehabilitation for rotator cuff defects is frequently more rocky and the length of treatment significantly longer than for shoulder impingement syndrome.[44]

There are several exceptions to this basic treatment philosophy. The first is the young, 20- to 30-year-old, active patient with an acute tear and severe functional deficit resulting from violent trauma. The second exception is the middle-aged, 30- to 50-year-old, active patient who has an acute tear of the rotator cuff secondary to violent trauma. Patients from these two scenarios presenting with suspected acute rotator cuff tears should initially be evaluated with an arthrogram and are best treated with early operative rotator cuff repair. The third exception is the highly competitive athlete, particularly one who is involved in overhead or throwing sports. They should also be treated more aggressively, because repair is essential for restoration of the normal strength required to return these athletes to the same competitive level as prior to a rotator cuff injury. A fourth exception is the middle-aged or elderly patient who does not respond to the conservative rehabilitation program outlined. Secondary studies of the rotator cuff are not necessary in this group, as the performance of an adequate acromioplasty to relieve impingement is the most important step of the operative procedure. Excision of the bursa allows evaluation of the rotator cuff after completion of the acromioplasty, and rotator cuff lesions in patients with satisfactory rotator cuff tendon tissue should be repaired if possible. Patients with poor quality tendons or massive, retracted defects that cannot be mobilized for repair are better treated with rotator cuff debridement in combination with an adequate acromioplasty. It has been the observation of the senior author that the results of surgery are more dependent upon the adequacy of the acromioplasty and the postoperative rehabilitation, than the handling of the rotator cuff lesion.

A specific rehabilitation protocol is the mainstay of our conservative treatment program. We personally instruct each of our patients in the exercise program described below, and each patient is given a home therapy kit which includes elastic bands (Therabands) of six different colors and strengths, a pulley set, and a three-piece, 1-meter-long stick (Fig. 19–1). To accompany the kit, patients receive a fully illustrated handbook with all the exercises, anatomical drawings, and definitions of related terms and a demonstration videotape to remind them how to perform the exercises. The program is tailored to each individual patient, altering the basic core program as necessary to fit the needs of that patient. We ask the patients to do all the work on their own while at home, at work, or when travelling. The simplicity of the therapy kit and its compact nature facilitate this process. We caution our patients never to push their therapy to the point of causing discomfort. The senior author has coined the term "Orthotherapy" to describe this program, which is an interactive exchange between the patient and the treating orthopaedic surgeon aimed at creating an exercise regimen that initially gently improves motion and then gradually improves strength in the shoulder girdle. We ask the patients to call us directly if problems arise during their rehabilitation, so that adjustments in the program can be made quickly, which avoids down-time and minimizes setbacks.

Nonsteroidal anti-inflammatory medications are generally used for a brief period of time (3 to 4 weeks) as an adjunctive treatment to help control inflammation and allow commencement of the exercise program without further aggravating the condition. We do not use other treatment modalities, such as phonophoresis or iontophoresis, for the treatment of impingement syndrome or rotator cuff lesions. These treatments necessitate visits to a therapy facility, and we have not found them to be essential in effective treatment. However, we do recommend that prior to each rehabilitation session all of our patients use moist heat. The rare patient that is unable to comfortably initiate the passive range of motion aspect of the treatment program may be a candidate for an injection of a local anesthetic and occasionally a corticosteroid preparation. Again, the sole purpose of this injection is to control local inflammation and allow for the conservative treatment program to be undertaken. We like to limit the total number of steroid injections to three, and we prefer to have at least a 2- to 3-month span between injections.

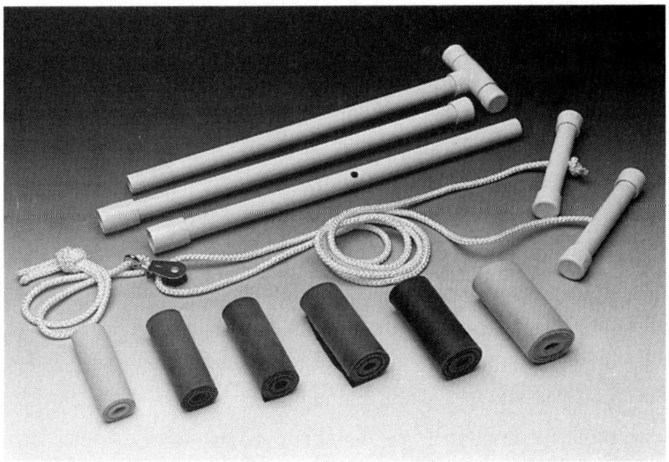

Fig. 19–1. The home-therapy kit is comprised of a pulley set, elastic Therabands, and a three-piece 1-meter stick. The pulley set includes a rope with two handles, whose length can be adjusted, plus a pulley and a hook that can be attached over the top of a door. Strips of six different elastic bands (Therabands) of variable resistance are included, and should have their ends tied together to form a loop that can be fitted around a fixed object, such as a door handle. The 1-meter stick is composed of three separate sections for easy storage, and one portion contains a "T" handle that fits into the palm of the affected extremity. A full set of exercise instructions is given to each patient, along with a videotape demonstrating the proper form for each exercise, and a fully illustrated text with anatomical drawings delineating each individual exercise.

THE ORTHOTHERAPY PROGRAM

PHASE ONE

The goal of the initial phase of our Orthotherapy program is to restore full, painless passive range of motion to the affected shoulder (Fig. 19–2). Codman pendulum exercises gently maintain glenohumeral motion and are supplemented by passive forward flexion, abduction, extension, internal rotation, and external rotation exercises using the 1-meter stick. Passive elevation is enhanced by the use of a pulley system, employing the unaffected extremity as the motor power. Forward flexion, abduction, and external rotation can be performed in the supine position to diminish the effects of gravity, or to use gravity to the patient's advantage for increasing passive range of motion. Other exercises initiated during this phase include wall walking, posterior capsular stretches, door hanging, and gentle stretching of the shoulder by hanging from the top of a door or from an overhead bar. Patients are asked to avoid actively using their affected extremity in the impingement arc, above 70° of elevation. However, they are encouraged to continue using their arm below shoulder level to perform simple activities of daily living. We have found moist heat, in the form of a hot shower or a hot and moist thick folded towel that is covered with a plastic wrap and placed beneath a heating pad, to be effective in enhancing patient comfort for the

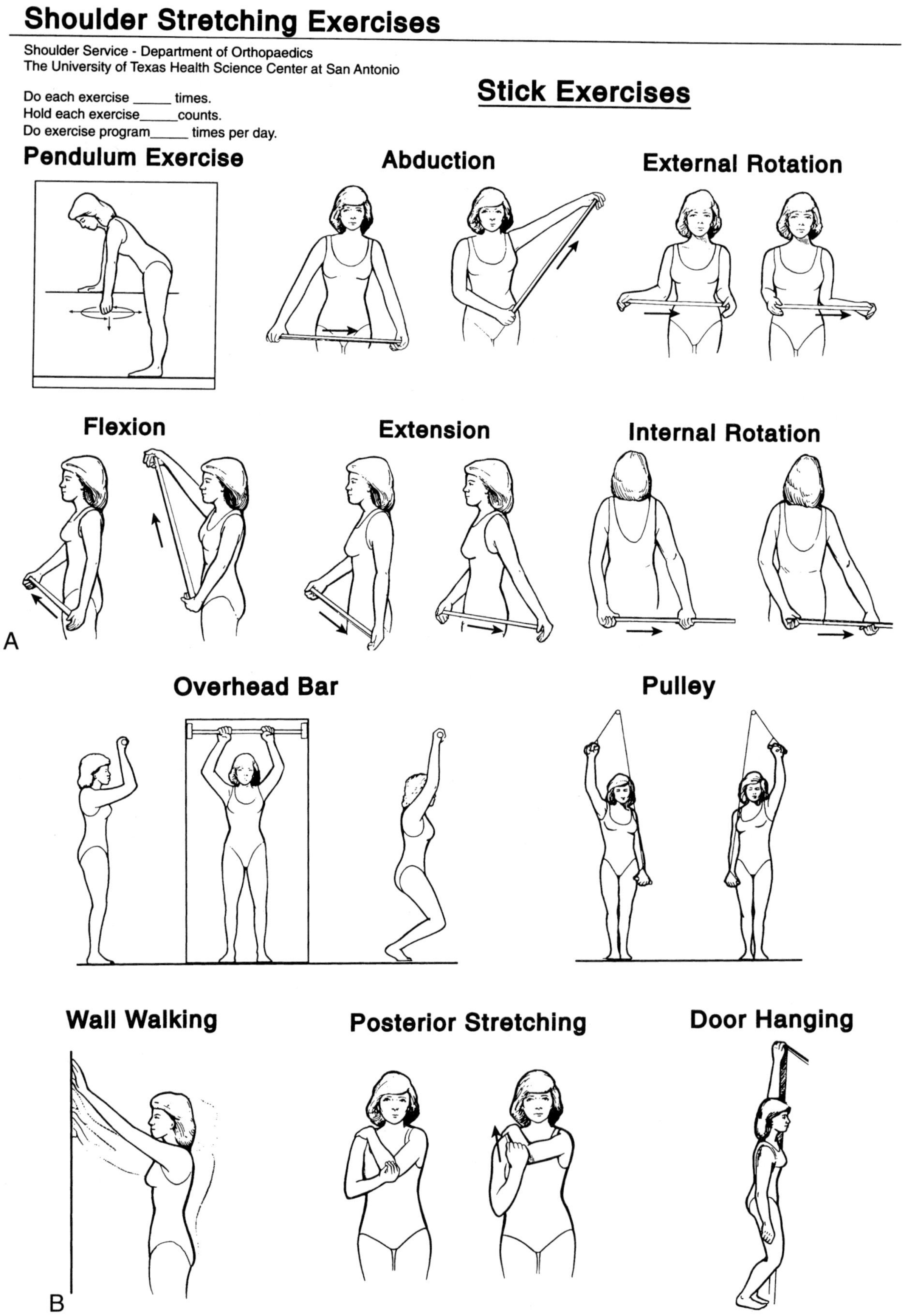

Fig. 19–2. The shoulder stretching exercises include the gentle pendulum exercises, stick exercises, use of the overhead pulley, the posterior capsular stretch, wall walking, and the more advanced stretching exercises using a door or an overhead bar.

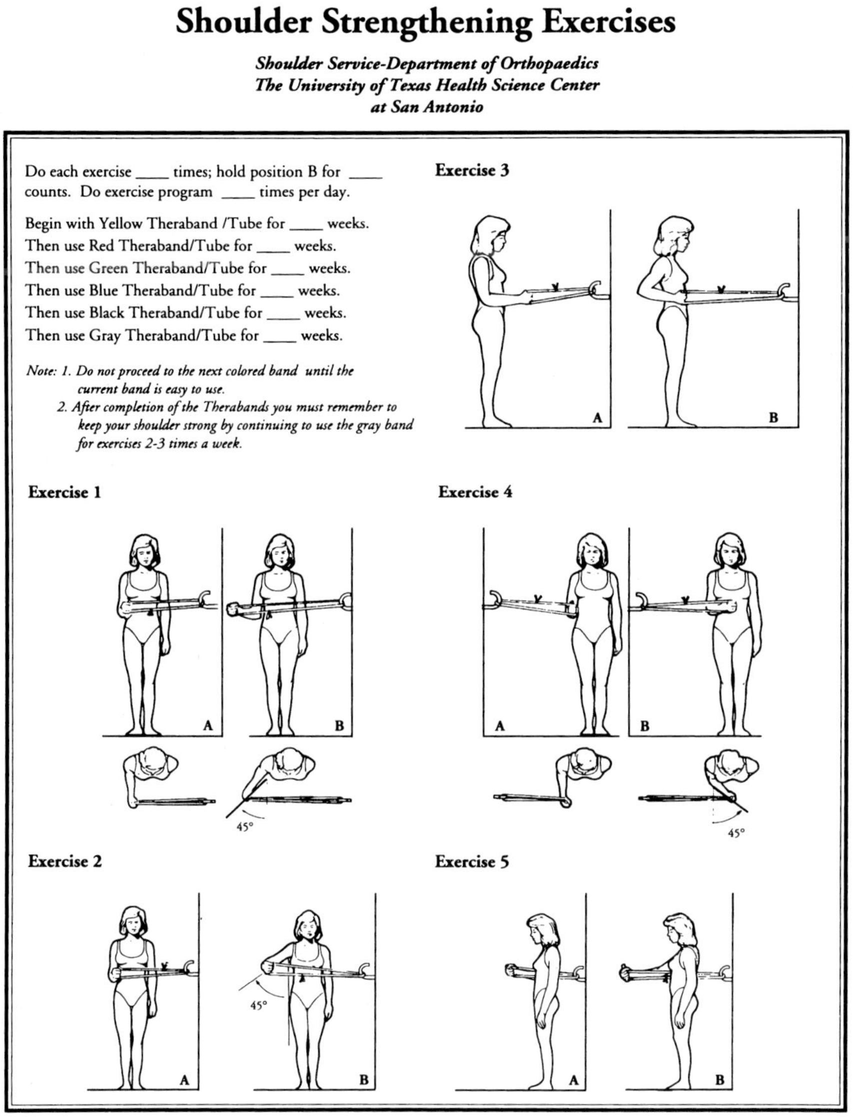

Fig. 19–3. The shoulder strengthening program is designed to improve strength in the remaining rotator cuff, as well as improving strength of the deltoid. The five Theraband exercises provide resistance against internal and external rotation, abduction, extension, and forward flexion in order to strengthen the rotator cuff muscles and the three distinct portions of the deltoid muscle. The pulley set can be wall mounted and used with free weights after patients have worked their way through all six levels of Therabands (see Fig. 19–4).

performance of the exercise program. Ice diminishes inflammation when applied to the sore shoulder after activities or therapy sessions. It is not unusual for patients to require 4 to 6 weeks to restore a functional passive range of motion.

PHASE TWO

When the passive range of motion is greatly improved, functional, or near normal and comfortable, patients are advanced to the second phase of the Orthotherapy program. A group of exercises designed to strengthen the remaining muscles of the rotator cuff, scapular stabilizers, and the deltoid are added to the program (Figs. 19–3 through 19–5). These exercises are not a substitute for the range of motion exercises, and it is important that patients continue to work on maintaining their passive range of motion once it is achieved. We have used Therabands (Hygenic, Akron, OH) to build strength in the muscle groups of the shoulder girdle. These are elastic bands that are manufactured in six different colors, representing six different levels of resistance. The elastic material is purchased in 6-inch-wide rolls that are cut into strips 5 feet long and 3 inches wide. The ends of each strip are tied in a knot to form a loop that the patient can place over a fixed object (e.g., a door handle). The patient can then pull or push against the resistance of the band to perform each of the five exercises shown in Figure 19–3. These bands provide resistance against active external rotation, internal rotation, abduction, extension, and forward flexion. Each of these exercises is started with the elbow flexed 90° and the shoulder in the neutral position of 0° forward flexion, abduction, and external rotation. The exercises move through an arc of approximately 45° in each of the five planes of motion. Some patients are unable to perform one specific exercise comfortably from 0 to 45°, so the exercise range may have to be modified (e.g., from 0 to 15°). If one specific exercise is too painful even after modification, it can be eliminated entirely. The anterior deltoid is the most im-

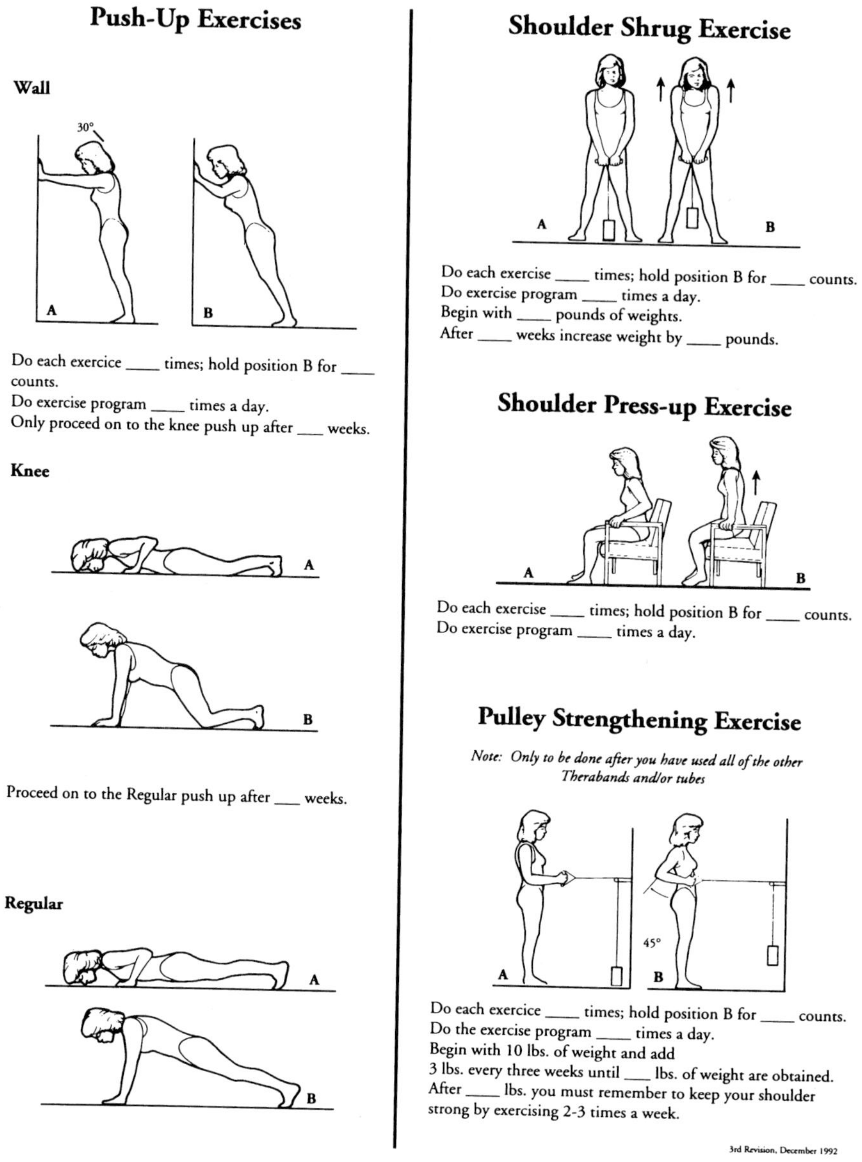
Push-Up Exercises
Wall
30°
A
B
Do each exercice ___ times; hold position B for ___ counts.
Do exercise program ___ times a day.
Only proceed on to the knee push up after ___ weeks.
Knee
A
B
Proceed on to the Regular push up after ___ weeks.
Regular
A
B
Shoulder Shrug Exercise
A
B
Do each exercise ___ times; hold position B for ___ counts.
Do exercise program ___ times a day.
Begin with ___ pounds of weights.
After ___ weeks increase weight by ___ pounds.
Shoulder Press-up Exercise
A
B
Do each exercise ___ times; hold position B for ___ counts.
Do exercise program ___ times a day.
Pulley Strengthening Exercise
Note: Only to be done after you have used all of the other Therabands and/or tubes
45°
A
B
Do each exercice ___ times; hold position B for ___ counts.
Do the exercise program ___ times a day.
Begin with 10 lbs. of weight and add
3 lbs. every three weeks until ___ lbs. of weight are obtained.
After ___ lbs. you must remember to keep your shoulder strong by exercising 2-3 times a week.
3rd Revision, December 1992

Fig. 19–4. The scapular stabilizer muscles are strengthened with the use of push-ups, shoulder shrugs, and shoulder press-ups.

portant muscle of the shoulder girdle, and special emphasis must be placed on strengthening this muscle. Decreased anterior deltoid strength greatly limits function of the shoulder, and any activity in front of the patient becomes extremely difficult. Anterior deltoid dysfunction, in combination with rotator cuff deficiency, allows the humeral head to migrate anteriorly and superiorly during forward flexion, which causes severe impingement and pain. Therefore emphasis is also placed on strengthening the scapular stabilizers (serratus anterior, rhomboids, latissimus dorsi, and trapezius), as these muscles play a very important role in the rotator cuff deficient shoulder.

Exercises to improve the strength of the scapular stabilizers include shoulder press-ups, shoulder shrugs, and push-ups. Shoulder press-ups are performed in an arm chair, raising the torso off the seat of the chair. These exercises improve strength in the latissimus dorsi muscles, which have a depressive effect on the humerus. Shoulder shrugs are performed initially with 10 lbs of weight, and the weight can gradually be increased. This gives improved strength in the trapezius, which allows for better compensatory scapular rotation, thereby protecting the humeral head from impingement in abduction. Push-ups progress from wall push-ups to knee push-ups, and then military push-ups. The improved serratus anterior and rhomboid strength gained from these exercises prevents scapular winging, which can accompany any chronic shoulder disorder. Patients with specific weakness of the anterior deltoid will benefit from a special supine exercise. These exercises gradually increase the strength of the anterior deltoid.

We emphasize to our patients that we do not believe in the "no pain, no gain" theory of therapy and stress that we follow a "no pain" theory of treatment. Patients should perceive a stretching sensation while performing the exercises, but should not experience pain during the routine performance of the exercise program. If the pa-

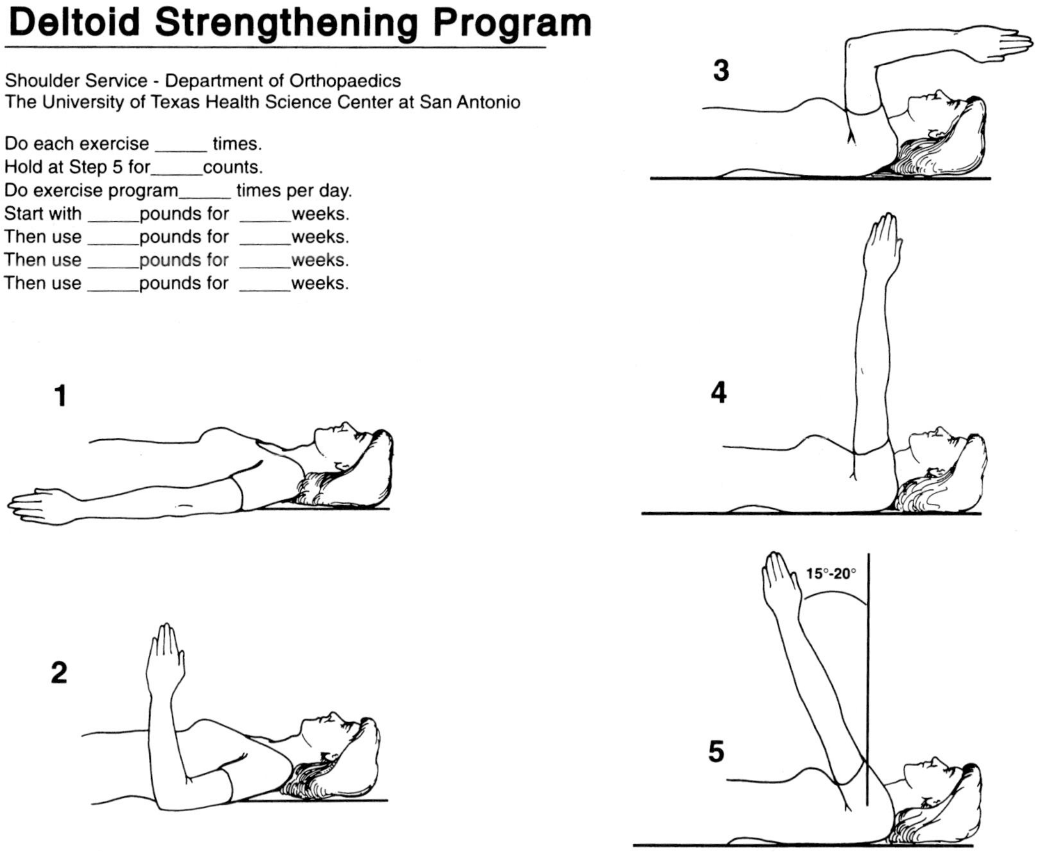

Fig. 19–5. Good anterior deltoid strength is required for functional use of the shoulder, so patients with specific weakness of the anterior deltoid are given a supine exercise designed to improve their strength with minimal discomfort, by diminishing the effect of gravity.

tients complains of pain, their exercise program must be modified to eliminate the pain. Patients are initially asked to perform the complete set of exercises 3 times per day, doing one set of five repetitions for each exercise. Spreading the exercises out over the entire day helps patients avoid overuse and allows them to complete the entire program in about 15 minutes. We give our patients guidelines with respect to time for the progression from one level of band to the next, but we tell the patients that they should not advance to the next level unless the level they are working at has become easy for them. If they progress to the next level and experience pain during exercise, we ask them to drop back down a level. Most patients with rotator cuff defects require a minimum of 3 months to complete the second phase of therapy.

PHASE THREE

The last phase of the treatment program involves the reintegration of patients back into their normal activities including work, hobbies, and sports. Patients should be gradually reimmersed in these activities and monitored closely during their return for recurrence of symptoms. When patients feel better and return to normal activities, there is a natural tendency to gradually abandon the rehabilitation program. Patients must be encouraged to remain on a maintenance exercise program, and occasional emphatic reminders are often necessary. This maintenance program should be performed 3 times per week, and it should include both the range of motion and strengthening exercises.

SUMMARY

Differences in success rates for conservative treatment of rotator cuff tears have largely been attributed to differences in selection criteria for operative intervention. It is expected that more stringent criteria for conservative treatment would lead to a larger percentage of satisfactory final outcomes. However, our clinical experience has shown us that strict attention to the details of a program specifically designed to treat rotator cuff pathology can give successful end results without significant deterioration over time for the vast majority of middle-aged and elderly patients with rotator cuff defects. We attribute our success to initiating and maintaining our patients on the Orthotherapy program, which has been designed for patient compliance. It is a simple yet effective program and requires a minimal amount of patient effort and time commitment in order to obtain satisfactory results. The control of the rehabilitation by the treating orthopaedic surgeon eliminates the need for the patient to leave their home or job to receive rehabilitation, allows the surgeon to customize the program to attain the desired goals for each individual patient, and is cost effective.

A well-designed, conservative treatment program will provide satisfactory return of function and alleviation of pain for the vast majority of patients with rotator cuff tears secondary to chronic impingement. Surgeons should not be hasty to commit their patients to operative treatment for rotator cuff tears, unless the tear is the result of violent trauma in a young, active adult, and a massive avulsion of the rotator cuff is suspected and then documented. The conservative Orthotherapy treatment program outlined in this chapter has been highly successful in the handling of this clinical condition in our patient population.

We have used this Orthotherapy program for the past 12 years and have been extremely satisfied with the results. A recent review of our patients has reinforced the senior author's philosophy that strengthening of the deltoid and scapular stabilizers and the remaining muscles of the rotator cuff can provide a successful result without surgery.

ACKNOWLEDGMENT

This research was performed by the Shoulder Service at the University of Texas Health Science Center in San Antonio.

REFERENCES

1. Neer CS. Anterior acromioplasty for the chronic impingement syndrome in the shoulder. *J Bone Joint Surg Am.* 1972;54:41–50.
2. Neer CS. Impingement lesions. *Clin Orthop.* 1983;173:70–77.
3. Neer CS. Cuff tears, biceps lesions, and impingement. In: Neer CS, ed. *Shoulder Reconstruction.* Philadelphia: WB Saunders; 1990:41–142.
4. Ogata S, Uhthoff HK. Acromial enthesopathy and rotator cuff tear. A radiologic and histologic postmortem investigation of the coracoacromial arch. *Clin Orthop.* 1990;254:39–48.
5. Cotton RE, Rideout DF. Tears of the humeral rotator cuff: A radiological and pathological necropsy survey. *J Bone Joint Surg Br.* 1964; 46:314–328.
6. DePalma AF. *Surgery of the Shoulder.* 3rd ed. Philadelphia: JB Lippincott; 1983.
7. DePalma AF, Callery G, Bennett GA. Variational anatomy and degenerative lesions of the shoulder joint. In: *Instructional Course Lectures.* Ann Arbor: JW Edwards; 1949:255–281.
8. DePalma AF, White JB, Callery G. Degenerative lesions of the shoulder joint at various age groups which are compatible with good function. In: *Instructional Course Lectures.* Ann Arbor: JW Edwards; 1950:168–180.
9. Grant JCB, Smith CG. Age incidence of rupture of the supraspinatus tendon. *Anat Rec.* [abstract] 1948;100:666.
10. Keyes EL. Observations on rupture of the supraspinatus tendon: Based upon a study of 73 cadavers. *Ann Surg.* 1933;97:849–856.
11. Pettersson G. Rupture of the tendon aponeurosis of the shoulder joint in anterior inferior dislocation. *Acta Chir Scand.* (Supp.) 1942; 77:1–184.
12. Uhthoff HK, Loer J, Sarkar K. The pathogenesis of rotator cuff tears. In: Takagishi N, ed. *The Shoulder.* Tokyo: Professional Postgraduate Services; 1987:211–212.
13. Wilson CL. Lesions of the supraspinatus tendon: Degeneration, rupture, and calcification. *Arch Surg.* 1943;46:307–325.
14. Wilson CL, Duff GL. Pathologic study of degeneration and rupture of the supraspinatus tendon. *Arch Surg.* 1943;47:121–135.
15. Zuckerman JD, Kummer FJ, Cuomo F, et al. The influence of coracoacromial arch anatomy on rotator cuff tears. *J Shoulder Elbow Surg.* 1992;1:4–14.
16. Burkhart SS. Arthroscopic treatment of massive rotator cuff tears. Clinical results and biomechanical rationale. *Clin Orthop.* 1991; 267:45–56.
17. Burkhart SS. Fluoroscopic comparison of kinematic patterns in massive rotator cuff tears. A suspension bridge model. *Clin Orthop.* 1992;284:144–152.
18. Burkhart SS. Arthroscopic debridement and decompression for selected rotator cuff tears. Clinical results, pathomechanics, and patient selection based on biomechanical parameters. *Orthop Clin N Am.* 1993;24:111–123.
19. Burkhart SS, Esch JC, Jolson RS. The rotator crescent and rotator cable: an anatomic description of the shoulder's "suspension bridge." *Arthroscopy.* 1993;9:611–616.
20. Basamania C, Seltzer DG, Kechele P, Rockwood CA. The conservative management of rotator cuff tears. Manuscript in preparation, 1994.
21. McLaughlin HL. Rupture of the rotator cuff. *J Bone Joint Surg Am.* 1962;44:979–983.
22. Rowe CR. Ruptures of the rotator cuff: Selection of cases for conservative treatment. *Surg Clin N Am.* 1963;43:1531–1540.
23. Cofield RH. Current concepts review. Rotator cuff disease of the shoulder. *J Bone Joint Surg Am.* 1985;67:974–979.
24. Matsen FA, Arntz CT. Rotator cuff tendon failure. In: Rockwood CA, Matsen FA, eds. *The Shoulder.* WB Saunders; Philadelphia, 1990:647–677.
25. Itoi E, Tabata S. Conservative treatment of rotator cuff tears. *Clin Orthop.* 1992;275:165–173.
26. Samilson RL, Binder WF. Symptomatic full thickness tears of the rotator cuff: An analysis of 292 shoulders in 276 patients. *Orthop Clin N Am.* 1975;6:449–466.
27. Wolfgang GL. Surgical repair of tears of the rotator cuff of the shoulder. Factors limiting the result. *J Bone Joint Surg Am.* 1974; 56:14–26.
28. Tabata S, Kida H, Takahara M, et al. A comparative study of nonsurgical treatment and surgical treatment of complete tears of the rotator cuff. In: Takagishi S, ed. *The Shoulder.* Tokyo: Professional Postgraduate Services; 1987:241.
29. Takagishi N. Conservative treatment of ruptures of the rotator cuff. *J Jpn Orthop Assn.* 1978;52:781–787.
30. Brown JT. Early assessment of supraspinatus tears. Procaine infiltration as a guide to treatment. *J Bone Joint Surg Br.* 1949;31:423–425.
31. Neer CS, Craig EV, Fukuda H. Cuff-tear arthropathy. *J Bone Joint Surg Am.* 1983;65:1232–1244.
32. Williams GR, Rockwood CA. Massive rotator cuff defects in glenohumeral arthritis. In: Friedman RJ, ed. *Arthroplasty of the Shoulder.* New York: Thieme; 1994:204–214.
33. Altchek DW, Schwartz E, Warren RF, et al. Radiologic measurement of superior migration of the humeral head in impingement syndrome. *Orthop Trans.* 1990:14:250.
34. Matsen FA, Arntz CT. Subacromial impingement. In: Rockwood CA, Matsen FA, eds. *The Shoulder.* Philadelphia: WB Saunders; 1990: 623–646.
35. Speer KP, Garrett WE. Muscular control of motion and stability about the pectoral girdle. In: Matsen FA, Fu FH, Hawkins RJ, eds. *The Shoulder: A Balance of Mobility and Stability.* Rosemont: American Academy of Orthopaedic Surgeons; 1993: 159–172.
36. Rockwood CA, Williams GR, Burkhead WZ. Management of Patients with massive rotator defects by acromioplasty and rotator cuff debridement. *Orthop Trans.* 1988;12:190–191.
37. Rockwood CA, Lyons FR. Shoulder impingement syndrome: Diagnosis, radiographic evaluation, and treatment with a modified Neer acromioplasty. *J Bone Joint Surg Am.* 1993; 75:409–424.
38. Levy HJ, Gardner RD, Lemak LJ. Arthroscopic subacromial decompression in the treatment of full-thickness rotator cuff tears. *Arthroscopy.* 1991;7:8–13.
39. Zvijac JE, Lemak LJ, Levy HJ. Arthroscopic subacromial decompression in the treatment of full thickness rotator cuff tears: a three to six year follow-up. Presented at American Academy of Ortho-

paedic Surgeons annual meeting. San Francisco, CA, February, 1993.

40. Blauth W, Gartner J. Postoperative results of arthrography following suturing of ruptured rotator cuff. *Orthopade.* 1991;20:262–265.
41. Harryman DT, Mack LA, Wang KA, et al. Repairs of the rotator cuff: Correlation of functional results with integrity of the cuff. *J Bone Joint Surg Am.* 1991;73:982–989.
42. Wulker N, Melzer C, Wirth CJ. Shoulder surgery for rotator cuff tears. Ultrasonographic three-year follow-up of 97 cases. *Acta Orthop Scand.* 1991;62:142–147.
43. Bloom RA. The active abduction view: A new manoeuvre in the diagnosis of rotator cuff tears. *Skel Radiol.* 1991;20:255–258.
44. Frogameni AD, Morrison DS, Woodworth P. *Conservative treatment for subacromial impingement syndrome.* Presented at American Academy of Orthopaedic Surgeons annual meeting. San Francisco, CA, February, 1993.

Section 6

Arthroscopic Management of Rotator Cuff Disease

Chapter 20

Arthroscopic Subacromial Decompression, Arthroscopic-Assisted (Mini-Open) Rotator Cuff Repair, and Arthroscopic Cuff Repair

Evan J. Bachner and Stephen J. Snyder

The field of shoulder arthroscopy has undergone a rapid evolution over the past 20 years. Shoulder arthroscopy was first described by Burman[1] as early as 1931 and again by Takagi[2] in 1935. Wiley and Older developed arthroscopic techniques on cadaver shoulders in 1972 and 1973 and subsequently used these techniques on patients.[3] The arthroscope was initially used in this joint for diagnostic purposes only. However, with the explosion of technology used for surgical arthroscopy in the knee, there has been a corresponding increase in operative arthroscopy of the shoulder as well.

Numerous investigators have published techniques and results of various arthroscopic procedures in the shoulder. Arthroscopic subacromial decompression was popularized by Ellman[4] and has been studied and refined by others.[5–13] Subacromial decompression and debridement of labral tears and rotator tears are now widely performed arthroscopically. More recently, subacromial decompression has been accomplished arthroscopically followed by a mini-open repair of the rotator cuff with a lateral deltoid-splitting incision.[8,13–16] Johnson has pioneered arthroscopic fixation of rotator cuff tears;[17] his technique employs a metallic staple. Bioabsorbable staples are now available. Although Wilson has recently reported excellent results in his series,[18] he is discontinuing his use of a metal staple, because a second operation was often required to remove the implant. Wolf[19] has used a suture anchor with a suture hook for arthroscopic repair of rotator cuff tears with absorbable sutures, performing a tendon-to-tendon repair and at times supplementing that with a tendon-to-bone repair. Bartlett has used a suture anchor with a permanent suture that is placed through the cuff into bone.[20]

We have been using a new technique for arthroscopic fixation of rotator cuff tears, which involves suture screw anchors placed into bone with permanent mattress sutures. For partial-thickness flap tears, we have been repairing these arthroscopically as well.

There are obviously numerous good techniques described for performing arthroscopic shoulder surgery. We will however, confine this chapter to the techniques that we are currently using.

Anatomy

Prior to operating on the shoulder for impingement syndrome and rotator cuff lesions, it is imperative to understand both the bony anatomy and the soft-tissue anatomy. In our patient population, most patients have a MRI performed preoperatively (see Chapter 5) and all patients have a supraspinatus outlet or arch view to carefully assess the shape and of the acromion, as well as its thickness, particularly in the anterior third. We use the classification system proposed by Morrison and Bigliani,[21] which includes three acromial types based on the contour of the anterior inferior surface.

ACROMION GEOMETRY

Type I: flat acromial undersurface (Fig. 20–1).
Type II: curved acromial undersurface paralleling the humeral head.
Type III: hooked acromion, one with an anterior osteophyte or beak that narrows the supraspinatus outlet.

In addition, we feel that a preoperative assessment of the acromial thickness of the anterior third is critical to performing an adequate decompression without risking acromial fracture. The modified acromial classification of Snyder and Wuh[22] considers the thickness of the anterior third of the acromion measured at the intersection of the anterior and middle thirds in addition to the morphology of the undersurface. The letters A, B, and C supplement the Morrison and Bigliani types I, II, and III.

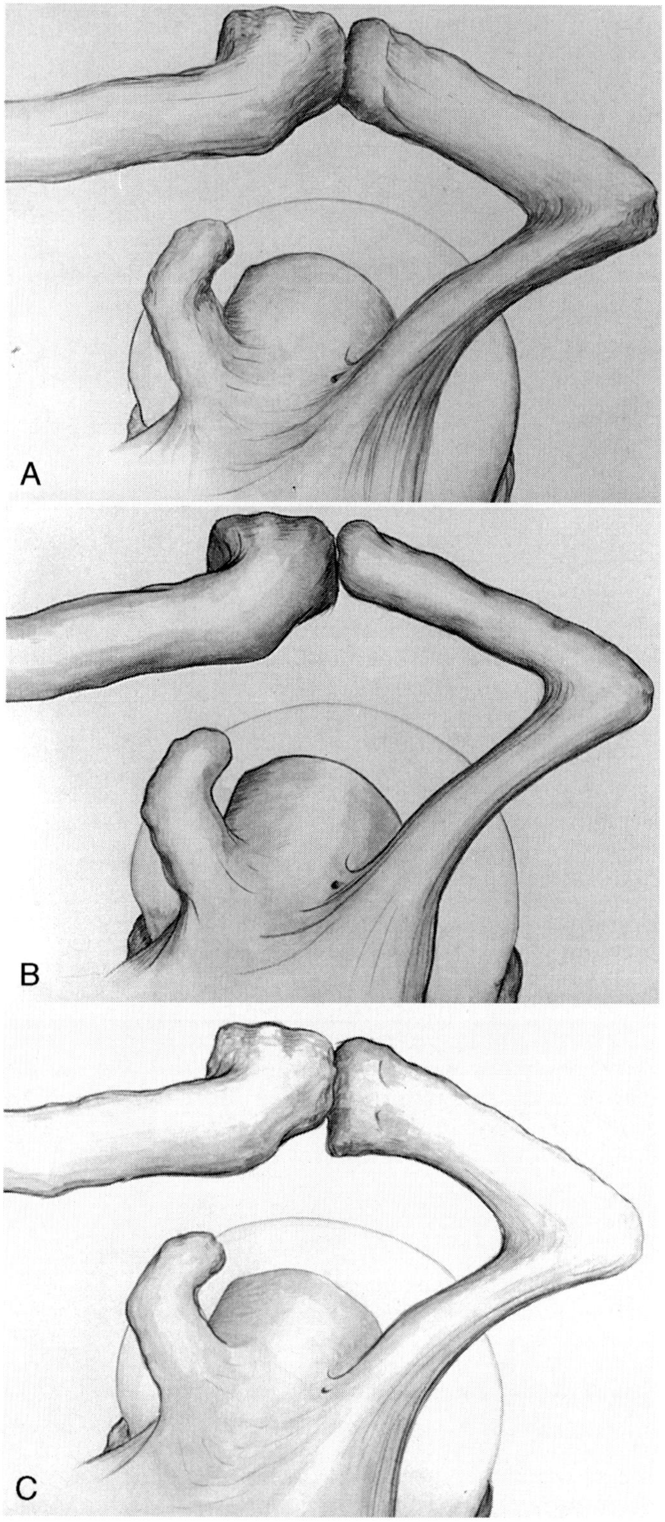

Fig. 20–1. Acromial arch morphology: *A,* type I arch, flat *B,* type II arch, curved; and *C,* type III arch, hooked with the presence of an anterior spur.

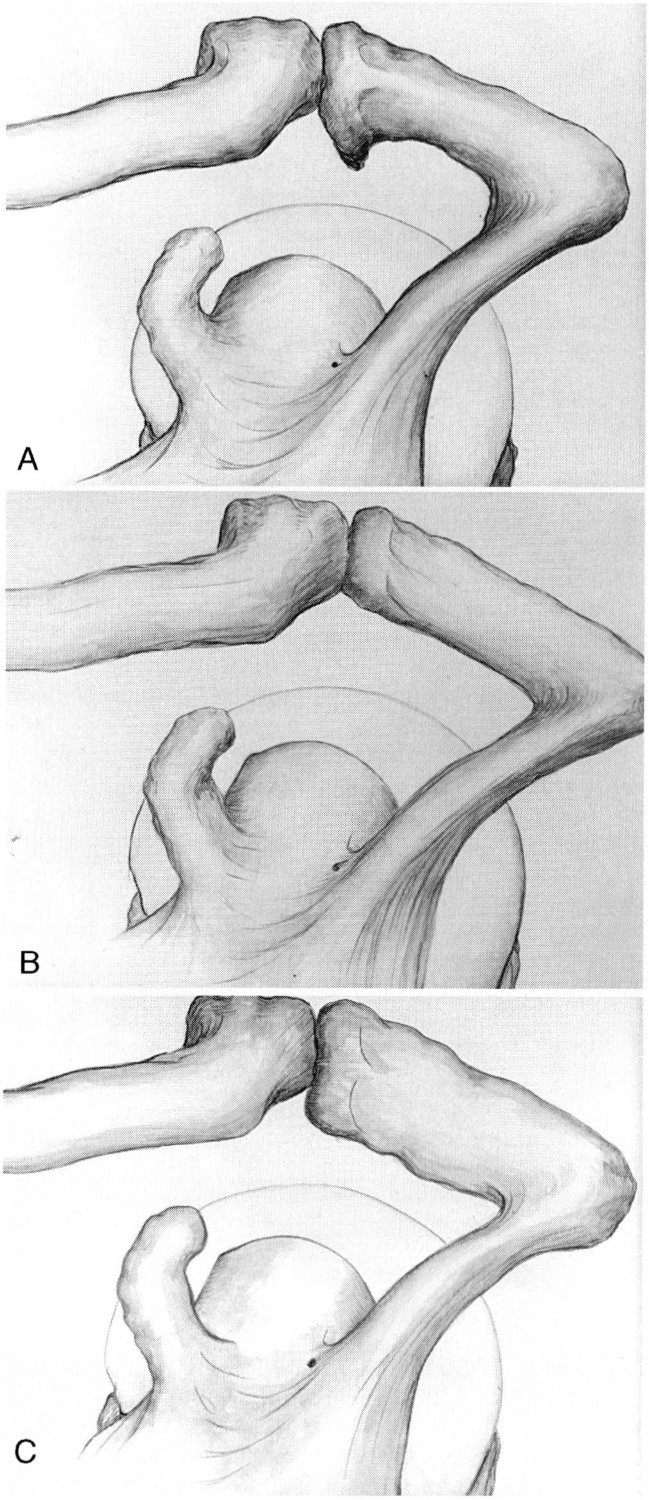

Fig. 20–2. Acromial thickness: *A,* type A arch, acromion less than 8-mm thickness. *B,* type B arch, acromion between 8- and 12-mm thickness, and *C,* type C arch, acromion greater than 12-mm thickness.

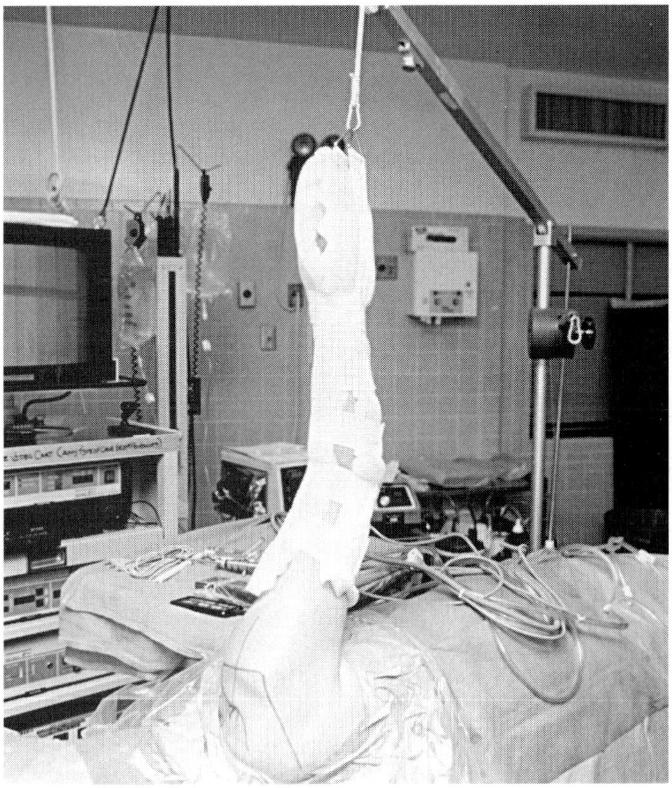

Fig. 20–3. The standard lateral decubitus arthroscopic position with the torso tilted 30° posteriorly. The arm is in 70° of abduction, 20° of forward flexion, and supported with the sterilized foam traction unit (STaR Sleeve, Arthrex, Naples, FL) attached to the shoulder suspension device (Arthrex).

ACROMION THICKNESS

Type A: thin acromion, < 8 mm thick at the intersection of the anterior and middle thirds (Fig. 20–2)
Type B: average thickness, between 8 to 12 mm
Type C: thick acromion, > 12 mm

Extra care must be taken in a patient with a thin acromion to avoid iatrogenic acromial fracture.

GLENOHUMERAL JOINT EVALUATION

Positioning

The patient is placed in the lateral position, tilted 30° posteriorly from the vertical (Fig. 20–3). The arm is positioned in 70° of abduction and 20° of forward flexion, with 10 lbs of traction applied through a sterile STaR foam sleeve (Arthrex, Naples, FL). All bony prominences are padded and the patient is secured in this position with a bean bag and kidney rests.

Portals

Three standard portals for shoulder arthroscopy are used: posterosuperior, anterosuperior, and lateral (Fig. 20–4). We create a posterior portal in the soft spot approximately 2 cm inferior and 1 to 2 cm medial to the posterolateral corner of the acromion after distending the joint with saline. The anterior portal is created by visualizing the area just inferior to the biceps tendon. A portal is made by removing the arthroscope while holding the cannula in place and inserting a taper-tipped rod

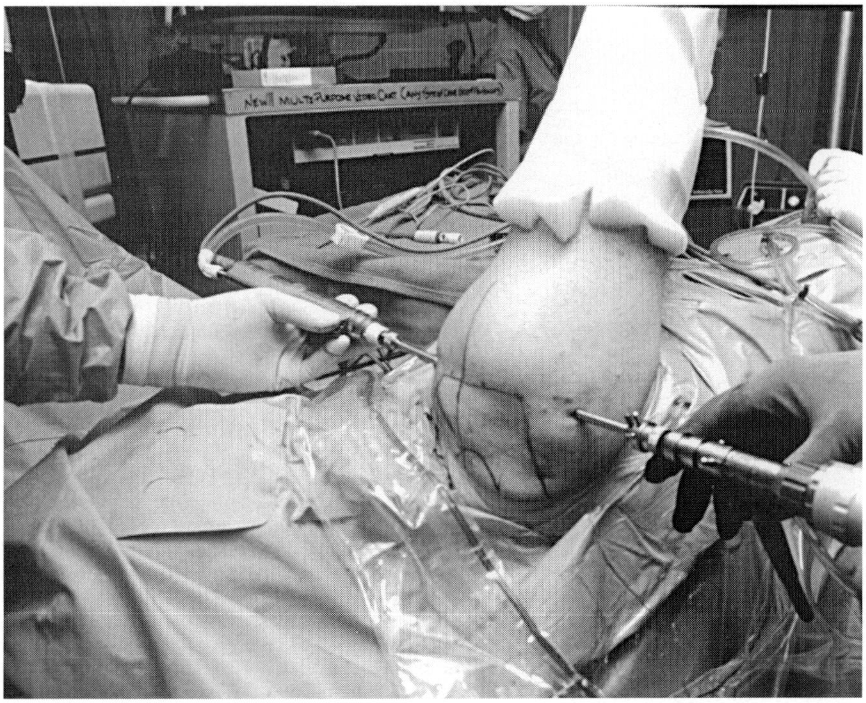

Fig. 20–4. Standard portals for glenohumeral arthroscopy include the posterosuperior (right) and anterosuperior (left).

Table 20–1. Anatomic Review

Posterior Portal Placement
1. Biceps tendon—from the rotator cuff interval to the attachment at the superior glenoid tubercle
2. Posterior labrum and posterior capsule
3. Inferior recess
4. Glenoid articular surface
5. Supraspinatus tendon portion of the rotator cuff and its insertion into the humerus.
6. Posterior cuff tendons in the humeral head bare area
7. Articular surface of the humeral head including the area of Hill-Sachs lesions
8. Subscapularis recess, superior glenohumeral ligament, subscapularis tendon, and the middle glenohumeral ligament crossing it at a 45° angle
9. Middle glenohumeral ligament attachment to the anterosuperior labrum
10. Inferior glenohumeral ligament and inferior labrum
Anterior Portal Placement
11. Posterior capsule and labrum
12. Posterior rotator cuff both superior and inferior to the biceps tendon including the infraspinatus and teres minor tendons
13. Anterior glenoid labrum and glenohumeral ligaments
14. Subscapularis tendon, bursa, and recess (a hiding spot for loose bodies)
15. Attachment of the subscapularis tendon to the humeral head, anterior humeral articular cartilage and anterior surface of the biceps tendon.

through the cannula, tenting the anterior skin, and making a skin incision near the rod. The anterior cannula is then inserted over the rod. The lateral portal is usually established at the time of bursoscopy in line with the supraspinatus tendon. The portal is made approximately 2 cm lateral to the midlateral border of the acromion on a line beginning at the posterior edge of the AC joint and extending perpendicular to the lateral border of the acromion. The operating cannula, with a blunt trochar, is directed through the deltoid muscle and underlying submuscular bursal layer into the subacromial space.

Arthroscopic Examination

A complete systematic examination of the glenohumeral joint space is performed using a 15-point evaluation system previously described[23] (Table 20–1 and Fig. 20–5). The insertion of the supraspinatus tendon located posterior to the passage of the biceps tendon is visualized. If a cuff lesion is noted, then a 4.5-mm shaver is inserted through the anterior portal to debride frayed edges of the rotator cuff. This technique aids in the visualization of the remainder of the joint and allows further assessment of the cuff lesion. The cuff is palpated from the articular side and can also be palpated from the bursal side with a blunt probe inserted through the lateral portal. Additionally, a suture marker can be placed through an area of pathology. An 18-gauge spinal needle is inserted percutaneously near the lateral border of the acromion into the area of the visualized articular cuff defect. A monofilament absorbable suture is then passed

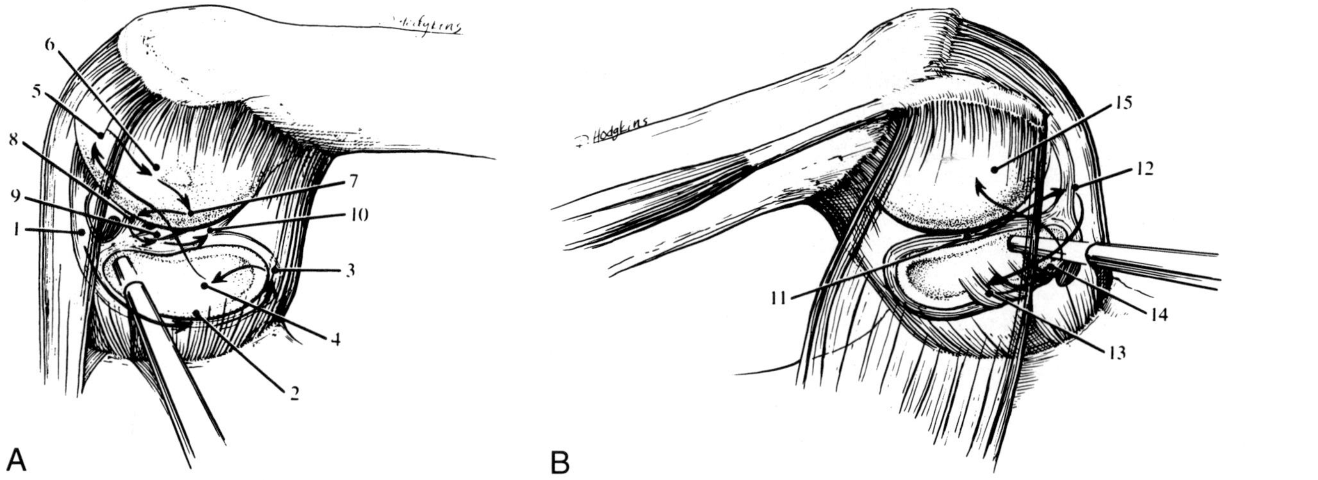

Fig. 20–5. ***A,*** **The 10 steps for the complete evaluation of the shoulder joint from the posterior portal: position 1, biceps tendon; position 2, posterior labrum and posterior capsule attachment to the posterior glenoid; position 3, inferior recess; position 4, glenoid articular surface; position 5, supraspinatus tendon of the rotator cuff and its insertion into the humeral neck; position 6, posterior cuff tendons and the bare area of the humeral head; position 7, articular surface of the humeral head, especially the area of the Hill-Sachs lesion; position 8, subscapularis recess, including the superior glenohumeral ligament, the subscapularis tendon and the middle glenohumeral ligament crossing it at a 45° angle; position 9, middle glenohumeral ligament attachment and the anterosuperior labrum; and position 10, inferior glenohumeral ligament and the inferior labrum.** ***B,*** **The five steps for evaluation of the shoulder from the anterior portal: position 11, posterior capsule and posterior labrum; position 12, posterior aspect of the rotator cuff, both superior and inferior to the biceps tendon; position 13, anterior glenoid neck, labrum, and the glenohumeral ligaments; position 14, subscapularis tendon, subscapularis bursa, and recess; and position 15, attachment of the subscapularis tendon to the humeral head, the anterior humeral articular cartilage, and the anterior surface of the biceps tendon.**

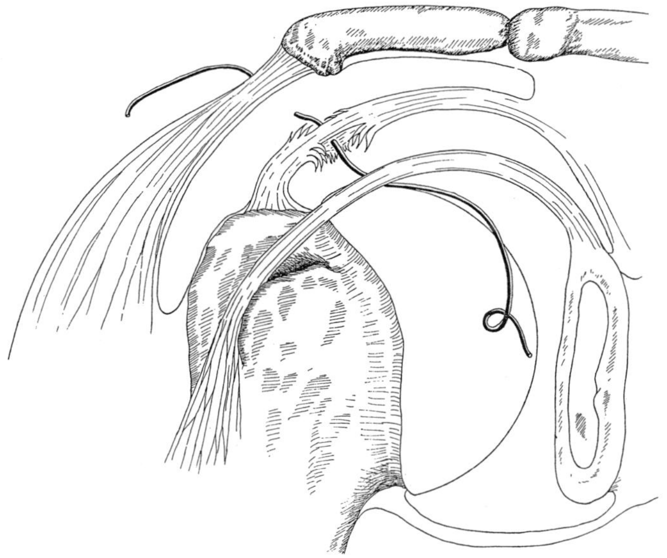

Fig. 20–6. A marker suture of heavy absorbable material, inserted via a percutaneous spinal needle, is used to correlate the articular and bursal surfaces of the rotator cuff.

through the needle and the needle is removed, leaving the suture to help identify the corresponding bursal area of the cuff lesion (Fig. 20–6).

SUBACROMIAL BURSOSCOPY

Positioning

The patient's torso is left in the same position, however the arm is repositioned with the shoulder holder to approximately 15° of abduction and 0° of flexion. The suspension weight is increased to between 12 and 15 lbs (Fig. 20–7).

Bursal Entry

The posterior skin incision is used to gain entry into the bursal space. This is accomplished by advancing the cannula with a blunt trochar subcutaneously to the pos-

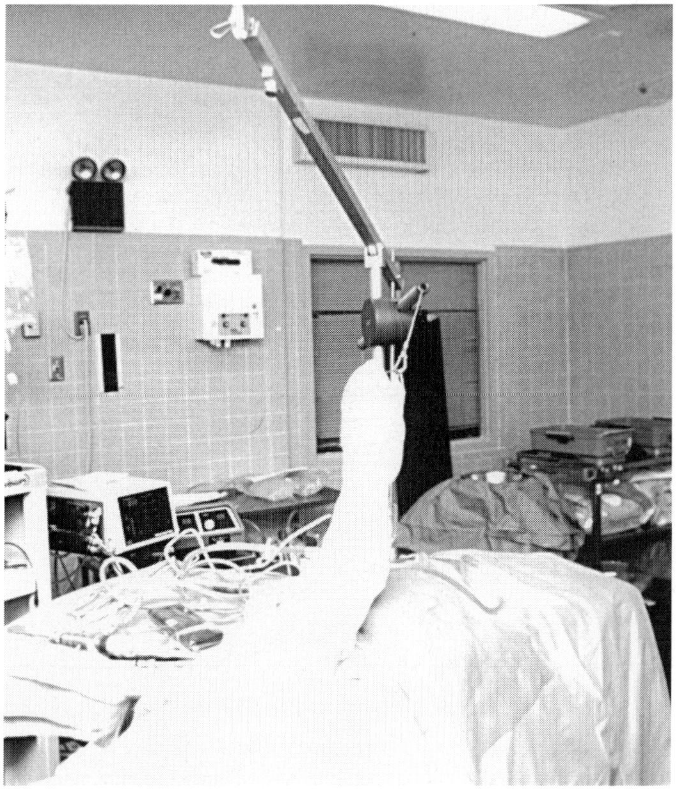

Fig. 20–7. Positioning of the patient for bursoscopy: the arm is moved to 15° abduction and 0° flexion.

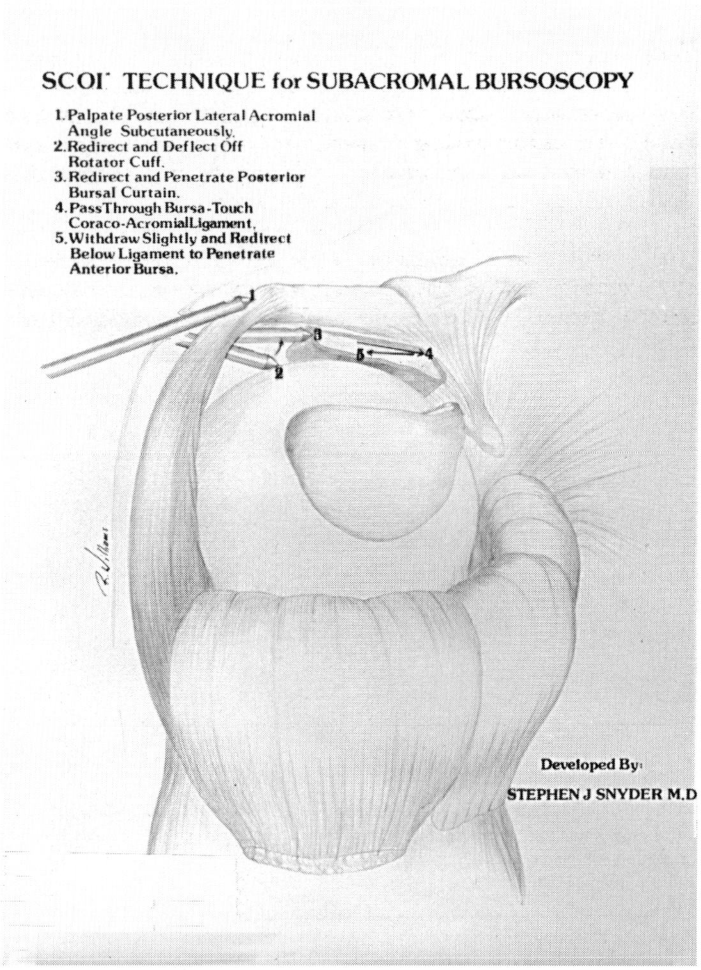

Fig. 20–8. Five steps necessary to ensure accurate placement of the arthroscope in the bursal space.

terolateral edge of the acromion. It is then redirected away from the acromion toward the rotator cuff. Once the cuff is palpated, the cannula is then redirected to penetrate the posterior bursal curtain midway between the cuff and acromion. The cannula is then directed toward the coracoacromial ligament, which is palpated with the trochar tip. It is then withdrawn slightly and advanced toward the anterolateral corner of the acromion to reach the anterior limit of the bursal space (Fig. 20–8). The trochar is removed and a blunt rod is used to puncture the bursal wall anteriorly and exit the original anterior skin incision. An anterior cannula is then inserted over the guide rod.

BURSOSCOPY

A complete bursal anatomy review is then performed as previously described (Table 20–2 and Fig. 20–9). An arthroscopic subacromial decompression and mini-Mumford or Mumford procedure is performed as needed.[16] Excess bursal tissue is removed with a shaver to visualize the cuff surface. The previously placed suture marker is identified, and this area of the cuff is carefully evaluated. If significant fraying or fragmentation is present, debridement is performed to evaluate the extent of the injury.

ROTATOR CUFF TEAR CLASSIFICATION

We use a classification system to methodically document rotator cuff lesions as follows (Fig. 20–10):[13]

SURFACE

A Articular surface tears of the rotator cuff.
B Bursal surface tears.
C Complete tears of the cuff connecting the articular and bursal surfaces.

TEAR SEVERITY

0 Normal cuff with smooth covering of synovium or bursa
1 Superficial synovial or bursal irritation with fraying of the capsule without tendon fiber failure
2 Minimal tendon tearing with capsular fraying < 2 cm in size
3 Moderate disruption of tendon fibers with fraying and fragmentation in an area of up to 2 to 3 cm

Table 20–2. Bursal Anatomy

Posterior Portal
1. Anterior-inferior surface of the acromion and coracoacromial ligament
2. Lateral subdeltoid shelf
3. Tuberosity insertion of the rotator cuff
4. Supraspinatus tendon musculotendinous junction and "critical zone"
5. Medial fat pad beneath the acromioclavicular joint
Anterior Portal
6. Posterior bursal curtain
7. Posterior superior surface of the supraspinatus and infraspinatus tendons
8. Rotator cuff anterior and superior border of the subscapularis tendon

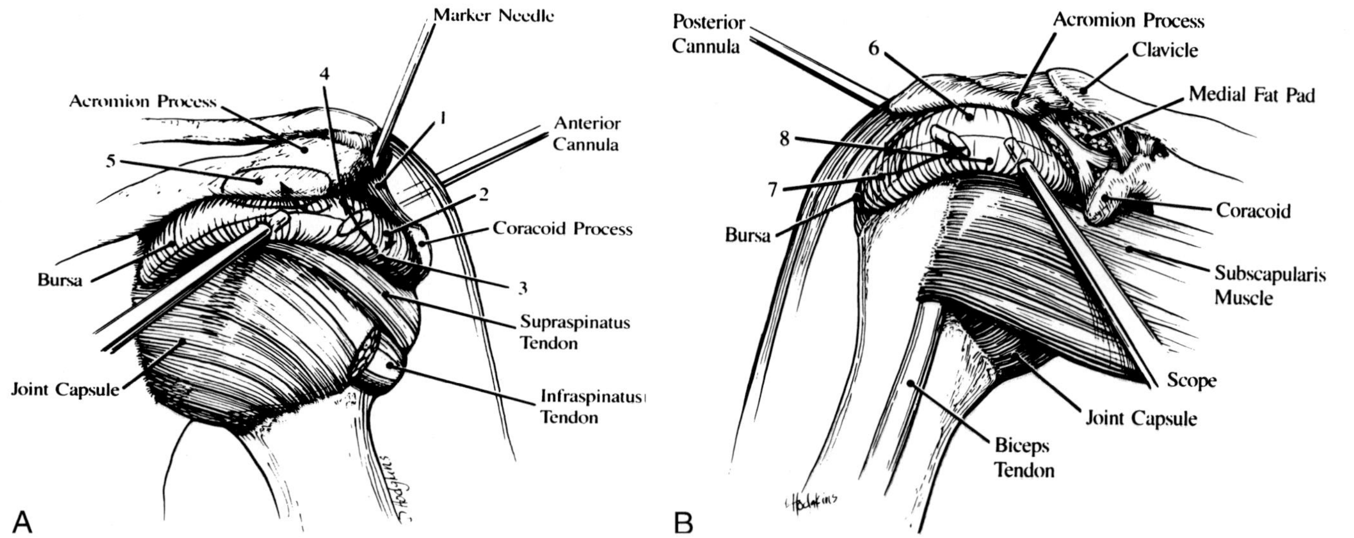

Fig. 20–9. ***A,*** **The five steps for bursoscopic evaluation of the shoulder from the posterior portal: (1) the anterior inferior surface of the acromion and the coracoacromial ligament attachment; (2) the lateral subdeltoid shelf; (3) the tuberosity insertion of the rotator cuff; (4) the supraspinatus tendon "critical zone" and the musculotendinous junction; and (5) the medial fat pad beneath the AC joint.** ***B,*** **The three steps of bursoscopic evaluation of the shoulder from the anterior portal: (6) the posterior bursal curtain; (7) the posterior superior surface of the supraspinatus tendon and the infraspinatus tendon; and (8) the rotator interval area anteriorly and the superior border of the subscapularis tendon.**

4 Severe fraying and fragmentation often with flap formation of cuff tendon in an area of > 3 cm

TEAR LOCATION

SS Supraspinatus tendon
IS Infraspinatus tendon
RI Rotator interval
SbS Subscapularis tendon

ARTHROSCOPIC SUBACROMIAL DECOMPRESSION

The patient is maintained in the bursal position with the body tilted 30° posteriorly from a lateral decubitus position. The body remains in a bean bag with the arm held by a sterile foam traction sleeve in 15° of abduction and neutral flexion. A weight of 12 to 15 lbs is used for suspension of the arm.

Following a complete bursal evaluation, the arthroscope is returned to the posterior portal. An anterior bursal portal is used for an outflow drain. A third bursal portal is developed approximately 2 to 3 cm distal from the lateral acromion in line with the posterior aspect of the AC joint and perpendicular to the lateral border of the acromion (Fig. 20–11). Any debris or bursal tissue that obstructs viewing is removed with a 4.5-mm shaver inserted through an insulated operating cannula with a diaphragm. If not already doing so, the irrigation fluid is switched to a nonconductive irrigant. This can be glycine or glycerol (Synovisol, Baxter Travenol, Deerfield, IL, 2.6% glycerol). While viewing from the posterior portal, an electrosurgical tool is introduced through the lateral portal with a subacromial electrode tip (Linvatec-Concept, Largo, FL). The coracoacromial ligament and other soft tissues are removed first by creating a series of parallel cuts with the electrode starting at the posterior edge of the AC joint extending to the lateral border of the acromion. Perpendicular to these cuts, additional cuts are made with the electrode to create a checkerboard pattern on the undersurface of the acromion (Fig. 20–12). This facilitates removal of the soft tissues with the shaver. An aggressive high-speed shaving blade is then introduced through the lateral operating portal to remove all soft tissue remnants from the anterior undersurface of the acromion. The electrode is then reinserted to coagulate any bleeding vessels and release any remnants of the coracoacromial ligament and bursa from the anterior and lateral edges of the acromion. If necessary, the shaver is reintroduced to further debride the anterior and lateral margins of the anterior third of the acromion to clearly delineate the area of intended decompression. While using the shaver, the outflow through the anterior bursal portal is clamped closed. This is then opened while using the high-speed acromionizer burr with suction off. The bony resection is begun with a high-speed acromionizer or barrel-shaped burr introduced through the lateral operating cannula. The amount of acromial resection is determined based on the arch thickness, with obviously less bone resected for a thinner anterior acromion. The burr is first used to thin the lateral edge of the acromion extending from the area of the operating cannula to the anterolateral corner of the acromion (Fig. 20–13).

A second cut is then made which we call the "orientation trough." This is started at the lateral border of the acromion and is extended medially across the undersurface of the acromion to the posterior aspect of the AC joint. The depth of the orientation trough is again determined by the preoperative arch view. If the acromion is < 8 mm (type A thickness), the trough should be < 1 mm deep. With increasing thickness of the acromion, the trough is deepened appropriately. With a Type C acromion, a trough measuring 3 to 4 mm can be made. During the bony abrasion, outflow through the handpiece is not used. A 5.5-mm cannula connected to a gravity drainage is used to drain all the bony chips from the subacromial space. This provides for maintaining good visualization throughout the decompression without tangling soft tissue in the burr or causing additional bleeding by over-suctioning the space.

After the orientation trough is made, the arthroscope is placed in the lateral portal and the operating cannula is placed in the posterior border. The portal changes are accomplished with switching sticks. First, the shaver is used to remove any bursal tissue obstructing the view and to remove any remaining coracoacromial ligament adjacent to the posterior edge of the orientation trough. The acromionizer burr is then used to flatten the posterior edge of the orientation trough. The burr is used in a sweeping motion from medial to lateral, resecting additional layers of bone in the area in front of the trough. It is helpful to return to the orientation trough in order to assure an appropriate depth of resection and achieve a smooth undersurface of the acromion. The bony resection is continued toward, but not through, the anterior acromial edge. An estimation of the width of anterior bone resection can be made by comparing the known thickness of the acromionizer burr to the remaining anterior acromial lip. The anterior spur is then removed beginning at the inferior edge, and the surface is then smoothed until flat.

The arthroscope is then returned to the posterior portal for a final visual inspection, and any bone or soft tissue still overhanging from the anterolateral corner of the acromion can be removed with a shaver or burr inserted in the lateral portal.

ARTHROSCOPIC MINI-MUMFORD RESECTION OF THE DISTAL CLAVICLE

If either preoperatively or during the subacromial decompression, a bone spur is seen on the undersurface of the AC joint; it should be removed at this time (Fig. 20–14). While viewing from the posterior portal, the electrosurgical tool inserted through the lateral operating cannula is used to incise the AC joint capsule. The shaver is then used to remove the surrounding soft tissue. This is

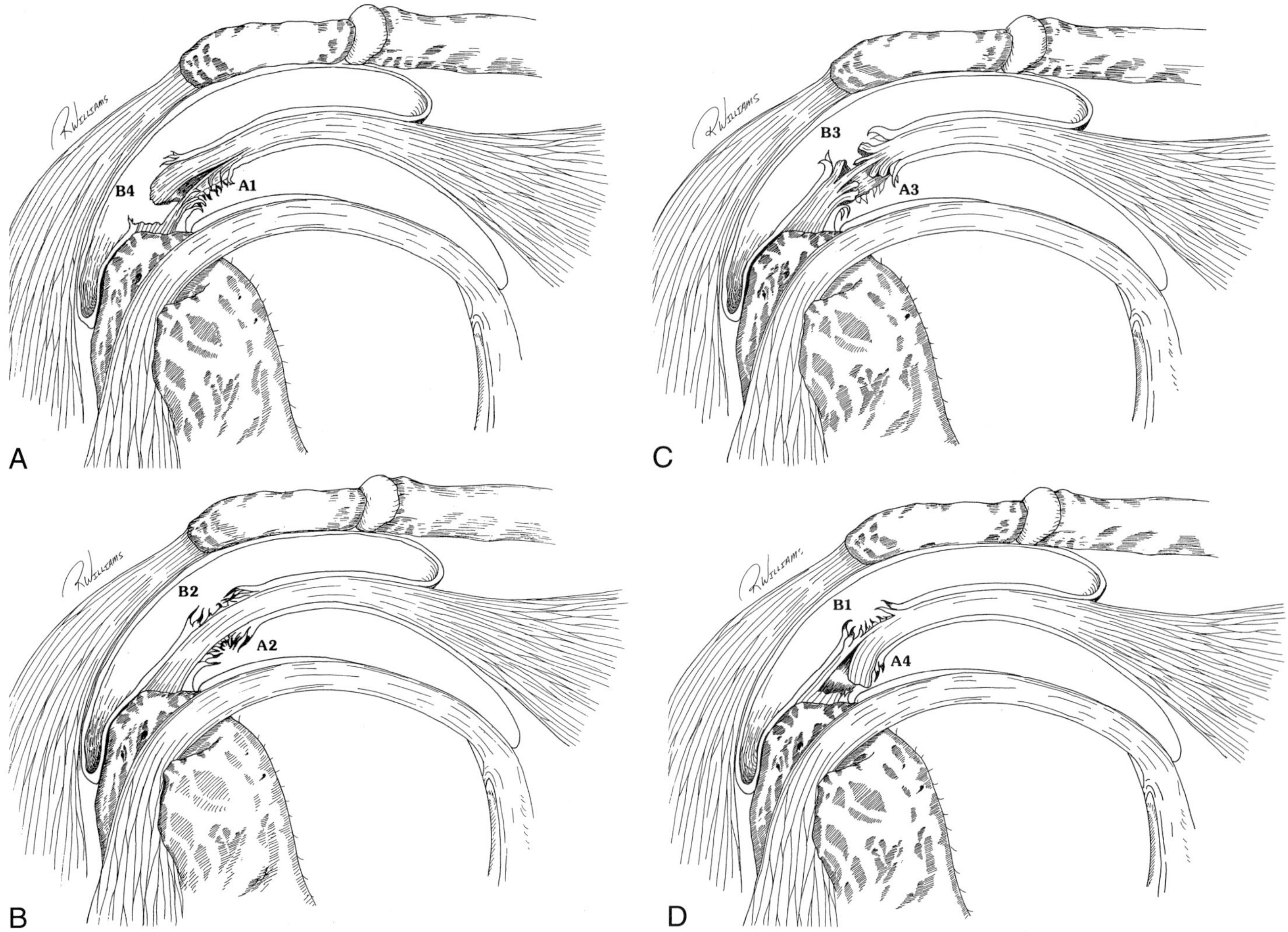

Fig. 20–10. Diagrammatic representation of partial-thickness rotator cuff tears, anterior view: *A,* A1B4C0 rotator cuff tear; *B,* A2B2C0 rotator cuff tear; *C,* A3B3C0 rotator cuff tear; and *D,* A4B1C0 rotator cuff tear. Diagrammatic representation of full-thickness rotator cuff tears, lateral view: *E,* A0B0C1 rotator cuff tear; *F,* A0B0C2 rotator cuff tear; *G,* A0B0C3 rotator cuff tear; and *H,* A0B0C4 rotator cuff tear.

then exchanged for an acromionizer burr, and while draining through the anterior gravity cannula, the clavicular facet of the AC joint can be abraded until it is flush with the undersurface of the acromion. The mini-Mumford resection must extend both anteriorly and posteriorly to the cortices of the clavicle in order to provide for an adequate decompression. The resection is continued medially for approximately 1 cm. Care must also be taken not to stray too far medially to avoid bleeding or division of the coracoacromial ligaments or clavicle fracture.

ARTHROSCOPIC EXCISION OF THE DISTAL CLAVICLE (MUMFORD PROCEDURE)

Resection of the distal 2 cm of the distal clavicle is a well accepted treatment for disease of the AC joint. Traditionally, the distal clavicle resection has been performed through an incision above the AC joint. The muscular fascia is divided and the periosteum is elevated. An osteotome or saw is used to remove the distal clavicle and the soft tissues are repaired as tightly as possible over the defect. The results of this procedure are quite good; however, certain morbidity does exist. The surgical scar can be painful and less than cosmetically ideal. Dimpling or a defect in the area of AC joint resection has been noted. Because of the open procedure and dissection, there may be significant postoperative discomfort and an overnight hospital stay may be required. Additionally, deltoid and trapezius weakness may occur because of detachment during the exposure.

The potential benefits of an arthroscopic resection are smaller, more cosmetic incisions; the capsular ligaments, deltoid attachments, and trapezius attachments are not detached from the superior aspect of the joint, which lessens the risk of instability and defects. This procedure can usually be done as an outpatient, saving time, money, and adding to patient comfort and convenience.

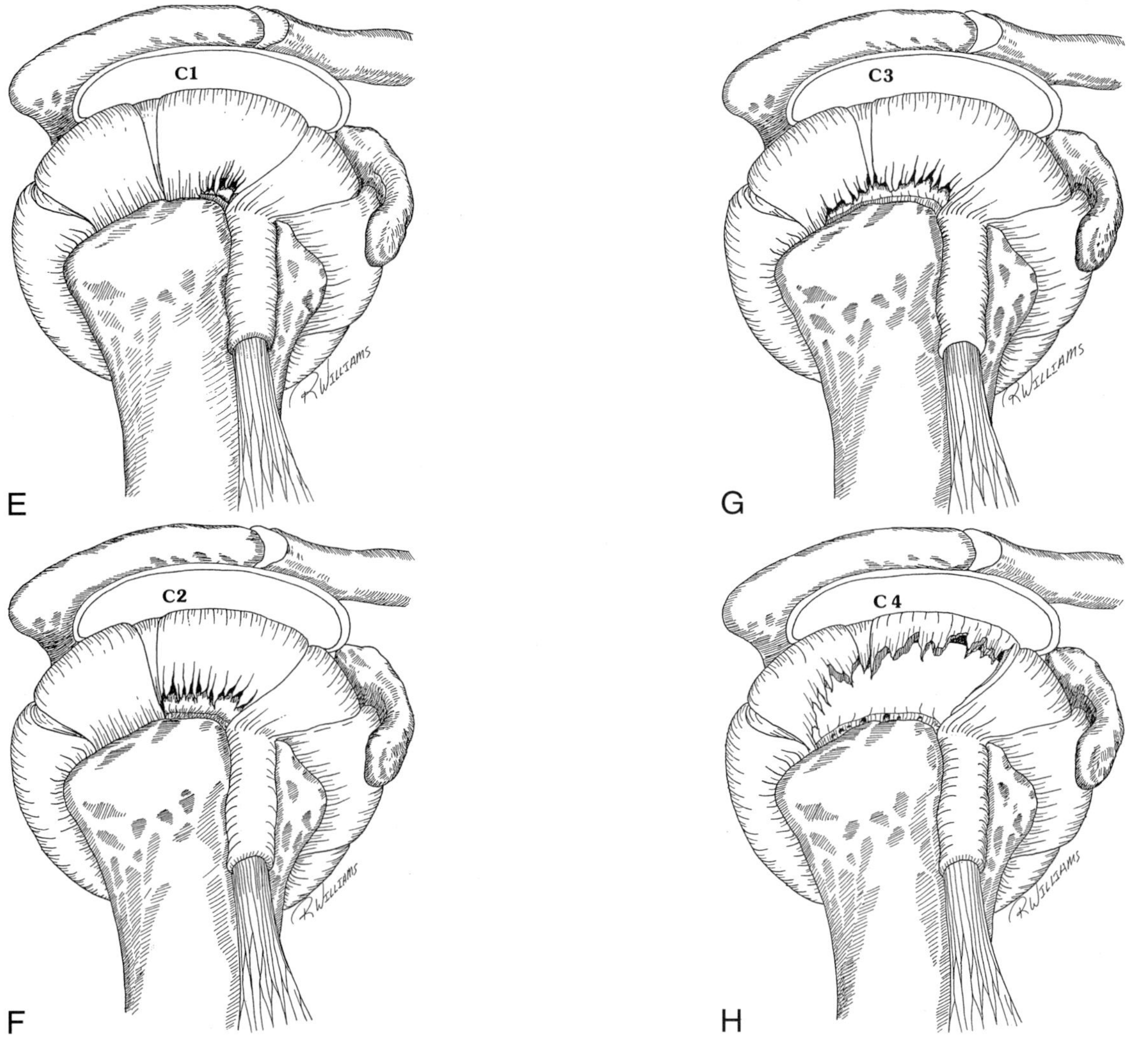

Fig. 20–10—*continued*

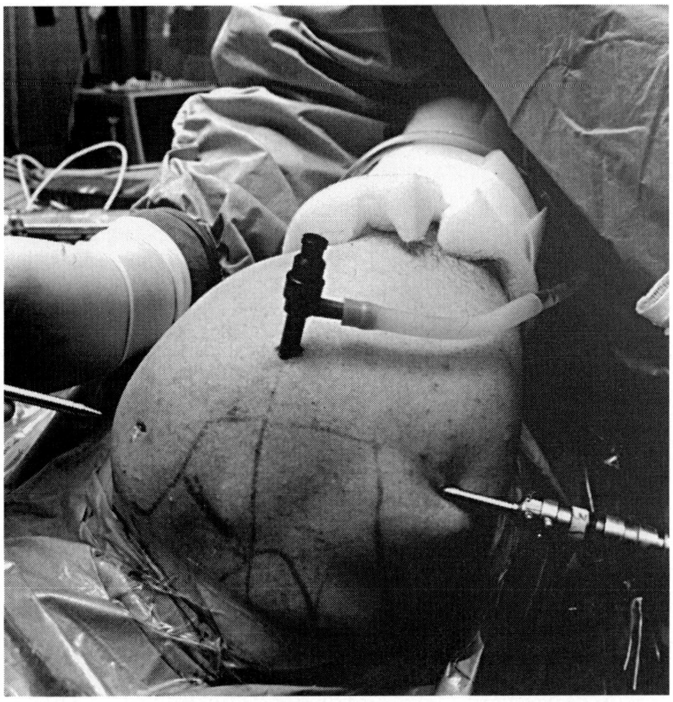

Fig. 20–11. Lateral bursal portal is established 2 to 3 cm distal to the lateral acromion, in line with the posterior aspect of the AC joint, and perpendicular to the lateral acromial border.

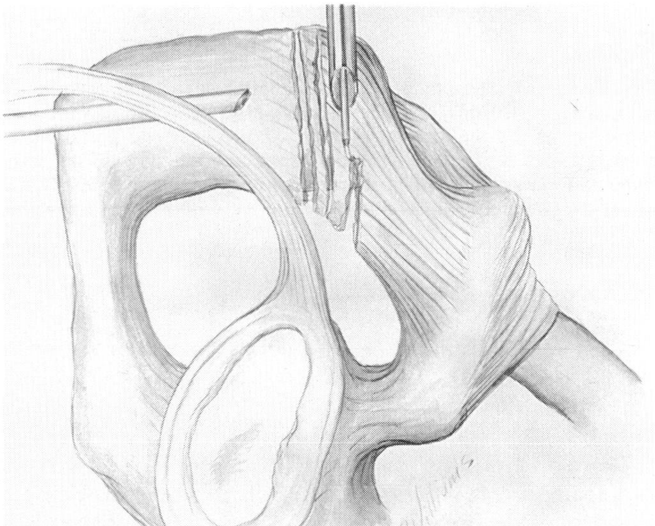

Fig. 20–12. The electrosurgical tool is inserted through the lateral portal to transect and checkerboard the coracoacromial ligament beneath the acromion.

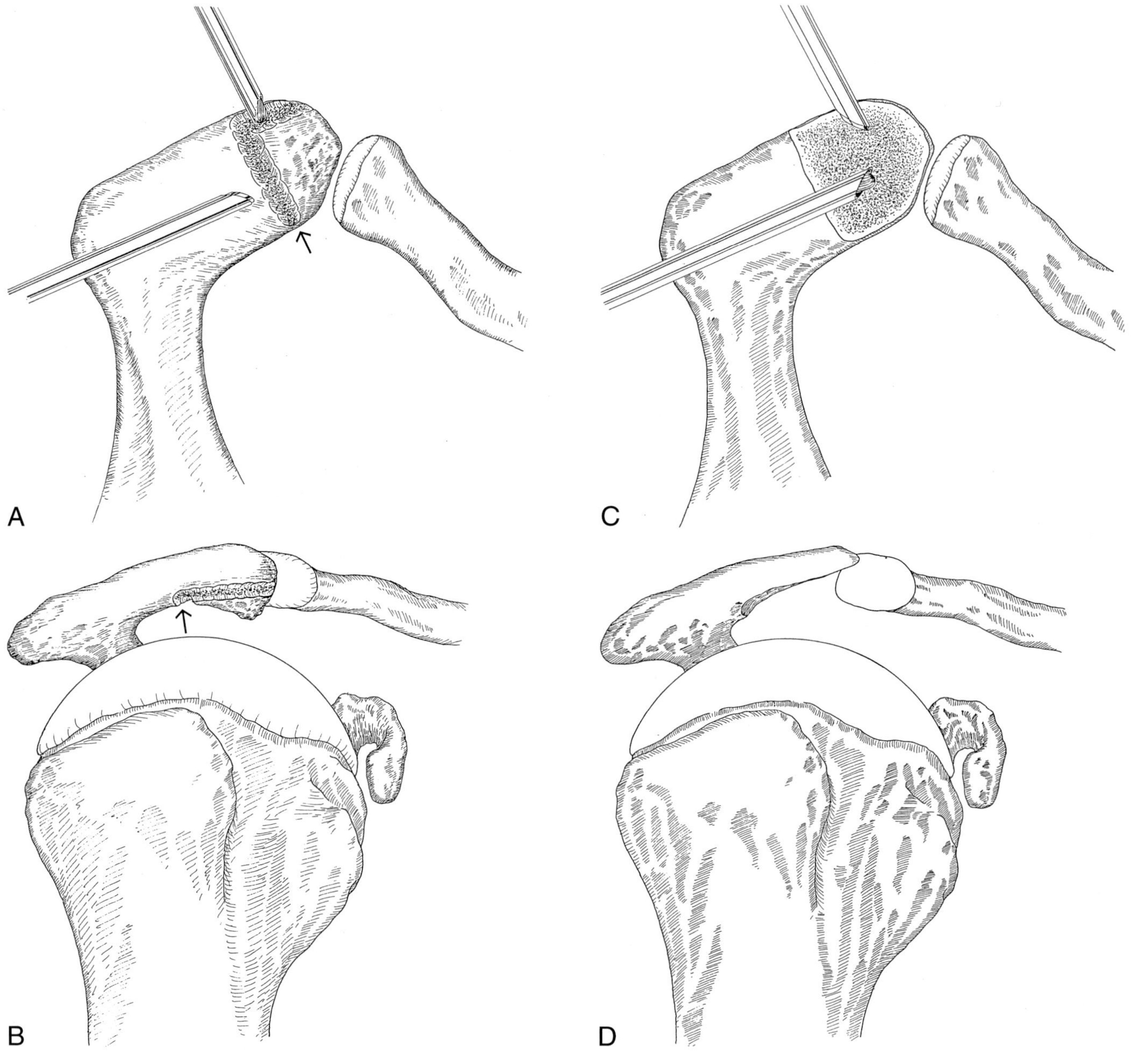

Fig. 20–13. ***A,*** **Technique for arthroscopic subacromial decompression. With the arthroscope viewing within the bursa through the posterior portal and the acromioplasty blade in the lateral portal, an L-shaped trough is developed, beginning at the lateral edge of the acromion and extending to the posterior edge of the AC joint medially and along the lateral edge of the acromion to the anterolateral corner.** ***B,*** **Lateral view of the acromion following the initial L-shaped trough.** ***C,*** **The acromioplasty is completed, visualizing with the arthroscope in the lateral portal and flattening the remaining undersurface of the acromion with the abrader in the posterior portal.** ***D,*** **Lateral view of the acromion demonstrating the completed acromioplasty with the perfectly flat acromial shape.**

TECHNIQUE

We use the three standard portals: posterior superior portal for posterior bursal viewing; anterior superior portal primarily for gravity drainage of the bursal space; and lateral subacromial portal, primarily for instrumentation.

Before beginning the Mumford procedure,[24] a complete subacromial decompression is performed. Using a posterior view, the electrosurgical tool with a subacromial electrode is used to resect the capsule and periosteum around the AC joint, extending from posterior to anterior. An aggressive shaver is then used to remove to all soft-tissue debris surrounding the joint. The Claviculizer (Dyonics, Andover, MA), a specially designed router-type burr used to rapidly resect the end of the inferior three-fourths of the clavicle, is inserted via the lateral portal to core out the central portion of the distal clavicle to a preset depth of 1.5 cm (Fig. 20–15). The remaining cortical shell can then be removed using the Claviculizer, or the Acromionizer, and a grasper. The burr and shaver

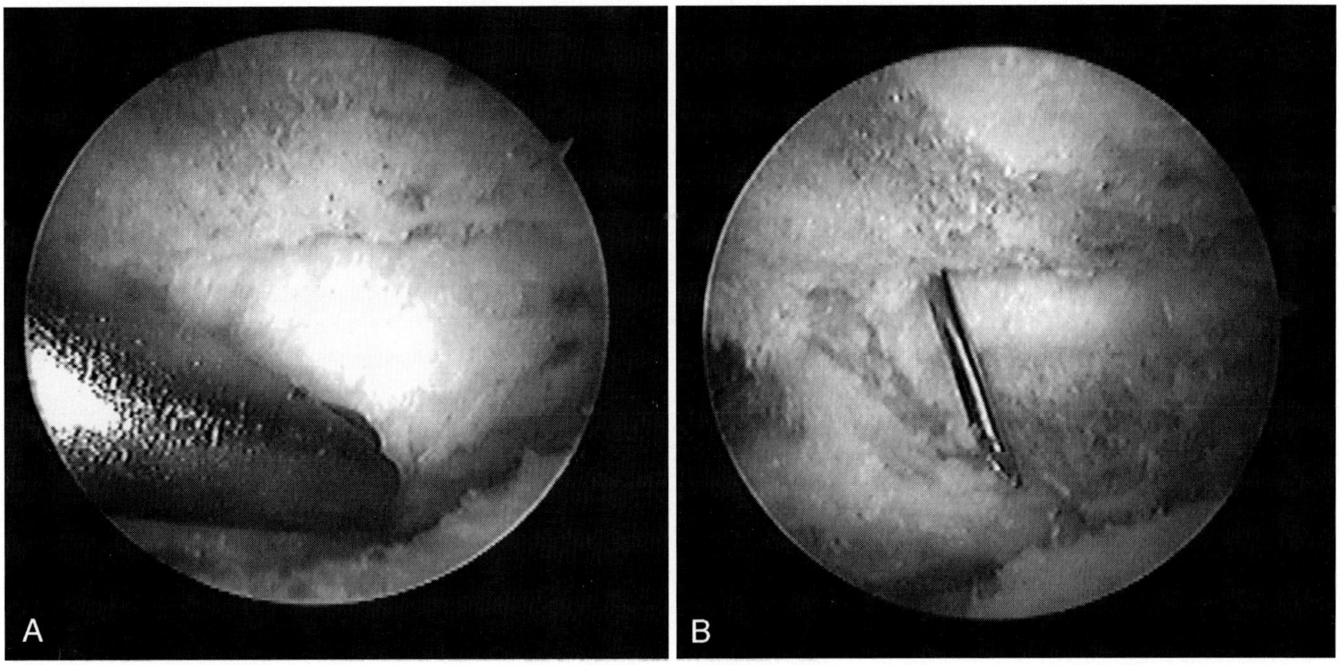

Fig. 20–14. Mini-Mumford procedure. *A,* The subacromial decompression has been completed (above), revealing a prominent distal clavicle that may impinge on the rotator cuff below. An acromionizer burr prepares to flatten the distal clavicle undersurface. *B,* A spinal needle marks the AC joint following resection of the inferior 30% of the distal clavicle.

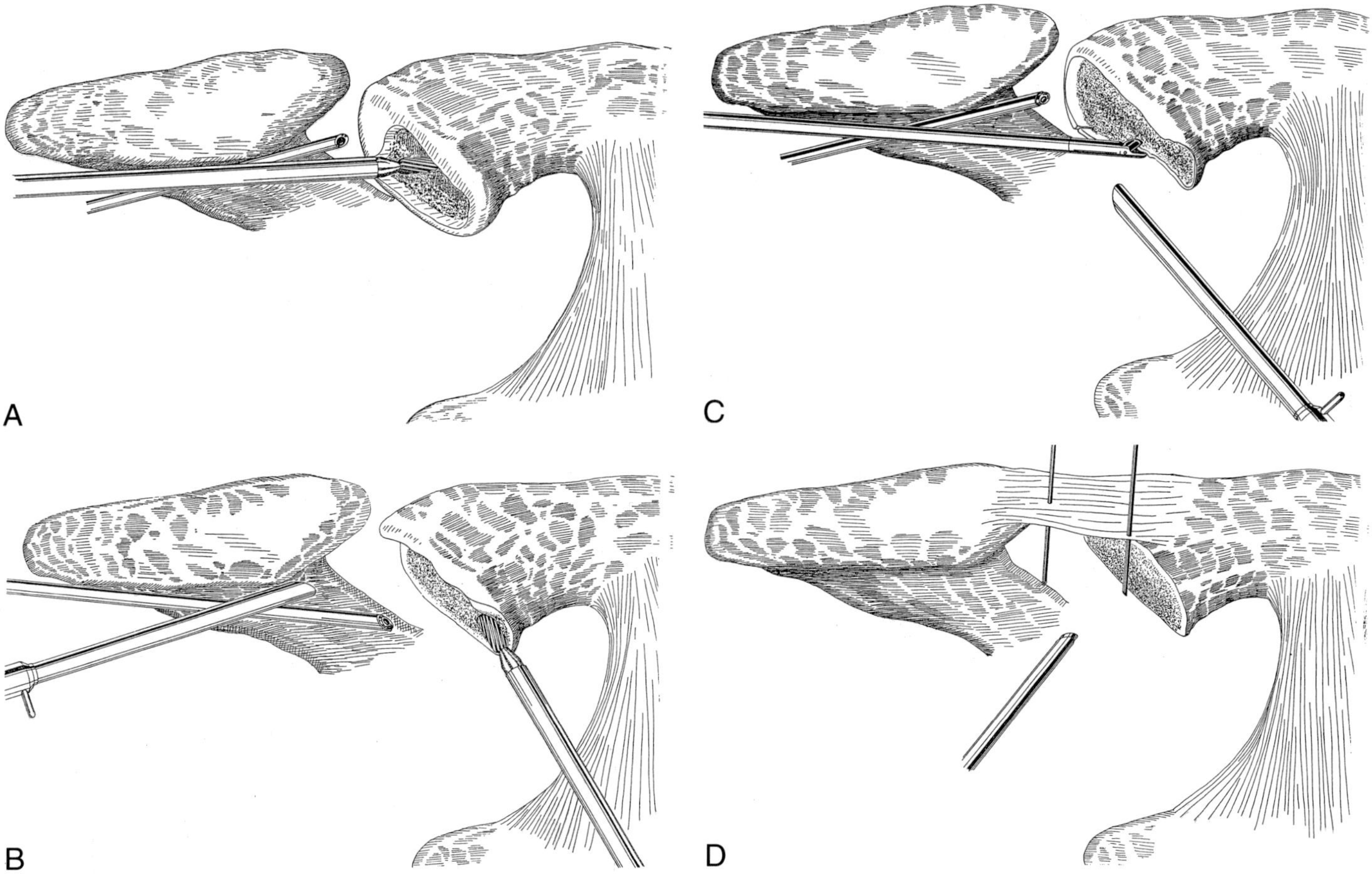

Fig. 20–15. Arthroscopic Mumford procedure. *A,* With the arthroscope in the posterior portal, the claviculizer is inserted via the lateral portal to core out the central portion of the distal clavicle to a depth of 1.5 cm. *B,* The arthroscope is moved laterally, a drainage cannula inserted posteriorly, and the burr is used from the anterior portal to remove the superior cortex and flatten the end of the resected distal clavicle. *C,* A suction punch removes the remaining cortical shell and periosteum from the distal clavicle. *D,* Viewing from posterior, two spinal needles are inserted percutaneously into the area of the resected distal clavicle to measure the amount of bone removed.

are then moved to the anterior portal to complete resection of the remaining superior clavicle and achieve a flat surface.

ARTHROSCOPIC-ASSISTED (MINI-OPEN) ROTATOR CUFF REPAIR

Prior to surgery, a discussion concerning the possible need to progress with a mini-open rotator cuff repair is held with the patient. If the patient consents to open surgery as needed, and a repairable lesion is encountered, we will proceed. We have found that almost all repairable rotator cuff tears can be addressed with a mini-open approach.

The mini-open technique is performed while maintaining the patient in the lateral decubitus position with the arm in the bursal position. If a mini-open repair is intended, during the arthroscopic portion of the procedure the torn cuff edge can be debrided, and if the tendon has retracted significantly, a superior capsular release is performed. This can be done with a thin, sharp elevator (we use the Liberator Elevator, Linvatec-Concept, Largo, FL). The superior capsule is released from the superior glenoid, extending from a point just anterior to the biceps tendon to the posterior-superior portion of the glenoid. The elevator is inserted through the lateral portal, passing through the rotator cuff tear, and is directed into the glenohumeral joint. We prefer to use the sharp blade on the end of the elevator to make multiple punctures in the capsule that are then connected, working around the periphery of the superior glenoid in order to completely release the capsule and cuff from the bone. The retracted cuff can then be mobilized more easily in a lateral direction.

Following completion of the subacromial decompression and Mumford or mini-Mumford procedure, an attempt is made to mobilize the cuff toward the greater tuberosity with a grasper. It is sometimes useful to place one or more traction sutures in the free edge of the tendon with a suture punch. We have found that the suture Shuttle Relay is useful in this situation to help pass a nonabsorbable heavy suture. It is at this point that a final decision is made as to whether the cuff is repairable to the greater tuberosity.

Following the extra-articular and bursal work, the traction weight is changed to 10 lbs. The operative field is then prepared again with povidone-iodine solution. Gloves and instruments are then changed for the open procedure. A modified Kessel incision is used on the previously drawn orientation line (which extends from the posterior aspect of the AC joint to the lateral border of the acromion and distally down the lateral aspect of the arm). The skin incision is approximately 5 cm long, starting just medial to the lateral border of the acromion, extending to the lateral operating portal (Fig. 20–16). This incision is applicable for most tears; if the tear is closer to the rotator interval, the incision can be placed 2 cm anterior to the orientation line. Full-thickness skin flaps are created and elevated from the deltoid fascia. This facilitates the closure. The deltoid is split in line with its fibers, starting 1 cm posterior to the anterolateral corner of the acromion. The fascia is sharply divided and the muscle bluntly divided with a large elevator. The deltoid can be safely split 4 to 5 cm distal to the lateral border of the acromion. Any further splitting may endanger the axillary nerve. A gloved finger can be introduced into the subacromial space to assess the quality of the decompression. The subdeltoid bursa is then divided and adequate bursal tissue excised to allow complete visualization of the rotator cuff and greater tuberosity. An electrosurgical tool is used to make several parallel cuts in the bursa overlying the greater tuberosity, and a large elevator with a sponge is used to remove the remaining bursal tissue and expose the bone adequately.

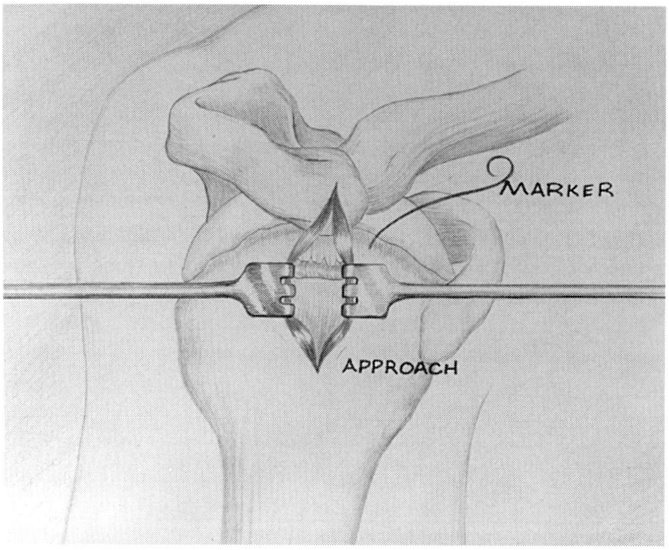

Fig. 20–16. The surgical incision for the mini-open rotator cuff repair is 5 cm long, beginning on a line from the posterior edge of the AC joint to the lateral subacromial portal.

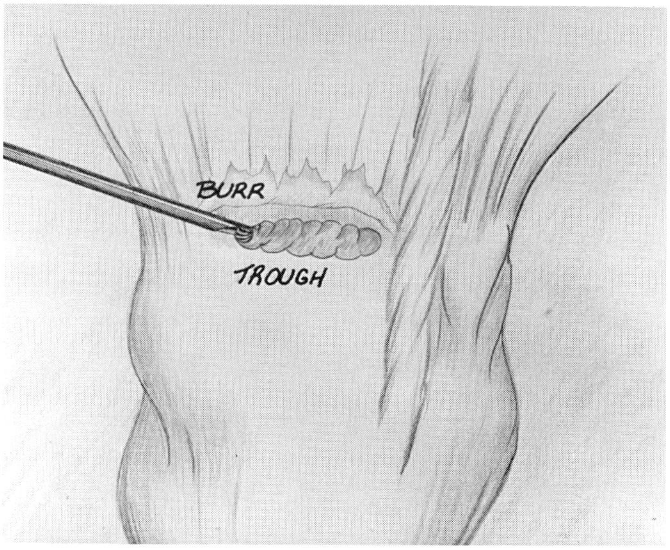

Fig. 20–17. A trough is created, using a high-speed burr, with enough depth to expose underlying cancellous bone.

If the biceps tendon was noted to be significantly damaged at the time of arthroscopy, a biceps tenodesis can be performed at this time.

The leading edge of the rotator cuff should be debrided back to healthy tissue. If traction sutures were placed prior to opening, these can be used to help deliver the edge of the cuff into the wound. A high-speed burr is used to prepare a trough into cancellous bone adjacent to the articular cartilage (Fig. 20–17). The length of the trough is determined by the size of the cuff tear. The remaining cuff and biceps tendon should be protected while using the burr.

SUTURE TECHNIQUE

We prefer to repair the cuff with multiple nonabsorbable No. 2 sutures, using alternating colors to facilitate identification. Although any good suture technique can hold healthy tendon, the use of a nonstrangulating grasping suture is often helpful for most cuff tears. We often use a modified Kessler suture weaving technique called a SCOI (Southern California Orthopaedic Institute) stitch (Fig. 20–18). This technique will close delaminations in the tendon, roll the free edge of the cuff into bone once tied, and distribute the traction forces on the cuff into the better quality tissue. The number of sutures required depends on the size and quality of the tear.

BONY TUNNELS AND SUTURE PASSAGE

It is important for the sutures in the cuff to be firmly attached to good quality bone to avoid failure of the repair. To facilitate this, we currently use the rotator cuff instruments manufactured by the Linvatec-Concept Company. These instruments are helpful in preparing bony tunnels and passing the sutures through the bony trough toward the greater tuberosity in order to be tied. There are three basic instruments used, including a gauge punch, a circular rasp, and a curved suture passer, which are all available in small, medium, and large sizes (Fig. 20–19). The choice of size varies according to the surgical exposure and bone quality. Whenever possible, we prefer the larger instruments to achieve maximal size bony bridges, alternating between the medium and large sizes so that tuberosity holes are placed in a different line, thereby avoiding a stress riser in the tuberosity.

The gauge punch is used first (Fig. 20–20). The sharp

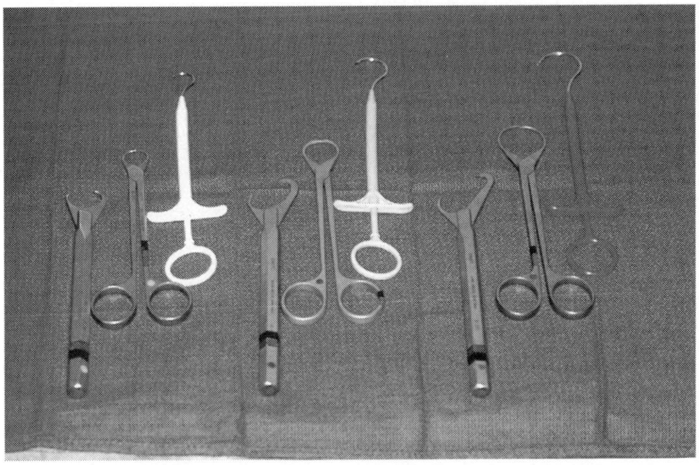

Fig. 20–19. The Concept rotator cuff repair system includes three sizes of three individual instruments (cortical gauge punch, circular rasp, and suture passer) in addition to the rotator cuff Liberator Elevator. (Courtesy of Linvatec-Concept, Largo, FL.)

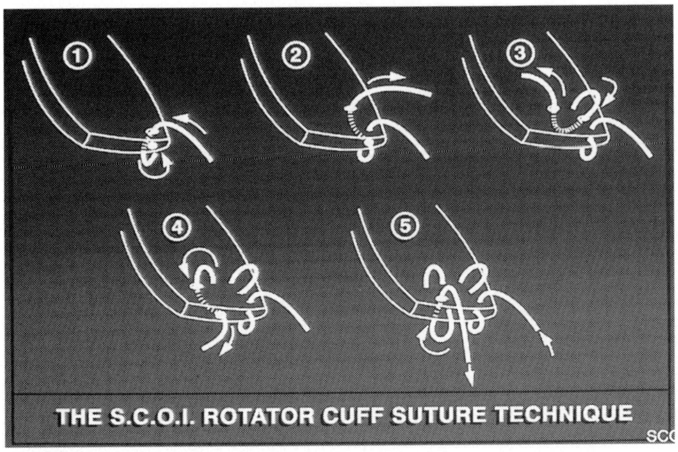

Fig. 20–18. The SCOI rotator cuff weave stitch: (1) pass the needle superiorly to inferiorly through the free end of the tendon; (2) pass through the center of the free edge and medially 1 to 1.5 cm, to exit on the bursal surface; (3) pass the needle vertically from the bursal to the articular surface; (4) it passes directly from the articular to the bursal surface of the tendon again; this creates a 1 cm loop of suture on the articular surface of the joint, which closes laminations; (5) it passes from the bursal surface through the substance of the tendon and exits at the free edge, 1 to 1.5 cm from the original entry point; and (6) finally, it is passed from the articular to the bursal surface, 3 mm medial to the edge. (Courtesy of Linvatec-Concept, Largo, FL.)

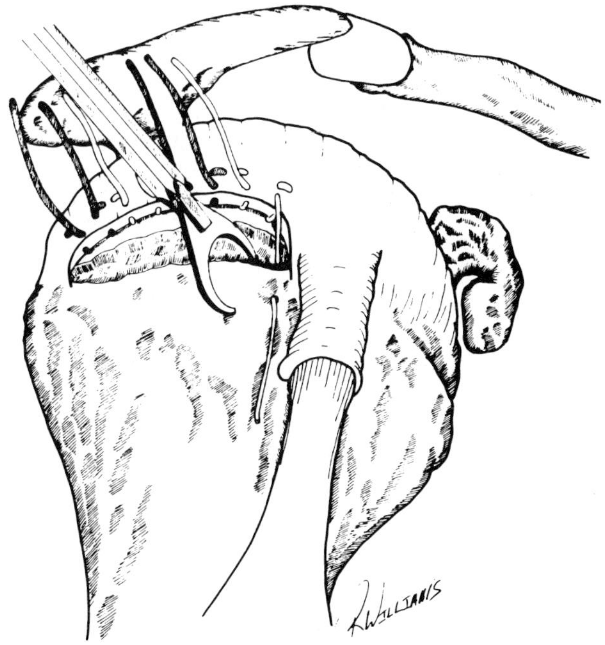

Fig. 20–20. The cortical gauge punch is used first to create a hole in the bone trough and then the greater tuberosity. (Courtesy of Linvatec-Concept, Largo, FL.)

end of the punch starts a hole in the center of the bone trough. The punch is rotated 180° so that the blunt tip of the measuring arm is placed just above the original hole in the trough. The punch is then impacted into the proper position in the tuberosity. After the cortex has been perforated, the handle of the punch is lowered so that the curve of the instrument heads in the appropriate direction toward the hole in the bone trough. This instrument is then replaced by the circle rasp. This is first inserted into the tuberosity hole (Fig. 20–21). Care must be taken to guide the rasp into the same path as the punch; applying thumb pressure on the convex arm of the rasp in the tuberosity hole will avoid breaking through the tuberosity. The second side of the circle rasp is then easily seated into the trough hole. While maintaining some downward pressure on the rasp, the handles are gently closed with an alternating back-and-forth motion. The circular rasp can then smooth the bony tunnel.

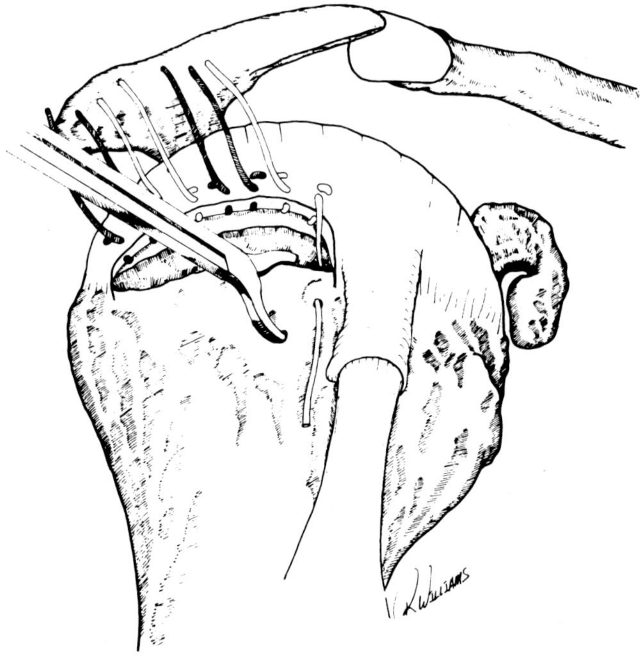

Fig. 20–21. The circle rasp is used to connect the holes in the tuberosity and the bone trough. (Courtesy of Linvatec-Concept, Largo, FL.)

The suture passer is inserted through the tuberosity hole and should easily follow the tunnel to the trough hole. Depression of the plunger on the handle will expose the wire loop for passage of the suture (Fig. 20–22). Adjacent suture limbs are paired for passage through the bony trough. The wire loop is retracted back into the passer and the sutures can then be retrieved through the greater tuberosity. Additional bony tunnels are made anterior and posterior to the central hole. It is preferable to use a different size instrument for adjacent holes, so that the holes will be at different levels on the tuberosity. Additional holes are made to accommodate the number of sutures placed in the rotator cuff. Each suture limb is then paired with its partner after passage through different holes.

In preparation for tying the sutures, the arm is abducted and all the sutures are pulled in a lateral direction to bring the edge of the rotator cuff into the trough. While maintaining traction on the remaining sutures, each suture is tied in sequence over a bone bridge with multiple square knots (Fig. 20–23).

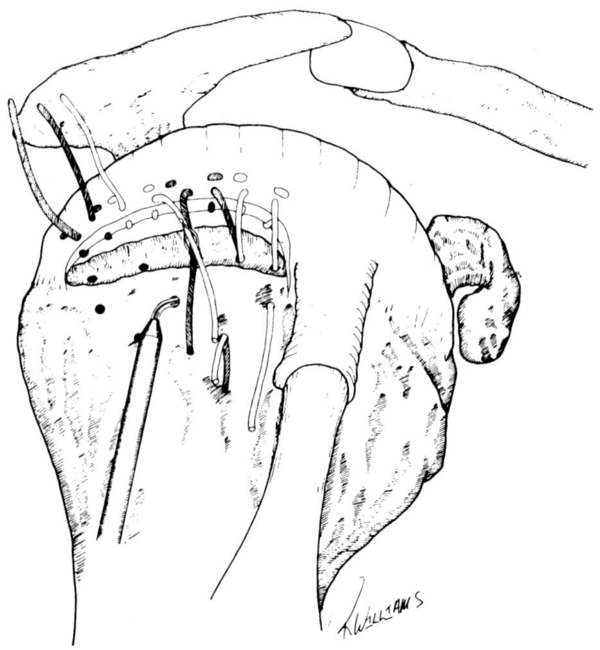

Fig. 20–22. The appropriate size suture passer is inserted into the tuberosity hole and retrieves the rotator cuff sutures from the trough. (Courtesy of Linvatec-Concept, Largo, FL.)

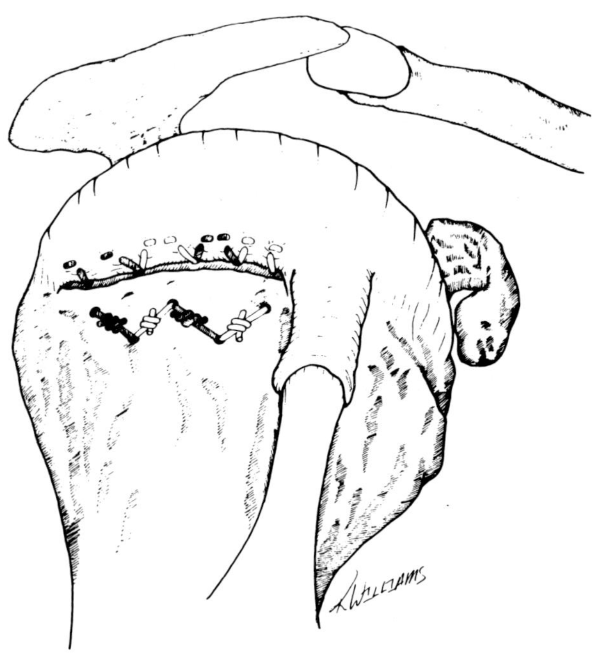

Fig. 20–23. The sutures are tied over the bone bridges, securing the rotator cuff tendon into the bony trough. (Courtesy of Linvatec-Concept, Largo, FL.)

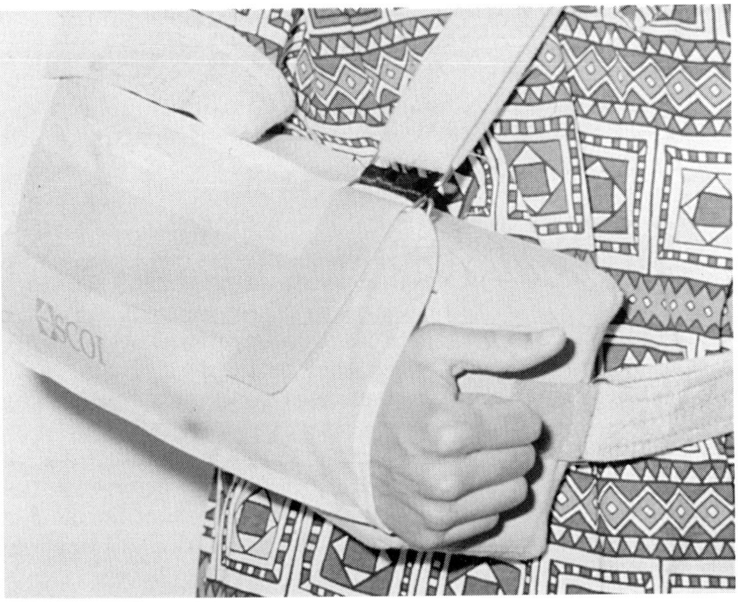

Fig. 20–24. Pillow sling (Ultra Sling, Smith & Nephew DonJoy, Carlsbad, CA).

In most cases, the bone bridges are quite solid. However, in the case of poor bone quality, the surgeon may be concerned that a suture may cut through the bone. To reduce this risk, a small soft-tissue patch (e.g., Gore-Tex, WL Gore & Associates, Flagstaff, AZ) can be placed under each knot over the bony bridges. Pledglets should be trimmed so that there is no excess material present after the knot is tied. After the final suture is tied, the arm is taken through a range of motion and is assessed for the possible need for abduction bracing.

The deltoid is closed in two layers with No. 1 absorbable suture. The subdeltoid bursal layer is closed, followed by the superficial deltoid fascia. The subcutaneous layer is closed with an undyed absorbable suture and, if necessary, a subcuticular skin closure is performed with a 4–0 clear monofilament absorbable suture. Skin closure strips and a sterile dressing are applied.

POSTOPERATIVE PROTECTION

For cuff repairs that can be performed with minimal tension into good quality bone, the shoulder is protected for 3 to 4 weeks with a shoulder immobilizer that includes a small abduction pillow (Fig. 20–24). This takes some tension off the repair while providing for additional comfort and ease of axillary hygiene. In addition, a velcro flap allows the sling to open so the patient can exercise the elbow and hand periodically during the day.

In cases in which either the tendon or bone quality is poor, or if the repair is performed under tension, a functional abduction brace is used for the first few weeks, followed by an Ultra Sling for an additional 2 to 3 weeks. We prefer the SCOI Shoulder Brace (Smith & Nephew DonJoy, Carlsbad, CA) (Fig. 20–25). A clean tank top shirt is put on prior to the application of the brace. This brace permits flexion and extension of the elbow, as well as early hand and wrist exercises. Passive abduction of the arm between 30 and 70° begins after 1 week. The brace does remain on continuously for the 3- to 4-week period, but the tank top can be changed provided reliable help is available.

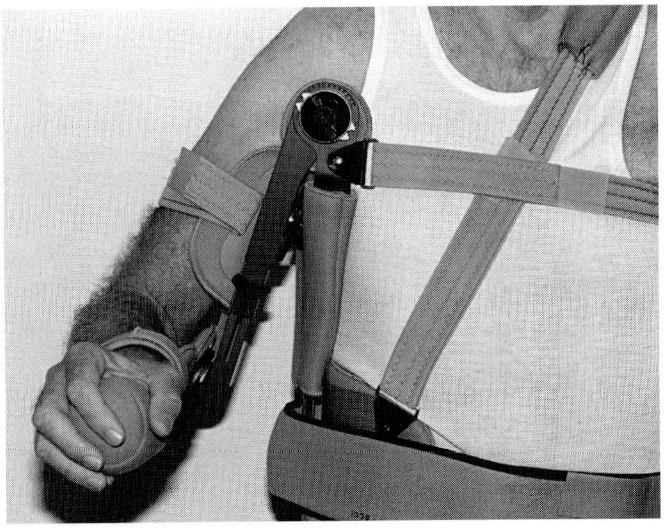

Fig. 20–25. The DonJoy-SCOI brace is a functional postoperative shoulder support that allows active flexion and extension of the elbow. (Courtesy of Smith & Nephew DonJoy, Carlsbad, CA.)

ARTHROSCOPIC REPAIR OF THE ROTATOR CUFF

In our initial series of patients, no tears larger than CII (2-cm complete tear) were judged appropriate for arthroscopic repair. However, it now appears that some larger tears that can be mobilized or partially closed with side-to-side sutures may be amenable to arthroscopic fixation as well. If judged appropriate for arthroscopic fixation, the following technique is used. The arm is kept in the bursoscopy position using 10 lbs of traction in 15 to 20° abduction. After the subacromial decompression is completed, a shaver and suction punch are used through the lateral or anterior operating cannula to debride the rough edges of cuff tendon and the remaining soft tissue on the greater tuberosity distal to the site of intended reattachment of the cuff to bone (Fig. 20–26). An arthroscopic burr inserted through the lateral or anterior cannula is used to create a small trough adjacent to the articular cartilage of the humeral head, below the torn rotator cuff edge (Fig. 20–27). A spinal needle placed lateral to the edge of the acromion is used to determine the appropriate position for drilling or punching the pilot holes and inserting suture anchors. A drill bit or bone punch is inserted through a small stab incision and 2 or 3 holes are made into good quality bone either in or adjacent to the bony trough. The holes are directed obliquely to pass below the subchondral bone at an angle of approximately 270° to the cuff tendon (Fig. 20–28).

A 5.5-mm operating cannula with a diaphragm is inserted into the bursal space through the anterior portal and a 9-mm cannula is placed in the lateral portal. Via the same lateral stab incision that was used for drilling, the suture screw anchors (we prefer Revo Screws, Linvatec-Concept, Largo, FL) preloaded with No. 2 braided nonabsorbable suture, are advanced through the skin and deltoid muscle without need of a cannula (Fig. 20–29). Each screw is advanced into bone to the seating mark on the driver. Traction on the suture tests the stability of the anchors. Both limbs of the first suture are withdrawn through the anterior cannula using a crochet hook. One or two additional suture anchors are then inserted into the drill holes. After the final anchor is implanted, one limb of the most anterior suture is brought out laterally and one anteriorly (Fig. 20–30). To avoid confusion, we use alternating colored sutures on the suture anchors. In addition, in order to avoid inadvertent

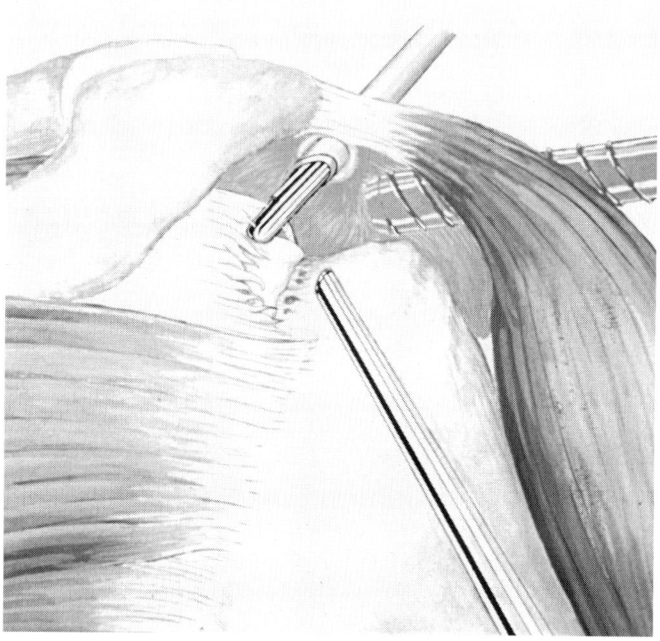

Fig. 20–26. Posterior view of the right shoulder showing a moderate size cuff tear in the supraspinatus region. A shaver is brought in through the anterior portal.

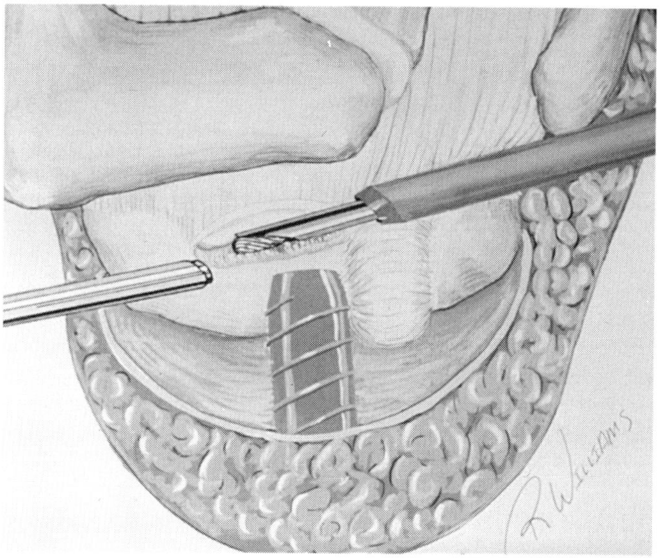

Fig. 20–27. Dorsal view of the shoulder demonstrating the burr through the anterior portal preparing a trough adjacent to the articular cartilage.

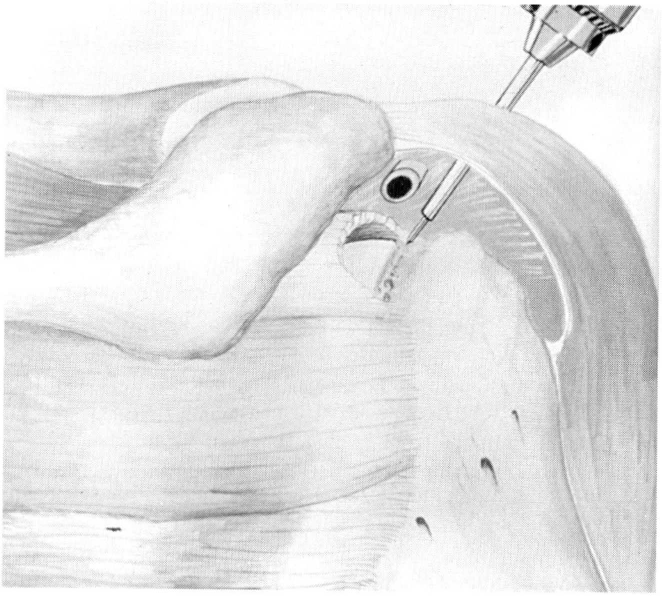

Fig. 20–28. Posterior view of the shoulder demonstrating a drill or punch placed percutaneously through the deltoid into the prepared trough to create 2 or 3 pilot holes. No cannula is needed.

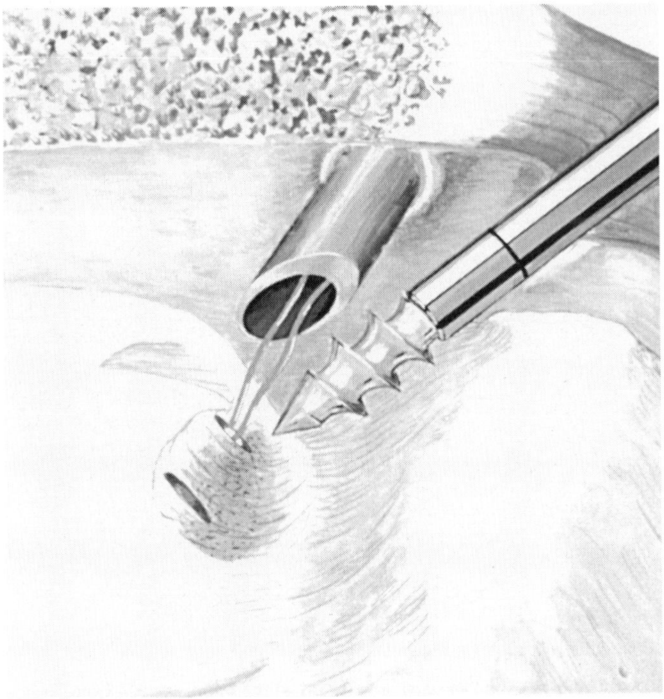

Fig. 20–29. Posterior view of the shoulder demonstrating a Revo miniature suture screw anchor going through the deltoid toward the pilot hole in the humerus. The anterior anchor has already been inserted; its suture exits the anterior cannula.

tangling of the sutures, the anterior cannula is removed and replaced over a guide rod through the anterior portal, thereby placing all the sutures outside the cannula except for the one being passed.

A modified Caspari suture punch is inserted through the lateral operating cannula to achieve a healthy bite into the edge of the rotator cuff (Fig. 20–31). This punch has been modified by the manufacturer by cutting a 2-mm slot in the end of the upper jaw. A Shuttle Relay (Linvatec-Concept, Largo, FL) is passed with the punch through the cuff from inferior to superior where it is grasped and removed through the anterior cannula. The limb of suture in the lateral cannula is threaded through the eyelet of the Shuttle Relay. By pulling on the anterior limb of the Shuttle, the suture is carried through the cuff, from bottom to top, and out the anterior cannula with the Shuttle Relay (Fig. 20–32). The second limb of the suture is then retrieved through the lateral cannula with a crochet hook. A Shuttle Relay is again passed through the cuff from bottom to top, with the suture punch approximately 7 mm from the first puncture site, creating a broad mattress stitch. The second limb is brought through the rotator cuff in a similar fashion with the Shuttle. The sutures are left untied through the anterior portal. This process is repeated for the second and, if necessary, third set of sutures depending upon the size of the cuff tear. If only two suture anchors have been used, both limbs of the more posterior suture are retrieved through the lateral operating cannula with a crochet hook (Fig. 20–33).

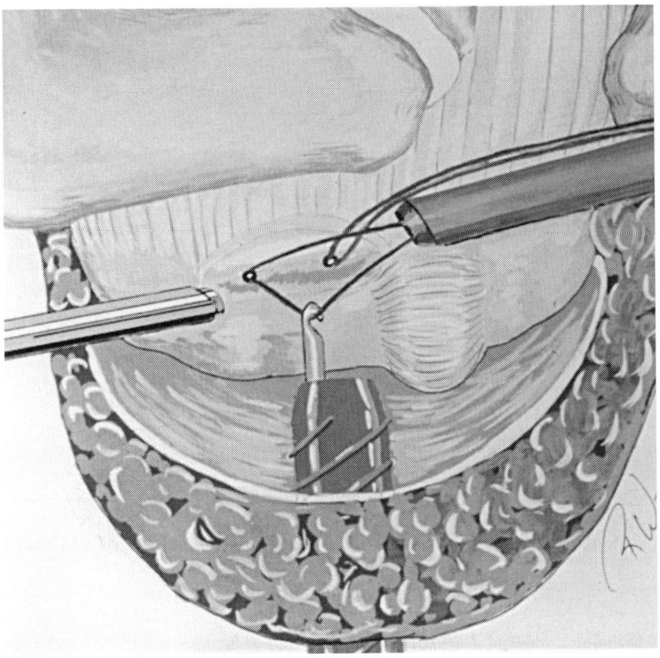

Fig. 20–30. Dorsal view of the shoulder, with arthroscope in the posterior portal; crochet hook in the lateral portal is retrieving one limb of suture where the corresponding limb is exiting the anterior portal. Both limbs of the other suture lie outside the anterior cannula to avoid tangling.

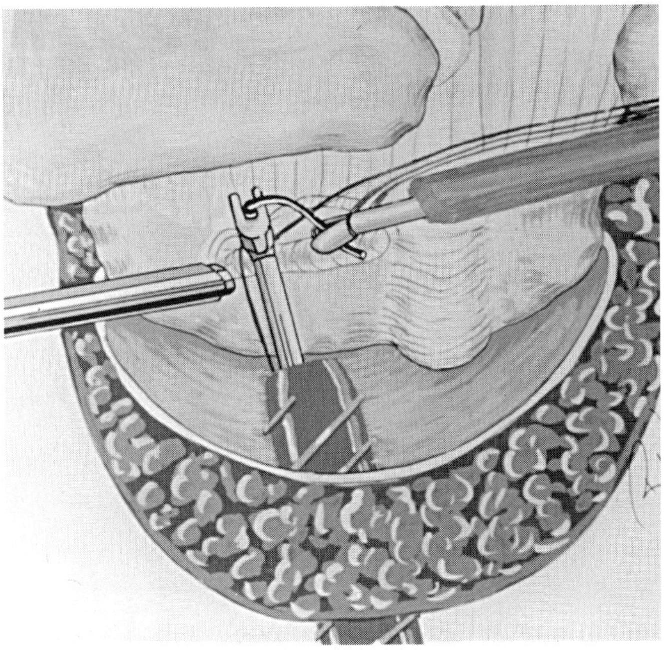

Fig. 20–31. Dorsal view of the shoulder, with arthroscope in the posterior portal. The modified Caspari punch is introduced through the lateral operating portal to pass the suture Shuttle Relay through the torn cuff. An arthroscopic grasper through the anterior portal retrieves the Shuttle. Three suture limbs lie outside the anterior cannula waiting to be passed.

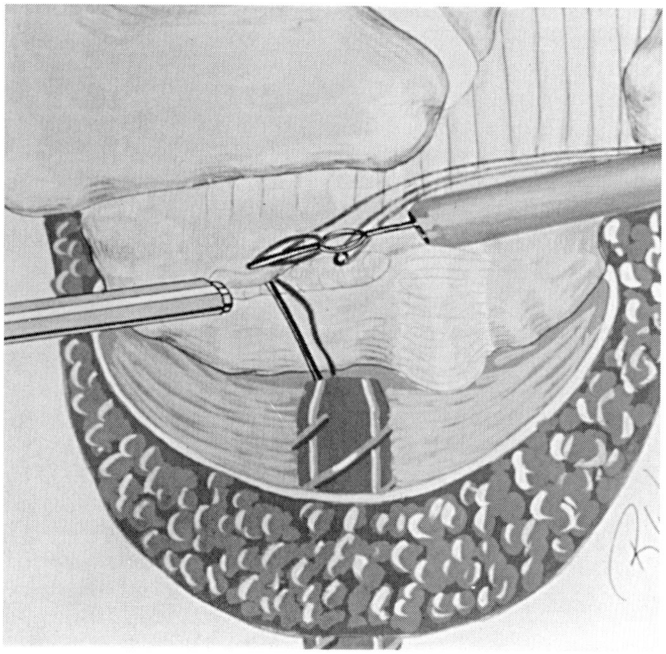

Fig. 20–32. Dorsal view of the shoulder; one limb of suture from the lateral portal is being transported via the Shuttle through the rotator cuff from below to above as the Shuttle is retrieved and pulled through the anterior portal.

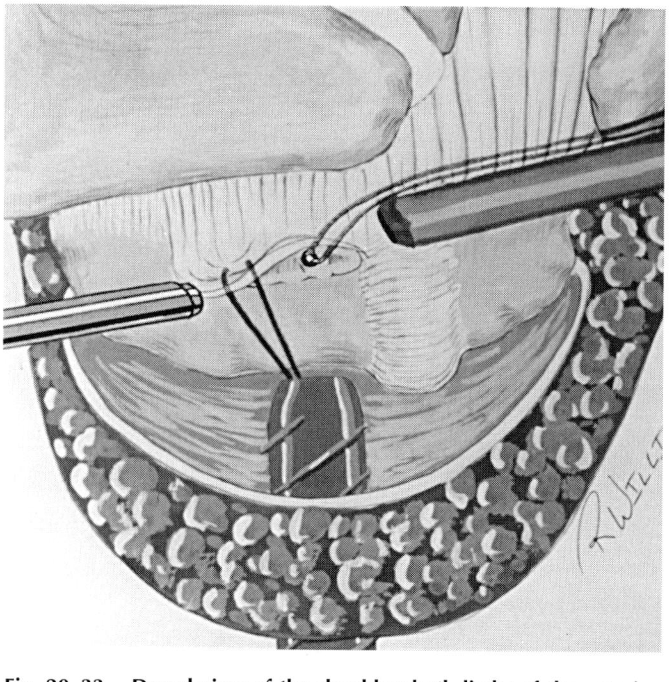

Fig. 20–33. Dorsal view of the shoulder; both limbs of the anterior suture lie outside the anterior cannula to avoid twisting. Both limbs of the posterior suture lie in the lateral portal in preparation for knot tying.

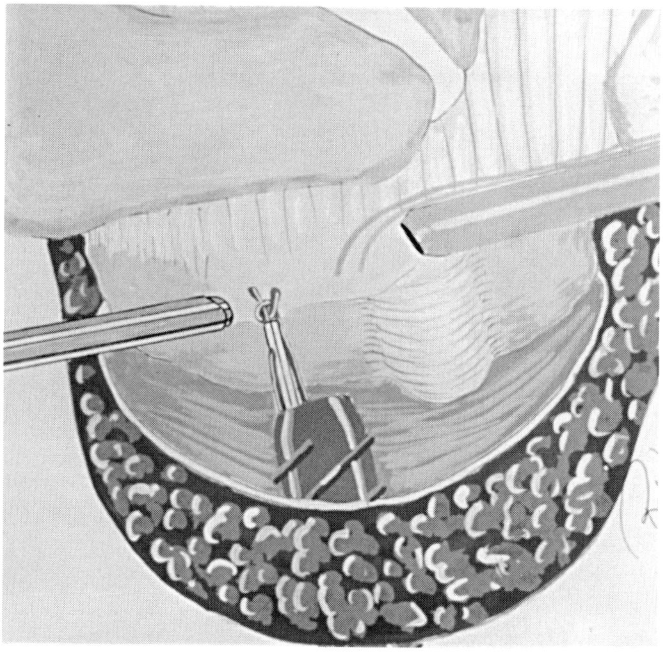

Fig. 20–34. Dorsal view of the shoulder; the arthroscopic knot pusher is tying the sutures through the lateral operating cannula. Two sutures lying outside the anterior cannula will be tied later.

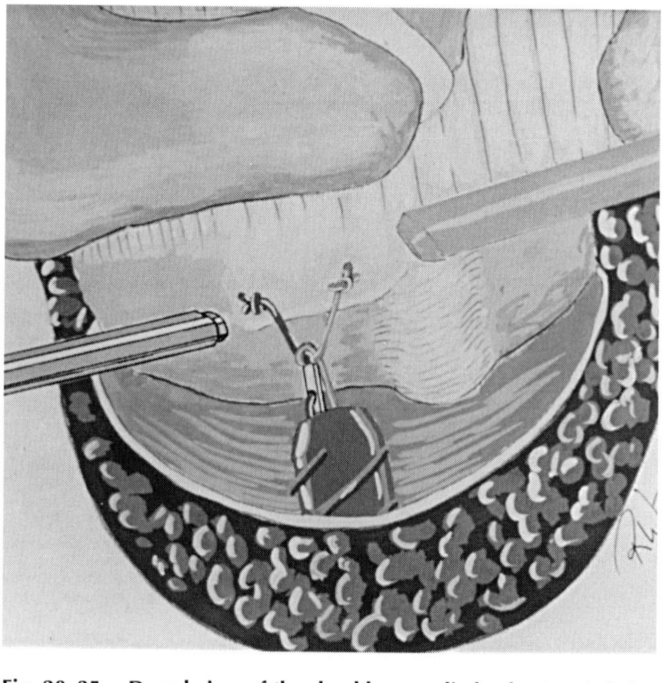

Fig. 20–35. Dorsal view of the shoulder; one limb of suture is being tied together with the knot pusher through the lateral portal. An arthroscopic basket placed through the anterior portal is used to cut the sutures.

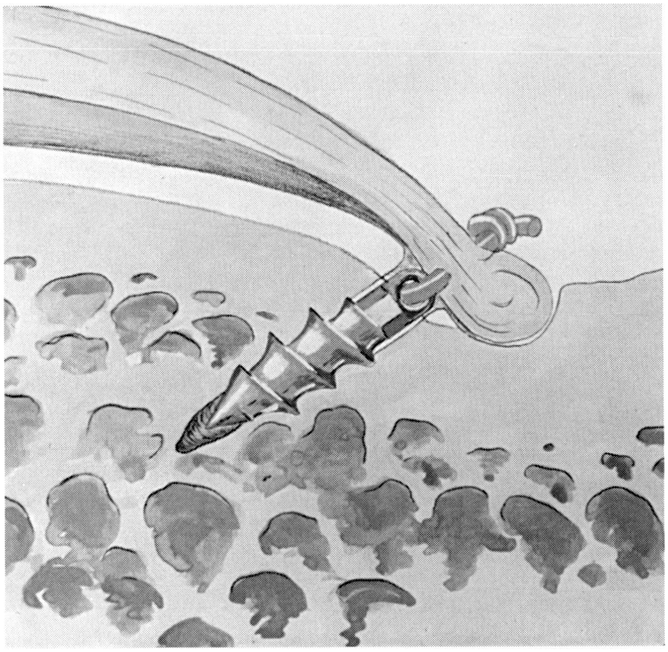

Fig. 20–36. A coronal view demonstrates completion of the fixation.

An arthroscopic knot pusher is used through the lateral portal to tie multiple stacked knots (Fig. 20–34). One limb of the suture is then cut and the other limb left to tie to one limb of the adjacent suture. This remaining limb is brought out the anterior portal. The next suture pair is similarly tied with an arthroscopic knot pusher. One limb is then cut. Finally, the two remaining limbs are both brought out through the lateral cannula and tied to one another to achieve a bridging mattress suture between the two anchors (Fig. 20–35). A basket punch is used to cut all the suture ends (Fig. 20–36). If the suture accidently breaks during knot tying, the Revo Screw can be easily removed and reinserted using the screw driver.

An arthroscopic probe is used to palpate the cuff and the stability of the sutures. The arthroscopic incisions are closed with subcutaneous absorbable sutures and/or paper skin tapes. A sterile dressing is applied followed by an Ultra Sling with a small abduction pillow.

REFERENCES

1. Burman MS. Arthroscopy or the direct visualization of joints: An experimental cadaver study. *J Bone Joint Surg Am.* 1931;13:669–695.
2. Watanabe M. Arthroscopy of the shoulder joint. In: Watanabe M, ed. *Arthroscopy of Small Joints.* Tokyo: Igaku-Shoin; 1985; 44–56.
3. Wiley AM, Older MB. Shoulder arthroscopy. Investigations with a fibro-optic instrument. *Am J Sports Med.* 1980;8:18.
4. Ellman H. Arthroscopic subacromial decompression. *Arthroscopy.* 1987;3:173.
5. Esch JC, Ozerkis LR, Helgager JA, Keene N, Lilliott N. Arthroscopic subacromial decompression: Results according to the degree of rotator cuff tear. *Arthroscopy.* 1988;4:241.
6. Ellman H. *Arthroscopic decompression: Two to five year results.* Presented at the AAOS Specialty Day Meeting, American Shoulder and Elbow Surgeons. Las Vegas, NV, 1989.
7. Andrews JR, Broussard TS, Carson WG. Arthroscopy of the shoulder and the management of partial tears of the rotator cuff: A preliminary report. *Arthroscopy.* 1985;1:117.
8. Snyder SJ. Rotator cuff lesions. Acute and Chronic. *Clin Sports Med.* 1991;10:595–614.
9. Snyder SJ, Pachelli AF, Del Pizzo W, Friedman MJ, Ferkel RD, Pattee G. Partial thickness rotator cuff tears: Results of arthroscopic treatment. *Arthroscopy.* 1991;7:1–7.
10. Ellman H. Arthroscopic subacromial decompression. Analysis of 1 to 3 year results. *Arthroscopy.* 1987;3:173. UCLA shoulder rating scale.
11. Gartsman GM. Arthroscopic acromioplasty for lesions of the rotator cuff. *J Bone Joint Surg Am.* 1990;72:169.
12. Paulos LE, Horner CD, Parker RD. Arthroscopic subacromial decompression for impingement syndrome of the shoulder. *Tech Orthop.* 1988;3:33.
13. Snyder SJ, Pattee GA. Shoulder arthroscopy in the evaluation and treatment of rotator cuff lesions. *Tech Orthop.* 1988;3:47.
14. Levy HJ, Uribe JW, Delaney LG. Arthroscopic-assisted rotator cuff repair. Preliminary results. *Arthroscopy.* 1990;6:55.
15. Snyder SJ, Wuh HCK. Arthroscopic evaluation and treatment of rotator cuff and superior labral anterior posterior lesions. *Oper Tech Orthop.* 1991;1:207–220.
16. Snyder SJ. Evaluation and treatment of the rotator cuff. *Orthop Clin North Am.* 1993;24:173.
17. Johnson LL. *Diagnostic and Surgical Arthroscopy of the Shoulder.* St. Louis: Mosby-Year Book, 1993:391.
18. Wilson FD. *Arthroscopic fixation of full-thickness rotator cuff tears: Staple technique.* Presented at the Arthroscopy Association of North America Specialty Day Meeting. San Francisco, CA, February 1993.
19. Wolf E. Personal communication.
20. Bartlett E. *Arthroscopic evaluation and treatment of rotator cuff pathology.* Presented at Arthroscopy Association of North America Annual Meeting Instructional Course. Palm Desert, CA, April 1993.
21. Morrison DS, Bigliani LU. *The clinical significance of variation in acromial morphology.* Presented at AAOS Specialty Day Meeting, American Shoulder and Elbow Surgeons, San Francisco, CA, January 1987.
22. Snyder SJ, Wuh HCK. *Modified classification of the supraspinatus outlet view based on the configuration and anatomic thickness of the acromion.* Presented at the Arthroscopy Association of North America Specialty Day Meeting. San Francisco, CA, February 1993.
23. Snyder SJ. A complete system for arthroscopy and bursoscopy of the shoulder. *Surg Rounds Orthop.* 1989;July:57.
24. Snyder SJ. Arthroscopic acromioclavicular joint debridement and distal clavicle resection. *Tech Orthop.* 1988;3:41–45.

Suggested Reading

Snyder SJ, Karzel RP, eds. Shoulder arthroscopy and related surgery. *Orthop Clin North Am.* 1993:24.

Section 7

Surgical Management of Massive Cuff Tears and Degeneration

Chapter 21

A Unified Biomechanical Rationale for the Treatment of Rotator Cuff Tears: Debridement Versus Repair

Stephen S. Burkhart

Codman[1] was the first modern surgeon to advocate repair of the torn rotator cuff. His concept of rotator cuff repair appealed to one's sense of order. By restoring the anatomy, one restored the mechanics of the cuff.

As the field of shoulder surgery matured, the concept of "repairing the tear" became translated into "covering the hole" in the cuff. Unfortunately, it lost something in the translation. What it lost was an overriding respect for the mechanics of the shoulder. A number of techniques have been devised to "cover the hole" in the rotator cuff, including supraspinatus muscle slide,[2] fascial graft,[3] freeze-dried allograft,[4] and tendon transposition.[5,6] Unfortunately, most of these techniques either ignore or openly violate the mechanics of the shoulder.

My goal in this chapter is to present a logical concept of treatment of rotator cuff tears based on sound biomechanical principles. This concept uses both repair and debridement in different situations. This may sound paradoxical, but the paradox can be resolved. Allow me to explain.

THE PAINFUL ROTATOR CUFF

Why are shoulders with rotator cuff tears painful? Numerous scientific articles have provided evidence that a hole in the cuff, as an isolated entity, is not painful. Many patients with known rotator cuff tears have been successfully treated by nonoperative means, leaving the hole in the cuff unrepaired.[7–9] There are reports of good pain relief from rotator cuff debridement and decompression, despite leaving an unrepaired hole in the cuff.[10–12] Even after open rotator cuff repair, residual cuff defects have been shown by ultrasonography[13] and by arthrography[14] in shoulders with good clinical results.

If the hole in the cuff is not painful, then what causes the pain in a shoulder with a rotator cuff tear? The causes can be either mechanical or biological (Table 21–1).

Table 21–1. Causes of Pain in Rotator Cuff Tear

Mechanical
Edge instability
Impingement
Biological
Synovitis
Secondary to edge instability of cuff tear
Secondary to other shoulder pathology (e.g., instability or synovial disease)
Intra-articular pathology
SLAP lesion
Bicipital tendinitis
Loose bodies
Adhesive capsulitis

The common mechanical causes of pain are impingement and edge instability (the situation in which the tear has an unstable redundant margin). Arthroscopic examination has confirmed that a small cuff tear with a nonretracted margin may act as a flap that can catch under the acromion. If this "unstable edge" is stabilized by rotator cuff repair, the catching in the shoulder should no longer be a source of pain. Alternatively, the unstable edge of a large medially-retracted tear may be stabilized by debriding the edge to a stable margin. This configuration leaves an arching free margin to a tension structure. This is a biomechanically favorable situation, because such a margin minimizes stress risers and bending moments along the free margin (see discussion under "Edge Stability").

Biological sources of pain can exist in the form of synovitis, adhesive capsulitis, and associated intra-articular pathology (SLAP lesion, bicipital tendinitis or biceps tendon tear, and loose bodies). The synovitis itself may be caused by chronic irritation secondary to "edge instability." It should be emphasized that the hole in the cuff is not in itself a cause of pain.

BIOMECHANICS: DEFINING THE FUNCTIONAL ROTATOR CUFF TEAR

I propose the term "functional rotator cuff tear" to define a tear that is anatomically deficient yet biomechanically intact. In order to be a functional cuff tear,

Table 21–2. Criteria for Functional Cuff Tear

Intact force couples (coronal and transverse planes)
Stable-fulcrum kinematic pattern
Intact suspension bridge
Tear within minimal surface area
Edge stability

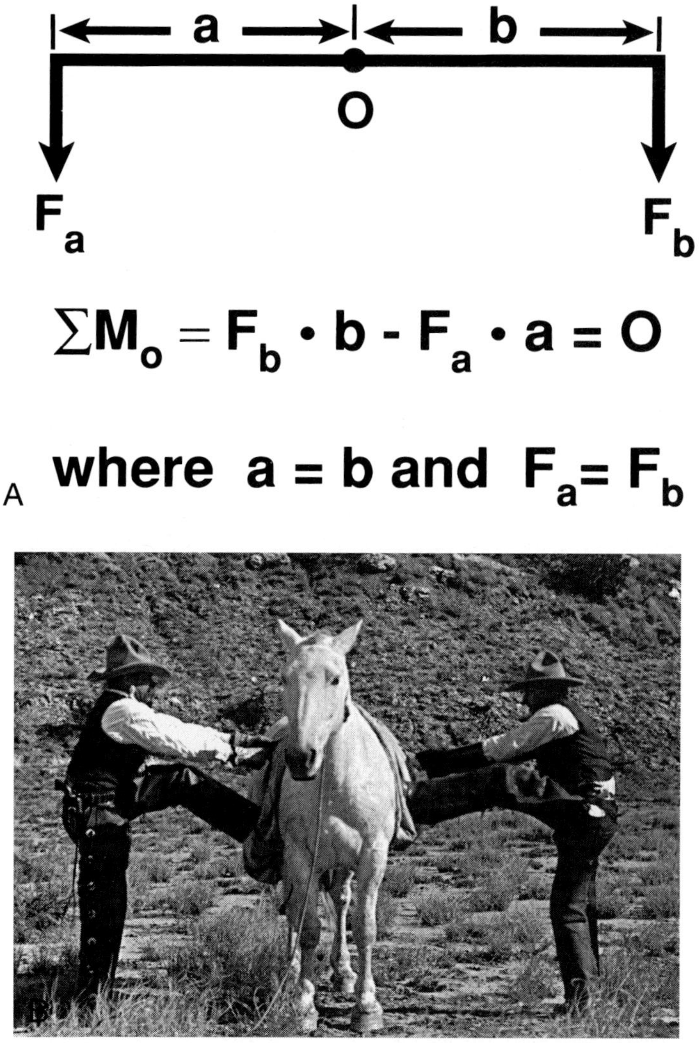

Fig. 21–1. *A,* **Force couple in which the forces are applied at equal distances from the center of rotation, creating moments that are equal and opposite.** *B,* **Balanced force couple created by two cowboys tightening the cinch on a pack horse. By applying equal and opposite forces at equal distances from the center of rotation, the cowboys tighten the cinch without rotating the pack.**

the tear must satisfy five biomechanical criteria (Table 21–2).

1. Force couples must be intact in the coronal and transverse planes.
2. A stable-fulcrum kinematic pattern must exist.
3. The shoulder's "suspension bridge" must be intact.
4. The tear must occur through a "minimal surface area."
5. The tear must possess "edge stability."

FORCE COUPLES OF THE SHOULDER

A force couple consists of a pair of forces acting on an object that tends to rotate that object. For the object to be in equilibrium, the forces must create moments that are equal and opposite in direction. This can occur (1) with two forces of equal magnitude that are at equal radii from the center of rotation (Fig. 21–1) or (2) with two unequal forces at different radii from the center of rotation such that their moments (force × distance) are equal and opposite (Fig. 21–2).

The coronal plane force couple was first described by Inman et al.[15] as consisting of the deltoid being counterpoised against the inferior portion of the rotator cuff (Fig. 21–3). The more important force couple in clinical application is the transverse plane force couple in which the anterior cuff (subscapularis) is balanced against the posterior cuff[16] (infraspinatus and teres minor) (Fig. 21–4).

The integrity of the posterior rotator cuff is easily tested on exam by resisted external rotation (Fig. 21–5). A useful test for subscapularis function is the lift-off test[17] (Fig. 21–6). The lift-off test places the shoulder in a starting position of extreme internal rotation so that the pectoralis major's insertion is so rotated that it can no longer function as an internal rotator in that position. This position (with the hand behind the back) isolates the subscapularis as the only internal rotator of the shoulder, and additional internal rotation (from subscapularis contraction) will cause the hand to "lift off" the lower back.

In order to have a stable fulcrum of glenohumeral joint motion, the force couples must be intact in both the coronal and transverse planes.

KINEMATIC PATTERNS

I performed fluoroscopic triplane imaging on 14 patients with massive unrepaired cuff tears of known location.[18] In this way, I was able to correlate the observed kinematic patterns with the known location of the cuff tears. Four kinematic patterns of glenohumeral motion were identified.

Type I—Stable Fulcrum Kinematics

Patients in this category had tears of the superior rotator cuff and part of the posterior cuff, comprising the supraspinatus and part of the infraspinatus (Fig. 21–7). This pattern of tear permitted preservation of essential force couples in the coronal and transverse planes such that the patients had normal motion and near normal strength.

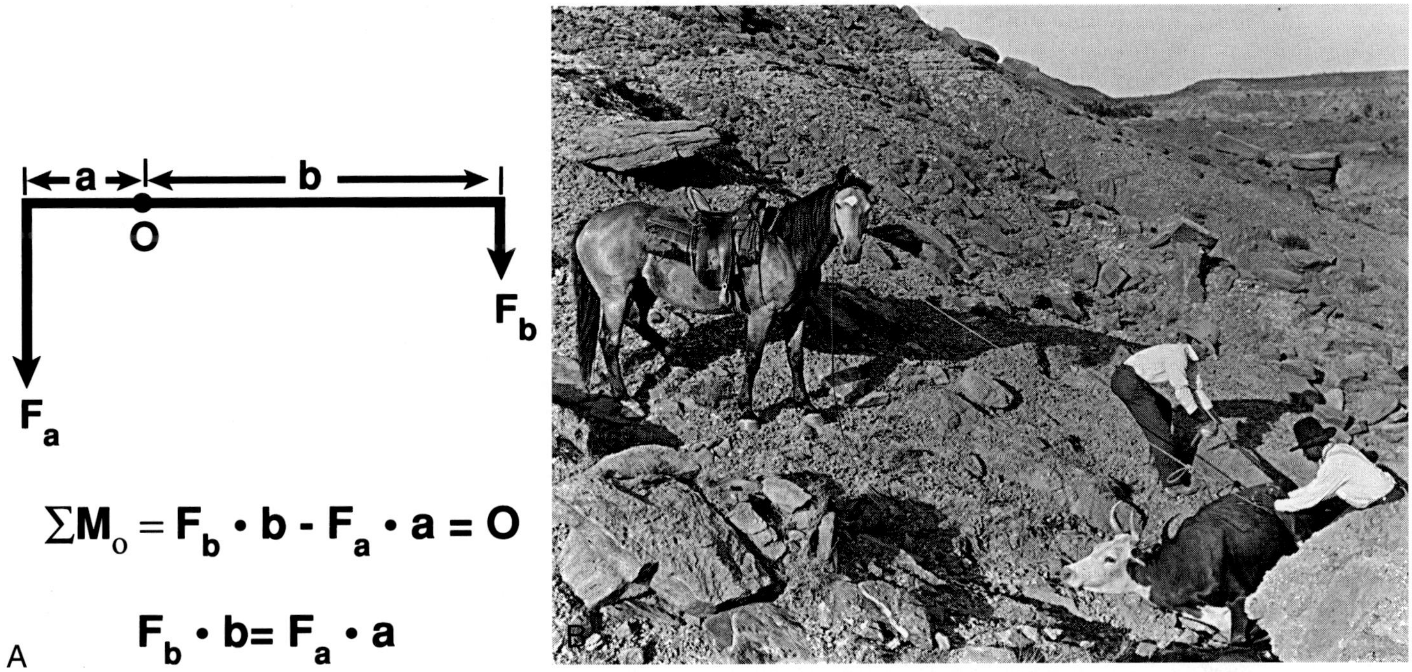
a
b
O
F_b
F_a
$\Sigma M_O = F_b \cdot b - F_a \cdot a = O$
$F_b \cdot b = F_a \cdot a$
A
B

Fig. 21–2. *A,* Force couples with unequal forces acting at different radii from the center of rotation, such that the moments created by the forces (force × distance) are equal and opposite. *B,* Cowboy creates balanced force couple by pulling on the cow's tail to prevent the pull of the horse from spinning the cow.

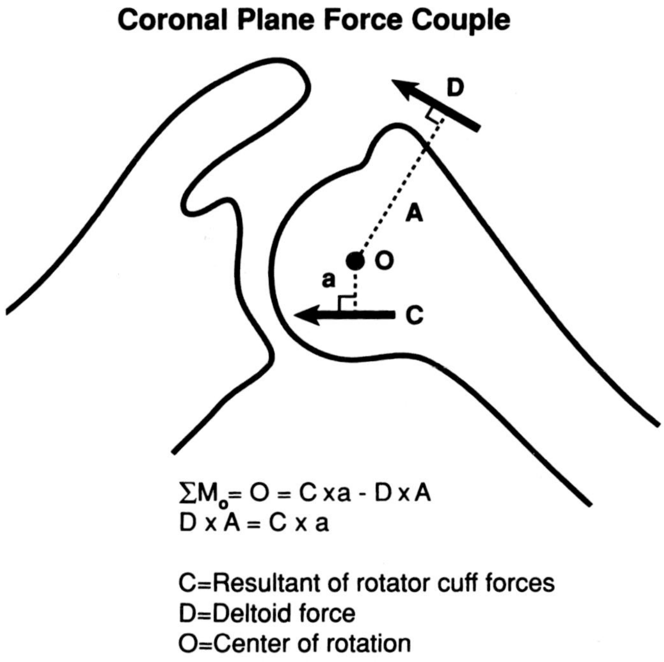

Fig. 21–3. Coronal plane force couple. The inferior portion of the rotator cuff (below the center of rotation) creates a moment that must balance the deltoid moment: (C) = resultant of rotator cuff forces, (D) = deltoid force, and (O) = center of rotation.

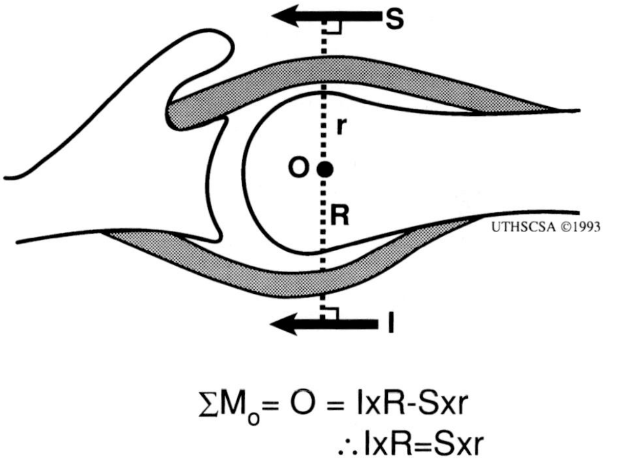

Fig. 21–4. Transverse plane force couple (axillary view). The subscapularis anteriorly is balanced against the infraspinatus and teres minor posteriorly: (I) = infraspinatus and (S)= subscapularis.

Type II—Unstable Fulcrum Kinematics: Posterior Cuff Tear Pattern

These patients had massive tears that involved virtually all of the superior and posterior rotator cuff (Fig. 21–8). Their active motion consisted of little more than a shoulder shrug. This pattern exhibited uncoupling of the essential force couples in the coronal and transverse planes, with the inability to create a stable fulcrum for glenohumeral motion.

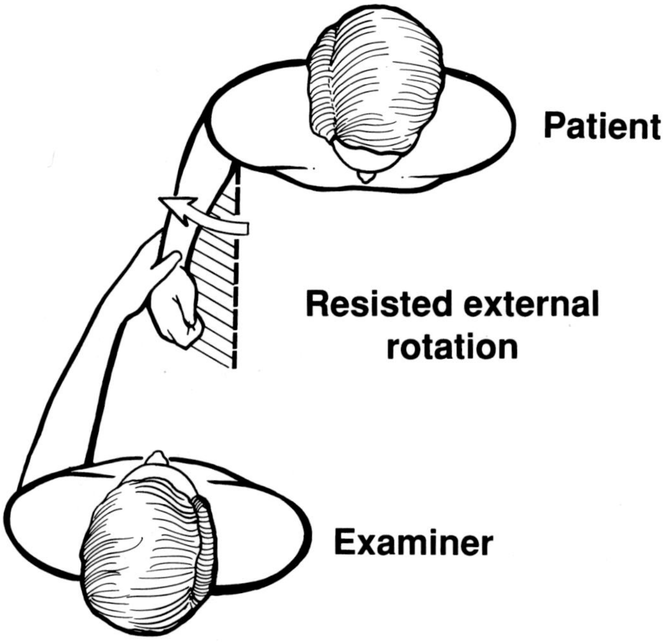

Fig. 21–5. Strength of resisted external rotation is the best test for external rotator function. The starting position is neutral shoulder rotation with the elbow flexed 90°. The patient actively performs external rotation of the shoulder against the examiner's resistance.

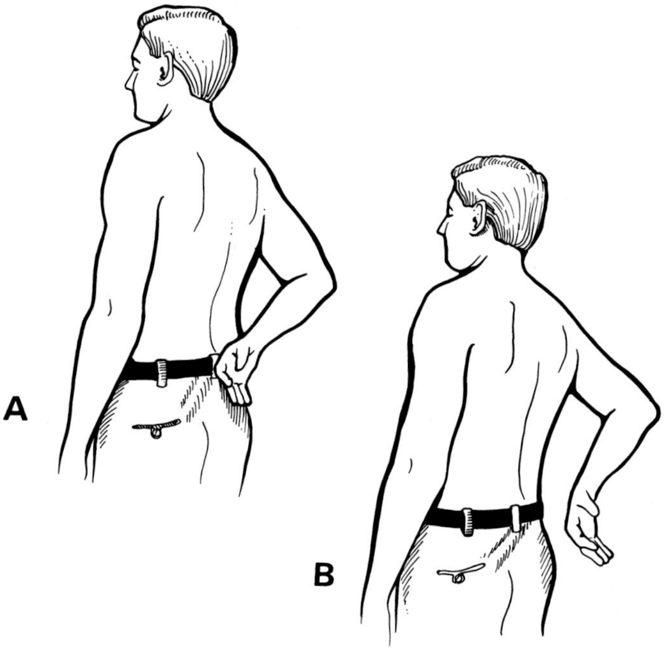

Fig. 21–6. *A,* This is the starting position for the lift-off test, with the shoulder internally rotated and the elbow flexed so that the back of the hand rests on the lower lumbar area. *B,* The patient actively lifts the hand away from the lower back. The starting position is one of approximately 100° internal rotation of the shoulder, and the only internal rotator in this position is the subscapularis. Inability to perform the lift-off test implies a nonfunctional subscapularis muscle.

SUBSCAPULARIS TEAR PATTERNS

The final two kinematic patterns involved subscapularis tears. Type III kinematics occurred with partial subscapularis tears and displayed good clinical motion, whereas type IV kinematics were associated with complete subscapularis tears and displayed poor motion.

Type III—Captured Fulcrum Kinematics

These patients had massive cuff tears that involved all of the supraspinatus, a major portion of the posterior cuff, and at least one-half of the subscapularis (Fig. 21–9). There was enough sparing of the posterior cuff that the patients had fair strength of resisted external rotation. In addition, there was enough intact subscapularis that the lift-off test was negative. However, the coronal plane force couple was not balanced enough to keep the humeral head centered in the glenoid, and the humerus subluxed superiorly to establish an acromiohumeral fulcrum. The deltoid was strong enough to allow elevation of the shoulder about this acromiohumeral fulcrum.

Patients with captured (acromiohumeral) fulcrum kinematics could be classified into two groups that were distinguished by the amount of anterosuperior coverage of the humeral head by the acromion. In both groups, the acromion acted as an "awning" over the top of the humeral head. Patients with a short awning obtained a fulcrum of motion at the anterior border of the acromion or on the soft-tissue sling in front of the acromion that allowed full forward elevation (Fig. 21–10). In contrast, the fulcrum of motion in patients with a long awning was posterior to the front edge of the acromion, such that it would impinge on the anterior acromion with attempted elevation and full forward elevation could not be achieved (Fig. 21–11).

This awning effect has important implications in patients with captured fulcrum kinematics. Patients with a short awning have significantly better forward elevation than those with a long awning. In fact, the limit of forward elevation that can be expected in a patient with an acromiohumeral fulcrum and a long overhanging acromion is equal to the angle that the slope of the acromion makes with a vertical line. At that point, the proximal humerus impinges on the anterior acromion, mechanically restricting further forward elevation.

Type IV—Unstable Fulcrum Kinematics: Subscapularis Tear Pattern

Patients in this category had a lesion that was the reverse of the type II lesion. The tear involved all of the superior cuff (supraspinatus) and all of the anterior cuff (subscapularis) (Fig. 21–12). The posterior cuff was intact. Shoulder elevation was poor. Fluoroscopy revealed subluxation in the coronal and transverse planes, with an inability to create a fulcrum for glenohumeral motion.

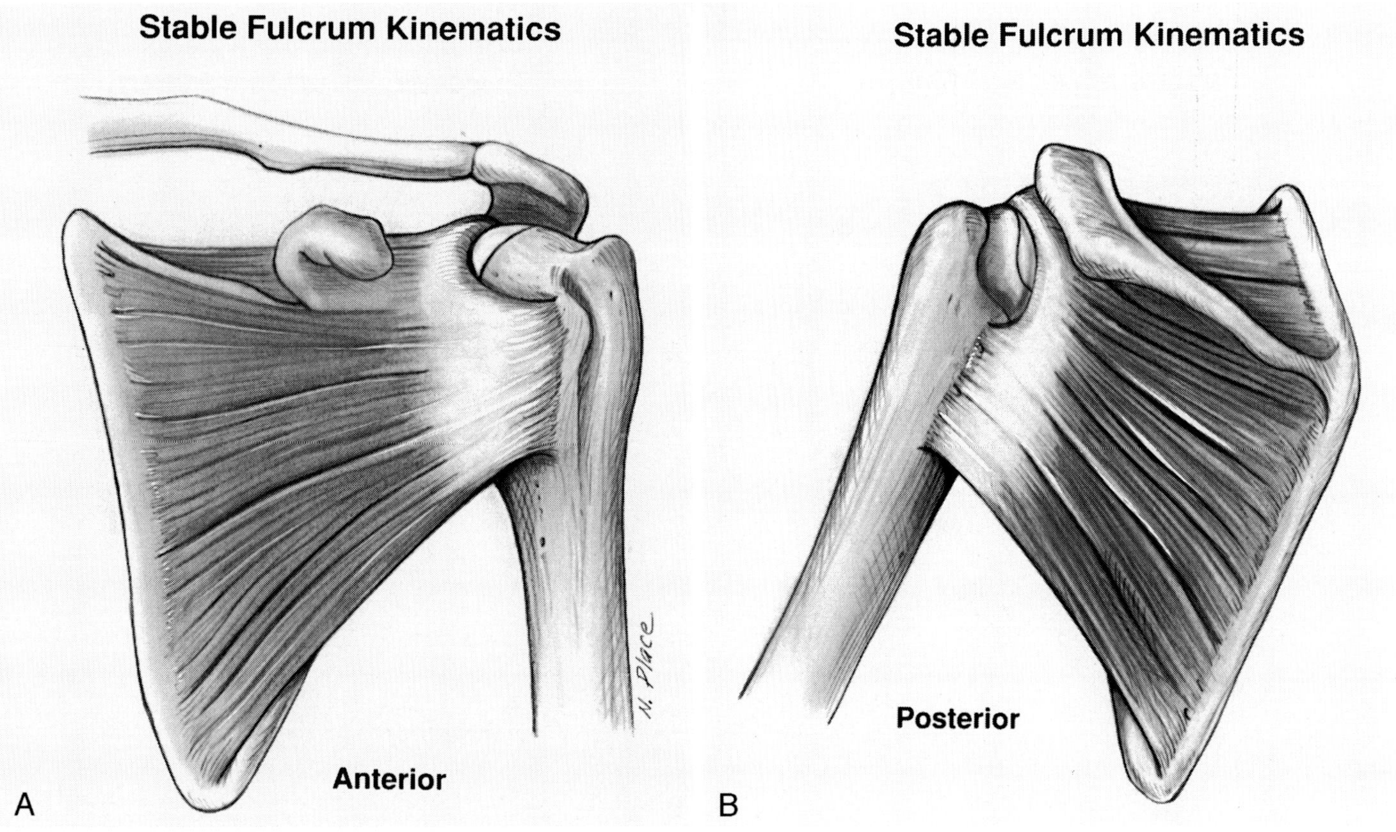

Fig. 21–7. ***A and B,*** **Stable fulcrum kinematics. The tear involves the supraspinatus and a portion of the infraspinatus.**

This group was initially confusing because the external rotators were intact and strong. However, the lift-off test was positive in each instance, indicating a complete tear of the subscapularis as the reason for the loss of the transverse plane force couple. The two patients with poor results in this clinical series had complete tears of the subscapularis.

This fluoroscopic investigation confirmed that the location of the rotator cuff tear is a key element in shoulder kinematics, and the location is much more important than the size of the tear.

The only tear pattern that displayed stable-fulcrum kinematics was the pattern that involved supraspinatus plus a portion of infraspinatus, the type I pattern, so that there was still enough posterior cuff to balance the subscapularis. This cuff tear pattern was associated with a stable fulcrum of glenohumeral motion, satisfying the second requirement of a functional rotator cuff tear.

SUSPENSION BRIDGE MODEL

A suspension bridge is a loaded cable, and as such it makes an excellent biomechanical model for a rotator cuff tear.[18] The free margin of the tear corresponds to the cable, and the anterior and posterior attachments of the tear correspond to the supports at each end of the cable's span (Fig. 21–13). The supraspinatus, which is not a depressor of the humerus, can still exert its effect as a compressor of the humeral head by means of its distributed load along the span of the suspension bridge configuration even though its insertion into the humerus is torn. The critical parameter in a complete rotator cuff tear is the force (both axial and shear) present at the two supports (Fig. 21–14), and the critical issue is whether the force is sufficient to cause extension of the tear.

Free-body analysis of a tear involving the supraspinatus plus half the infraspinatus can be performed.[19] This analysis predicts a maximal axial force of 169.79 N and maximal shear force of 124.65 N at the margins of the tear. We have completed an experimental study[20] on seven cadaver shoulders in which we created the above tear (supraspinatus plus half of infraspinatus) and symmetrically loaded the tear to a maximum of 684.0 N, with an average of 497.6 N ultimate load on each cuff tear by means of a MTS Model 810 (Materials Testing System, Minneapolis, MN). In this way, we were able to isolate a distributed load to the suspension bridge. These experimental loads were well above the predicted marginal loads for a maximal contraction of the supraspinatus and infraspinatus,[18] yet they caused no extension of the tear either anteriorly or posteriorly. Failure always occurred through the soft tissues of the suspension bridge rather

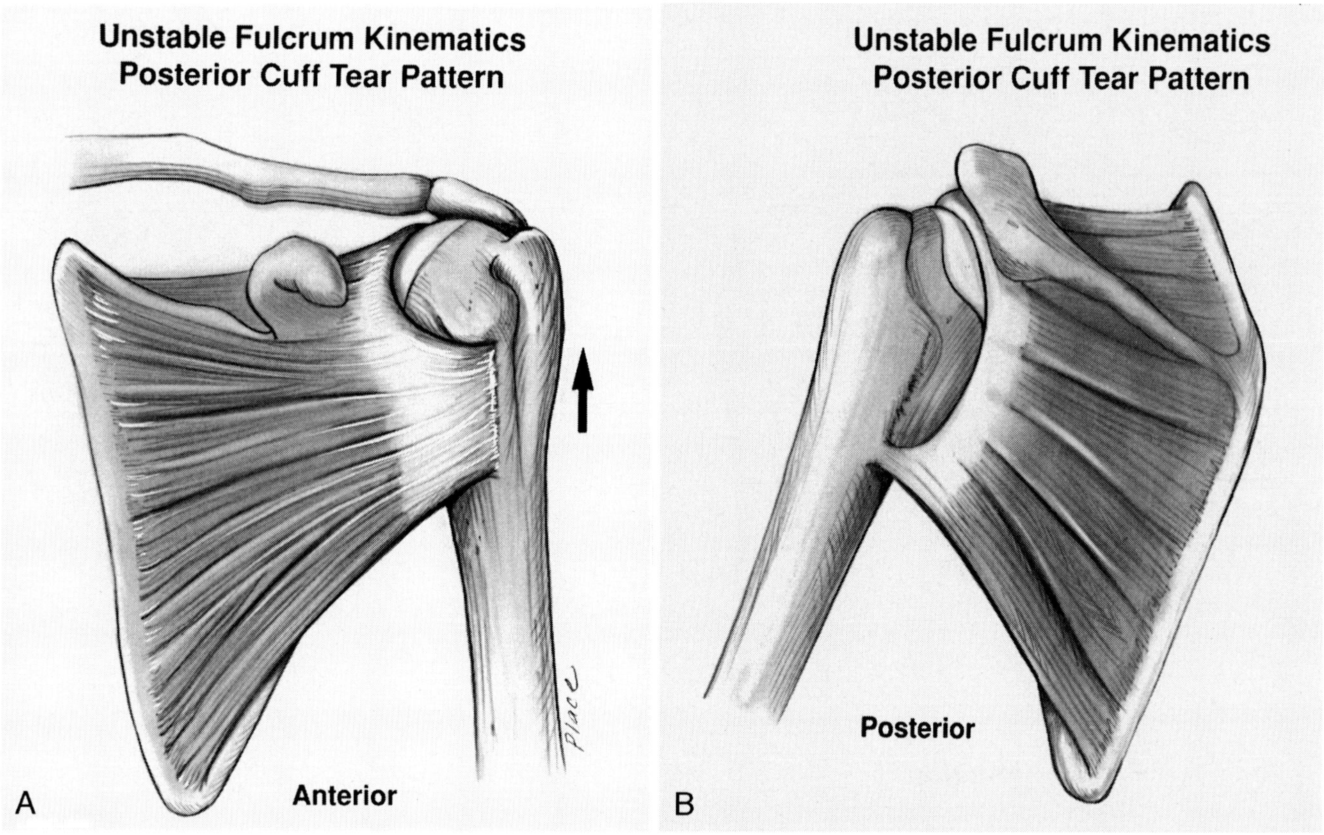

Fig. 21–8. *A and B,* **Unstable fulcrum kinematics, posterior cuff tear pattern. The tear involves the supraspinatus and all the posterior cuff. The anterior cuff (subscapularis) is intact.**

than through the bone insertions of the rotator cuff fibers. Therefore, one would not expect unrepaired tears to propagate anteriorly or posteriorly on a mechanical basis alone; significant biologic weakening of these cuff attachments would have to occur before fiber failure would be anticipated.

Arthroscopic visualization of the articular surface of an intact rotator cuff reveals a cablelike transverse thickening of the capsule surrounding a much thinner crescent of tissue (distal to the cable) that inserts onto the greater tuberosity (Fig. 21–15). This cablelike structure is consistently located at the margin of the avascular zone and subtends the insertions of the supraspinatus and infraspinatus. This cable has an anterior attachment adjacent to the biceps tendon and a posterior attachment at the inferior border of infraspinatus[19] (Fig. 21–16). Two previous studies[21,22] suggest that this thickened structure is an extension of the coracohumeral ligament.

We dissected the rotator crescent and cable in 20 cadaver shoulders (aged 60 to 85 years) and measured the thickness of the crescent and the cable by digital micrometer[19] (Fig. 21–17). The average thickness of the cable was 4.72 mm, whereas the crescent averaged only 1.82 mm in thickness (Fig. 21–18). This marked discrepancy in thickness suggests a protective function for the cable, with stress transfer along the cable and stress-shielding of its enclosed rotator crescent.

To test the hypothesis of stress-shielding of the rotator crescent by the rotator cable, we performed an experiment in which we symmetrically loaded the supraspinatus and infraspinatus attachments to the rotator cable and crescent in four cadaver shoulders (all greater than 60 years old) by means of a MTS Model 810.[23] Hall-effect transducers were placed in the rotator cable and the rotator crescent to measure the relative strain, or percentage elongation, of these two structures under load. In general, the cable showed significant elongation before the crescent underwent any elongation at all (Fig. 21–19). This experiment confirmed the hypothesis that the rotator cable can play a significant role in stress transfer from the supraspinatus and infraspinatus muscles by direct transfer along the cable to its terminal insertions, bypassing the distal insertions of the rotator crescent. It also demonstrated that the rotator cable can stress-shield the rotator crescent in a manner analogous to a load-bearing "suspension bridge." This stress-shielding, coupled with the location of the rotator crescent in the avascular zone, sets the stage for potential cuff failure on a biological basis rather than a mechanical basis. In other words, rotator cuff failure is more likely a result of simple aging than of tensile overload. As long as the rotator cable is stress-shielding the rotator crescent, tensile overload of the crescent would be unlikely based on our biomechanical findings.[23]

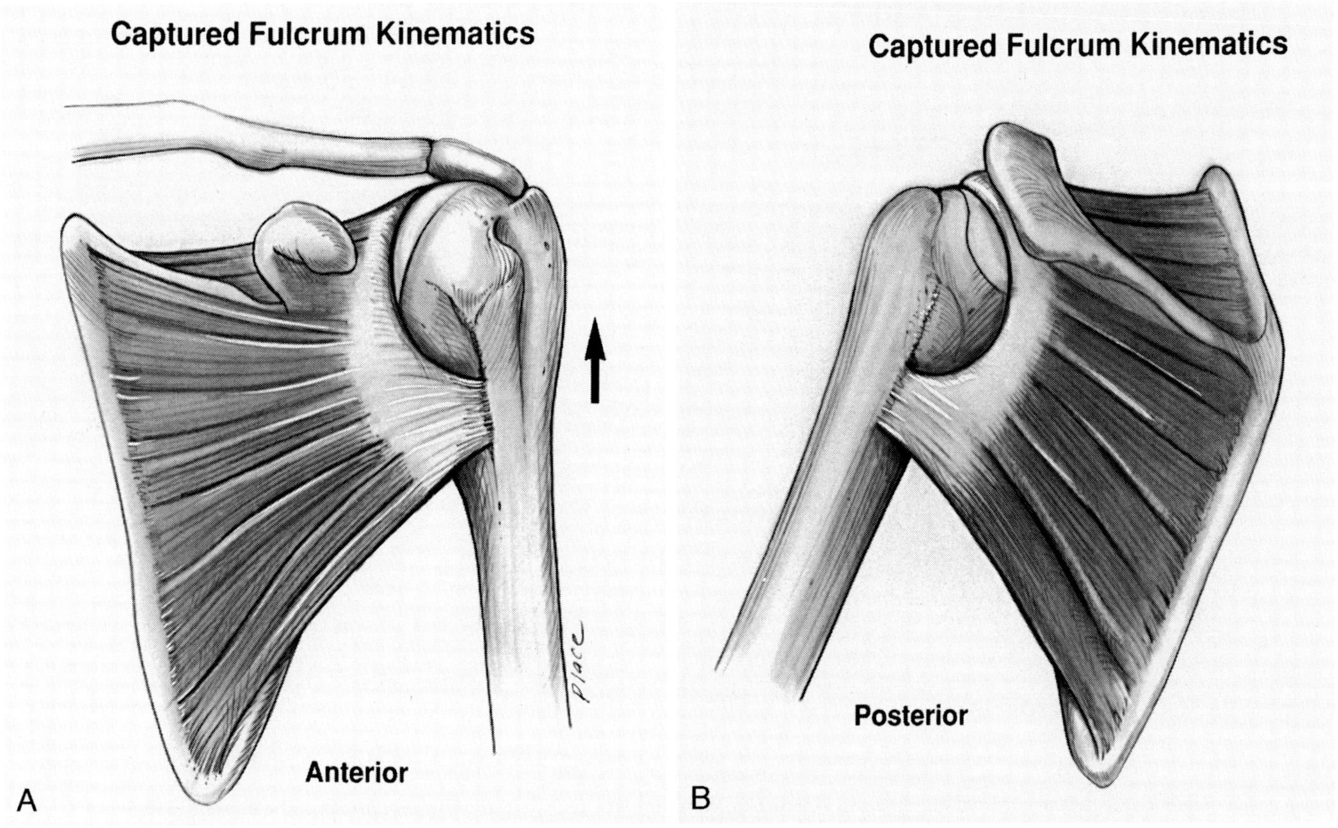

Fig. 21–9. *A and B,* Captured fulcrum kinematics. The tear involves the supraspinatus, at least 50% of the subscapularis, and a major portion of the posterior cuff. There is proximal humeral migration with an acromiohumeral fulcrum of motion.

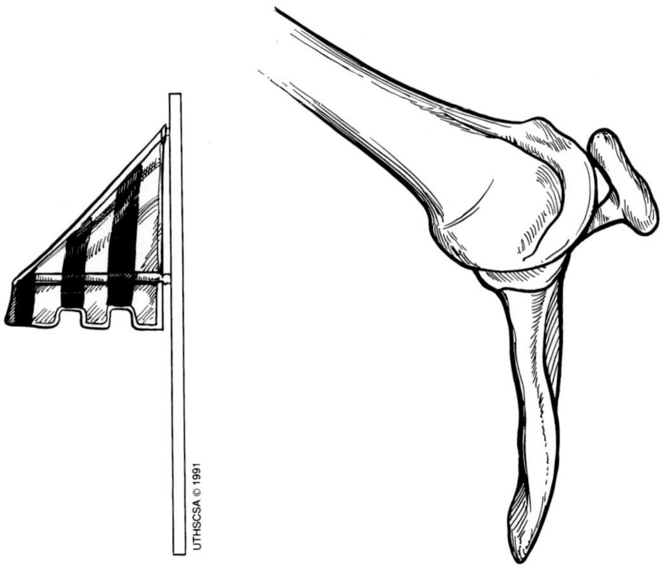

Fig. 21–10. Short awning (short anterior acromion). The fulcrum of motion is so far anterior that there is no impingement with forward elevation, and motion is full.

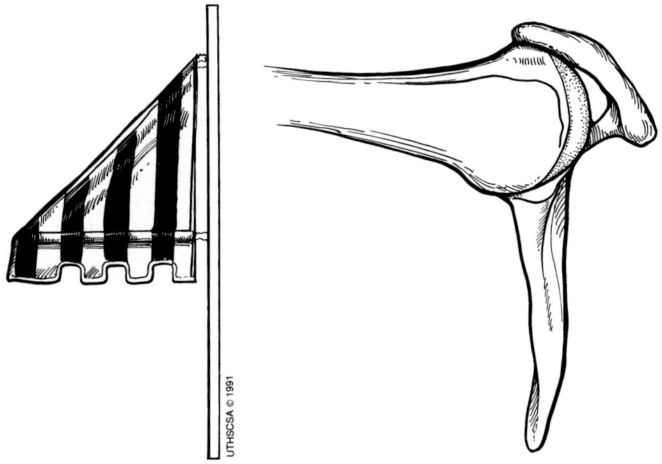

Fig. 21–11. Long awning (long anterior acromion). With forward elevation of the humerus, the overhanging anterior acromion impinges on the humerus, mechanically restricting motion.

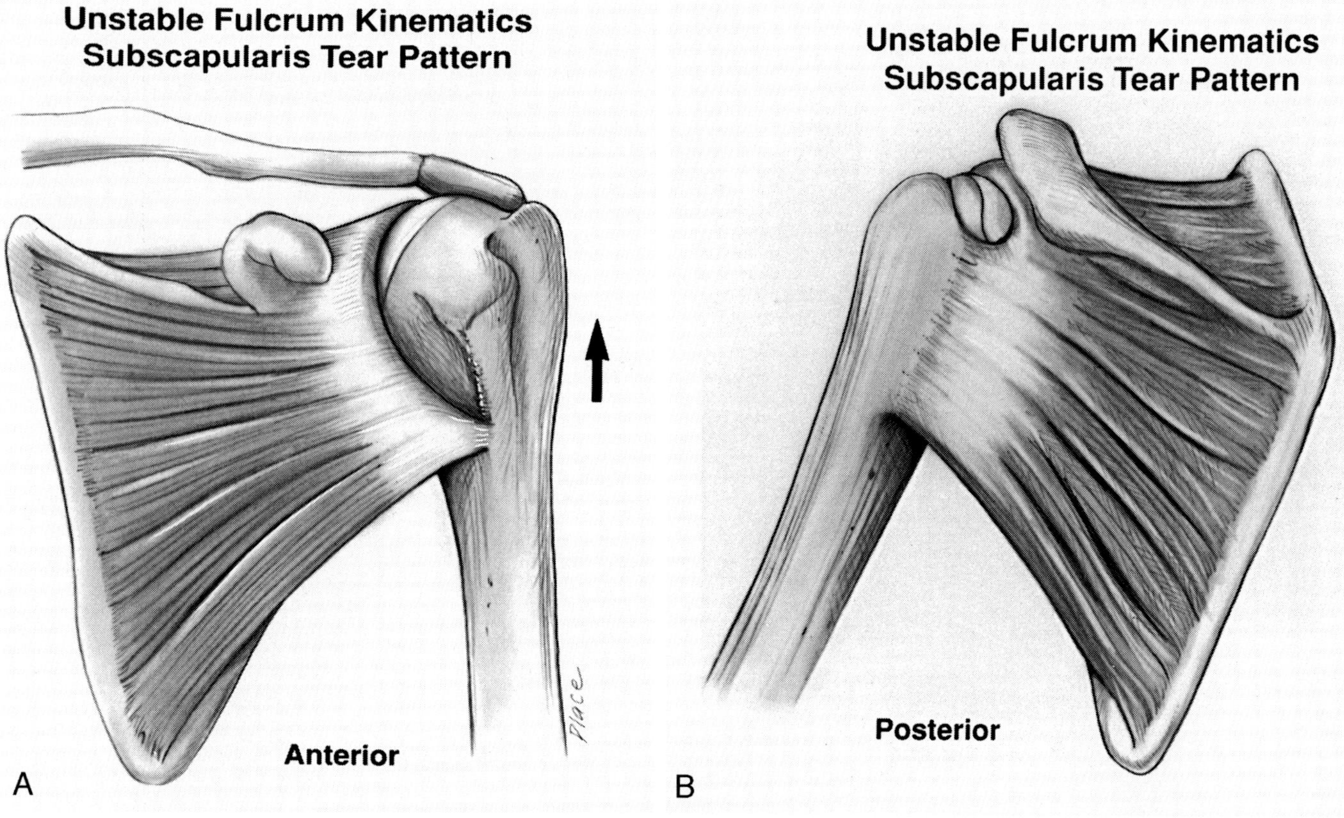

Fig. 21–12. ***A and B,*** **Unstable fulcrum kinematics, subscapularis tear pattern. The tear involves the supraspinatus and all the subscapularis. The posterior cuff muscles (external rotators) are intact.**

We recently tested an additional group of cadaver shoulders in a similar manner.[24] In this study, elongation (strain) was measured by a Differential Variable Reluctance Transducer (MicroStrain, Burlington, VT). Two of these shoulders, which were in a younger age group and had thick rotator crescents, did not demonstrate stress-shielding of the crescent by the cable. The older shoulders, with thin crescent tissue, again demonstrated stress-shielding of the crescent by the cable. These preliminary findings suggest that there may be two functional classes of rotator cuff based on the behavior of the cable-crescent complex under load. These two functional classes may be categorized as cable-dominant shoulders (in which the crescent is stress-shielded by the cable) and crescent-dominant shoulders (in which there is no stress-shielding of the crescent by the cable).[19]

It is intriguing to postulate that crescent-dominant shoulders may become cable-dominant shoulders with advancing age. Most of the shoulders we have tested have been greater than 60 years old and have been cable dominant. However, we do not know if people are born with cable-dominant shoulders or if they develop as a result of adaptive changes over time. One may speculate that progressive thinning of the relatively avascular crescent tissue may be an inevitable consequence of aging, and that hypertrophy of the cable may gradually develop as the cable takes on increasing loads with age because of crescent thinning.

MINIMAL SURFACE AREA

"Minimal surface area" is a structural engineering term that applies to tension structures such as tents, fabric-covered airplane wings, and various saddle-shaped roof designs.[24] By definition, a minimal surface area is the smallest geometric area that can span the space between two adjacent frames. An important property of a minimal surface area is that tension is equal in all directions on its surface.

Nature has provided us with a number of naturally occurring minimal surface areas. The simplest example is that of a soap bubble in a bubble wand. Consider the case of a bubble wand composed of two arches at right angles to each other. The bubble assumes a saddle shape, which is the minimal surface area between the two arches of the wand (Fig. 21–20). Because this is a minimal surface area, tension is equal in all directions as one would expect, or else the bubble would burst.

I submit that nature has created a functional equivalent to a minimal surface area in the shoulder in the form of the stress-shielded rotator crescent. In this case, the two arches that form the "frame" for this minimal surface area are (1) the rotator cable and (2) the arching bony attachments of the supraspinatus and infraspinatus onto the greater tuberosity of the humerus (the rotator crescent insertion) (Fig. 21–21). The intervening sheet

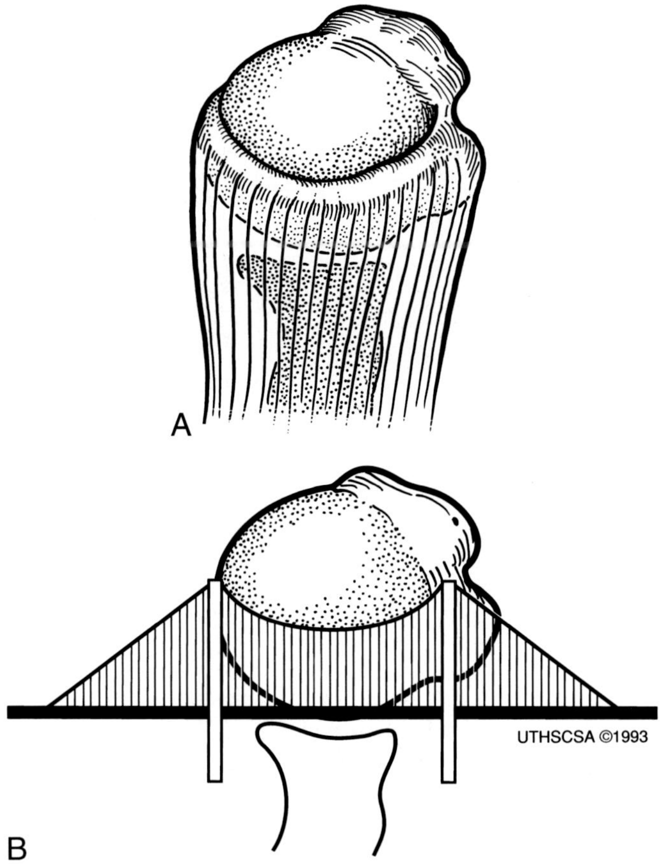

Fig. 21–13. *A and B,* A rotator cuff tear can be modeled after a suspension bridge. The free margin of the tear corresponds to the cable, and the anterior and posterior attachments of the tear correspond to the supports at each end of the cable's span.

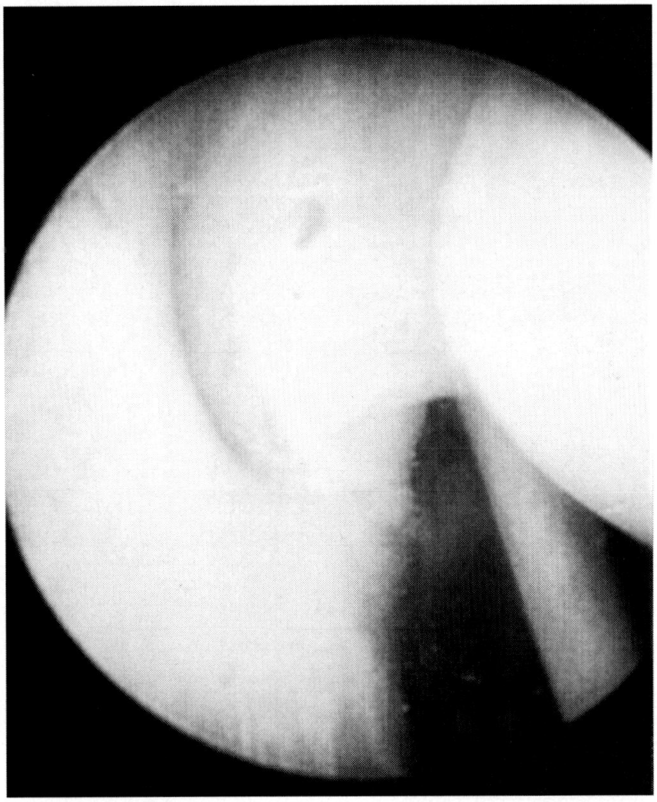

Fig. 21–15. Arthroscopic view of the rotator cable and rotator crescent in a right shoulder viewed through a posterior portal. The crescent lies between the cable and the humeral head. Note the distinct invagination at the junction of the rotator crescent with the rotator cable.

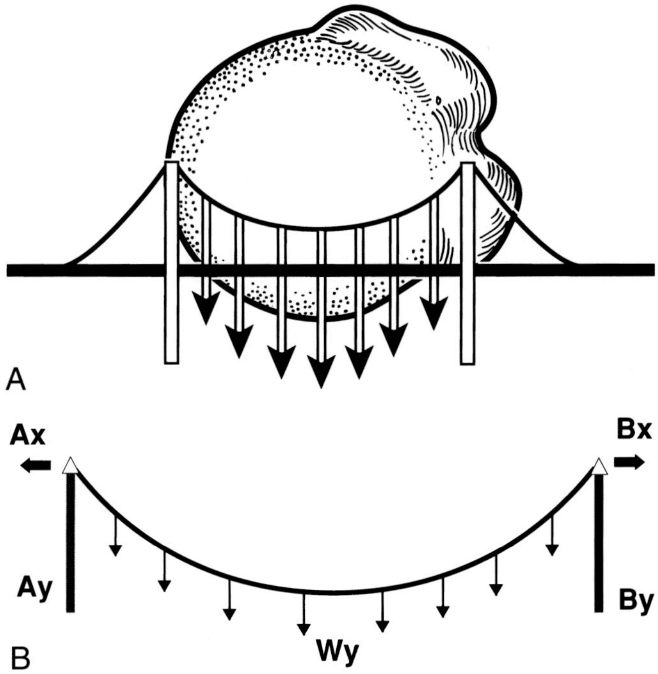

Fig. 21–14. *A,* Rotator cuff tear modeled after a uniformly loaded cable. *B,* Free-body diagram used to calculate the maximal axial forces (A_y and B_y) and the maximal shear forces (A_x and B_x).

of fibrous tissue, the rotator crescent, would then be a minimal surface area. Realizing that the rotator crescent tissue is not strictly isotropic, we must consider the minimal surface area analogy an approximation. Nonetheless, this model is useful and demonstrates an excellent way for nature to stress-shield and protect these rotator cuff insertions.

I have noted at arthroscopy that virtually all rotator cuff tears, both partial and complete, begin in the rotator crescent. We have tried experimentally to load intact "cable-crescent complex" attachments to failure at loads up to 1343.0 N and have been unable to cause failure of an intact cable-crescent insertion at these extremely high loads.[25] Therefore, I do not think that most rotator cuff tears are initiated as a result of mechanical tensile overload. I submit that some rotator cuff tears within the crescent occur because these relatively avascular tissues are stress-shielded and undergo degeneration as a result of a relative absence of physiologic stress, much as one sees bone resorption in the proximal femur because of stress-shielding after total hip replacement.

If we envision a stress-shielded crescent with a degenerative tear surrounded by a strong cable that is unlikely to undergo tensile failure (assuming there is no ongoing biologic process to weaken the tendon attachments), then we have a biomechanical basis to consider debridement rather than repair of the torn tissues in selected older individuals.

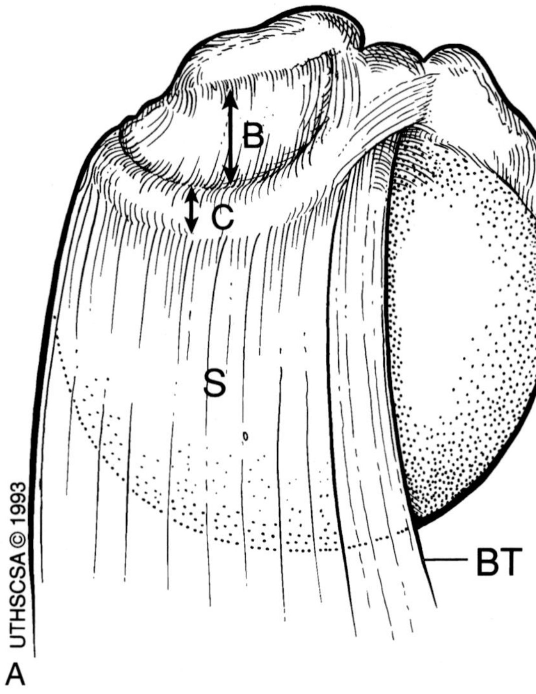

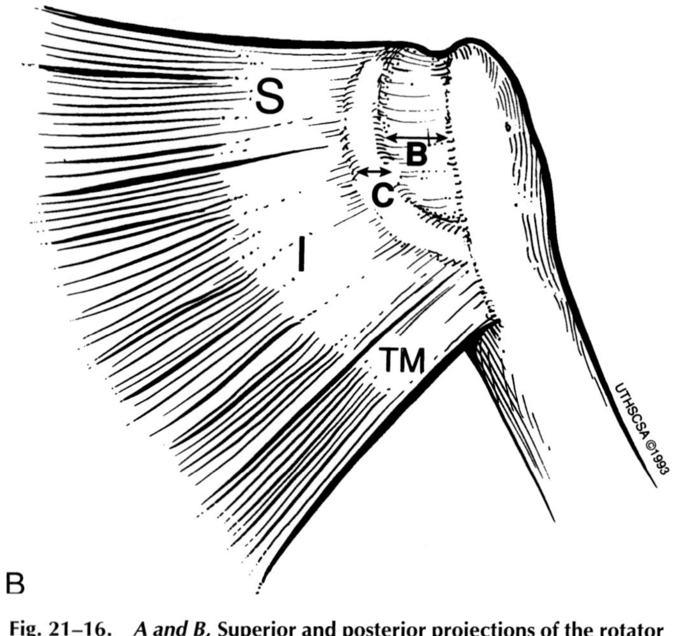

Fig. 21–16. *A and B,* **Superior and posterior projections of the rotator cable and crescent. The rotator cable extends from the biceps to the inferior margin of infraspinatus, spanning the supraspinatus and infraspinatus insertions: (C) = width of rotator cable, (B) = medial-lateral diameter of rotator crescent, (S) = supraspinatus, (I) = infraspinatus, (TM) = teres minor, and (BT) = biceps tendon.**

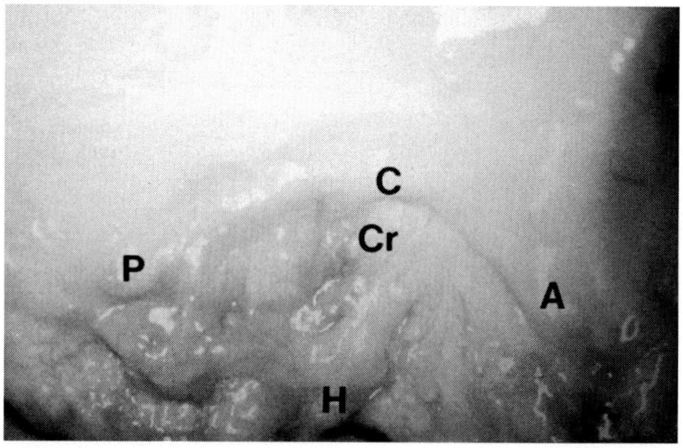

Fig. 21–17. Anatomical specimen of the rotator cuff after dissecting its insertions from the humerus: (H) = humeral attachment of rotator cuff, (C) = rotator cable, (Cr) = rotator crescent, (A) = anterior attachment of rotator cable, and (P) = posterior attachment of rotator cable.

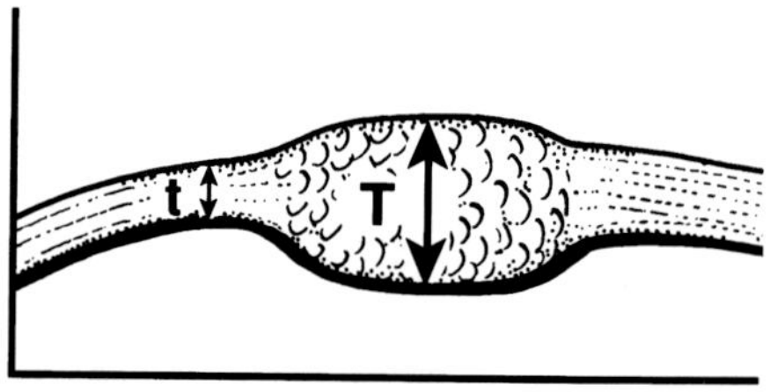

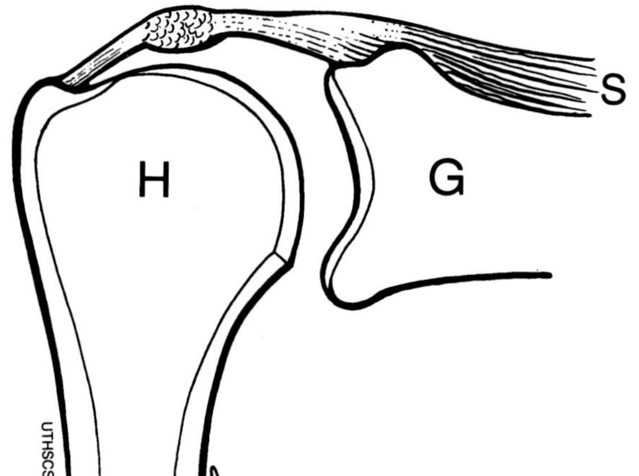

Fig. 21–18. Coronal section of rotator crescent and cable. Note the thickened rotator cable in comparison to the thin rotator crescent. Inset: (T) = thickness of rotator cable and (t) = thickness of rotator crescent.

EDGE STABILITY

The free edge of a tension structure should be smooth, without redundant margins, in order to avoid localized marginal stress concentrations and to avoid tensile entrapment of the redundant edge. Tension structures based on minimal surface areas are often designed with arching free margins (Fig. 21–22), because this configuration minimizes stress risers and bending moments along these free margins.[24] This arching margin is mechanically strong and efficiently resists failing from repetitive loading.

In the case of a rotator cuff tear with a redundant edge, one can imagine that with shoulder motion this edge may

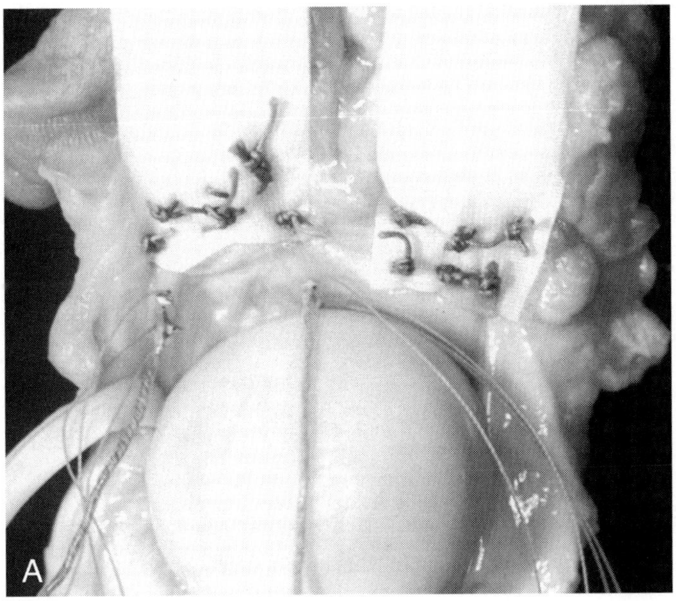

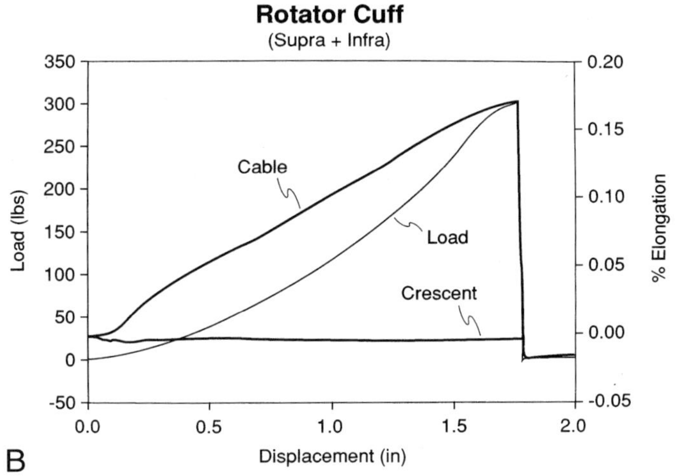

Fig. 21–19. *A,* **A test specimen is uniformly loaded by the MTS machine through nylon straps. Transducers have been placed in the rotator cable and rotator crescent.** *B,* **Graphic representation of percentage elongation of cable and crescent as increasing load is applied to the cable-crescent complex. The cable underwent significant elongation while the crescent did not elongate at all up to the 300-lb load at which the fixation of the construct was lost. This graphically demonstrates stress-shielding of the crescent by the cable.**

undergo a tensile entrapment, causing pain as well as localized stress concentrations within the rotator cable. This type of rotator cuff tear displays edge instability (Fig. 21–23). Smaller tears have unstable subacromial edges that tend to catch under the acromion (subacromial edge instability). Larger tears have unstable articular edges, because these large redundant edges extend more medially and tend to catch intra-articularly between the humeral head and the edge of the rotator cable (articular edge instability).

In a tear with an unstable edge, there are two ways to create edge stability. One way would be to repair the rotator cuff tear to bone (Fig. 21–24), so that one restores

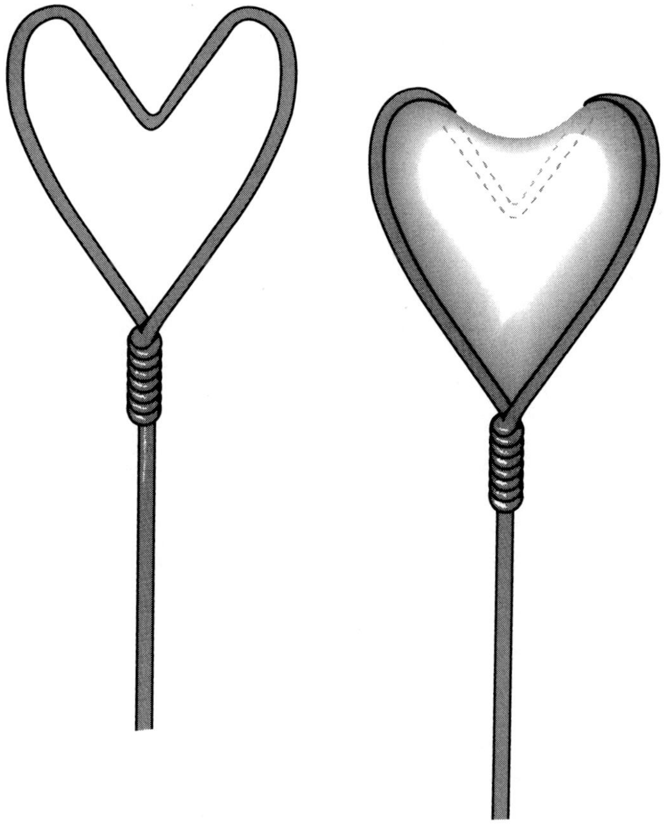

Fig. 21–20. *A and B,* **Bubble wand is composed of two arches at right angles to each other. The bubble automatically assumes the shape of a minimal surface area, which in this case is a saddle shape.**

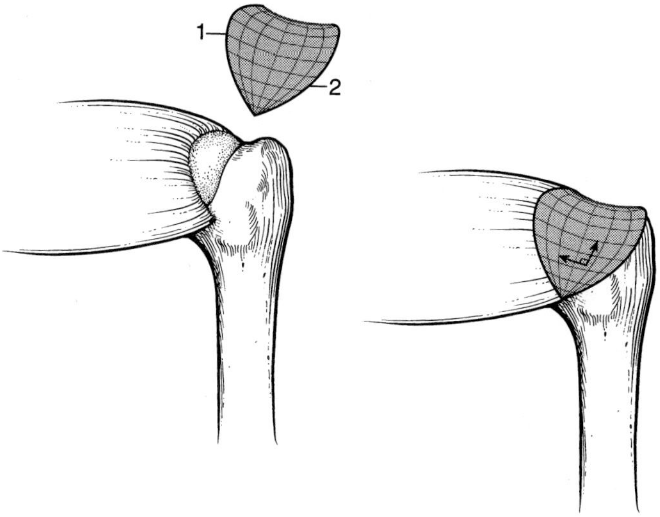

Fig. 21–21. The two arches for the rotator crescent's minimal surface area are (1) the rotator cable and (2) the arching bony attachments of the supraspinatus and infraspinatus onto the greater tuberosity of the humerus (the rotator crescent insertion).

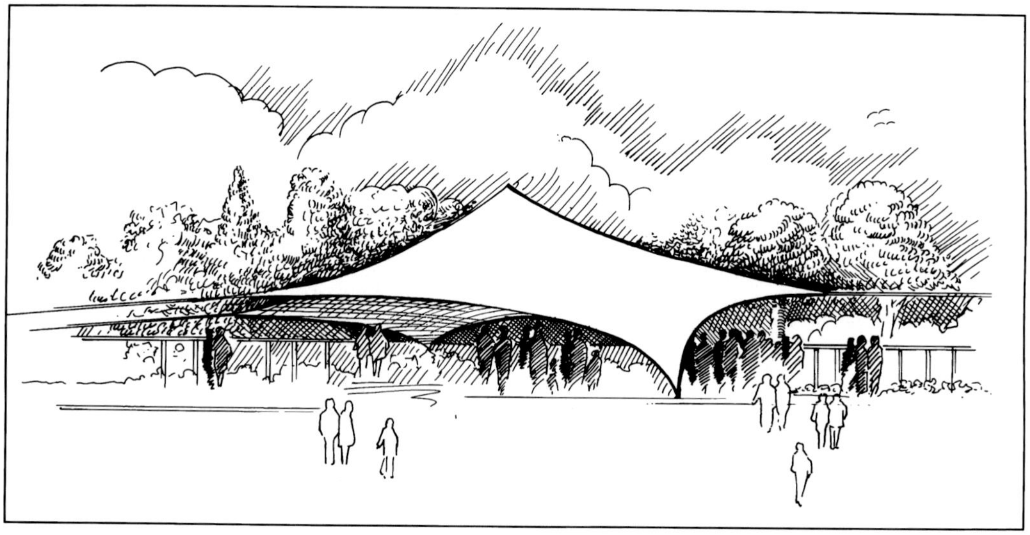

Fig. 21–22. Example of a tension structure with arching free margins designed to minimize stress risers and bending moments along the free margins.

the cuff's double-arched system with an intervening minimal surface area. In this configuration, there are no free edges that can catch and become subject to tensile entrapment.

The second way to create edge stability is to debride the redundant margins of the tear to a stable edge (Fig. 21–25). In the case of a massive tear, the debridement would likely extend to the free margin of the rotator cable. A shoulder that has had a decompression combined with debridement of torn redundant cuff margins to achieve edge stability is not likely to experience painful tensile entrapment. In addition, the arching free margin of the tear minimizes stress risers and bending moments at the margin. Therefore, if this shoulder meets the criteria for having a "functional cuff tear" and achieves edge stability to provide pain relief, the results of cuff debridement plus decompression can be quite good.

Shoulders with functional cuff tears typically have good motion and good strength despite a hole in the cuff. Rather than thinking in terms of "covering the hole" in functional cuff tears, we need to direct our attention to "stabilizing the edge," either by repair or by debridement.

Clinical implications: Repair versus debridement versus partial repair

There are three main clinical implications of the foregoing biomechanical discussion. The first implication is that functional tears with an unstable but minimally retracted edge may gain edge stability by simple repair. Rotator cuff repair adds a set of suspenders to the requisite belt (rotator cable) of the functional cuff tear and is the preferred treatment (in conjunction with subacromial decompression) of tears that can be easily repaired. Repair is especially important in younger active people, because they may have a crescent-dominant rotator cuff that does not have a stress-shielded crescent.

The second implication is that unrepaired rotator cuff tears with intact force couples and an intact rotator cable may have normal function if the patient can obtain satisfactory pain relief. Therefore, these tears may be amenable to arthroscopic debridement and decompression in selected individuals who can obtain edge stability, thereby obviating the need for a more extensive open procedure with its increased morbidity and prolonged rehabilitation. Bear in mind that these tears may be quite large, because the rotator cable extends to the lower border of infraspinatus. Arthroscopic decompression and cuff debridement can yield good results only if the patient has reasonably strong external rotators and a negative lift-off test, ensuring a balanced force couple in the transverse plane.

The third clinical implication is that some massive irreparable tears with poor function might best be treated by partial repair of the rotator cuff tear to balance the force couples. The reason that these tears have such poor function is that they are so extensive that the force couples are no longer balanced and they do not have stable fulcrum kinematics. These tears do not have intact mechanics and therefore are "dysfunctional tears." Typically these are tears that involve all the posterior rotator cuff, although a tear of most of the subscapularis can also cause an imbalance of the force couples. Testing resisted external rotation in a patient with a massive posterior cuff tear will reveal that he has little (if any) strength with resisted external rotation. The lift-off test is a specific test for subscapularis function and is far superior to testing resisted internal rotation.

If the patient is not able to externally rotate the shoulder or if he has a positive lift-off test, his force couples are not balanced. In this case, active elevation is poor. If arthroscopy confirms the clinical impression of a massive

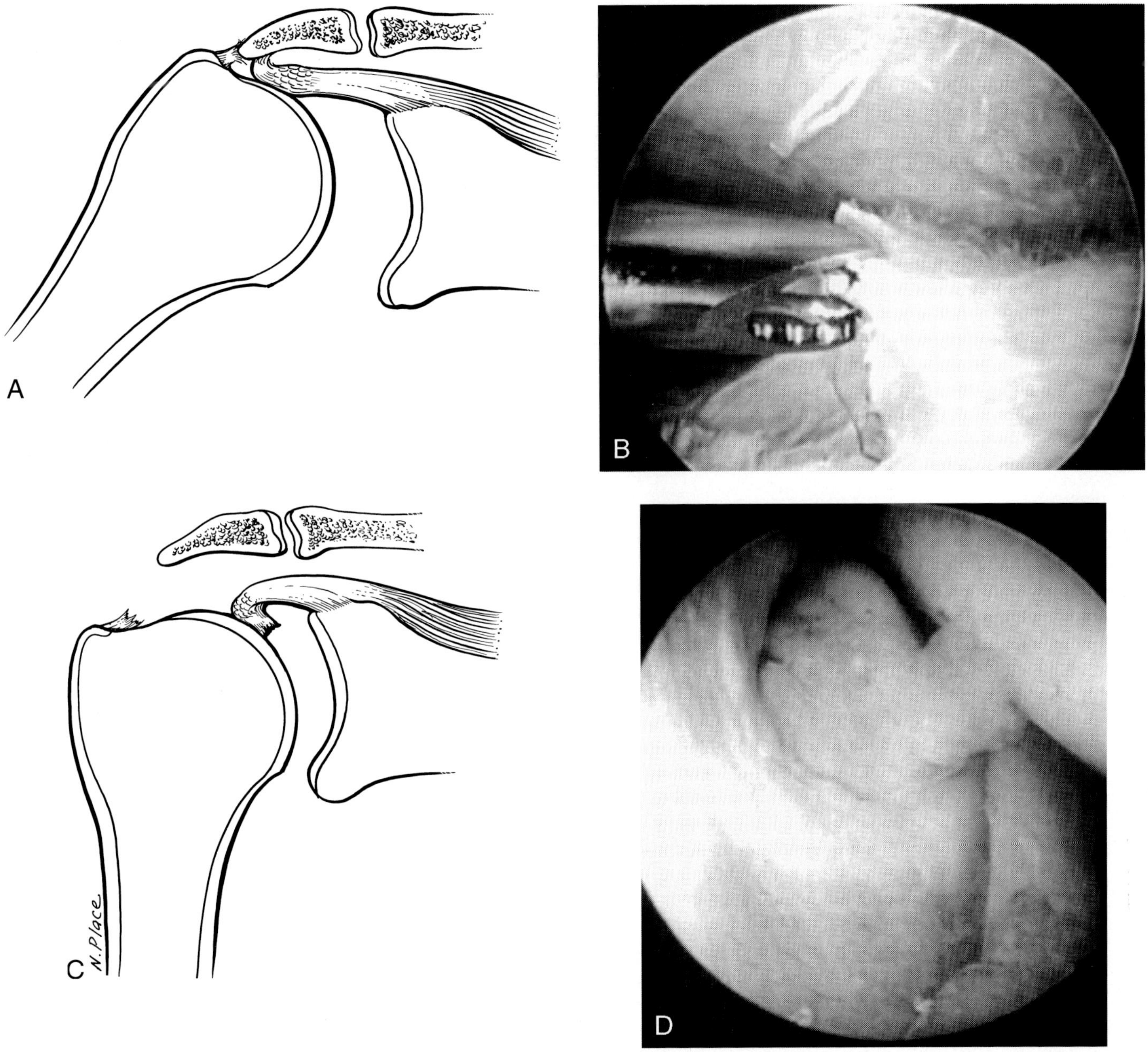

Fig. 21–23. *A,* Subacromial edge instability; the redundant subacromial edge can become entrapped under the acromion. *B,* Arthroscopic subacromial view (through posterior viewing portal) of a left shoulder with a rotator cuff tear that demonstrates subacromial edge instability. *C,* Articular edge instability; the redundant articular edge can become entrapped intra-articularly between the rotator cable and the humeral head. *D,* Arthroscopic view of a right shoulder (through posterior viewing portal) with a rotator cuff tear that catches between the rotator cable and the humeral head, demonstrating articular edge instability (patient's head is to the left).

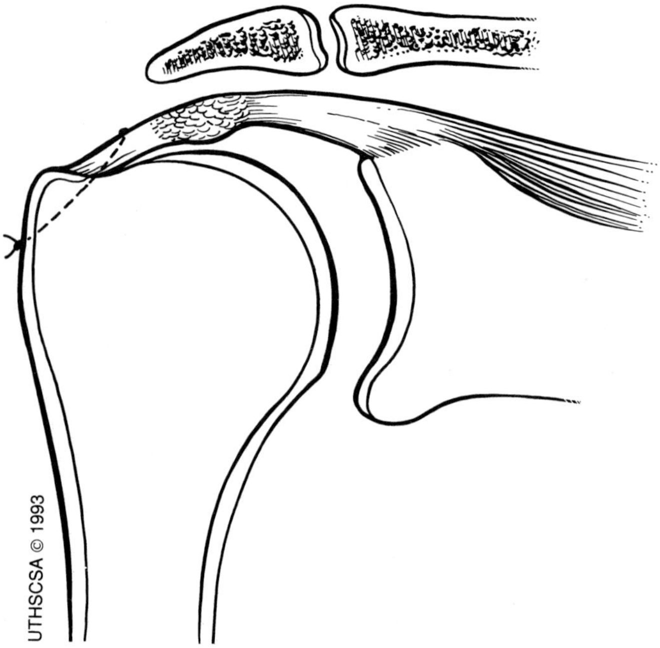

Fig. 21–24. Rotator cuff repair stabilizes the edge of a reparable tear.

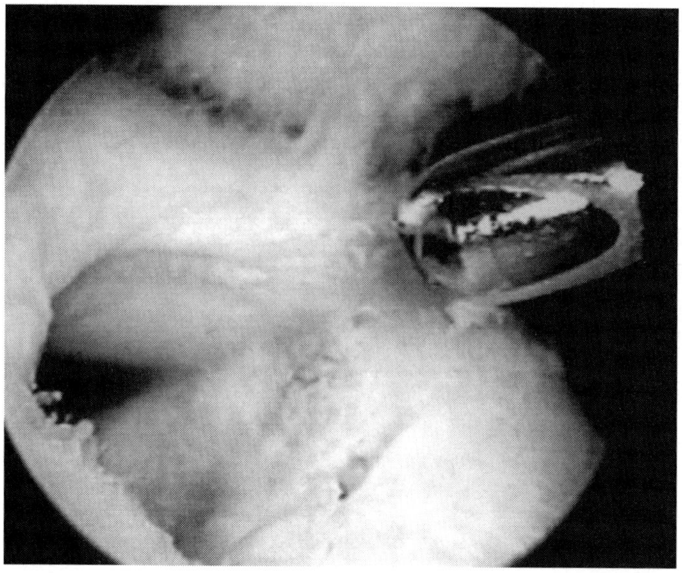

Fig. 21–25. Arthroscopic view through posterior subacromial portal of a tear in a right shoulder that has been given edge stability by debridement to a thick arching margin without redundancy.

"dysfunctional cuff tear" in an active individual who requires a strong shoulder, I proceed with an open partial repair of the torn posterior or anterior cuff to balance the force couples. The superior cuff is generally too retracted to repair in these massive tears, so I leave a hole in the top of the cuff.

Congenital Subacromial Stenosis

Congenital subacromial stenosis is a previously undescribed entity that causes a decrease in the height of the subacromial space without proximal migration of the humerus.[26] I first noted congenital subacromial stenosis in 1988 as a contributing factor to an impingement syndrome. Since that time, I have identified 25 patients with this condition (Fig. 21–26).

Several investigators have concluded that narrowing of the acromiohumeral interval to less than 7 mm on a standard AP radiograph signified a complete rotator cuff tear.[27–33] My 25 patients had an average acromiohumeral interval of 4.7 mm in association with a normal glenohumeral relationship (i.e., the inferior humeral articular margin was at the same level as the inferior glenoid articular margin) (Fig. 21–27).

Fifteen of the 25 shoulders (60%) with congenital subacromial stenosis had rotator cuff tears. Patients requiring surgery comprised a bimodal age distribution: those with an impingement syndrome requiring decompression had an average age of 42, whereas those with rotator cuff tears requiring surgical treatment had an average age of 66. The natural history seems to be a relentless progression to complete rotator cuff tear as a result of abrasion within this narrowly confined subacromial space. Therefore, an aggressive approach toward subacromial decompression may be indicated in younger symptomatic individuals to prevent late cuff tear.

Congenital subacromial stenosis seems to cause tears of the superior cuff through repetitive abrasion in older individuals. The posterior and anterior cuff are typically not involved. Therefore, the coronal and transverse plane force couples are usually intact, and these tears are functional cuff tears. For that reason, many of these patients make ideal candidates for cuff debridement and decompression.

Clinical Results of Arthroscopic Debridement and Decompression for Massive Rotator Cuff Tears

I have previously reported good results in selected patients with massive (> 5 cm diameter) rotator cuff tears who underwent arthroscopic debridement and decompression.[10] I have expanded that review to 25 patients with long-term follow-up[34] (average 54 months; range 39 to 72 months), and had 88% good and excellent results by Ellman's criteria.[35] A similar study by Zvijac et al.[36] showed that their initial good results from arthroscopic debridement and decompression deteriorated with time. Unlike the series by Zvijac et al., the good results in my series have not deteriorated with time. One must assume that the reason for the lack of deterioration with time is that care was taken in most cases to select patients with functional cuff tears.

My personal series of arthroscopic debridement and decompression for rotator cuff tears now totals 72 patients, with follow-up ranging from 6 months to 72 months.[34] This group had good and excellent results of 90% by Ellman's criteria. There were seven failures. Of

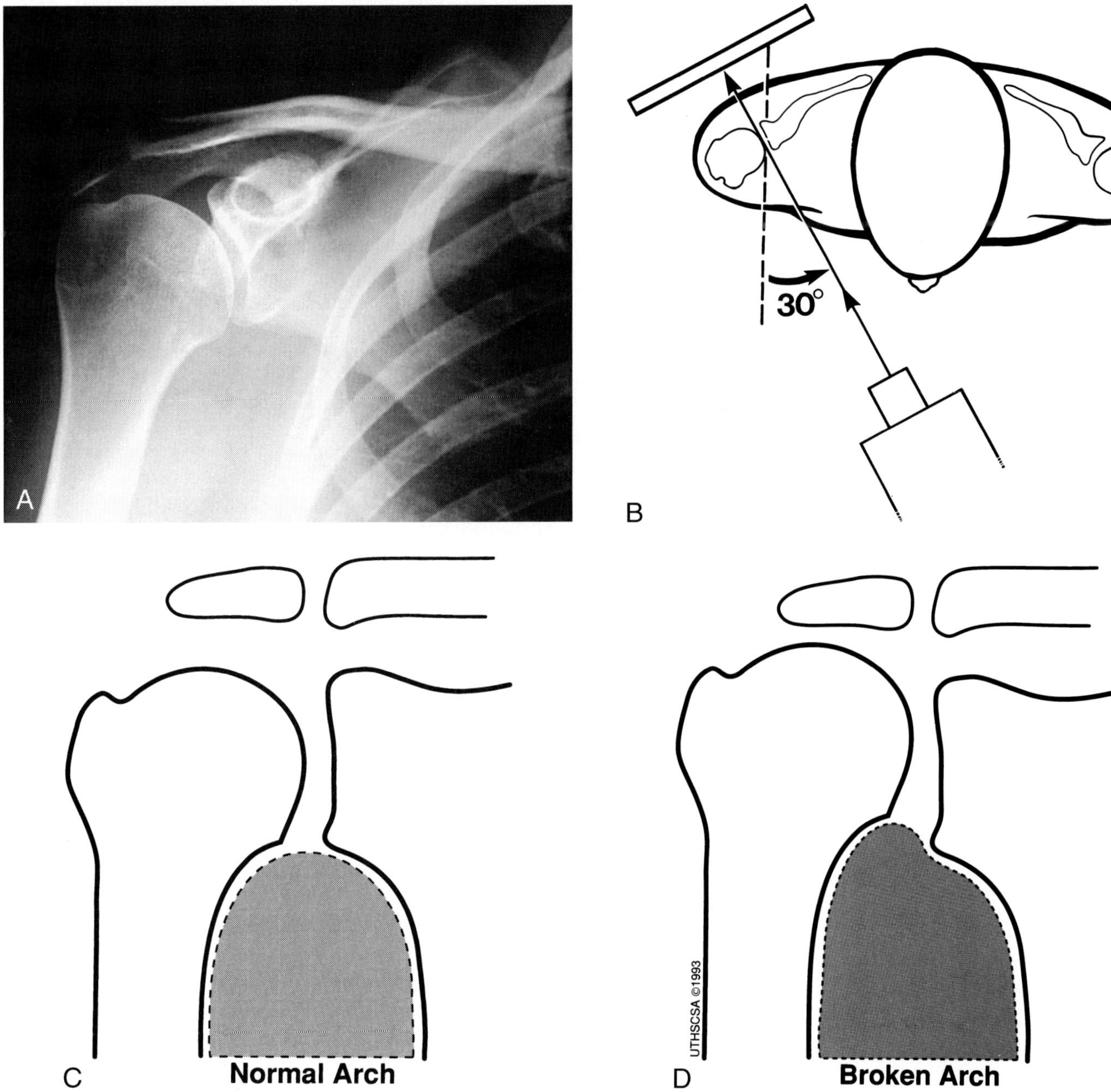

Fig. 21–26. *A,* The scapulohumeral arch is well demonstrated on a 30° posterior oblique radiograph in which the beam is parallel to the joint line. *B,* Technique of taking 30° posterior oblique radiograph. *C,* A small acromiohumeral interval with a smooth unbroken scapulohumeral arch signifies congenital subacromial stenosis. *D,* A decreased acromiohumeral interval with a "broken arch" signifies a rotator cuff tear.

these, four were complete posterosuperior tears with no intact external rotators; two were complete subscapularis tears; one was a worker's compensation case in which the cause of failure was never determined.

One must be particularly cognizant of the poor prognosis associated with complete subscapularis tears. These patients may mislead the examiner into thinking that the transverse plane force couple is intact because the external rotators are strong. It is crucial that the examiner perform the lift-off test for subscapularis function prior to consideration of any surgery. For the massive posterosuperior tears and the complete subscapularis tears with poor motion, partial cuff repair to restore the force couples may be preferable to arthroscopic debridement and decompression.

Author's Indications for Arthroscopic Debridement and Decompression

The ideal candidate for arthroscopic debridement and decompression would have a ''functional cuff tear'' as

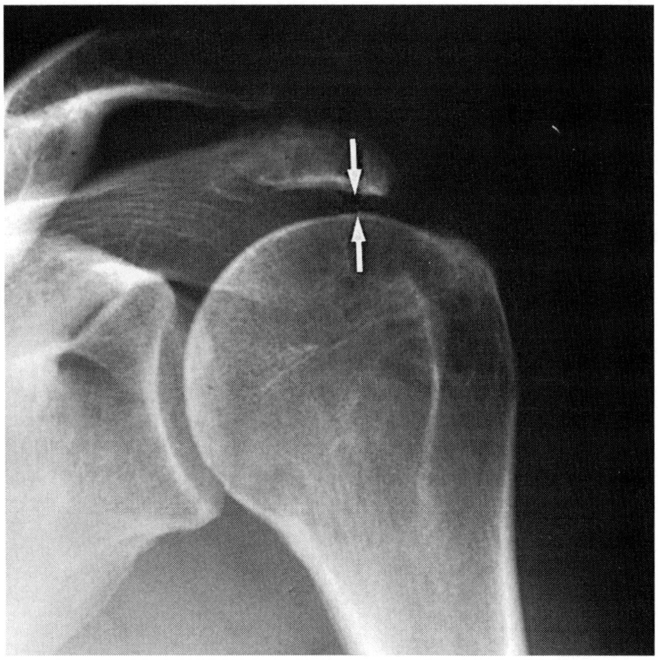

Fig. 21–27. **The acromiohumeral interval is measured on the standard AP view as the distance from the dome of the acromion to the top of the humeral head. Note that the inferior articular margins of the humerus and the glenoid are at the same level, implying congenital subacromial stenosis as the etiology of the narrowed acromiohumeral interval in this patient. This patient has an unrelated AC joint separation.**

defined earlier in this review. In addition, he should meet the following criteria (Table 21–3):

1. no improvement after 4 months of nonoperative treatment
2. age greater than 60 years
3. large tear that is not easily reparable
4. active forward elevation of at least 100°, even though painful
5. strong external rotators
6. subscapularis intact (negative lift-off test)
7. balanced force couples

As a special case, the older patient with congenital subacromial stenosis and a cuff tear is usually an excellent candidate. In addition, I think it is important to discuss the option of surgical repair with the patient and let him decide if he wants that or an arthroscopic debridement.

I agree with Ellman et al.[12] that there is a definite place for a ''limited goals'' group. This would include patients with poor function but low demands who desire only pain relief. This would include elderly patients, usually involving a nondominant extremity, with massive posterosuperior or complete subscapularis tears. In such patients, arthroscopic debridement and decompression can relieve pain, but motion and strength will not improve.

Clinical Results of Partial Rotator Cuff Repair

Some patients have massive tears that either extend posteriorly to involve all or most of the posterior cuff or anteriorly to involve all or most of the subscapularis. Such patients have limited shoulder elevation because of a loss of the transverse plane force couple. These are ''dysfunctional cuff tears.'' In high-demand patients with irreparable cuff tears, one should consider partial repair of the posterior or anterior cuff to restore the force couple, even though the superior cuff is generally too retracted to repair. This requires that the surgeon leave a hole in the top of the cuff. Anatomic dissections have shown that the rotator cable inserts into the humerus at the lower border of infraspinatus (Fig. 21–16). Therefore, in order to restore the cable and restore the force couples, I try to repair at least the inferior half of the infraspinatus (Fig. 21–28). Anteriorly, the cable inserts alongside the biceps tendon, above the subscapularis, so that subscapularis tears have to be repaired completely in order to restore the rotator cable and restore the force couples.

I have participated in a combined study comprising 14 patients who underwent partial repair for massive retracted rotator cuff tears, with an average follow-up of 20.8 months.[37] The average age of the patients was 56. Forward elevation improved from a preoperative average of 59.6° to a postoperative average of 150.4°, for an average gain of 90.8° forward elevation. Strength gained an average of 2.2 grades (on a 0 to 5 scale). The UCLA score improved from a preoperative average of 9.8 to a postoperative average of 27.6. Despite the impressive improvement in function, the average residual defect in the cuff was 1 cm by 3 cm ($3cm^2$). Once again, this study has shown that good function is possible despite a residual hole in the rotator cuff.

Partial Repair versus Tendon Transposition

Tendon transposition to cover rotator cuff defects in massive tears has been advocated.[5,6,38–40] In this procedure, all or a portion of an intact subscapularis or infraspinatus tendon is transferred superiorly to cover the hole in the cuff, with subscapularis transfer being the most popular. However, the mechanics of the shoulder are unfavorably altered by this transfer. Ordinarily, the centroid (line of action) of the subscapularis passes inferior to the center of rotation of the humeral head. In this position, the subscapularis forms an important coronal plane force couple with the deltoid (Fig. 21–29). By transferring this muscle superiorly to cover the defect in the cuff, the centroid of the transferred portion of

Table 21–3. Criteria for Arthroscopic Debridement and Decompression

No improvement after 4 months of nonoperative treatment
Age greater than 60 years
Large irreparable tear
Active forward elevation of at least 100°
Strong external rotators
Subscapularis intact
Balanced force couples

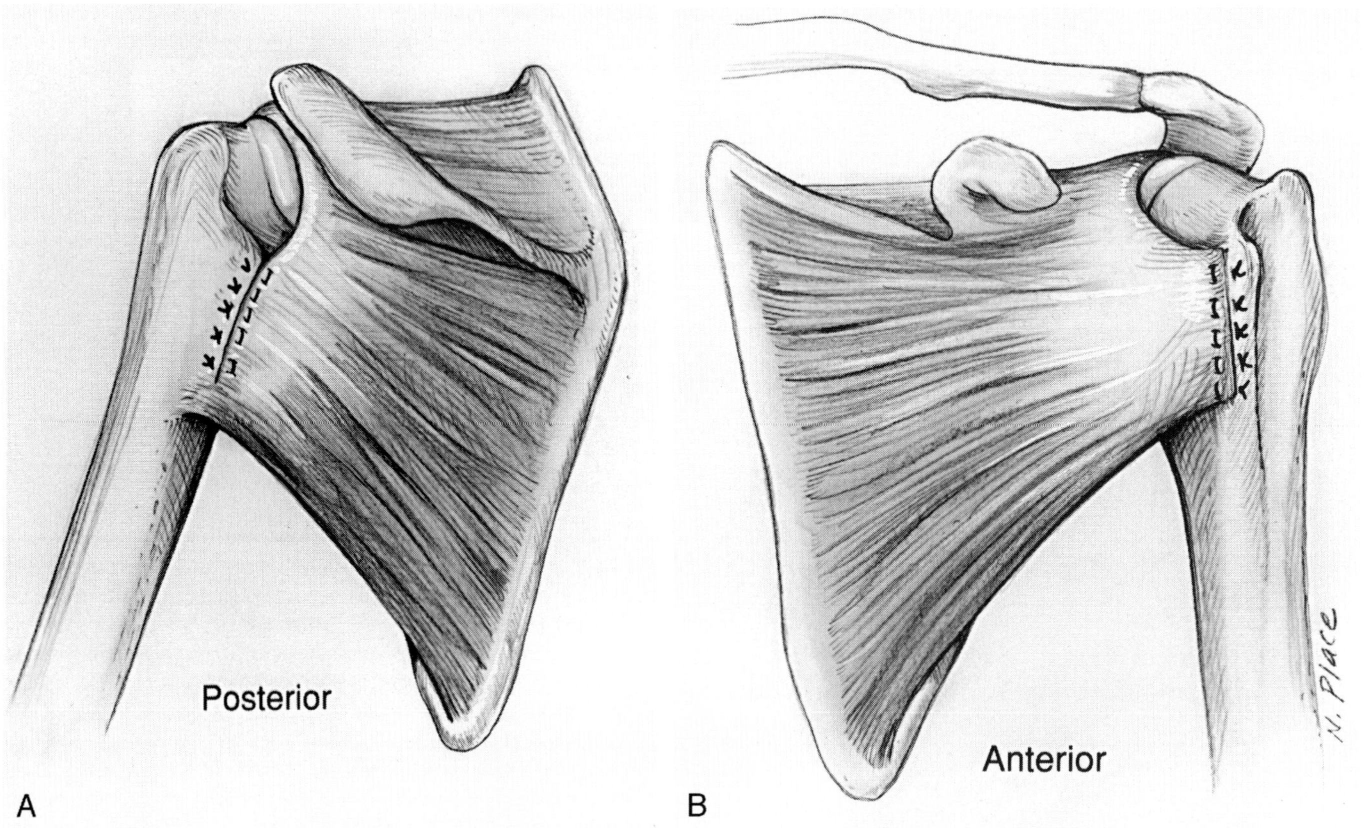

Fig. 21–28. ***A,*** **Partial repair of a massive irreparable posterior cuff tear should include at least the lower half of infraspinatus in order to repair the rotator cable and restore force couples.** ***B,*** **Massive anterior cuff tears demand complete repair of the subscapularis.**

subscapularis passes superior to the center of rotation. In this position, the moment produced by the subscapularis is in the same direction as the moment created by the deltoid, and the force couple is destroyed. This destruction of the coronal plane force couple, which is responsible for maintaining a stable fulcrum of motion for the shoulder, can contribute to superior migration of the humerus.

Partial repair of massive tears is a biomechanically sound procedure, in contradistinction to tendon transposition. In partial cuff repair, we restore the force couples, restore the suspension bridge, and do not violate an intact depressor of the humeral head.

The Logic of Rotator Cuff Debridement

Is arthroscopic debridement and decompression a rational approach to the torn rotator cuff? Certainly it makes biomechanical sense in the properly selected patient, and I have been extremely satisfied with my clinical results. The key is patient selection, and the patients must have functional cuff tears that are biomechanically intact.

Three recent studies addressed the issue of rotator cuff debridement versus repair.[12,36,41] Zvijac et al.[36] followed 25 patients with full-thickness rotator cuff tears treated by debridement and decompression. They concluded that the results of debridement deteriorated with time and were inferior to rotator cuff repair. However, this study was weighted toward a younger age group (average age was 53.5 and ranged as low as 25 years of age) and made no attempt to relate function or patient selection to the location of the tear. As I have stated, the location of the tear is the single most critical issue in choosing candidates for debridement. Also, I wish to emphasize that almost everyone that I consider for rotator cuff debridement and decompression is over 60 years of age. Montgomery et al.[41] performed a prospective study on 88 patients comparing arthroscopic debridement to open repair. They concluded that the results of open repair were superior to arthroscopic debridement, but this study also did not correlate results with cuff tear location. Despite these conclusions, the senior investigator of that study (FHS) still does arthroscopic cuff debridements for indications similar to those that I have set forth in this review, and he has stated that he believes there is a definite place for debridement in selected patients.[42] Ellman et al.[12] arthroscopically debrided and decompressed 40 shoulders and concluded that cuff debridement and decompression was useful in selected older patients with small tears (< 2 cm). They stated that cuff repair was better than debridement for tears in the 2 to 4 cm size

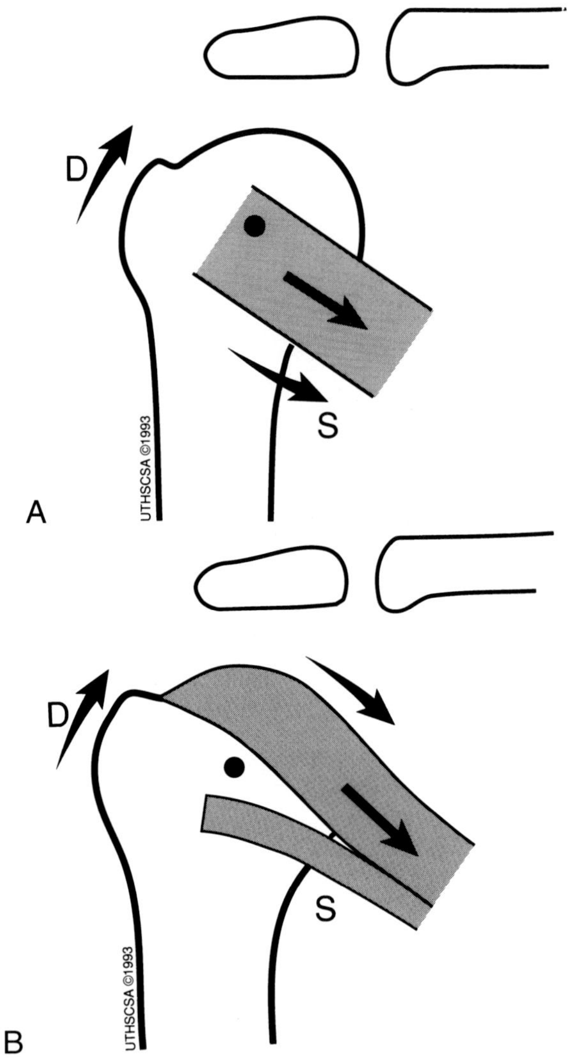

Fig. 21–29. ***A,*** **The centroid (line of action) of the subscapularis lies inferior to the center of rotation, forming a force couple with the deltoid. These two muscles have moments that are opposite in direction.** ***B,*** **The subscapularis in its transferred position now has its centroid above the center of rotation, and its moment is in the same direction as the deltoid moment. This muscle transfer destroys the important coronal plane force couple; (D)= deltoid moment and (S)= subscapularis moment.**

range. They applied the useful concept of a "limited goals" category for patients who were predestined to have a poor UCLA score by virtue of their poor function. These patients had massive tears with poor UCLA scores caused by poor motion and strength; yet 86% were satisfied with their pain relief.

Table 21–4. Unifying Treatment Concepts

Identify or create a functional cuff tear
Stabilize the edge of a functional cuff tear

Table 21–5. Treatment Guidelines for Rotator Cuff Tears

Cuff repair
Young patients
Selected high-demand older patients
Cuff debridement and decompression*
Older patients with functional cuff tears
Older patients with congenital subacromial stenosis
Partial repair of rotator cuff tears
High-demand patients with irreparable tears
Goals
Create functional cuff tears
Restore force couples
Tendon transposition *never* done
Limited-goals category
Goal is pain relief
Patient acceptance of poor function

*Older patients are those > 60 years of age.

In my opinion, none of these studies provided data sufficient to universally condemn rotator cuff debridement. The study by Ellman et al.[12] points out the fact that we could preselect a 100% failure rate by UCLA criteria if we only operated on dysfunctional tears. Arthroscopic debridement and decompression has a place in the treatment of rotator cuff tears. A primary goal of this review is to define that place.

One objection to debridement that is frequently raised is that unrepaired rotator cuff tears will lead relentlessly to cuff-tear arthropathy. However, the highest estimate of cuff tear arthropathy in the literature is that of Neer et al.,[43] who estimated that it occurs in only 4% of their patients with unrepaired rotator cuff tears.

We have shown experimentally that rotator cuff tears are unlikely to extend on a purely mechanical basis. Therefore, if unrepaired cuff tears are unlikely to extend, and if cuff-tear arthropathy is unlikely to occur in patients with unrepaired tears, the purported advantages of heroic open cuff reconstruction over arthroscopic debridement and decompression begin to look meager indeed.

Repair versus Debridement: Reconciling the Paradox

My task now is to assimilate all the foregoing data, conclusions, and opinions into a rational system of guidelines for the treatment of rotator cuff tears. We have to consider preoperative function, the age of the patient, and the demands that will be placed on the shoulder. The two unifying concepts are (Table 21–4):

1. identify or create a functional cuff tear
2. stabilize the edge of a functional cuff tear.

These broad treatment concepts have led to the development of specific treatment guidelines as follows (Table 21–5):

1. repair cuff tears when possible in young patients and selected high-demand older patients (older patients are those greater than 60 years of age)
2. arthroscopically debride and decompress tears in

older patients with functional cuff tears and in older patients with congenital subacromial stenosis
3. perform open or arthroscopic partial repair of massive dysfunctional tears in order to restore the force couples and create functional tears in high-demand patients with irreparable tears
4. never transfer an intact rotator cuff tendon from its anatomic position in order to cover a hole in the top of the cuff; and
5. consider a ''limited goals'' category of elderly patients with dysfunctional cuff tears in whom arthroscopic debridement and decompression may be done for pain relief only, accepting the fact that the pre-existing poor function will not improve.

The paradox of rotator cuff debridement versus repair is easily resolved by a treatment concept that is based on biomechanical principles (''restore the force couples'') rather than intuitive conjecture (''cover the hole''). This approach may be unorthodox, but it is logical and rational. And logic dictates that a rational approach will ultimately confirm its orthodox nature.

ACKNOWLEDGMENT

The author wishes to thank Smith and Nephew DonJoy Inc. (Carlsbad, CA) for their generosity in providing their Biomechanics Research Lab and personnel to help conduct the experiments cited in references 20, 23, and 25.

References

1. Codman EA. *The Shoulder: Rupture of the Supraspinatus Tendon and Other Lesions In or About the Subacromial Bursa.* Boston: G Miller; 1934:173.
2. Debeyre J, Patte D, Emelik E. Repair of ruptures of the rotator cuff with a note on advancement of the supraspinatus muscle. *J Bone Joint Surg Br.* 1965;47:36–42.
3. Heikel HVA. Rupture of the rotator cuff of the shoulder. Experiences of surgical treatment. *Acata Orthop Scand.* 1968; 39:477–492.
4. Neviaser JS, Neviaser RJ, Neviaser TJ. The repair of chronic massive ruptures of the rotator cuff of the shoulder by use of a freeze-dried rotator cuff. *J Bone Joint Surg Am.* 1978;60: 681–684.
5. Cofield RH. Subscapular muscle transposition for repair of chronic rotator cuff tears. *Surg Gynecol Obstet.* 1982;154: 667–672.
6. Cofield RH. Current concepts review: Rotator cuff disease of the shoulder. *J Bone Joint Surg Am.* 1985;67:974–979.
7. Takagishi N. Conservative treatment of ruptures of the rotator cuff. *J Jpn Orthop Assoc.* 1978;52:781–787.
8. Samilson RL, Binder WF. Symptomatic full thickness tears of the rotator cuff: An analysis of 292 shoulders in 276 patients. *Orthop Clin North Am.* 1975;6:449–466.
9. Wolfgang GL. Surgical repair of tears of the rotator cuff of the shoulder, factors influencing the result. *J Bone Joint Surg Am.* 1974; 56:14–26.
10. Burkhart SS. Arthroscopic treatment of massive rotator cuff tears: Clinical results and biomechanical rationale. *Clin Orthop.* 1991; 267:45–56.
11. Rockwood CA Jr, Williams GR, Burkhead WZ. *Debridement of irreparable, degenerative lesions of the rotator cuff.* Presented at the American Shoulder and Elbow Surgeons Seventh Open Meeting. Anaheim, CA, March 10, 1991.
12. Ellman H, Kay SP, Wirth M. Arthroscopic treatment of full-thickness rotator cuff tears: 2- to 7-year follow-up study. *Arthroscopy: J Arth Rel Res.* 1993;9:195–200.
13. Harryman DT II, Mach LA, Wang KA, et al. Repairs of the rotator cuff: Correlation of functional results with integrity of the cuff. *J Bone Joint Surg Am.* 1991;73:982–989.
14. Calvert PT, Packer NP, Stoker DJ, et al. Arthrography of the shoulder after operative repair of the torn rotator cuff. *J Bone Joint Surg Br.* 1986;68:147–150.
15. Inman VT, Saunders JB, Abbott LC. Observations on the function of the shoulder joint. *J Bone Joint Surg Am.* 1944;26:1–30.
16. Burkhart SS. Arthroscopic debridement and decompression for selected rotator cuff tears: Clinical results, pathomechanics, and patient selection based on biomechanical parameters. *Orthop Clin North Am.* 1993;24 1:111–123.
17. Gerber C, Krushell R. Isolated rupture of the tendon of the subscapularis muscle: Clinical features in 16 cases. *J Bone Joint Surg Br.* 1991;73:389–394.
18. Burkhart SS. Fluoroscopic comparison of kinematic patterns in massive rotator cuff tears: A suspension bridge model. *Clin Orthop.* 1992;284:144–152.
19. Burkhart SS, Esch JC, Jolson RS. The rotator crescent and rotator cable: An anatomic description of the shoulder's ''suspension bridge.'' Accepted for publication in *Arthroscopy: J Arth Rel Res.* Publication pending.
20. Burkhart SS, Cawley PW, Pflaster DS, Thomas TD, Esch JC, Nottage WM. The ultimate strength to failure of rotator cuff tears involving the rotator crescent. Unpublished data.
21. Clark JM, Sidles JA, Matsen FA. The relationship of the glenohumeral joint capsule to the rotator cuff. *Clin Orthop.* 1990;254:29–34.
22. Clark JM, Harryman DT II. Tendons, ligaments, and capsule of the rotator cuff. *J Bone Joint Surg Am.* 1992;74:713–725.
23. Burkhart SS, Cawley PW, Pflaster DS, Thomas TD, Esch JC, Nottage WM. Symmetric tensile loading of the rotator cable: Demonstration of a stress-shielding effect on the rotator crescent. Unpublished data.
24. Roland C. Frei Otto: *Tension Structures.* New York: Praeger; 1970: 9.
25. Burkhart SS, Cawley PW, Pflaster DS, Thomas TD, Esch JC, Nottage WM. Biomechanical testing of the intact rotator cable-crescent complex. Unpublished data.
26. Burkhart SS. *Congenital subacromial stenosis.* Presented at the American Shoulder and Elbow Surgeons Ninth Closed Meeting. Vail, CO, Sept 11, 1992.
27. Cotton RE, Rideout DF. Tears of the humeral rotator cuff. *J Bone Joint Surg Br.* 1964;46:314–332.
28. DeSmet AA, Ting YM. Diagnosis of rotator cuff tear on routine radiographs. *J Can Assoc Radiol.* 1977;28:54–57.
29. Ellman H, Hanker G, Bayer M. Repair of the rotator cuff. *J Bone Joint Surg Am.* 1986;68:1136–1144.
30. Golding SC. The shoulder: The forgotten joint. *Brit J Radiol.* 1962; 35:149–158.
31. Harrison SH. The painful shoulder. *J Bone Joint Surg Br.* 1949; 31:418–422.
32. Kotzen LM. Roentgen diagnosis of rotator cuff tear. *AJR.* 1971; 112:507–511.
33. Weiner DS, Macnab I. Superior migration of the humeral head. *J Bone Joint Surg Br.* 1970;52:524–527.
34. Burkhart SS. Long-term follow-up of arthroscopic decompression and debridement of full-thickness rotator cuff tears: Clinical results and biomechanical rationale. Presented at Arthroscopy Association of North America Fall Course. Monterey, CA, November 20, 1992.
35. Ellman H. Arthroscopic subacromial decompression: Analysis of one- to three-year results. *Arthroscopy: J Arth Rel Res.* 1987; 3:173–181.
36. Zvijac JE, Lemka LJ, Levy HJ. *Arthroscopic subacromial decompression in the treatment of full-thickness rotator cuff tears: A three- to six-year follow-up.* Presented at Arthroscopy Association of North America 12th Annual Meeting. Palm Desert, CA, April 3, 1993.
37. Burkhart SS, Nottage WM, Ogilvie-Harris DJ, Kohn HS, Pachelli A. *Partial repair of massive rotator cuff tears.* Presented at Symposium on Arthroscopic Shoulder Surgery. Laguna Beach, CA, March 19, 1993.
38. Cofield RH. Tears of the rotator cuff. *Instr Course Lect.* 1981; 30:258–273.
39. Neer CS II. Impingement lesions. *Clin Orthop.* 1983;173:70–77.

40. Neviaser RJ, Neviaser TJ. Transfer of subscapularis and teres minor for massive defects of rotator cuff. In: Bayley I, Kessel L, eds. *Shoulder Surgery.* Berlin: Springer-Verlag; 1982: 60–63.
41. Montgomery T, Yerger B, Savoie FH. *A comparison of arthroscopic debridement versus open surgical repair of full-thickness tears of the rotator cuff.* Presented at Arthroscopy Association of North America 1993 Specialty Day Meeting. San Francisco, CA, February 21, 1993.
42. Savoie FH. Personal communication.
43. Neer CS II, Craig EV, Fukuda H. Cuff-tear arthropathy. *J Bone Joint Surg Am.* 1983;65:1232–1244.

Chapter 22

Open Debridement of the Massive Degenerative Cuff Tear

Gerald R. Williams, Jr.

The surgical management of chronic, irreparable rotator cuff defects most likely generates more controversy than any other topic in shoulder surgery. The controversy arises largely because of insufficient data. Many investigators[1–12] have documented the success of acromioplasty and rotator cuff repair in patients with reparable defects. However, discriminating data regarding various surgical techniques used for irreparable defects are lacking.

Many surgical techniques have been described for reconstructing massive, irreparable rotator cuff defects. These techniques include repair at or near the normal anatomic insertion site with the arm held in abduction with a brace while healing takes place,[13] reattachment of the cuff to bone at a more proximal position on the humerus,[6,7] advancement of the supraspinatus origin,[14,15] and superior transposition of the subscapularis and/or teres minor.[16–18] In addition, tendon transfer techniques have been described using the anterior deltoid,[19] the trapezius,[20] and the latissimus dorsi.[21] Tendon substitution techniques using autograft biceps tendon,[8,22] autograft coracoacromial ligament,[13,23] autograft fascia lata,[13,16,23,24] allograft rotator cuff,[25] and prosthetic material[26–29] have also been reported. Rockwood and colleagues[30–33] have documented good results in patients with chronic massive irreparable defects who have undergone acromioplasty and partial debridement of the rotator cuff.

Acromioplasty with partial rotator cuff debridement is a viable option in the management of these difficult cases. First, it can offer excellent pain relief and a high degree of patient satisfaction. Secondly, the technique is much easier and perhaps more reproducible than the other reconstructive techniques that have been described. Lastly, in spite of the criticism that is often levied against this technique, there is little long-term follow-up data of truly similar patients documenting better results with any of the above mentioned reconstructive techniques.

SURGICAL RATIONALE

It is well known that a full-thickness rotator cuff defect is compatible with asymptomatic shoulder function. Several cadaver and autopsy studies have documented a relatively high, age-related incidence of partial and full-thickness rotator cuff defects.[34–38] At least one of these studies documented asymptomatic shoulder function prior to death.[36] Pettersson[39] documented arthrographically proven partial-thickness or full-thickness rotator cuff defects in 13 (48%) of 27 asymptomatic shoulders ranging in age from 55 to 85 years. Finally, McLaughlin[6,7] and others[10,40–42] have documented successful nonoperative management of full-thickness rotator cuff defects in spite of the persistent cuff defect.

The pain relief associated with acromioplasty and rotator cuff repair may primarily be the result of the acromioplasty rather than the cuff repair. Many investigators have reported good pain relief following acromioplasty and cuff repair for chronic rotator cuff defects.[1–12] However, Packer and colleagues[43] compared the results of acromioplasty and cuff repair in 30 patients, with cuff repair alone in 26 patients. Twenty-six (87%) of the 30 patients who had undergone combined subacromial decompression and cuff repair experienced good pain relief, whereas only 14 (54%) of the 26 patients treated with cuff repair alone experienced similar results. Packer and colleagues[43] concluded that an "adequate decompression" should be an integral part of any rotator cuff operation.

Several studies[44–46] have documented a relatively high incidence of postoperative recurrent rotator cuff defects in patients who had undergone prior acromioplasty and rotator cuff repair. Lundberg[44] documented arthrographically proven recurrent cuff defects in 33% of 21 shoulders that had undergone cuff repair. Blauth and Gartner[45] also used arthrography to document recurrent rotator cuff defects in 12 of 41 operatively repaired rotator cuffs. Blauth and Gartner[45] could document no correlation between the quality of the postoperative result and the arthrographic findings. Calvert and associates[46] performed arthrography on 21 patients who had undergone acromioplasty and rotator cuff repair an average of 30 months prior to follow-up. Ninety percent of the 20 patients demonstrated full-thickness rotator cuff defects on the postoperative arthrogram, and 85% of the 20 patients were asymptomatic. Active shoulder elevation was 180° in 14 patients, 170° in 1 patient, 140° in 1 patient, and 90° or less in the remaining 4 patients.

Ultrasonography has also been used in the postoperative setting to document the status of the rotator cuff. Wulker and associates[47] examined 97 shoulders at an average of 37 months following rotator cuff repair. Ultrasound revealed recurrent full-thickness rotator cuff defects in 29 (30%) shoulders. There was poor correlation between clinical outcome and sonographic results. The investigators recommended that the rotator cuff be repaired only if repair can be accomplished without undue tension. If "extensive mobilization" or coverage with "alloplastic material" or "regional muscle flaps" are required, the investigators recommended acromioplasty and debridement.

More recently, Harryman and colleagues[48] used ultrasound to evaluate 105 operatively repaired rotator cuffs at an average of 5 years postoperatively. Patients who underwent repair of tears involving two and three tendons had an incidence of postoperative recurrent defects of 43% and 68% respectively. The investigators documented better postoperative results in patients with an intact cuff. However, in patients with the largest recurrent defects (three tendon involvement) there was 91% patient satisfaction.

Burkhart[49] has shown the importance of balanced anterior and posterior rotator cuff force couples in patients with chronic massive rotator cuff defects who have good overhead elevation. Poor overhead function in a patient with a chronic massive rotator cuff defect may be secondary to pain or to unbalanced force couples. If subacromial injection of lidocaine provides pain relief for this patient and restores overhead elevation, it seems reasonable to assume that acromioplasty and partial rotator cuff debridement (assuming that the tear is not reparable) would be successful.

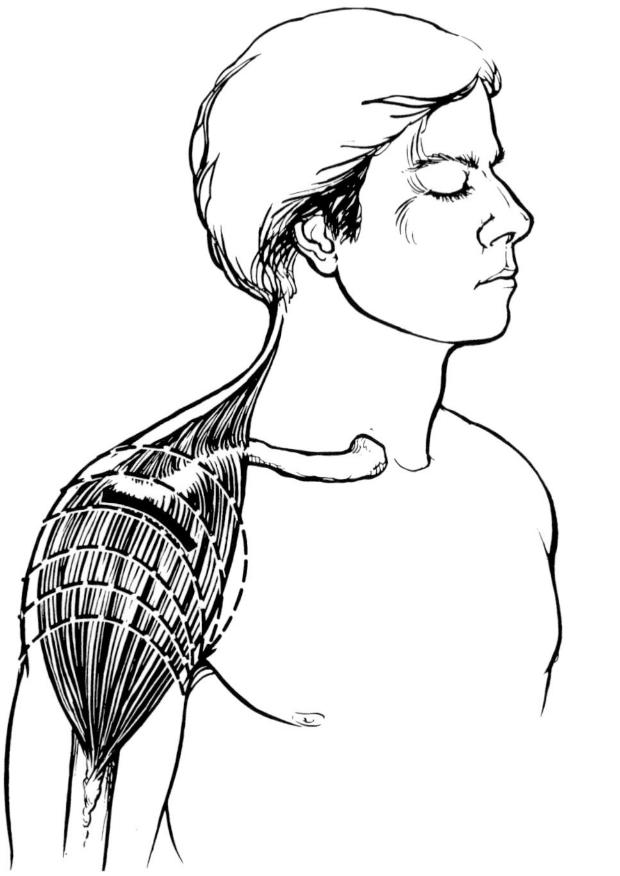

Fig. 22–1. The skin incision used parallels the lateral border of the acromion and is placed in Langer's skin lines.

SURGICAL TECHNIQUE

A standard anterosuperior acromioplasty incision is performed. The incision should be in Langer's skin lines and should parallel the lateral border of the acromion (Fig. 22–1). Full-thickness skin flaps are developed medially and laterally to expose the AC joint and the proximal aspect of the anterior and lateral deltoid. The deltoid fibers are split longitudinally along an imaginary line extended laterally from the anterior cortical border of the clavicle. This split is slightly more posterior than the junction of the anterior and lateral thirds of the deltoid.[3] The muscle is split in line with its fibers approximately 3 to 3.5 cm distal to the lateral edge of the acromion in order to expose the white, glistening roof of the underlying subdeltoid/subacromial bursa. In most patients the deep surface of the deltoid can be bluntly separated from the roof of the bursa. However, occasionally this is not possible and the deltoid is reflected along with the roof of the subacromial bursa.

The split in the lateral deltoid is continued onto the dorsal surface of the acromion as far medially as the AC joint. The incision in the deltotrapezius fascia should be approximately 1 to 1.5 cm posterior to the anterior border of the acromion. This allows for a strong cuff of deltotrapezius fascia, periosteum, and Sharpe's fibers for the subsequent reattachment of the anterior deltoid. If greater posterior exposure is required, a small portion of the lateral deltoid can be removed from the lateral edge of the acromion. This is accomplished by making a second incision in the deltotrapezius fascia on the dorsal aspect of the acromion, parallel to the lateral edge of the acromion and perpendicular to the anterior previously placed incision in the deltotrapezius fascia. This results in an L-shaped incision, with the apex near the anterior lateral corner of the acromion (Fig. 22–2).

With the anterior and lateral portions of the deltoid retracted the roof of the subacromial bursa and the coracoacromial ligament are visualized. The roof of the subacromial bursa is incised from the under surface of the acromion anteriorly and posteriorly. The coracoacromial ligament is grasped and incised from its attachment on

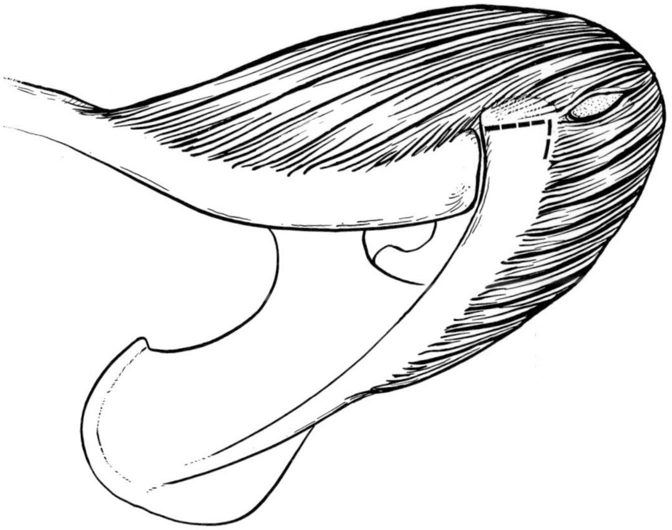

Fig. 22–2. The deltotrapezius fascia is incised on the dorsal surface of the acromion in line with the anterior cortical border of the clavicle. A second incision in the deltotrapezius fascia parallels the lateral border of the acromion and is used to release any lateral deltoid if necessary. This results in an L-shaped incision with the apex at the anterolateral corner of the acromion.

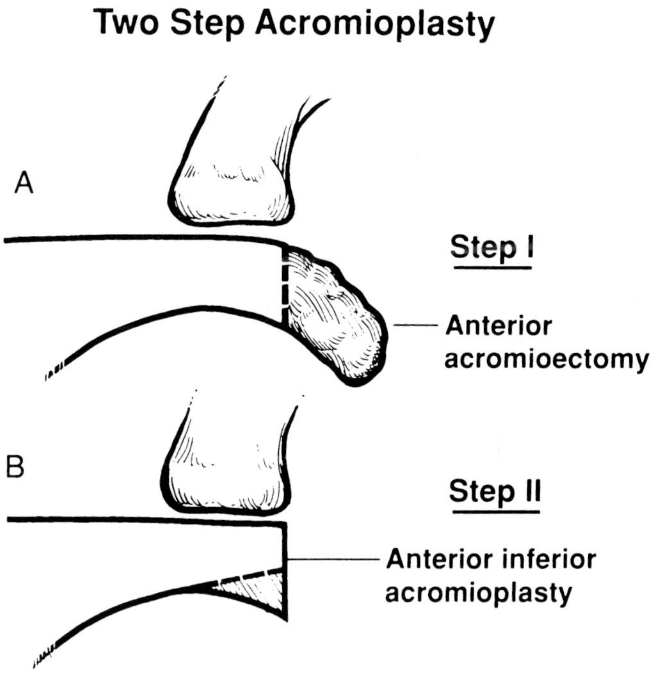

Fig. 22–3. The two-step modification of the Neer acromioplasty includes (*A*) an anterior acromionectomy followed by (*B*) an anterior inferior acromioplasty.

the acromion. The acromial branch of the thoracoacromial artery is often encountered at the most medial extent of the coracoacromial ligament and is controlled with electrocautery. The coracoacromial ligament is then excised.

The two-step modification of the Neer acromioplasty as described by Rockwood and Lyons[50] is then performed. In the first step, any of the anterior acromion extending anterior to a line projected laterally from the anterior cortical border of the clavicle is vertically removed. In the second step, an inferior acromioplasty is performed in order to remove any inferior prominence from the acromion (Fig. 22–3). A hand-held rasp is then used to contour the corners and to remove any irregularities, which are prominent on the anteroinferior cancellous surface of the acromion (Fig. 22–4). A thorough debridement of all hypertrophied subacromial bursa is then carried out.

The undersurface of the AC joint is then palpated. Any significant downward projecting osteophytes are removed with a rongeur or an osteotome. If possible, concomitant distal clavicle excision should be avoided because of the potential for proximal migration of the humerus into the defect created. Excision of the distal clavicle should only be performed if three preoperative conditions have been met: (1) there must be tenderness to palpation of the AC joint and pain with hyperadduction; (2) there must be significant radiographic changes of degenerative arthritis within the AC joint; and (3) there must be significant pain relief obtained with isolated injection of the AC joint with a local anesthetic.

In the presence of longstanding massive rotator cuff defects, the long head of the biceps, the humeral head, and the greater tuberosity are easily visualized. The long head of the biceps is frequently hypertrophied and

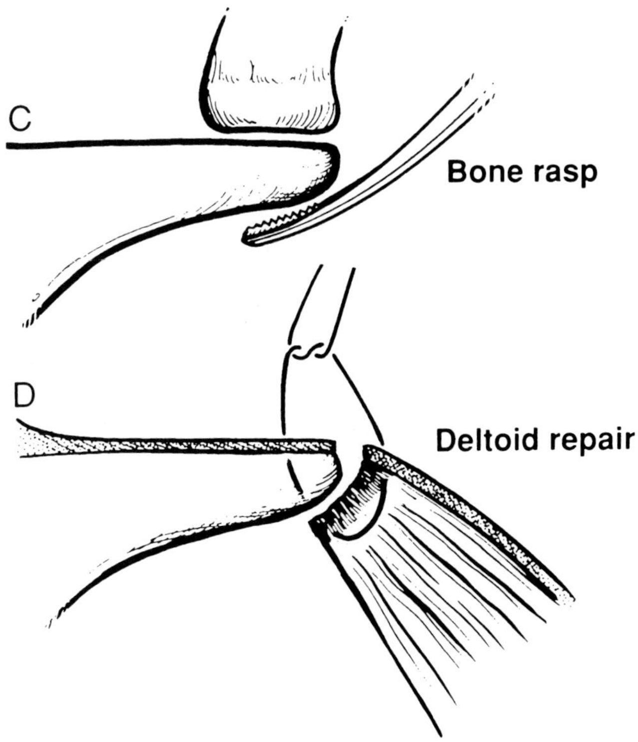

Fig. 22–4. The cancellous undersurface of the acromion is contoured using a bone rasp (*C*) and the deltoid is reattached to bone as well as to the deltotrapezius fascia (*D*).

should be preserved as a secondary humeral head depressor. The greater tuberosity should be inspected for a reactive exostosis from chronic impingement with the acromion. If this exostosis is present, the prominence should be removed using a rongeur or an osteotome.

The boundaries of the rotator cuff tear should then be identified in preparation for mobilization and attempted repair. Traction sutures are first placed in the anterior and posterior edges of the tear. Blunt and sometimes sharp dissection are required to lyse any superficial adhesions between the posterior rotator cuff and the overlying bursa and acromion and spine of the scapula. Complete mobilization of the cuff may also require incision of the coracohumeral ligament and (rarely) release of the glenoid capsular attachment. If after mobilization any portion of the posterior cuff can be repaired to its anatomic insertion site, it should be repaired to cancellous bone and tied over the lateral cortex. Any remaining portions of the rotator cuff that cannot be reattached and that impinge between the acromion and humeral head when the arm is passively flexed should be debrided.

The most important part of the procedure is secure reattachment of the anterior deltoid. In the presence of a massive rotator cuff tear that has not been repaired, good anterior deltoid function is mandatory for overhead elevation. The strong cuff of periosteum, deltotrapezius fascia, and Sharpe's fibers that accompany the anterior deltoid are securely reattached to the cancellous bone of the anterior acromion. If any lateral deltoid has been removed, it also is repaired to bone. The split in the deltoid fibers is repaired with interrupted nonabsorbable suture. The subacromial space is infiltrated with a long-acting local anesthetic. This provides early postoperative pain relief and will facilitate early rehabilitation.

POSTOPERATIVE REHABILITATION

Postoperative rehabilitation is as important as the surgery itself. Consequently, the surgeon should be actively involved. The primary objectives are (1) to restore passive

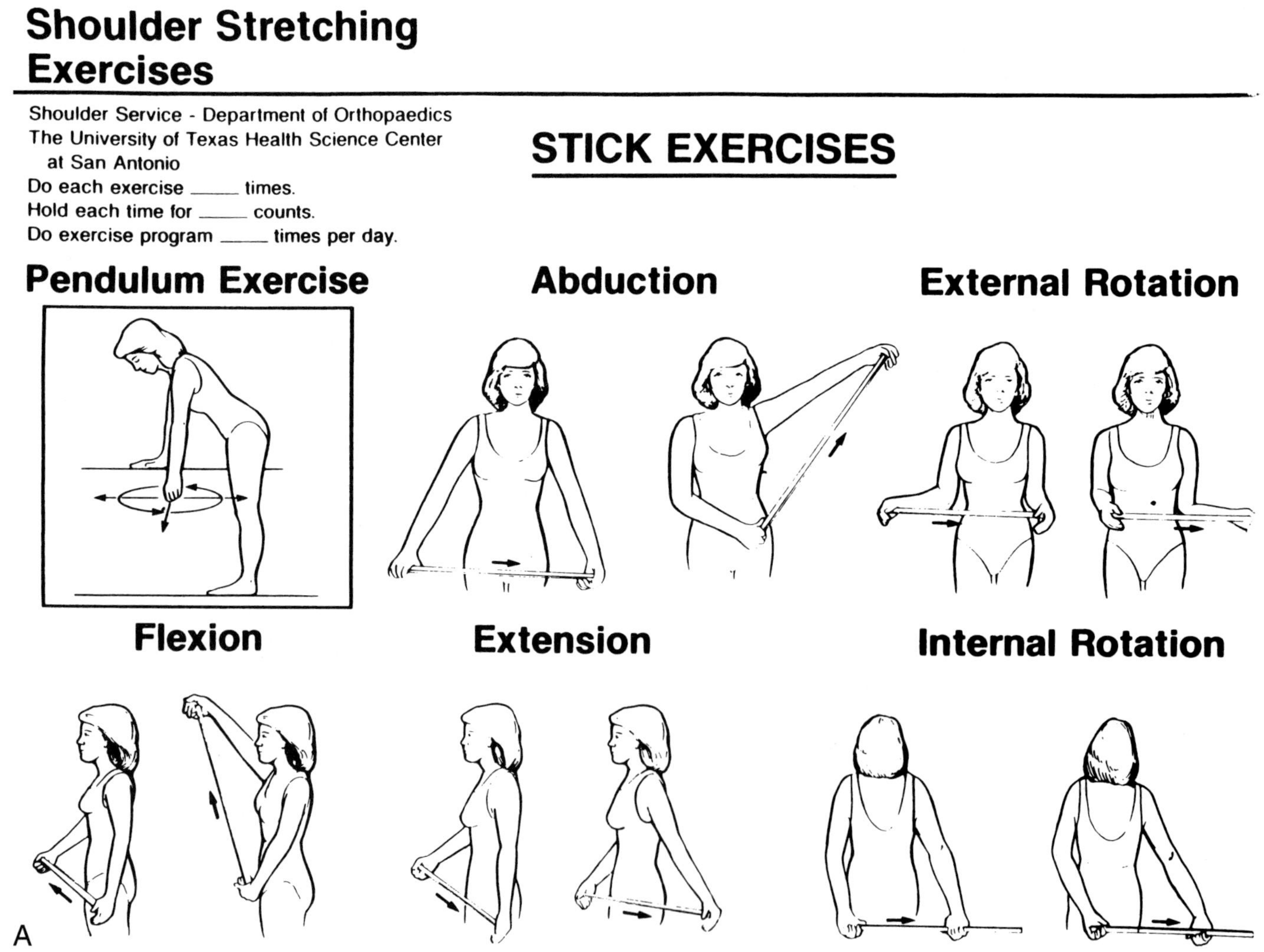

Fig. 22–5. Patients are instructed in a home shoulder stretching program (*A and B*). A home strengthening program for the remaining rotator cuff muscles and the three portions of the deltoid (*C*), as well as for the scapular stabilizing muscles (*D*), is also used.

range of motion to the glenohumeral joint while the deltoid is healing to the acromion and (2) to strengthen the scapular stabilizers, three portions of the deltoid, and remaining portions of the rotator cuff.

Passive range of motion begins on the afternoon or evening of surgery while the subacromial anesthetic is still effective. The operated arm is removed from the shoulder immobilizer and passively flexed to 90 or 120°. On the first postoperative day, the patient is instructed to perform pendulum exercises, supine passive flexion using the motor power of the opposite arm, and passive external rotation exercises using an exercise wand. Upon discharge, the patient is instructed to continue these exercises. However, active shoulder flexion is discouraged for 2 weeks to protect the anterior deltoid repair. The patient is given a take-home rehabilitation kit consisting of a two-piece 3-foot exercise wand, an overhead pulley kit system, and a fully illustrated and descriptive exercise program (Fig. 22–5). The skin suture is removed at 2 weeks postoperatively and the shoulder immobilizer is discontinued. During the third postoperative week, the patient is encouraged to use his shoulder for activities of daily living and is instructed to refrain from lifting. When the range of motion has been restored to a functional level, isokinetic strengthening exercises with resistive rubber tubing are instituted to strengthen the three parts of the deltoid and the remaining rotator cuff muscles. Specific exercises are used to strengthen the scapular stabilizing muscles. In the case of persistent or profound anterior deltoid weakness, a specific strengthening program for the anterior deltoid is used (Fig. 22–6). If any portion of the posterior cuff has been repaired, active use of the shoulder, as well as strengthening exercises, are withheld for 6 to 8 weeks postoperatively.

RESULTS

In general, acromioplasty and rotator cuff debridement provides good pain relief and overall function. However, results are best in patients with a good functioning anterior deltoid muscle, an intact long head of

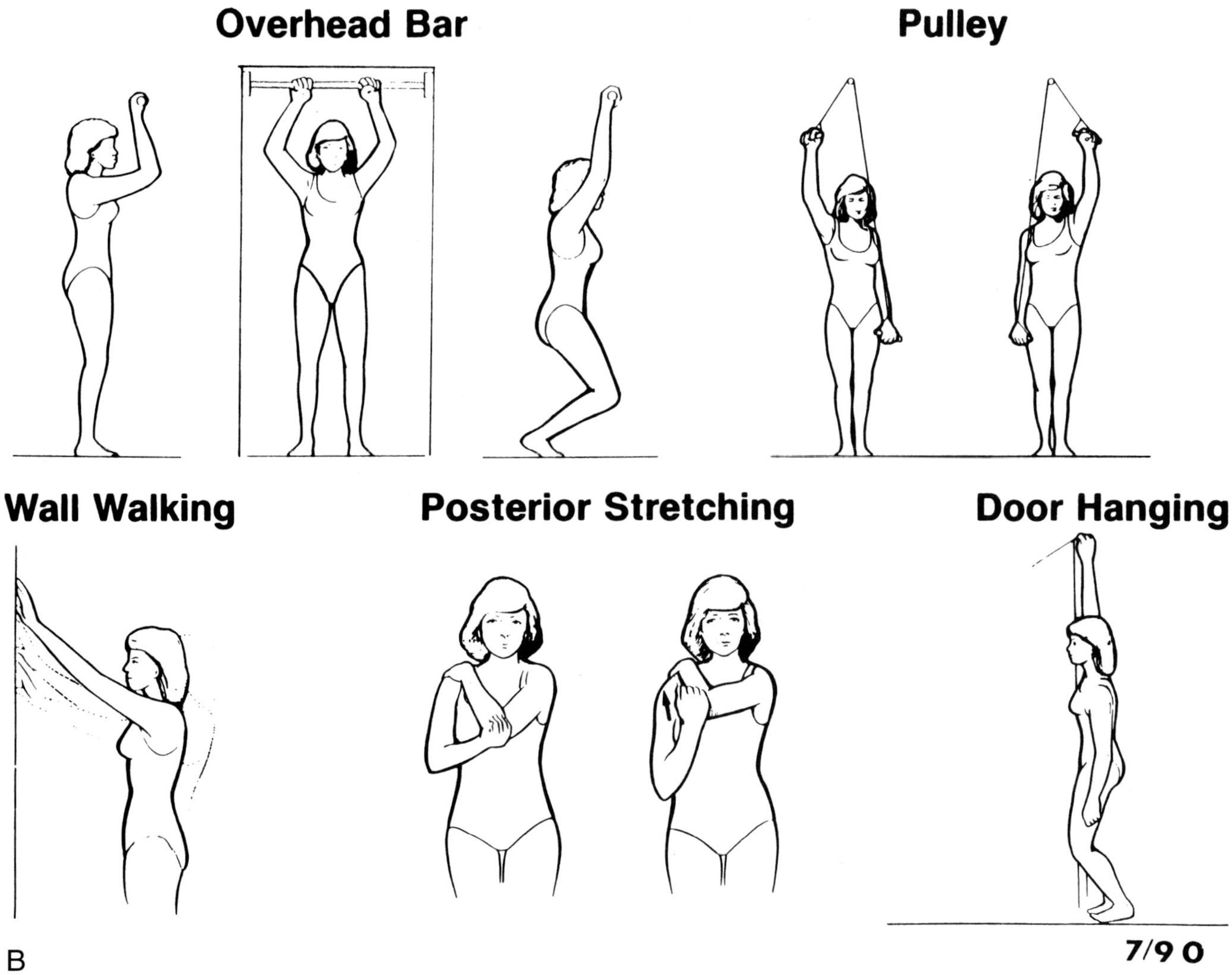

Fig. 22–5—*continued*

the biceps, and no history of prior surgery. Rockwood and colleagues[33] reported 85% of shoulders with no pain or mild pain at an average follow-up of 6.5 years. This was increased to 94% in patients with a strong deltoid, functioning long head of the biceps, and no history of prior surgery. Average active overhead elevation improved from a preoperative value of 105° to a postoperative value of 140°. Active postoperative overhead elevation in patients with an intact and functioning anterior deltoid was 165°. Most patients demonstrated weakness with overhead activities but continued to be satisfied with their overall functional level. There was no deterioration of the postoperative results with time (Fig. 22–7).

DISCUSSION

Acromioplasty and partial rotator cuff debridement should be considered only after complete mobilization of the rotator cuff and every attempt at repair has been made. Consequently, comparison of the results of this procedure with the results following acromioplasty and

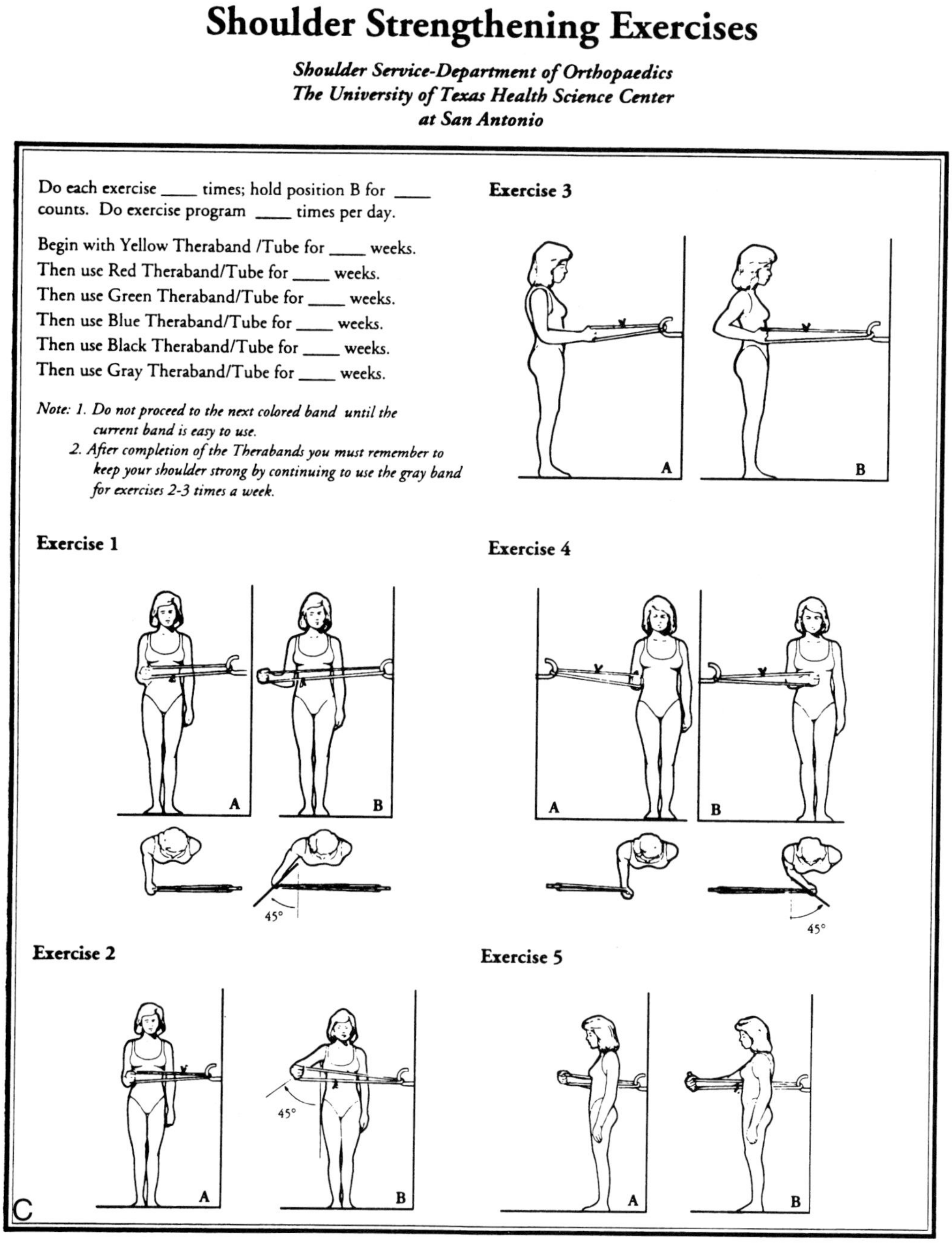

Fig. 22–5—*continued*

rotator cuff repair lack statistical validity. In reality, acromioplasty and partial rotator cuff debridement would best be compared with the other surgical techniques that have been described for situations in which the rotator cuff defect is not reparable. These techniques would include advancement of the supraspinatus origin, transposition of the subscapularis and/or teres minor, muscle transfer techniques, and tendon substitution techniques. Unfortunately, surgical results following many of the above techniques have been reported in small numbers of patients or have been included among the results of patients who underwent surgery for reparable defects in the same series.

Rockwood and colleagues[33] report some residual weakness in most patients undergoing acromioplasty and partial rotator cuff debridement in spite of a high degree of patient satisfaction and significant pain relief. These results compare favorably to the sparse results reported with other methods of managing irreparable rotator cuff defects. However, the controversy surrounding this technique cannot ultimately be answered until standardized, prospective data with this technique are compared with

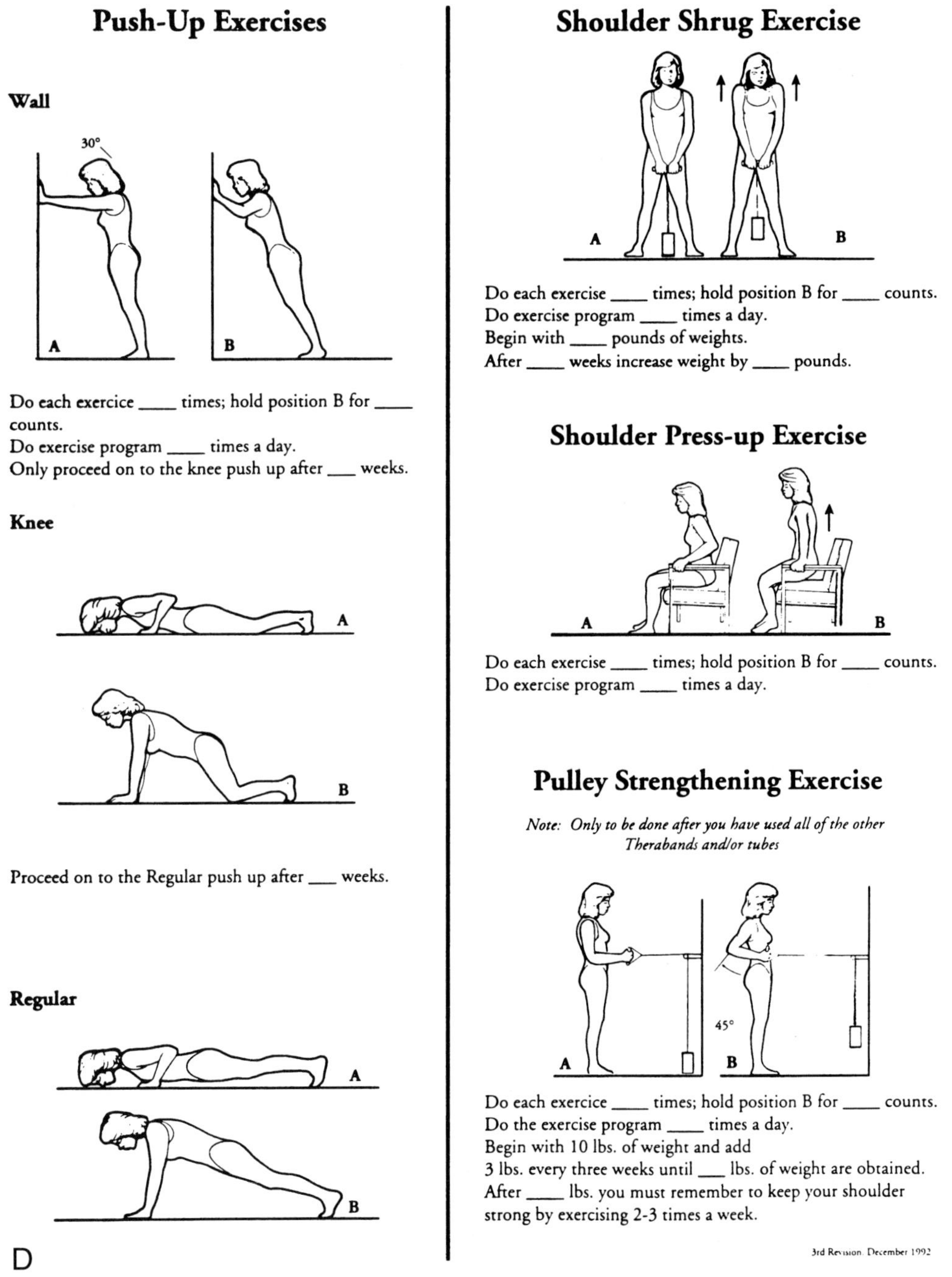

Fig. 22–5—*continued*

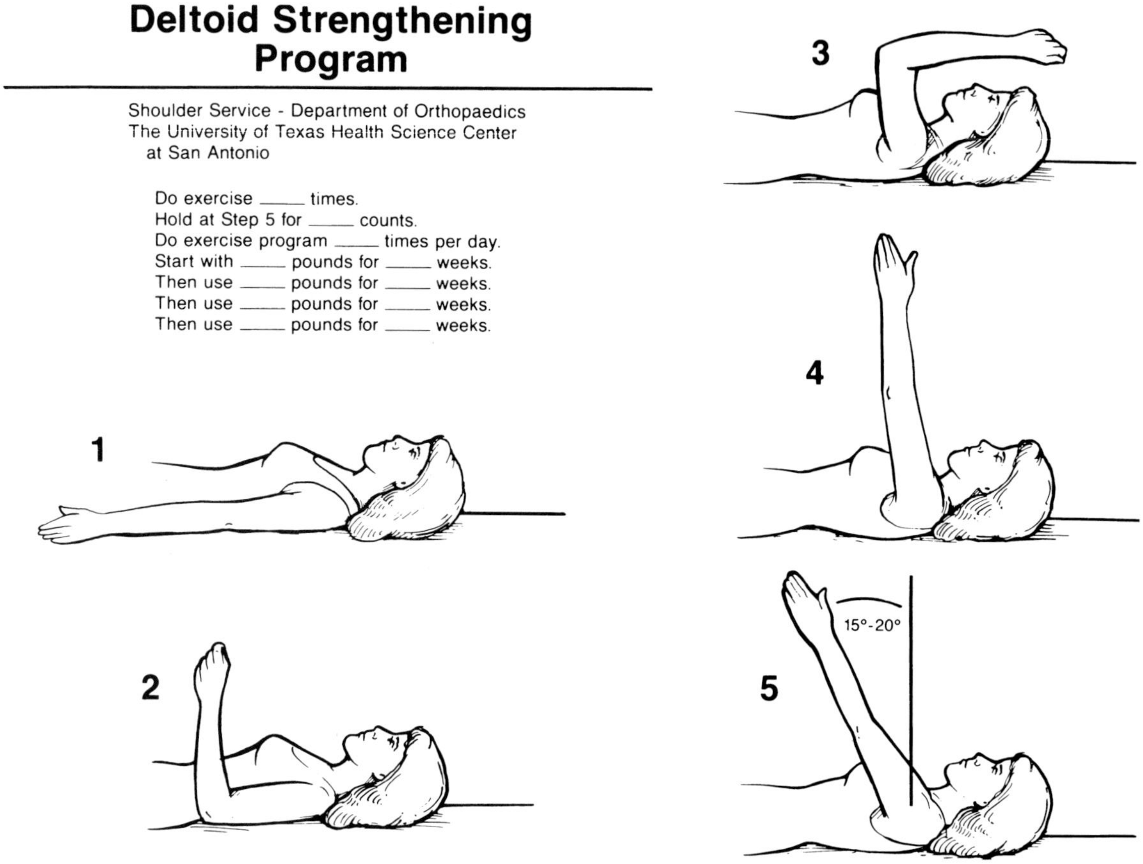

Fig. 22–6. In cases of anterior deltoid weakness, a specific home exercise program for strengthening the anterior deltoid is used.

other techniques in similar patients who have been controlled for tear size. Because pain relief seems to be obtained with most of the procedures, functional scoring of shoulder results with particular emphasis on strength must be obtained.

Apoil[51,52] began performing a procedure that he called "superior arthrolysis" in patients with irreparable lesions of the rotator cuff in 1953. His technique consisted of a deltopectoral incision, excision of the coracoacromial ligament and hypertrophied subacromial bursa, tenodesis of the long head of the biceps, and debridement of any portion of the rotator cuff that impinged between the acromion and the humeral head. Postoperatively the patient was placed in a "thoracobrachial" cast (i.e., a modified shoulder spica cast) with the arm in 90° of abduction for 45 days. The cast was bivalved to allow "physical therapy" in the form of "gentle functional movement such as hand to mouth, to head, and to neck." Its aim was not to increase muscle power. After cast removal, abduction was gradually decreased over 15 days. At this time, muscle strengthening was begun. Apoil[51,52] reported the results with this procedure in 100 patients with an average follow-up of 45 months. Pain relief was excellent in 95% of the cases. However, 19 of the patients had 125° or less of flexion.

The early positive results with "superior arthrolysis" reportedly have not been maintained with time.[19] This has been used as a potential argument against acromioplasty and partial rotator cuff debridement. However, the technique described by Apoil[51,52] differs in several important ways from the technique of acromioplasty and partial rotator cuff debridement as described by Rockwood and colleagues.[33] First, the impingement process must be relieved by performing an adequate acromioplasty and subacromial decompression. This includes excision of the coracoacromial ligament, hypertrophied subacromial bursa, partial rotator cuff debridement, and excision of any existing greater tuberosity exostoses. The most important component of this process, which differs from Apoil's procedure, is the acromioplasty. Secondly, the biceps tendon functions as an important secondary "humeral head depressor." As a result, according to Rockwood and colleagues,[33] it should be preserved. Lastly, the key to overhead function following acromioplasty and partial rotator cuff debridement is a strong and functioning deltoid. Therefore, rather than immobilizing the shoulder in a cast for 45 days and reserving muscle strengthening for 60 days following the surgery, Rockwood and colleagues[33] emphasize early, aggressive deltoid and shoulder muscle rehabilitation that begins

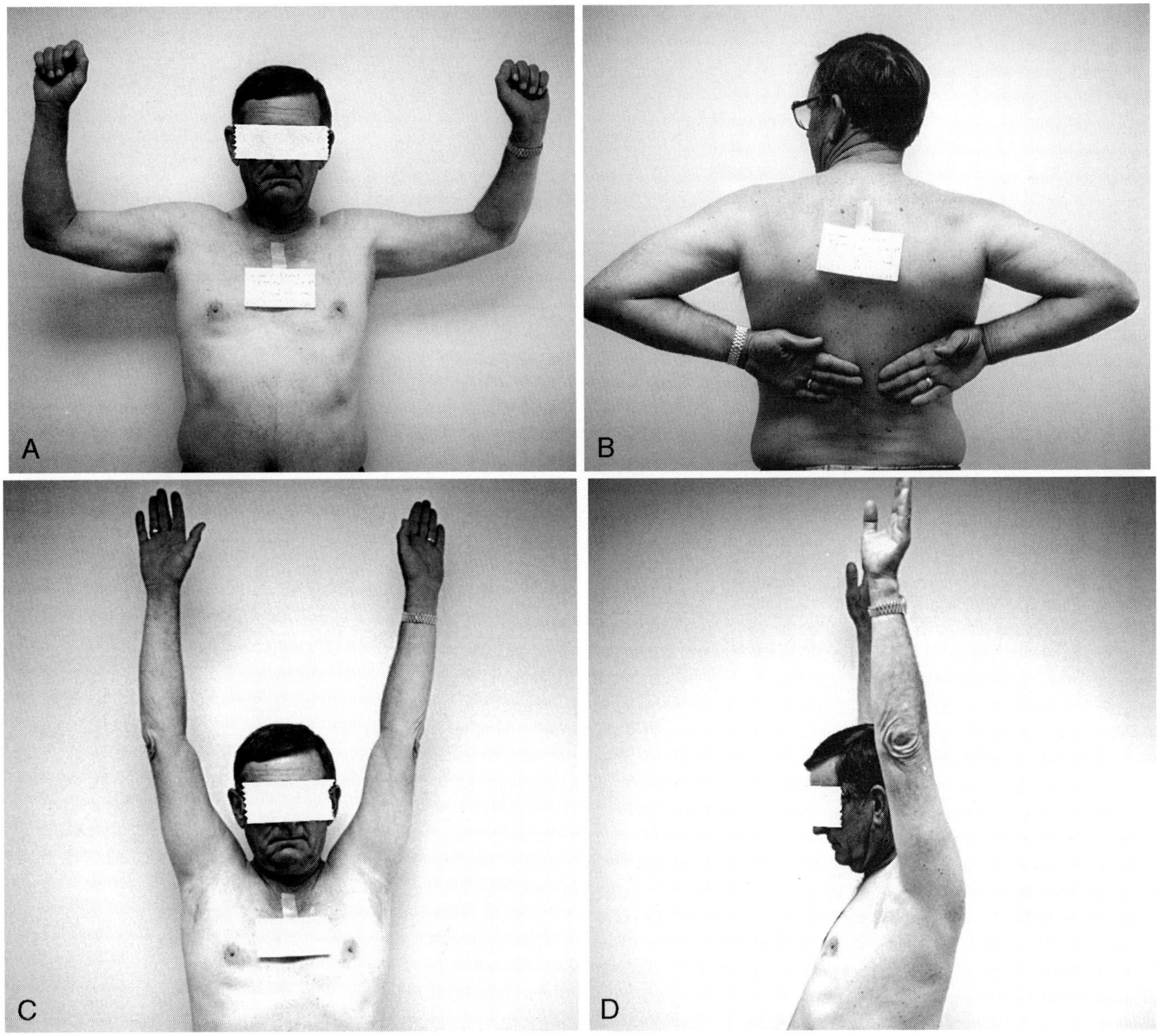

Fig. 22–7. ***A through D,*** **Long-term (8.5 years) functional results in a patient who underwent bilateral rotator cuff debridement.**

on the day of surgery. It is conceivable that these important differences in technique may explain any differences in outcome between the two procedures.

CONCLUSION

The two-step modified Neer acromioplasty, when combined with subacromial decompression and partial debridement of the necrotic remnants of the irreparable supraspinatus and infraspinatus tendons, can provide excellent pain relief and acceptable overhead function in patients with chronic impingement syndrome in association with an irreparable rotator cuff defect. This is particularly true in the presence of an intact biceps tendon, a strong anterior deltoid, and a negative history of prior surgery. The improved function following this procedure is secondary not only to pain relief but also to aggressive rehabilitation of the anterior deltoid, scapular stabilizers, and the remaining portions of the rotator cuff. As Neer[1] stated in his now classic article on anterior acromioplasty, "The rare patient with an irreparable tear can be made more comfortable if impingement is relieved and can gain surprising function if the deltoid is permitted to remain strong."

REFERENCES

1. Neer CS II. Anterior acromioplasty for the chronic impingement syndrome in the shoulder. *J Bone Joint Surg Am.* 1972;54:41–50.
2. Neer CS II, Flatow EL, Lech O. Tears of the rotator cuff. Long term results of anterior acromioplasty and repair. *Orthop Trans.* 1988; 12:673.
3. Bigliani LU, Cordasco FA, McIlveen SJ, Musso ES. Operative repair of massive rotator cuff tears: Long term results. *J Shoulder Elbow Surg.* 1992;1:120–130.
4. Cofield RH. Rotator cuff disease of the shoulder. *J Bone Joint Bone Joint Surg Am.* 1985;67:974–979.
5. Hawkins RJ, Misamore GW, Hobeika PE. Surgery for full thickness rotator cuff tears. *J Bone Joint Surg Am.* 1985;67:1449–1455.
6. McLaughlin HL. Lesions of the musculotendinous cuff of the shoulder: I, The exposures and treatment of tears with retraction. *J Bone Joint Surg Am.* 1944;27:31–51.
7. McLaughlin HL. Rupture of the rotator cuff. *J Bone Joint Surg Am.* 1962;44:979–983.
8. Neviaser JS. Ruptures of the rotator cuff of the shoulder. *Arch Surg.* 1971;102:483–485.
9. Watson M. Major ruptures of the rotator cuff: The results of surgical repair in 89 patients. *J Bone Joint Surg Br.* 1985;67:618–624.
10. Wolfgang GL. Rupture of the musculotendinous cuff of the shoulder. *Clin Orthop.* 1978;144:230–243.
11. Post M, Silver R, Singh M. Rotator cuff tear. Diagnosis and treatment. *Clin Orthop.* 1983;173:78–91.
12. Ellman H, Hanker G, Bayer M. Repair of the rotator cuff. End result study of factors influencing reconstruction. *J Bone Joint Surg Am.* 1986;68:1136–1144.
13. Bateman JE. The diagnosis and treatment of ruptures of the rotator cuff. *Surg Clin North Am.* 1963;43:1523–1530.
14. Debeyre J, Patte D, Elmelik E. Repair of ruptures of the rotator cuff of the shoulder. *J Bone Joint Surg Br.* 1965;47:36–42.
15. Ha'eri GB, Wiley AM. Advancement of the supraspinatus muscle in the repair of ruptures of the rotator cuff. *J Bone Joint Surg Am.* 1981; 63:232–238.
16. Cofield RH. Subscapularis muscle transposition for repair of chronic rotator cuff tears. *Surg Gynecol Obstet.* 1982;154:667–671.
17. Neer CS II. Impingement lesions. *Clin Orthop.* 1983;173:70–77.
18. Neviaser RJ, Neviaser TJ. Transfer of subscapularis and teres minor from massive defects of the rotator cuff. In: Bayley I, Kessel L, eds. *Shoulder Surgery.* New York: Springer-Verlag; 1982:60–63.
19. Augereau B. Rekonstruktion massiver rotatoren manschetten rupturen mit einem deltoid lappen. *Orthopade.* 1991;20:315–319.
20. Mikasa M. Trapezius transfer for global tear of the rotator cuff. In: Bateman JE, Welsh RP, eds. *Surgery of the Shoulder.* Philadelphia: BC Decker; 1984:196–199.
21. Gerber C, Vinh PS, Hertel R, Hess CW. Latissimus dorsi transfer for the treatment of massive tears of the rotator cuff. *Clin Orthop.* 1988; 232:52–61.
22. Bush LF. The torn shoulder capsule. *J Bone Joint Surg Am.* 1975; 57:266–269.
23. Heikel HVA. Rupture of the rotator of the shoulder-experiences of surgical treatment. *Acta Orthop Scand.* 1968;39:477–492.
24. Bayne O, Bateman J. Long term results of surgical repair of full thickness rotator cuff tears. In: Bateman JE, Welch RP eds. *Surgery of the Shoulder.* Philadelphia: BC Decker; 1984:167–171.
25. Neviaser RJ, Neviaser TJ. The repair of chronic massive ruptures of the rotator cuff of the shoulder by use of a freeze dried rotator cuff. *J Bone Joint Surg Am.* 1978;60:681–684.
26. Post M. Rotator cuff repair with carbon filament. *Clin Orthop.* 1985; 196:154–158.
27. Ozaki J, Fugimoto S, Masuhara K. Repair of chronic massive rotator cuff tears with synthetic fabrics. In: Bateman JE, Welch RP, eds. *Surgery of the Shoulder.* Philadelphia: BC Decker; 1984:185–191.
28. Ozaki J, Fugimoto S, Masuhara K, Tamai S, Yoshimoto S. Reconstruction of chronic massive rotator cuff tears with synthetic materials. *Clin Orthop.* 1986;202:173–183.
29. Parrish F, Murray J, Urkuhart B. The use of polyethylene mesh (Marlix) as an adjunct in reconstructive surgery of the extremities. *Clin Orthop.* 1978;147:276–286.
30. Rockwood CA. Shoulder function following decompression of irreparable cuff lesions. *Orthop Trans.* 1984;8:92.
31. Rockwood CA. The management of patients with massive rotator cuff defects by acromioplasty and rotator cuff debridement. *Orthop Trans.* 1986;3:622.
32. Rockwood CA, Burkhead WZ. Management of patients with massive rotator cuff defects by acromioplasty and rotator cuff debridement. *Orthop Trans.* 1988;12:190–191.
33. Rockwood CA, Williams GR, Burkhead WZ. *Debridement of massive, degenerative lesions of the rotator cuff.* Presented at the Seventh Open Meeting of the American Shoulder and Elbow Surgeons. Anaheim, CA, March 10, 1991.
34. Cotton RE, Rideout DF. Tears of the humeral rotator cuff. *J Bone Joint Surg Br.* 1964;46:314–328.
35. Grant JCB, Smith GC. Eight incidents of rupture of the supraspinatus tendon. *Anat Rec.* 1948;100:666.
36. DePalma AF, Gallery G, Bennett GA. Variational anatomy in degenerative lesions of the shoulder joint. In: Blount WP, ed. *American Academy of Orthopaedic Surgeons Instructional Course Lectures.* Ann Arbor: JW Edwards; 1949;6:265–281.
37. Ozaki JF, Nakagawa Y, Masuhara K, Itami S. Tears of the rotator cuff of the shoulder associated with pathological changes in the acromion. *J Bone Joint Surg Am.* 1988;70:1224–1230.
38. Ogata S, Uhthoff HK. Acromial enthesopathy and rotator cuff tear. *Clin Orthop.* 1990;264:39–48.
39. Pettersson G. Ruptures of the tendon aponeurosis of the shoulder joint in anterior/inferior dislocation. *Acta Chir Scand Supp.* 1942; 77:1–184.
40. DePalma AF. *Surgery of the Shoulder.* 3rd ed. Philadelphia: JB Lippincott; 1983:246.
41. Rowe CR. Ruptures of the rotator cuff: Selection of cases for conservative treatment. *Surg Clin North Am.* 1963;43:1531.
42. Nixon JE, DiStefano V. Ruptures of the rotator cuff. *Orthop Clin North Am.* 1975;6:423–447.
43. Packer NP, Calvert PT, Bayley JIL, Kessel L. Operative treatment of chronic ruptures of the rotator cuff of the shoulder. *J Bone Joint Surg Br.* 1983;65:171–175.
44. Lundberg BJ. The correlation of clinical evaluation with operative findings and prognosis in rotator cuff rupture. In: Bayley I, Kessel L, eds. *Shoulder Surgery.* Berlin: Springer-Verlag; 1982;26–38, 1982.
45. Blauth W, Gartner J. Postoperative results of arthrography following suturing of ruptured rotator cuff. *Orthopade.* 1991;20:262–265.
46. Calvert PT, Packer NP, Stoker DJ, Bayley JIL, Kessel L. Arthrography of the shoulder after operative repair of the torn rotator cuff. *J Bone Joint Surg Br.* 1986;68:147–150.
47. Wulker N, Melzer C, Wirth CJ. Shoulder surgery for rotator cuff tears. Ultrasonographic three year follow-up of 97 cases. *Acta Orthop Scand.* 1991;62:142–147.
48. Harryman DT, Mack LA, Wang KW, Jackins SE, Richardson ML, Matsen FA III. Repairs of the rotator cuff. Correlation of functional results with integrity of the cuff. *J Bone Joint Surg Am.* 1991;73:982–989.
49. Burkhart SS. Arthroscopic treatment of massive rotator cuff tears: Clinical results and biomechanical rationale. *Orthop Trans.* 1990; XIV:173.
50. Rockwood CA, Lyons F. Shoulder impingement syndrome: Diagnosis, radiographic evaluation and treatment with a modified Neer acromioplasty. *J Bone Joint Surg Am.* 1993;75:409–424.
51. Apoil A, Augereau B. Antero-superior arthrolysis of the shoulder for rotator cuff degenerative lesions. In: Post M, Morrey B, Hawkins R, eds. *Surgery of the Shoulder.* St. Louis: Mosby-Year Book; 1990:267–270.
52. Apoil A, Dautry P, Koechlin P, Hardy J. The surgical treatment of rotator cuff impingement. In: Bayley I, Kessel L, eds. *Shoulder Surgery.* New York: Springer-Verlag; 1982:22–27.

Chapter 23

Anterior Acromioplasty, Tendon Mobilization, and Direct Repair of Massive Rotator Cuff Tears

Timothy P. Codd and Evan L. Flatow

Tears of the rotator cuff were first described in 1835 by J. G. Smith.[1] However, he first noted the injury in 1832 in a cadaver specimen "removed" (i.e., by grave robbing) before the passage of laws allowing anatomic dissection. In 1833 the passage of laws permitting procurement of cadaver specimens allowed Smith to dissect shoulders. He found a consistent pattern of injury of the rotator cuff in many shoulders, and reported these findings first in the *London Medical Gazette* and then more widely in the *American Journal of Medical Sciences.* This knowledge languished for the better part of a century.

It was left to Codman to revive interest in the rotator cuff and in shoulder in general as a joint that had "been held in little interest by the general surgeons."[2] In 1911 Codman reported the first repair of the rotator cuff.[3] Early acceptance of Codman's ideas met with resistance. Bosworth in 1940 reported his early attempts to repair three massive rotator cuff tears. He achieved such poor results that he advised his fourth patient with a massive tear to undergo a shoulder fusion.[4] However, Bosworth's results improved later in his series, and since that time operative repair of the rotator cuff has become a common shoulder procedure with many repair techniques describe.[2,5–11,12–30]

Neer introduced anterior acromioplasty in 1972.[31] Although there is disagreement as to whether subacromial impingement is the primary etiology or just a secondary phenomenon in rotator cuff tears, by the time surgical repair is performed impingement is usually present and responsible for pain and progressive tendon damage.[13] The addition of routine anterior acromioplasty at the time of tendon repair has been associated with an improvement in clinical results.[32–35] Many techniques have been described to repair large tendon defects. We have preferred tendon mobilization and repair with transposition of existing tissue,[24,36] rather than distant tendon transfers or the use of synthetic or cadaver tendon grafts. In this chapter, we review our approach to the surgical management of massive full-thickness rotator cuff tears.[37–40]

PRINCIPLES

Restore Motion

Although it is often surprising how much passive motion shoulders with rotator cuff tears can have, stiffness does occur.[24] If the shoulder does not have full passive motion under anaesthesia, it should be gently manipulated to break up inferior capsular adhesions that are not easily reached from a superior surgical approach. This is usually performed before draping, but if full motion cannot be achieved, manipulation is deferred until after an open release. Often the coracohumeral ligament is shortened, tethering external rotation, and must be divided.[3] Excessive force should not be used, especially because the humerus in a shoulder with chronic pain may be predisposed to fracture by disuse osteoporosis.

It is important to realize that shoulders with large cuff tears may have good passive motion even though the rotator cuff tendons are retracted and adherent to surrounding structures, because motion may occur through the tear. If the tendons are reattached to the humerus but not released from the coracoid and glenoid rim, a stiff shoulder will result that cannot be mobilized by postoperative therapy except through disruption of the repair.

Decompress Impingement

An anterior acromioplasty is performed to decompress impingement and to prevent continuing wear on the repaired tendons.[41,42] If the AC joint is enlarged, then the undersurface of the joint is beveled to remove any osteophytes that are projecting down and contributing to impingement. Only if the AC joint is tender and painful preoperatively is the distal clavicle excised.

Mobilize Tendons

There is a tendency in the literature on rotator cuff repair to dwell on techniques for "covering the head," underemphasizing methods of tendon mobilization. This is unfortunate, because the aim of repair is to restore a functioning muscle-tendon unit that can move and stabilize the shoulder. The vast majority of tears, even though massive, can be repaired by mobilization and transposition of existing tissue.[24,36] Thus the emphasis should be less on deciding what type of graft to sew into the defect and more on releasing the tendons to close the defect and to allow muscle "pull" and tendon gliding.

Repair Tendons

The goal of repair is to provide dynamic stability, restore strength of external rotation, improve head depression, and seal the synovial cavity for articular nutrition. Subacromial decompression and cuff debridement has been advocated for patients with irreparable, massive tears.[43] However, Apoil and Augereau have noted only 40% good results, progressive glenohumeral arthritis, and superior humeral subluxation with follow-up greater than 10 years after debridement of large tears.[44] Two separate reports of arthroscopic acromioplasty with long-term follow-up noted inferior results in the presence of an unrepaired full-thickness rotator cuff tears, and both investigators concluded that open repair was preferable for the majority of these cases.[46] Furthermore, in two separate reports, Ellman and coworkers found better results after open rotator cuff repair than after arthroscopic debridement of full-thickness tears;[16,45] however, this was not a direct comparison. Montgomery and coworkers performed a randomized, prospective comparison of open surgical repair and arthroscopic debridement and acromioplasty for full-thickness tears of the rotator cuff.[47] The open repair group did significantly better. Finally, we and others have noted that the coracoacromial arch has a passive, stabilizing effect against superior humeral translation, and that removal of this arch by generous surgical decompression, without repair of a massive cuff tear to restore active head depression, can lead to superior head subluxation and a loss of function.[48,49] For all of these reasons, we believe that an active, healthy patient deserves an attempt to repair the cuff to restore a functioning muscle-tendon unit.

Preserve Deltoid

The rotator cuff and deltoid muscles are the prime movers of the shoulder, and if the cuff is torn and damaged, it is imperative that surgical reconstruction not jeopardize the deltoid, which is often the only remaining good muscle. Although it is tempting to detach the deltoid origin for exposure of large tears, with experience this is not necessary and may lead to deltoid pull-off, weakness, and joint sinuses. Damage to the deltoid can be a significant factor in the failure of rotator cuff repair and is associated with poorer results after attempts at revision surgery.[50–53]

Diamond and later Neviaser commented on the value of longitudinal splits in the deltoid in the direction of its fibers combined with subperiosteal exposure of the acromion.[54,55] Our original use of a "T" take-down of the anterior deltoid was changed to a split extending from the anterior aspect of the AC joint, similar in principle to Nevaiser's approach.[56] Bigliani and coworkers advocated moving the split posteriorly, improving access to the posterior cuff tendons.[36] This is our current approach.

Individualized Rehabilitation

Rehabilitation after rotator cuff repair must be carefully supervised by the surgeon who performed the repair. Only he or she can know the quality of the tissues, the strength of the repair, and the precise geometry of the reconstruction. The surgeon must communicate with all those participating in the patient's care. Institution of exercises with weights before tendon healing has been shown to be a common cause of failure,[52] and failure can also occur if the therapist does not know the precise limits dictated by the operative findings.

TECHNIQUE

Examination and Preoperative Planning

A thorough history should be obtained. The precise nature of the patient's chief complaint is vital. Pain is more reliably improved with rotator cuff surgery than weakness and functional loss. It is important that the surgeon and the patient agree on the goals of surgery, and this process begins with understanding why the patient is seeking treatment in the first place.

The mechanism of any injury, as well as the nature of exacerbating activities, should be documented. A history of a sudden loss of strength and function after an accident or trauma in a patient subsequently shown to have a large cuff tear would lead us to recommend timely repair.[57] In such cases, there is often far less muscle scarring and atrophy, and much less difficulty mobilizing the tendons at repair, than in chronic, longstanding cases with the same size tendon defect. A careful evaluation for other sources of shoulder pain and weakness, especially cervial radiculopathy, is mandatory.

Also important in the history is any prior treatment that patients have received. Several studies have shown that receiving more than three cortisone injections weakens remaining cuff tissue and has an adverse affect on surgical outcome.[57,59,60,61]

The physical exam can yield important information. Muscle atrophy, especially of the spinati, should be recorded. The AC joint should be examined for tenderness. Failure to treat a symptomatic AC joint is a significant cause of failure of rotator cuff repairs.[50,51,24] External rotation weakness can be impressive and suggests involvement of the infraspinatus and posterior cuff. If the arm is held at the side by the physician and then falls into internal rotation when released ("drop sign"), the patient must be warned that some weakness will likely persist despite cuff repair and rehabilitation. Testing for subscapularis involvement is best achieved with the test described by Gerber,[62] the subscapular rupture "lift off" test. Asymmetry of the biceps caused by rupture of the long head should be assessed. The examiner should also be alert to the possibility of neurological disease. Axillary nerve palsy can accompany cuff tears, especially those occurring after glenohumeral dislocation.[58,63,64]

Provocative tests for impingement[31,65] evaluate irritation of the rotator cuff and biceps tendon beneath the coracoacromial arch. Although multiple steroid injections can be detrimental to the outcome after repair, injections of local anesthetics into the subacromial space and the AC joint can determine the need for AC joint resection[66] and can confirm that the shoulder (and not the neck, for example) is the source of the patient's symptoms.

Imaging studies can be extremely helpful. Standard radiographic views may show degenerative changes in the greater tuberosity, including cyst formation, sclerosis, and excrescences.[67] The axillary view may demonstrate an os acromiale. Superior migration of the humeral head on anteroposterior radiographs can be an indicator of a massive rotator cuff tear.[68] Special radiographic views are also helpful.[69] The supraspinatus outlet view best demonstrates acromial morphology as described by Bigliani.[70,71] Other studies will depend on the physician's preference and the quality of studies available to him or her. Ultrasonography in particular seems to be significantly dependent on the interest and skill of the radiologist performing the study.[58] Although arthrography is highly accurate for the diagnosis of full-thickness rotator cuff tears,[20,21,58,72] our preferred imaging study is MRI, which is highly accurate in determining tear size, muscle retraction, acromial shape, and the presence of os acromiale. MRI has been especially helpful in raising the suspicion of neurologic disease in patients whose tear seems too small on MRI to explain their clinical weakness.

Setup

We perform rotator cuff repairs under regional anaesthesia (interscalene brachial plexus block). This avoids many of the unpleasant effects associated with general anaesthesia and also aids in postoperative pain control. Appropriate perioperative antibiotics are administered. The patient is placed in the semisitting or "beach-chair" position. The patient is placed high on the table, with the operative shoulder over the corner of the table. Towels are placed under the medial border of the scapulae, and the arm is positioned to allow extension of the operative shoulder for improved visualization of the posterior cuff. The patient's bony prominences are protected, and hyperextension of the neck is avoided. The patient is then shaved and prepped with a standard antimicrobial scrub and prep.

Approach

The incision is made in the direction of the skin creases in order to provide the most cosmetically appealing scar. It starts over the lateral third of the acromion and extends to the lateral tip of the coracoid (Fig. 23–1). This skin incision can be adjusted medially to allow better AC access in those patients with preoperative AC tenderness. Adequate undermining and mobilization of the skin flaps allows visualization of the entire anterior acromion and upper deltoid. Proper placement of the deltoid split allows access to even massive rotator cuff tears with minimal, if any, removal of the deltoid origin from the acromion. A substantial cuff of deltoid is then left on the bone. A small amount of deltoid is subperiostially dissected to allow an adequate acromioplasty. This preservation of deltoid cuff significantly improves closure. Occasionally, if deltoid origin is removed, or if a sufficient soft-tissue cuff is not available, drill holes should be placed in the acromion to ensure a secure repair of the deltoid.

The deltoid split is begun with needle-tip electrocautery just anterior to the AC joint. The split is continued straight laterally past the antero-lateral corner of the acromion. The incision is then carried distally 3 to 4 cm, centered on the middle part of the greater tuberosity. A stay suture is placed at the distal extent of the incision to prevent distal propagation of the deltoid split, which might injure the axillary nerve (Fig. 23–2). This modified deltoid split is more lateral and posterior than previously described incisions.[31,73] By centering the deltoid split over the middle portion of the greater tuberosity, better posterior exposure is obtained and mobilization of the rotator cuff is facilitated. Rotation of the humerus under the split provides excellent anterior and posterior exposure. With this modified exposure, a second posterior

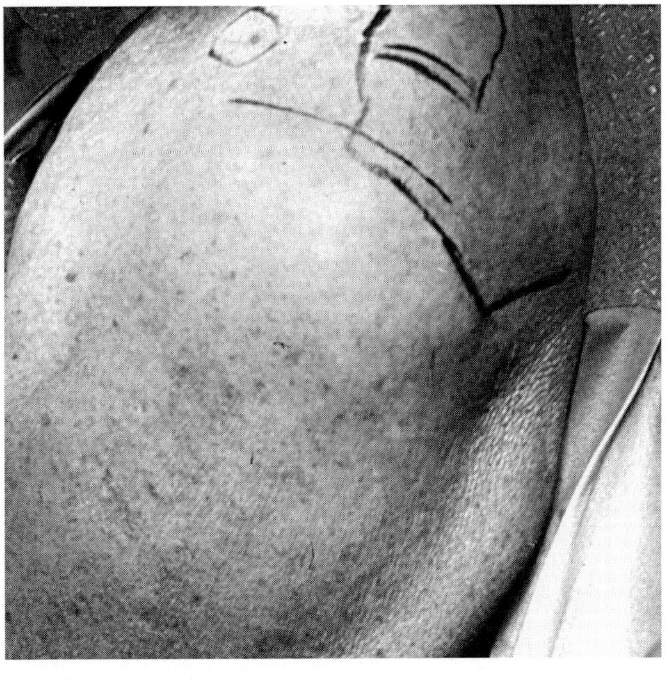

Fig. 23–1. The skin incision is placed in Langers lines for cosmesis. The incision starts over the lateral third of the acromion and extends toward the coracoid.

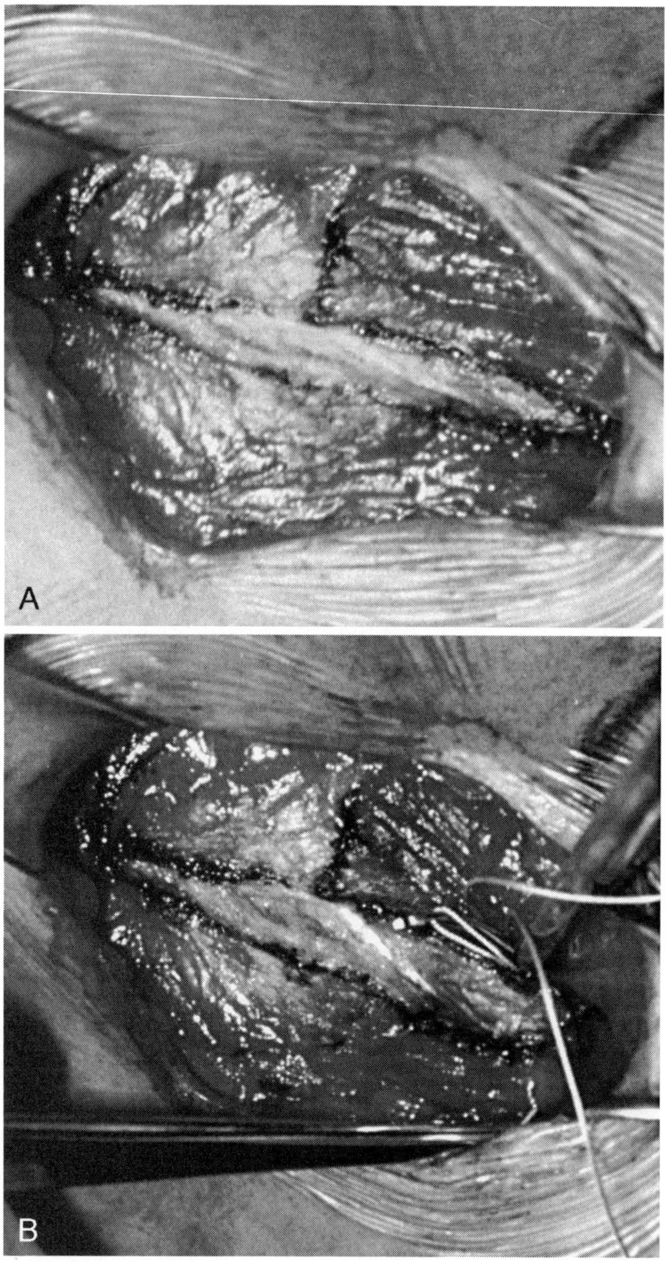

Fig. 23–2. *A,* The deltoid is split for about 4 cm from the anterolateral corner of the acromion. The split is centered over the greater tuberosity. The incision is continued along the anterior aspect of the acromion to the AC joint. *B,* The stay suture is placed at the distal extent of the deltoid split. This prevents propagation of the split and possible injury to the axillary nerve.

approach is not necessary for access to the posterior cuff, even in massive tears.

Anterior Acromioplasty

As noted by several investigators, achieving adequate subacromial decompression seems to be a crucial step in eliminating pain and avoiding postoperative wear on the

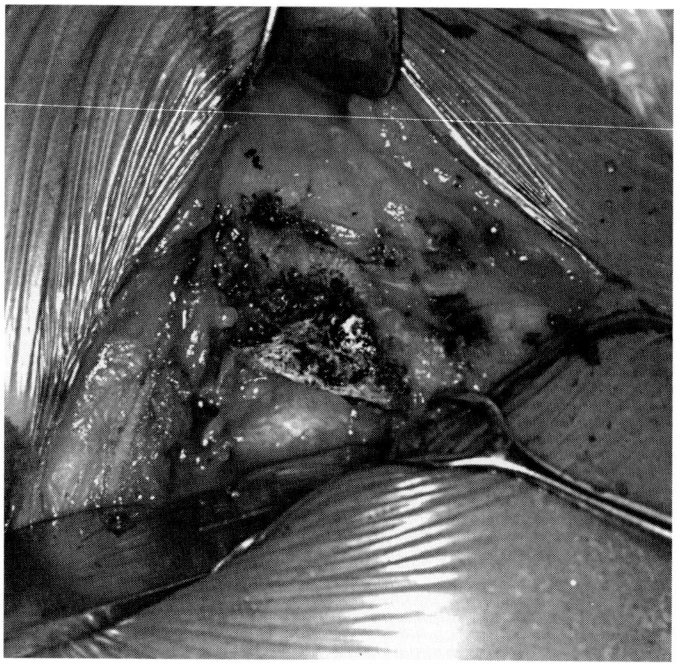

Fig. 23–3. The deltoid is subperiostially elevated from the anterior acromion, and the coracoacromial ligament is excised. A flat retractor levers the head down. These maneuvers allow good visualization of the anteroinferior acromion.

repaired cuff tendon.[74–76] Residual subacromial impingement has been identified as a source of failure after rotator cuff surgery.[35,50,51,65,75] For these reasons, as well as to provide increased exposure of the rotator cuff, a formal anterior acromioplasty[31] is performed routinely at the time of repair of massive rotator cuff tears. Slight abduction of the arm will release tension on the deltoid and facilitate exposure. The coracoacromial ligament is then dissected sharply from its insertion on the undersurface of the acromion and excised (Fig. 23–3). Preserving the coracoacromial ligament and reattaching it at the time of deltoid closure may have a role in providing a buffer and superior stabilizer in some patients with rotator cuff deficiency,[48] but this is a developmental procedure with little follow-up, and we do not currently recommend it for general use. The subacromial space is then cleaned of bursal adhesions and scar. Care must be taken in cleaning the subacromial space, as the torn edge of the rotator cuff may be adherent to the undersurface of the acromion.

With the acromion now exposed, its width is palpated with the thumb and forefinger. A blunt flat retractor (Darrach or similar type) is then placed under the acromion to protect the torn cuff and humeral head. While pressure is applied to the posterior acromion, an A-O osteotome is used (bevel up) to remove an adequate wedge of anterior acromion (Fig. 23–4). We prefer this technique, as it minimizes the possibility of over resection of the acromion and the disastrous complications of acromial fracture. The acromioplasty is then completed and smoothed with a power-burr, rasp, or ronguer. In those patients without preoperative AC tenderness, a modified AC arthroplasty is performed to remove excrescences from the inferior part of the clavicle that may contribute to impingement. Again, this is performed with the burr, rasp, or ronguer.

Acromioclavicular Arthroplasty

In patients with preoperative AC tenderness and pain, the distal clavicle is resected. This procedure is performed with a technique derived from arthroscopic procedures. The AC joint is palpated on its superior aspect. An incision is then made in the inferior joint capsule and a power burr is used to resect the distal clavicle from below, leaving the superior and posterior capsule intact for stability. Rasps are used to ensure that the resection is even and that the edges are smooth. An adequate quantity of bone, generally 6 to 8 mm, is resected (Fig. 23–5). Care must be taken with this approach to ensure that the posterior and superior cortical rims of the distal clavicle are removed, as residual bone can result in failure. With this approach (preserving much of the AC joint capsule), problems are avoided that occur when the joint is destabilized.[66] Only 6 to 8 mm of distal clavicle needs to be removed in our experience.

Tendon Mobilization

Rotator cuff tendon mobilization is performed with blunt dissection above and below the cuff. The tendon edge is freshened and nonabsorbable stay sutures are placed to allow mobilization (Fig. 23–6). Mobilization starts anteriorly and progresses to the posterior aspect of the cuff. Care must be taken not to dissect below the level of the teres minor tendon to avoid injury to the axillary nerve as it exits the quadrilateral space. Likewise, care should be directed while bluntly mobilizing the supra-

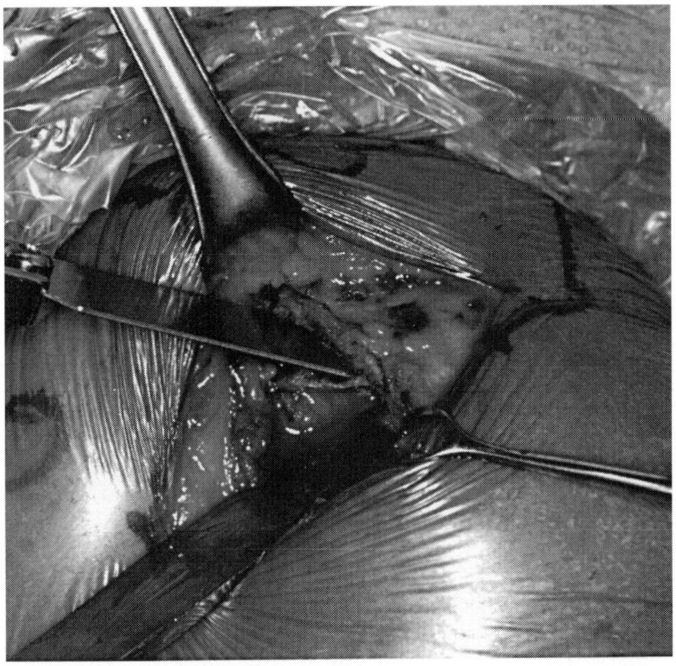

Fig. 23–4. An osteotome is used to perform the acromioplasty.

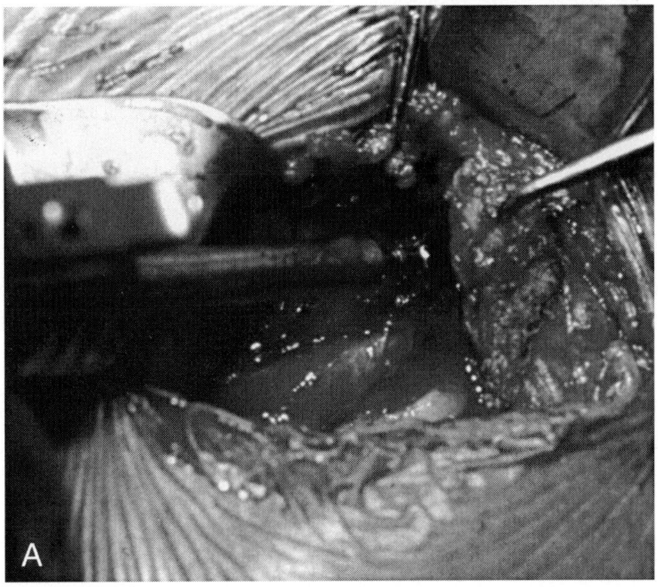

A

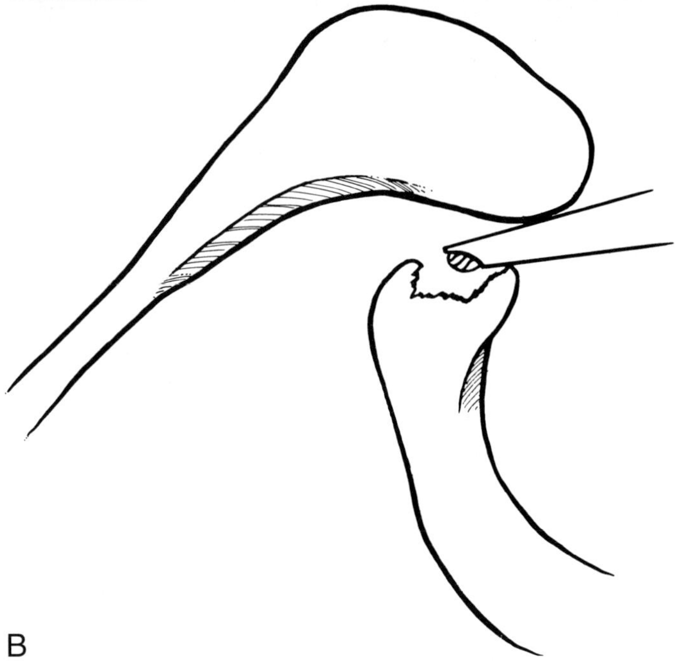

B

Fig. 23–5. *A*, If the AC joint is enlarged and contriuting to impingement, its inferior osteophytes are trimmed. Only if there is preoperative AC tenderness and pain is the distal clavicle completely resected. If this is indicated, a minimal (6 to 8 mm) but even resection is performed from below with a power burr, preserving the posterior and superior AC capsule for stability. *B*, A complete AC resection must include the posterior and superior cortical rims. Inadequate removal of bone, especially posteriorly, can result in failure.

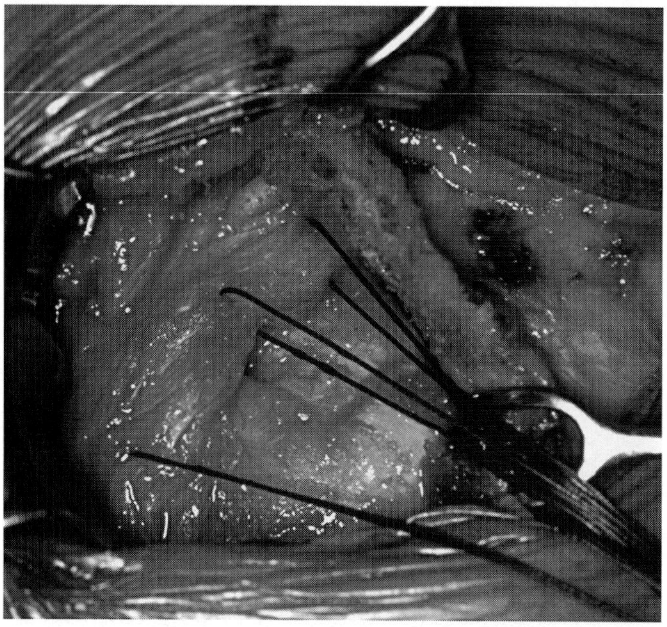

Fig. 23–6. Nonabsorbing sutures, seen here passed through the edges of the torn rotator cuff, allow mobilization while minimizing trauma to the cuff tissue.

spinatus tendon retracted in its fossa, to avoid injury to the suprascapular nerve.[77,78]

If the coracohumeral ligament is shortened, tethering the tendon to the coracoid, it is released.[79] The coracoid base can be released 270° anteriorly, laterally, and posteriorly. The medial side is avoided for fear of injuring the suprascapular nerve. If the retracted tendons are scarred to the glenoid rim and tethered by a shortened glenohumeral capsule, the capsule is divided within the joint (working through the tear), avoiding the biceps origin. Although this essentially creates a lesion similar in principle to a Bankart lesion, instability has not been a result. Filling in the cuff defect with a graft without releasing the tendons from the glenoid rim and coracoid would make as little sense as grafting an old flexor tendon laceration in the hand while leaving it scarred and adherent in its bed. Mobilizing the tendons not only facilitates repair, but allows them to glide and function.

Often the free edge of the supraspinatus tendon is retracted to the glenoid rim and scarred to the adjacent more medial aspect of the subscapularis tendon and contracted rotator interval (and coracohumeral ligament). Dividing the rotator interval allows realignment of the supraspinatus laterally, an ''interval slide.''[36] This is accomplished by performing a complete release of the coracohumeral ligament and the rotator interval (Fig. 23–7).[79] This may allow the contracted supraspinatus tendon now freed anteriorly (interval slide), inferiorly (capsular release), and superiorly (bursal release) to slide laterally to facilitate reattachment to the greater tuberosity. Occasionally, the posterior cuff is also released, freeing the interval between the infraspinatus and the supraspinatus. This is necessary if the tendons are bunched at the glenoid rim by scar; to pull them up over the larger circumference head a releasing incision is needed (like stretching the collar of a turtle neck sweater to pull it off). Care is taken to avoid the suprascapular artery and nerve, which run lateral to the acromial base.

Specialized Techniques

If the cuff is still unable to be repaired without tension while the arm is at the side, the biceps or subscapularis may be rerouted. Transposition of the upper portion of the subscapularis tendons to aid in the repair of massive tears is performed by detaching the superior 40 to 60% of the subscapularis at its insertion and transferring it superiorly[41,45,56,80,81] (Fig. 23–8). Transfer of other muscles, in particular the teres minor,[82] is not performed out of concern that weakness of external rotation may occur.

The biceps can be incorporated between the anterior and posterior cuff edges to provide a ''bridge'' as described by McLaughlin.[23] Alternatively, J.S. Nevaiser[60] has proposed excising the intra-articular portion and using this as a free graft. This is probably not an acceptable technique if the biceps is intact, as the biceps performs an important function as a humeral stabilizer and depressor.

Other heroic methods have been advocated, in particular the use of fascial grafts and synthetic substitutes,[24,60,84,83] latissimus dorsi transfer[85] and deltoid flaps.[86] These have not been necessary for the repair of primary tears in our experience. The majority of massive cuff tears can be mobilized and repaired to the tuberosity with the arm at the side with the techniques of transposition and repair of existing tissue described above.

Tendon Repair

The humerus is prepared by removing any excrescences from the greater tuberosity. A shallow bone trough in the anatomic neck of the humerus just distal to the edge of the cartilage is created with a ronguer or burr. This location is slightly proximal to the normal insertion on the tuberosity, facilitating repair. Bone holes are then created through the tuberosity, exiting in the trough. Bone sutures are then passed (Fig. 23–9). A variety of instruments are available for this purpose.

The rotator cuff tissue is prepared. In the past, investigators[87] have suggested the need to debride the ''avascular edges'' of the torn cuff. This reduces the tissue available and increases the difficulty of repair of massive rotator cuff tears. More recent studies by Uhthoff[61] and Swintosky and coworkers.[88] have concluded that the edges of the torn cuff are well vascularized. Indeed there is significant neovascularization and granulation of the cuff edges. Thus in most instances tendon edges have good blood supply and should only be ''freshened'' to provide a clean edge to hold sutures.[89]

Prior to repair of the cuff, sutures are placed in the realigned rotator intervals (anterior and posterior) but not tied down. The arm is placed at the side (not in ab-

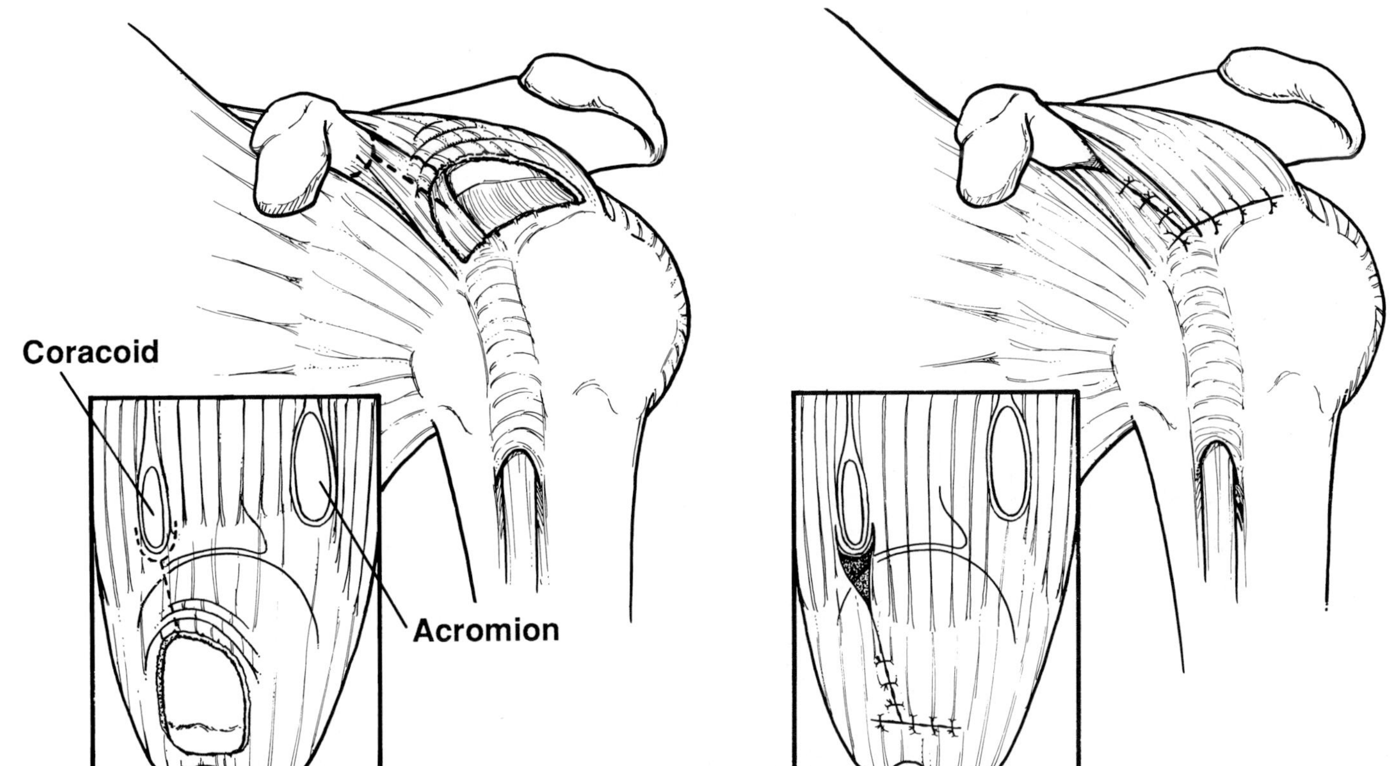

Fig. 23–7. *A,* In a large tear with a shortened and retracted supraspinatus tendon, the anterior edge of the retracted supraspinatus tendon is scarred to the medial subscapularis, which is not retracted, and the coracoid base. An "interval slide" divides the supraspinatus from these structures and realigns it laterally to facilitate tendon repair. *B,* Supraspinatus tendon shown before an interval slide is performed. The tendon is retracted and unable to be mobilized. Scissors are along the rotator interval directed toward the base of the coracoid. *C,* Interval slide complete. Tendon is now able to be pulled laterally. *D,* Illustration of a massive rotator cuff tear. Arrows indicating direction of pull of the retracted cuff tendons. After interval slide and posterior cuff release, cuff is now lateralized and mobilized to allow repair. *E,* An interval slide has already been performed, but the cuff can still not be completely mobilized. *F,* Scissors shown in the direction of the "posterior" interval between the infracspinatus and supraspinatus in preparation for a posterior cuff release. Care is taken to avoid damage to the suprascapular nerve, which lies at the medial extent of this interval. *G,* After the posterior cuff release, the tendons can be realigned and repaired.

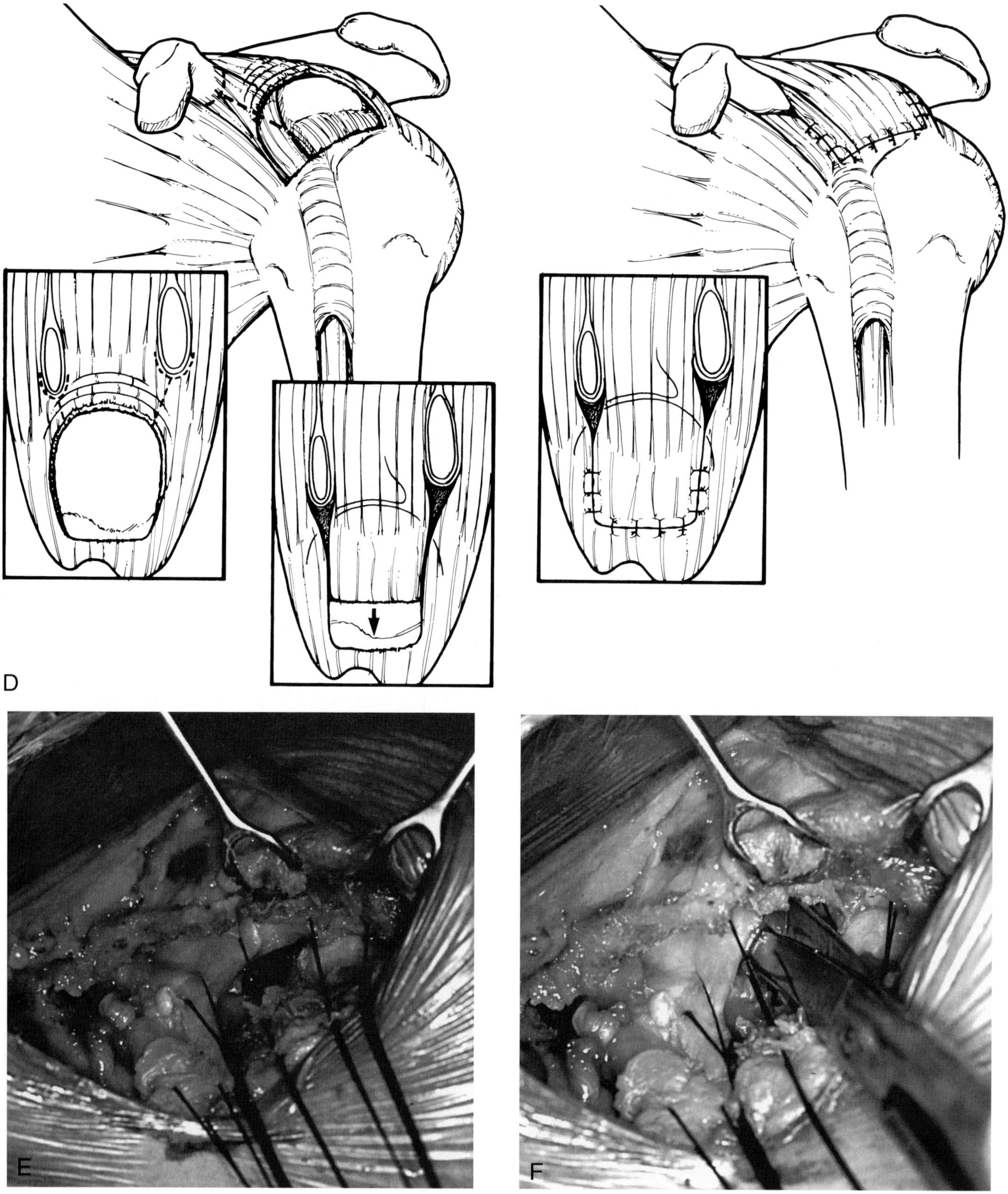

Fig. 23–7—*continued*

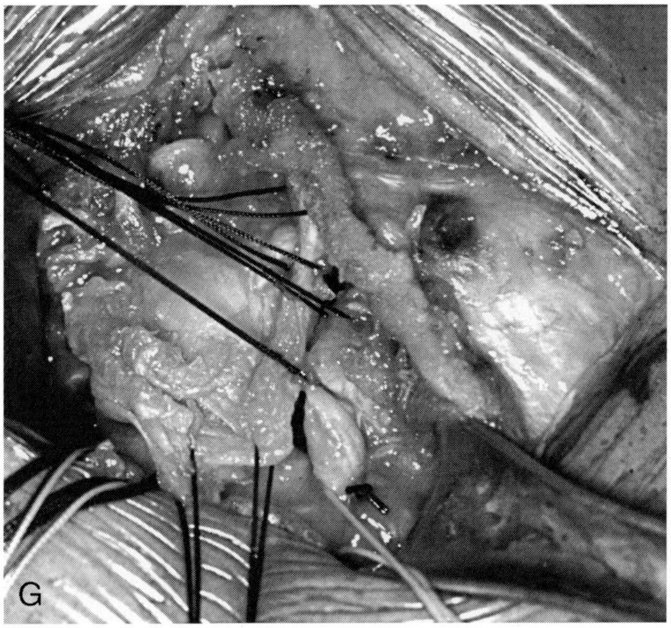

Fig. 23–7—*continued*

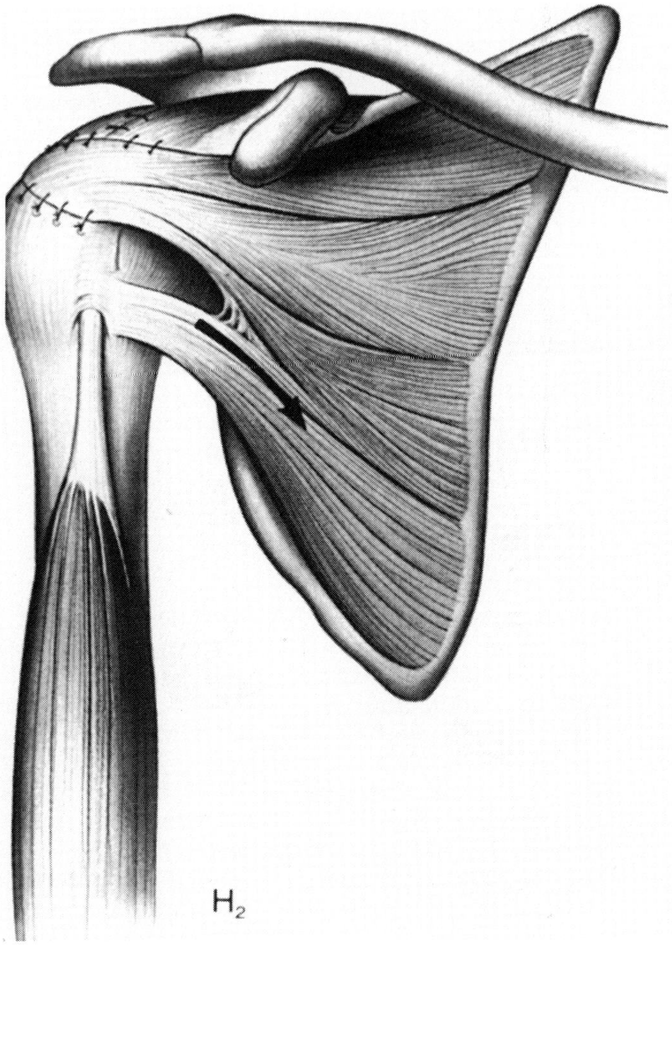

Fig. 23–8. The upper portion of the subscapularis tendon may be transposed by detaching the superior 40 to 60% at this insertion and transferring it superiorly. This is rarely performed.

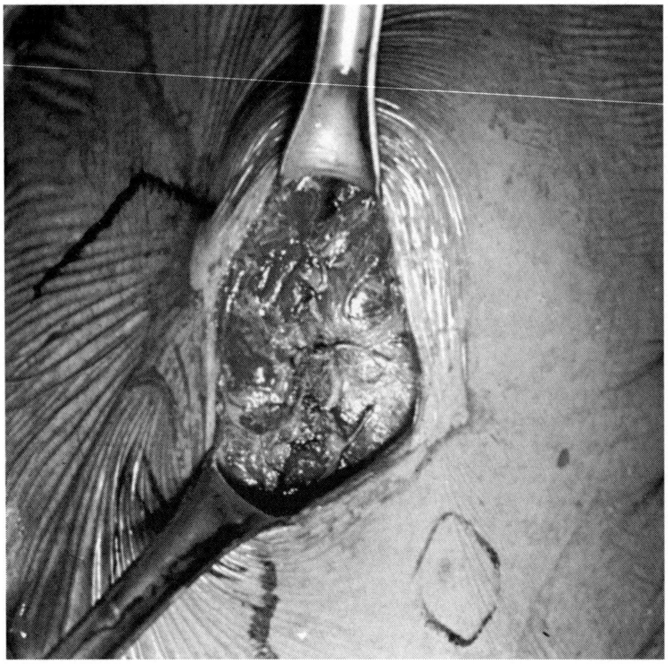

Fig. 23–9. The deltoid split is repaired with heavy, non-absorbable sutures.

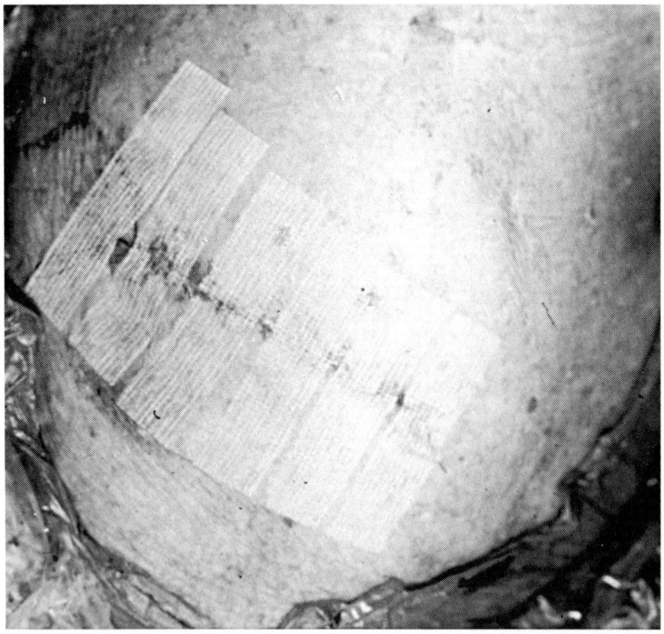

Fig. 23–10. The skin is repaired with subcuticular sutures for a cosmetically pleasing scar.

duction). The optimum position is approximately 10° flexion, 10° abduction, and slight internal rotation. The cuff is then repaired by tying down the tendon to bone sutures (No. 1 nonabsorbable) and the tendon to tendon interval sutures. Simple sutures, alternating with modified Mason-Allen sutures,[90] are used to repair the tendon to the bone trough. The repair must then be tested by rotating internally and externally and elevating to at least 100°. The repair should be strong enough to maintain this motion, as the motion will be needed for postoperative rehabilitation. It should be noted that in massive rotator cuff tears a watertight repair may not be possible.[91] However, Packer and associates[26] and Calvert et al.[92] have demonstrated that complete watertight closure is not essential for good results. Rather, the primary goal of the repair is to restore mechanical continuity of the musculotendinous unit of the rotator cuff. Finally, the deltoid is repaired to the cuff of tendon on the acromion and distal clavicle with heavy braided nonabsorbable sutures. If needed, bone sutures are used through drill holes in the acromion.[93] As we have mentioned, the importance of a good deltoid repair cannot be overemphasized (Fig. 23–10).

Rehabilitation

In the immediate postoperative period, patients are placed in a sling and swathe until the regional anaesthesia has worn off. These patients are maintained in a sling. As all repairs are performed at the side, this is the only support necessary. We do not routinely use an abduction brace, as it allows the arm to slide into extension, which creates tension across the site of repair rather than relieving it. Passive elevation in the scapular plane is started on the first postoperative day, performed by the physician or therapist. Elbow and hand motion, and pendulum exercises are also performed. These exercises are the only ones recommended for the first 6 to 8 weeks. Pulley exercises involve some muscle activity,[94] and in massive tears we avoid assistive exercises during this period. At 6 to 8 weeks assistive exercises such as pulley elevation and external rotation with a stick are added. Active and resisted exercises are started when bone and tendon healing are more advanced, usually at about 3 months. Earlier introduction of weights in the exercise program has been reported as a factor leading to failure.[52] Also, it is important to emphasize to the patient that rotator cuff rehabilitation is a prolonged process, as demonstrated by Brems,[11] and that the rehabilitation process can continue as long as 12 to 18 months postsurgery.[95]

CONCLUSIONS

Using the techniques outlined above, we have been able to achieve consistently satisfactory results in treating massive rotator cuff tears.[24,36] This can be accomplished without tendon transfers,[82] allografts,[83] synthetic material,[84] or sacrifice of the deltoid.[86] What is important is a systematic approach to the massive tear, with attention to technical details. Proper patient selection, careful surgical technique, and meticulous rehabilitation are all important. The skills necessary to treating these difficult cases improve with experience, so that the proportion of tears which are ''irreparable'' becomes quite low.

REFERENCES

1. Smith JG. Pathological appearances of seven cases of injury of the shoulder joint with remarks. *Am J Med Sci.* 1835;16:219.
2. Codman EA. *The Shoulder. Rupture of the Supraspinatus Tendon and Other Lesions In or About the Subacromial Bursa.* Malabar, FL: RE Krieger; 1984.
3. Codman EA. Complete rupture of the supraspinatus tendon. Operative treatment with report of two successful cases. *Boston Med Surg J.* 1911;164:708–710.
4. Bosworth DM. An analysis of 28 consecutive cases of incapacitating shoulder lesions radically explored and repaired. *J Bone Joint Surg Am.* 1940;22:369–392.
5. Bassett RW, Cofield RH. Acute tears of the rotator cuff. The timing of surgical repair. *Clin Orthop.* 1983;175:18–24.
6. Bakalim G, Pasila M. Surgical treatment of rupture of the rotator cuff tendon. *Acta Orthop Scand.* 1975;46:751–757.
7. Bateman JE. The diagnosis and treatment of ruptures of the rotator cuff. *Surg Clin North Am.* 1963;43:1523–1530.
8. Bayne O, Bateman JE. Long Term Results of Surgical Repair of Full Thickness Rotator Cuff Tears. In: Bateman JE, Walsh RP, eds. *Surgery of the Shoulder.* Philadelphia: BC Decker; 1984:167–171.
9. Bigliani LU, Kimmel J, McCann PD, Wolfe IN. Repair of rotator cuff tears in tennis players. *Am J Sports Med.* 1992;20:112–117.
10. Bjorkenheim J, Paavolainen P, Ahovuo J, and Slatis, P. Surgical repair of the rotator cuff and surrounding tissues: Factors influencing the results. *Clin Orthop.* 1988;236:148–153.
11. Brems JJ. Digital muscle strength measurement in rotator cuff tears. *Orthop Trans.* 1987;1:235; 1988;12:757–758.
12. Codman EA. Rupture of the supraspinatus, 1834–1934. *J Bone Joint Surg.* 1937;19:643–652.
13. Cofield RH. Current concepts review: Rotator cuff disease of the Shoulder. *J Bone Joint Surg Am.* 1985;67:974–979.
14. Constant CR. Shoulder function after rotator cuff tears by operative and nonoperative means. In: Post M, Morrey BF, Hawkins RJ, eds. *Surgery of the Shoulder.* St. Louis: Mosby-Year Book; 1990:231–233.
15. Earnshaw P, Desjardins D, Sarkar K and Uhthoff, HK. Rotator cuff tears: The role of surgery. *Can J Surg.* 1982;25:60–63.
16. Ellman H, Hanker G, Bear M. Repair of the rotator cuff. End results study of factors influencing reconstruction. *J Bone Joint Surg Am.* 1986;68:1136–1144.
17. Ellman H, Kay SP, Wirth M. Arthroscopic treatment of full-thickness rotator cuff tears: Two to seven year follow-up study. *Arthroscopy.* 1993;9:195–200.
18. Godsil RD, Linscheid RL. Intratendinous defects of the rotator cuff. *Clin Orthop.* 1970;69:181–188.
19. Heikel HVA. Rupture of the rotator cuff of the shoulder. Experiences of surgical treatment. *Acta Orthop Scand.* 1968;39:477–492.
20. Lindblom K, Palmer L. Ruptures of the tendon aponeurosis of the shoulder joint. The so-called supraspinatus ruptures. *Acta Chir Scand.* 1939;82:133–142.
21. McLaughin BL. Reconstruction of the shoulder joint. *Instr Course Lect AAOS.* 1944;2:343.
22. McLaughlin BL. Lesions of the musculotendinous cuff of the Shoulder: 1. The exposure and treatment of tears with retraction. *J Bone Joint Surg.* 1944;26:31–51.
23. McLaughlin HL, Asherman EG. Lesions of the musculotendinous cuff of the shoulder. IV. Some observations based upon the results of surgical repair. *J Bone Joint Surg Am.* 1951;33:76–86.
24. Neer CS, Flatow EL, Lech, O. Tears of the rotator cuff. Long term results of anterior acromioplasty and repair. *Orthop Trans.* 1988; 12:673.
25. Cofield RH. Tears of the rotator cuff. *Instr Course Lect AAOS.* 1981; 30:258.
26. Packer NP, Calvert PT, Bayley JIL, Kessel L. Operative treatment of chronic ruptures of the rotator cuff of the shoulder. *J Bone Joint Surg Br.* 1983;65:171–175.
27. Post M, Silver R, Singh M. Rotator cuff tear. Diagnosis and treatment. *Clin Orthop.* 1983;173:78–91.
28. Watson M. Major ruptures of the rotator cuff. The results of surgical repair in 89 patients. *J Bone Joint Surg Br.* 1985;4:618–624.
29. Weiner DS, MacNab, L. Ruptures of the rotator cuff. Follow-up evaluation of operative repairs. *Can J Surg.* 1970;13:219–227.
30. Wilson PD. Complete rupture of the supraspinatus tendon. *JAMA.* 1931;96:433–438.
31. Neer CS. Anterior acromioplasty for the chronic impingement syndrome in the shoulder: A preliminary report. *J Bone Joint Surg Am.* 1972;54:41–50.
32. Flatow EL. Technique of anterior acromioplasty. In: Kohn D, Wirth CJ, eds. *Die Schulter: Aktuelle Operative Therapie.* Stuttgart: Thieme; 1992:100–105.
33. Flatow EL, Fischer RA and Bigliani LU. Results of Surgery. In: Ianotti JP, ed. *Rotator Cuff Disorders: Evaluation and Treatment.* Park Ridge, IL: American Academy of Orthopaedic Surgeons. 1991:53–63.
34. McShane RB, Leinberry CF, Fenlin JM. Conservative open anterior acromioplasty. *Clin Orthop.* 1987;223:137–144.
35. Neer CS, Marberry TA. On the disadvantages of radical acromionectomy. *J Bone Joint Surg Am.* 1981;63:416–419.
36. Bigliani LU, Cordasco FA, McIlveen SJ, Musso ES. Operative repair of massive rotator cuff tears: Long-term results. *J Shoulder Elbow Surg.* 1992;1:120–139.
37. Bigliani LU, Craig EV, Flatow EL. Shoulder reconstruction. In: *Orthopaedic Knowledge Update 3.* Chicago: American Academy of Orthopaedic Surgeons. 1990:313–326.
38. Bigliani EL, Flatow EL. History, physical examination, and diagnostic modalities. In: McGinty JB, Caspari RB, Jackson RW, Poehling GG, eds. *Operative Arthroscopy.* Raven: New York; 1991:453–464.
39. Bigliani LU, Steinmann SP, Flatow EL. Complications. In: Ianotti JP, ed. *Rotator Cuff Disorders: Evaluation and Treatment.* Park Ridge, IL: American Academy of Orthopaedic Surgeons; 1991:63–74.
40. Flatow EL. Technique of rotator cuff repair. In: Kohn D, Wirth CJ, eds. *Die Schulter: Aktuelle Operative Therapie.* Stuttgart: Thieme; 1992:90–95.
41. Cofield RH. Subscapular muscle transposition for repair of chronic rotator cuff tears. *Surg Gynecol Obstet.* 1982;154:667–672.
42. Cofield RH, Hoffmeyer P, Lanzar WH. Surgical repair of chronic rotator cuff tears. *Orthop Trans.* 1990;14:251–252.
43. Rockwood CA Jr, Williams GR Jr, Burkhead WZ Jr. Debridement of irreparable, degenerative lesions of the rotator cuff. *Orthop Trans.* 1993;16:740.
44. Apoil A, Augereau B. Antero-superior arthrolysis of the shoulder for rotator cuff degenerative lesions. In: Post M, Morrey BF, Hawkins RJ, eds. *Surgery of the Shoulder.* St. Louis: Mosby; 1990:257–260.
45. Flatow EL, Neer CS II. Transfer of the Upper Portion of the Subscapularis for Large and Massive Tears of the Rotator Cuff. Presented at The Fifth International Conference on Surgery of the Shoulder, Paris, France, July, 1992.
46. Gartsman GM. Arthroscopic acromioplasty for lesions of the rotator cuff. *J Bone Joint Surg Am.* 1990;72:169–180.
47. Montegomery TJ, Yerger B, Savoie F. *Management of full thickness rotator cuff tears of the rotator cuff: A comparison of arthroscopic debridement with open repair.* Presented at the 59th Annual Meeting of the American Academy of Orthopaedic Surgeons, Washington DC, 1991.
48. Flatow EL, Weinstein DM, Duralde XA, Compito CA, Pollock RG, Bigliani LU. *Coracoacromial ligament preservation in rotator cuff surgery.* Presented at American Shoulder and Elbow Surgeons, Twelfth Annual Closed Meeting. Williamsburg, Virginia, November, 1993.
49. Wiley AM. Superior humeral dislocation. A complication following decompression and debridement for rotator cuff tears. *Clin Orthop.* 1991;263:135–141.
50. Bigliani LU, Cordasco FA, McIlveen SJ, Musso ES. Operative treatment of failed repairs of the rotator cuff. *J Bone Joint Surg.* 1992; 74:1505–1515.
51. DeOrio JK, Cofield RH. Results of a second attempt at surgical repair of a failed initial rotator cuff repair. *J Bone Joint Surg Am.* 1984; 66A:563–567.
52. Nevaiser RJ, Nevaiser TJ. Reoperation for failed rotator cuff repair: Analysis of fifty cases. *J Shoulder Elbow Surg.* 1992:1:283–286.
53. Wolfgang GL. Surgical repair of tears of the rotator cuff of the shoulder. Factors influencing the result. *J Bone Joint Surg Am.* 1974; 56:14–26.
54. Diamond B. *The Obstructing Acromion.* Springfield, IL: Charles C. Thomas; 1964.

55. Neviaser TJ, Neviaser RJ, Neviaser JS. The four-in-one arthroplasty for the painful arc syndrome. *Clin Orthop.* 1982;163:107–112.
56. Neer CS II. *Shoulder Reconstruction.* Philadelphia: WB Saunders; 1990.
57. Arntz CT, Matsen FA II, Jackins S. Surgical management of complex irreparable rotator cuff deficiency. *J Arthroplasty.* 1991;6:363–370.
58. Ianotti JP, ed. In: *Rotator Cuff Disorders, Monograph Series.* Park Ridge, IL: American Academy of Orthopaedic Surgeons; 1991.
59. Nasca RJ. Surgical treatment of complete rotator cuff tears. In: Bateman JE, Welsh RP. *Surgery of the Shoulder.* Philadelphia: BC Decker; 1984;149–153.
60. Neviaser JS. Ruptures of the rotator cuff of the shoulder. New concepts in the diagnosis and operative treatment of chronic ruptures. *Arch Surg.* 1971;102:483–485.
61. Uhthoff HK, Sarkar K, Lohr J. Repair in rotator cuff tendons. In: Post M, Morrey BF, Hawkins RJ, eds. *Surgery of the Shoulder.* St. Louis: Mosby-Year Book; 1990;216–219.
62. Gerber C, Krushnell RJ. Isolated rupture of the tendon of the subscapularis muscle. *J Bone Joint Surg Br.* 1991;73:389–394.
63. Bush LF. The torn shoulder capsule. *J Bone Joint Surg Am.* 1975; 57:256–259.
64. Ozaki J, Kugai A, Tomita Y, Tamai S. Tear of an ossified rotator cuff of the shoulder. A case report. *Acta Orthop Scand.* 1991;63:339–340.
65. Hawkins RJ, Chris AD, Kiefer GN: Failed anterior acromioplasties. *Orthopaedic Transactions.* 1987;11:233.
66. Flatow EL. The biomechanics of the acromioclavicular, sternoclavicular, and scapulothoracic joints. In: Heckman JD, ed. *Instructional Course Lectures.* Rosemont, IL: American Academy of Orthopaedic Surgeons. 1993;42:237–245.
67. Neer CS, Craig EV, Fukuda H. Cuff tear arthropathy. *J Bone Joint Surg Am.* 1983;65:1232–1244.
68. Weiner DS, MacNab L. Superior migration of the humeral head. A radiological aid in the diagnosis of tears of the rotator cuff. *J Bone Joint Surg Br.* 1970;52:524–527.
69. Burkhart SS. Fluoroscopic comparison of kinematic patterns in massive rotator cuff tears. *Clin Orthop.* 1992;284:144–152.
70. Bigliani LU, Morrison DS, April EW. The morphology of the acromion and Its relationship to rotator cuff tears. *Orthop Trans.* 1986; 10:216.
71. Neer CS, Poppen N. Supraspinatus outlet. *Orthop Trans.* 1987; 11:234.
72. Craig EV. The geyser sign and torn rotator Cuff. Clinical significance and pathomechanics. *Clin Orthop.* 1984;191:213–215.
73. Hawkins, RJ, Missnore, GW, Hobecka, PE. Surgery for full-thickness rotator cuff tears. *J Bone Joint Surg Am.* 1985;67:1349–1355.
74. Burkhart SS. Arthroscopic debridement and decompression for selected rotator cuff tears. Clinical results, pathomechanics and patients selection based on biomechanical parameters. *Orthop Clin North Am.* 1993;24:111–123.
75. Flugstad D, Matsen FA, Larry L, Jackins SE. Failed acromioplasty. Etiology and prevention. *Orthop Trans.* 1986;10:229.
76. Neer CS. Impingement lesions. *Clin Orthop.* 1983;173:70–77.
77. Bigliani LU, Dalsey RM, McCann PD. An anatomical study of the suprascapular nerve. *Arthroscopy.* 1990;6:301–305.
78. Warner JP, Krushnell RJ, Masquelet A, Gerber C. Anatomy and relationship of the suprascapular nerve: Anatomical constraints to mobilization of the supraspinatus and infraspinatus muscles in the management of massive rotator cuff tears. *J Bone Joint Surg.* 1992; 74:36–45.
79. Neer CS, Satterlee CC, Dalsey RM, Flatow EL. The anatomy and potential effects of contracture of the coracohumeral ligament. *Clin Orthop.* 1992;280:13–16.
80. Debeyre J, Patte D, Elmelik E. Repair of ruptures of the rotator cuff of the shoulder with a note on advancement of the supraspinatus muscle. *J Bone Joint Surg Br.* 1965;47:36–42.
81. Ha'Eri GB, Wiley AM. Advancement of the supraspinatus in the repair of ruptures of the rotator cuff. *J Bone Joint Surg Am.* 1981; 63A:232–238.
82. Neviaser RJ, Neviaser TJ. Transfer of the subscapularis and teres minor for massive defects of rotator cuff. In: Bayley JL, Kessel L, eds. *Shoulder Surgery.* Berlin: Springer-Verlag; 1982.
83. Neviaser JS, Neviaser RJ, Neviaser TJ. The repair of chronic massive ruptures of the rotator cuff of the shoulder by use of a freeze dried rotator cuff. *J Bone Joint Surg Am.* 1978;60:681–684.
84. Ozaki J, Fujimoto S, Masuhara K, Tamai S, Yoshiomoto S. Reconstruction of chronic massive rotator cuff tears with synthetic materials. *Clin Orthop.* 1986;202:173–183.
85. Gerber C. Latissimus dorsi transfer for the treatment of irreparable tears of the rotator cuff. *Clin Orthop.* 1992;275:152–160.
86. Vandenbussche E, Augereau B, Naouri JF, Apoil A. Repair of major rotator cuff ruptures: Eight years experience with 121 deltoid grafts. *J Bone Joint Surg Br.* 1993;75:189.
87. Rathburn JB, MacNab I. The microvascular pattern of the rotator cuff. *J Bone Joint Surg Br.* 1970;52:540–553.
88. Swiontkowski MF, Iannotti JP, Boulas HJ, et al. Intraoperative assessment of rotator cuff vascularity using Laser Doppler Flowmetry. In: Post M, Morrey BF, Hawkins RJ, eds. *Surgery of the Shoulder.* St. Louis: Mosby-Year Book; 1990:202–212.
89. Walker SW, Couch WH, Boester GA, Sprowl DW. Isokinetic strength of the shoulder after repair of a torn rotator cuff. *J Bone Joint Surg.* 1987;69:1041–1044.
90. Gerber C, Beck M, Schneeberger AG. *The immediate in-vitro stability of different techniques of repair of the supraspinatus tendon to bone.* Presented at the Fifth Congress of the European Society for Surgery of the Shoulder and Elbow, Wurzburg. Germany, June, 1991.
91. Harryman DT, Mack LA, Wang KY, Jackins SE, Richardson ML, Matsen FA. Repairs of the rotator cuff. Correlation of functional results with integrity of the cuff. *J Bone Joint Surg Am.* 1991;73:982–989.
92. Calvert PT, Packer NP, Stoker DJ, et al. Arthrography of the shoulder after operative repair of the torn rotator cuff. *J Bone Joint Surg Br.* 1986;68:147–150.
93. Watson-Jones R. *Fractures and Joint Injuries.* 4th ed. Baltimore: Williams & Wilkins; 1962;2:449–454.
94. McCann PD, Wootten ME, Kadaba MP, Bigliani LU. A kinematic and electromyographic study of shoulder rehabilitation exercises. *Clin Orthop.* 1993;288:179–188.
95. Gore DR, Murray MP, Sepic SB, Gardner GM. Shoulder muscle strength and range of motion following surgical repair of full-thickness rotator cuff tears. *J Bone Joint Surg Am.* 1986;68:266–272.

Chapter 24

Subscapularis Transfer for Management of Massive Rotator Cuff Tears

Sumner E. Karas

Since Neer's report on subacromial decompression with rotator cuff repair in 1972, many studies have confirmed that subacromial decompression and reconstruction of chronic full-thickness rotator cuff tears provides excellent pain relief and improved function in a large percentage of patients. However, the results for repair of larger tears have been reported to be less favorable than those for smaller ones. Larger tears which are not amenable to tendon-to-bone or tendon-to-tendon repair remain problematic. New methods have evolved in an effort to overcome this surgical challenge. Several techniques have been largely discarded because of generally unsatisfactory results, including those which incorporate synthetic materials,[1] devascularized fascial grafts,[2] and allografts.[3] Other alternatives include muscle advancement,[4–6] "interval slide,"[7] latissimus dorsi transfer,[8] partial cuff repair,[8a] decompression with rotator cuff debridement alone,[9] and subscapularis transfer.[7,10–15] This last technique is particularly useful in closing troublesome superior defects, which occur when there is supraspinatus scarring and retraction.

HISTORY OF SUBSCAPULARIS TRANSFER

There is no single accepted reconstructive technique that can be considered the "gold standard" for dealing with massive tears of the rotator cuff, as evidenced by the number of different techniques that are reported in this textbook. Cofield[10] first described the surgical technique of subscapularis transposition in 1982. Initially he reported the results of 26 operations, but half of these patients had rotator cuff repairs combined with glenohumeral prosthetic arthroplasties. Only 10 operations in his initial series were performed for "degenerative tendonitis." Half of the patients with degenerative cuff disease were reported to be "much better" after subscapularis transposition. The remaining half considered themselves "improved." Although one patient continued to have moderate pain, none of the patients considered themselves worse as a result of the operation. The average postoperative active elevation among these patients was 130°. The investigator concluded that subscapularis transposition was an acceptable alternative for repairing large or massive rotator cuff tears in which there was tendon substance loss. More recently, Cofield[11] reported that a few of these patients had disruption of their surgical repairs in the early postoperative period, resulting in significant loss of active movement.

In 1982, RJ and TJ Neviaser[14] reported on 17 patients who had transfer of the subscapularis and teres minor for repair of massive cuff defects. Although they mentioned that some defects were amenable to closure by transfer of a single tendon, the reported results did not distinguish between those patients who had subscapularis transfer alone and those who had a second tendon used in the repair. They described five patients with excellent results and seven patients with good results. Another five patients were graded as poor, although three of the failures were attributed to deltoid dysfunction secondary to previous surgery. The investigators concluded that transfer of the subscapularis and teres minor was a satisfactory salvage procedure for relieving pain and improving motion so long as deltoid function was unimpaired.

There have been other references to using the subscapularis for closure of massive cuff defects. Bigliani et al.[7] reported that it was necessary to transfer the subscapularis in 11 of 61 patients with massive rotator cuff tears. These 11 patients were described as having superior defects on account of retracted and deficient supraspinatus tendons. Unfortunately, the investigators did not report the results of this subset of patients separately from the 50 other patients in their series of massive cuff reconstructions. In 1983 Neer[12] reported his preference for shifting the upper half of the subscapularis for closing large superior defects. In his text on shoulder reconstruction,[13] he describes transferring the upper 70% of the subscapularis for closing massive cuff defects. In a more recent review, 33 of these patients were studied at an average of 4.5 years follow-up. Overall, there were 16 excellent, 9 satisfactory, and 9 unsatisfactory results. The unsatisfactory results were generally attributed to lack of strength rather than pain, and the investigators considered transfer of the subscapularis a good technique for repair of massive cuff tears.[13a]

In spite of the initial enthusiasm for this procedure, recently there have been several anecdotal reports suggesting that postoperative deterioration of function can occur following transfer of the subscapularis.[8a,16,17] Some surgeons have abandoned this procedure because of occasional loss of active elevation and overhead function following surgery.

My own experience with subscapularis transfer[18] confirms the need for caution and clinical judgement when considering transfer of this muscle. Among 20 patients with massive degenerative cuff tears who underwent subscapularis transfer, 85% were satisfied with the results of surgery, despite the fact that some patients continued to complain of difficulty with heavy lifting or performing repetitive overhead activities. Excellent pain relief was achieved in most patients, consistent with other contemporary reports of cuff repairs combined with subacromial decompression. Although the average postoperative active elevation was 152° (range = 70 to 180°), 2 patients (10%) had significant deterioration of active shoulder elevation following surgery despite substantial relief of pain, and neither was satisfied with the results of surgery. Thus, the recommendation that surgeons exercise caution when considering transfer of the subscapularis in patients who have full active overhead elevation preoperatively.

INDICATIONS

When the surgeon is confronted with a large or massive rotator cuff tear, he must first define the defect and then mobilize the component tendons of the cuff. The simplest solution to a large tear is still a primary tendon-to-bone or tendon-to-tendon repair. In spite of one's best efforts, however, some tears cannot be reattached with the arm by the side and without excessive tension. Under these circumstances, the surgeon may consider progressing to a more complex reconstructive alternative to deal with tissue deficiency rather than settling for a compromised direct repair. Subscapularis transfer is one such alternative that is particularly useful for closing troublesome superior defects.

Patient selection for subscapularis transfer is important. In light of recent reports documenting deterioration of active elevation in some patients undergoing this transfer, the procedure should not be used indiscriminately. The operation is best performed on individuals who are either unable to elevate their arms overhead or who have markedly compromised overhead function preoperatively.

In most instances the surgeon should be able to anticipate a larger tear. There are telltale signs: wasting in both of the spinatus fossae, weakness of external rotation, and significant scapulothoracic substitution as the arm is elevated through mid range elevation. Sometimes there are definitive preoperative studies that indicate the presence of a larger tear, such as plain radiographs demonstrating upward migration of the humeral head (Fig. 24–1) or an MRI which shows a massive tear with retraction. However, just because a tear is large, this does not mean that the surgeon will be unable to perform a primary closure. The ability to repair the cuff is dependent on the quality and mobility of the soft tissues. However, if the surgeon is sensitive to the fact that a patient is likely to have a massive tear, he can discuss the possibilities of more complex reconstructive solutions with the patient preoperatively. A patient who has functional overhead elevation, even with poor mechanics and/or with pain, should be advised about the possibility of loss of active

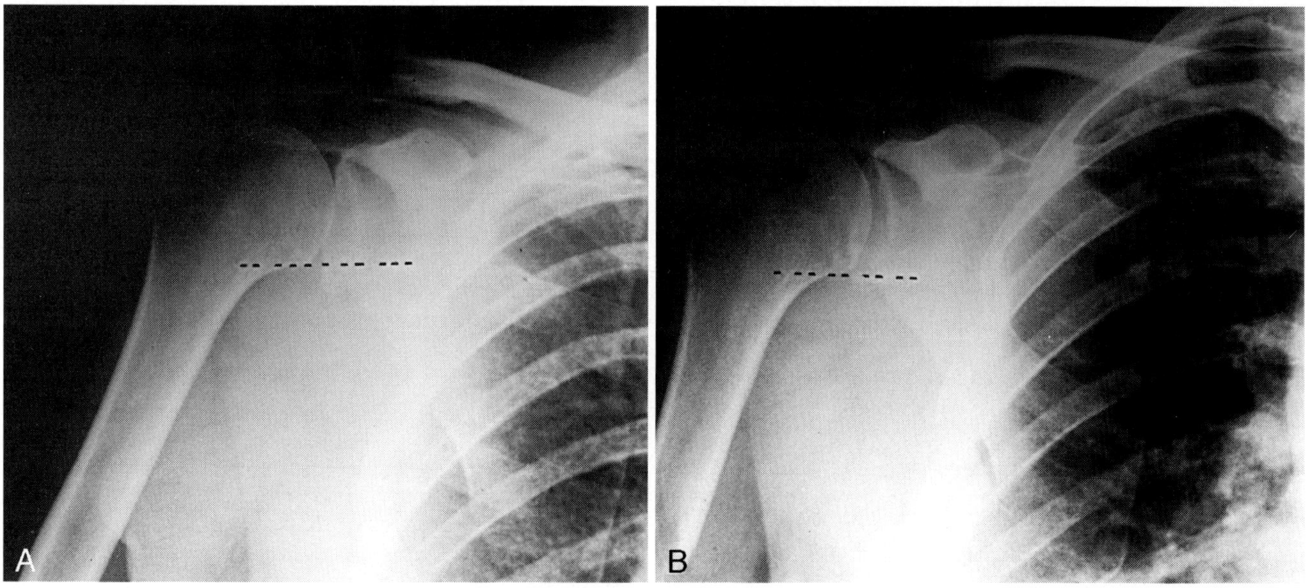

Fig. 24–1. ***A,*** **Preoperative radiograph demonstrates superior migration of the humeral head with respect to the glenoid in a patient with a massive rotator cuff tear and early arthropathy.** ***B,*** **Glenohumeral relationship improved after rotator cuff repair, which necessitated subscapularis transfer.**

elevation following subscapularis transfer, if the surgeon is contemplating such a procedure for reconstruction of a probable massive defect.

The quality of the subscapularis tendon itself is important in the decision making process. If there is evidence of attritional wear in its upper half or if the substance and quality of the musculotendinous structure is suboptimal, this may preclude an effective transfer.

Thus, the ideal patient for subscapularis transfer is one who cannot elevate his arm overhead preoperatively, has a massive tear that cannot be closed primarily in spite of maximal soft-tissue mobilization, and whose subscapularis is of good quality. The transfer must be reparable so that complete and secure closure of the cuff defect can be accomplished without excessive tension; this allows the institution of early rehabilitation.

OPERATIVE TECHNIQUE

The operation is usually done through an anterior deltoid-splitting approach. Just enough deltoid is elevated from the anterior acromion to afford exposure for an anterior acromioplasty and resection of the coracoacromial ligament. The deltoid, as always, warrants the utmost respect; care should be taken in the initial dissection to preserve a good soft-tissue sleeve to facilitate a secure repair. When splitting the fibers of the deltoid, one must not extend the longitudinal split more than 4 to 5 cm, in order to avoid injury to the axillary nerve.

If the patient has symptomatic AC arthritis, the distal clavicle should be excised. If there are osteophytes on the undersurface of the AC joint but no clinical findings to suggest derangement of this joint, only the undersurface of the distal clavicle needs to be resected in order to complete the decompression of the subacromial space and supraspinatus outlet. Although the bursa has been implicated in the healing of rotator cuff tears, it is often necessary to resect bursal tissue to clearly define the extent of the rotator cuff tear and to eliminate any potential for mechanical nonoutlet impingement.

When dealing with larger cuff tears, it is helpful to place traction sutures in the component tendons of the cuff. An exhaustive effort is made to mobilize the rotator cuff so that its torn edges can be advanced to a bone trough just lateral to the anatomic neck. Release of the coracohumeral ligament, release of superficial adhesions, and capsular releases along the undersurface of the rotator cuff at the level of the glenoid rim may aid in cuff mobilization.

Recent studies suggest that the torn edges of the rotator cuff are well vascularized and should be incorporated in the surgical repair.[19] However, these free edges are frequently friable and often do not hold sutures well. A limited debridement of the edges often results in better quality tissue being available for repair, thereby resulting in a more secure reattachment of tendon to bone. Thus, concern for optimizing tissue quality is often justification for limited tendon edge debridement.

If the mobilized cuff cannot be secured with the arm held at the side and without excessive tension on the repair, then subscapularis transfer should be considered for closure of a superior defect (Fig. 24–2).

Depending on the size of the defect, anywhere from

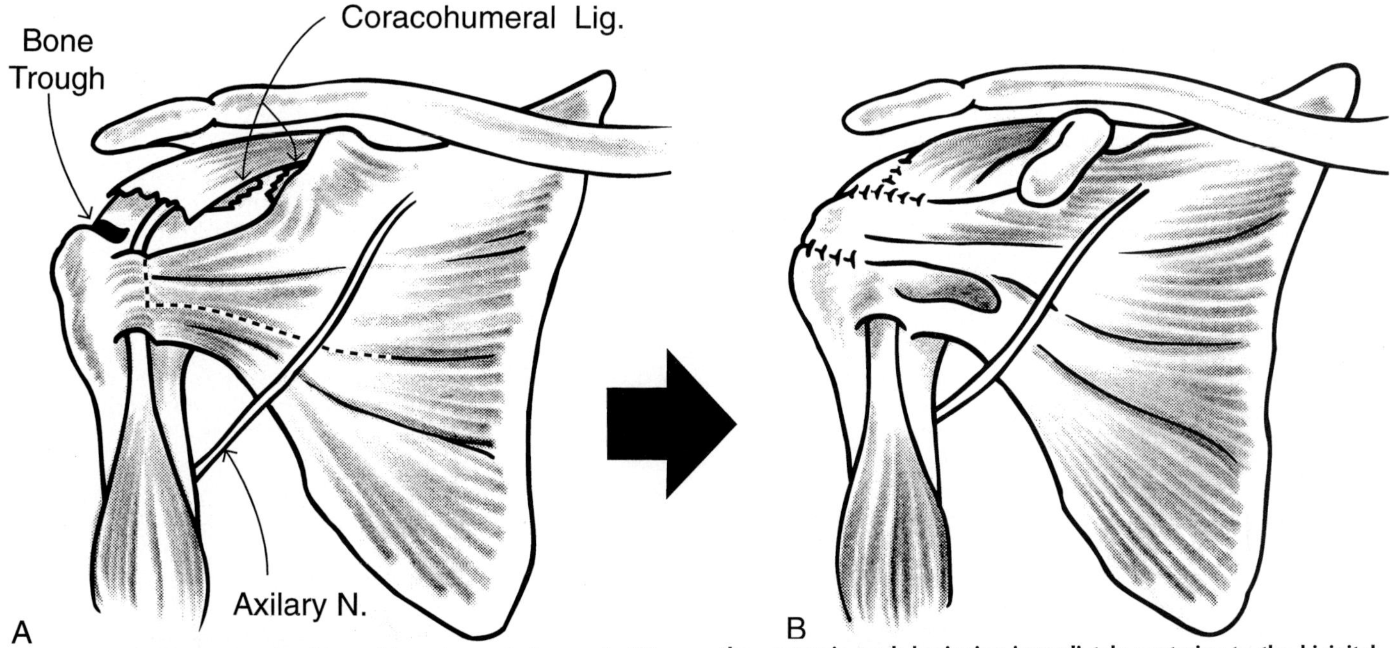

Fig. 24–2. ***A,*** **The surgeon should consider subscapularis transfer if he is unable to affect a primary tendon-to-bone or tendon-to-tendon repair in spite of optimal tendon mobilization, including release of the coracohumeral ligament and capsular releases along the glenoid rim.** ***B,*** **The inferior border of the subscapularis is sutured to a bone trough along the anatomic neck beginning immediately posterior to the bicipital groove. The leading edge of the subscapularis and it's superior border are then approximated to the free edges of the supraspinatus and infraspinatus tendons to close the defect.**

the upper half to two-thirds of the subscapularis will need to be detached from its insertion and dissected free from the underlying capsule. The musculotendinous junction and the muscle are incised obliquely downward and medially. Soft-tissue attachments between the subscapularis and the coracoid process are released. One must be mindful of the nearby musculocutaneous and axillary nerves while mobilizing the subscapularis. The transverse humeral ligament should be preserved. If the soft-tissue sleeve enclosing the bicipital groove is severed while mobilizing the tendon, this stabilizing ligament must be reconstructed in order to prevent biceps tendon subluxation and further loss of head depressor function. When subscapularis mobilization is complete, the anterior capsule should still be intact. The upper part of the subscapularis should be freely mobile. This is then advanced superiorly and laterally. The lower border of the transferred portion of tendon is secured to a cancellous trough just medial to the greater tuberosity. It's free edge is then secured to the trimmed edges of the infraspinatus and supraspinatus tendons to close the superior defect. When the repair is complete, range of motion is tested. The degree of tension on the repair will determine how cautious or aggressive to be in the early phases of rehabilitation.

POSTOPERATIVE MANAGEMENT

The role of abduction splints and other postoperative arm-supporting devices following cuff repair remains controversial. Some surgeons prefer to "protect" larger cuff repairs, as well as those cases which incorporate poor quality tendon. However, an abduction orthosis is not a substitute for inadequate soft-tissue mobilization or a tenuous cuff repair. A cuff repaired under tension is likely to yield an unsatisfactory result, even if the patient uses an abduction orthosis following surgery. It is the author's practice not to employ such devices after cuff repair, even if the repair necessitates subscapularis transfer. Only a sling is used, and it is removed several times daily for exercises and personal hygiene; it is discarded 5 to 6 weeks after surgery. If an abduction splint is employed, it should not interfere with the usual rehabilitative program. Although there is no universal agreement regarding postoperative arm support, the important role of postoperative therapy is not controversial.

One cannot overemphasize the importance of carefully supervised physiotherapy in obtaining optimal results from surgical repairs of rotator cuff tears. A technically well performed reconstruction can yield an unsatisfactory result unless a well conceived, progressive rehabilitative program is undertaken. The variability in the extent of cuff tears and in the techniques employed to repair them demands that the therapy programs be individualized. These considerations are of utmost importance when one considers the added biological and mechanical complexities inherent in subscapularis transfer. When subscapularis transfer is used in the reconstruction of a massive rotator cuff tear, the surgeon must test the range of motion when the transfer is complete. The degree of tension on the repair will help to determine guidelines for the early phases of rehabilitation.

Passive range of motion exercises are instituted within a few days after surgery in an effort to prevent the development of adhesions and contractures. If a cuff repair with subscapularis transfer is so tenuous that the surgeon is reluctant to initiate these exercises, one must seriously question the wisdom of the initial decision to risk the added morbidity of mobilizing the subscapularis to begin with. On the other hand, if the surgeon is able to achieve a secure closure, it is reasonable to initiate pendulums and passive elevation in the plane of the scapula within a week of the procedure. Specific restrictions are determined individually at the end of the operation, although in general when the subscapularis is advanced superiorly, one would like to avoid any external rotation until some early tendon healing has occurred. Passive elevation often can be done by a family member under the guidance of a physiotherapist. In our protocol for rehabilitation following subscapularis transfer, we initiate supine active assisted range of motion 6 weeks after surgery. Patient comfort and shoulder mechanics determine the progression to supine active range of motion, active range of motion on a gradually increasing incline, and finally elevation against gravity. Gentle assisted external rotation is never initiated until 2 to 3 months after surgery. External rotation should not be performed forcefully. Although light weights are added to supine elevation 8 to 10 weeks after surgery to facilitate the transition to elevating the arm against gravity, more formal muscle strengthening exercises are not initiated until 4 months after surgery.

COMPLICATIONS

It is often said that bigger surgery begets bigger complications. When dealing with massive rotator cuff tears, the surgeon must be mindful of all of the potential complications associated with subacromial decompression and rotator cuff repair in general. If, in addition, it is necessary to transfer the subscapularis to close the cuff defect, several additional problems unique to this procedure need also be considered.

The common pitfalls of more routine cuff surgery include (1) inadequate subacromial decompression, (2) deltoid dysfunction (either from detachment of the muscle origin or from axillary nerve injury), (3) suprascapular nerve injury, and (4) failure of the cuff repair itself. These problems can be avoided by adhering to certain basic principles. An adequate acromioplasty must be performed, and any bony excrescences compromising the supraspinatus outlet (including any osteophytes along the undersurface of the AC joint) must be removed. The deltoid muscle must be handled with the utmost respect; a minimum amount of deltoid should be detached in a manner that preserves a good soft-tissue sleeve to facilitate subsequent repair. The deltoid must be securely reattached to the acromion. A split in the deltoid cannot extend distally so far as to jeopardize the axillary nerve. Knowledge of the anatomy of the suprascapular nerve, particularly as it courses around the base of the scapular spine after exiting the scapular notch, will prevent nerve injury that might occur while mobilizing the supraspinatus tendon. Disruptions of cuff repairs can be minimized by clearly defining the anatomy of cuff tears, securely repairing the cuff without excessive tension, and carefully supervising the rehabilitative program following repair.

Additional complications which can occur with subscapularis transfer include (1) deterioration of function in active elevation; (2) proximal injury to the axillary nerve as it courses over the subscapularis; and (3) (theoretical problems with) anterior instability.

The initial enthusiasm for subscapularis transfer has been tempered by recent reports documenting that certain patients have experienced a deterioration of function and particularly loss of active elevation after surgery, despite substantial relief of pain.[18] Preoperatively, some patients have had the ability to use their arms in a functional manner for overhead activities, although with pain. After reconstruction a few have lost the ability to actively elevate their arms above shoulder height against gravity (Fig. 24–3).

There is no proven explanation for this deterioration of shoulder function. A major force vector of the subscapularis is below the center of rotation of the humerus (Fig. 24–4). Therefore, the subscapularis acts as an important head depressor and as a force couple with the deltoid. One possible explanation for the observed deterioration of function is that many patients with larger cuff tears have marginal head depression; with the remaining functioning tendons, there is little functional reserve. When musculotendinous units are transferred, they frequently drop a grade level in strength. A weak-

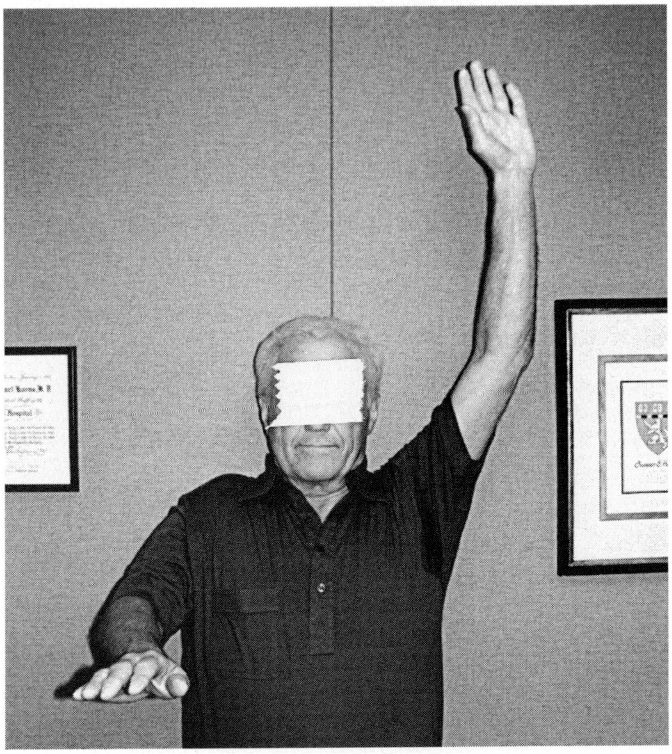

Fig. 24–3. This 66-year-old right-handed man underwent subacromial decompression and debridement of an irreparable cuff tear of his left shoulder in 1987. In 1989, a massive defect in his right shoulder was reconstructed with a subscapularis transfer. He had deterioration of function after right shoulder surgery in spite of good compliance with postoperative protocols. Although both shoulders are free of pain, he is more satisfied with the shoulder that was debrided.

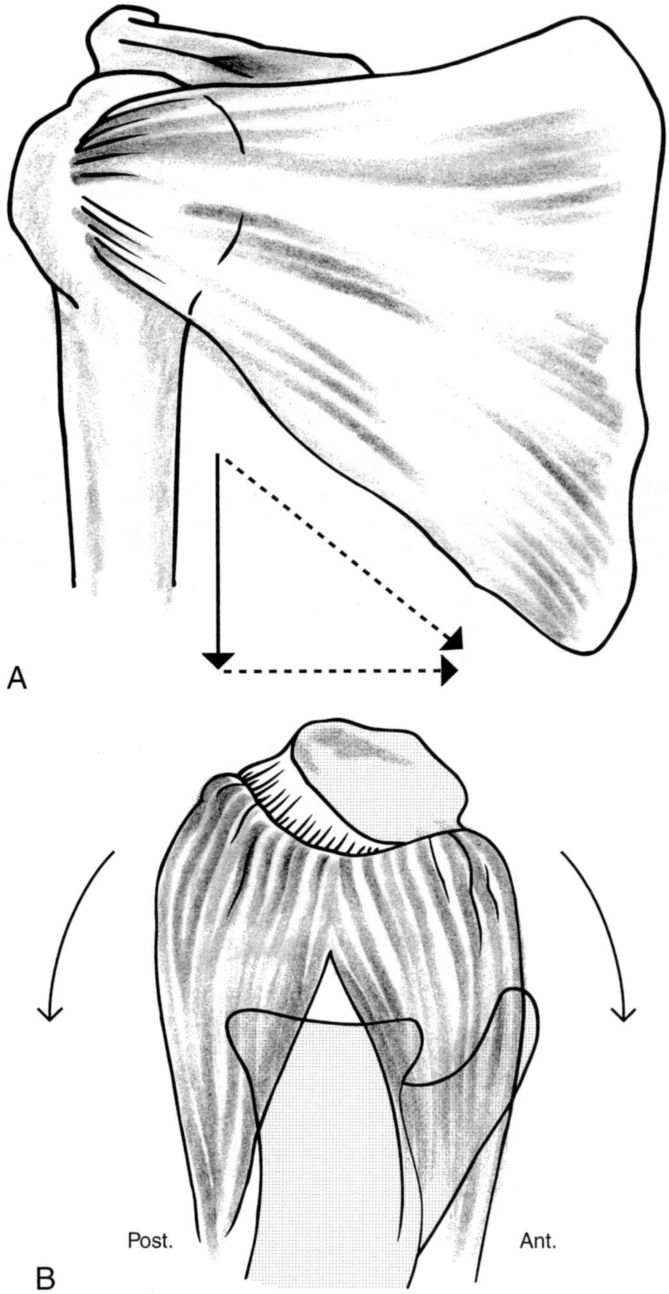

Fig. 24–4. *A,* A major force vector of the subscapularis is below the center of rotation of the humerus. A failed or weakened subscapularis transfer may adversely affect this force couple with the deltoid. *B,* A second possible explanation for deterioration of active elevation after subscapularis transfer may be the disruption of balanced force couples created by the anterior and posterior aspects of those portions of the rotator cuff that remain intact.

ened or failed transfer may shift the balance of a compromised system to a point where there is inadequate depressor function to allow the deltoid to effectively elevate the arm.

A second possible biomechanical explanation is based upon the force couples created by the anterior and posterior aspects of the cuff. Patients can have large cuff tears with a stable fulcrum if there is a good balance between the force moments of the anterior and posterior cuff musculature. If the subscapularis is transferred superiorly, it's force vector is altered. The anterior cuff may then be insufficient to balance the posterior cuff moment. The uncoupling of these forces could cause loss of a stable glenohumeral joint fulcrum, thus leading to humeral head translation, and ineffective deltoid function.[8a,20]

Given these circumstances, the surgeon must be selective when considering subscapularis transfer as an option for closure of massive cuff defects. Two prerequisites for transfer should be a healthy subscapularis tendon and the ability to achieve a secure and complete cuff closure with the transferred segment of the subscapularis tendon. However, one might want to think twice before transferring the subscapularis in a patient who preoperatively has full overhead elevation and good functional use of his arm for overhead activities. In such individuals, the surgeon might want to consider alternative reconstructive options.

A second potential complication unique to a repair that requires mobilization of the subscapular is proximal injury to the axillary nerve. Nerve injury can be prevented as long as the surgeon has a thorough understanding of the anatomy of the axillary nerve–after it arises as one of the terminal branches of the posterior cord, it drapes over the subscapularis before it enters the quadrilateral space. When mobilizing the subscapularis, the musculocutaneous nerve may also be at risk in those individuals who have branches entering the conjoined muscle group proximally. Once again, a thorough understanding of the anatomy and the anatomical variants of the musculocutaneous nerve will prevent injury.

Investigators have expressed a theoretical concern for the development of anterior instability after subscapularis transfer.[13,21] Although there have been no reported instances of anterior subluxation or dislocation occurring after this reconstruction, it would seem prudent to preserve the anterior capsule in the process of mobilizing the subscapularis. For the same reason, one should leave at least the lower one third of the subscapularis intact. The small number of reported subscapularis transfers is most likely the only reason why this complication has not yet been described.

FINAL CONSIDERATIONS

A number of reports have now established subscapularis transfer as a useful adjunct in the armamentarium of techniques available for closing difficult rotator cuff defects.[7,10–13] Although the technique has been referred to as a muscle transposition, considering the changes in tendon insertion (as well as the alterations in its vector), it seems more appropriate to refer to this operation as a muscle transfer.

Considering the superior and lateral advancement of the subscapularis, the surgeon might justifiably be concerned about the potential loss of external rotation with this procedure. In light of recent reports documenting the development of degenerative arthritis in shoulders that have been made excessively tight after repairs for instability (secondary to posterior subluxation and translation), such concerns certainly merit attention. However, from a practical standpoint, loss of external rotation has not proven to be a problem. The amount of external rotation achieved after this operation is not significantly different from what has been reported in other contemporary series of more routine rotator cuff repairs.

Subscapularis transfer should be reserved for those situations in which cuff closure cannot be achieved by simpler methods. The surgeon should be selective when considering transferring the subscapularis in individuals with full active range of motion preoperatively. Because of the potential added morbidity of causing weakness of external rotation, I have been reluctant to simultaneously transfer the teres minor.

Pain relief and overall patient satisfaction after subscapularis transfer have been comparable to what has been reported in other recent series of rotator cuff repairs. This is consistent with previous reports that pain relief after rotator cuff repair is independent of cuff tear size. This undoubtedly reflects the importance of adequate subacromial decompression and the prevention of cuff impingement in achieving such results. These results reinforce the presumption that the primary indication for rotator cuff reconstruction remains relief of pain.

REFERENCES

1. Ozaki J, Fujimoto S, Masuhara K, Tamai S, Yoshimoto S. Reconstruction of chronic massive rotator cuff tears with synthetic material. *Clin Orthop.* 1986;202;173–183.
2. Bayne O, Bateman JE. Long term results of surgical repair of full thickness rotator cuff tears. In: Bateman JE, Walsh RP, eds. *Surgery of the Shoulder.* Philadelphia: BC Decker; 1984:167–171.
3. Neviaser JS, Neviaser RJ, Neviaser TJ. The repair of chronic massive ruptures of the rotator cuff of the shoulder by use of a freeze-dried rotator cuff. *J Bone Joint Surg Am.* 1978;60;681–684.
4. Debeyre J, Patte D, Elmelik E. Repair of ruptures of the rotator cuff and the shoulder with a note on advancement of the supraspinatus muscle. *J Bone Joint Surg Br.* 1965;47:36–42.
5. Ha'eri GA, Wiley AM. Advancement of the supraspinatus in repair of ruptures of the rotator cuff. *J Bone Joint Surg Am.* 1981;63:236–238.
6. McLaughlin L. Lesions of the musculotendinous cuff of the shoulder, I: The exposure and treatment of tears with retraction. *J Bone Joint Surg Am.* 1944;26:31–51.
7. Bigliani L, Cordasco F, McIlveen S, Musso E. Operative repair of massive rotator cuff tears: Long-term results. *J Shoulder Elbow Surg.* 1992;3:121–130.
8. Gerber C, Vinh T, Hertel R, Hess C. Lattisimus dorsi transfer for the treatment of massive tears of the rotator cuff. *Clin Orthop.* 1988; 232:51–61.
8a. Burkhart S, Nottage W, Oglivie-Harris D, Kohn H, Pachelli A. Partial repair of irreparable rotator cuff tears. *Arthroscopy.* 1994;4:363–370.
9. Rockwood CA, Williams G, Burkhead W. *Debridement of irrepairable,*

degenerative lesions of the rotator cuff. Seventh Annual Meeting of the American Shoulder and Elbow Surgeons. Anaheim, CA, March 3, 1991.

10. Cofield R. Subscapular muscle transposition for repair of chronic rotator cuff tears. *Surg Gynecol Obstet.* 1982;154:667–672.
11. Cofield R. Subscapularis tendon transposition for large rotator cuff tears. In: Paulos L, Tibone J, eds. *Operative Techniques in Shoulder Surgery.* Gaithersburg, MD: Aspen Publishers; 1991:155–160.
12. Neer C. Impingement lesions. *Clin Orthop.* 1983;173;70–77.
13. Neer CS II. *Shoulder Reconstruction.* Philadelphia: WB Saunders; 1990:106–136.

13a. Flatow E, Neer C. *Transfer of the upper portion of the subscapularis for large and massive tears of the rotator cuff.* Fifth International Conference on Surgery of the Shoulder. Paris, France, July 12, 1992.

14. Neviaser RJ, Neviaser TJ. Transfer of the subscapularis and teres minor for massive defects of rotator cuff. In: Bayley JL, Kessel L, eds. *Shoulder Surgery.* Berlin: Springer-Verlag; 1982;60–69.
15. Neviaser RJ, Neviaser TJ. Reconstruction of chronic tears of the rotator cuff. In: Batemen, Walsh CV, eds. *Surgery of the Shoulder.* St. Louis: Mosby; 1984:172–179.
16. Cofield R. Personal communication, 1990.
17. Bigliani L. *Shoulder problems in the throwing athlete.* Discussion at AAOS Instructional Course. New York, NY, December 6, 1992.
18. Karas S, Giachello T. *Subscapularis transfer for reconstruction of rotator cuff tears.* Ninth Annual Meeting of American Shoulder and Elbow Surgeons. San Francisco, CA, February 21, 1993.
19. Kumagai J, Uhthoff H, Sarkar K, Murnaghan J. Collagen type III in rotator cuff tears: An immunohistochemical study. *J Shoulder Elbow Surg.* 1992;1:187–192.
20. Burkhart S. Flouroscopic comparison of kinematic patterns in massive rotator cuff tears. *Clin Orthop.* 1992;284:144–152.
21. Bigliani L, Rodosky M. Techniques of repair of large rotator cuff tears. *Techniques Orthop.* 1994;9:133–140.

Chapter 25

Teres Minor Transfer

Pekka Paavolainen

A tear of the rotator cuff is a common orthopaedic problem that leads to pain and disability. Massive tears of the rotator cuff usually entail complete loss of the supraspinatus and infraspinatus tendon and may be associated with considerable secondary retraction and scarring of the ruptured muscles. Reconstruction of a torn rotator cuff can be successful in a high percentage of shoulders. Small and moderate size defects are fairly easy to correct, but chronic, massive, and badly retracted tears are a real challenge for the orthopaedic surgeon. Although most previously published techniques for repair stress the importance of watertight seals with complete coverage of the humeral head, it may not be possible to achieve this ideal goal.[1–4]

Conditions affecting the success of repairs of the rotator cuff include (1) poorly vascularized, retracted tendons; (2) relative upward migration of the proximal humerus; and (3) the lack of a suitable stump at the insertion area eliminating the possibility of end-to-end reconstruction. In addition, degenerative changes in the glenohumeral joint, as well as concomitant lesions of the anterior cuff or biceps tendon,[5] may compromise the result.

An accurate clinical diagnosis may be made preoperatively in most patients from the past medical history, physical examination, plain radiography, and arthrography. However, the surgeon may encounter a rupture that is larger than expected, as neither single-contrast nor double-contrast arthrograms are consistently accurate in estimating the size or extent of the tear.

One aspect of the current debate centers on whether conservative or operative treatment is preferable for rotator cuff impingement lesions and ruptures. The degenerative nature of the disease is evident; among the elderly some degree of defect in the rotator cuff is common, and its incidence increases with age. For this reason, many investigators advocate initial conservative treatment for rotator cuff tears, emphasizing that surgery is a second option. The reported overall success rate with conservative treatment has varied from 30 to 60%. If there is no response to conservative treatment within a few months, arthrographic or sonographic evaluation should be used to exclude the possibility of the presence of a more extensive lesion than was first diagnosed. The old maxim, "the diagnosis can be aggressive, although the treatment is conservative," is still valid.

To surgically repair a rotator cuff tear, the tendon defect must first be defined and the tendon edges mobilized. The surgeon is often confronted with large tears in which there is real loss of tendon substance, making it difficult to proceed with primary tendon-to-tendon or tendon-to-tuberosity repair.[6] Many surgeons have observed that the degree of scarring and inelasticity of the musculotendinous tissue may be more important in determining the mobility of the tissues than is the size of the gap or tear. If sufficient mobilization is not obtained, alternative techniques of muscle rotation and transposition or advancement of the supraspinatus from its fossa have been advocated to obtain a watertight repair.[1–4] Poor quality tendons pose a difficult problem, because there is no adequate substitute for the rotator cuff; the use of fascial grafts and synthetic substitutes has not been uniformly successful.[7–9]

There have been several attempts to classify the size and patterns of cuff ruptures, but there is no universal agreement on the definition of massive tears. According to Patte,[10] an accurate classification system takes into account the extent of the tear, its topography in the sagittal and frontal planes, the trophic quality of the muscle, and the integrity of the long head of the biceps; all these factors influence the success of surgical repair. In the sagittal plane, the extent of the lesion should be measured at the level of the bony detachment.[10]

There is no universal agreement on either the definition or treatment of a "massive" rotator cuff tear. Cofield[6] and Post et al.[12] used this term for any tear with a diameter of more than 5 cm. More detailed surgical definitions have been suggested, but there is no consistent correlation between the size of the tear and the technical difficulties encountered during the repair procedure; this is because of the fact that most of the classifications contain no description of the tear from the frontal plane. In this dimension, the simple measurement of the gap should be replaced by two determinations: (1) the elasticity of the muscle and (2) an assessment of the possibility of direct tendon reinsertion into bone after excision of the necrotic ends. If direct reinsertion is not possible, a plastic procedure is required.[10]

In our experience, tears of 5 cm or larger can sometimes be repaired easily, whereas some smaller tears may demand elaborate surgical procedures in order to achieve coverage of the head. The technical difficulties of the operation are more dependent on the time lapse between the injury and the eventual surgical reconstruction than the absolute size of the rupture in the rotator cuff. A careful search should be made for concomitant lesions, because luxation or tendinitis of the biceps brachii might affect both the operative procedure and its final outcome.[5,10,13]

The main aims of the reconstruction of the torn rotator cuff are to reestablish continuity, restore the soft-tissue spacer function, center the head in the glenoid, make an adequate correction of concomitant lesions of the joint, and relieve impingement. Major studies of the results of surgical treatment of cuff tears have indicated that resection of the anterior of the undersurface of the acromion, release of the coracoacromial ligament and (in some patients) resection of the outer end of the clavicle will increase the rate of success of surgical repair. Resection of the lateral acromion is no longer recommended.[2–5]

There are three basic methods or repairing cuff tears. The first is to attach the proximal edge of the ruptured tendon to the underlying cancellous bone at the most distal point to which it can be advanced without tension. The second is to advance local tissues to replace the deficient tendon.[14–18] The third is to use a free graft of local or distant tissue, either an allograft or xenograft, or prosthetic material to repair the defect.[7,8,19] The tissue advancement techniques depend largely on the mobilization and trophic quality of the musculotendinous units of the supraspinatus and infraspinatus.[11] If sufficient mobilization of these muscles cannot be obtained, alternative procedures, such as those proposed by DeBeyre et al.[14] and Ha'Eri and Wiley,[15] have been used to allow closure of the rotator cuff. The problem with these techniques is the risk of neurovascular injury of the pedicle. Warner et al.[20] demonstrated in cadavers that even when an extensive, modified disinsertion advancement technique was used, neither the supraspinatus nor the infraspinatus muscle could be advanced laterally by more than about 3 cm. In all shoulders, the limiting factor for lateral mobilization was tension on the motor branches of the suprascapular nerve. Clinically, when a tendon has retracted in a chronic tear of a rotator cuff, the neurovascular bundle may be tethered by scar tissue and may not be safely mobilized even this much, so that other alternatives might need to be considered.[20]

In such cases, advancement of surrounding tissues can be achieved with a rotational flap of the remaining part of the cuff tendon, using either the subscapularis tendon (from the anterior aspect of the cuff)[6] or the teres minor (from the posterior aspect),[18] or by simultaneous advancement of both the subscapularis and the teres minor.[16,17] As a last resort, even more advanced transpositions of the surrounding muscle can be tried, such as the trapezius (from the scapular region)[21] or the latissimus dorsi (from the humeral shaft).[22]

Although there is some controversy over the role played by the biceps brachii as a stabilizer of the humeral head, transection of the biceps tendon should be avoided unless pathological changes in tendon function are present (i.e., a badly frayed or totally luxated tendon). In such cases, a bookleaf-like opened proximal biceps tendon can be incorporated into the repair to help bridge tissue defects.[13]

For the transfer of the teres minor, we have developed a new surgical technique in which tendons adjacent to the tear have been detached from their insertions with a block of cancellous bone and relocated into new positions. The cancellous blocks have been secured with cancellous screws to promote bone-to-bone healing.

SURGICAL TECHNIQUE

An anterosuperior approach, with the patient in a semi-sitting position, is used. The technique is illustrated in Figures 25–1 and 25–2. An incision is made down to the fascia over the deltoid. The deltoid is then sharply incised to reflect it from its attachment to the acromion, up to the level of the AC joint; it is then split between its anterior and medial portions, 3 to 4 cm distally, to provide access to the rotator cuff.[9] The subacromial bursa and coracoacromial ligament are excised and an anterior acromioplasty performed according to the technique of Neer. The entire medial to lateral width of the undersurface of the acromion is removed, as well as any possible bony prominence on the undersurface of the AC joint. The status of the cuff is determined by positioning the arm. The size of the cuff tear is determined after debridement of necrotic tendinous tissue of the margins. Mobilization of the retracted cuff is then done, including extra-articular lysis of adhesions and division of the coracohumeral ligament, as well as intra-articular release of the capsular attachments, and blunt dissection beyond the rim of the glenoid. Care must be taken not to disrupt the stabilizing structures of the long head of the biceps tendon in so-called lateral lesions.[13] In cases in which these elements have already been lost (anterior or combined lesions) and the tendon is found to be luxated or badly frayed, tenodesis is recommended.[13] In such cases, a more extensive release of the rotator interval may be performed ("interval slide") to laterally mobilize the supraspinatus. In global tears in which all the lateral facets of the cuff are lost (i.e., teres minor) and the cuff is badly retracted and scarred, no attempts at reconstruction of the cuff are made. In these cases, anterior acromioplasty is considered to be enough for the relief of pain.

In all cases in which this new technique has been used, the presence of a massive tear that included attachments of both the supraspinatus and infraspinatus was confirmed during surgery (i.e., Patte's classification: group III, segments 4 and 5). These tendons were so severely retracted that sufficient mobilization without neurovascular injury was impossible (Patte's stage 3), making it necessary to consider other alternatives.

Once a decision has been made to perform the transposition, the edges of the remaining tendon and muscle

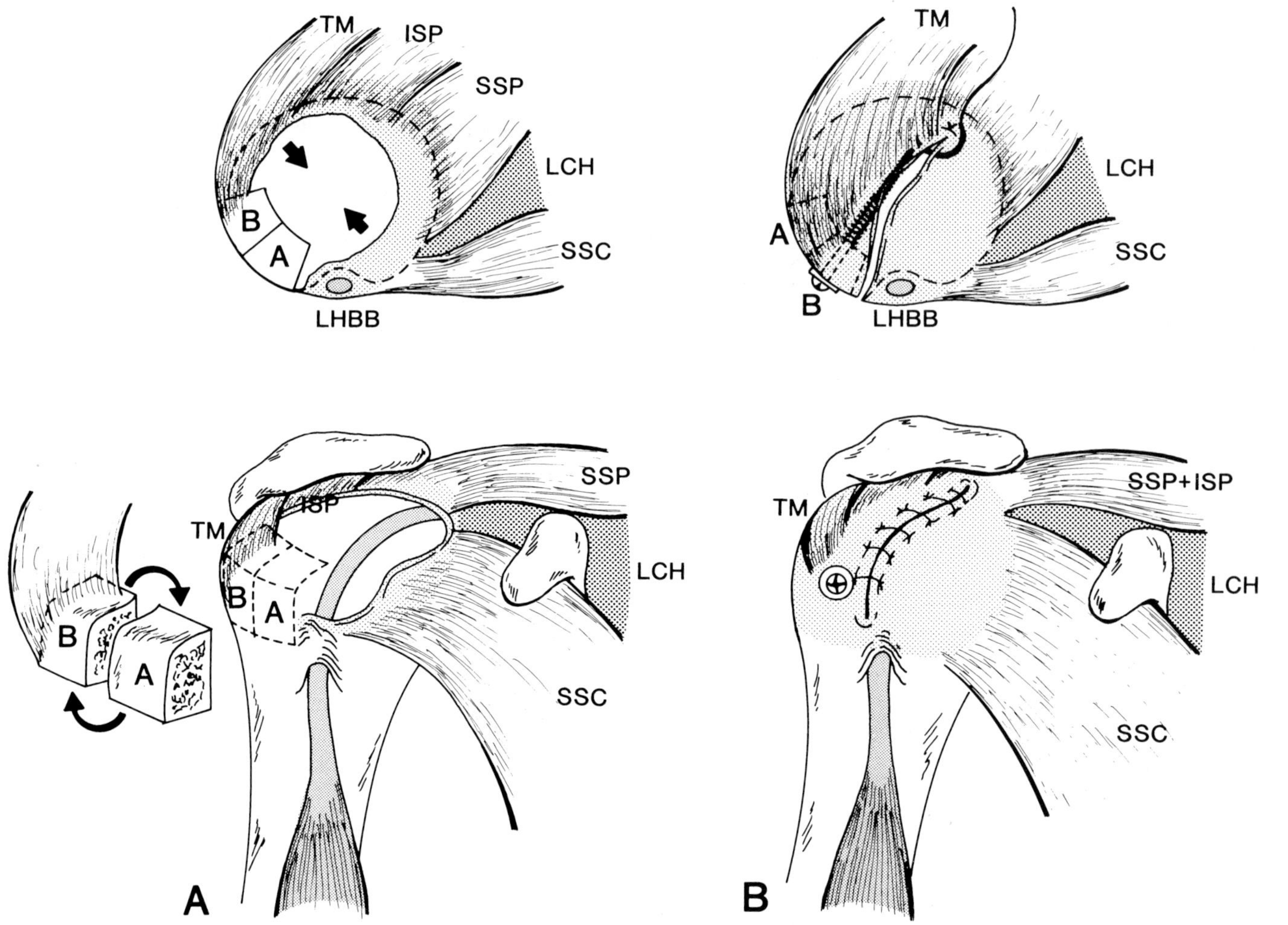

Fig. 25–1. Schematic representation of the teres minor transfer procedure. *A*, The posterior muscle insertions are released with a block of cancellous bone (Block B) and exchanged with a similar block removed from the inlay bed (Block A). *B*, The transferred block is fixed with a screw, and the remaining gap on the top of the humeral head is closed by suturing the released margins of the remaining rotator cuff together.

components are mobilized, taking extreme care not to damage the axillary nerve, which is the motor nerve of the deltoid and the teres minor. With the arm maximally internally rotated, the posterior muscle insertions can be released, along with a block of cancellous bone (1 to 1.5 cm × 1 cm), using a small oscillating saw and chisel. The capsule then has to be released along the posterior glenoid rim, allowing the transfer of the muscle, its tendon, and the capsule en bloc. The tendon, along with the bone block (see Block B in Fig. 25–1), is advanced anteriorly toward the lateral margin of the intertubercular groove. A second block of bone (see Block A in Fig. 25–1) is removed in a similar fashion and is used to fill the space left in the posterior aspect of the humeral head. The teres minor bone block is then secured into its prepared new position with a cancellous screw after temporary fixation. The massive cuff tear, now considerably reduced, is then closed by suturing the margins of the tear together. The holding capacity of the suture line can be increased by using the proximal end of the biceps tendon as an overlay graft on that site. No fixation is required for bone graft A, as it will be held in place by the repaired rotator cuff.

Excessive tendon loss in the suture area can also be reduced by a more extensive release in the rotator interval, performed so that the supraspinatus can be mobilized laterally (''an interval slide''). In this maneuver the entire rotator interval is sharply released to the base of the coracoid. The incision is made on the inferior aspect of the coracohumeral ligament, so that it still remains attached to the supraspinatus tendon. This incision allows 1 to 1.5 cm of lateral mobilization of the torn and retracted supraspinatus tendon. Alternatively, a subscapularis transfer can be performed to close an upper gap left by a retracted, deficient supraspinatus tendon. Usually only the upper third of the subscapularis tendon should be transferred (the lower part of the subscapularis tendon is still muscular at its bony insertion and should not be released), and to prevent anterior instability of the glenohumeral joint, the capsule should not be disturbed.[6]

Postoperatively, the arm is placed in a Velpeau dressing for 6 weeks. An abduction pillow or splint is used only in those cases in which closure could not be achieved without unfavorable tension. The rehabilitation program consists of passive assisted exercises on the first postop-

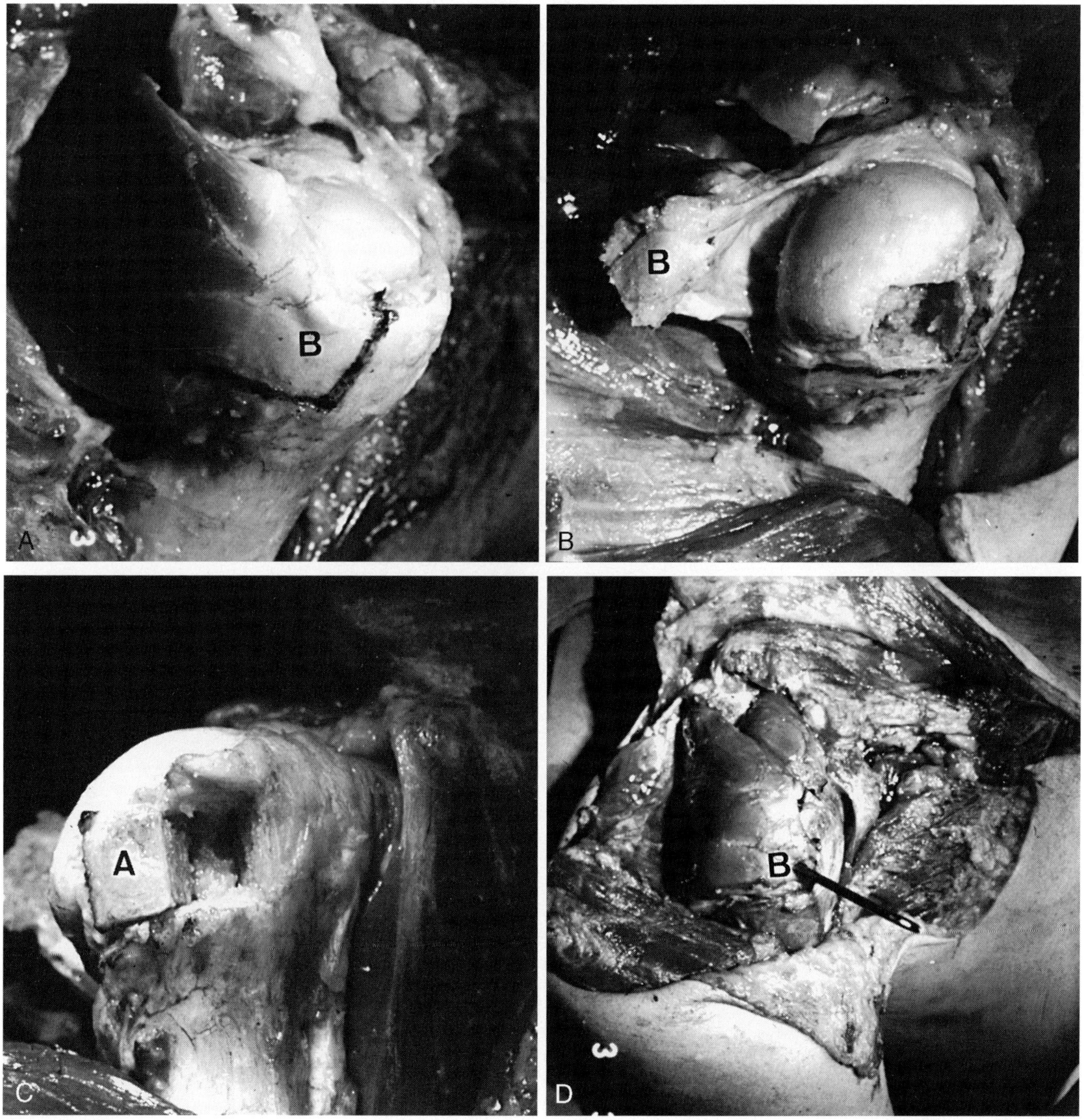

Fig. 25–2. *A,* A cadaver dissection demonstration of the procedure. Block B with the remaining posterior elements of the rotator cuff with line of dissection marked. *B,* The capsule has been released along the posterior glenoid rim, thus enabling the transfer of both the muscle, its tendon, and capsule en bloc. *C,* Block A has been released from the recipient area and transposed posteriorly into the space left on the posterior aspect of the humeral head. *D,* Temporary fixation of bone Block B, along with its musculotendinous elements, into its new position.

erative day (i.e., pendulum exercises and assisted forward elevation in the scapular plane). Active exercises are begun after 6 weeks and resistance is gradually increased. A continuous interscalene block with bupivacaine is used as an analgesic during the first postoperative days. To avoid chronic impingement against the acromion, removal of the cancellous screw under local anesthesia is recommended 3 to 6 months postoperatively.

RESULTS

The preliminary results of the first 31 patients operated with this method were published in 1990.[18] We concluded that relief of pain, including night pain and pain associated with activity, was evident in 93% of the cases. The overall function in daily activities was objectively and subjectively improved in 90% of the cases. The average

Neer's Functional Assessment Score increased to 72.5 points; in 11 patients, the increase was to 80 points or more. The range of postoperative abduction was 40 to 180°, with 15 patients having more than 170° of abduction (Fig. 25–3). In three cases, the postoperative Functional Assessment Scores were lower than the preoperative. However, these patients were satisfied with the relief of their nocturnal pain.[18]

Since the 1990 study, this maneuver has been added to the normal repertoire of surgical procedures for ruptured rotator cuffs in our unit. It is now often used in combination with some other advancement of the surrounding muscles (subscapularis, interval slide, or biceps interposition).

Transposition of tendons in massive cuff tears may be regarded as a salvage procedure. Advancement or transposition of the tendons for rotator cuff repair can be used to restore the soft-tissue spacer function between the humeral head and the acromion. Unfortunately, there are few studies that focus on the quality of the cuff tissue after reconstruction of a cuff tear;[23,24] however, those that do show quite clearly that in many cases, es-

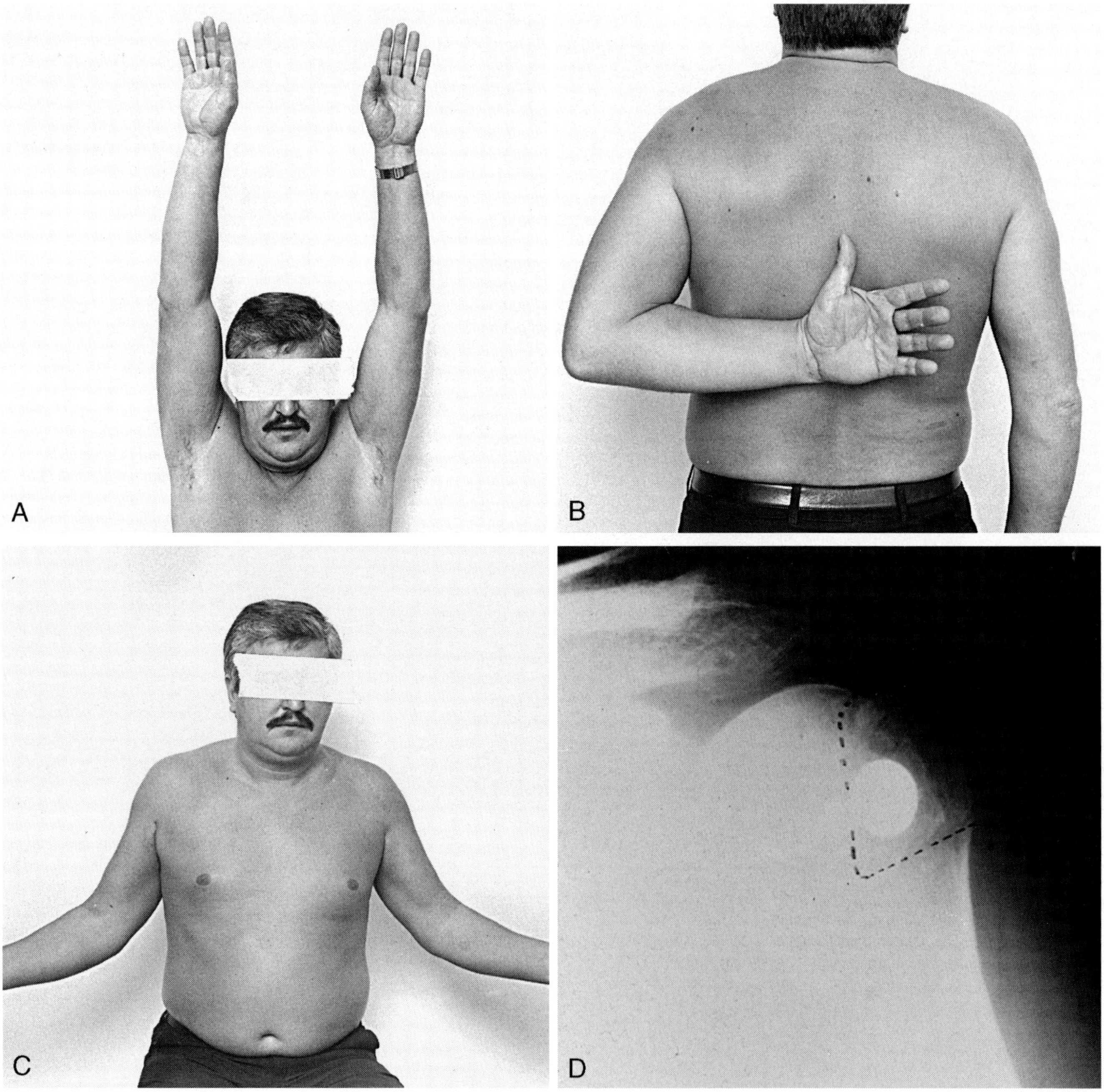

Fig. 25–3. Functional result in flexion (*A*), internal rotation (*B*), and outward rotation (*C*) of a patient 2.5 years after the operation. Post operative radiographs of the shoulder with the transposed block encircled with dots. The screw was removed 3 months after the operation.

pecially after massive rupture, the quality and endurance of the tissue between the acromion and the head of the humerus is poor.[49,25] These results also suggest that the surgeon should be quite hesitant to propose a second attempt at rotator cuff repair.[9] The best opportunity for surgical reconstruction, if a good result is to be achieved, is the first time that repair is attempted.[25] That is why our new technique was devised to combine the properties of the remaining vital tendons and to secure fixation of the transposed insertion—the better the interposition material, the better the pain relief and the better the functional results.

Several different methods for tendon transfer, including the use of the teres minor with tendon-bone suture, have been described previously. This modification of those transfers using a bone block has not been previously reported. This is only one modification of those earlier methods.[17,25]

In the literature, the most important argument against transposition of the posterior elements is the fear that weakness of external rotation and loss of dynamic stability might result. The center of the humeral head has been shown to coincide with the center of rotation of the glenohumeral joint. Keating et al.[26] determined the percentage each rotator cuff muscle contributed to the total moment of all four muscles. It appeared that the subscapularis contributed 53% of the moment about the humeral head, the supraspinatus contributed 14%, the infraspinatus contributed 22%, and teres minor contributed 10%. The force-generating capacity of the subscapularis was equal to that of the other three muscles combined.[26] Burkhart et al.[27] described the force couples of the glenohumeral joint in the transverse and coronal plane (i.e., the role of the supraspinatus and infraspinatus in the transverse plane and the deltoid and infraspinatus/teres minor in the coronal plane). Uncoupling of either essential force couple results in loss of the ability to maintain a fulcrum for motion at the glenohumeral joint.[27]

Massive tears, however, tend to involve the posterior rotator cuff rather than the anterior cuff (i.e., sectors 4 to 6 in Patte's classification).[10,13] In these cases, the necessary force couples are no longer maintained. The glenohumeral fulcrum has already been lost and motion is poor. If we cannot restore the normal fulcrum through conventional repair techniques, sacrificing the teres minor (only 10% of the total moment) seems justified, especially if a painless shoulder is the result. In addition, the motor function of the muscle is preserved intact, and only the insertion of the muscle and therefore its vector have been changed.

The lack of histologic data on the healing capacity and longevity of the tendon-to-bone junction led us to modify this technique to a bone-to-bone interface. The muscular nature of the insertion of the teres minor muscle also lends itself well to such a modification.[10] The healing capacity of bone to bone is secure, especially in this type of reconstruction in which fairly heavy forces are acting against the new insertion area. A bone-to-bone interface also allows the combination of subscapularis advancement in massive tears.[6,16,17] Temporary screw fixation of the transferred bone block further secures the junction, and the screw can easily be removed later under local anesthesia.

Anterior acromioplasty is an essential part of this type of reconstruction, not only to relieve impingement but also to improve surgical exposure and to protect the rotator cuff from residual impingement during the healing period. Too often residual anterior subacromial impingement has been identified as a source of failure after rotator cuff surgery.[4,5] Biceps tendinitis can be related to luxation of the tendon or a narrow and degenerated intertubercular groove with attrition of the tendon. Tenodesis was performed in all cases with luxation tendinitis, whereas in cases of attrition tendinitis, tenodesis was done only when the gliding surface of the tendon had been destroyed.[13]

Although studies show that larger defects correspond to poor clinical end results, there is no significant correlation between the final outcome and the technique used in reconstructing the rotator cuff.[2,3,5,25] Adequate correction of the basic pathological condition (i.e., relief of impingement and restoration of the soft-tissue spacer function between the humeral head and the acromion) guarantees flexibility of the ball-to-socket interlock. This, along with adequate correction of the concomitant lesions of the joint, leads to a good end result independent of the reconstruction method used. This finding supports the view that perhaps even "nonorthodox" methods can also be used successfully to achieve the basic goal of a surgical repair, resulting in healthy, well-vascularized tissue that is not under tension.

We do not recommend this technique as a routine for fresh massive tears, which often can be repaired with more conventional techniques with good results. It should be reserved for those cases with badly frayed, retracted ruptures with extensive contractures, scarring, and poor quality of the rotator cuff tendons (group III, stage 3 in Patte's classification).[10] The patient's good cooperation is absolutely necessary, because of the demanding, active, long-term rehabilitation program following surgery. Although reconstruction of the rotator cuff using our method led to successful relief of pain and improvement in daily activities, several recent reports have pointed out that, especially in elderly patients with a massive tear but with nearly normal function, arthroscopic decompression and debridement may produce comparable results with less risk and effort.[27]

REFERENCES

1. Wolfgang GL. Rupture of the musculotendinous cuff of the shoulder. *Clin Orthop.* 1978;134:230–243.
2. Watson M. Major ruptures of the rotator cuff. *J Bone Joint Surg Br.* 1985;67:618–624.
3. Bigliani LU, Cordasco FA, McIlveen SJ, Musso ES. Operative repair of massive rotator cuff tears: long-term results. *J Shoulder Elbow Surg.* 1992;1:120–130.
4. Bigliani LU, Cordasco FA, McIlveen SJ, Musso ES. Operative treatment of failed repairs of the rotator cuff. *J Bone Joint Surg Am.* 1992; 74:1505–1515.
5. Björkenheim J-M, Paavolainen P, Ahovuo J, Slätis P. Surgical repair

of the rotator cuff and surrounding tissues: factors influencing the results. *Clin Orthop.* 1988;236:148–153.
6. Cofield RH. Subscapular muscle transposition for repair of chronic rotator cuff tears. *Surg Gynecol Obstet.* 1982;154:667–672.
7. Nasca RJ. The use of freeze-dried allografts in the management of global rotator cuff tears. *Clin Orthop.* 1988;228:218–226.
8. Ozaki J, Fujimoto S, Masuhara K, Tamai S, Yoshimoto S. Reconstruction of chronic massive rotator cuff tears with synthetic materials. *Clin Orthop.* 1986;202:173–183.
9. DeOrio JK, Cofield RH. Results of a second attempt at surgical repair of a failed initial rotator cuff repair. *J Bone Joint Surg Am.* 1984; 66:563–567.
10. Patte D. Classification of rotator cuff lesions. *Clin Orthop.* 1990; 254:81–86.
11. Patte D, DeBeyre J, Goutallier D. Rotator cuff repair by muscle advancement. In: Bateman JE, Welsh RP, eds. *Surgery of the Shoulder.* St. Louis: BC Decker; 1984:49–59.
12. Post M, Silver R, Singh M. Rotator cuff tear: Diagnosis and treatment. *Clin Orthop.* 1983;173:78–91.
13. Paavolainen P, Slätis P, Ahuvuo J. Anterior vs. lateral lesion of the rotator cuff. In: Takagishi N, ed. *The Shoulder.* Proceedings of the Third International Conference on Surgery of the Shoulder. Tokyo: Professional Postgraduate Services; 1987:225–230.
14. DeBeyre J, Patte D, Elmelik E. Repair of the rotator cuff of the shoulder. *J Bone Joint Surg Br.* 1965;47:36–42.
15. Ha'Eri GB, Wiley AM. Advancement of the supraspinatus muscle in the repair of ruptures of the rotator cuff. *J Bone Joint Surg Am.* 1981; 63:232–238.
16. Neviaser RJ, Neviaser TJ. Transfer of subscapularis and teres minor for massive defects of the rotator cuff. In: Bayley JI, Kessel L, eds. *Shoulder Surgery.* Berlin: Springer-Verlag; 1982:60–63.
17. Neviaser RJ, Neviaser TJ. Reconstruction of chronic tears of the rotator cuff. In: Bateman JE, Welsh RP, eds. *Surgery of the Shoulder.* St. Louis: BC Decker; 1984:172–179.
18. Paavolainen P, Slätis P, Björkenheim J-M. Transfer of the tuberculum majus for massive ruptures of the rotator cuff. In: Post M, Morrey BF, Hawkins RJ, eds. *Surgery of the Shoulder.* St. Louis: Mosby-Year Book;1990:252–256.
19. Solonen K, Vastamäki M. Reconstruction of the rotator cuff. *Int Orthop.* 1983;7:49–53.
20. Warner JJP, Krushekk RJ, Masquelet A, Gerber C. Anatomy and relationships of the suprascapular nerve: Anatomical constraints to mobilization of the supraspinatus and infraspinatus muscles in the management of massive rotator-cuff tears. *J Bone Joint Surg Am.* 1992; 74:36–45.
21. Mikasa M. Trapezius transfer for global tear of the rotator cuff. In: Bateman JE, Welsh RP, eds. *Surgery of the Shoulder.* St. Louis: BC Decker; 1984:196–199.
22. Gerber C, Vinh TS, Hertel R, Hess C. Latissimus dorsi transfer for the treatment of massive tears of the rotator cuff. *Clin Orthop.* 1988; 232:51–61.
23. Calvert PT, Packer NP, Satoker DJ, Bayley JIL, Kessel L. Arthrography of the shoulder after operative repair of the torn rotator cuff. *J Bone Joint Surg Br.* 1986;68:147–150.
24. Crass JR, Craig EV, Feinberg SB. Sonography of the postoperative rotator cuff. *Am J Radiol.* 1986;146:561–564.
25. Ellman H, Hanker G, Bayer M. Repair of the rotator cuff. *J Bone Joint Surg Am.* 1986;68:1136–1144.
26. Keating JF, Waterworth P, Shaw-Dunn J, Crossan J. The relative strengths of the rotator cuff muscles. *J Bone Joint Surg Br.* 1993; 75:137–140.
27. Burkhart SS. Arthroscopic treatment of massive rotator cuff tears. *Clin Orthop.* 1991;267:45–56.

Chapter 26

Biceps Transfer Interposition Grafting in Massive Rotator Cuff Tears

Phillip E. Hansen

Massive rotator cuff tears are defined as those tears being generally larger than 5 cm and involving more than two of the major rotator cuff tendons, with the remaining tendinous material frequently being retracted and of relatively poor quality.[1] The humeral head herniates upward through the remnants of the rotator cuff and comes to lie under the acromion. Active elevation causes the humeral head to impinge upon the acromion and subacromial arch with pain and limitation of active range of motion.[2]

The surgical management of massive rotator cuff tears remains somewhat controversial. The majority of rotator cuff tears, even those defined as massive, can be repaired by a standard technique as originally described by McLaughlin.[3] This technique involves mobilization of rotator cuff remnants, closure of the defect beginning at the apex medially, progressing laterally, and then suturing the lateral edge of the rotator cuff into a trough in the humeral head.

A relatively small percentage of massive rotator cuff tears cannot be repaired in this fashion.[4] Failure to reestablish appropriate rotator cuff tension produces a loss of the normal head depressing effect, causing an upward herniation of the humeral head with respect to the glenoid and resulting in sheer stresses that can lead to early degenerative changes in the glenohumeral joint itself (Fig. 26–1). In addition, as the rotator cuff and its associated capsuloligamentous thickenings are not able to stabilize the humeral head in the glenoid, the humeral head can also translate anteriorly and posteriorly producing additional sheer stresses.[5] Synovial fluid is no longer contained within a watertight capsule but is free to go into the subacromial area and is, therefore, relatively unavailable for nutrition to the articular surfaces of the glenohumeral joint.[6] These combined factors are thought to play a role in the development of cuff tear arthropathy seen in some patients with unrepaired massive rotator cuff tears.

There have been multiple techniques described to close an otherwise irreparable rotator cuff tear: (1) muscle transfer procedures, including subscapularis,[7] teres minor,[8] latissimus dorsi,[1] pectoralis major, and supraspinatus slide;[9,10] (2) free avascular autologous tissue grafts, including fascia lata and also the avascular intra-articular portion of the long head of the biceps tendon;[12] (3) cadaveric materials, including freeze-dried rotator cuff preparations;[13,14] (4) artificial substitutes, including a carbon-fiber composite[15] as well as a Teflon felt replacement;[16] and (5) resection of the rotator cuff itself combined with complete or partial acromionectomy.[5,17]

A useful technique originally described by Bush[18] in 1975 incorporates an intact but transferred long head biceps tendon into the defect remaining following maximal mobilization of the rotator cuff itself. In this original report, the results in 14 patients were described. There was limited follow-up of as little as 9 months. Subacromial decompression was not routinely performed. An acromial osteotomy was used for visualization. Good and excellent results of 79% were reported. There has been only limited further mention of this technique in the literature; specifically, no series incorporating more modern shoulder principles has been reported.

I have used a modification of the Bush biceps transfer interposition graft technique since 1984. Because other standard repair techniques are typically used in most rotator cuff repairs, only 32 out of 363 rotator cuff repairs during this period have required this technique.

Indications for its use include a massive, otherwise unreconstructible, rotator cuff tear in which the free margins of the rotator cuff are retracted and the overall quality of tissue is relatively poor. The long head of the biceps must be intact and of suitable quality for transfer. Generally this means at least 80% of the tendinous cross-sectional area is intact. Some tenosynovitis and some fraying is acceptable. Patients must also have a relatively normal glenohumeral joint on radiograph. Minor ring osteophyte formation is acceptable. At the time of surgical exploration, the articular surfaces must be smooth and of relatively normal appearance. The patient must be motivated and otherwise a good candidate not only to withstand the surgical procedure but also to understand, cooperate, and attend rehabilitation postoperatively.

Contraindications to this procedure would include paralysis of the remaining rotator cuff and/or the deltoid

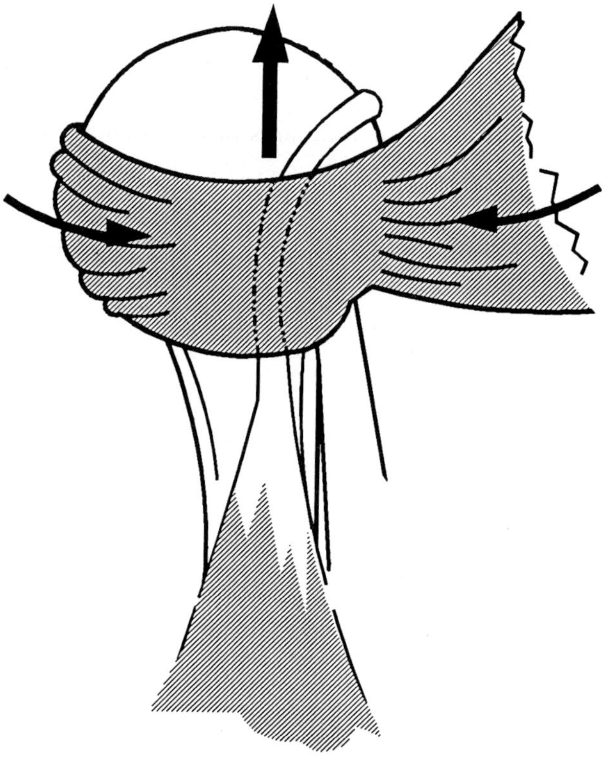

Fig. 26–1. Absent superior rotator cuff allows superior head migration unopposed by the remaining rotator cuff.

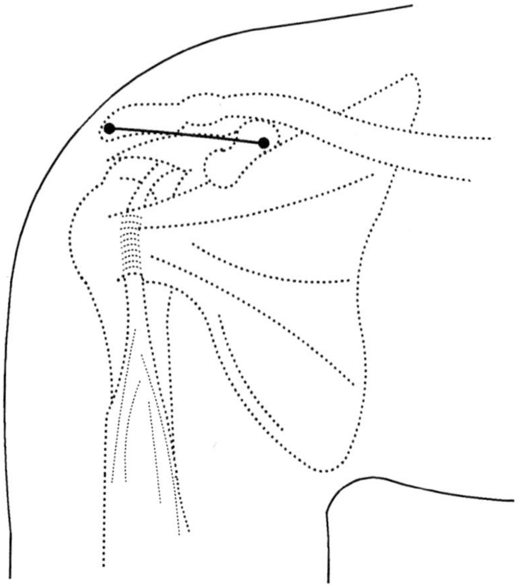

Fig. 26–2. Modified Gardner incision.

muscle. In addition, significant degenerative changes within the glenohumeral joint itself would probably require additional procedures such as total joint replacement. This procedure could be performed in conjunction with such a procedure. To date I have not used this procedure in conjunction with total shoulder replacement. This technique should not be used if the rotator cuff is otherwise repairable by standard techniques. Obviously this technique cannot be used in the absence of an intact intra-articular portion of the long head biceps tendon. Recent sepsis and/or poor patient motivation or poor general patient health are relative contraindications to this procedure.

TECHNIQUE

Because most patients requiring this procedure are relatively elderly (usually over 50 years old) and may have other underlying medical conditions, a complete history and physical examination combined with appropriate medical consultation should be obtained. The patient is placed in a modified beach chair position with two folded towels holding the scapula anteriorly. The patient is given intravenous antibiotics preoperatively. The skin is cleansed for 10 minutes with a chlorhexidine gluconate (Hibiclens) prep followed by an ethanol wash. The arm is then draped freely using iodoform adhesive skin drapes.

In a modification of the Gardner[19] technique, an anterior skin incision is used following the lines of Langer from the anterior portion of the lateral acromion progressing medially to a point just above and just lateral to the coracoid process (Fig. 26–2). Following cutaneous hemostasis, subcutaneous flaps are elevated above and below to allow for wide exposure subcutaneously. A stay suture is place in the deltoid approximately 3 cm inferior to the most anterior portion of the acromion. The deltoid is split from the anterior acromion down to this stay stitch, which prevents a more distal dissection with possible axillary nerve injury. Approximately 1 cm of deltoid is detached off the anterior acromion laterally from this vertical split. Using a Darrach retractor, the humeral head is held down away from the acromion while a generous anterior and inferior acromionectomy is performed according to the technique of Neer.[20] The acromion is made flat completely back and medially.

Routinely in these patients with massive tears, there is coexisting pathology in the AC joint.[21] This is manifest by pain preoperatively, radiographic changes of narrowing and/or spur formation, and most importantly prominence of the inferior area of the acromion at the clavicular joint by the palpating surgical finger at the time of acromioplasty. Therefore, a separate periosteal incision is made over the distal clavicle. Great care is taken that this does not communicate with the incision in the deltoid more laterally used for acromionectomy (Fig. 26–3). The distal clavicle is exposed subperiosteally, taking care not to dissect medially enough to detach any of the trapezoid ligament. One centimeter of distal clavicle is excised. It is typically not necessary to detach the deltoid off of the entire anterior acromion across to the clavicle for exposure. By retaining this intact section of deltoid, deltoid problems during the postoperative period have been avoided. The deltoid then is reapproximated to the remnants of the acromioclavicular capsular complex, trapezius muscle, and periosteum. It is imperative to obtain good stability of the distal clavicle by this repair.

The subacromial space is explored. Redundant bursa is excised. Some of the bursal material may be quite thick and may initially appear to be rotator cuff. By close examination at the lateral-most attachments of this material, the rotator cuff remnants (if any) can be differentiated from thickened bursal material, as the latter will have no lateral attachments to the humeral head. Redundant bursal material is excised to allow for better visualization and to avoid its inadvertent incorporation into the rotator cuff repair.

A careful and meticulous mobilization of the remaining rotator cuff is performed. This is done with a combination of traction sutures, sharp and blunt dissection, and digital manipulation. The coracohumeral ligament is frequently sectioned to provide additional mobilization. The apex of the rotator cuff tear is identified. The anterior and posterior remnants of the rotator cuff are then brought together, beginning at the apex, with vertical mattress sutures of No. 1 Tevdek material. Progressing from medial to lateral, additional sutures are placed to restore tension to the rotator cuff anteriorly and posteriorly. It is in those cases in which the remaining cuff material is insufficient to allow for closure all the way to the bony humerus laterally that the biceps transfer interposition graft technique is indicated (Fig. 26–4).

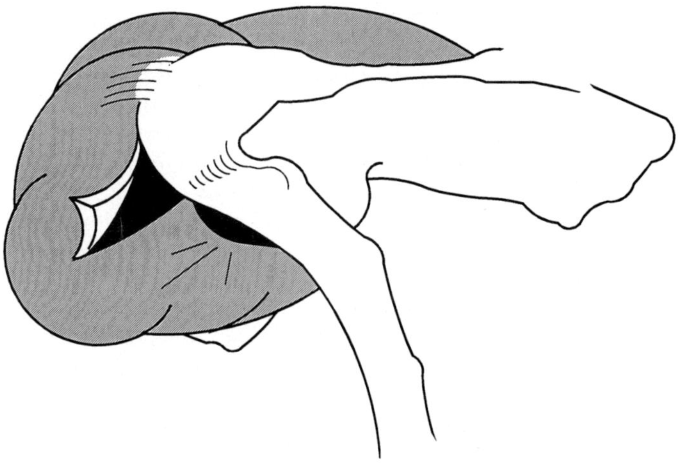

Fig. 26–3. Separate deltoid incisions for subacromial decompression and distal clavicular excision. Note intact portion of deltoid between the incisions.

The transverse humeral ligament is incised and the biceps is mobilized by means of an umbilical tape passed around it. A trough 1.5 cm posterior and lateral to the bicipital groove is made using a ¼-inch curved gouge. Great care is taken not to fracture the greater tuberosity into the bicipital groove. The groove is of sufficient depth and is smoothed superiorly onto the articular surface and is routed inferiorly towards the original bicipital groove so that the biceps tendon can then be mobilized into the groove. It should remain intrinsically stable both in internal and external rotation of the humeral head. The biceps must be mobilized fully from its original location in order to allow for full external rotation with the elbow at the side, while the biceps tendon remains seated in its newly formed groove. The posterior rotator cuff remnant is then sutured to the posterior portion of the biceps tendon. The anterior rotator cuff remnant is sutured to the anterior-most portion of the biceps tendon. At the greater tuberosity, the rotator cuff remnant is then sutured into a shallow groove made in the humeral head

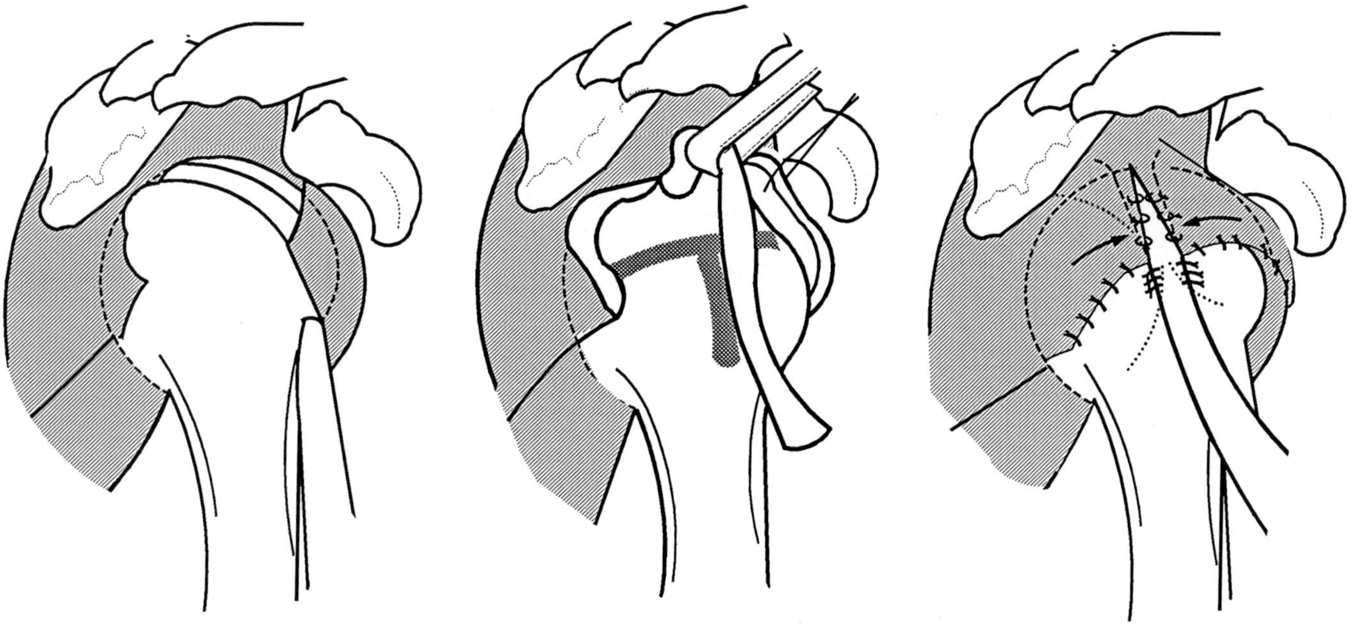

Fig. 26–4. ***A,*** **Rotator cuff edges are freshened and mobilized maximally.** ***B,*** **The biceps tendon is mobilized from its original groove. A new longitudinal groove is fashioned 1.5 cm posteriorly. Troughs are made to correspond into the lateral-most advancement of the rotator cuff remnant anteriorly and posteriorly.** ***C,*** **The biceps is placed in its new groove and the posterior rotator cuff remnant is sutured to the biceps posteriorly, while the anterior cuff remnant is sutured to the biceps anteriorly.**

both anteriorly and posteriorly to the newly made groove in which the biceps long head has come to reside. The rotator cuff is then sutured down into the shallow groove using No. 1 Tevdek sutures through drill holes in bone, again taking great care that fracture of the tuberosity does not occur. The bone here can be quite osteoporotic. Incorporation of any remaining rotator cuff tissue at the tuberosity helps to decrease the probability of sutures tearing through this soft bone. A watertight repair is typically achieved. The repair is done with the arm at the side. The repair will allow the arm to externally rotate to at least 45°. Care is taken that none of the sutures pass in a circumferential manner about the biceps tendon, as these might serve to strangulate the tendon. The goal here is to provide for a vascularized, immediately stable support to the repaired rotator cuff tissue that will allow for relatively early mobilization. Physiologic tension of the remaining rotator cuff with the arm at the side should be achieved.[15] There is a theoretical advantage that the vascularized biceps tendon will provide additional blood supply to the poorly vascularized rotator cuff tissue,[22] aiding healing and decreasing the frequency of recurrent tearing.

A meticulous deltoid repair is performed, suturing it to the acromion with nonabsorbable No. 1 Tevdek suture through drill holes that incorporate both the anterior acromion and its overlying osteo-periosteal tissue. The vertical split in the deltoid is repaired with absorbable Vicryl suture. The skin is repaired with a subcuticular pull-out suture technique.

I have used an abduction pillow postoperatively but have emphasized to the patient the importance of avoiding extension forces on the shoulder caused by the pillow sliding posteriorly on the chest wall.

Postoperatively, the patients are maintained in the hospital until they are comfortable on oral pain medications, averaging 3 days with a range of 2 to 5 days. They are allowed to flex forward at the waist and perform pendulum exercises off of the pillow beginning after 2 to 3 days. The pillow is maintained at all other times for 4 weeks. The patient's arm is then removed from the pillow and placed in a sling, which is worn for two additional weeks. Passive range-of-motion exercises consisting of passive pendulum, passive flexion with a pulley, external rotation with a stick, and internal rotation exercises are performed 3 times a day out of the sling. Patients are encouraged to avoid active overhead flexion of the arm for at least 12 weeks, and no weights are allowed for at least 6 months. Patients are encouraged to continue with their exercise regimen for at least 1 year postoperatively.

CLINICAL RESULTS

Since 1984 this surgical technique has been used in 32 shoulders in 31 patients. Twenty-six patients have been followed for 2 or more years. Two patients died of unrelated causes. Three patients have been lost to follow-up. This leaves 21 patients with 22 shoulders available for greater than a 2-year follow-up, and these patients will comprise the basis for the clinical results reported here. There were 5 female and 16 male patients with the dominant arm involved in 13 cases and the nondominant involved in 9 cases. One female patient had this procedure performed on both shoulders. Average patient age at time of surgery was 59 years, with a range of 44 to 74 years. The average length of symptoms was 27 months, with range of 1 month to 132 months. Two patients had a prior documented anterior dislocation as the initial injury. One patient had prior surgery; this was an attempted rotator cuff repair that was aborted in favor of a debridement and anterior-inferior acromionectomy. The patient remained painful even at rest and desired an additional attempt at repair.

The primary indication for surgical intervention was pain (Table 26–1). Preoperatively, 19 out of 22 shoulders had significant rest pain, and all but one patient had significant pain with use. No patient performed all the activities of daily living used to evaluate results (Table 26–2). These included lifting overhead, lifting 10 lbs, sleep-

Table 26–1. Pain (0–4)

	Rest Pain		*Pain With Use*	
	No. Patients	*No. Patients*	*No. Patients*	*No. Patients*
0 (None)	3(14%)	19(86%)	1(5%)	14(64%)
1	5(23%)	2(9%)	0	7(32%)
2	12(55%)	1(5%)	4(18%)	1(5%)
3	2(9%)	0	12(55%)	0
4 (Most)	0	0	5(23%)	0
Average	1.6	0.2	2.9	0.4

Table 26–2. Activities of Daily Living

	Sleep		*Raise Arm*		*10 lbs*	
	Pre-op	*Post-op*	*Pre-op*	*Post-op*	*Pre-op*	*Post-op*
Yes (%)	1(5%)	22(100%)	2(10%)	19(63%)	4(18%)	21(95%)
No (%)	21(95%)	0	20(90%)	3(27%)	18(82%)	1(5%)
	Comb Hair		*Back Pocket*		*All 5*	
	Pre-op	*Post-op*	*Pre-op*	*Post-op*	*Pre-op*	*Post-op*
Yes (%)	8(36%)	20(90%)	17(77%)	21(95%)	0	19(86%)
No (%)	14(64%)	2(10%)	5(23%)	1(5%)	22(10%)	3(14%)

Table 26–3. Active Elevation

	Pre-op	*Post-op*
0–45°	4(18%)	1(5%)
45–90°	9(41%)	1(5%)
90–135°	2(9%)	0
135–180°	7(32%)	20(90%)
AVERAGE	97°	166°

Table 26–4. Subjective Satisfaction

Fully satisfied	20(90%)
Mostly satisfied	1(5%)
Somewhat satisfied	0
Not satisfied	1(5%)

Table 26–5. Subjective Overhead Strength

	Pre-op	*Post-op*
0(None)	0	0
1	11(50%)	3(14%)
2	10(45%)	4(18%)
3	1(5%)	11(50%)
4(Normal)	0	4(18%)
Average	1.6	2.7

ing on the shoulder without pain, combing of the hair, and reaching in the back pocket. Only two shoulders could be actively lifted overhead, and the average active elevation was 97°, with a range from 10 to 180° (Table 26–3). Only one patient had no difficulty sleeping and only six patients could lift 10 lbs comfortably. The average pain score preoperatively was 2.9.

The average postoperative follow-up was 44 months, with a range of 24 to 86 months. All patients are now sleeping comfortably at night. All but two patients are able to perform all five activities of daily living used in this report for evaluation of results. All but one patient was pleased with the operative result and would have the operation performed again (Table 26–4). Nineteen of 22 patients had no pain at rest. Two had mild pain and one had moderate pain. Fourteen of 22 shoulders had no pain with use. Seven had mild pain not requiring analgesics and one had moderate pain that interfered significantly with activities of daily living. The average pain score was 0.4. All but three patients could now lift the arm above the head, although only four patients felt they had normal overhead strength (Table 26–5). One patient had weaker than normal strength, but his opposite arm, also known to have a rotator cuff tear, has become so painful that he now uses the operative arm for most of his activities of daily living. He is planning to undergo a repair of his rotator cuff on that shoulder in the near future.

There are many systems reported for grading results in shoulder surgery (Table 26–6).[20,23] Using Neer's criteria,[20] there were 20 satisfactory and 2 unsatisfactory results. Using criteria described by Bigliani for results following rotator cuff tear repair,[23] there were 19 excellent results, 1 good result, 1 fair result, and 1 poor result. Using the criteria of Post et. al.,[2] there were 13 excellent results, 8 good results, 0 fair results, and 1 poor result.

These results compare favorably with reports of large series of rotator cuff tear repairs, as well as with other alternative means of closure of massive rotator cuff tears that are otherwise unreconstructible (Table 26–7).[10,14,17,24–27]

The one fair result was in a patient who was disabled from a previous on-the-job back injury. He had undergone a previous attempt at rotator cuff repair in another institution. This was aborted in favor of a cuff debridement and decompression. He was disappointed in that his pain and function were no better than prior to his biceps transfer procedure, but his strength, pain, and function were no worse, and his active flexion increased by 30°. The one poor result was in a 74-year-old female patient who had an obvious re-rupture postoperatively. Radiographs demonstrated a humeral-acromial distance[28,29] of 2 mm postoperatively, and she had only 45° of active forward flexion. There is no clinical information to indicate when this recurrent rupture may have occurred. This was the only case in which there was an actual loss of active forward flexion. However, her pain was greatly relieved. She had complete resolution of both moderate rest pain and severe pain with use. She has remained happy with her result, despite her lack of improvement in functional activities. This same patient underwent this same operative procedure on her opposite dominant arm 6 months later with an excellent result that she describes as "normal" in all respects.

Table 26–6. Overall Result (%)

	Neer[19]	*Bigliani*[22]	*Post*[2]
Excellent	90	86	59
Good		5	36
Fair	10	5	0
Poor		5	5

Table 26–7. Results Compared With Other Series (%)

	Biceps Transfer Graft	*Mixed Series Cuff Repair*[24]	*Massive Tears*[23]
Excellent	86	84	65
Good	5		20
Fair	5	16	7
Poor	5		8
	Supraspinatus Advancement[10]	*Allograft*[14]	*Resection Cuff*[17]
Excellent	78	50	82
Good		31	
Fair	22	6	18
Poor		13	

In this series there have been no infections, acromial fractures, or other complications noted. There has been one rupture of the long head biceps tendon, clinically evident by enlargement of the biceps anteriorly and inferiorly in the upper arm. This occurred 10 weeks postoperatively in association with activities of daily living. At the patient's request, this rupture was not repaired. This patient has been followed for 52 months. He performs full activities of daily living. He has no pain at rest or with use. He has an excellent range of motion. His only complaint is that he still has mild weakness with overhead use for an extended period. He is extremely pleased with his result.

DISCUSSION

The excellent results reported in this series are particularly gratifying in light of results previously reported using other techniques for closure of otherwise irreparable tears of the rotator cuff. Although it is not always possible to compare on a case-by-case basis other reports in the literature, in general these other reports have used the same or similar descriptions for their definitions of massive rotator cuff tears and the same or similar methods of calculating results.

Meticulous attention to detail is required for this technique to be effective. The importance of a complete and thorough subacromial decompression cannot be overly emphasized. This is probably the primary factor in providing pain relief in these patients,[26] even in the patient who has an apparent rupture of the repair.

Mobilization of the remaining rotator cuff is essential. The interposition of the biceps graft is not a replacement for rotator cuff tissue; it is simply a vascularized anchored graft which allows the re-establishment of a yoke mechanism between anterior and posterior rotator cuff tendons, so that a net resultant inferior head depressor effect can be re-established (Fig. 26–5). This helps to stabilize the humeral head both in the superior/inferior and in the anterior/posterior planes. It provides for compressive rather than sheer forces at the glenohumeral joint. It also provides a watertight repair, which allows for the confinement of synovial fluid intra-articularly in the glenohumeral joint providing maximal articular nutrition. This theoretically may help to decrease the risk of developing cuff tear arthropathy.

This technique does not preclude the biceps from continuing to be functional as a head depressor. The biceps is not sutured into its new groove and has the potential to once again become a gliding tendon. The biceps has been shown to be an important head stabilizer in an otherwise normal glenohumeral joint.[30] It is probably of even greater importance in a shoulder with a deficient rotator cuff. By not detaching the biceps but by simply moving it to a new groove, its previous function is not necessarily destroyed.

The biceps is autologous material and of a local nature. No additional incisions nor, indeed, any additional preoperative planning is required. Should a massive tear which is otherwise unreconstructible be encountered at the time of exploration, the biceps can be rapidly mobilized and incorporated into this repair. No intact cuff tissue is detached from the humerus and therefore is not rendered potentially less functional. The subscapularis and teres minor are usually left attached laterally and are simply mobilized superiorly to the biceps tendon, which has been mobilized into its new groove. Only one patient required an associated subscapularis advancement in addition to the biceps transfer to achieve rotator cuff closure. The result in this patient was graded good with no pain at rest or with use, forward flexion actively to 165°, and full ability to do activities of daily living. Overhead strength was graded as moderately weak.

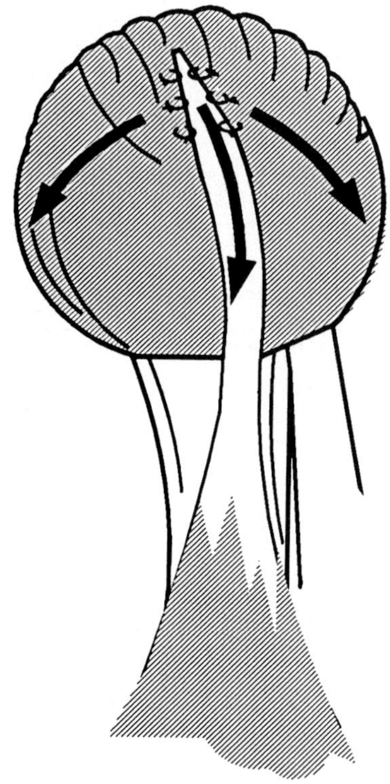

Fig. 26–5. The intact biceps acts as a stabilizing yoke mechanism, allowing the anterior and posterior cuff remnants to become head depressors providing for immediate vascularized stabilization of the rotator cuff repair.

There is no apparent additional morbidity associated with this technique. Despite the 4-week period of immobilization on the abduction pillow, 80% of the shoulders achieved normal or near normal active forward flexion, and only one shoulder lost any active forward flexion. Maximum active range of motion was achieved at approximately one year postoperatively, but additional strength was developed up to 2 years following the operative procedure. No patient experienced a demonstrable deterioration of their clinical result once obtained at 2 years.

Using this technique since 1984, there have been no massive rotator cuff tears that have not been repairable as long as the biceps tendon was available for use. In the four cases in which the biceps was not available, other techniques were used to achieve cuff closure. As this represents a small number of the cases, no significant conclusion can be drawn, but my impression is that these patients tended to have reliable pain relief but overall had a lesser functional result because of less active forward elevation as well as less strength in use, both overhead and in the forward flexed position.

There have been no significant complications encountered with this procedure. There was one biceps rupture, occurring relatively late following the surgical procedure, that resulted in no significant deterioration in the clinical result.

Only 10 shoulders have had adequate comparable preoperative as well as postoperative radiographs at final follow-up to evaluate radiographic changes[28] over time. However, none of these patients has demonstrated any progression of those radiographic changes noted in the preoperative films.

Although not appropriate in most rotator cuff repairs, in those instances in which standard techniques have failed to allow closure of a massive rotator cuff tear, this technique has proven to be reliable and effective in providing for pain relief and a durable, predictable improvement in functional activities of daily living. It should remain one of a variety of techniques available in the surgeon's armamentarium for the treatment of these difficult problems.

REFERENCES

1. Gerber C, Viuh TS, Hertel R, Hess CW. Latissimus dorsi transfer for the treatment of massive tears of the rotator cuff. *Clin Orthop.* 1988;232:51–61.
2. Post M, Silver R, Singh M. Rotator cuff tear diagnosis and treatment. *Clin Orthop.* 1983;173:78–91.
3. McLaughlin HL. Lesions of the musculotendinous cuff of the shoulder. I. The exposure and treatment of tears with retraction. *J Bone Joint Surg.* 1944;26:31–51.
4. Hawkins RJ, Misamore GW, Hobeika PE. Surgery for full-thickness rotator cuff tears. *J Bone Joint Surg.* 1985;67:1349–1355.
5. Burkhart SS. Arthroscopic treatment of massive rotator cuff tears. *Clin Orthop.* 1991;267:45–56.
6. Neer CS, Craig EV, Fukuda H. Cuff-tear arthropathy. *J Bone Joint Surg Am.* 1983;65A:1232–1244.
7. Cofield RH. Subscapular muscle transposition for repair of chronic rotator cuff tears. *Surg Gynecol Obstet.* 1982;154:667–672.
8. Neviaser RJ, Neviaser TJ. Transfer of subscapularis and teres major for massive defects of the rotator cuff. In: Bayley I, Kessel L, eds. *Shoulder Surgery.* Berlin: Springer-Verlag; 1982:60–63.
9. Debeyne J, Patte D, Elmelik E. Repair of ruptures of the rotator cuff of the shoulder. *J Bone Joint Surg Br.* 1965;47:36–42.
10. Ha'eri GB, Wiley AM. Advancement of the supraspinatus muscle in the repair of ruptures of the rotator cuff. *J Bone Joint Surg Am.* 1981; 63:232–238.
11. Nirschl RP. Rotator cuff surgery. In: Barr JS, ed. *Instructional Course Lectures.* St. Louis: AAOS; 1989;38:447–461.
12. Neviaser RJ, Neviaser TJ. Lesions of musculocutaneous cuff of shoulder: Diagnosis and management. In: Murray DG, ed. *Instructional Course Lectures.* St. Louis: CV Mosby; 1981;30:239–249.
13. Nasca RJ. The use of freeze-dried allografts in the management of global rotator cuff tears. *Clin Orthop.* 1988;228:214–226.
14. Neviaser JS, Neviaser RJ, Neviaser TJ. The repair of chronic massive ruptures of the rotator cuff of the shoulder by use of a freeze-dried rotator cuff. *J Bone Joint Surg Am.* 1978;60:681–684.
15. Post M. Rotator cuff repair with carbon filament. *Clin Orthp.* 1985; 196:154–158.
16. Ozaki J, Fujimoto S, Masuhara K, Tamai S, Yoshimoto S. Reconstruction of chronic massive rotator cuff tears with synthetic materials. *Clin Orthop.* 1986;202:173–183.
17. Rockwood CA, Williams GR, Burkhead WZ. Debridement of irreparable degenerative lesions of the rotator cuff. *Orthop Trans.* 1992–1993;16:74.
18. Bush LF. The torn shoulder capsule. *J Bone Joint Surg Am.* 1975; 57:256–259.
19. Gardner RC. A simple, rapid, and esthetic exposure of the shoulder joint. *Surg Gynecol Obstet.* 137:99, 1973.
20. Neer CS. Anterior acromioplasty for the chronic impingement syndrome in the shoulder. *J Bone Joint Surg Am.* 1972;54:41–50.
21. Watson M. Major ruptures of the rotator cuff. *J Bone Joint Surg Br.* 1985;67:618–624.
22. Wolfgang GL. Surgical repair of tears of the rotator cuff of the shoulder. *J Bone Joint Surg Am.* 1974;56:14–26.
23. Bigliani LU, Cordasco FA, McIlveen SJ, Musso ES. Operative treatment of failed repairs of the rotator cuff. *J Bone Joint Surg Am.* 1992; 74:1505–1515.
24. Bigliani LU, Cordasco FA, McIlveen SJ, Musso ES. Operative repair of massive rotator cuff tears: Long-term results. *J Shoulder Elbow Surg.* 1992;1:120–130.
25. Cofield RH. Rotator cuff disease of the shoulder—current concepts review. *J Bone Joint Surg Am.* 1985;67:974–979.
26. Ellman H, Hanker G, Bayer M. Repair of the rotator cuff. *J Bone Joint Surg Am.* 1986;68:1136–1144.
27. Packer NP, Calvert PT, Bayley JIL, Kessel L. Operative treatment of chronic ruptures of the rotator cuff of the shoulder. *J Bone Joint Surg Br.* 1983;65:171–175.
28. Hamada K, Fukuda H, Wikasa M, Kobayashi Y. Roentgenographic findings in massive rotator cuff tears. *Clin Orthop.* 1990; 254:92–96.
29. Weiner DS, Macnab I. Superior migration of the humeral head: A radiological aid in the diagnosis of tears of the rotator cuff. *J Bone Joint Surg Br.* 1970;52:524–527.
30. Kumar VP, Satku K, Balasubramaniam P. The roll of the long head of biceps brachii in the stabilization of the head of the humerus. *Clin Orthop.* 1989;244:172–175.

Chapter 27

Deltoid Muscular Flap Transfer for Massive Defects of the Rotator Cuff

Dominique F. Gazielly

In old, chronic retracted rotator cuff tears with loss of tendinous substance the choice of therapy or surgical technique is a difficult one, as these tears are, by definition, irreparable with conventional surgical techniques using direct or transosseous suturing with the arm at the side. In a certain number of patients, specific rehabilitation that concentrates on strengthening the humeral head depressor muscles can lead to satisfactory recovery of function with reduced pain and subnormal active movement. For some active patients (especially manual workers), however, results achieved relating to pain may be insufficient. Also, these patients continue to suffer from muscular fatigue in anterior elevation, which prevents normal return to work. In such cases, our policy since 1986 has been to compensate for the loss of musculotendinous cuff by transplanting a deltoid muscular flap, a technique initially described by Takagishi[1] and later modified by Augereau.[2]

The surgery is simple, of short duration, and reproducible; but success is dependent on the scrupulous following of indications and contraindications, meticulous operative technique, and to a large extent specific postoperative rehabilitation.

BIOMECHANICAL FUNCTION OF THE DELTOID FLAP

The basic principle is to cover the humeral head when exposed through the loss of tendinous substance with a neo-cuff, whose muscular structure offers several advantages.

The first advantage obtained by placing a deltoid flap in the subacromial space is the insertion of a thick layer of tissue that will act as a pillow between the bald humeral head and the acromion, after removal of any bony prominence by antero-inferior acromioplasty. This is the so-called "cushioning" effect of deltoid flap repair.

The second advantage is a contractile property that is not lost after transplantation. Care is taken when the flap is removed to ensure that it remains innervated and vascularized of its underlying surface. This contractile force is exerted between two fixed points: a lower fixed point that is the base of the flap, which remains attached to the middle deltoid, and an upper fixed point formed by the suture line joining the free border of the flap to the edge of the remaining cuff. During the first few degrees of active anterior elevation, the deltoid flap contracts at the same time as the deltoid muscle, because the innervation is the same (Fig. 27–1). However, when the medial deltoid is about to cause the humeral head to rise (force D), the previously described fixed points cause the contraction of the flap to exert a downward force on the greater tuberosity and the humeral head, which will offset the elevating force of the deltoid during the first 60° of active anterior elevation. The elevation exerted by the deltoid will be less strong if a portion of the medial deltoid has been diverted to use in this flap. In this way, the action of the deltoid flap reinforces the action of the intrinsic and extrinsic depressor muscles of the humeral head (force A). A new equilibrium occurs between the elevating force "D" of the deltoid and force "A" exerted by the depressors reinforced by the deltoid flap. A new resultant "R" is thus created, permitting full active anterior elevation with the restored scapulo-humeral rhythm.

Two points need stressing. First, the biomechanical action of the deltoid flap is more effective with better muscular quality of the deltoid and a stronger contractile force. A thin deltoid muscle showing signs of fatty degeneration is obviously a surgical contraindication for this method. Second, at this time no EMG study, either in vitro or in vivo, has been carried out to confirm this theory. Certain studies, such as that made by Howell,[3] however, indicate that the medial deltoid, even after transplantation, might have a synchronous action with the supraspinatus muscle, thereby initiating anterior elevation by its depressor action upon the greater tuberosity.

PREOPERATIVE MANAGEMENT

We have always stressed[4] the importance of preparing a patient before considering surgical repair of the rotator cuff, especially when tears are massive. The preoperative period is used for specific rehabilitation and for precise imaging of the extent of lesions.

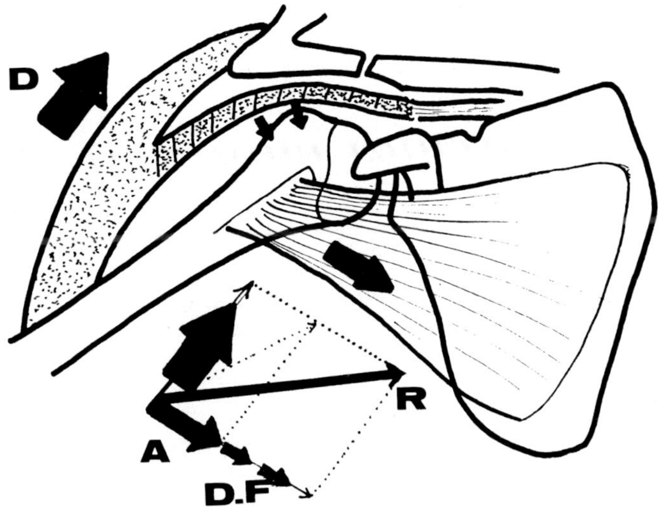

Fig. 27–1. The deltoid flap (DF) reinforces the action of the depressor muscles (A) to oppose the elevating force (D) of the deltoid, causing a new resultant (R) which permits full, active anterior elevation.

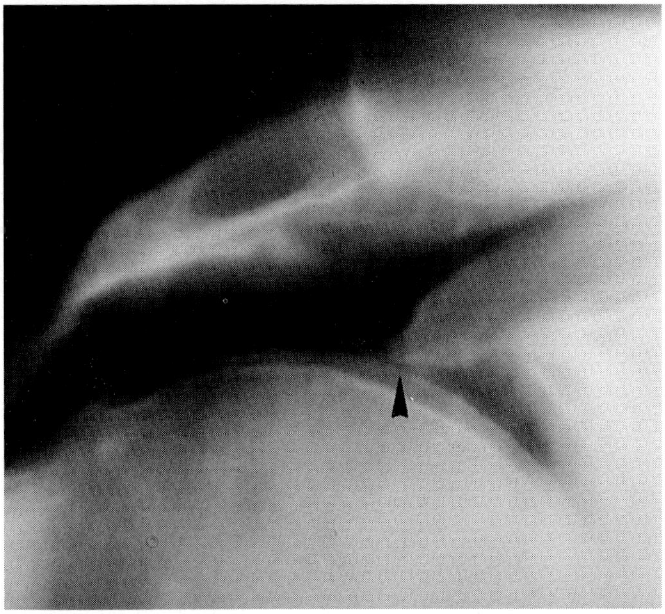

Fig. 27–2. Chronic massive rotator cuff tear on frontal view of preoperative air-constant arthrography: supraspinatus tendon is retracted above the superior rim of glenoid (arrow).

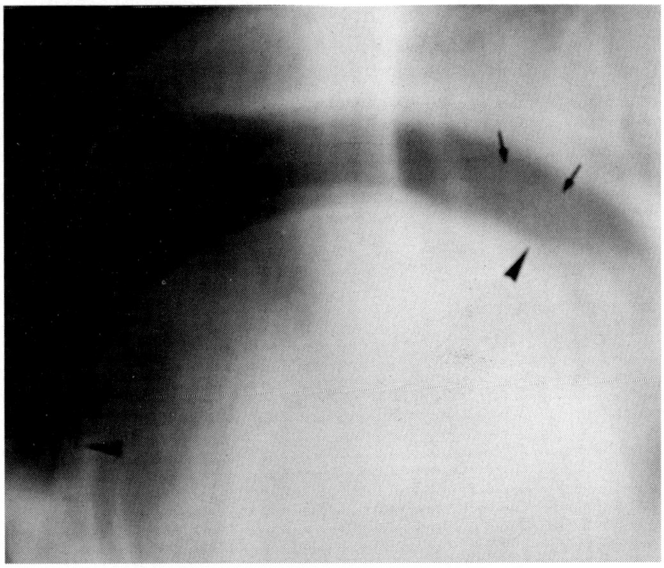

Fig. 27–3. Sagittal view of the same tear: posterior extension of the defect to the infraspinatus tendon.

The aim of preoperative rehabilitation is threefold. The first goal is to overcome joint stiffness with daily passive, assisted exercises in all ranges of movement. A stiff shoulder joint is an absolute contraindication for deltoid flap repair, as early exercising of the flap would not be possible with a stiff joint and results for active mobility would be disappointing. The second goal is to strengthen the deltoid muscle, which is to be partly transplanted, so that optimum local trophicity can be achieved before surgery. The third goal is equally important, because this period is used to teach the patient the exercises to be performed immediately after surgery, particularly early exercising of the flap. This period is also a time of mental preparation, in which the purpose of surgery is explained to the patient who is informed of the importance of postoperative rehabilitation, of the consequences on his personal and occupational life, and of the length of time that may be required before he can return to work. Because patients often are manual workers, they need to be fully aware of any financial problems that may arise.

Precise, reproducible imaging will demonstrate the extent of lesions and whether or not they are repairable (Figs. 27–2 and 27–3). Such information must be obtained preoperatively and should not be a surprise finding at surgery, in which case deltoid flap repair will have to be improvised under poor technical conditions. A massive cuff tear must be demonstrated by frontal and sagittal views using reliable imaging performed on a supple shoulder. Before repair it is necessary to know whether the tear is an isolated one of the supraspinatus retracted around the glenoid and whether the tear extends either anterior or posterior.

Since 1985 we have used an air contrast arthrography technique described by Bernageau.[5] This technique has always been fully satisfactory, especially with regard to clinical and radiographic correlation. Our definition of a massive tear includes not only a retracted tendon but also a time correlate. In patients who have been suffering from discomfort for a long time and have no history of recent trauma, the retraction of the tendon under such conditions is definitive. Sagittal scans demonstrate any posterior extension of the tear to the infraspinatus. Tears extending anterior to the subscapularis can be determined by systematic arthroscanning, which as described by Goutaillier and Bernageau[6] also demonstrates any signs of fatty degeneration of the rotator cuff muscles that may oppose the decision to perform deltoid flap repair. It is also possible, of course, to use MRI for this preoperative imaging.

SURGICAL TECHNIQUE

Patient Positioning

The patient is placed sitting or in the beach chair position, arm at the side, with the elbow resting on a support. The surgeon stands opposite the shoulder to be operated with the chief assistant next to the patient's head.

Surgical Approach

An anterosuperior lateral approach is used starting from the lateral segment of the clavicle, passing over the AC joint and the acromion, and finishing approximately 4 cm under the lateral edge of the acromion (Fig. 27–4). The subcutaneous layer is detached at the front and back. A vertical incision is made in the anterior deltoid along the axis of the AC joint, which is left undisturbed, to the junction between the internal and medial bundles of the anterior deltoid. The deltoid muscle fibers are then divided across their full thickness over a distance of 3 to 4 cm, starting from the acromioclavicular space. The antero-lateral bundle of the deltoid is then detached from the antero-superior edge of the acromion. It is important to perform this detachment subperiosteally, in order to provide firm tissue for suturing between the edges of the remaining cuff and the medial border of the flap that is attached at the acromial border. The anterior medial deltoid is not detached at the clavicle. A retractor is placed under the anterior lateral deltoid that has been detached from the acromion, taking care not to damage the future deltoid flap. Anterior acromioplasty with resection of the coracoacromial ligament is systematically carried out; it is of prime importance to achieve adequate bone decompression, thus giving a flat acromion that will not be a source of harm for the underlying deltoid flap.

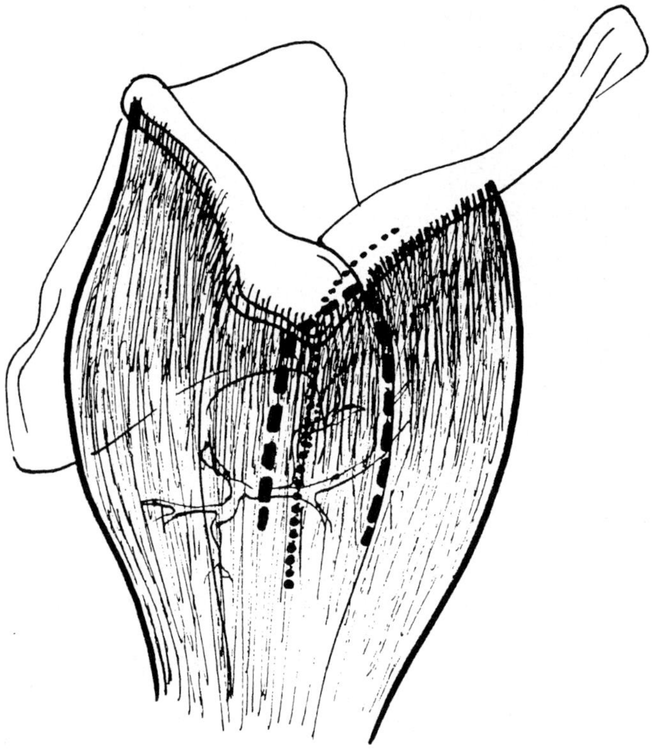

Fig. 27–4. Surgical technique of deltoid flap. Antero-supero-lateral approach (.....) design of deltoid flap (-----).

Assessment of Lesions

The cuff tear is now fully visible and the long head of the biceps tendon usually is exposed. After total excision of the subacromial bursa, precise assessment is made of the remaining tendinous cuff. In our experience, intraoperative data have, in most cases, confirmed the information given by preoperative arthrography. At the very least, in chronic massive tears the supraspinatus tendon has disappeared entirely and its retracted sleeve overhangs the upper rim of the glenoid by a few millimeters. The tear may extend back towards the infraspinatus, whose upper edge will appear worn and thinned; it might have disappeared altogether, in which case the upper tip of the teres minor can be seen at the back of the operative field. The tear also may extend anterior towards the subscapularis. The head of the long biceps is examined for signs of dislocation or subluxation, and its degenerative lesions are assessed. The tendinous tissues of the remaining cuff that appear fragile and devascularized are resected to leave a vascularized, bleeding edge so that the flap can be solidly anchored. Also, a complete capsulotomy is required around the superior and posterior rims of the glenoid to free the sleeve of the remaining cuff and to facilitate suturing the deltoid flap.

Flap Size

The width of the flap ultimately depends on the width of the tear in the sagittal plane. The anterior border is formed by the initial incision between the anteromedial head and the anterolateral head, and the medial border is the former acromial insertion. The deltoid flap is cut outwards into the medial deltoid, and its length relates to the anteroposterior extension of the tear. The posterior border of the flap is formed by the posterior incision, which must not be cut lower than 4 cm away from the lateral edge of the acromion to avoid possible damage to axillary nerve branches. The muscle fibers are divided throughout the entire thickness of the deltoid around this posterior lateral incision. The underlying surface of the flap is freed from the subdeltoid bursa plane. The base of the flap needs to be sufficiently wide, approximately 2 to 3 cm, to maintain its vascularization and innervation.

Associated Surgical Procedures

At this stage, a certain number of associated procedures can be performed, particularly ablation of an inferior clavicular osteophyte or detachment of the coracohumeral ligament in the event of reduced external rotation.

Suturing the Deltoid Flap

Nonabsorbable sutures are sewn from the upper to the lower surface along the edges of the remaining cuff, taking a firm hold (Fig. 27–5). The sutures must be passed first through the posterior segment of the tear at the upper part of the teres minor or infraspinatus, then taken gradually down towards the midportion at the free end of the supraspinatus sleeve and down as far as the upper part of the subscapularis tendon. Six to eight sutures can be made along the edges of the remaining cuff; the needle used is not discarded. Each suture is then drawn upwards from the undersurface to the corresponding surface of the flap, taking care to include the superficial aponeurosis. All the sutures are held by forceps. Each suture is knotted by hand ties, with the deepest-lying sutures in the posterior corner of the tear. It is most important that the suture knots rest against the aponeurosis of the deltoid flap to avoid having to make muscular knots that are less resistant. The strongest sutures are those joining the acromial segment and the adjacent anterior and posterior parts of the flap, where the superfi-

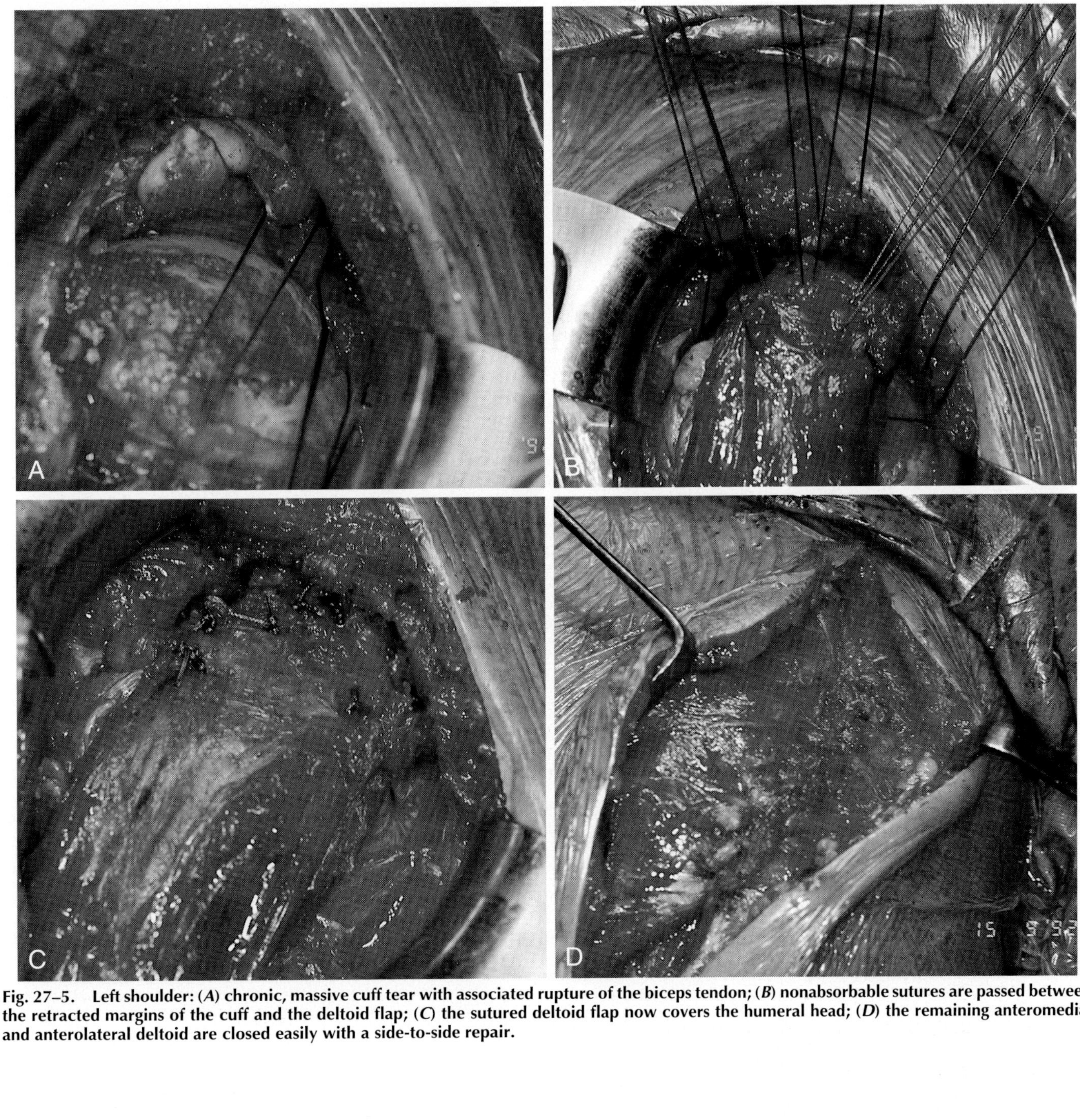

Fig. 27–5. Left shoulder: (*A*) chronic, massive cuff tear with associated rupture of the biceps tendon; (*B*) nonabsorbable sutures are passed between the retracted margins of the cuff and the deltoid flap; (*C*) the sutured deltoid flap now covers the humeral head; (*D*) the remaining anteromedial and anterolateral deltoid are closed easily with a side-to-side repair.

cial aponeurosis is strongest. The other anterior and posterior sutures are muscular sutures on a thin aponeurosis, which are relatively weaker.

Closing the Tear

The closing stage is problem free, provided two technical conditions have been followed: the deltoid has not been detached from the clavicle and the acromial dissection is subperiosteal. The upper, medial edge of the initial deltoid incision is sutured to the trapeziodeltoid cap over the acromion and the lower medial edge to the anterior border of the medial deltoid. In this way the flap is covered easily by the anteromedial deltoid, thus avoiding any subcutaneous trough that would be unaesthetic. Care must be taken not to strangulate the base of the flap around the lower part of the incision. A suction drain is put in place and left for 48 hours.

Postoperative Care

The operated upper limb is placed in a light, removable abduction wedge adjusted at 70° while the patient is still anesthetized on the operating table. Postoperative rehabilitation is started the day after surgery.

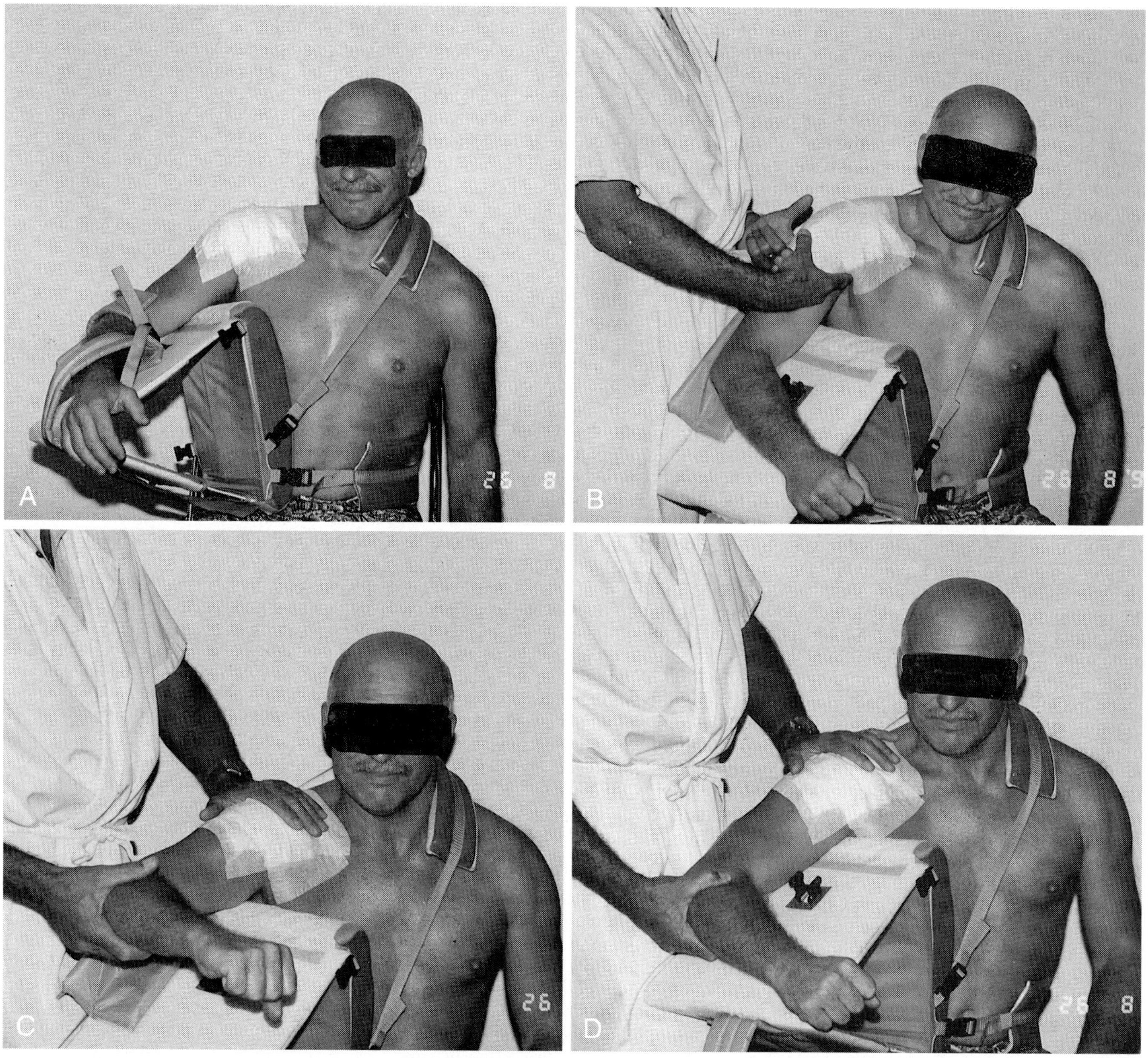

Fig. 27–6. Postoperative rehabilitation of deltoid flap: (*A*) abduction wedge at 70° first 6 weeks; (*B*) isometric resistance; (*C*) passive elevation off pillow; (*D*) passive external rotation off pillow; (*E*) pendulum exercises; (*F*) passive flexion using opposite arm; (*G*) assisted external rotation; (*H*) assisted elevation; (*I*) early goals achieved of active flexion, abduction, and external rotation; (*J*) assisted flexion with stick; (*K*) adduction exercises with elastic band; (*L*) rotation exercises with elastic band; and (*M*) press-up exercise.

POSTOPERATIVE SHOULDER REHABILITATION

Immediate postoperative rehabilitation is of vital importance and must be strictly followed to ensure a good functional result within a reasonable period of time. The upper limb is rested in an abduction wedge set at 70° abduction. This wedge is worn night and day for 30 days and then during the daytime only from day 30 to day 45 postoperatively (Fig. 27–6).

Postoperative rehabilitation has two main goals.

First, to protect the flap against subacromial compression and tensioning. This protection is obtained by active shoulder-stump depressor exercises with the humerus carrying out an external piston movement. Any tensioning is avoided by permanent wearing of the wedge. Second, early exercising of the flap is indispensable to maintain its contractile property and to avoid its atrophy.

The rehabilitation program is as follows:

Day 1 — Mobilization of elbow, wrist, and fingers on the wedge.

Day 2 — With the patient sitting, active depressor exercises of the shoulder are performed, external piston movement of the humerus against physiotherapist's manual resistance. Passive raising of the upper limb is added by the physiotherapist, with the patient attempting to hold this position by isometric contraction of the deltoid. The arm is returned to the wedge against manual resistance. Passive mobilization in external rotation within the limit set by pain.

Day 3 — Pendulum exercises are added with the torso leaning over 90°.

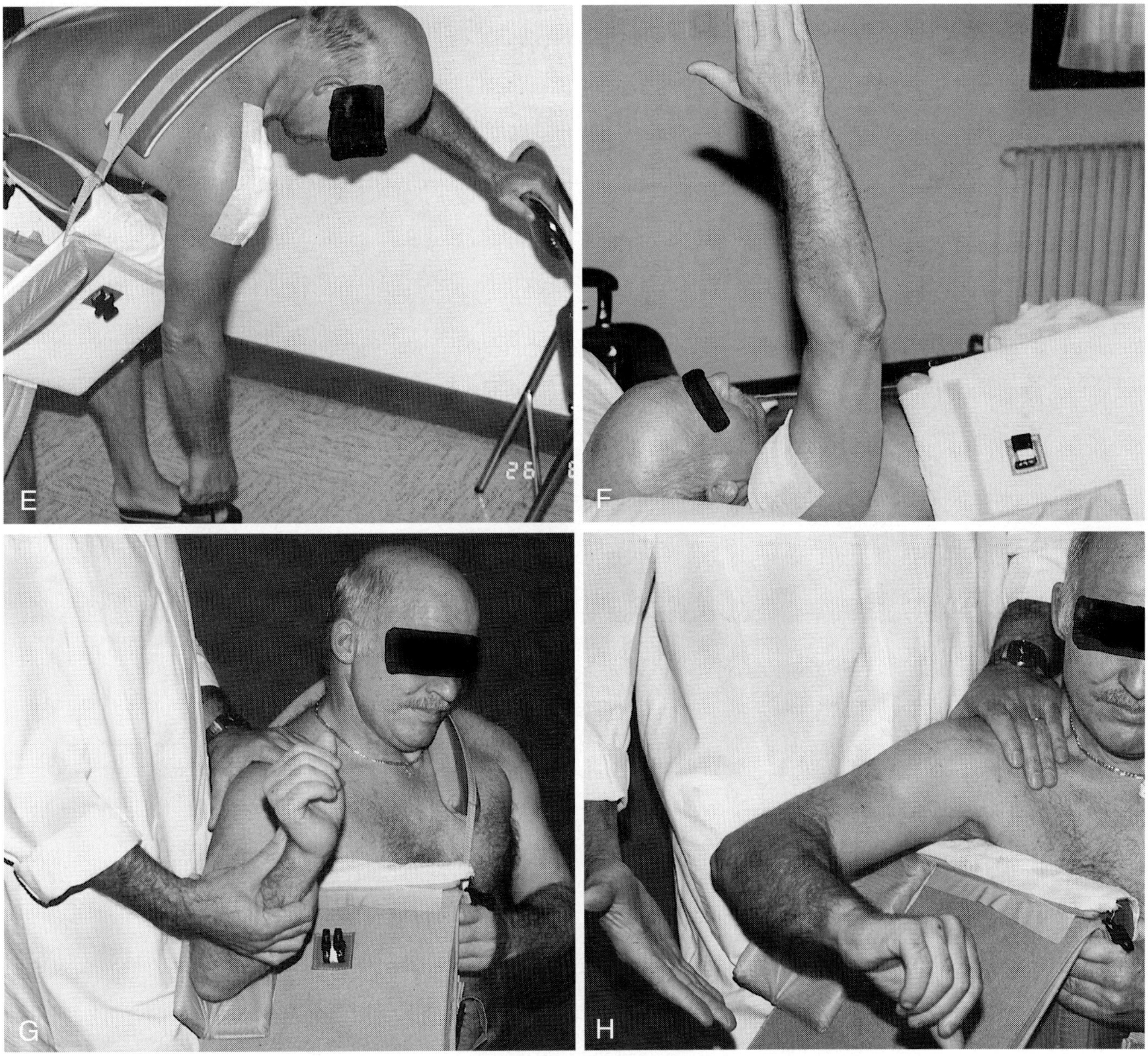

Fig. 27–6. ***continued***

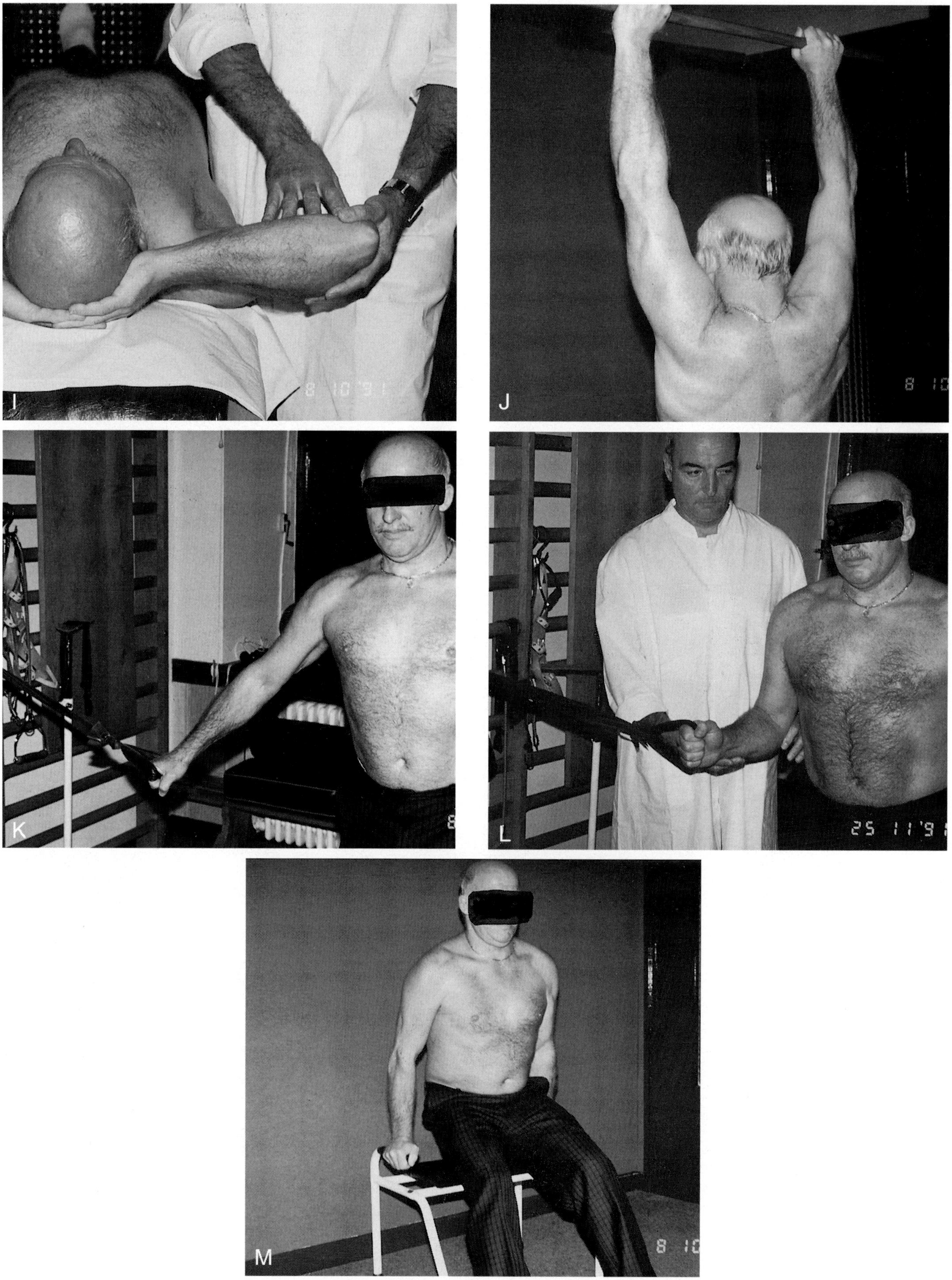

Fig. 27–6. *continued*

Day 4 — Passive flexion exercises are added using the opposite arm with the patient lying on his/her back.
Day 5 — With the patient sitting, assisted active external rotation is performed followed by nonassisted rotation on the wedge.
Day 15 — When the patient leaves the Shoulder Unit, he/she should be able to (1) lying, achieve passive flexion in line with the plane of the bed (about 160°) and (2) sitting, be able to hold his arm actively at 90° flexion with the elbow bent and achieve 45° active external rotation on the wedge. The patient must perform rehabilitation exercises on his/her own 3 times a day, carrying out pendulum and passive flexion exercises. Three times a week, the patient must attend physiotherapy; the physiotherapist will teach the patient shoulder depressor movements and will carry out isometric exercises of the deltoid.
Day 45 — The wedge is removed and replaced by a cushion worn over the shoulder. Assisted active flexion, extension, and internal rotation exercises are performed holding a stick. Assisted by the physiotherapist, active external rotation is carried out with the elbow at the side and the arm in abduction. Depressor exercises adducting the upper limb against elastic resistance are added.
Day 50 — The cushion is removed.
Day 60 — Exercises to strengthen the internal and external rotators (with elbow at the side) against elastic resistance are added.
Day 90 — Deltoid strengthening occurs under close supervision of the physiotherapist to prevent elevation of the shoulder stump.
Day 120 — Readaption to exertion is added: press-ups, ball games, proprioceptive exercises, and balneotherapy.

CONCLUSIONS

The postoperative rehabilitation of a deltoid flap is critical and must be followed with strict care; it is also long, and the patient must be informed beforehand. This rehabilitation is both manual and individual. Postoperative rehabilitation using pulleys, mechanotherapy, or arthromotors is contraindicated.

RESULTS

Clinical Results

During the period from 1986 to 1991, 95 patients were treated in our Shoulder Unit for chronic, massive cuff tears revealed by contrast arthrography made by the same radiographic unit. Medical treatment based on rehabilitation to overcome stiffness and strengthen the humeral head depressor muscles proved to be sufficient in 140 patients (72%) whose recovery of function met their expectations. Arthroscopic debridement was suggested for 35 patients (18%) who had recovered normal active movement but who still suffered from pain, usually caused by impingement between an overhanging anteroinferior acromion and a degenerative biceps tendon. Deltoid flap repair was suggested in 20 patients (10%), 16 men and 4 women of average age 58 (range = 47 to 73 years). Fourteen of these patients were active manual workers, of which 11 (79%) were off work for massive cuff tear and resulting functional disability. Six of these patients were industrial injuries. Five other patients were retired, and one patient worked at home. Functional disability had lasted an average of 21 months (range = 6 months to 10 years). Deltoid flap repair was suggested to these 20 patients, as they still suffered functional discomfort after a 6-month period of specific rehabilitation based on strengthening the humeral head depressor muscles. This functional discomfort prevented 11 of the 14 manual workers from returning to work. All 14 patients suffered from pain and muscular fatigue. After this preoperative rehabilitation, active anterior elevation attained was 120° in 55% of patients and was less than 90° in 45%, although normal passive movement was recovered in all patients. No patient with a stiff shoulder had surgery, stiffness being a surgical contraindication for deltoid flap repair. In our experience, the lesions found at surgery confirmed preoperative imaging data. In four patients (20%), the tear involved the supraspinatus retracted at the glenoid; in seven patients (35%), both the supraspinatus and the infraspinatus retracted at the glenoid were involved; in six patients (30%), the tear involved the supraspinatus retracted at the glenoid with extension to the upper third of the subscapularis; and in three patients (15%), the tear involved both the supraspinatus and the infraspinatus retracted at the glenoid with extension to the upper third of the subscapularis. The long head of the biceps tendon was normal in eight patients, degenerate five times, dislocated four times, and torn in three patients. Tenodesis was required in seven patients, given the extent of the degenerate lesions.

The 20 patients were seen at follow-up by a rehabilitation specialist other than the surgeon after an average period of 40 months (range = 14 to 52 months). Results (Table 27–1) regarding pain were noteworthy, because

Table 27–1. Clinical Results of Deltoid Flap (20 Cases) of Pain, Active Forward Elevation, Muscular Strength, and Constant's Score

No. of Cases Preoperative		*Pain*	*No. of Cases Postoperative*
		None	9
2		Slight	11
16		Moderate	
2		Severe	
		Active Forward Elevation	
7		>150°	13
4		120–150°	1
		90–120°	1
4		60–90°	1
3		30–60°	4
2		0–30°	
		Muscular Strength (lbs)	
		>10	
		5 to 10	6
9		1 to 4	8
11		0	6
		Constant's Score/100 Pts	
	80–100 pts	5	25%—Excellent results
	65–79 pts	7	35%—Good results
6	51–64 pts	3	15%—Fair results
14	0–50 pts	5	25%—Poor results

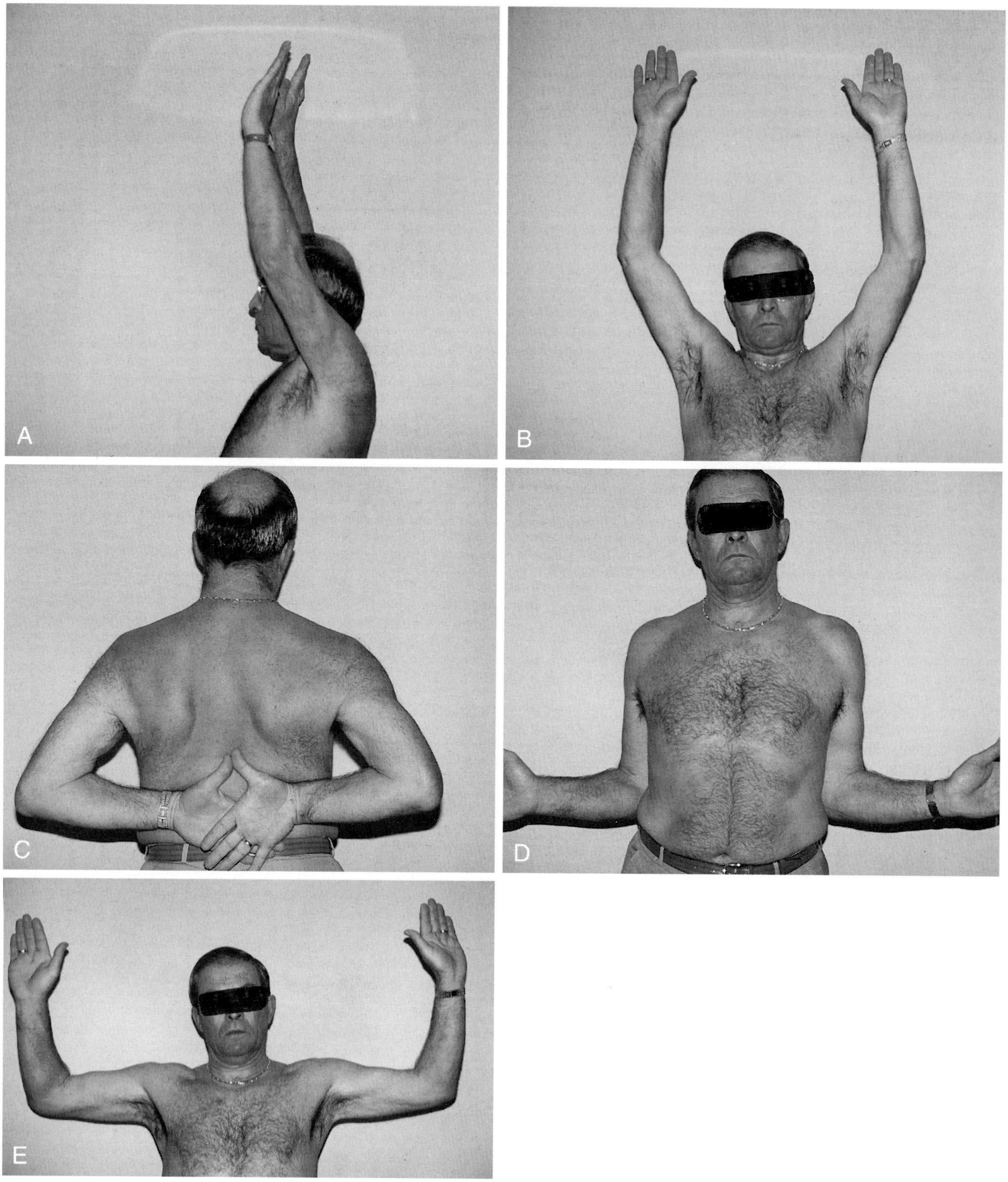

Fig. 27–7. Clinical result with 2-year follow-up of bilateral deltoid flap on a 62-year-old man (*A*); (*B*) forward elevation; (*C*) internal rotation; and (*D and E*) external rotation.

45% of those patients undergoing operation no longer suffered from pain, and 55% suffered slight pain on exertion. The level of activity achieved postoperatively was satisfactory in 65% of patients. Thirteen (65%) patients had recovered full active anterior elevation, which ranged between 90 and 150° in four patients but was less than 90° in five patients (Fig. 27–7). Internal rotation with the hand behind the back was normal in over 80%; external rotation, with the arm abducted at 90°, reached 70° in 14 patients (70%). Of the 10 patients who were unable to abduct the arm in lateral rotation preoperatively, six (60%) recovered this movement after surgery, of whom three had surgery for a tear involving both the supraspinatus and the infraspinatus. Muscular strength was improved in 14 patients (70%), but on average the improvement was low. However, these 14 patients no longer complained of muscular fatigue. Postoperative muscular strength scored a zero rating in six patients (30%). Jobe's test was positive in all patients, regardless of the score achieved for muscular strength. Constant's nonweighted score showed a total increase from 41/100 points preoperatively (range, 11 to 58) to 63/100 postoperatively (range = 32 to 83). Objective overall results assessed using Constant's scale were excellent (25%), good (35%), average (15%), and poor (25%). Seventeen of the 20 patients were satisfied (85%). Eleven of the 14 active workers were able to return to work at the 12th postoperative month (4 of the 6 industrial injuries).

With regard to postoperative complications, there were no cases of infection, flap necrosis, or damage to the axillary nerve. No cosmetic deformities occurred. One patient required subsequent arthroscopic acromioplasty to treat pain resulting from insufficient anterio-inferior acromioplasty.

The clinical results observed in this personal series were fully comparable with those reported previously by two other European investigators, Augereau and Saragaglia.[7] It is difficult to compare results from different series, especially for a surgery such as this in which the indication for deltoid flap repair may vary according to surgeon, tear size, and the patient population. However, two basic concepts emerge from these two publications: (1) deltoid flap repair has a remarkable effect on pain, and (2) postoperative strength is often fairly weak. A period of 12 to 18 months is required before maximum muscular strength can be recovered. This figure, although never exceeding an average of 6 lbs, fortunately is enough that muscular fatigue pain is overcome, thus enabling active patients to return to work.

Overall objective results, assessed using Constant's scoring method and reported by the three investigators who have published their work on the deltoid flap, are summarized in (Table 27–2).[8–10]

Table 27–2. Objective Reported Results of Deltoid Flap

	Postoperative Constant's Score/100 pts				
	Average	*80–100 pts Excellent*	*65–79 pts Good*	*51–64 pts Fair*	*0–50 pts Poor*
Augereau (76 cases)	61 pts	26%	45%	10%	19%
Gazielly (20 cases)	63 pts	25%	35%	15%	25%
Saragaglia (28 cases)	68 pts	19%	51%	11%	19%

Radiographic Results

The postoperative acromiohumeral space measured 7 mm or more in 60% of the patients in our series. Of the 10 patients in which preoperative imaging showed an acromiohumeral space of less than 7 mm, two were increased to exceed 7 mm. In no case did flap repair cause acromiohumeral impingement. Augereau reported 17 patients (37%) whose humeral heads were recentered.

Anatomical Results

We used ultrasonography (performed by a doctor with a long experience in rotator cuff ultrasonography, especially after cuff surgery) to analyze the anatomical results of these 20 deltoid flap repairs. A 7.5-mHz transducer was used. All 20 flaps were seen after a minimum follow-up period of 12 months. Eighteen flaps (90%) appeared continuous on postoperative ultrasonographs; 13 flaps were thick (5 to 9 mm) with a striated structure in half of this number (Fig. 27–8). These 13 continuous, thick flaps related to 12 excellent or very good functional results and one fair result. Five flaps (25%) were continuous but thinner (4 mm) and more importantly, showed a fibrous appearance on postoperative ultrasonographs. These five thinner continuous flaps related to four poor results and one fair result. In one patient, the flap had disappeared and functional results were poor. Finally, in one case the flap was visible but discontinuous, appearing torn in the front portion with a fair functional result.

Augereau[2] reported 22 flaps assessed by MRI after an average follow-up period of 2.5 years. Eighteen were continuous with an intact cuff. Twelve of these showed homogenous stroma and thickness of 2 mm or more, which yielded nine excellent and five good results. Four flaps appeared discontinuous and gave two very good and two poor results.

Generally speaking, it would appear that there is a certain parallel between anatomical and clinical results. We endeavored to ascertain whether there was a good anatomo-clinical correlation for the three fair results (15%) and the five poor results (25%). The purpose of analyzing these fair and poor results for the correlation between anatomical and clinical results in our series was to determine more precisely the indications and contraindications for deltoid flap repair in massive, irreparable cuff tears with a tendinous defect.

The three fair results, which obtained a postoperative constant score of between 51 and 64/100, included two male patients and one female patient. Functionally, all three patients no longer suffered pain and achieved active flexion of 110° and average lateral rotation of 60° in abduction, but muscular strength was poor in the two

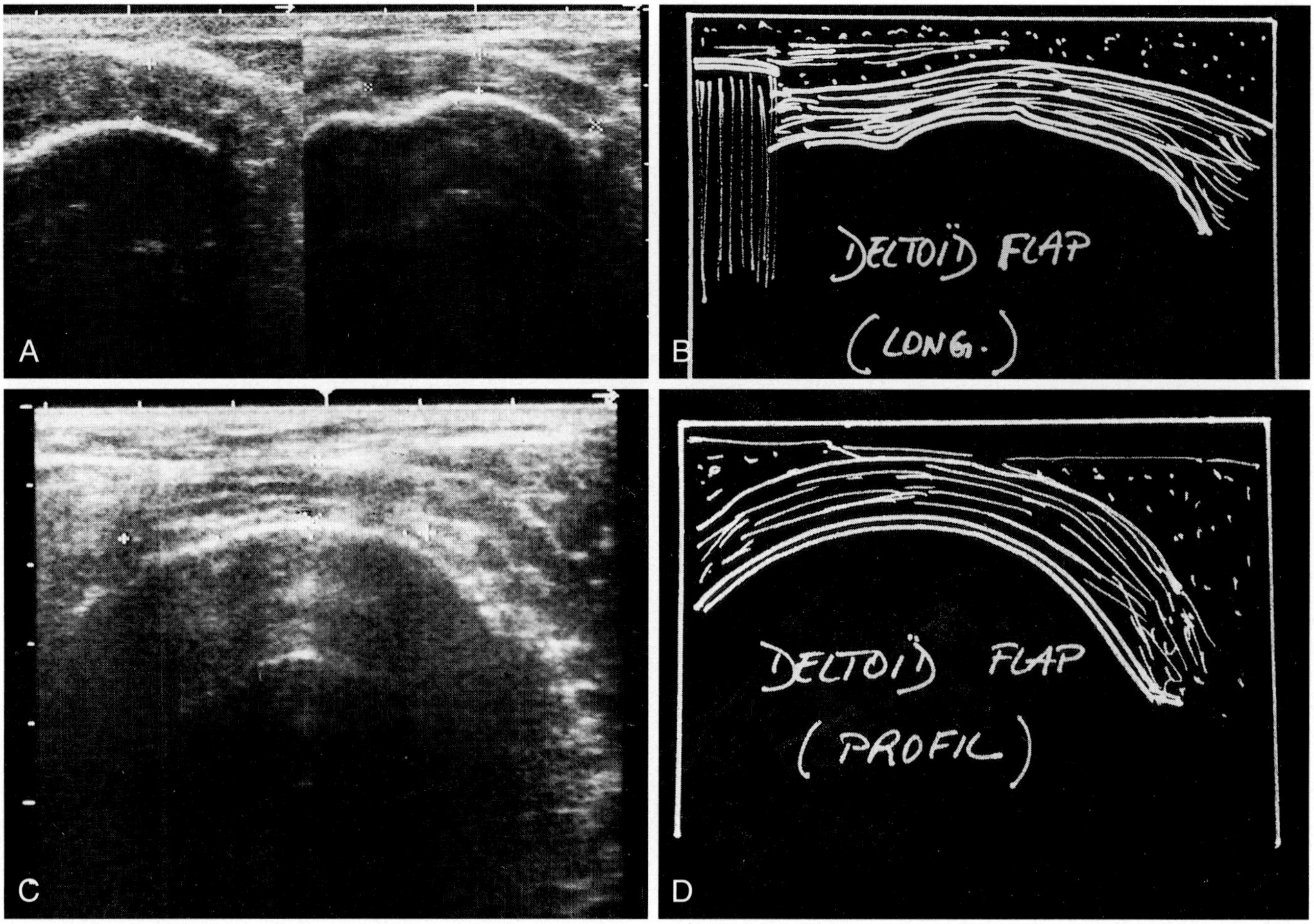

Fig. 27–8. ***A,*** **Postoperative ultrasound confirms the integrity of the flap in the longitudinal plane.** ***B,*** **Graphic representation of ultrasound depicted in** ***A. C,*** **Ultrasonographic evaluation in the sagittal plane allows visualization of the deltoid flap covering the humeral head.** ***D,*** **Graphic representation of ultrasound depicted in** ***C.***

male patients and rated zero in the female patient. Postoperative ultrasonographs showed a thin, fibrous flap in one of the male patients, aged 63 years, who had undergone surgery twice previously for recurrent cuff tear. The female patient, aged 50 years, also showed a thin, fibrous cuff; initial general muscular quality in this patient was poor, especially the deltoid muscle. Finally, the third patient was a young male patient, aged 45 years, in whom the deltoid flap appeared torn in its front portion. Early overuse at the third postoperative month against medical advice accounted for this fair result.

The five poor results obtained postoperative constant scores of between 0 and 50/100 points. In four cases, patients were over the age of 65 and had thin deltoid muscles. In all four cases, preoperative active movement was reduced, even after a specific rehabilitation period of 6 months. Results were good regarding pain but poor for active movement, which did not recover, and muscular strength, which remained poor. In two patients the flap had disappeared, and two other patients showed fibrous involution. Finally, in the fifth case (a farmer) the poor result was caused by a fall 3 years after surgery, whereas the objective functional result before the fall had been good. The deltoid flap at ultrasonography was thin and fibrous.

CONCLUSIONS

Considering the results published for different series of deltoid flap repair and our own personal experience, it would appear that this type of surgery offers a reliable alternative for treating chronic, massive rotator cuff tears. It is a surgical technique with practically no morbidity and is effective for pain relief and restoration of active movement. In most cases, muscular fatigue is overcome, thus allowing active patients to return to work. However, these results are only possible provided five conditions are met.

The first concerns the indications that we believe are most specific: deltoid flap repair is indicated in active, motivated adults with good muscular quality who have managed to recover near normal active movement after specific rehabilitation but who continue to suffer from pain and muscular fatigue, preventing their return to work. Deltoid flap repair requires advance programming, as postoperative leave from work lasts an average of 6 to 12 months depending upon the type of work involved.

The second condition is to take full heed of contraindications. In our experience, this type of surgery is contraindicated in patients over 65 with signs of fatty muscular degeneration on preoperative imaging, with a thin deltoid muscle, who do not manage to recover satisfactory active movement after a specific rehabilitation program.

Third, accurate surgical technique is required. In our opinion, deltoid flap repair cannot be improvised intraoperatively and requires a specific surgical approach. Subperiosteal detachment from its acromial insertion of the antero-lateral bundle alone is of fundamental importance, as is subacromial bone decompression which must be adequate. The sutures joining the flap borders and the cuff edges must be solidly anchored to allow immediate postoperative rehabilitation.

Fourth, postoperative rehabilitation is unavoidable if deltoid flap repair is to be successful. This rehabilitation must be carried out by a team of specialists; it is meticulous, manual, and of long duration, requiring strict discipline and strong patient motivation. The main objectives of this rehabilitation, it is recalled, are to protect the flap and to allow early mobility and strengthening.

Finally, the fifth condition for success is to allow the flap to fulfill its biomechanical role while avoiding excessive demand on its capacity. The deltoid flap appears to complete or to take over the action of the intrinsic and extrinsic depressors of the humeral head and contributes to the dynamic repositioning of the humeral pivot.

If these five conditions are fulfilled, deltoid flap repair is, in our opinion, a totally satisfactory form of surgery that warrants use whenever simple suturing or transosseous reattachment with the arm at the side is not possible.

REFERENCES

1. Takagishi N. The new operation for the massive rotator cuff rupture. *J Jap Orthop Assoc.* 1978;52:775–780.
2. Augereau B. Traitement chirurgical des ruptures de la coiffe des rotateurs, Cahiers d'Enseignement SOFCOT. *Expansion Scientifique Francaise.* Paris. 1989;161.
3. Howell SM, Imobersteg AM, Seger DH. Clarification of the role of the supraspinatus muscle in shoulder function. *J Bone Joint Surg Am.* 1986;68.
4. Gazielly DF. Preoperative management and rehabilitation of rotator cuff tears. In: Post M, Morrey BF, Hawkins RJ, eds. *Surgery of the Shoulder.* St. Louis: Mosby-Year Book; 1990:234–237.
5. Bernageau J, Patte D. Bilan radiologique pre-operatorie de la periarthrite scapulo-humerale. Interet de l'arthro- pneumotomographie. *J Radio Electromyogr.* 1972;53:432–437.
6. Goutallier D, Bernageau J, Patte D. L'evolution par scanner de la trophicite des muscles de la coiffe des rotateurs. *Rev Chir Orthop.* 1989 (supplement 1):126.
7. Saragaglia D, Cambuzat A, Tourne Y, et al. Transfer of the deltoid muscular flap for massive defects of the rotator cuff: 27 patients. Presented at the Fifth International Conference on Surgery of the Shoulder, Abstract No. 26, in *J Shoulder Elbow Surg.* 1993;2, Part 2.
8. Constant CR, Murley AMG. A clinical method of functional assessment of the shoulder. *Clin Orthop.* 1987;214:160–164.
9. Gazielly DF. Deltoid muscular flap transfer for treatment of massive rotator cuff tears. Presented at the 10th Annual Meeting of American Shoulder and Elbow Surgeons. Seattle, WA, September 4–7, 1991.
10. Gazielly DF, Jully JL, Montagnon C. Deltoid muscular flap transfer for the treatment of massive rotator cuff tears. Presented at the Fifth International Conference on Surgery of the Shoulder, Abstract No. 25, in *J Shoulder Elbow Surg.* 1993; vol. 2.

Chapter 28

Latissimus Dorsi Transfer for Massive Cuff Defects

Marybeth Ezaki

Massive defects of the rotator cuff that cause in the patient loss of function or disabling pain are a difficult challenge. Operative repairs of tears of the rotator cuff do not always succeed or are not possible because of the size of the tear or deficiency or poor quality of cuff tissues. Tight closure of the rotator cuff using local tissues resulted in only 68% favorable outcomes in Debeyre's series cited by Patte.[1] In his review of repeat repairs of rotator cuff defects, Bigliani found that 10 of the 11 patients with deficient tissues had a poor result.[2] Not all tears of the rotator cuff need to be repaired. Burkhead and Rockwood have shown that debridement of the rotator cuff may be a reasonable option if extrinsic muscle control is adequate.[3] This has also been noted by Gschwend who reported that in cases of defective rotator cuffs with no signs of ''pseudoparalysis'' good function was maintained.[4] Other factors such as coordinating intrinsic and extrinsic muscles of the shoulder are as important as the condition of the rotator cuff tendon itself.

TREATMENT OPTIONS

The options for the surgical treatment of large defects in the rotator cuff have included tissue augmentation with local muscle advancement, ''distant'' muscle substitution, use of substances such as freeze-dried allograft cuff tissue, and synthetic cuff prostheses such as Marlex (Davol, Cranston, RI). Mobilization of the subscapularis muscle and tendon was described by Cofield,[5] the infraspinatus and subscapularis by Neer,[6] subscapularis and teres minor by R.J. Neviaser and J.J. Neviaser,[7] the supraspinatus muscle by Ha'eri and Wiley,[8] and both the supraspinatus and infraspinatus muscles by Debeyre.[1]

Use of the biceps tendon or the coracoacromial ligament as local sources of tissue or free fascia lata graft have been described. Bigliani states that there is no adequate substitute for the rotator cuff and does not recommend allografts and synthetic prostheses as a reconstructive option.[2] Only one investigator writes about transfer of the latissimus dorsi tendon to supplement the tissues of the deficient rotator cuff in the adult. Gerber has shown encouraging results with this technique that are comparable to other series in the treatment of a selected group of patients with massive cuff tears.[9–11] He relates the functional loss in the patient with massive rotator cuff deficiency to the patient with a brachial plexus injury with loss of suprascapular nerve function. Transfer of the latissimus dorsi tendon to the cuff in paralytic conditions partially restores motor function to assist in abduction of the shoulder, as well as stabilizing the humeral head-glenoid fulcrum. The depressor force of the latissimus theoretically can limit cranial migration of the humeral head and further impingement.

LATISSIMUS DORSI: ANATOMY AND FUNCTION

The latissimus dorsi is a large, flat muscle that takes origin from the dorsal spines of T7 through L5, the sacrum and the crest of the ilium. It may also have origins on the lowest three or four ribs and an attachment on the inferior pole of the scapula. Its insertion is into the medial crest and floor of the bicipital groove of the proximal humerus, providing a strong internal rotational moment. The innervation of the latissimus dorsi is through the thoracodorsal nerve, which is mainly from the C7 root via the posterior cord of the brachial plexus. The blood supply is through the long, constant thoracodorsal pedicle that lies on the anterolateral surface of the muscle in the axilla (Fig. 28–1).

The latissimus dorsi muscle may be used for many different soft-tissue problems. It is thin, broad, and has a long dependable neurovascular pedicle. Its presence in situ is not necessary for shoulder function. All or part of it can be transferred as a unipolar transplantation, moving only the insertion, as done by Zachary,[12] into an externally rotating position on the humerus, or as a Clark-type transfer with a prolongation graft to motor elbow flexion. It can be used as a bipolar transfer, moving both the origin and insertion such as in the procedures to restore elbow flexion or extension following neurologic injury.[13] The latissimus can also be transferred to a distant site using microvascular technique to cover a number of defects, either with or without a skin paddle.

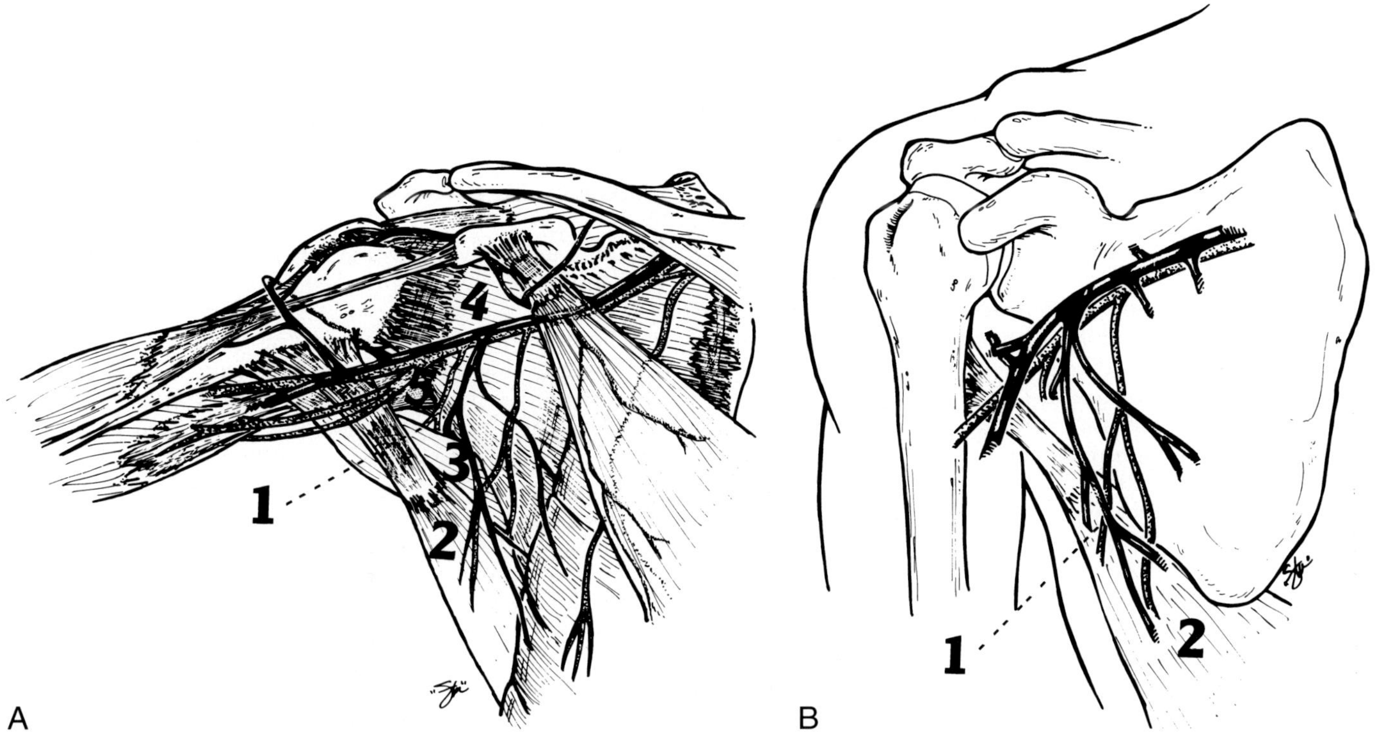

Fig. 28–1. *A,* **Relationship of thoracodorsal neurovascular bundle (1) to the anterior aspect of the latissimus dorsi (2), the teres minor (3), and the quadrangular space (4).** *B,* **Close-up view of thoracodorsal artery, nerve (1), and latissimus dorsi (2).**

LATISSIMUS DORSI: REVIEW OF BIOMECHANICS AS APPLIED TO THE SHOULDER

The shoulder is a multiaxial and multiarticular joint. The instant center of rotation of the shoulder changes with motion, and the actions of muscles change depending on the position in relation to the center of rotation.[14] Saha studied shoulder muscle biomechanics and noted that the "action of all axio-scapulo-humeral group of muscles acting on the gleno-humeral joint changes continuously during elevation."[15] He divided the shoulder girdle musculature into three functional groups. The "prime movers" include the deltoid and the clavicular head of the pectoralis major. The components of the rotator cuff comprise the "steering group." The "depressor group" includes the sternal head of the pectoralis major, the latissimus dorsi, and the teres major and minor.

Two systems participate in shoulder abduction or elevation: the "intrinsic" supraspinatus-subscapularis-long head of biceps system and the "extrinsic" deltoid system.[14] The superior portion of the rotator cuff functions to stabilize the fulcrum for abduction of the glenohumeral joint. The long head of triceps, long head of biceps, coracobrachialis, and pectoralis minor all provide a longitudinal compressive force that permits superior subluxation of the humeral head. This "impinging" force must be counteracted by a humeral head depressor force.

Although there is debate over the exact role of the supraspinatus, its participation as a humeral head depressor is argued by Jones, Winslow, and Duchenne.[14] As is seen clinically, if the function of the supraspinatus is lost either by cuff deficiency or functional paralysis, cranial migration of the humeral head can occur and increase impingement. Although the latissimus dorsi functions as an extrinsic shoulder adductor, internal rotator, and depressor, electromyographic action potentials are present throughout the abduction range of the shoulder. The actual force vector applied by the latissimus changes with the position of the shoulder, so that at maximum shoulder abduction, the latissimus exerts almost pure glenohumeral compressive force. Saha found, by needle electrode, that the latissimus is maximally active at 180° of abduction.[15]

HISTORY OF USE OF LATISSIMUS DORSI IN TRANSFERS ABOUT THE SHOULDER

Much of the literature describing musculotendinous transfers to the rotator cuff deals with the clinical indications of poliomyelitis and other paralyzing conditions such as brachial plexopathy. The history of muscle transfer to the shoulder area largely begins with L'Episcopo, who in 1934 described a technique to rebalance the external and internal shoulder rotators in children affected by obstetrical traction injuries to the brachial plexus.[16]

He reported six cases in which he detached the teres minor tendon and reinserted it into the humerus in the interval between the long head of the triceps and the deltoid. Prior to his report only release of the internal rotation contracture had been reported. The specific use of the latissimus tendon as a transfer about the shoulder was reported in one case by Zachary;[12] this also was a child with a brachial plexopathy in whom he transferred both the latissimus dorsi and the teres major tendons to the posterior aspect of the humerus, attaching the tendon transplant to the periosteum and the lateral head of the triceps to provide external rotation. Saha described transferring the latissimus to the posterior portion of the greater tuberosity at the inferior attachment of the infraspinatus tendon in a case of poliomyelitis with shoulder imbalance.[15] Harmon used the latissimus in conjunction with multiple muscle transfers to provide motor function to the paralyzed shoulder.[17] Hoffer reported 11 cases of children with brachial plexopathy in which the latissimus and pectoralis major tendons were transferred to the posterior-superior aspect of the rotator cuff "as high as possible." This procedure was designed specifically to overcome the internal rotation contracture of the shoulder. No release of contractures were done concomitantly. The latissimus strength had to be a grade 4 or greater for the procedure to be considered.[18]

Gerber in 1988 reported the technique and preliminary results of latissimus dorsi transfer in 14 patients with loss of external rotation control and superior migration of the humeral head caused by massive tears in the rotator cuff.[9] In these patients, repair of the cuff to a bony trough on the humerus was not possible. He likens the functional loss to the patient with a brachial plexus injury with loss of suprascapular nerve function. Successful latissimus dorsi transfer provides abduction, external rotation, and depressor force to the shoulder. The indications for latissimus transfer were the presence of pain with decreased function and the inability to reconnect the cuff to a bony trough with the arm in 60° of abduction.

SURGICAL TECHNIQUE

The transfer of the latissimus dorsi muscle to the rotator cuff respects the principles of tendon transplantation surgery: a donor muscle of sufficient strength, a direct line of pull from the origin of donor to insertion of recipient, and adequate excursion of the muscle tendon unit. The latissimus has been shown to be active throughout the range of motion so that synergy with the new functional need is not an important consideration in this situation. The latissimus will function primarily as a tenodesis and not as a prime mover of the shoulder. The surgical technique is described by Gilbert[19] and Gerber[9] with several personal modifications.

The skin incisions used by Gerber are detailed in Figure 28–2. Alternatively, a transverse posterior axillary incision is made long enough to permit visualization of the inferior border of the latissimus muscle. The muscle is mobilized extensively along its superficial margins, inferiorly and posteriorly from its attachments to the inferior pole of the scapula and the overlying dorsal soft-tissue envelope. Along the anterior-inferior margin, the neurovascular pedicle is identified and carefully protected during the dissection of the tendon and its insertion onto the medial border of the humerus. The latissimus tendon is approximately 3 to 5 cm in width and 6 to 8 cm in length. It is very thin compared to the thickness of a healthy rotator cuff and must be handled with some care.

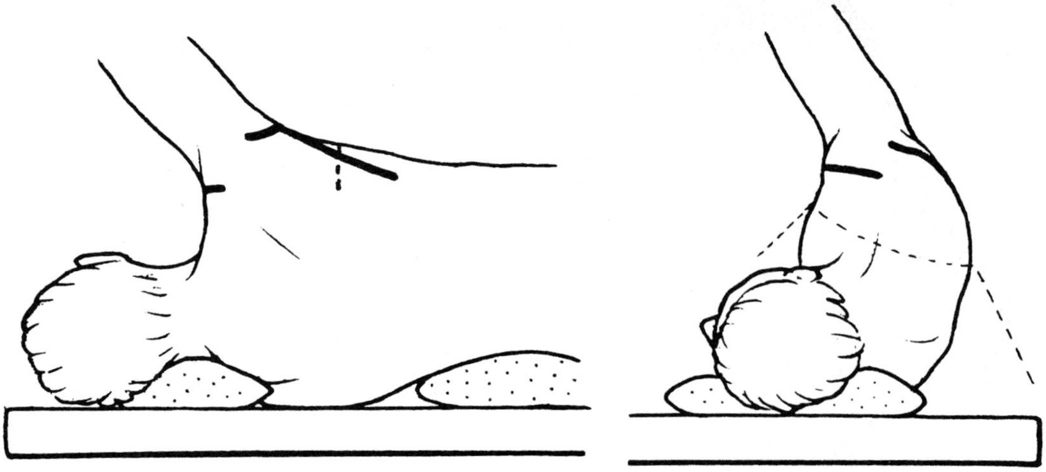

A B

Fig. 28–2. ***A and B,*** **Rear and axial views of the skin incision. Gerber recommends a longitudinal incision for exposure and harvesting of the latissimus dorsi (solid line A). Alternatively, a transverse incision can be used (broken line). A second superior approach is required for the decompression and anastomosis (solid line B). (From Gerber C, Vinh TS, Hertel R, Hess CW. Latissimus dorsi transfer for the treatment of massive tears of the rotator cuff. A preliminary report. *Clin Orthop.* 1988;232:51–61.)**

The tendon insertion can be visualized by abduction and internal rotation of the shoulder and the tendon is divided right at the bony insertion (Fig. 28–3). Great care is taken not to injure the posterior humeral circumflex artery at the superior edge of the tendon (Fig. 28–4). The latissimus sometimes shares a portion of tendon with the teres major, and it may be necessary to sharply separate the two. The latissimus tendon and muscle are mobilized to gain enough excursion to reach the postero-superior aspect of the rotator cuff with the shoulder at 60° of abduction (Fig. 28–5). This requires the extensive mobilization of the muscle from its investing fascia posteriorly and inferiorly as described.

The tract through which the latissimus tendon will pass must be medial to the instant center of rotation of the shoulder joint throughout its arc of motion; if it slips lateral to this point, it will act as a primary adductor of the shoulder. In order to maintain this path, the edge of the inferior enveloping fascia of the posterior deltoid is developed and used as a "pulley" (Fig. 28–6). A separate incision exposes the superior and posterior portion of the rotator cuff. Several anchoring sutures are woven into

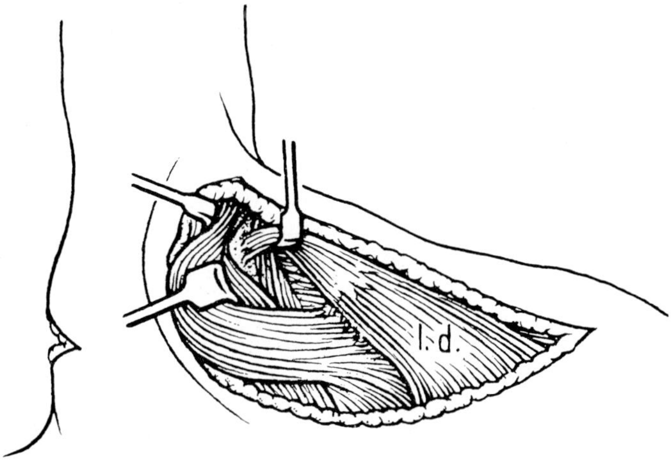

Fig. 28–3. The latissimus dorsi tendon is identified and released from the humeral shaft. Protection is given to the axillary nerve, which lies immediately adjacent to the proximal end of the tendon, and to the radial nerve, which curves around the humerus immediately distal to the tendon. (From Gerber C, Vinh TS, Hertel R, Hess CW. Latissimus dorsi transfer for the treatment of massive tears of the rotator cuff. A preliminary report. *Clin Orthop.* 1988;232:51–61.)

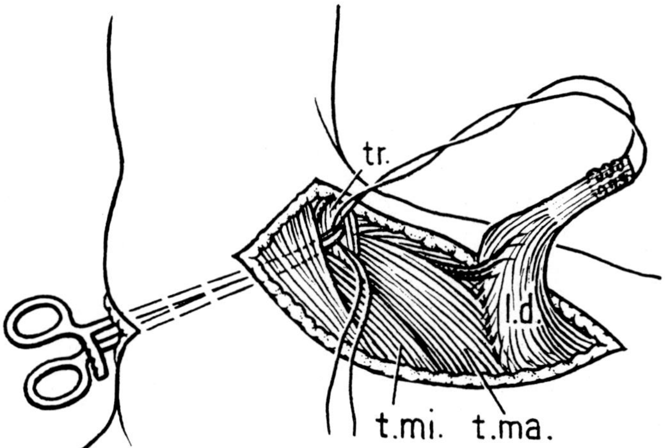

Fig. 28–5. The latissimus is mobilized distally to provide sufficient length for transfer. (From Gerber C, Vinh TS, Hertel R, Hess CW. Latissimus dorsi transfer for the treatment of massive tears of the rotator cuff. A preliminary report. *Clin Orthop.* 1988;232:51–61.)

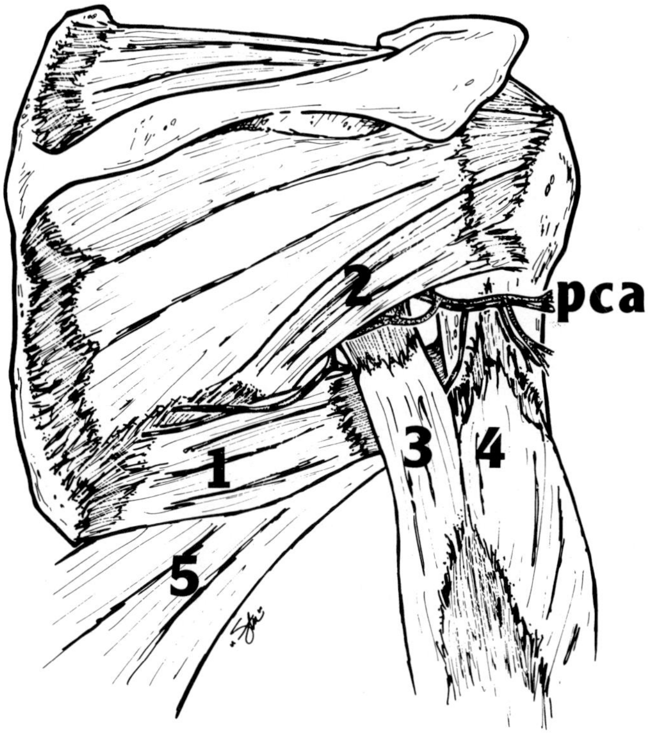

Fig. 28–4. Posterior view of quadrangular space. Posterior humeral circumflex (PCA) is seen exiting between the long (3) and lateral heads (4), below the teres minor (2), and above the teres major (1).

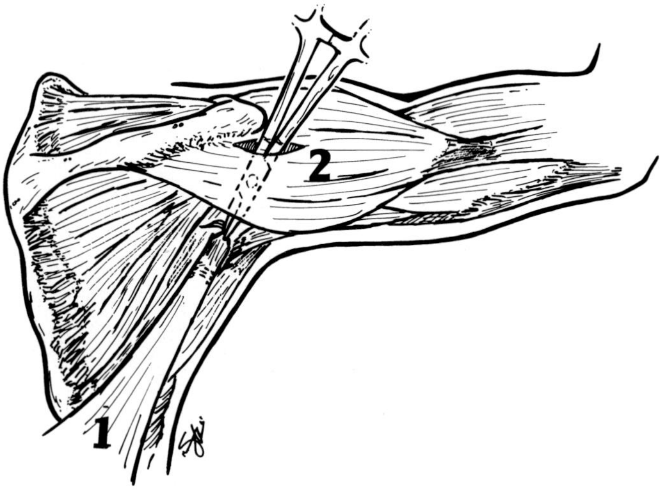

Fig. 28–6. A button hole must be created in the deltoid so that the deltoid edge will serve as a pulley for the transferred latissimus.

the latissimus tendon before it is passed to the superior wound. The path of the latissimus tendon lies superficial to the teres major and deep to the posterior third of the deltoid, using the edge of the deltoid fascia to prevent lateral subluxation of the tendon (Fig. 28–7). The thoracodorsal neurovascular pedicle is checked for kinking or compression. The tendon can then be sutured to existing cuff tissue to augment reconstruction of the rotator cuff or be anchored to bone to close a cuff defect (Fig. 28–8). Postoperative care is the same as that for rotator cuff reconstruction, with protected range of motion in an abduction brace for 6 weeks followed by graded range of motion and strengthening. Limited but functional, comfortable range of motion and humeral head depression are the goals.

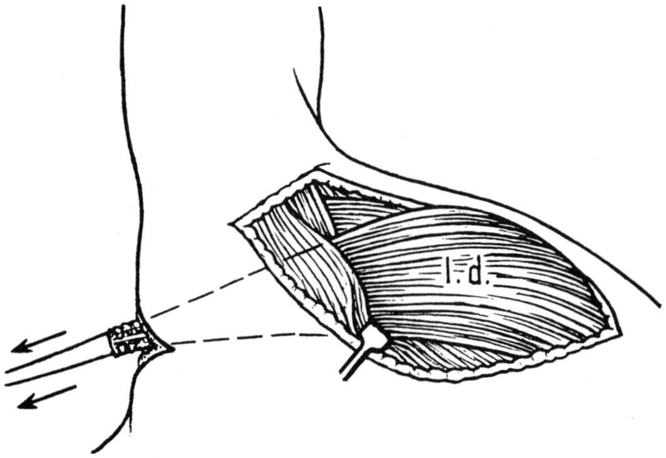

Fig. 28–7. The transferred tendon is pulled through the plane between the external rotators and the deltoid, then through the button hole seen in Figure 28–6 and into the superior wound. (From Gerber C, Vinh TS, Hertel R, Hess CW. Latissimus dorsi transfer for the treatment of massive tears of the rotator cuff. A preliminary report. *Clin Orthop.* 1988; 232:51–61.)

RESULTS

My experience with transfer of the latissimus dorsi to the rotator cuff has been largely in patients with brachial plexopathy; I have found, like Gerber in his series, that the presence of a functional deltoid is necessary for gain in shoulder abduction. The strength of the latissimus dorsi muscle in my patients appeared to correlate best with the strength of the triceps. The latissimus dorsi was not readily retrained in its role as an active transfer but functioned well as a tenodesis.

Gerber reported his results in 1992. Ninety-four percent of his 16 patients had satisfactory pain relief. For those patients with a functional subscapularis, range of motion improved. Gerber stresses that the subscapularis must be functional to balance the latissimus transfer and to prevent further superior migration of the humeral head. Other causes of shoulder dysfunction need to be addressed at the same time. There was no increase in osteoarthrosis in 14 of the 16 patients and only mild progression in the remaining two patients.

In the most recent follow-up with a minimum of 5 years, 9 of 16 patients were completely asymptomatic. Seven patients had improved pain relief. Flexion averaged 125° abduction and external rotation averaged 23°. This represented a gain of 42, 39, and 13° respectively. Constants score was 73% of normal. While the humeral head remained superiorly migrated, functional restoration of external rotation was achieved. Gerber reiterated the importance of an intact subscapularis for good results.

SUMMARY

The problem of the deficient rotator cuff, the surgical alternatives, the history of latissimus dorsi muscle transfers about the shoulder, the anatomy, and surgical technique of transfer of the latissimus dorsi to the rotator cuff are reviewed. The latissimus dorsi muscle is an adjunct

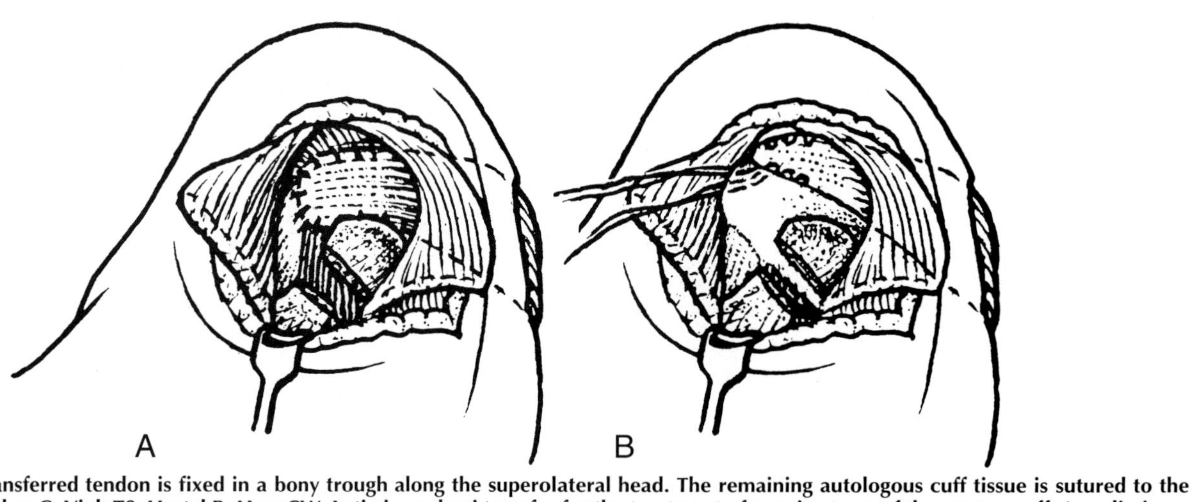

Fig. 28–8. The transferred tendon is fixed in a bony trough along the superolateral head. The remaining autologous cuff tissue is sutured to the transfer. (From Gerber C, Vinh TS, Hertel R, Hess CW. Latissimus dorsi transfer for the treatment of massive tears of the rotator cuff. A preliminary report. *Clin Orthop.* 1988;232:51–61.)

in the reconstruction of rotator cuff defects. It is available without significant donor morbidity, it is readily mobilized, and can be considered an alternative source of vascularized tissue with the appropriate biomechanical and physiological properties to augment reconstruction of massive defects of the rotator cuff. Results are comparable to cuff reconstruction with local muscle transfers in less challenging cases.

REFERENCES

1. Patte D, Goutallier D, Scheffer JC. Large cuff ruptures: Repair results by muscle advancement. In: Post M, Morrey, BF, Hawkins RJ, eds. *Surgery of the Shoulder.* St. Louis: Mosby-Year Book; 1990:248–251.
2. Bigliani LU, Cordasco FA, McIlveen SJ, Musso ES. Operative treatment of failed repairs of the rotator cuff. *J Bone Joint Surg Am.* 1992; 74:1505–1515.
3. Rockwood CA, Burkhead WZ. Management of patients with massive rotator cuff defects by acromioplasty and rotator cuff debridement. *Orthop Trans.* 1988;12:190.
4. Gschwend N, Rubeli M, Pidermann M. Rotator cuff tears: Relationship between clinical picture, operative findings, and results. In: Post M, Morrey BF, Hawkins HJ, eds. *Surgery of the Shoulder.* St. Louis: Mosby-Year Book; 1990:238–242.
5. Cofield RH. Subscapular muscle transposition for repair of chronic rotator cuff tears. *Surg Gynecol Obstet.* 1982;154:667.
6. Neer CS III. Impingement lesions. *Clin Orthop.* 1983;173:70–77.
7. Neviaser RJ, Neviaser JJ. Transfer of subscapularis and teres minor for massive defects of the rotator cuff. In: Bayley I, Kessel L, eds. *Shoulder Surgery.* Berlin: Springer-Verlag; 1982:60–63.
8. Ha'Eri GB, Wiley AM. Advancement of the supraspinatus muscle in the repair of ruptures of the rotator cuff. *J Bone Joint Surg Am.* 1981; 63:232–238.
9. Gerber C, Vinh TS, Hertel R, Hess CW. Latissimus dorsi transfer for the treatment of massive tears of rotator cuff, a preliminary report. *Clin Orthop.* 1988;232:51.
10. Gerber C. Latissimus dorsi transfer for the treatment of irreparable tears of the rotator cuff. *Clin Orthop.* 1992;275:152–160.
11. Gerber C, Rossier J. *Latissimus dorsi transfer for irreparable tears of the rotator cuff: A prospective study from concept to end results.* Presented at the American Shoulder and Elbow Surgeons' 10th Open Meeting. New Orleans, LA, February 27, 1994.
12. Zachary RB. Transplantation of teres major and latissimus dorsi for loss of external rotation at shoulder. *Lancet.* 1947;2:757.
13. Schottstaedt ER, Larsen LJ, Bost FC. Complete muscle transposition. *J Bone Joint Surg Am.* 1955;37:897.
14. Comtet JJ, Herzberg G, Al Naasan I. Biomechanical basis of transfers for shoulder paralysis. *Hand Clin.* 1989;5:1–14.
15. Saha AK. Surgery of the paralysed and flail shoulder. *Acta Orthop Scand.* (Supp) 1967;97:5–90.
16. L'Episcopo JB. Tendon transplantation in obstetrical paralysis. *Am J Surg.* 1934;25:122.
17. Harmon PH. Surgical reconstruction of the paralytic shoulder by multiple muscle transplantations. *J Bone Joint Surg Am.* 1950; 32:583.
18. Hoffer MM, Wickenden R, Roper B. Brachial plexus birth palsies: Results of tendon transfer to the rotator cuff. *J Bone Joint Surg Am.* 1978;60:691–195.
19. Gilbert A, Romana C, Ayatti R. Tendon transfers for shoulder paralysis in children. *Hand Clin.* 1988;4:633.

Chapter 29

Trapezius Transfer

Kaoru Yamanaka and Motohiko Mikasa

The torn rotator cuff is one of the most common injuries that causes shoulder dysfunction. However, treatment of massive rotator cuff tears remains both difficult and controversial.[1–5] The definition of a massive rotator cuff tear used in this chapter is a rotator cuff tear in which more than two components of the short rotators are avulsed.

We have employed three operations for the massive rotator cuff tear. These include (1) the McLaughlin procedure,[2] (2) the Debeyre procedure,[3] and (3) the trapezius transfer[6,7,8] to the greater tuberosity. The choice of the surgical procedures in our hands is individualized and is based on the intraoperative pathology encountered. Especially important factors in this decision making process are the size of the tear and the quality of the residual tendon. If the proximal stump could be approximated to the greater tuberosity with the arm abducted less than 60°, we performed the McLaughlin procedure. If the proximal stump could not be approximated to the greater tuberosity with an abduction angle of 90° and the stump was tendinous, we used the Debeyre procedure. If the proximal stump could not be approximated to the greater tuberosity and the stump was not tendinous, we elected to perform trapezius transfer to the greater tuberosity. It is this operation, the trapezius transfer to the greater tuberosity for treating a massive rotator cuff tear, that will be discussed based on our experience.

FUNCTIONAL ANATOMY

The trapezius is the largest of the suspensory muscles of the shoulder girdle. It is divided into three parts: the upper, intermediate, and lower fibers.[9]

The trapezius has a broad origin from the medial one third of the superior nuchal line of the occipital bone, the inion, as well as the tips of the spines of all the cervical and thoracic vertebrae. Its attachment to the cervical spine is to the ligamentum nuchae. The upper fibers of the trapezius pass inferolaterally to the lateral one third of the clavicle. The intermediate fibers of the trapezius pass horizontally to the acromion, as well as to the upper lip of the crest of the spine of the scapula; the lower fibers converge as they pass superolaterally and form an aponeurosis along the crest of the spines.

The upper fibers elevate the scapula along with the levator scapula and the intermediate fibers adduct the scapula. The lower fibers depress and adduct the scapula. The trapezius is innervated by (1) the accessory nerve (external branch) and by (2) the ventral rami of C3 and C4. In the trapezius transfer for a massive rotator cuff tear, the upper and intermediate fibers of the trapezius are partially used.

INDICATION

Any patient with a rotator cuff tear, in which the proximal remnant is not tendinous and cannot be approximated to the greater tuberosity, even if the shoulder is abducted to 90°, is considered a candidate for trapezius transfer. Clues that a massive rotator cuff tear may be encountered include preoperative radiographs demonstrating narrowing of the acromiohumeral interval to less than 6 mm, as well as an arthrogram demonstrating continuity of the contour of the subacromial bursa and that of the humeral head on orthogonal views.

OPERATIVE PROCEDURE

Under endotracheal anesthesia, the patient is placed in the beach chair position with the arm draped free. Initially, a 7-cm transacromial incision is made from 1 cm posterolateral to the AC joint to 1 cm inferolateral to the coracoid process (Fig. 29–1). After dividing the subcutaneous tissue, 4 cm of the deltoid muscle is split parallel to its fibers from the AC joint. Then the subacromial bursa is incised to investigate the size and repairability of the rotator cuff tear.

After inspecting the cuff tear, a decision is made whether or not to perform a McLaughlin or Debeyre repair or to proceed to the more extensive exposure required for trapezius transfer. If there is a massive tear involving more than two components of the short rotators and the stump end is not tendinous and cannot be approximated to the greater tuberosity, despite abducting the shoulder to 90° after mobilizing the tendon, neither the McLaughlin procedure or the Debeyre proce-

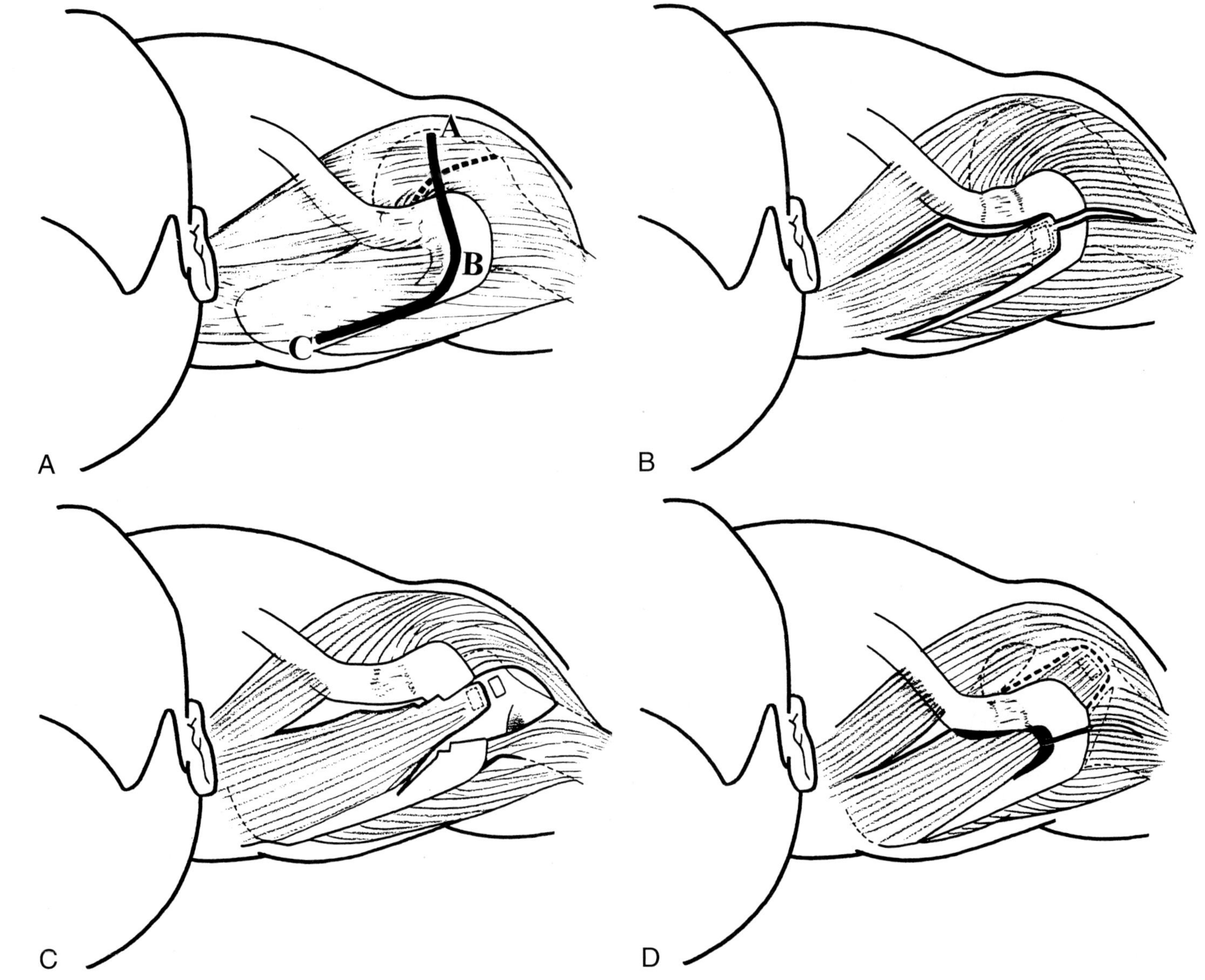

Fig. 29–1. *A,* A schema of the shoulder girdle viewed from the upper side. The skin incision starts 1 cm posterolateral to the AC joint and extends to 1 cm inferolateral to the coracoid process (Line A to B). A 4-cm deltoid-splitting incision at the AC joint is made (dotted line) and the cuff observed. If trapezius transfer is indicated, the position of the patient is changed to the recumbent position. The skin incision is elongated to the medial border of the scapula, along and 1 cm superior to the spine of the scapula (Line B to C). *B,* The trapezius is detached from the spine of the scapula (about 10 cm length) and also detached from the distal clavicle (about 4 cm). Then the upper trapezius is incised from this point, parallel with its fiber about 8 cm to make a trapezius flap with 1 *ts* 1 *ts* 0.8-cm bone block of the acromion. *C,* The acromion is osteotomized at the middle of the acromion in the scapular plane and retracted with self-retaining retractor. After confirming that the trapezius flap reaches the greater tuberosity by elevating the arm about 90°, make an appropriate size of trough just proximal to the greater tuberosity. *D,* The posterior part of the distal clavicle, the caudal surface of the acromion, and the anterior part of the neck of the acromion are partially resected to make easy to pass the bulky trapezius (black area). Holding the arm elevated, the flap of the trapezius is anchored by non-absorbable sutures. The acromion is reduced and fixed by Kirschner wires with tension band wiring.

dure are deemed appropriate. The trapezius transfer to the greater tuberosity is then performed.

To perform the trapezius transfer, using our technique, the patient is transferred to the decubitus position. The shoulder is re-prepped and draped sterilely. The skin incision is elongated medially from a point 1 cm posterolateral to the AC joint to the medial border of the scapula, along a line approximately 1 cm superior to the spine of the scapula. A skin flap is created anteriorly to visualize the trapezius muscle belly.

About 10 cm of the trapezius is detached from the spine of the scapula, while 4 cm of the trapezius is detached from the distal clavicle. The acromial insertion is maintained intact. The muscle belly of the trapezius is elevated and about 8 cm of the trapezius is separated, parallel to the trapezius muscle fibers. Along with these releases, the muscle belly of the trapezius is elevated. The insertion of the trapezius at the acromion is detached widely and carefully with a 1 × 1 × 0.8-cm bone block of the acromion using an air driven osteotome.

Following this, the deltoid muscle is split from the midlateral point of the acromion caudalward for 4 cm. The acromion is then osteotomized with a bone saw at the midlateral point of the acromion along the axis of the spine of the scapula. The subacromial space is visualized by retracting the anterior part of the acromion anteriorly and the posterior part of the acromion posteriorly with a self-retaining retractor. Debridement of the subacromial bursa and the osteophyte of the acromion are performed. The supraspinatus, subscapularis, infraspinatus, and (when involved) the teres minor tendons are trimmed back to fresh tendon tissue and mobilized as much as possible using traction sutures.

The shoulder is elevated about 90° in the scapular plane. After confirming that the small bony block at the end of the trapezius muscle flap reaches the greater tuberosity, a small bony groove (1 × 1 × 1 cm) is made in the tuberosity for an anchor site. Keeping the shoulder elevated in the scapular plane, the small bony fragment of the trapezius muscle flap is sutured into the groove with three nonabsorbable sutures. The suture line is augmented by suturing the trapezius to surrounding periosteum. The supraspinatus tendon is pulled out distally and sutured to the trapezius for lining. The residua of the infraspinatus and subscapularis tendons are both sutured to the trapezius.

The posterior part of the distal clavicle, the caudal surface, and the anterior part of the neck of the acromion are bevelled to make it easy to pass the bulky trapezius muscle beneath the acromion. The osteotomized acromion is reduced and fixed with the tension band wiring technique (2.0-mm Kirschner wires and 1.25-mm wire are used). Suction drainage is generally required. The deltoid split is approximated and the skin sutured. An abduction brace is immediately applied.

POSTOPERATIVE PROTOCOL

Passive elevation and passive rotation are started on the fifth postoperative day. Four weeks after the operation, active assisted exercises are started, and the degree of abduction in the brace is gradually decreased beginning 6 weeks after the operation. A sling is applied until bony union of the acromion is achieved.

ANALYSIS OF OUR CASES

From 1982 to 1993, we have treated 122 rotator cuff tears. Of these cases, 21 tears met the criteria previously outlined for a massive tear (i.e., greater than two tendon tears).

The McLaughlin procedure was performed in four cases, the Debeyre procedure in nine cases, and the tra-

Table 29–1. Shoulder Assessment Scoring System, Japanese Orthopaedic Association (JOA)

	Points
I Pain	30
II Function	20
III ROM	30
IV X-ray findings	5
V Joint stability	15
Total	100

Table 29–2. Clinical Cases of Trapezius Transfer

Case Age (Years)	*Side Sex*	*Spontaneous Pain*		*Abduction*		*External Rotation*		*Weakness of Abduction*		*Weakness of External Rotation*		*JOA Score (pts)*	
		Preop	*Postop*	*Preop*	*Postop*	*Preop*	*Postop*	*Preop*	*Postop*	*Preop*	*Postop*	*Preop*	*Postop*
Y. N. 72	l* m	++	−	40°	180°	30°	80°	+	+	+	−	45	90
M. S. 66	r* f	+	−	180°	145°	80°	30°	+	−	+	−	74	79
Y. K. 72	r* m	++	−	130°	160°	60°	35°	+	−	+	−	60	90
T. M. 59	r m	++	+−	135°	55°	75°	80°	+	+	+	+	55	44
T. O. 79	l m	++	−	40°	40°	0°	80°	+	+	+	+	26	41
T. M. 50	r* m	++	−	80°	140°	40°	70°	+	+	+	−	59	87
K. T. 73	r m	++	+−	30°	75°	0°	45°	+	−	+	+−	30	54

*Indicates dominant side.

pezius transfer to the greater tuberosity in seven cases. Shoulder function was evaluated by the Japanese Orthopaedic Association (JOA) scoring system for the shoulder. Shoulders were evaluated during the initial visit to the hospital and in follow-up examinations, as outlined in Table 29–1.

In the seven cases in which the trapezius transfer was employed, the average age of the patients at the time of their first visit to the hospital was 66 years of age. The right shoulder was involved in five cases and the left shoulder in two. The dominant side was involved in four cases. The average symptomatic period prior to the procedure was 17 months. Episodes of trauma were noted in four cases. The average follow-up period was 3 years and 9 months.

Preoperative pain at rest with nocturnal-related and motion-related exacerbation was evident in all cases. Preoperative range of motion averaged 77° in flexion and 43° in external rotation. Weakness in abduction was demonstrated in all cases, and weakness in external rotation was demonstrated in all but one case. The average JOA shoulder evaluation score was 50 points preoperatively (Table 29–2).

At the end of the follow-up period (44.8 months), no patient had pain at rest. Pain on motion and night pain were noted in one case. The average flexion increased to 109° and external rotation to 60°. Weakness of abduction persisted in six cases and weakness of external rotation was noted in two cases. The average JOA shoulder score was 69 points postoperatively.

CASE REPORT

A 66-year-old woman suffered from pain in her right shoulder for 4 months after bruising the shoulder in a car accident. The range of motion of the involved shoulder was almost normal, but the shoulder pain and the weakness of abduction and external rotation were persistent. Plain radiographs showed narrowing of acromiohumeral interval and osteophyte of the humeral head (Fig. 29–2). Shoulder arthrography demonstrated a massive rotator cuff tear. Because of continued shoulder pain, the operation was performed. During the procedure, the supraspinatus and infraspinatus tendons were discovered to be torn, and the stump retracted to near the rim of the glenoid. The subscapularis and teres minor tendons were preserved. The long head of the biceps was hypertrophied and slightly edematous. The articular cartilage of the humeral head was eroded and discolored. The trapezius muscle flap with a 1 × 1 × 0.8-cm bone fragment was prepared; then it was tightly anchored to the groove near the greater tuberosity with nonabsorbable sutures in 90° of abduction. The teres minor and subscapularis tendons could not be sutured to the trapezius muscle flap. Suction drainage was inserted and the wound was closed. An abduction brace was immediately applied.

Now, 4.5 years later, the patient can elevate her arm to 145°, but she complains of barometric pressure related pain in her shoulder and her muscle strength of abduction remains poor.

DISCUSSION

The massive rotator cuff tear is a difficult problem to resolve in rotator cuff surgery, because there remains no cuff to repair and the residual cuff is markedly attenuated. The long head of the biceps is often torn. The operative methods of treatment of the massive rotator cuff tear can be divided into three groups:

1. Tendon advancement (McLaughlin Procedure[2])
2. Muscle transfer (supraspinatus,[3] subscapularis,[8] teres minor,[9] deltoid,[10] and trapezius[6,7])
3. Augmentation by synthetic tissue transplantation[11]

The trapezius transfer is a salvage operation and, in our opinion, must not be employed if the McLaughlin procedure or the Debeyre procedure can be performed. The attractiveness of trapezius transfer lies in its potential advantages, which are (1) the trapezius is the synergist of the deltoid muscle, therefore, little re-education is necessary;[8] (2) the direction of the trapezius muscle fibers is similar to that of the supraspinatus, providing a straight line of pull; (3) the trapezius is strong enough to be transferred and act as an active participant in motion and not just provide a tenodesis effect; (4) the trapezius transfer can be adopted to a more severe cuff tear than the supraspinatus advancement, because the trapezius flap can be mobilized farther than the supraspinatus flap; and (5) the trapezius muscle transfer avoids artificial materials.

In our seven cases, pain relief was noted in 86%, improvement of range of motion in flexion was present in 71%, improvement of muscle power in abduction in 14%, and improvement in external rotation in 43%. Improvement of JOA shoulder score was 19 points higher on the average. The reduction of pain by the trapezius transfer is satisfactory; however, the improvement of range of motion and muscle strength in abduction are not spectacular.

Massive rotator cuff tears are divided into two groups, according to the preservation of the biceps. The end results of the trapezius transfer partially depend on preservation of the long head of the biceps. If the long head of the biceps is preserved, the end results are better.[8]

The long-term results of trapezius transfer as we have described are not as good as expected. We hope that a single coronal plane osteotomy and improved anchoring techniques of bone to bone suturing will lead to improved healing of the trapezius and that our results will improve; we still recommend its use when conventional suture techniques are not possible, in order to avoid the use of synthetic material.

Editor's Note

Although the use of the trapezius is somewhat attractive from a theoretical point of view (i.e., it is a large

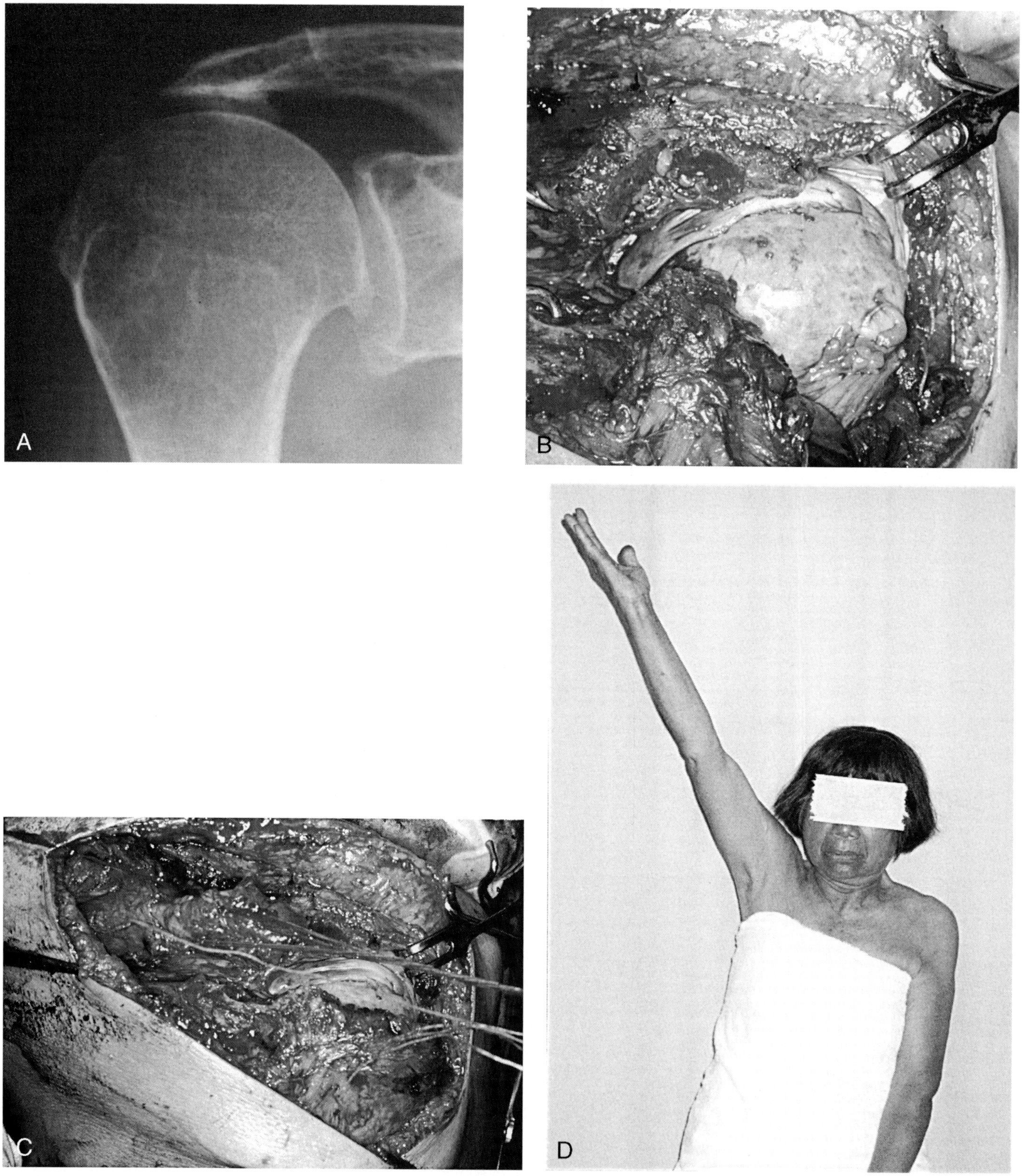

Fig. 29–2. *A,* A 66-year-old woman suffered from right shoulder pain after injuring her shoulder in a car accident. Plain shoulder radiographs showed narrowing of the acromiohumeral interval and osteophyte of the humeral head, suggesting a massive rotator cuff tear. *B,* At operation, the supraspinatus and the infraspinatus were torn and their stump ends were retracted to the glenoid rim; they were not tendinous but membranous. The long head of the biceps was flattened and degenerated. The rotator interval was widely opened. The articular cartilage was slightly eroded and discolored. *C,* The flap of trapezius with bone block was pulled by traction sutures. *D,* About 4.5 years later her range of motion was 145° in abduction, but her muscle strength of her shoulder abduction remained poor.

muscle synergistic with the deltoid), unless a stable pulley effect is achieved from a healed acromion osteotomy, it becomes (like the deltoid) a head elevator. This operation can be performed without acromial osteotomy obviating the concern about nonunion. Lingering concern about using the trapezius, however, is that if the patient goes on to develop rotator cuff tear arthropathy or the transfer fails for whatever reason and a fusion is the only option open to a patient, you have sacrificed the prime mover of scapulothoracic motion and burned a major bridge.

REFERENCES

1. Wilson PD. Complete ruptures of the supraspinatus tendon. *JAMA.* 1931;96:433–439.
2. McLaughlin HL. Lesions of the musculotendinous cuff of the shoulder. *J Bone Joint Surg Br.* 1944;26:31–51.
3. Debeyre J, Patte D, Elmelik E. Repair of ruptures of the rotator cuff of the shoulder. *J Bone Joint Surg Br.* 1965;47:36–42.
4. Bateman JE. *The Shoulder and Neck.* 2nd ed. Philadelphia: WB Saunders; 1978:306–307.
5. Neviaser JS, Neviaser RJ, Neviaser TJ. The repair of chronic massive ruptures of the rotator cuff of the shoulder by use of a freeze dried rotator cuff. *J Bone Joint Surg Am.* 1978;60:681–684.
6. Mikasa M, Yamanaka K. Experience of the trapezius transfer for the massive rotator cuff tear. *The Shoulder Joint.* 1979;3:77–80 (In Japanese).
7. Mikasa M. Trapezius transfer for global tear of the rotator cuff. *Surgery of the Shoulder.* Burlington: BC Decker Ink; 1984;196–199.
8. Mikasa M. Long-term results of surgical treatment for massive rotator cuff tears. With special reference to trapezius transfer. *Rinsho Seikei Geka (Clinical Orthopaedic Surgery).* 1989;24:38–45 (In Japanese).
9. Basmajian JB. *Grant's Method of Anatomy.* 8th ed. Baltimore: Williams & Wilkins; 1972;94–95.
10. Cofield R. Subscapularis muscle transfer for repair of chronic rotator cuff tears. *Surg Gynecol Obstet.* 1982;154:667–672.
11. Neviaser RJ, Neviaser TJ. Transfer of subscapularis and teres minor for massive defects of the rotator cuff. *Shoulder Surgery.* Berlin: Springer-Verlag; 1982;60–63.
12. Takagishi N. The new operation for the massive cuff rupture. *J Jpn Orthop Assoc.* 1978;52:775–780.
13. Bateman JE. The diagnosis and treatment of ruptures of the rotator cuff. *Surg Clin North Am.* 1963;43:1523–1530.
14. Ozaki J, Fujimoto S, Masuhara K, et al. Reconstruction of chronic massive rotator cuff tears with synthetic materials. *Clin Orthop.* 1986; 202:173–183.

Chapter 30

Allograft Repairs

Thomas P. Goss and Sanjay S. Desai

The term "massive rotator cuff tear" has been used rather freely in the orthopaedic literature. Several definitions have been offered, most of which center around the size of defect and/or the number of musculotendinous units involved. This is somewhat misdirected, because with rotator cuff surgery the procedure required and the functional outcome are more dependent upon whether the retracted tendons can be mobilized and satisfactorily reattached to the articular margin of the proximal humerus. Some large tears have mobile musculotendinous units and can be closed quite nicely producing a good to excellent result. Consequently, for the purposes of this chapter a "massive rotator cuff tear" is one which cannot be closed with the arm at the side, even after maximal mobilization of the musculotendinous units and use of the biceps tendon (if present), or one in which the repair would be extremely tenuous.

Preoperatively, it may be difficult to predict whether a patient has a massive rotator cuff tear. Suggestive signs and symptoms include (1) radiographic documentation of a high riding humeral head and a narrowed impingement space; (2) profound difficulty actively elevating the arm; (3) obvious spinatus atrophy; (4) a large palpable gap in the rotator cuff or palpable free fluid; (5) severe crepitus on shoulder range of motion; and (6) shoulder symptoms of long duration or a cuff tear documented arthrographically well in the past. Even when signs and symptoms are relatively mild to moderate, however, a massive tear may occasionally be present. Consequently, the surgeon must always be prepared to deal with this possible eventuality, because when encountered a massive tear is always a formidable surgical challenge.

The goals of rotator cuff surgery are to decompress the impingement interval and close the tendinous defect, thereby alleviating pain, restoring function, and preventing further deterioration of the glenohumeral articulation even to the point of "cuff-tear arthropathy."[1] If a massive tear is present (less than 5% of cases) the surgeon has three basic options: (1) decompress and debride the subacromial space without repair of the rotator cuff; (2) mobilize the musculotendinous units maximally, reattach the retracted edges to the articular margin of the humerus, incorporate the biceps tendon (if present) into the repair, and immobilize the arm in an abduction brace adjusted to take tension off the repair; and (3) use synthetic or biologic interpositional material to close the defect without undue tension (after maximal mobilization of the musculotendinous units and incorporation of the biceps tendon) with the arm at the patient's side.

Option One

Simply decompressing and debriding the subacromial space as advocated by Rockwood et al.[2] fails to address the problems caused by the torn rotator cuff: (a) pain caused by bony contact between the proximal humerus and undersurface of the acromion; (b) the continuing enlargement of the cuff defect resulting in a worsening clinical situation; and (c) the physiologic process that can lead to "cuff tear arthropathy." Despite favorable results reported by Rockwood et al., the experience of other investigators has been far less positive. Mansat and Bonnevaille[3] abandoned simple debridement of the rotator cuff, because a significant number of their patients went on to develop glenohumeral degenerative joint disease. Neer[4] observed that some individuals with rotator cuff tears develop "cuff tear arthropathy." Consequently, he could not "agree with the principle of debridement of massive rotator cuff tears since it disregards the function of the rotator cuff not only as a stabilizer of the head against ascent but also in the nutrition of the glenohumeral joint." Certainly in the intraoperative setting, having some technique to close a massive rotator cuff tear makes more sense, at least empirically.

Option Two

Maximal mobilization (including slides of the individual musculotendinous units) and repair of the torn rotator cuff (incorporating the biceps tendon, if present) followed by postoperative immobilization in a tension-relieving abduction brace is technically demanding; the repair often remains rather tenuous and the patient is immobilized for 6 weeks in an awkward, uncomfortable position. In addition, it is difficult to believe that a tear that can only be reattached to the articular margin of the proximal humerus with the arm in an elevated position will remain intact when the arm is eventually brought to the side.

Option Three

The use of synthetic material to close the rotator cuff defect, although appealing theoretically, certainly remains in the experimental stage.[5,6] The use of local autologous biologic material (transfers of the trapezius, latissimus dorsi, and pectoralis major and minor) is technically demanding, alters normal anatomy, and does not improve dynamic shoulder function. [4] The use of autologous material from a distant site (e.g., fascia lata graft) has received limited attention. Bateman[7,8] reported good results with fascial sutures of autogenous fascia lata in the management of large and massive tears. DeOrio and Cofield[9] used a combination of fascial grafts and subscapularis/supraspinatus transfers in seven patients with massive tears; they had five poor and two fair results.

There are two reports in the literature describing the use of biologic allograft material. In 1978 Nevaiser et al.[10] reported on the use of freeze-dried rotator cuff allograft (FDRCA) to close massive rotator cuff tears. They found no evidence of rejection, and their goals of pain relief and functional improvement were usually obtained. They reported excellent results in 8 of 16 patients, good results in 5 patients, a fair result in 1 patient, and poor results in 2 patients (both had previously undergone complete acromionectomies). Two shoulders were later re-explored and the repairs were noted to be intact. Microscopically, small specimens obtained from the graft and the recipients' own rotator cuff were indistinguishable. In 1988 Nasca[11] reported on his experience with FDRCA in seven patients with documented massive rotator cuff tears. Five of the seven patients had their pain relieved, but only two individuals had significant improvement in shoulder function. Nasca attributed pain relief to the surgical decompression/debridement and the postoperative immobilization. He felt that "the less favorable results in his series could reflect more stringent end result evaluation criteria as well as larger cuff defects of lower quality tissue." One patient explored 9 months postoperatively was found to have detachment and avascularity of the allograft. Nasca felt it was "reasonable to speculate that significant revascularization of the freeze dried allograft cuff tissue fails to occur and that with time the suture line will fail." His final conclusion was that FDRCA was not of significant value in the treatment of the patient with a massive rotator cuff tear.

SURGICAL TECHNIQUE AND POSTOPERATIVE MANAGEMENT

The patient is placed on the operating room table in the standard beach chair position with a roll under the vertebral border of the scapula and the shoulder over the edge of the table to allow access to the anterior, lateral, posterior, and superior aspects of the shoulder region (see Chapter 20). An incision is made over the anterosuperior aspect of the shoulder in Langer's lines, running from the most superior aspect of the acromion to a point just distal and lateral to the palpable coracoid process. The deltoid muscle is exposed, split in the line of its fibers from the AC joint distally a distance of 4 cm, and dissected sharply off the anterior margin of the acromion (Fig. 30-1). This portion of the middle deltoid is retracted laterally. The coracoacromial ligament is excised and a standard anterior acromioplasty is performed (see Chapter 20 for details of acromioplasty technique). Spurs over the inferior aspect of the distal clavicle are removed; if the AC joint is degenerated, the distal 1.5 cm of the clavicle is removed. A complete subacromial bursectomy is performed to allow visualization of the rotator cuff. At this point, it will be clear that either a large or massive tear of the rotator cuff is present. For the necessary exposure, the incision is extended back over the posterior aspect of the acromion, and the deltoid muscle is taken sharply off its lateral and posterolateral margin. The superficial surface of each of the four musculotendinous units is cleared of adhesions. The glenohumeral capsule is incised along the anterior, superior, and posterior margins of the glenoid, and a periosteal elevator is used to lift the infraspinatus/teres minor units off the infraspinatus fossa, the supraspinatus unit off the supraspinatus fossa, and the subscapularis unit off the ventral aspect of the scapula. "Tagging" sutures are placed in each of the musculotendinous units so that traction may be applied, aiding in their mobilization. Incisions are

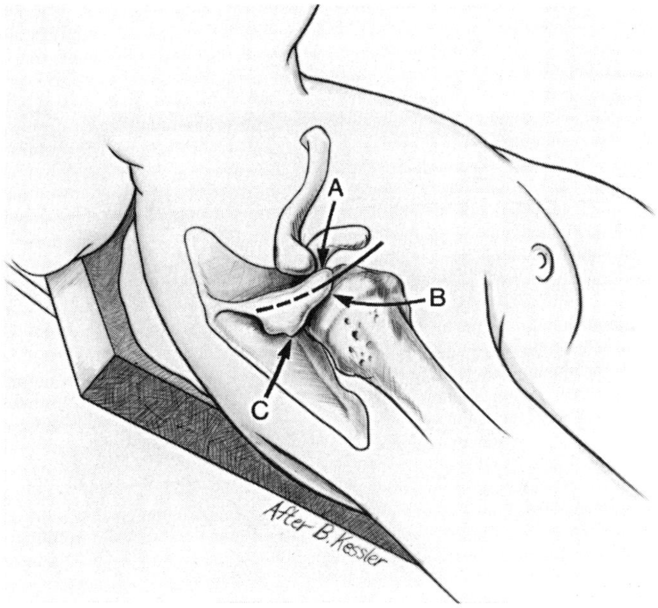

Fig. 30–1. The surgical incisions for patients undergoing rotator cuff surgery (solid line: the standard incision; dotted line: posterior extension for patients with large and massive tears). Deltoid detachment: (*A and B*) standard area of deltoid detachment; (*B and C*) posterior extension of deltoid detachment for patients with large and massive tears. (Modified from Bigliani LU. Anterior acromioplasty and repair of a torn rotator cuff. *Strategies Ortho Surg.* 1989;8.)

made along the superior and inferior aspects of the subscapularis musculotendinous unit, which can then be advanced superiorly and laterally. Although described by other investigators, I have found little advantage to performing a similar "slide" of the supraspinatus and infraspinatus/teres minor units. The long head of the biceps tendon, if present, is divided sharply at its origin over the superior aspect of the glenoid and tagged. The free margin of the rotator cuff is "freshened up," and using a Hall drill a bony trough is fashioned along the articular margin of the proximal humerus in the area of cuff detachment. Drill holes 1 cm apart are made distal to this trough. No. 1 nonabsorbable sutures are then passed through each drill hole and out through the trough (Fig. 30-2). The rotator cuff is then repaired as best as possible by (a) sewing the musculotendinous units to each other in a side to side fashion with multiple No. 1 nonabsorbable figure of eight sutures, (b) suturing as much of the free margin of the cuff as possible into the bony trough, using the previously placed No. 1 nonabsorbable sutures passed in a horizontal mattress fashion, and (c) incorporating the long head of the biceps tendon into the repair using No. 1 nonabsorbable figure of eight sutures. At this point a defect of variable size remains (usually not terribly large). FDCRA (Fig. 30-3) (which can be obtained from a number of tissue banks around the country) is reconstituted by immersing the graft in saline for 30 minutes. Firm tissue within the graft is then removed. The specimen may be folded upon itself and its margins sewn together with a running No. 1 absorbable simple suture to create a "double thickness" graft (Fig. 30-4). The graft is then sewn to the free rotator cuff margin with multiple No. 1 nonabsorbable figure of eight sutures. The allograft is drawn distally and sewn into the bony trough using the previously placed No. 1 nonabsorbable sutures passed in a horizontal mattress fashion (Fig. 30-5). The goal should always be to close the rotator cuff completely with the patient's arm at the side, avoiding undue tension and using as little allograft as possible. The deltoid muscle is then carefully reattached using multiple No. 1 nonabsorbable sutures placed in a horizontal mattress fashion, either through the soft tissues overlying the acromion or through drill holes in the acromial margin. The split in the deltoid muscle running from the AC joint distally is closed with a running 2-0 absorbable simple suture. The subcutaneous tissues and

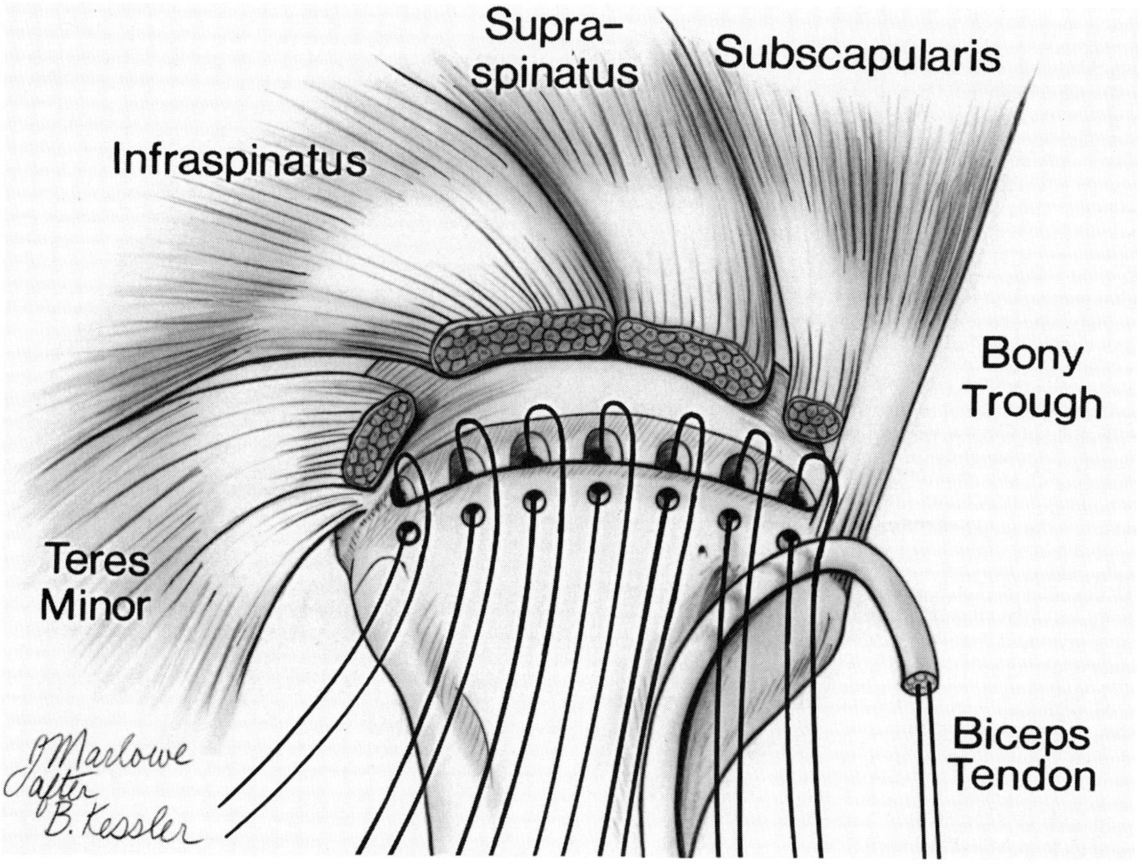

Fig. 30–2. A massive rotator cuff tear with detachment and retraction of the subscapularis, supraspinatus, infraspinatus, and teres minor musculotendinous units. Note the bony trough fashioned along the articular margin of the proximal humerus in the area of cuff detachment and the No. 1 nonabsorbable sutures passed through drill holes distal to the trough and exiting out through the trough. Also note the detached and "tagged" long head of the biceps tendon. (Modified from Bigliani LU. Anterior acromioplasty and repair of a torn rotator cuff. *Strategies Ortho Surg.* 1989;8.)

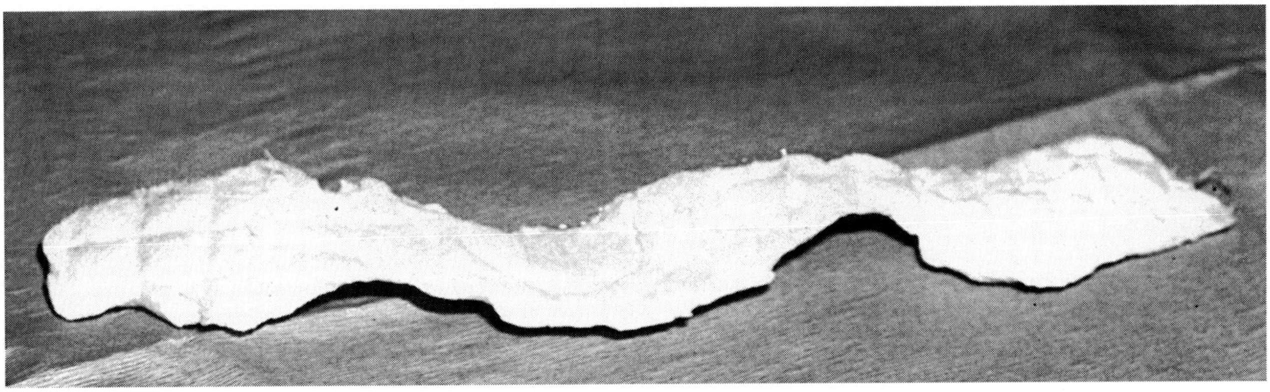

Fig. 30–3. Unreconstituted freeze-dried rotator cuff allograft.

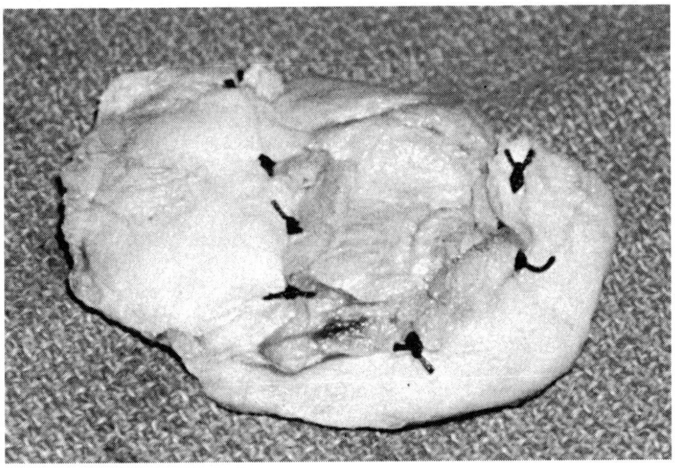

Fig. 30–4. Reconstituted "doubled" rotator cuff allograft prior to defect closure.

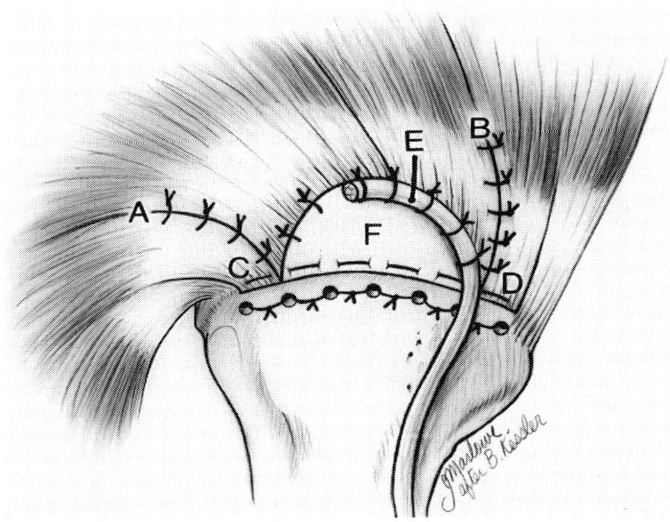

Fig. 30–5. Repair of a massive rotator cuff tear: (*A and B*) musculotendinous units repaired in a side to side fashion; (*C and D*) cuff margins sewn into the bony trough; (*E*) biceps tendon incorporated into the repair; and (*F*) allograft sewn to the rotator cuff margin/biceps tendon and into the bony trough. (Modified from Bigliani LU. Anterior acromioplasty and repair of a torn rotator cuff. *Strategies Ortho Surg.* 1989;8.)

skin are then reapproximated in the usual fashion. A routine sterile orthopedic dressing is applied, followed by a sling and swathe bandage. Because freeze-dried allografts tend to be incorporated at a slower rate than autogenous grafts, a period of 6 weeks of immobilization is desirable to ensure good healing. At the end of the 6 weeks, progressive functional use of the shoulder/upper extremity is encouraged. An intensive, closely monitored physiotherapy program is begun, focusing initially on regaining shoulder range of motion followed by strength. The patient's functional end result is not realized for at least 1 year postoperatively, and heavy manual physical use of the extremity is permanently prohibited.

THE UNIVERSITY OF MASSACHUSETTS MEDICAL CENTER EXPERIENCE

At our institution from 1981 to 1988, 10 patients (11 shoulders) underwent repair of a massive rotator cuff tear using FDRCA. Five patients (one patient underwent bilateral procedures) were less than or equal to 65 years of age, and five patients were over 65 years old. All patients noted significant but incomplete relief of pain, with a change of 6.8 preoperative pain to 2.3 postoperative pain (with a scale of 10 = maximal and 0 = none). Patients less than or equal to 65 years of age maintained their preoperative active and passive range of motion. Patients over the age of 65 lost an average of 35° of active forward flexion and 61° of passive forward flexion. Subjectively, all patients reported having less than the desired amount of shoulder strength postoperatively. Using Nevaiser's rating scale, there were no excellent, three good, four fair, and four poor results. The fair and poor results were generally caused by limited or loss of active/passive shoulder range of motion, and all of the poor results were in individuals over 65 years of age. Seventy-eight percent of the patients rated their shoulder better or much better overall (decreased pain and subjectively increased function) and would undergo the procedure again. One individual felt that his shoulder was the same, and one felt it was worse. There were no complications (no evidence of graft rejection and no infections). It was not possible to evaluate the integrity of the cuff repair, because none of the shoulders had to be re-explored and none of the patients would consent to a postoperative arthrogram. These results were clearly not as good as those of Neviaser et al.; in fact, they were similar to those of Nasca. However, we were more satisfied than Nasca in what we were able to achieve in this extremely difficult group of patients. For those individuals less than or equal to 65 years of age with a massive rotator cuff tear, decompression of the subacromial space, maximal mobilization and repair of the musculotendinous units (incorporating the biceps tendon, if present), and closure of any remaining defect with FDRCA seems to provide significant, although incomplete pain relief, maintains preoperative active and passive shoulder range of motion, and provides the patient with a subjective sense of improved function. In addition, there seem to be no adverse effects associated with the use of allograft material, and hopefully by restoring an intact soft-tissue cuff around the glenohumeral joint, further deterioration (even to the point of "cuff tear arthropathy") will be avoided.

The advantages are less clear in those patients over the age of 65. Although these individuals noted a clear reduction in pain and subjective improvement in shoulder function, they lost a significant amount of active and passive shoulder elevation, probably as a result of the prolonged period of postoperative immobilization. In addition, there is less concern that "cuff tear arthropathy" will develop during these older patients' remaining years. Perhaps in this group if it is clear preoperatively that a massive tear is present, an arthroscopic decompression and debridement of the subacromial space (acknowledging the experience of Rockwood et al. but preserving the deltoid attachment to avoid post operative immobilization) would be more appropriate. Wiley[12] found arthroscopic debridement and irrigation to be useful in treating chronic symptoms, especially in older patients. Gartsman[13] reported unsatisfactory results in patients with massive cuff tears; however, his rating system included shoulder function as well as pain relief. If unsuccessful, in regard to providing satisfactory pain relief, closure of the cuff defect with the aid of allograft can still be performed. Finally, the ultimate fate of the allograft and the long-term integrity of the repair remain unanswered questions.

CONCLUSIONS

1. Full-thickness rotator cuff tears should be treated expeditiously with a subacromial decompression and closure of the defect, provided the patient is willing and medically acceptable.
2. The more mobile the retracted musculotendinous units and the less dissection required to restore the integrity of the cuff, the better the final result with regard to pain relief, as well as shoulder range of motion, strength, and overall function.
3. Massive rotator cuff tears are those in which the defect cannot be closed with the arm at the side, even after maximal mobilization of the musculotendinous units and use of the biceps tendon (if present), or one in which the repair would be quite tenuous.
4. For those individuals with a massive rotator cuff tear, all surgical options are basically salvage procedures. The goals are pain relief, maintenance of function, and prevention of further glenohumeral deterioration. Because of the severe retraction and scarring of the musculotendinous units, improvement in dynamic function is rarely possible.
5. Although far from ideal, use of FDRCA seems to satisfy these goals as well as, if not better than, the other options. The surgical procedure is relatively simple without excessive soft- tissue dissection, restores the integrity of the cuff, and does not seem to be associated with any adverse consequences. Individuals realize significant pain relief, maintain their active and passive range of motion (those less than or equal to 65 years of age), and note significant subjective improvement in shoulder function.
6. Individuals over the age of 65 in whom it is clear preoperatively that a massive tear is present may be better served with a simple arthroscopic subacromial decompression/debridement, reserving a formal open repair using allograft for those in whom pain relief is insufficient.

REFERENCES

1. Neer CS II, Craig EV, Fukuda H. Cuff-tear arthropathy. *J Bone Joint Surg Am.* 1983;65:1232.
2. Rockwood CA Jr, Burkhead WZ. Management of patients with massive rotator cuff defects by acromioplasty and rotator cuff debridement. *Orthop Trans.* 1988;12:190.
3. Mansat M, Bonnevaille P. Impingement syndrome—surgical treatment of stage III [Abstract]. *Orthop Trans.* 1986;10:229.
4. Neer, C.S. II. *Shoulder Reconstruction.* Philadelphia: WB Saunders; 1990:117–118.
5. Ozaki J, Fujimoto S, Masuhara K, Tamai S, Yoshimota S. Reconstruction of chronic massive rotator cuff tears with synthetic materials. *Clin Orthop.* 1986;202:173.
6. Post M. Rotator cuff repair with carbon filament: A preliminary report of five cases. *Clin Orthop.* 1985;196:154.
7. Bateman JE. The diagnosis and treatment of ruptures of the rotator cuff. *Surg Clin North Am.* 1963;43:1523.
8. Bateman JE. *The Shoulder and Neck.* 2nd ed. Philadelphia: WB Saunders; 1978.
9. DeOrio JK, Cofield RH. Results of a second attempt at surgical repair of a failed initial rotator cuff repair. *J Bone Joint Surg Am.* 1984; 66:563.
10. Neviaser JS, Neviaser RJ, Neviaser TJ. The repair of chronic massive ruptures of the rotator cuff of the shoulder by use of freeze-dried rotator cuff. *J Bone Joint Surg Am.* 1978;60:681.
11. Nasca RJ. The use of freeze-dried allografts in the management of global rotator cuff tears. *Clin Orthop.* 1988;228:218.
12. Wiley AM. Arthroscopic evaluation and surgery for rotator cuff disease. In: Jackson, ed. *Shoulder Surgery in the Athlete.* Rockville, MD: Aspen Systems; 1985:83–91.
13. Gartsman GM. Arthroscopic acromioplasty for lesions of the rotator cuff. *J Bone Joint Surg Am.* 1990;72:169.

Chapter 31

Repair of Chronic Massive Rotator Cuff Tears with Teflon Felt

Jiro Ozaki

Every surgeon has encountered a rotator cuff tear that is longstanding and may be technically difficult to repair, secondary to tendon retraction and muscular contracture. The quality of rotator cuff tendons and muscles may be poor. In order to surgically repair a rotator cuff tear, the tendon defect must be defined, and a subacromial decompression in combination with cuff mobilization is essential. However, after these measures have been carried out, the surgeon is often confronted with tears of a greater size in which there is an apparent or real loss of tendon substance and an inability to effect primary tendon-to-tendon or tendon-to-tuberosity suture. This situation occurs in the chronic condition, because of intramuscular contractures of the rotator cuff and absolute loss of tendon substance caused by impingement of the cuff between the acromion[1] and the upper part of the humerus, in addition to the attrition of the torn edges. Specific techniques have been suggested to deal with this situation.[2–7] In 1980, we began using synthetic materials such as Marlex mesh, Teflon fabric, and Teflon felt for repairing chronic massive or global cuff defects.[8] In our most recent series, 3-mm-thick Teflon felt (USCI, CR Bard, Mullayhill, NJ) has been used. This thickness was chosen because the implanted synthetic materials should become as thick as the normal rotator cuff after implantation.[8] This chapter describes the current technique of cuff repair with Teflon felt (''Teflon felt cuff plasty'') and the long-term results in a series of 47 patients.

INDICATIONS AND CONTRAINDICATIONS

Teflon felt cuff plasty is indicated mainly for patients with chronic massive or global rotator cuff tears that cannot be repaired with conventional techniques and for augmentation of chronic small or moderate cuff tears in which tendon durability is suspect. Further indications include rotator cuff tears that occur in combination with humeral head damage, such as rheumatoid arthritis and traumatic injuries, at the time of prosthetic humeral head replacement.

The advantages of this procedure are the technical ease with which it can be performed, the minimal loss of shoulder motion involved, and the patient's usual ability to return to daily living activities in the early postoperative period. However, patients must be aware of the long healing time that follows repair and of the necessity of careful postoperative management.

Teflon felt cuff plasty is contraindicated in patients with previous or chronic infection.

SURGICAL PROCEDURE AND TECHNIQUES

Since our first publication, several improvements have been developed in the technique of this procedure.

Patient Position

The patient is placed in the supine position with a small pillow or half of a surgical sheet beneath the involved scapula. The anesthesiologist's equipment should be on the uninvolved side of the patient. The involved extremity is draped freely to permit movement during the procedure.

Skin and Deltoid Incision

The skin incision is illustrated in Figure 31–1. An anterior deltoid incision is made one finger-breadth lateral to the palpable coracoid process. A 5- to 6-cm incision is begun at the tip of the acromion and extends along the anterior deltoid margin. The deltoid muscle is detached from the anterior tip of the AC joint and acromion over a length of 1 cm. This cut extends straight out laterally past the lateral tip of the acromion. The fascia is opened in line with the interval of the anterior deltoid portion, and the interval is separated by blunt dissection over the humerus, with care not to injure the axillary nerve (Fig. 31–2). If firm, fibrous bands are encountered deep below the muscles, sharp dissection is necessary to provide adequate mobility of these tissues. Once the interval of the anterior deltoid muscle is reflected, the subacromial bursa and greater tuberosity can be exposed easily.

Anterior Acromioplasty and Decompression of the AC Undersurface

An anterior acromioplasty (described by Neer[5]) is performed. In addition, spurs present on the undersurface of the AC joint are removed by the osteotome.

Management of Diseased Subacromial Bursa and The Long Head of the Biceps Brachii (LHBB)

Enough thick-walled, diseased subacromial bursal tissue is resected to allow adequate exposure of the rotator cuff tear (Fig. 31–3). Evaluation and management of the LHBB tendon is extremely important. The long head of the biceps must be visualized before the torn cuff is repaired to ensure that it is not stenosed, subluxated, dislocated, or deformed. In my experience, instability or attrition of the LHBB tendon is always related to chronic cuff tears of the anterior portion. If the biceps is stenosed, it should be decompressed by incision of the transverse humeral ligament or resection of spur formation of the groove.

Mobilization of the Torn Cuff With Release of the Coracohumeral Ligament

Traction sutures are inserted for mobilizing the rotator cuff and the capsule, pulling at reversed directions from the deforming forces (Fig. 31–4). The contracted and shortened coracohumeral ligament is released from the

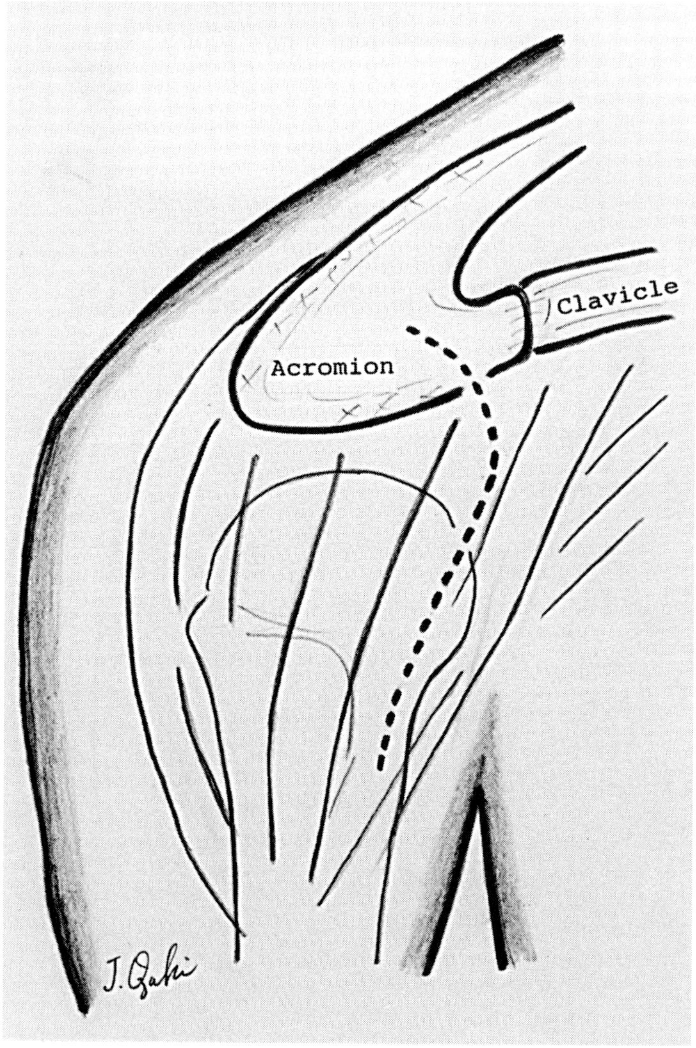

Fig. 31–1. A skin incision (dashed line) that follows the anterior fibers of the deltoid muscle.

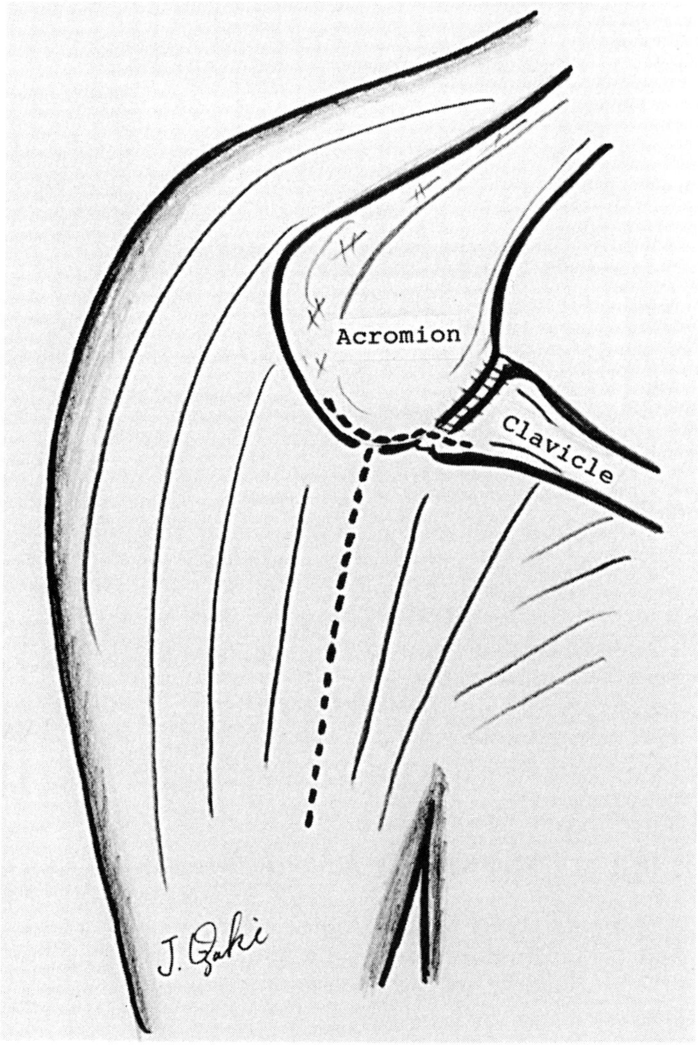

Fig. 31–2. Anterior deltoid incision (dashed line). The anterior deltoid interval is incised off the anterior acromion. This transverse incision is made to bone along the front of the acromion over a length of 1 cm.

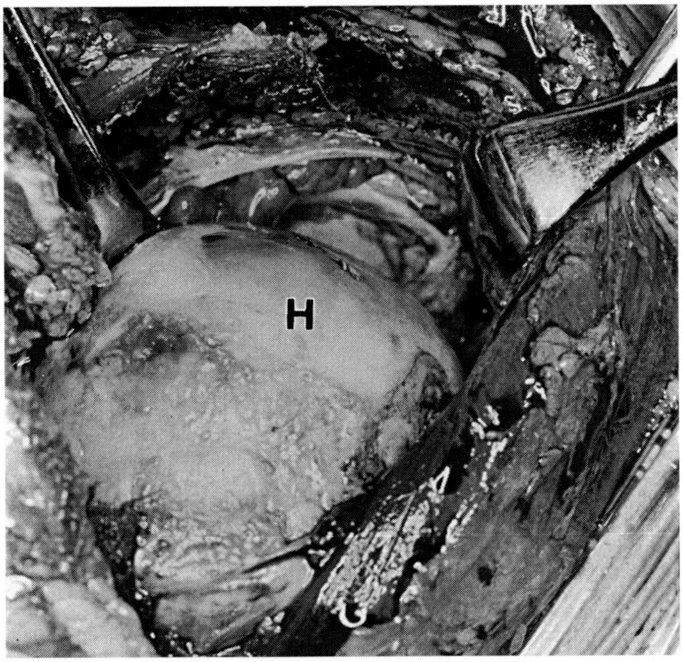

Fig. 31–3. A massive rotator cuff tear: the humeral head is exposed, and the torn rotator cuff edge is retracted. If a defect remains after cuff mobilization, Teflon felt cuff plasty is indicated (H = exposure of the humeral head).

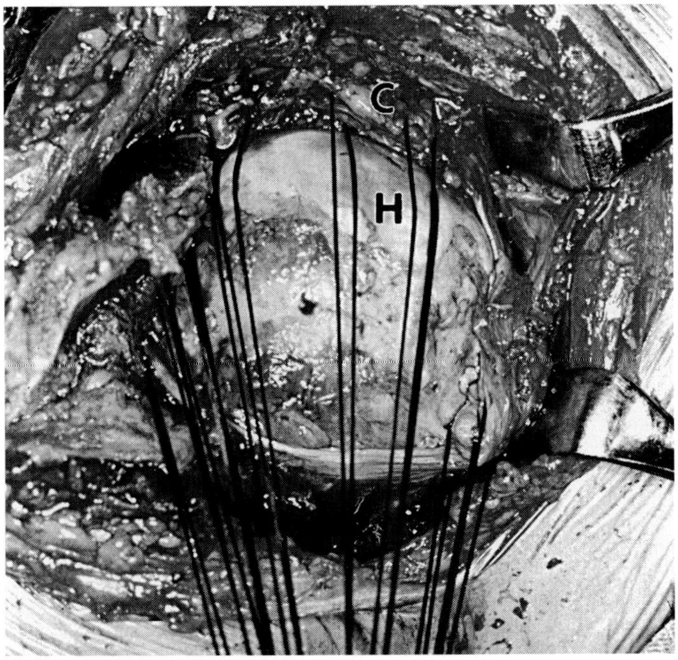

Fig. 31–4. Traction sutures for mobilizing the rotator cuff (C = torn cuff end; H = humeral head).

base of the coracoid process as described previously (Fig. 31–5).[9] Furthermore, the contracted and shortened capsule is released from the glenoid, while traction is maintained on the stay suture. These procedures allow adequate mobilization of the contracted rotator cuff.

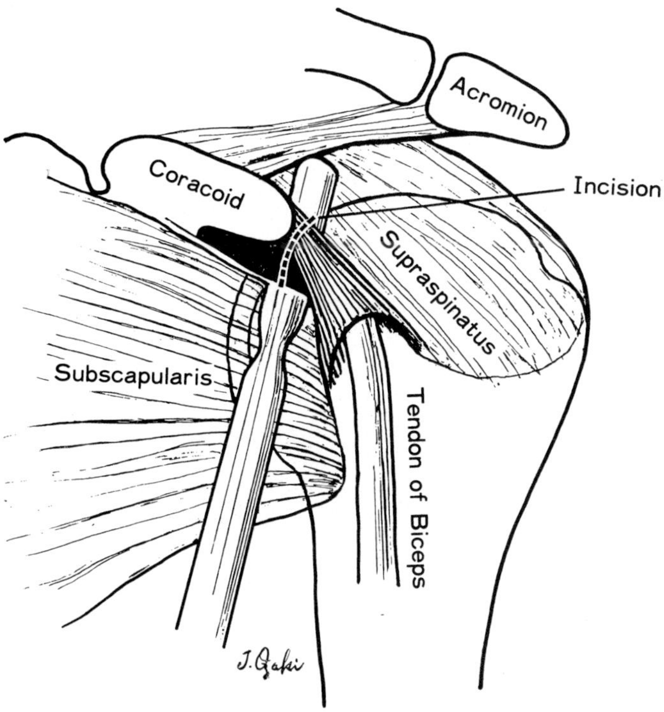

Fig. 31–5. Operative procedure of release of the contracted structures, including the coracohumeral ligament and rotator interval. A smooth retractor is placed beneath the contracted coracohumeral ligament, and the rotator interval is bluntly dissected with care being taken not to injure the long head of the biceps brachii. (From Ozaki J, et al. Recalcitrant chronic adhesive capsulitis of the shoulder. Role of contracture of the coracohumeral ligament and rotator interval in pathogenesis and treatment. *J Bone Joint Surg Am.* 1989;71:1511–1515.)

Closing Massive Cuffs With Teflon Felt

When the cuff has been mobilized, a shallow trough is made in the neck area of the humerus for tendon-to-bone repair. However, if the torn cuff edge cannot be pulled out or if the defect over the humeral head remains,[10] Teflon felt cuff plasty is indicated. Scissors are used to trim 3-mm-thick Teflon felt to the desired size. Using a knitted nylon suture, the Teflon felt is sutured to the undersurface of the torn cuff edges, creating a slight overlap of the cuff (Figs. 31–6 and 31–7).

The method of anchoring the graft to the tuberosity should be individualized, based on the bone quality of the humeral head and the size of Teflon felt graft used. A bony trough is not recommended if the humeral head is osteoporotic and replaced with fatty marrow. In these cases, we suture the graft to tendinous tissue near the tuberosities (Fig. 31–8). If the humeral head is of good quality, a shallow groove is made at the humeral neck for suturing the Teflon felt to bone. Some tension must be kept on the graft in all shoulder positions when selecting the site of the trough, and the suture line must not impinge against the residual acromion. The detached deltoid muscle then is sutured firmly to the strong fibrous tissues of the acromial superficial surface using a knitted nylon suture.

Postoperative Management

Following Teflon felt cuff plasty, the arm is maintained in 75° elevation in the scapular plane with an abduction orthosis of my design during the first 4 to 8 weeks following the surgery. One to 2 weeks following surgery, the arm is passively elevated slightly from the orthosis to the overhead position by the therapist. Four to 5 weeks following surgery, with the arm supported in 45 or 60° elevation with the orthosis, a self-assistive program is instructed by the therapist, including external rotation, elevation, and the use of a pulley. Five to 6 weeks following surgery, the arm is lowered to 30°, and the self-assistive exercises are continued. About 1 week before the orthosis is removed, the patient begins letting the arm come down to the side. Isometrics and strengthening exercises usually are deferred until after the sixth week following surgery. The patient learns that improvement in strength overhead can occur throughout the first year.

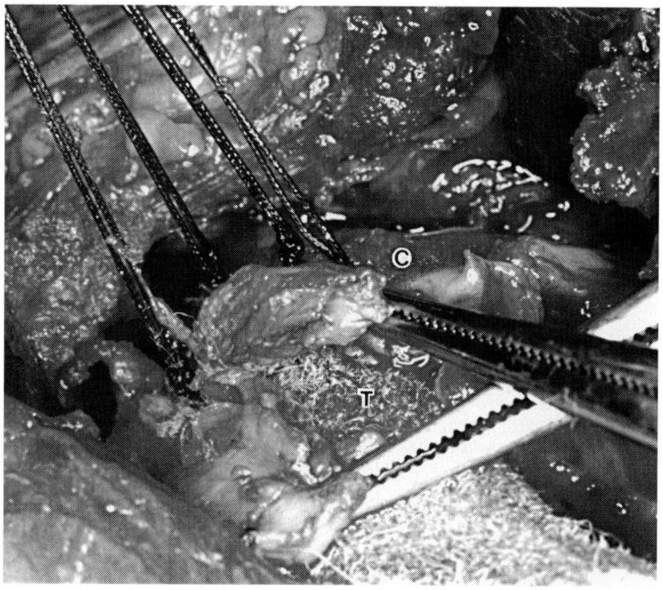

Fig. 31–6. Suturing the cuff end to the 3-mm-thick Teflon felt. The felt can be firmly sutured enough to create a slight overlap of the cuff (C = torn cuff end; T = Teflon felt).

CLINICAL MATERIALS AND RESULTS

Between 1982 and 1993, 110 shoulders with chronic large or massive cuff tears were treated with Teflon felt cuff plasty. The predominant complaints were prolonged dysfunction and pain in the involved shoulder. The extent of the cuff defects ranged from 4 × 3 cm to 9 × 8 cm (average = 5.4 × 4.1 cm).

Minimal foreign-body reactions occurred in all patients; transient subacromial effusion was seen in seven patients. In the present study, 50 shoulders were available with greater than 2 year follow-up; the mean follow-up period was 4.1 years. The patients were evaluated in terms of pain, range of motion, and muscle strength. The relief of pain was significant. Forty-five shoulders were free of pain; while five shoulders with cuff-tear arthropathy or axillary neuropathy were less improved. The improvement of abduction was satisfactory. Forty-five shoulders ranged from 120 to 180° of abduction. In five shoulders with cuff-tear arthropathy or axillary neuropathy, improvement of abduction and muscle strength was poor; however, none of the patients showed reduction of mobility or muscle strength. Forty-five shoulders (90%) had satisfactory functional results.

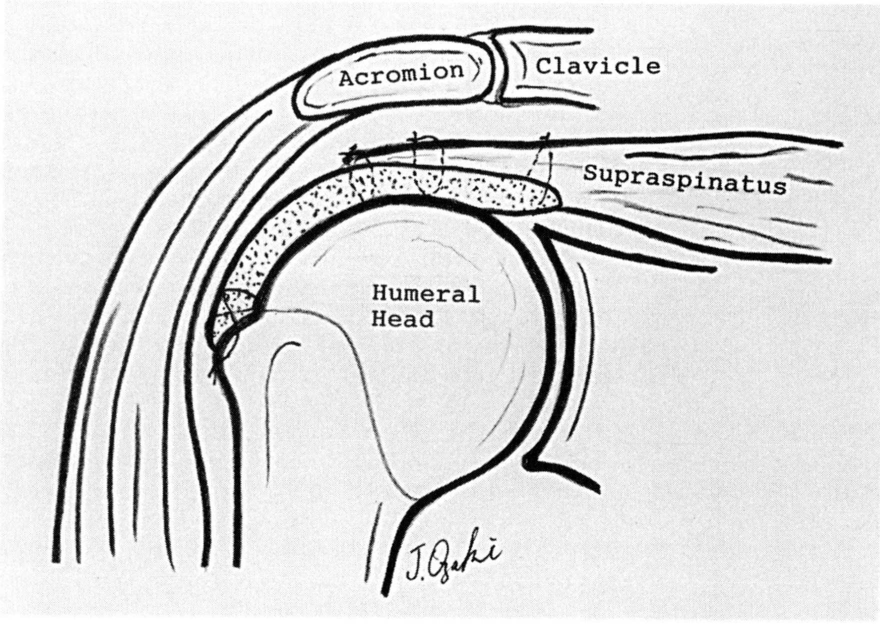

Fig. 31–7. Teflon felt graft in place, as seen from the lateral view. Moderate tension on the graft is essential when the sutures are tied. The graft edge can be fixed firmly near the tuberosities of the humerus (with the tendinous tissues) or less commonly into a bony groove.

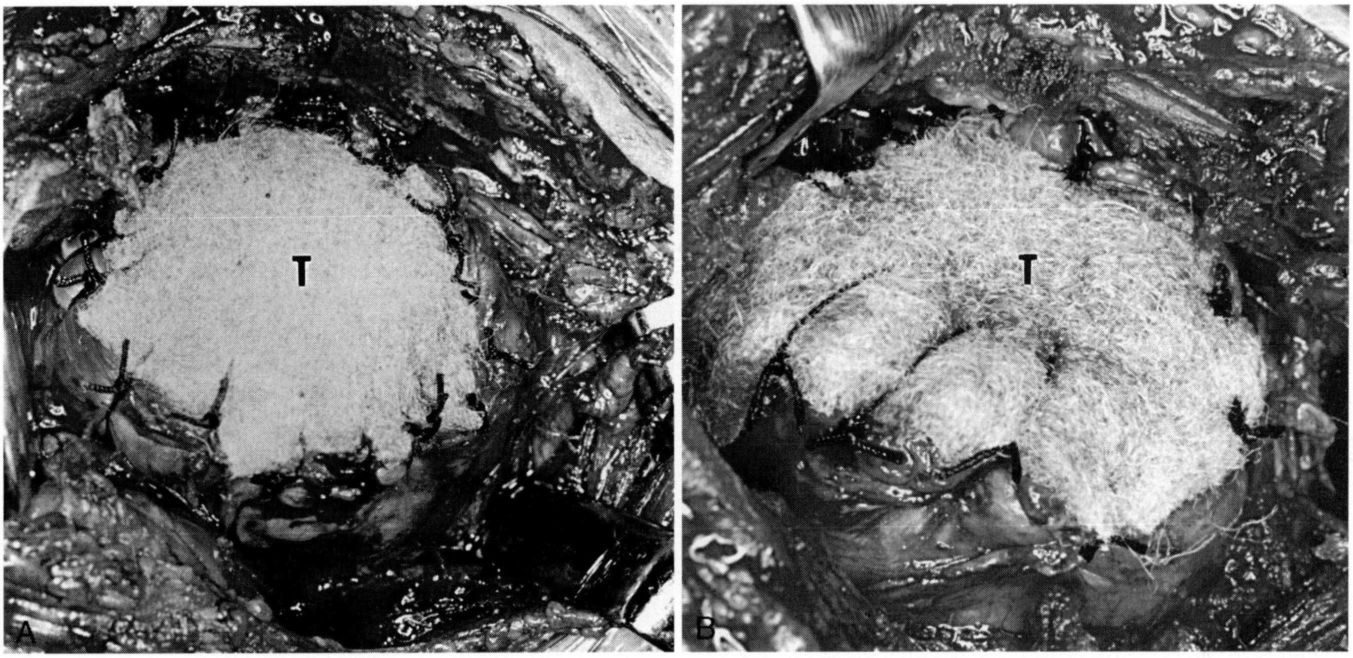

Fig. 31–8. *A,* **The felt edge is sutured into bursal and tendinous scar tissues near the tuberosities. In the shoulder with porotic humeral heads replaced by fatty marrow, a groove should not be made (T = Teflon felt).** *B,* **The felt edge is sutured at the shallow groove of the humeral neck (T = Teflon felt).**

Postoperative MRI

Postoperative MRI (GE: 1.5 T with surface coils) was performed on 21 shoulders of 21 patients who had undergone Teflon felt cuff plasty between 1985 and 1993. Thirteen patients had a low or relatively high-signal area (T2) in the region of the Teflon felt cuff-bone interval. It is believed that this region represents a new rotator cuff of Teflon felt (Fig. 31–9). While the thickness of the rotator cuff remained, the muscular atrophy of the supraspinatus and infraspinatus was unchanged on postoperative MRI scans. The remaining eight shoulders showed a high intensity lesion (T2).

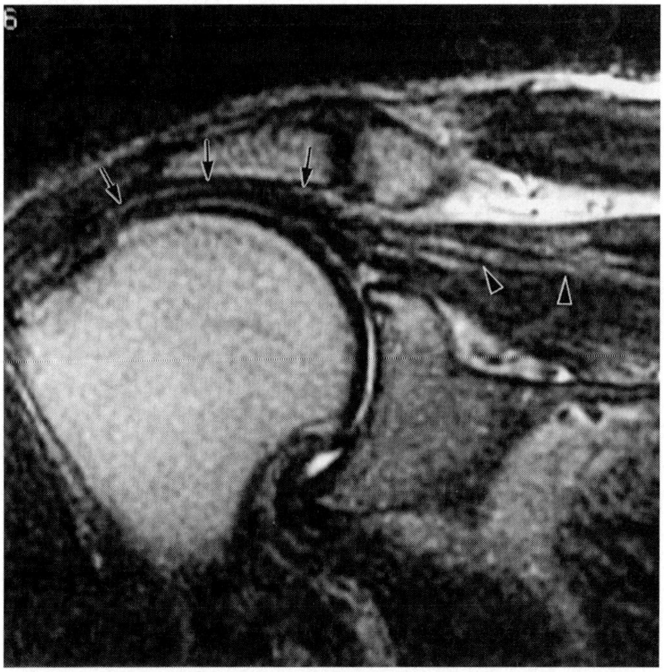

Fig. 31–9. MRI at 3 years after Teflon felt cuff plasty. The new rotator cuff of Teflon graft (arrows) is confirmed. The degeneration of the supraspinatus muscle (arrow heads) remained.

SHOULDER ARTHROPLASTY USING THE PROSTHETIC HUMERAL HEAD AND TEFLON FELT CUFF PLASTY

As described above, Teflon felt cuff plasty has also been used with prosthetic humeral heads at the time of glenohumeral reconstruction of shoulders with damaged humeral heads and massive cuff defects. This procedure is indicated for shoulders with rotator cuff arthropathy or other conditions in which humeral head destruction and massive cuff tissue loss coexist in the presence of a functional deltoid muscle.

A deltopectoral incision is used, and the damaged humeral head is resected with the osteotomy line at an angle of 45° to the long axis of the humerus, with the humerus in 35° of internal rotation. Before the massive cuff defects are repaired, all of the adhered subacromial scar tissue is released. The humeral component of the Neer prosthesis is inserted at an angle of 40° retrotorsion, and Teflon felt cuff plasty is performed (Fig. 31–10).

The shoulders are moved with assisted exercises within the first few days postoperatively. The postoperative man-

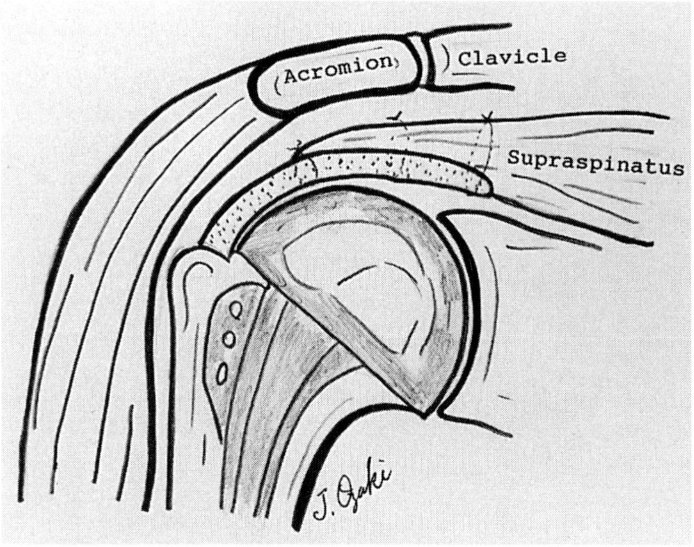

Fig. 31–10. **Shoulder arthroplasty using a prosthetic humeral head and Teflon felt cuff plasty.**

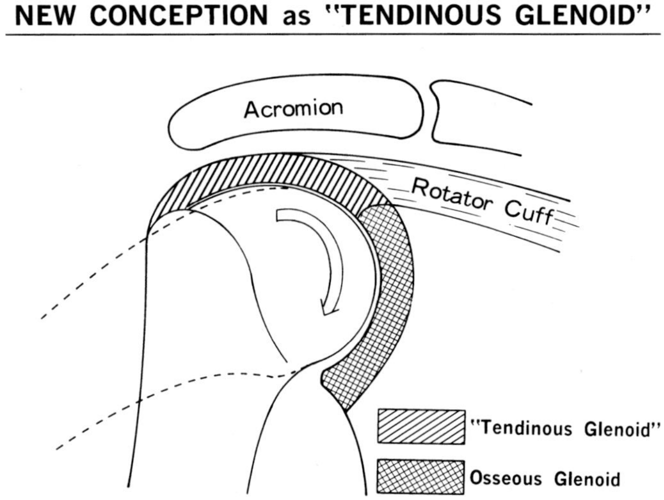

Fig. 31–11. The rotator cuff acts as a "tendinous glenoid" to compensate the small and shallow osseous glenoid. (From Ozaki J, et al. Reconstruction of chronic massive rotator cuff tears with synthetic materials. *Clin Orthop.* 1986;202:173–183.)

agement is similar to that described for rotator cuff repair without humeral replacement.

From 1982 to 1986, this procedure was performed on seven shoulders of seven patients. The diagnoses included osteoarthritis, posttraumatic arthritis, tumor, and rheumatoid arthritis. There were no complications, and the relief of pain and improvement of passive range of motion were significant at an average 6-year follow-up. Improvement in active motion and muscle strength were less spectacular, possibly because of prolonged disuse of the deltoid muscle. Mobility was not reduced in any of the patients.

Arthroplasty using a prosthetic humeral head and Teflon felt cuff plasty is a valuable procedure for the shoulders, even when both the articular surface of the humeral head and the rotator cuff are damaged.

DISCUSSION

The surgical treatment of a rotator cuff tear was first performed by Codman in 1909. Since then, many investigators have devised their own methods for the repair of chronic global or massive rotator cuff tears.

In the case of moderate rotator cuff tears that could not be sutured end-to-end without tension, McLaughlin attempted in 1962 to freshen the torn cuff and attach it to the humeral head at whatever point it could reach without tension.[4] However, for repair of some chronic massive or global tears of the rotator cuff, McLaughlin's technique cannot be applied. In 1965 Debeyre et al. devised a procedure of supraspinatus muscle advancement.[3] In 1978 Neviaser et al. incised the intra-articular portion of the long head of the biceps, producing a sheet that was used to close the defect. These methods, however, have not always been applied successfully, because the supraspinatus muscle or biceps tendon may be too small to bridge a massive or global cuff defect of the rotator cuff.

In biomechanical considerations of the rotator cuff, the action of the rotator cuff has been a subject of controversy. According to Codman (1934), the supraspinatus muscle acts as a fulcrum to furnish power for the deltoid muscle.[2] Kapandji (1970) described the supraspinatus as a "starter" muscle of abduction at the beginning of the shoulder motion.[11] Conversely, Linge and Mulder (1963) concluded that the role of the supraspinatus muscle is only of a quantitative nature, with no specific function of its own.[12]

By 1981 it was clear that the rotator cuff acts as a glenohumeral joint stabilizer that compensates for the small and shallow osseous glenoid. Later, in 1987 my colleagues and I analyzed the role that the rotator cuff plays in stabilization of the glenohumeral joint. Using a two-dimensional computer simulation, we showed that the contact stresses were distributed widely on the rotator cuff during the early and middle phase of abduction.[13] It was concluded that the rotator cuff muscles act as the "tendinous glenoid," which, collaborating with the "osseous glenoid," holds the humeral head stable so that the deltoid muscle can abduct the upper extremity. However, some patients with massive rotator cuff tears have been shown to have complete active overhead motion if the deltoid is functioning. In these cases, the acromion appears to serve as a compression mechanism (i.e., as an "acetabulum-like" acromion).

Concerning reconstruction of the rotator cuff with synthetic materials, two functions of the rotator cuff mechanism must be noted: (1) the rotator cuff conducts the power of short rotator muscles to the tuberosities of the humerus and (2) acts as the tendinous glenoid. This

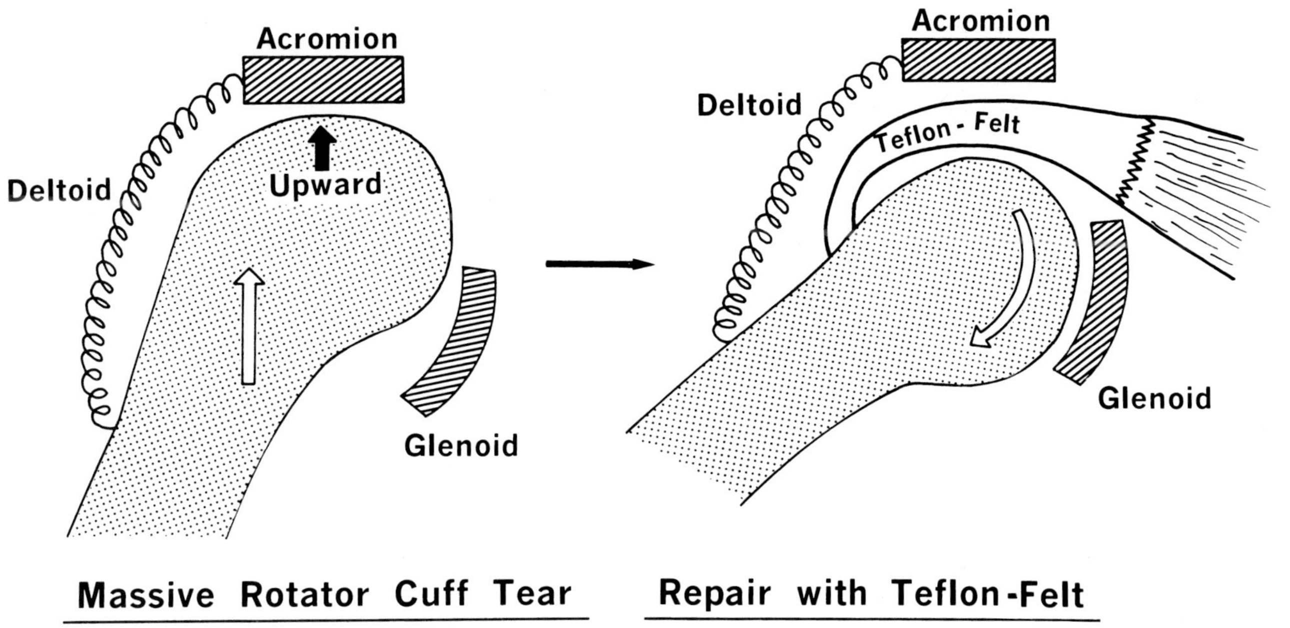

Fig. 31–12. The use of Teflon felt to bridge the cuff defects leads to functional results. (From Ozaki J, et al. Reconstruction of chronic massive rotator cuff tears with synthetic materials. *Clin Orthop.* 1986;202:173–183.)

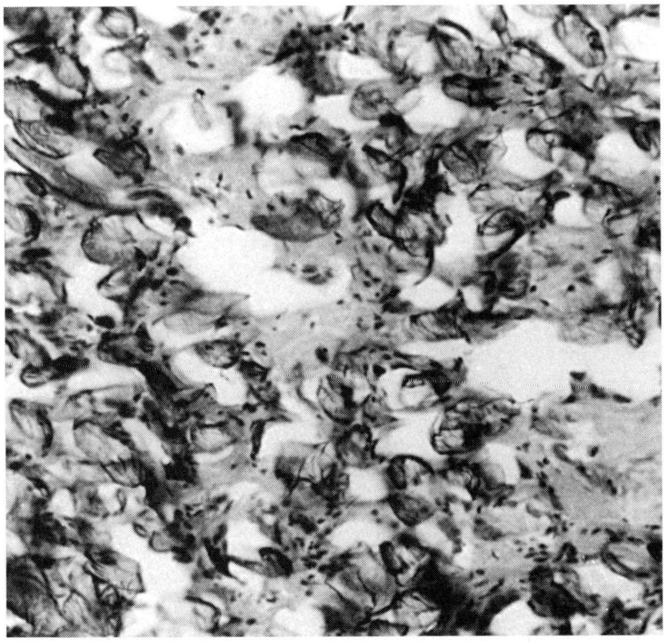

Fig. 31–13. Histology of Teflon felt at 3 months after implant of the experiment on rat (hematoxylin-eosin, original magnification ×200).

mechanism holds well for the reconstruction of degenerated short rotator muscles that have undergone myostatic contracture following chronic massive rotator cuff tears. Figure 31–11 shows the function of the rotator cuff as a tendinous glenoid. The deltoid alone tends to press the humeral head upward to the acromion, and a sliding fulcrum cannot be made on the glenoid. The action of the rotator cuff as a tendinous glenoid is to steer the humeral head on the glenoid and make the deltoid work effectively. Therefore, it is believed that the use of appropriate synthetic materials to bridge the cuff defect leads to satisfactory functional results (Fig. 31–12).

We have been using synthetic materials such as Marlex mesh and Teflon felt for repairing chronic massive or global cuff defects since 1980. In our recent series, 3-mm-thick Teflon felt has been used; the implanted synthetic materials should become as thick as the normal rotator cuff after implantation Fig. 31–13.[8] shows the histologic finding of the experiment on Teflon felt graft to the musculotendinous defect of the rat knee.

Reconstruction of the tears of the rotator cuff can be called "spherical tendon plasty." The advantages of Teflon felt cuff plasty include (1) technical ease, (2) minimal loss of shoulder motion, and (3) the ability of patients to return to daily living activities in the early postoperative period. However, the patients are informed of the long healing time after Teflon felt cuff plasty and the necessity of postoperative management.

REFERENCES

1. Ozaki J. Tears of the rotator cuff of the shoulder associated with pathological changes in the acromion. A study in cadavera. *J Bone Joint Surg Am.* 1988;70:1224–1230.
2. Codman EA. *The Shoulder.* Boston: Thomas Todd; 1934.
3. Debeyre J, Patte D, Elmelik E. Repair of rupture of the rotator cuff of the shoulder. With a note on advancement of the supraspinatus muscle. *J Bone Joint Surg Br.* 1965;47:36–42.
4. McLaughlin HL. Rupture of the rotator cuff. *J Bone Joint Surg Am.* 1962;44:979–983.
5. Neer CS II. Anterior acromioplasty for the chronic impingement syndrome in the shoulder. *J Bone Joint Surg Am.* 1972;54:41–50.
6. Neviaser JS, Neviaser RJ, Neviaser TJ. The repair of chronic massive

ruptures of the rotator cuff of the shoulder by use of a freeze-dried rotator cuff. *J Bone Joint Surg Am.* 1978;60:681–684.
7. Neviaser RJ, Neviaser TJ. Transfer of the subscapularis and teres minor for massive defects of the rotator cuff. In: Bayley I, Kessel L, eds. *Shoulder Surgery.* Berlin: Springer; 1982:60–69.
8. Ozaki J, Fujimoto S, Mashuhara K, Tamai S, Yoshimoto S. Reconstruction of chronic massive rotator cuff tears with synthetic materials. *Clin Orthop.* 1986;202:173–183.
9. Ozaki J, Nakagawa Y, Sakurai G, Tamai S. Recalcitrant chronic adhesive capsulitis of the shoulder. Role of contracture of the coracohumeral ligament and rotator interval in pathogenesis and treatment. *J Bone Joint Surg Am.* 1989;71:1511–1515.
10. Ozaki J. Pathogenesis of the loose shoulder. *Rinsho Seikei Geka.* 1981; 16:1161–1171 (in Japanese).
11. Kapandji IA. *The Physiology of the Joints.* Edinburgh: Churchill Livingstone; 1970.
12. Linge B, Muller JD. Function of the supraspinatus and its relation to the supraspinatus syndrome. An experimental study in man. *J Bone Joint Surg Am.* 1962;44:979–983.
13. Ozaki J, Ohneda Y, Nakagawa Y, Mashuhara K. Glenohumeral stabilizing mechanism. A two-dimensional computer simulation study based on Pauwel's stress distribution theory of a concave articular joint. In: Takagishi N, ed. *The Shoulder.* Tokyo: Professional Postgraduate Services; 1987:39–43.

Chapter 32

The End Result: Functional Assessment of Rotator Cuff Repair

Michael D. Ciepiela and Wayne Z. Burkhead, Jr.

The end result was merely the common sense notion that every hospital should follow every patient it treats, long enough to determine whether or not the treatment has been successful and then to inquire if not, why not, with a view to preventing similar failures in the future. This routine tracing of every case, interesting or uninteresting, brings to our attention many things in which our knowledge, our technique, our organization, our own skill or wisdom, and perhaps even our care and our consciences needed attention.

Codman[1]

The practical goal of rotator cuff repair is to provide the patient with a painless functional shoulder that endures over time. Scientifically, one would like to evaluate the effectiveness and durability of repair technique at progressive time intervals. Correlation of the functional result with the anatomic result following operative treatment of a rotator cuff tear can be difficult. A question of the integrity of the repair itself may be suspected after clinical evaluation; however, adjunctive testing is relatively expensive and its value is variable.

Although the ''gold standard'' in diagnosing primary cuff tears, arthrography has been shown to have little value in diagnosing the failure of a repaired rotator cuff.[2] This is because of the contrast leakage that invariably occurs despite an intact functional repair. Calvert and Kessel et al. performed arthrography on 20 patients at an average of 30 months postoperatively following open repair of rotator cuff tears. Of the 20 patients, 18 showed leakage of dye into the subacromial space. Of these 18 patients, 17 had complete relief of pain and 15 had full range of motion.[2]

MRI was shown to be accurate in predicting 90% (6 of 7) of full- thickness retears in a series of 31 patients by Owen, Ianotti, et al.[3] They ignored all potential normal postoperative findings, using the presence of a fluid-like signal intensity on T2-weighted images that extends through an area of the rotator cuff or the nonvisualization of a portion of the rotator cuff as their diagnostic criteria. Even more recently, Haygood et al. defined the expected and unexpected MRI observations after surgical procedures on the shoulder, including impingement, rotator cuff surgery, and instability corrective surgery. They noted that MRI could be diagnostic of full-thickness rotator cuff tears but that this modality could not distinguish between partial-thickness tears, tendinitis, and normal postoperative changes. They indicated additional study is needed to further define the value of MRI in diagnosing postoperative rotator cuff tears.

Ultrasonography has been reported as 90% accurate in detecting large retorn rotator cuffs, provided certain criteria are met. The postoperative rotator cuff has an echogenic appearance for at least 6 months after surgery. Therefore, the presence of a gap or defect in the tendon, and not just echogenicity, is the criteria recommended in order to diagnose a retorn rotator cuff. The value of ultrasonography, being an operator dependent modality, must be weighed from center to center.[5]

Recently, Harryman et al. correlated the functional evaluation of a rotator cuff repair to the integrity of the cuff. Ultrasonography was used to evaluate the cuff integrity, categorizing the findings as type 0–1A as no tear or a partial-thickness defect in the supraspinatus tendon, type 1B as a full-thickness defect of the supraspinatus, type 2 as a full-thickness defect in the supraspinatus, and type 3 as a full-thickness defect in the supraspinatus, infraspinatus, and subscapularis. Muscle testing was done isometrically using a hand-held dynamometer. They tested internal rotation, external rotation, and extension with the arm at the side and the elbow flexed 90°. Forward flexion and abduction were evaluated at 90°. The results of their efforts showed an ultrasonographically intact cuff as the most important factor in attaining a good functional outcome.[6]

Information from the above data can be invaluable to the clinician. This data does not, however, determine what value the treatment mode had for the patient (i.e., an elderly patient whose strength is restored but still has disabling pain at night).

Pain, as subjective as it may be, has been the major criteria used to classify an excellent, good, or poor result of rotator cuff tear treatment. Many direct their treatment plan toward the goal of pain relief, primarily because the outcome with this goal in mind will be readily evident as it is generally first and foremost on the patient's mind.

Methods for evaluation of functional improvement have been proposed in the literature, but no single method has yet to gain uniform acceptance. There is a renewal toward looking at functional results of treatment; either compared to a pretreatment change or compared to a normal shoulder.

Muscle measurement of strength was advocated by Moseley. [7] He tested his patients both preoperatively and postoperatively, and tested the unaffected side as well. Moseley used a spring balance or tension meter to provide a numerical representation of power in pounds of force (Figs. 32–1 and 32–2).

He measured patients at 90° abduction and 90° forward flexion, as well as maintenance of abduction (isometric) at 90° abduction. This method of strength testing was reproducible, reliable, and inexpensive. The other criteria he used were pain and active range of motion. An excellent result was obtained within his system if (1) pain was resolved or mildly present with prolonged use; (2) the patient was able to maintain abduction at 90° nearly as well as the opposite side; (3) the patient's range of motion was at least 145° in abduction and forward flexion; (4) the patient's power, as tested by the tensiometer, was at least 70% of the unaffected side; and (5) the patient had the capacity to return to work. No points were assigned in his system. Rather, if a result was not excellent, then subjectively it could be termed fair or good. Although not complete in objectivity, this early attempt to quantify results showed the value and necessity of a system.

A shoulder scoring system was published by Neer in 1970 to assess functional recovery following proximal humerus fractures (Table 32–1).[8] Neer stated, "An objective system that can be generally accepted for the future judging of long-term results is needed." His system weighs components of the result based on Neer's perception of their importance to the patient. Pain, being the most important component, is worth 35 points, function is worth 30 points, range of motion is worth 25 points, and anatomy is worth 10 points. A perfect score is 100 points, with excellent results scoring 90 to 100 points, satisfactory results scoring 80 to 90 points, unsatisfactory results scoring 70 to 79 points, and failure results scoring below 70 points.

The Japanese Orthopaedic Association has adapted a scoring system similar to Neer's. In addition, stability and radiographic evaluation are weighed as well (Table 32–2).

Constant and Murley, in their 1986 publication, describe a useful method of functional assessment of the shoulder. [9] This system, like Neer's, had a maximum of 100 points. The primary differences lie in the relative value of the various parameters, as well as their method of strength testing. They de-emphasized the importance of subjective pain, assigning it a 15-point value. Activities of daily living, also a subjective parameter, were valued at a maximum of 20 points. Range of motion and strength, being objective data, were valued more significantly and were assigned a maximum of 40 and 25 points, respectively (Table 32–3). Pain is defined as the most severe degree of pain the patient exhibits during their

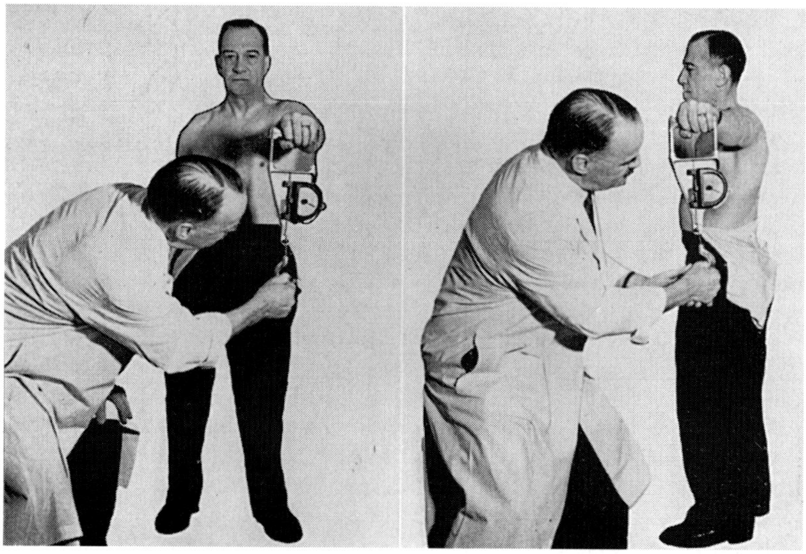

Fig. 32–1. The use of a tension meter is an effective, objective method of testing muscle strength.

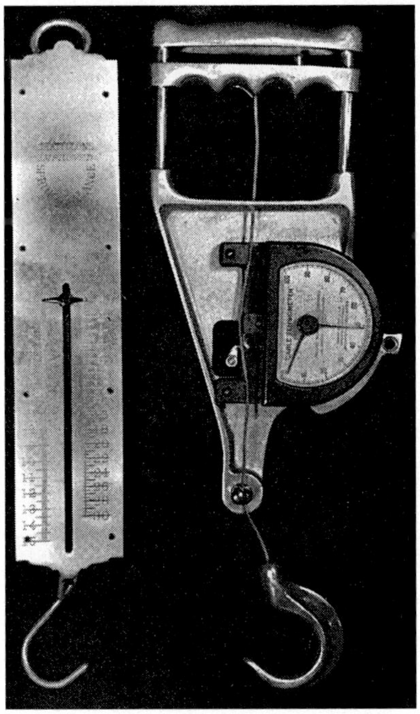

Fig. 32–2. The above depicts a spring balance on the left and a tension meter on the right, similar to the ones used by Moseley in his description of objective muscle testing.

Table 32–2. Shoulder Assessment Scoring System, Japanese Orthopaedic Society

Pain	30
Function	20
ROM	30
X-ray Findings	5
Joint Stability	15
Total	100

activities of daily living, with no pain worth 15 points to severe pain having 0 point value. Activities of daily living such as work capacity, recreational capacity, and ability to sleep are valued at 10 points. An additional 10 points is available dependent upon the maximum level of the body the patient can position his hand.

Active and not passive range of motion is used for their assessment. Forward flexion and lateral elevation are worth a maximum of 10 points each, depending on the degree from 0 to 180° obtained. External rotation is worth a maximum of 10 points. Internal rotation is also worth a maximum of 10 points, depending on the level of the spine that can be reached.

Strength is tested using the isometric method described by Moseley with a spring balance at 90° abduction (or the maximum degree of abduction the patient can actively attain). They stated that isokinetic testing by a Cybex II Dynamometer (Lumex, Bayshore, NY) is reliable and reproducible. The practicality of using this device in most clinical situations is questionable in their opinion, because of the expense of the equipment. They, therefore, incorporated the spring balance as a reasonable test of strength offering portability and economy to the clinician. They evaluated both shoulders for comparative purposes. To test the reliability of their method, three observers evaluated 100 abnormal shoulders. The observer error averaged 3% (range = 0 to 8%), showing their system to be quite reliable.

Table 32–1. Neer Rating Scale

Pain	35
Function	25
Range of Motion	25
Anatomy	10
Excellent 90–100	Satisfactory 80–90
Unsatisfactory 70–79	Failure <70 points

Constant and Murley noted the use of a Cybex II Dynamometer would be a more accurate method of testing shoulder strength. Several investigators have shown the efficacy of this equipment in testing shoulder strength.[10,11] The deltoid, supraspinatus, subscapularis, and internal rotators can be isolated and tested individually in a reliable reproducible manner. Recently the use of a fixed spring balance has been found to be as reliable and reproducible as Isobex testing.[12]

One of us (MDC), with Bernasek and Leffers, used the Biodex Dynamometer in a recent study that defined the normal strength ratios of the individual rotator cuff components to the deltoid muscle.[12] The normal ratio of supraspinatus to deltoid was approximately 1.0, external rotators to deltoid 0.33, and subscapularis to deltoid 0.50. Similar testing was done on shoulders diagnosed with impingement syndrome. The average ratio of supraspinatus to deltoid was 0.58, external rotators to deltoid 0.26, and subscapularis to deltoid 0.60. All subjects were then placed in a 6-week standard rotator cuff strengthening program providing deltoid maintenance. All subjects were then re-examined and retested on the Biodex Dynamometer with the subsequent ratios calculated. As the abnormal ratios approach the normal values, the patients clinically improved; this occurred in 92% of subjects.

The value of incorporating strength testing and active range of motion into the postoperative functional assessment is apparent throughout the literature.[6–9,13–15] Many investigators incorporate manual muscle testing grading strength on a 0 to 5 scale.[6,8,15] Recognizing the inconsistency of this approach, the comparative value of this data is given less weight than other components of the evaluation. The proposed standardized evaluation form of the American Shoulder and Elbow Surgeons independently evaluates pain, motion, strength, stability, and function, with strength being tested by the manual muscle method.

The evaluation system employed by Gore et al. individually graded the subjective data from pain, occupational status, and functional capacity following cuff repair.[14] They also individually scored radiographic findings, active and passive range of motion, and isometric muscle strength. To test muscle strength, a device was created using U-shaped deflection beam force gauges with connections at the arms and wrists of patients, seating the patient in a stabilized position (Fig. 32–3). They measured internal rotation, external rotation, and abduction at 45°. They also measured abduction at 90°, if the patient

Table 32–3. Constant and Murley Functional Assessment

	Right	Left	
Pain			
None	15	15	
Mild	10	10	
Moderate	5	5	
Severe	0	5	Total
Activities of daily living			
Activity level	*Right*	*Left*	
Full work	4	4	
Full recreation/sport	4	4	
Unaffected sleep	2	2	Total
Positioning	*Right*	*Left*	
Up to waist	2	2	
Up to xiphoid	4	4	
Up to neck	6	6	
Up to top of head	8	8	
Above head	10	10	Total
Range of motion			
Forward flexion	*Right*	*Left*	
0–30°	0	0	
31–60°	2	2	
61–90°	4	4	
91–120°	6	6	
121–150°	8	8	
151–180°	10	10	Total
Lateral elevation	*Right*	*Left*	
0–30°	0	0	
31–60°	2	2	
61–90°	4	4	
91–120°	6	6	
121–150°	8	8	
151–180°	10	10	
External rotation	*Right*	*Left*	
Hand behind head with elbow held forward	2	2	
Hand behind head with elbow held back	2	2	
Hand on top of head with elbow held forward	2	2	
Hand on top of head with elbow held back	2	2	
Full elevation from on top of head	2	2	Total
Internal rotation	*Right*	*Left*	
Dorsum of hand to lateral thigh	0	0	
Dorsum of hand to buttock	2	2	
Dorsum of hand to lumbosacral junction	4	4	
Dorsum of hand to waist (L3)	6	6	
Dorsum of hand to T12	8	8	
Dorsum of hand to T7	10	10	
Power	*Right*	*Left*	
Resist 0 lbs	0	0	
Resist 5 lbs	5	5	
Resist 10 lbs	10	10	
Resist 15 lbs	15	15	
Resist 20 lbs	20	20	
Resist 25 lbs	25	25	Total
Shoulder Junction	*Right*	*Left*	
Pain			
Activities of daily living			
Work			
Recreation			
Sleep			
Position			
Range	*Right*	*Left*	
Abduction			
Flexion			
Internal rotation			
External rotation			
Power			
	______		Total

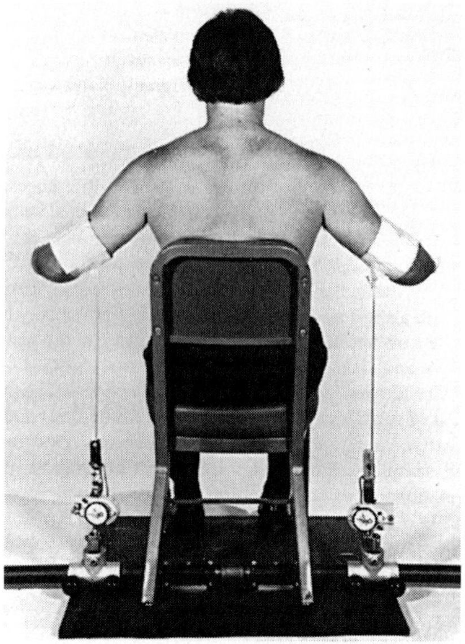

Fig. 32–3. The U-shaped flexion beam force gauge, as described by Gore, is another effective objective method of muscle testing. The abduction strength of both shoulders is being simultaneously tested in the above figure.

Table 32–4. University of California at Los Angeles End-Result Scores

	Points
Pain	
Present all of the time and unbearable; strong medication frequently	1
Present all of the time but bearable; strong medication occasionally	2
None or little at rest, present during light activities; salicylates frequently	4
Present during heavy or particular activities only; salicylates occasionally	6
Occasional and slight	8
None	10
Function	
Unable to use limb	1
Only light activities possible	2
Able to do light housework or most activities of daily living	4
Most housework, shopping, and driving possible; able to do hair and dress and undress, including fastening brassiere	6
Slight restriction only; able to work above shoulder level	8
Normal activities	10
Active forward flexion	
150 or more	5
120 to 150	4
90 to 120	3
45 to 90	2
30 to 45	1
Less than 30	0
Strength of forward flexion (manual muscle-testing)	
Grade 5 (normal)	5
Grade 4 (good)	4
Grade 3 (fair)	3
Grade 2 (poor)	2
Grade 1 (muscle contraction)	1
Grade 0 (nothing)	0
Satisfaction of the patient	
Satisfied and better	5
Not satisfied and worse	0

Table 32–5. Shoulder-Rating Score Sheet of the Hospital for Special Surgery

	No. of Points
Pain (30 points)	
None = 6 points, mild = 3, moderate = 2, severe = 0 during:	
1. Sports	______
2. Non-sports overhead reaching	______
3. Activities of daily living	______
4. Sitting at rest	______
5. Sleeping	______
Total	______
Functional limitation (28 points)	
None = 7 points, mild = 4, moderate = 2, severe = 0 during:	
1. Sports with hand overhead	______
2. Sports not involving use of the shoulder	______
3. Reaching overhead	______
4. Non-specific activities of daily living	______
Total	______
Tenderness (5 points)	
None = 5 points, at one or two sites = 3, at more than two sites = 0	
Total	______
Impingement maneuvers (32 points)	
Indicated numbers of points are assigned for each maneuver in an all-or-none fashion, 0 points being assigned if the maneuver is positive	
1. Impingement sign (15)	______
2. Abduction sign (12)	______
3. Adduction sign (5)	______
Total	______
Range of motion (5 points)	______
One point is assigned for each 20-degree loss of motion in any plane, to a maximum of 5 points	
Total	______

was capable of this motion. Their objective was to correlate the subjective to the objective data, as well as the data to the size of the rotator cuff tear. They found that postoperatively patients average 126° of active flexion and 130° of active abduction. Passive motion averaged 21° more than active. The postoperative shoulder strength was 86% of normal. They also correlated greater strength and range of motion postoperatively for tears less than 2.5 cm.

Ellman et al. developed the University of California at Los Angeles End Results Score System with a maximum score of 35 points.[16] Pain and function were the major emphases with a maximum score of 10 points each. Strength by manual muscle testing was maximally valued at 5 points, as were active forward flexion and patient satisfaction. They attempted to correlate the results of their system to others. With respect to Neer's definitions, a score of 28 points or less was unsatisfactory and a score of greater than 28 points satisfactory. To compare to systems rating excellent, good, fair, and poor, 34 to 35 points was excellent and 29 to 33 points was good (Table 32–4).

The Hospital for Special Surgery rating scale has been described by Altchek et al (Table 32–5).[17] Note that points are scored for the absence of tenderness as well as the obliteration of provocative maneuvers. However, no specific score for strength is given.

All assessment systems incorporate, to a certain extent, the guidelines present in the American Shoulder and Elbow Surgeons' Shoulder Evaluation Form (Table 32–6).

Table 32–6. American Shoulder and Elbow Surgeons' Rating Scale

Name ______________ Hosp. # ______________ Date ______________ Shoulder: R/L.

I. *PAIN:* (5 = none, 4 = slight, 3 = after unusual activity, 2 = moderate, 1 = marked, 0 = complete disability, NA = available) ______

II. *MOTION:*

A. Patient sitting

1. Active total elevation of arm: __________ degrees*
2. Passive internal rotation:
(Circle segment of posterior anatomy reached by thumb)
(Note if reach restricted by limited elbow flexion)

1 = Less than trochanter	5 = L5	9 = L1	13 = T9	17 = T5
2 = Trochanter	6 = L4	10 = T12	14 = T8	18 = T4
3 = Gluteal	7 = L3	11 = T11	15 = T7	19 = T3
4 = Sacrum	8 = L2	12 = T10	16 = T6	20 = T2

3. Active external rotation with arm at side: __________ degrees
4. Active external rotation at 90° abduction: __________ degrees
(Enter "NA" if cannot achieve 90° of abduction)

B. Patient Supine
1. Passive total elevation of arm: __________ degrees*
2. Passive external rotation with arm at side: __________ degrees

*Total elevation of arm measured by viewing patient from side and using goniometer to determine angle between *arm* and *thorax*.

III. *STRENGTH:* (5 = normal, 4 = good, 3 = fair, 2 = poor, 1 = trace, 0 = paralysis)
A. Anterior deltoid __________ C. External rotation __________
B. Middle deltoid __________ D. Internal rotation __________

IV. *STABILITY:* (5 = normal, 4 = apprehension, 3 = rare subluxation, 2 = recurrent sublaxation, 1 = recurrent dislocation, 0 = fixed dislocation, NA = not available)
A. Anterior __________ B. Posterior __________ C. Inferior __________

V. *FUNCTION:* (4 = normal, 3 = mild compromise, 2 = difficulty, 1 = with aid, 0 = unable, NA = not available)

A.	Use back pocket	______	I.	Sleep on affected side	______
B.	Perineal care	______	J.	Pulling	______
C.	Wash opposite axilla	______	K.	Use hand overhead	______
D.	Eat with utensil	______	L.	Throwing	______
E.	Comb hair	______	M.	Lifting	______
F.	Use hand with arm at shoulder level	______	N.	Do usual work	______
G.	Carry 10–15 lbs. with arm at side	______	O.	Do usual sport	______
H.	Dress	______			

Table 32–7. Simple Shoulder Test

Comfortable at side?
Sleep comfortably?
Tuck in shirt?
Hand behind head?
Place can on shelf at level of shoulder?
Lift 1 lb. to level of shoulder?
Lift gallon to head level?
Carry 20 pounds?
Toss softball underhand?
Throw softball overhand?
Wash opposite shoulder?
Work full time at regular job?

The primary discrepancies lie in the relative value of the various components, as well as the methodology of strength testing. Manual muscle testing is variable and is therefore valued less than other components of the evaluation. More recent literature advocates reproducible quantitative muscle strength measurements using reliable equipment that is not operator dependent. This can be performed either isometrically or perhaps even more indicative of true strength, isokinetically. These types of strength testing justify the increased emphasis of these values in the overall functional assessment. Recent literature emphasizes the importance of muscle strength as it correlates to pain, especially fatigue- type pain, the overall satisfaction of the patient, and the success of rotator cuff repair.

At the other end of the spectrum from elaborate isokinetic testing is the simple shoulder test.[18] This test designed by Matsen et al. consists of a brief questionnaire consisting of 12 simple yes or no questions related to activities of daily living including work and sport (Table 32–7). This evaluation scheme has a high test-retest reproducibility and allows the practitioner to not only determine pre- and postoperative status but also to map the patient's progress. Another functional questionnaire is the shoulder Pain and Disability Index (SPADI).[19] This visual analog scale was found to be the most sensitive to clinical change and was felt to be the best questionnaire when compared to the subjective shoulder rating scale, the simple shoulder test, the modified—ASES form, and the SF-36 by Beaton and Richards.[20]

Surgeons tend to base surgical results primarily on whether a patient is happy or unhappy with the result. As scientists, however, it is important for us to identify what constitutes the variability in the observed results. The use of objective testing allows one to sort through a potpourri of data including muscle strength, motion, repair integrity, and pain, and correlate that data with the type of tear, the technique of repair, and the degree to which the functional ability of the patient meets that particular patient's functional demands. We can then have the ability to evaluate our treatment technique more effectively and predict prognosis more accurately. Finally, repeated objective measurement follow-up can ensure maintenance of results, assist with outcome based analysis of treatment, and perhaps most important of all, increase our knowledge and improve our techniques.

REFERENCES

1. Codman EA. *The Shoulder: Rupture of the Supraspinatus Tendon and Other Lesions in or About the Subacromial Bursa.* Malabar, FL: RE Krieger; 1984.
2. Calvert PT, Packer NP, Stokes DJ, Bayley JIL, Kessel L. Arthrography of the shoulder after operative repair of the torn rotator cuff. *J Bone Joint Surg Br.* 1986;68:147–150.
3. Owen RS, Ianotti JP, Kneeland JB, Dalinka MK, Deren JA, Oleaga L. Shoulder after surgery: MR imaging with surgical validation. *Radiology.* 1993;186:443–447.
4. Haygood TM, Oxner KG, Kneeland JB, Dalinka MK. Magnetic resonance imaging of the postoperative shoulder. *MRI Clinics North Am.* 1993;1:143–155.
5. Cross JR, Craig EV, Feinberg SB. Sonography of the postoperative rotator cuff. *Am J Radiology.* 1986;146:561–564.
6. Harryman DT II, Mack LA, Wang KY, Jackins SE, Richardson ML, Matsen FA. Repairs of the rotator cuff. *J Bone Joint Surg.* 1991; 73:982–989.
7. Moseley HF. Examination of the shoulder. In: Moseley HF, ed. *Shoulder Lesions.* New York: Paul B. Hober. 1972;22–30.
8. Neer CS II. Displaced proximal humeral fractures. *J Bone Joint Surg Am.* 1970;52:1077–1103.
9. Constant CR, Murley AHG. A clinical method of functional assessment of the shoulder. *Clin Orthop.* 1986;214:160–164.
10. Callahan TD, Johnson ME, Chao EIS. Shoulder strength. Analysis using Cybex II isokinetic dynamometer. *Clin Orthop.* 1991;274: 249–257.
11. Magnusson SD, Glein GW, Nicholas JA. Subject variability of shoulder abduction strength testing. *Am J Sports Med.* 1990;18: 349–353.
12. Emery RJH, Banus MJK, Crossman JE. A standard method for strength measurement in the Constant score using a spring balance. Presented at the 6th International Congress of Shoulder Surgery, Helsinki, Finland, July 1, 1995.
13. Ciepiela MD, Bernasek TL, Leffers D. *The comparison of strength ratios, radiographs, and physical examination in normal shoulders versus shoulders of rotator cuff syndrome.* Presented at the Florida Orthopaedic Society, 1993. Submitted for publication.
14. Barrett WP, Franklin JL, Jackson SE, Wyss ER, Matsen FA. Total shoulder arthroplasty. *J Bone Joint Surg Am.* 1987;69:865–872.
15. Gore DR, Murray MP, Sepic SB, Gardner GM. Shoulder muscle strength and range of motion following surgical repair of full thickness rotator cuff tears. *J Bone Joint Surg Am.* 1986;68: 266–272.
16. Ellman H, Handler G, Bayer M. Repair of the rotator cuff: End results. Study of factors, influence, and reconstruction. *J Bone Joint Surg.* 1986;68:1136–1144.
17. Altchek BDW, Warren, RF, Wickiewicz TL, Skyhar MJ, Ortiz G, Schwartz E. Arthroscopic acromioplasty: Technique and results. *J Bone Joint Surg.* 1990; 72A:1198–1207.
18. Matsen FA, Lippitt SB, Sidles JA, Harryman DT. Evaluating the shoulder in practical evaluation and management of the shoulder. In Matsen FA et al. (eds): The Shoulder. Philadelphia: W. B. Saunders, pp 3–12, 1994.
19. Roach KE, Budiman ME, Songsiridej N, Lertrantanakul Y: Development of a shoulder pain and disability index. *Arth Care Res.* 1991; 4:143–149.
20. Beaton DE, Richards RR. Measuring shoulder function: A comparison of five shoulder questionnaires. Presented at the 6th International Conference on Shoulder Surgery. Helsinki, Finland, June 29, 1995.

Chapter 33

Management of Failed Rotator Cuff Repairs

Wayne Z. Burkhead, Jr. and Jeffery S. Cantrell

This lady has had 6 difficult operations; all were necessary except the first.

Alex Boune, Quoted by L. Kessel

Success and failure of rotator cuff repair, like success and failure in life, are perceived phenomenon based on objective and subjective impressions generated to a large degree by the subjects' and their observers' expectations. Therefore, patients who are given an unrealistic expectation of the results of rotator cuff surgery may have a problem reconciling what otherwise may be considered a good result by their surgeon. On the other hand, a surgeon may be dissatisfied with the postoperative motion following cuff repair, whereas the patient is delighted that they can rest well at night and perform activities of daily living. The objective criterion, as much as they are objective, are outlined in the chapter on functional evaluation after repair.

Prior to embarking on the course of treatment, one must first identify the cause of failure of the operation. Common causes of failure of the operation are listed in Table 33–1. These include (1) incorrect diagnosis, (2) poor patient selection, (3) incorrect operation, (4) inadequate operation, (5) uncorrected or unrecognized intraoperative complication, (6) uncorrected or unrecognized postoperative complication, (7) the painful stiff shoulder with scarring and adhesions, (8) reflex sympathetic dystrophy, (9) late degenerative arthritis, and (10) rotator cuff tear arthropathy. Although this algorithm or table is helpful in identifying potential causes, it is important to realize that one or more of these factors may be operational in any one patient, in contributing to what the physician or patient perceives as a failure.

INCORRECT DIAGNOSIS

We have all seen patients who have massive rotator cuff tears with no pain and reasonable function, even in the overhead position. Likewise, the shoulder is a watershed area and there are numerous conditions that can present with pain similar to rotator cuff disease (see Chapter 5). If the patient's other primary or secondary sources of pain are not considered and an arthrogram is done, revealing what may be in reality a silent rotator cuff tear, even the soundest of repairs will be perceived by the patient as a failure.

Ellman[1] has noted on arthroscopy that patients with impingement and sometimes small rotator cuff repairs may have significant underlying degenerative arthritis, seen at the time of their arthroscopy. A careful history, physical examination, and the judicious use of imaging and diagnostic arthroscopy will help keep this source of failure to a minimum.

INCORRECT OPERATION

To a large extent, the only way to perform an incorrect operation for rotator cuff tears is to make an incorrect diagnosis. However, specifically in young patients with minor degrees of rotator cuff tearing secondary to instability, an acromioplasty and decompression, even though adequate for most patients with rotator cuff disease, may well be the wrong operation for someone who needs capsulolabral reconstruction as described in Chapter 11. In other words, even if the correct diagnosis is made (i.e., rotator cuff tearing), the operation may be incorrect because it does not address the primary cause, which is underlying instability.

POOR PATIENT SELECTION

Personality—Intellectual Factors

Surgical judgement is a learned phenomenon garnered through years of experience. Part of that experi-

Table 33–1. Causes of Failed Rotator Cuff Repairs

- Incorrect diagnosis
- Poor patient selection
- Incorrect operation
- Inadequate operation
- Intraoperative complications
- Postoperative complications
- Adhesions
- Reflex sympathetic dystrophy
- Late DJD
- Rotator cuff-tear arthropathy

ence leads us to our ability to judge our patients' willingness and their ability to accept the hardships and frustrations that rotator cuff repair may present them. Patients who are unwilling to tolerate a certain degree of immobilization after surgery, are unable to comprehend the concepts of passive or active motion, or lack the discipline of doing the daily exercise regimen that are so important for a good result from rotator cuff repair will either (1) disrupt their repair or (2) develop excessive scarring, limited motion, and a painful stiff shoulder. Patients who have secondary gain in mind from personal or workmen's compensation injuries, frequently have subjective results, which are much lower than the objective results or the surgeon's expectations. I refer to these as the "someone to blame or something to gain" group of patients. When asked how their shoulders were injured, instead of simply describing the mechanism of injury, these symptom and event "magnifiers" often make comments like, "My foreman made me lift it," or "He dropped his end." Those patients who won't take some responsibility for their injury often won't feel responsible enough for their result to cooperate with your instructions. The passive aggressive employee becomes easily enough the passively aggressive patient and deals with their doctor in the same manipulative way that they deal with authority figures in their life. Hawkins has previously documented the paucity of good and excellent results in patients seeking workmen's compensation.[2] A successful person is generally a successful patient. Success does not necessarily imply monetary wealth, in fact it may be exclusive of this illusive ephemeral goal. The successful truck driver who is a successful father will do better and will often be more appreciative of your care than the person whose idea of success is writing a check from their trust fund.

Cigarette smokers with a low threshold of pain, anxiety, and cool sweaty hands may be candidates to develop reflex sympathetic dystrophy (RSD) following any kind of shoulder operation. Mallon[3] evaluated 57 patients who underwent rotator cuff repairs and analyzed nonsmokers versus smokers in workmen's compensation patients. Statistical analysis of the results showed that smokers did worse after rotator cuff repair than did nonsmokers in terms of range of motion, pain relief, and improvement in ability to perform activities of daily living. The worst group in his study were patients who both smoked and had workmen's compensation claims. Their conclusion suggested that cessation of smoking prior to rotator cuff repair would be recommended in all groups of patients, especially those with workmen's compensation claims, as a possible means of improving outcome of rotator cuff repair.

ASSOCIATED DISEASES

Although patients with diabetes may have some difficulty healing wounds, have tendency towards stiffness, and have frequent neural symptoms, most are compliant responsible patients having lived years with the discipline of regular lifesaving self-injection. Patients with Parkinsonism often have cogwheel rigidity, which inhibits their ability to exercise and increases the risk of developing postoperative adhesive capsulitis. Balance problems in the Parkinsonian patient also increases the likelihood of falling in the perioperative period. Several of these conditions are discussed in the chapter on adhesive capsulitis.

INADEQUATE OPERATION

Inadequate Decompression

Residual impingement is not an uncommon cause of failure. In fact, 20% of the patients in Neer's 1972 article[4] were revisions for failed lateral acromionectomy. It should be noted that residual impingement can occur despite rather aggressive acromionectomies, especially lateral acromionectomy in which a residual spike of medial bone, untreated AC joint arthritis, incomplete release of the coracoacromial ligament, or a combination of all three exist.

Both the studies by Bigliani et al.[5,6] and DeOrio[7] consider lateral acromionectomy or inadequate anterior acromionectomy to play a key role in failures seen in their series. Out of the 27 patients in DeOrio and Cofield's series that required a second attempt at surgical repair of failed rotator cuff, a partial lateral acromionectomy had been done in 13 shoulders, anterior acromioplasty had been done in 12 shoulders, and distal clavicle excision in 11. At second operation, anterior acromioplasty was done in five of these shoulders. A revision anterior acromioplasty was done in one shoulder, revision lateral acromioplasty was done in two shoulders, and distal clavicle excision was performed in one shoulder. Seven of the 15 patients that had not had an anterior acromioplasty at the time of initial attempt at repair had signs and symptoms of continuing subacromial impingement, in addition to a second rotator cuff tear.[7]

In Bigliani et al.'s series of 31 patients that required operative treatment of a failed repair of the rotator cuff, 16 patients had an anterior acromioplasty, 7 had a lateral acromionectomy, and 5 had no procedure performed on the acromion at all. Three patients had repair of an unfused os acromiale. All 31 patients had an anterior-inferior acromioplasty performed at the time of their second operation; a previous anterior acromioplasty was revised in 16 patients, and a previous lateral acromionectomy was revised in seven patients. The five patients that had no previous attempt at acromioplasty underwent anterior acromioplasty during the second procedure. The three patients with an unfused os acromiale also underwent anterior acromioplasty. Overall, 28 of the 30 patients (90%) in this series had a persistent subacromial impingement lesion after their first operation, because treatment of the acromion had been inappropriate or inadequate. Seven of these patients actually healed their large rotator cuff tear; however, the persistent impingement caused a second small or medium sized tear proximal to the suture line.[5,6]

The steps of Neer's acromioplasty and its modifications are presented in Chapter 23. An acromioplasty that addresses only the medial acromion limited to the ligamentous insertion of the coracoacromial ligament may result in a persistent lateral spike of bone with persistent impingement (Fig. 33–1). Likewise, an anterolateral acromioplasty results in residual anteromedial acromion and coracoacromial ligament tightness (Fig. 33–2).

Acromioplasties done only with a gauge, burr, or a curved osteotome may result in residual medial and lateral spike or a ''rat bite'' acromioplasty (Fig. 33–3). Residual impingement results in an acromion that is made flat but is still too long. This can be seen after both open and arthroscopic decompression in which only an inferior acromioplasty is performed. This complication can be avoided by the Esche technique[8] of arthroscopic acromioplasty or Rockwood's technique[9] of open anterior acromioplasty (see Chapter 22).

Packer and Kessel et al.[10] reported on 11 patients out of their series of 63 rotator cuff repairs that required a second attempt at operative rotator cuff repair. Out of these 11 failures, 6 had not been decompressed at the initial operation. Of these six, two had decompression alone which relieved their pain. In the other five patients who had previous decompression, one had a further decompression alone; subsequently, one had a second rotator cuff repair alone, and the other three had a combination of subacromial decompression and rotator cuff repair. The only 2 patients of these 11 failed rotator cuff repairs that did well were those that had repeat decompression alone. The other nine patients did poorly, with two eventually requiring hemiarthroplasty and one eventually requiring arthrodesis. That is, no second repair of the rotator cuff achieved a good result in their series.

Untreated AC Joint Disorders

Bigliani[6] has stressed the importance of including the AC joint in considering the source of symptoms and it's contribution to the impingement and it's role as a complicating factor in repair of the rotator cuff. Fifteen percent of their patients with a failed rotator cuff repair had persistent symptoms over the AC joint. The technique of AC joint excision and a more thorough treatment of its relationship to cuff disease can be found in Chapter 9.

Inadequate Repair of the Cuff

In the evaluation by Bigliani et al. of 31 patients with failed repairs of the rotator cuff, the fact that was most commonly associated with failure of the primary repair in their series was a massive or large tear. Thirty of their patients (97%) had their failure related to a tear greater than 3 cm. Inadequate mobilization of retracted rotator

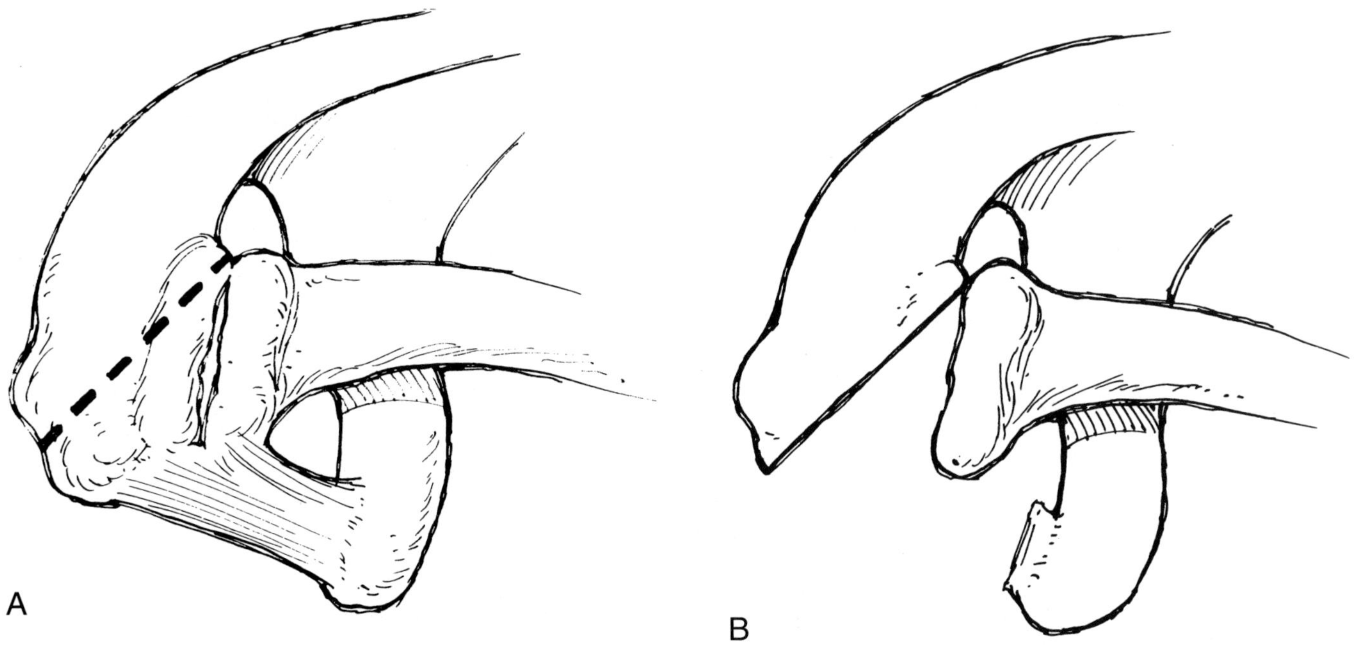

Fig. 33–1. ***A,*** **Acromioplasty that addresses only the medial acromion.** ***B,*** **This limited medial acromionectomy results in a persistent lateral spike of bone, which can cause persistent impingement.**

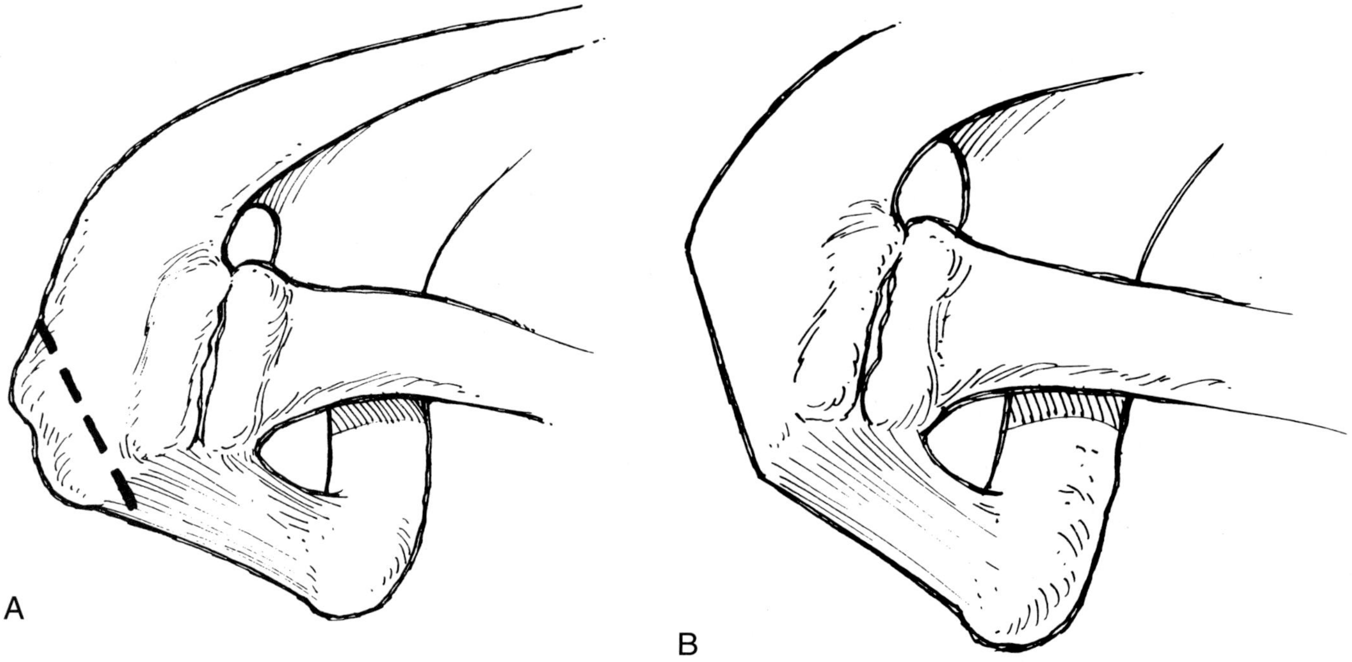

Fig. 33–2. ***A,*** **An anterolateral acromioplasty.** ***B,*** **Residual anteromedial acromion and coracoacromial ligament after an anterolateral acromioplasty can result in residual tightness.**

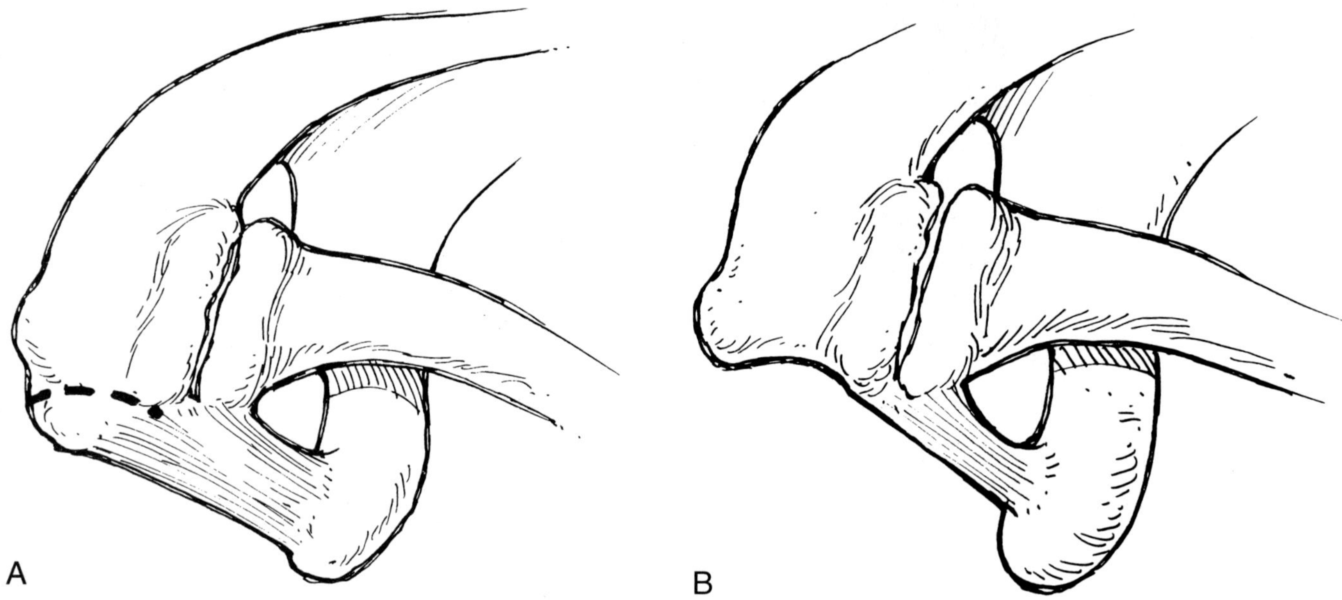

Fig. 33–3. ***A,*** **Acromioplasties done only with a gauge bur or curved osteotome may lead to what is referred to as a "rat bite" acromion.** ***B,*** **This may result in a residual medial and lateral spike and resultant persistent impingement**

cuff tendon and failure to fix the repair to a bony trough was also cited as reason for failure. Of the 15 patients in Bigliani's series that had an inadequate repair, 11 patients did not have adequate mobilization and reattachment into a bony trough. Eight of these patients had good quality cuff tissue at their second operation and did well after mobilization and anchoring into a bony trough.[5,6]

In DeOrio and Cofield's series, 18 of their 27 patients had initial cuff tears greater than 3 cm (large or massive tendon tears).[7] Kessel and Packer et al. also reported on 4 patients out of their 63 primary repairs for rotator cuff tears that failed, because staples had been used to reattach the rotator cuff to bone. All required staple removal and none of these had a good result.[10]

Post noted that at reoperation there was often found to be thickened, hypertrophied bursal tissue resembling diseased rotator cuff that had been closed over a cuff tendon defect. This had been mistakenly regarded as cuff tissue at the time of the initial repair.[11]

INTRAOPERATIVE COMPLICATIONS

Fracture of the Acromion

Intraoperative complications are clearly the most avoidable, including fracture of the acromion during acromioplasty.[12] Fracture of the acromion can occur with both open and arthroscopic techniques. Because the surgeon should be aware by visual inspection and palpation of a fracture which occurs at the time of an open procedure, these fractures are more readily recognized and treated. A fracture after arthroscopic decompression is harder to diagnose (Fig. 33–4) and requires a high index of suspicion. Theoretically (though this has not always been my experience) patients, after successful arthroscopic acromioplasty, should have less pain than those after open acromioplasty. One should be suspicious, therefore, if the patient, after an arthroscopic decompression and/or mini-open repair, has a tremendous amount of pain over and above what was expected with a routine rotator cuff repair.

Fracture of the acromion, arthroscopically, can occur through old unfused physeal lines in both the mesoacromial, metaacromial, and preacromial region. The most disabling fracture occurs at the base in the region of the old metaacromion. Fracture of the acromion during open acromioplasty results most commonly when the osteotome is placed at too oblique of an angle, fracturing through the superior cortex, or if the osteotome is driven too far back, fracturing the posterior inferior acromion. The Rockwood acromioplasty done in two stages allows one to judge the thickness of the acromion prior to the inferior acromioplasty. Also, Cofield and Bigliani both agree that unrecognized or unstable os acromiale lesions can lead to postoperative impingement.[5-7]

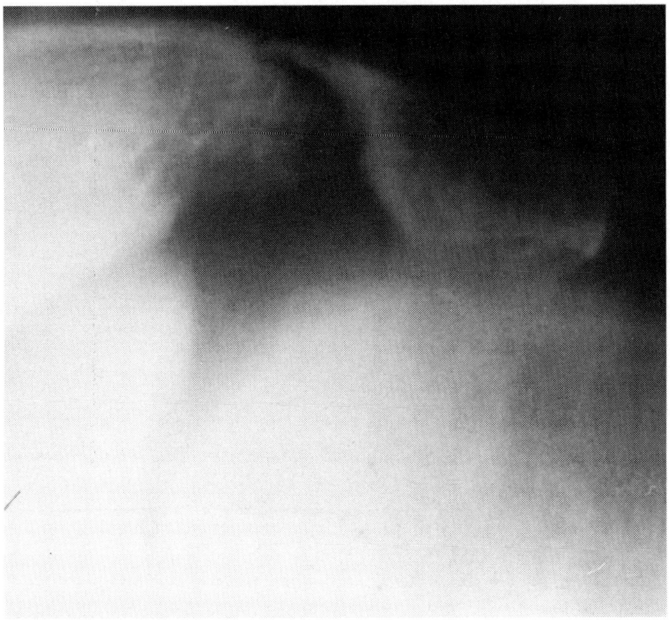

Fig. 33–4. ***A,*** **A 56-year-old woman, status post arthroscopic acromioplasty.** ***B,*** **A fracture at the base of the acromion with displacement and hinging at the AC joint is noted. This patient subsequently required acromionectomy after attempt at open reduction internal fixation.**

Fracture Greater Tuberosity

Fracture of the greater tuberosity can occur through drill holes for sutures in osteopenic bone. This can be avoided by placing the suture holes at differing levels along the diaphysis of the humerus. An overly aggressive trough may also put the tuberosity at risk. Short of frank fracture, the sutures can connect themselves through osteopenic bone in the metaphysis of the humerus and cause the suture to slide through and result in loss of fixation of the rotator cuff. One way to avoid this is with the use of Teflon felt (Bard Vascular Systems, Division C.R. Bard, Billerica, ME) or the coracoacromial ligament as a pledget.

Bigliani et al. illustrated a case in their analysis of 31 failures that cites and overly aggressive bony trough in the greater tuberosity leaving a defect at the time of initial repair. This precluded adequate repair to the bone at repeat operation, despite the presence of adequate rotator cuff tissue quality.[5,6]

Axillary Nerve Injury

Axillary nerve injury can occur from the injudicious splitting of the deltoid down the raphe. The degree of disability that can occur with this depends on two factors: (1) the degree of injury, (i.e., neuropraxia versus axonotmesis versus neurotmesis) and (2) the location of the injury (i.e., the farther around anteriorly and medially the nerve is injured the less the disability will be). It should be remembered that in smaller patients, the nerve may be closer than 5 cm to the lateral edge.[13]

Deltoid Compromise

Deltoid dehiscence, like axillary nerve palsy, is a devastating but largely avoidable complication of rotator cuff repair. The development of healthy deltotrapezial flaps, suture that "grabs" the muscle as well as the fascia, respect for the muscular nature of the lateral deltoid insertion, the judicious use of drill holes in the acromion when necessary, and the avoidance of radical acromionectomy (Fig. 33–5) can avoid this complication.

Bigliani et al. found that detachment of the deltoid origin from the acromion was thought to be a factor in the failure in 13 of the 31 patients in their series. Seven of these patients had a previous lateral acromionectomy.[5,6] Thirteen of 27 patients in DeOrio and Cofield's series had lateral acromionectomy done as part of the initial procedure.[7] Bigliani et al. related inadequate physical therapy for 5 of their 31 patients, with an additional 2 having postoperative trauma causing their failure of the deltoid.[5,6]

Deltoid dehiscence can be treated in a variety of ways. Most commonly it is the lateral deltoid that loses its grip before it heals. When this occurs the deltoid retracts to the upper brachium but usually maintains a thin layer of scar that is connected to the lateral acromion (Fig. 33–6). This scar can be folded back on the deltoid to create a thick fascial insertion (Fig. 33–7). A running suture is placed along the tissue to create a tendinous structure. With mobilization and abduction of the arm, the deltoid origin is approximated to the residual acromion. Then sutures can be placed behind this permanent suture so that the sutures are pulling against the suture and not the muscle or newly created tendon.

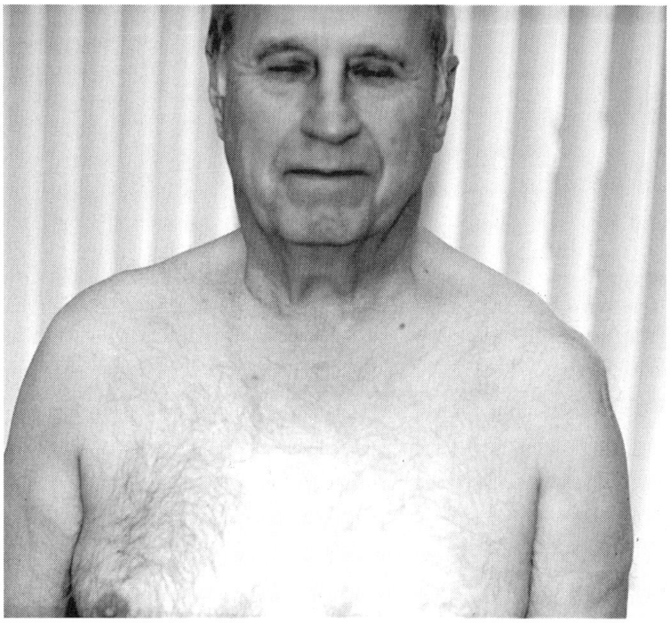

Fig. 33–5. Neither the clinical nor the cosmetic results of acromionectomy are pleasing if the deltoid fails to heal.

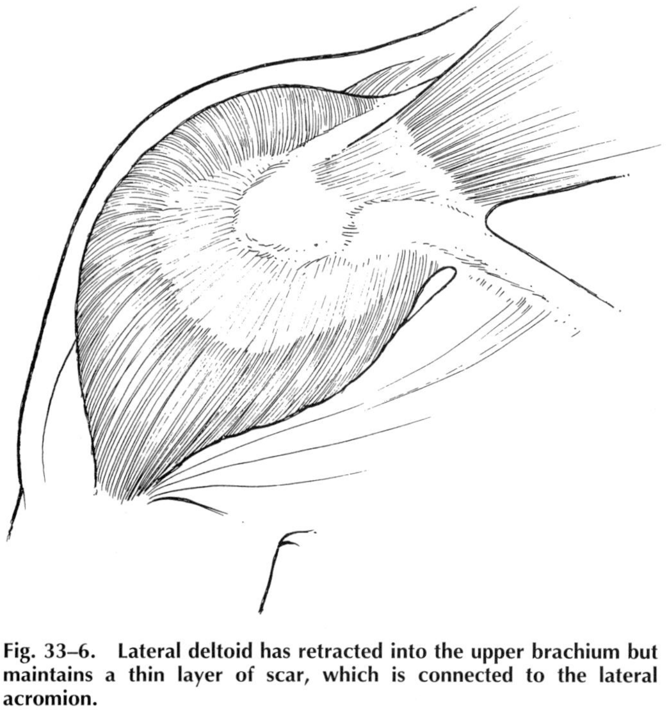

Fig. 33–6. Lateral deltoid has retracted into the upper brachium but maintains a thin layer of scar, which is connected to the lateral acromion.

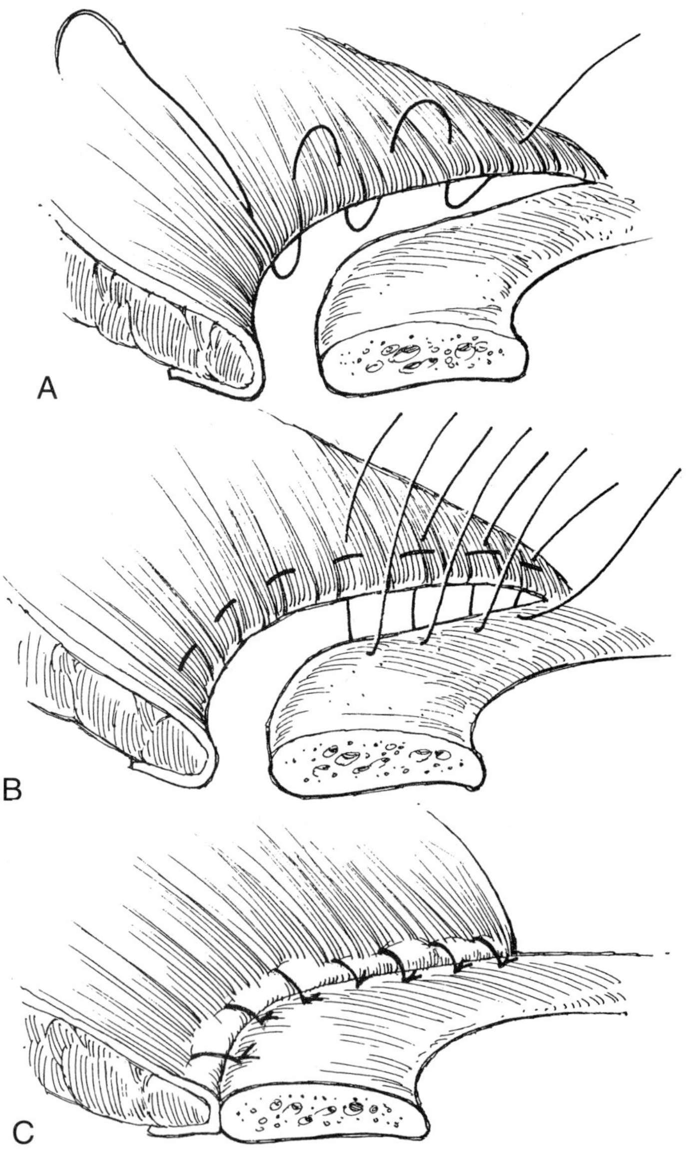

Fig. 33–7. ***A,*** **A thick fascial insertion can be created by folding the residual scar back onto the deltoid, then placing a running suture to hold it in place. The length of the new tendon can be altered based on the degree to which the underlying deltoid can be mobilized.** ***B,*** **With mobilization and abduction of the arm, the deltoid origin is approximated to the residual acromion. Note the sutures can be placed behind the permanent suture so that the pull is against the suture and not the muscle.** ***C,*** **Tying down the sutures via drill holes in the acromion.**

For patients in whom lateral acromionectomy has resulted in deltoid dehiscence, Neer has recommended a sliding osteotomy of the spine of the scapula to recreate, as best can be done, an acromion (Fig. 33–8).[14] Other techniques such as deltoid transfer have been recommended for the treatment of deltoid loss; however, the results of large numbers of these patients is not available and the investigators who have employed them describe them as unpredictable at best. My own experience with three deltoid transfers has been disappointing as well. Therefore, my preferred method of treatment of a ruptured deltoid that cannot be repaired is to perform a glenohumeral fusion.

Satterlee and Neer,[15] in a prospective study, reported on reoperation after failed attempts to repair tears of the rotator cuff in 72 shoulders. Two groups were compared, one with an intact deltoid and one with a damaged deltoid secondary to retraction scarring or denervation. Ninety percent of the patients in the group with normal deltoid had excellent or satisfactory results; however, less than 57% in the group with damaged deltoid had excellent or satisfactory results, leading them to believe that previous deltoid damage was a more important cause of failure than previously appreciated.

Post also addressed the importance of early recognition of deltoid dehiscence for immediate repair in order to salvage the function of the muscle.[11] Satterlee and Neer, in their review of 72 shoulders for failed rotator cuff repair, evaluated deltoid atrophy and retraction by clinical observation and palpation, as well as electromyography and nerve conduction velocity studies to detect evidence of denervation.[15]

Rockwood and Groh et al.[16] reported their series of 36 patients that had been referred to them for postoperative loss of anterior or anterolateral deltoid muscle following procedures about the shoulder secondary to either deltoid detachment or axillary nerve injury. All patients were significantly disabled, and all patients were dissatisfied with their result of the previous operation. Their conclusion was that loss of the anterior deltoid function secondary to denervation or detachment resulted in irrevocable pain and impairment of function. They stressed the importance of paying careful attention to the surgical technique of the deltoid reattachment to the bone and protection of the axillary nerve to prevent the dire consequences to shoulder function.

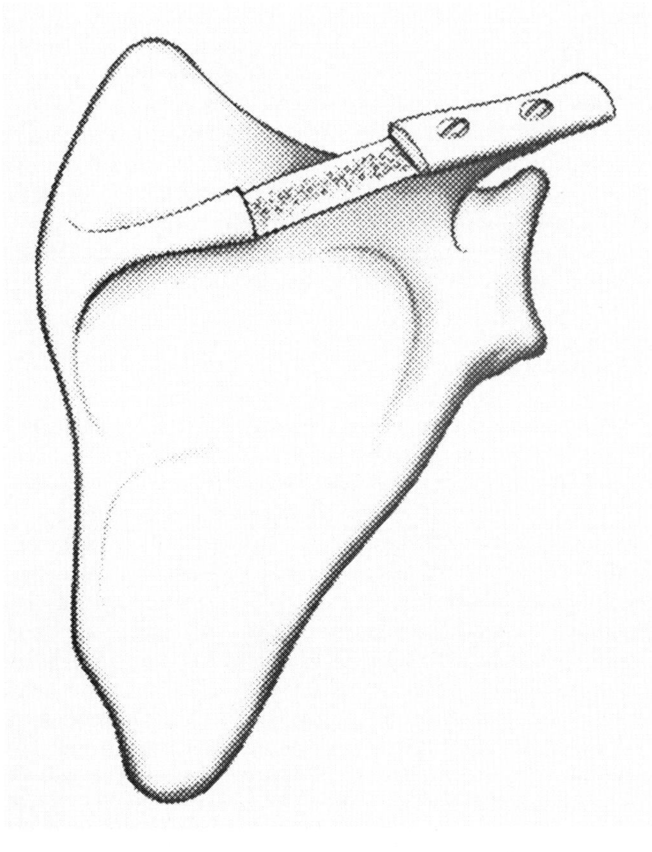

Fig. 33–8. Sliding osteotomy of the spine of the scapula to recreate an acromion, as recommended by Neer.

Other Intraoperative Complications

Post[11] addresses suprascapular nerve injury as a possible intraoperative complication. This usually occurs when the suprascapular nerve is damaged as it coursed the base of the scapular spine during attempted mobilization procedures. Dissection should not allow elevation from the bony floor more than 2 cm medial to the superior glenoid rim, otherwise nerve injury and additional weakening of the external rotator muscles can result.

POSTOPERATIVE COMPLICATIONS

DeOrio and Cofield[7] felt that appropriate postoperative immobilization tailored to the complexity of repair was important. They noted that in 14 of the 27 failed cuff repairs in their series, insufficient postoperative support played a role in the failure. This led them to recommend the judicious use of braces as dictated by the characteristics of the repair.

Bigliani et al.[6] used an abduction pillow or brace to protect the repair of the deltoid muscle only when the muscle was mobilized and repaired to the acromion again. They no longer use an abduction brace routinely, as it allows the arm to slide into extension, creating more tension across the site of repair.

Post[11] noted that sinus tract can occur as associated with postoperative wound infections. When wide surgical excision of infected tissues ensue, postoperative function is subsequently compromised, based on residual muscle power. One patient in the series by Bigliani et al. had failure of the initial cuff repair secondary to infection.[6]

The Painful Stiff Shoulder

In the series by Bigliani et al.,[6] a stiff frozen shoulder developed in five of their patients secondary to inadequate rehabilitation after the initial repair. They felt that pendulum exercises and passive elevation in the scapular plane should be performed early, even after the treatment of a massive tear. Active and resisted exercises are reserved for later time after healing of the tendon is performed.

Reflex Sympathetic Dystrophy

RSD can complicate any shoulder surgery. While there are certain patients who are perhaps doomed or destined to develop RSD, placement of skin incisions in the watershed area, away from the terminal branches of the superficial skin nerves, will avoid painful neuroma and at least that portion of RSD that is related to those factors. A detailed description of the treatment of RSD is beyond the scope of this chapter.

Late Degenerative Arthritis

Patients may have mild degenerative joint disease at the time of rotator cuff repair. Repair of the rotator cuff does not necessarily protect against the progression or indeed the development of late degenerative arthritis. Four of the six patients with persistent pain in Bigliani's series had developed glenohumeral arthritis.[6]

Rotator Cuff Tear Arthropathy

As in late degenerative arthritis, repair of the rotator cuff does not protect all patients from the development of an inexorable rotator cuff tear arthropathy.

Results of Repeat Operations for Failed Rotator Cuff Repairs

Rerupture, or perhaps more accurately failure of the cuff to heal, does not always result in the perception of failure. Prior to Neviaser's discussion[17,18] it was felt that repair of rotator cuffs at a second setting might improve pain but had little chance of improving motion. In a study of 46 cases of reoperation for failed repair, Neviaser and Neviaser found that in an average follow-up of 30 months, 42 of 46 patients had improvement in pain and 22 patients had gained motion. A 10% post revision dissatisfaction rate persisted; however, almost 90% were pleased with their results. They conclude that a generous anterior acromioplasty, as well as rerepair of the rotator cuff, gave encouraging results. Deltoid weakness from previous deltoid detachment, as in other studies, was a major determinant of return of motion and overall satisfaction with the result.

In a series by Bigliani et al.[6] the overall result of repeat repair was satisfactory in 52% of patients and unsatisfactory in 48%. However, 81% of these patients had satisfactory relief of pain, but 45% had persistent weakness. The factors that were associated with inferior results were previous lateral acromionectomy, previously detached origin of the deltoid, and the finding that the tissue of the rotator cuff available at the time of repeat operation was of poor quality. They mobilized and repaired the cuff to a bony trough in 26 patients, the other 5 patients had a longitudinal split in the cuff and only required repair of the tendon side-to-side. All the repairs were performed with the patient's arm at the side.

DeOrio and Cofield[7] reported 76% of the 21 patients operated on for failed initial rotator cuff repair had diminished pain. Overall, 17% had a good result, 25% had a fair result, and 58% reportedly had a poor result. Nine of their shoulders required additional tissue to be mobilized in order to repair the defect, including a subscapularis transposition, incorporation of the long head of the biceps, free fascia lata graft, or trapezius transfer. Even though 63% of the patients still had moderate to severe pain, 67% felt they had benefitted from the procedure, mainly from relieving residual subacromial impingement. Their results and findings led them to be quite leery of a second attempt at surgical repair of a failed rotator cuff, using pain as a primary indication for a second procedure.

Satterlee and Neer[15] evaluated 72 shoulders in 71 patients that underwent reoperation for failed rotator cuff repairs. As mentioned above, the most important irreparable lesion in their series was detachment or paralysis of the deltoid muscle. Not all these patients had a rotator cuff tear at reoperation. The results in the group with intact deltoid were excellent or satisfactory in over 90% of the patients they rerepaired (there were 33 shoulders). However, when the deltoid was damaged, the rate fell to 50% for excellent or satisfactory results, even with deltoidplasty or other salvage procedures (there were 39 shoulders). They concluded that it was critical to accomplish four objectives when addressing failed rotator cuffs: (1) careful release of adhesions and subacromial decompression, (2) adequate rotator cuff repair to preserve head depressor function, (3) as well as mechanical and nutritional functions, and (4) the preservation of restoration of the deltoid origin was also important.

CONCLUSIONS

Adherence to the general surgical principles outlined in Chapter 23 for primary repair of the rotator cuff is of utmost importance, because repeat repairs and reconstruction are noted to not yield the good results associated with primary repairs.[5,7] An intact deltoid and good quality rotator cuff tissue are factors associated with a good result, while previous lateral acromionectomy, insufficient deltoid, and poor quality cuff tissue are associated with inferior results after repeat repair and reconstruction.[6] Any of the previously described repair techniques from debridement to muscle transfer can be done to rerepair the cuff based on the patients' and physicians' expectations and needs. The patient with deltoid muscle loss remains the great challenge currently. In my hands at least, glenohumeral fusion provides the most likely satisfactory outcome, i.e., a painless shoulder which has some motion.

REFERENCES

1. Ellman H, Harris E, Kay SP. Early degenerative joint disease simulating impingement syndrome: Arthroscopic findings. *Arthroscopy.* 1992;8:482–487.
2. Hawkins RJ, Chris AD, Kiefer GN. Failed anterior acromioplasties. *Orthop Trans.* 1987;11:233.
3. Mallon WJ. *Smoking and worker's compensation: Relation to outcome after rotator cuff repair.* Presented at the American Shoulder and Elbow Surgeons' 10th Open Meeting. New Orleans, LA, February 27, 1994.
4. Neer CS. Anterior acromioplasty for the chronic impingement syndrome in the shoulder. A preliminary report. *J Bone Joint Surg.* 1972; 54:41–50.
5. Bigliani LU, McIlveen SJ, Cordasco FA, Musso ES. Operative management of failed rotator cuff repairs. *Orthop Trans.* 1988; 12:674.
6. Bigliani LU, McIlveen SJ, Cordasco FA, Musso ES. Operative treatment of failed repairs of the rotator cuff. *J Bone Joint Surg.* 1992; 74:1505–1515.
7. DeOrio JK, Cofield RH. Results of a second attempt at surgical repair of a failed initial rotator cuff repair. *J Bone Joint Surg.* 1984; 66:563–567.
8. Esche JC, Ozerkis LR, Helgager JA, Kane N, Lilliott N. Arthroscopic subacromial decompression: Results according to the degree of rotator cuff tear. *Arthroscopy.* 1988;4:241–249.
9. Rockwood CA, Lyons FR. Shoulder impingement syndrome: Diagnosis, radiographic evaluation, and treatment with a modified Neer acromioplasty. *J Bone Joint Surg.* 1993;75: 409–423.
10. Packer NP, Calvert PT, Bayley JIL, Kessel L. Operative treatment of chronic ruptures of the rotator cuff of the shoulder. *J Bone Joint Surg Br.* 1983;65:171–175.
11. Post M. Complications of rotator cuff surgery. *Clin Orthop.* 1990; 254:97–104.
12. Matthews LS, Burkhead WZ, Gordon S, Racanelli J, Ruland L. Acromial fracture complicating arthroscopic subacromial decompression—Report of six cases. Presented at American Shoulder & Elbow Surgeons Closed Meeting. Vail, Colorado, September, 1992.
13. Burkhead WZ, Scheinberg RR, Box G. Surgical anatomy of the axillary nerve. *J Shoulder Elbow Surg.* 1992;1:31–36.
14. Neer CS III. *Shoulder Reconstruction.* Philadelphia: WB Saunders; 1991.
15. Satterlee CC, Neer CS. Reoperation for failed rotator cuff repairs. *J Shoulder Elbow Surg Suppl.* 1993;2:S10.
16. Groh GI, Simoni M, Rolla P, Rockwood CA. Loss of deltoid following shoulder operations: An operative disaster. Presented at the American Shoulder and Elbow Surgeons' 10th Open Meeting. New Orleans, LA, February 27, 1994.
17. Neviaser RJ, Neviaser TJ. Restoration for failed rotator cuff repair: Analysis of 46 cases. *Orthop Trans.* 1989;13:241.
18. Neviaser RJ, Neviaser TJ. Reoperation for failed repairs: Analysis of 50 cases. *J Shoulder Elbow Surg.* 1992;1:283–286.

Index

Note: Page numbers in *italics* indicate figures; page numbers followed by t indicate tables.